The

Biologic

a

Basis of

# INFECTIOUS
# DISEASES

The

Biologic

and Clinical

Basis of

# INFECTIOUS
# DISEASES

## FIFTH EDITION

## STANFORD T. SHULMAN, M.D.
Professor of Pediatrics and
   Associate Dean for Academic Affairs
Northwestern University Medical School
Chief, Division of Infectious Diseases
The Children's Memorial Hospital
Chicago, Illinois

## JOHN P. PHAIR, M.D.
Professor of Medicine
Northwestern University Medical School
Chief of Infectious Diseases
Northwestern Memorial Hospital
Chicago, Illinois

## LANCE R. PETERSON, M.D.
Professor of Pathology and Medicine
Northwestern University Medical School
Director, Clinical Microbiology
Northwestern Memorial Hospital
Chicago, Illinois

## JOHN R. WARREN, M.D.
Professor and Vice Chairman
Department of Pathology
Northwestern University Medical School
Medical Director, Pathology Laboratory
Northwestern Memorial Hospital
Chicago, Illinois

W. B. SAUNDERS COMPANY
*A Division of Harcourt Brace & Company*
Philadelphia, London, Toronto, Montreal, Sydney, Tokyo

**W. B. SAUNDERS COMPANY**

*A Division of Harcourt Brace & Company*

The Curtis Center
Independence Square West
Philadelphia, Pennsylvania 19106

**Library of Congress Cataloging-in-Publication Data**

The biologic & clinical basis of infectious diseases / [edited by]
    Stanford T. Shulman — [et al.]. — 5th ed.
        p.    cm.
    Rev. ed. of: The biologic & clinical basis of infectious diseases.
4th ed. c1992.
    Includes bibliographical references and index.
    ISBN 0–7216–5948–9
    1. Communicable diseases.    I. Shulman, Stanford T.    II. Biologic
& clinical basis of infectious diseases.
    [DNLM: 1. Communicable Diseases.    WC 100 B616 1997]
RC111.B47  1997
616.9 — dc20
DNLM/DLC                                                    96-16760

THE BIOLOGIC AND CLINICAL BASIS OF
INFECTIOUS DISEASES, 5TH EDITION                    ISBN 0–7216–5948–9

Printed in the United States of America.

Last digit is the print number:     9    8    7    6    5    4    3    2    1

*The editors wish to dedicate this work to the pioneering efforts of the previous editors, Dr. Phil Paterson, Dr. Bert Sommers, and the late Dr. Guy Youmans; to our wives, Claire Shulman, Nancy Phair, LoAnn Peterson, and Deanna Warren, who provide continuing support; and to our children. A special acknowledgment goes to Sam Levitt and the late Esther Levitt for their love and encouragement, and to Debbie Shulman for her expert editorial assistance.*

## DOSAGE NOTICE

Every effort has been made by the authors, the editors, and the publisher of this book to ensure that dosage recommendations are precise and in agreement with the standards of practice accepted at the time of publication.

However, dosage schedules are changed from time to time in the light of accumulating clinical experience and continuing laboratory studies. This is most likely to occur in the case of recently introduced products.

We urge, therefore, that you check the package information data for the manufacturer's recommended dosage to be certain that changes have not been made in the recommended dose or in the contraindications for administration. In addition, there are some quite serious situations in which drug therapy must be individualized and expert judgment advises the use of a higher dosage or administration by a different route than is included in the manufacturer's recommendations. Throughout the text examples of such instances are indicated by a footnote.

THE EDITORS

# CONTRIBUTORS

**MOSHE ARDITI, M.D.**
Assistant Professor of Pediatrics, University of Southern California Medical School, Los Angeles, California; Division of Infectious Disease, Children's Hospital of Los Angeles, Los Angeles, California
*Introduction to Infections of the Central Nervous System; Common Etiologic Agents of Bacterial Meningitis*


**ELLEN GOULD CHADWICK, M.D.**
Associate Professor of Pediatrics, Northwestern University Medical School; Associate Director, Section of Pediatric and Maternal HIV Infection, The Children's Memorial Hospital, Chicago Illinois
*Human Immunodeficiency Virus Infection and AIDS*


**JOHN T. CLARK, M.D.**
Associate Professor of Medicine; Section of Geriatrics, Northwestern University Medical School, Chicago, Illinois
*Bone and Joint Infections: Septic Arthritis and Osteomyelitis*


**A TODD DAVIS, M.D.**
Professor of Pediatrics, Northwestern University Medical School; Head, Division of General Academic Pediatrics, The Children's Memorial Hospital, Chicago, Illinois
*Temperature Regulation, the Pathogenesis of Fever and the Approach to the Febrile Patient; Zoonoses; Exanthematous Diseases*


**JAMES L. DUNCAN, D.D.S., Ph.D.**
Associate Professor of Microbiology–Imunology, Northwestern University Medical School, Chicago, Illinois; Associate Dean of The Graduate School, Northwestern University, Evanston, Illinois
*Dental Infections and Other Diseases of the Oral Cavity*


**KRISTIN A. ENGLUND, M.D.**
Instructor of Medicine, Northwestern University Medical School; Consultant, Infectious Diseases, Northwestern Memorial Hospital, Chicago, Illinois
*Laboratory Evaluation of Infectious Diseases*


**DALE N. GERDING, M.D.**
Professor of Medicine, Northwestern University Medical School; Chief, Medical Services (III), Veteran's Administration Lakeside Medical Center, Chicago, Illinois
*Infections Caused by Anaerobic Bacteria; Antimicrobial Therapy*


**ROBERT J. HERCEG, M.D.**
Resident in Pathology, Northwestern University Medical School, Chicago, Illinois
*Normal Flora in Health and Disease*

**BETSY C. HEROLD, M.D.**
Assistant Professor of Pediatrics, University of Chicago Pritzker School of Medicine, Chicago, Illinois
*Virus–Host Interactions*


**STUART JOHNSON, M.D.**
Assistant Professor, Department of Medicine, Northwestern University Medical School; Staff Physician, Infectious Disease Section, Veteran's Administration Lakeside Medical Center, Chicago, Illinois
*Infectious Diarrhea*


**BEN Z. KATZ, M.D.**
Associate Professor of Pediatrics, Northwestern University Medical School; Attending Physician, The Children's Memorial Hospital, Chicago, Illinois
*Viral Infections of the Upper Respiratory Tract, Infectious Mononucleosis, and the Chronic Fatigue Syndrome; Viral Infections of the Lower Respiratory Tract*


**STEPHEN D. MILLER, Ph.D.**
Professor of Microbiology–Immunology, Director, Interdepartmental Immunobiology Center, Northwestern University Medical School, Chicago, Illinois
*The Immune System and Microbe-Induced Autoreactive Host Responses and Autoimmune Disease*


**ROBERT L. MURPHY, M.D.**
Associate Professor of Medicine, Division of Infectious Diseases, Northwestern University; Director, AIDS Clinical Treatment Unit, Northwestern Memorial Hospital, Chicago, Illinois
*Sexually Transmitted Diseases; Diagnosis and Management of Infection in the Immunocompromised Host*


**GARY A. NOSKIN, M.D.**
Assistant Professor of Medicine, Northwestern University Medical School; Associate Firm Chief, Patterson Firm, Northwestern Memorial Hospital, Chicago, Illinois
*Fungal Infections; Diagnosis and Management of Infection in the Immunocompromised Host; Nosocomial Infections*


**FRANK J. PALELLA, Jr., M.D.**
Instructor of Medicine, Division of Infectious Diseases, Northwestern University Medical School; Associate Director, HIV/STD Outpatient Treatment Center, Northwestern Memorial Hospital, Chicago, Illinois
*Sexually Transmitted Diseases*


**LANCE R. PETERSON, M.D.**
Professor, Medicine and Pathology, Northwestern University Medical School; Director, Clinical Microbiology, Consultant, Infectious Disease, Northwestern Memorial Hospital, Chicago, Illinois
*Normal Flora in Health and Disease; Infections Caused by Anaerobic Bacteria; Laboratory Evaluation of Infectious Diseases; Mechanisms of Microbial Susceptibility and Resistance to Antimicrobial Agents; Antimicrobial Agent Susceptibility Testing and Monitoring of Drug Therapy*


**JOHN P. PHAIR, M.D.**
Professor of Medicine, Northwestern University Medical School; Chief of Infectious Disease, Northwestern Memorial Hospital, Chicago, Illinois
*Temperature Regulation, the Pathogenesis of Fever, and the Approach to the Febrile Patient; Infections of the Lower Respiratory Tract: General Considerations; Community-Acquired Bacterial Pneumonia; Fungal Infections; Human Immunodeficiency Virus Infection and AIDS; Diagnosis and Management of Infection in the Immunocompromised Host; Infective Endocarditis; Antimicrobial Therapy*

## ROBERT J. POOLEY, Jr., M.D.

Resident in Pathology, Northwestern University Medical School, Northwestern Memorial Hospital, Chicago, Illinois
*Mechanisms of Microbial Susceptibility and Resistance to Antimicrobial Agents*

## BORIS E. REISBERG, M.D.

Assistant Professor of Medicine, Division of Infectious Diseases, Northwestern University School of Medicine; Consultant, Infectious Disease, Veteran's Administration Lakeside Hospital, Chicago, Illinois
*Common Intestinal Parasitic Infections; Malaria*

## ANTHONY J. SCHAEFFER, M.D.

Herman L. Kretschmer Professor and Chairman, Department of Urology, Northwestern University Medical School; Attending Physician, Northwestern Memorial Hospital, Chicago, Illinois
*Urinary Tract Infections: Cystitis and Pyelonephritis*

## STANFORD T. SHULMAN, M.D.

Professor of Pediatrics and Associate Dean for Academic Affairs, Northwestern University Medical School; Chief, Division of Infectious Diseases, The Children's Memorial Hospital, Chicago, Illinois
*Introduction to Infectious Diseases; Bacterial Infections of the Upper Respiratory Tract; Infectious Diarrhea; Viral Hepatitis; Rickettsial Diseases; Infective Endocarditis; Staphylococci, Staphylococcal Disease, and Toxic Shock Syndrome; Antimicrobial Therapy; Principles of Immunization*

## PATRICIA G. SPEAR, Ph.D.

Professor and Chairman, Department of Microbiology–Immunology, Northwestern University Medical School, Chicago, Illinois
*Virus–Host Interactions*

## TINA Q. TAN, M.D.

Assistant Professor of Pediatrics, Northwestern University Medical School; Attending Physician, Division of Infectious Diseases, The Children's Memorial Hospital, Chicago, Illinois
*Infections at the Extremes of Life, Bone and Joint Infections: Septic Arthritis and Osteomyelitis*

## RICHARD B. THOMSON, Jr., Ph.D.

Associate Professor of Pathology, Northwestern University Medical School, Chicago, Illinois; Director, Microbiology and Virology, Department of Pathology and Laboratory Medicine, Evanston Hospital, Evanston, Illinois
*Viral Infections of the Lower Respiratory Tract*

## MICHELE TILL, M.D.

Assistant Professor of Medicine, Northwestern University Medical School, Chicago, Illinois
*Viral Infections of the Central Nervous System*

## CARL WALTENBAUGH, Ph.D.

Associate Professor of Microbiology–Immunology, Northwestern University Medical School, Chicago, Illinois
*The Immune System and Microbe-Induced Autoreactive Host Responses and Autoimmune Disease*

## XUEDONG WANG, M.D., Ph.D.

Resident in Pathology, Northwestern University Medical School, Northwestern Memorial Hospital, Chicago, Illinois
*Antimicrobial Agent Susceptibility Testing and Monitoring of Drug Therapy*

## JOHN R. WARREN, M.D.

Professor and Vice Chairman, Department of Pathology, Northwestern University Medical School; Medical Director, Pathology Laboratory, Northwestern Memorial Hospital, Chicago, Illinois

*Bacteria–Host Interactions; Mycobacterial Infections; Infections at the Extremes of Life; Sepsis*

## RAM YOGEV, M.D.

Professor of Pediatrics, Northwestern University Medical School; Attending Physician, Division of Infectious Diseases; Director, Section of Pediatric and Maternal HIV Infection, The Children's Memorial Hospital, Chicago, Illinois

*Introduction to Infections of the Central Nervous System; Common Etiologic Agents of Bacterial Meningitis*

# PREFACE
## to the Fifth Edition

Expectations for the fifth edition of *The Biologic and Clinical Basis of Infectious Diseases* can be understood most readily from knowledge of the history of the textbook and the principles that have linked all previous editions.

About three decades ago, faculty of Northwestern University Medical School devised an interdepartmental course in Infectious Diseases for medical students. It was based on the premise that basic scientists and clinicians could collaborate in presenting information about medical microbiology and host-parasite relationships in a manner more relevant to clinicians than was traditionally the case. For nine years, course materials were expanded and refined continually as students responded enthusiastically to the efforts of the faculty.

Convinced that the premises behind the course were sound and emboldened by its success, Guy Youmans and his colleagues organized the course materials into the first edition of the textbook, which was published in 1975. It was received favorably not only by teachers and students of medicine but also by a diversity of audiences interested in the field of infectious diseases.

Despite changes in the editorial leadership in recent years, all subsequent editions have remained true to the concepts embodied in the initial text. These include emphasis on the microbe-host interrelationships and concentration on clinically relevant information. Each edition has incorporated information about newly recognized entities such as Legionnaires' disease or HIV infection and has included instructive case presentations. Of equal importance, they have catalogued the expanding concept of microbial infection as a direct and indirect cause of the diversity of human disease.

As was the case with the first edition, the material in each edition in succession has represented the core of information used in the Infectious Diseases course for medical students at Northwestern University Medical School. That tradition is also true for the fifth edition, even though the emphasis in the course of instruction of the medical school's preclinical curriculum has undergone major revision. This is possible because linkage to clinical problem solving, which is a major objective of the current curriculum, has been an important concept of this book from the outset. Reliance solely on faculty of Northwestern University for editorship and contributed text is another constant that has led to consistency in the quality and focus of the book.

Annual preparation for the Infectious Diseases course provides a unique signal to editors and contributors when a revision of the textbook is warranted. This edition was prepared because important new information is available about the ever expanding importance of microbial infection in the direct and indirect pathogenesis of human disease. All chapters have been revised and many are newly prepared for this edition. The utilization of instructive case presentations has been expanded, and there has been some reorganization of material included. The fifth edition of this book promises to continue the success of its predecessor editions.

The editors and contributors owe a special thanks to many people who helped in making this edition a reality.

HARRY N. BEATY
Dean
Northwestern University Medical School

# CONTENTS

## SECTION IX  TREATMENT AND PREVENTION OF INFECTIOUS DISEASES

# I HOST–MICROBE INTERACTIONS

# 1

# INTRODUCTION TO INFECTIOUS DISEASES

STANFORD T. SHULMAN, M.D.

**VIRULENCE**

**HISTORIC BEGINNINGS OF THE STUDY OF INFECTIOUS DISEASES**

**CURRENT STATUS OF THE DISCIPLINE**

The study of infectious diseases is a clinical specialty of medicine that is concerned with the pathogenesis, diagnosis, and management of illnesses directly caused by infectious microorganisms. This ever-widening spectrum of microorganisms includes bacteria, viruses, fungi, protozoa, helminths, and even algae. The specialty of infectious diseases rests firmly upon the broad scientific foundations of microbiology, epidemiology, and immunology. Indeed, from the historical perspective, the fields of microbiology and epidemiology, and more recently immunology, spawned the discipline of infectious diseases. In recent years, advances in the fields of molecular biology, including molecular genetics and molecular virology and bacteriology, have contributed to improving our understanding of the mechanisms of host–parasite interactions in ways that were unthinkable even a few years ago. Consequently, striking advances have occurred, for example, in elucidating the precise molecular basis for the interaction between adherence surface structures of an organism and corresponding specific surface receptors on a eukaryotic host cell, and in

unraveling the very complex relationship between the human immunodeficiency virus (HIV) and the various components of the immune system. Advances of these kinds are now occurring virtually on a weekly basis.

## VIRULENCE

All animals coexist with an indigenous microflora (see Chapter 2). We are each heavily *colonized* by, and live in a state of peaceful coexistence with, countless microorganisms that colonize our skin and most of our mucosal surfaces. We swim in a veritable sea of microbes. The mouth, pharynx, gastrointestinal tract, and other areas are heavily colonized by many different bacterial species, beginning shortly after birth. A classic symbiosis appears to have been established between host and parasite. This relationship is so close that it has been suggested that, from an evolutionary perspective, mitochondria (the important energy-generating intracytoplasmic organ-

1

elles) evolved phylogenetically from intracellular bacterial forms, representing actual fusion of microbe and host.

\ Under normal circumstances, a large number of host factors operate to maintain the delicate host–microbe balance. These include the normal physical barriers of intact skin and mucosal surfaces, as well as both nonspecific and highly specific aspects of the immune system (see Chapter 3). Any of a wide range of circumstances can disrupt this delicate balance between host and microbe. Examples include burns that disrupt the important skin barrier, enabling invasion by surface microbes; antibiotic therapy that alters the complex balance of microorganisms colonizing a mucosal surface, leading to overgrowth of certain species; surgery that breaches normal anatomic barriers or leaves behind foreign bodies such as sutures or tubes; malnutrition; physical and/or emotional stress; and countless others.

When the delicate balance between eukaryotic host and prokaryotic microorganism becomes disturbed in these or in other ways, *infection* of the host, rather than colonization, may ensue. The relative ability of a microorganism to produce infection is termed *virulence* and is related to a variety of complex mechanisms of disease induction. However, it is imperative to recognize that virulence is a *relative* term. That is, some organisms are highly virulent in that most or all normal hosts who become exposed to and colonized by them develop clinical illness. Examples may include organisms like *Yersinia pestis,* the cause of plague; *Salmonella typhi,* the agent of typhoid fever; and HIV, the virus causing acquired immunodeficiency syndrome (AIDS). On the other hand, when the normal host defenses are compromised, microorganisms that usually coexist symbiotically with the normal host can induce serious, even life-threatening infections. In this way, a normally harmless microorganism can demonstrate its virulence, or its potential to cause clinically apparent infection opportunistically. Examples are the coagulase-negative staphylococci that opportunistically cause infection of implanted foreign bodies such as shunts or prosthetic heart valves. Clearly the apparent virulence of a microorganism depends upon the host setting and the status of the host's normal defenses, which ordinarily hold microorganisms in check.

Thus, infection is generally a consequence of the interaction between a relatively highly virulent microorganism and a normal intact host, or between a relatively less virulent microbe and a host with some degree of transient or permanent impairment of host defense mechanisms.

In general, many important modern advances in medical therapy result also in the undesired effect of impairing the ability of the host to withstand infection. Examples include corticosteroid and cytotoxic medications that directly affect both specific and nonspecific components of the immune system, antimicrobial agents that modify the normal delicately balanced indigenous microflora, and drugs or procedures that lessen the gastric acidity that kills most ingested microorganisms. Common viral respiratory infections reduce transiently the respiratory tract's mucosal surface receptors for normal bacterial microflora, facilitating replacement of these normal flora by potentially more invasive, more virulent bacterial agents.

The 1980s saw the astonishingly dramatic worldwide emergence of a "new" infectious disease caused by HIV, an infection that ultimately debilitates host immune mechanisms, leading to vulnerability to a remarkable array of opportunistic infections. Most of these infections are caused by agents of low virulence with which uninfected individuals (those whose immune systems are intact) coexist peacefully. More than 13 million people worldwide are infected with HIV. It and resultant AIDS have become so widespread in certain areas of the world and of the United States that they have created a crisis in health care delivery. AIDS, even more than other illnesses, epitomizes the importance of understanding the delicate and precarious balance between host and microbe and of recognizing the consequences of disruption of this balance.

## HISTORIC BEGINNINGS OF THE STUDY OF INFECTIOUS DISEASES

The medical specialty of infectious diseases has its earliest beginnings in the descriptions by the Greeks, Romans, and Hebrews of epidemic afflictions—epidemics that reached particularly devastating proportions in the Middle Ages. Thucydides, a contemporary of Hippocrates, recognized the transmission of infection from one person to another, as occurred in the plague of Athens. Although Aretaeus in the second century A.D. was the first to allude to a doctrine of invisible infecting organisms, a variety of supernatural explanations were offered in the ancient and medieval worlds for smallpox and other epidemic disorders. The two great scourges of the Middle Ages were syphilis and bubonic plague; the latter was responsible for the black death, which appeared in Europe about 1348 and annihilated one fourth of the earth's population. Rather than being attributed to the crowded living conditions and poor sanitation of the walled medieval towns, these illnesses were blamed on comets or other astrologic features, crop failures, droughts or floods, or on poisoning of wells by Jews.

The spread of syphilis through Europe, which began around 1495, was recognized early on to be contagious by direct contact. Girolamo Fracastoro, a classmate of Copernicus and the man who gave syphilis its name in the 16th century, came impressively close to proposing a germ theory of disease, long before the existence of microorganisms was known. Reflecting upon his clinical experience with plague in Italy, Fracastoro wrote in 1546 that the disease is not caused by a "mysterious shadow or miasma, nor by obstructed humors but by a kind of seed." He indicated that these seeds were so minute that they were invisible and that when transmitted from one person to another they multiply and propagate themselves, soon producing in the second person the disease seen in the first. He proposed that spread of such agents occurred in three ways: by direct bodily contact, by fomites, and through the air.

After the invention of the microscope by Antony van Leeuwenhoek in the late 17th century and its further refinements, active speculation began regarding a possible relationship between disease states and the microorganisms seen through the microscope. Such speculation became even stronger by the 1830s when it was shown that both alcoholic fermentation and the process of putrefaction were the direct consequences of the activity of microscopic organisms. Both Fracastoro in the 16th century and Henle in 1840 emphasized the similarity between disease and putrefaction or decay. Robert Koch's isolation of the bacterial agent of anthrax in 1877, his development of techniques to culture microbes on solid media, and his most famous discovery of the tubercle bacillus in 1882 (an organism at that time responsible for one of every seven deaths) laid the groundwork for a flood of research aimed at the isolation and identification of the causative agents of many infectious diseases.

Two important landmarks in the *prevention* of infectious diseases were Jenner's demonstration, at the end of the 18th century, of the efficacy of vaccination against smallpox and Pasteur's production and utilization of a successful vaccine against rabies in 1885. On May 14, 1796, Jenner, a country physician in Gloucestershire, inoculated the arm of a lad named James Phipps with matter obtained from a cowpox lesion on the hand of a dairymaid, and on July 1, 1796, he challenged the boy with matter from a pustular smallpox lesion. In this scientific fashion, he demonstrated that a serious life-threatening infection could be prevented by a previous infection with an attenuated strain of the causative agent. Similarly, beginning on July 6, 1885, Pasteur's successful development and use of attenuated rabies virus to immunize a youngster named Joseph Meister, who had been bitten by a rabid dog, quickly revolutionized the approach to the prevention of infectious diseases. In fact, almost 2500 individuals were immunized against the previously invariably fatal rabies, many successfully, in the year following Joseph Meister's immunization.

*Therapeutic advances* that truly established the study of infectious diseases as a medical discipline date to von Behring's and Kitasato's discoveries in 1890 that animal antisera prepared by prior injection of toxins into the animal were useful in treating diphtheria and tetanus, classic toxin-mediated diseases. In 1909, Ehrlich produced the "magic bullet" salvarsan (arsphenamine), or 606, an arsenical that was highly effective in the treatment of syphilis. This ushered in the era of chemotherapy for infectious diseases. Of course, one of the key advances of the chemotherapeutic era was Fleming's serendipitous discovery of the antibacterial effect of penicillin in 1929 and the subsequent development of this material for human use by Chain and Florey in the early 1940s.

The accelerating pace of microbiologic and immunologic discoveries and advances in prevention and therapy has now extended into the 1990s, with the application to problem solving of such modern molecular biologic techniques as gene manipulation. The discipline of infectious diseases has moved far beyond the descriptive stage, with the continuing promise of rapidly paced advances.

## CURRENT STATUS OF THE DISCIPLINE

Despite the major technologic advances that have influenced (and will continue to influence) the field of infectious diseases, major concerns persist regarding the implementation of simple preventative and therapeutic measures. For example, as discussed in Chapter 40, about 70 million cases of measles still occur annually, producing considerable morbidity and 1–1.5 million deaths, the vast majority in underdeveloped areas of the world, where the measles mortality rate is 3–15%. These illnesses are clearly preventable but occur because of economic and logistic factors that hamper the successful implementation of immunization programs. Only 5% of the world's health research resources are devoted to the problems of developing countries, even though those countries suffer 93% of the early mortality among the world's population. Shockingly, large outbreaks of measles and pertussis occurred in the United States in the late 1980s and early 1990s, with most measles cases occurring in the underimmunized, primarily African-American and Hispanic school-aged children of the inner cities (particularly Los Angeles, Houston, Dallas, and Chicago). The interplay between infectious diseases and malnutrition must also be highlighted, as it accounts for the approximate 10% mortality from measles and excess mortality from other infections in some areas of the world. Thus, in the United States and elsewhere, the translation of the fruits of scientific progress and modern technology to the poorer segments of society remains a tremendous challenge. That is, the public health aspects of infectious diseases continue to be a challenge that requires great effort. Until these challenges can be met, children will continue to succumb to preventable diseases like measles, tuberculosis will continue to kill 10,000 people daily worldwide, and HIV will continue to be transmitted. That success in these endeavors is possible with the proper organization and commitment was demonstrated by the complete worldwide eradication of smallpox achieved in 1977 and by the complete eradication of paralytic poliomyelitis from the entire Western Hemisphere by August 1991.

In addition to focusing on improved control of the infectious diseases of childhood, the clinical practice of infectious diseases in Western society is increasingly involved with the prevention, diagnosis, and management of infections in the immunocompromised host. This patient population has grown dramatically as a consequence of increasing numbers of organ transplant recipients, AIDS patients, and individuals receiving immunosuppressive therapies for oncologic or other disorders. There is every indication that these populations will continue to increase. These immunocompromised individuals are highly susceptible to opportunistic infections caused by a very wide array of infectious agents (see Chapters 23 and 24), a fact that continues to stimulate the development of innovative preventative and therapeutic strategies.

A particularly exciting aspect of infectious diseases has been the recognition of "new" clinical syndromes during the past one to two decades, including AIDS in 1981, toxic-shock syndrome in 1981, Lyme disease in 1982, Kawasaki disease in 1967, Hantavirus pulmonary syndrome in 1993, and Legionnaires' disease in 1977. At the same time, other disorders have disappeared or are disappearing. Thus, there is a changing menu of problems that demand the attention of physicians who specialize in the exciting clinical field of infectious diseases. Indeed, all of clinical medicine is concerned with infectious diseases in some way, making this specialty one that is central to the entire discipline of medicine.

# 2

# NORMAL FLORA IN HEALTH AND DISEASE

ROBERT J. HERCEG, M.D. and LANCE R. PETERSON, M.D.

Every person provides a natural habitat for a large variety of microorganisms. These constitute the normal or indigenous flora of the body. Most act as commensal organisms; that is, they live with and generally derive benefit from the host, but neither harm nor benefit their selected host. In contrast, parasitic organisms derive their existence at the expense of the host, usually manifested as a clinical infection that interferes with normal human functioning.

Historically, most infections have been the result of pathogenic organisms originating outside the patient's own microbiotic environment. With the arrival of the acquired immunodeficiency syndrome (AIDS), post-transplant immunosuppression, and other problems of modern medicine, however, diseases caused by a patient's indigenous flora, usually defined as opportunistic infections, are increasingly important.

This chapter will describe the various "normal" or indigenous microorganisms, where they are found in the body, and how they are classified. In general, the normal flora is considered protective, since usual indigenous microorganisms can help prevent colonization or infection by more virulent pathogens. The host's interaction with its normal flora will also be discussed along with the clinical rele-

vance of these interactions. There are multiple scenarios where knowledge of normal flora is helpful. Several examples include:

1. A patient is injured causing a breach of the normal barriers separating sterile from nonsterile body compartments and from the surrounding environment. This can be due to trauma (e.g., gunshot wounds, compound fractures) or via a therapeutic procedure (catheterization, intubation) as depicted in Figure 2–1. Microorganisms are either inoculated directly or are provided with a path of decreased resistance through which to migrate. Knowledge of the usual flora at the site of infection can help in selecting appropriate empiric therapy when infection develops.

2. A patient is clinically septic. Knowing commensal organisms at clinically suspected sites of infection can help determine successful empiric therapy. For example, *Escherichia coli* is a gram-negative bacillus normally found in the colon. Thus *E. coli* bacteremia can result from a perforated bowel, or secondary to a serious urinary tract infection (that develops after colonization of the perineum resulting from contamination by anal flora).

3. A patient is given extended-spectrum antimicrobials. Patients given these drugs for more than 24–48 h experience shifts in their normal flora. Organisms that are susceptible

to the administered agent are eliminated, allowing resistant organisms to overgrow. For instance, patients given a potent cephalosporin for a gram-negative bacterial infection may experience colonic overgrowth of *Candida albicans*, a fungal organism that is resistant to these agents. *C. albicans* is a commensal inhabitant in 15–30% of the population and overgrowth may cause diarrhea in some elderly patients and infants.

4. Specimens for culture can be contaminated during collection by indigenous organisms. Interpretation of positive cultures thus requires knowledge of what precisely has been sampled and how the specimen was collected. This is particularly important when a culture becomes positive several days after the patient has spontaneously recovered and no longer appears clinically infected.

5. Shifts in usual susceptibility patterns of normal flora can be crucial in an era of increasing immunosuppression. Patients may become colonized with new drug-resistant flora during life. These organisms may be nonpathogenic at low levels, or during periods of normal health, but this new, drug-resistant indigenous flora can then cause serious illness and sepsis if the proper setting (e.g., immunosuppression) arises.

## TAXONOMY AND NOMENCLATURE

Microbes are assigned to a family, genus, and species according to rules and precedents set by the International Commission on Microbial Taxonomy defining a logical system of taxonomic organization that can confuse and elude the beginning student. Groups of organisms sharing important global properties are members of the same family. The family name is capitalized and ends in -aceae. For example, the Enterobacteriaceae includes those bacteria that are glucose-fermenting, gram-negative bacilli that do not express cytochrome oxidase. Subsets of organisms within a family that share some biochemical properties but differ from other subsets in the same family are assigned different genus names (the genus name is capitalized, italicized, and often abbreviated with a single capital letter).

Bacterial species were traditionally organized according to morphologic and biochemical characteristics. Final speciation is now most commonly determined by similarities and differences in their genomic DNA. Due

to the high mutability and adaptation seen in many kinds of bacteria, isolates of the same pathogen seen in different hospitals (or even in different patients) may appear to react variably to biochemicals during identification, and may even express different antigens, making phenotypic classification less reliable than genotypic-based nomenclature. The gold standard for species identification is therefore now recognized as DNA analysis. If the DNA content of two different strains shows more than 80% similarity, the organisms are considered to be part of the same species, and are more precisely called different strains of that same species.

Advances in molecular biology and increasing usage of these techniques have led to many name changes and species reassignments over the years, and this is unfortunately likely to continue. It is helpful for laboratories to report the old name, if one exists, particularly if the change is recent. Examples include *Enterococcus faecalis* (formerly *Streptococcus faecalis*), *Helicobacter pylori* (formerly *Campylobacter pylori*), *Moraxella catarrhalis* (formerly *Branhamella catarrhalis* or *Neisseria catarrhalis*), *Burkholderia cepacia* (formerly *Pseudomonas cepacia*), and *Stenotrophomonas maltophilia* (formerly *Xanthomonas maltophilia*). These changes, though sometimes frustrating, do reflect a better understanding of the ge-

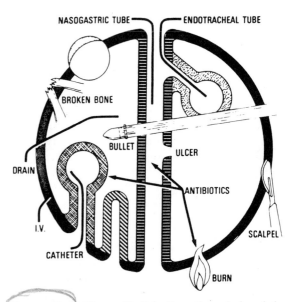

**FIGURE 2–1.** The epithelial disruptions induced by trauma, disease, and therapy that permit microbial invasion. (From Meakins, J. L. Host defenses. In: Simmons, R. L., and Howard, R. J., eds. *Surgical Infectious Diseases.* New York: Appleton-Century-Crofts, 1982. With permission.)

netic properties of these bacteria. A listing of current nomenclature, accompanied by older names, can be found in the paper by Bruckner and Colonna. Standard microbiology reference texts, such as the recent (1995) 6th edition of the *Manual of Clinical Microbiology*, also list current taxonomy.

## COLONIZATION AND PATHOGENICITY

### Mechanisms of Colonization

One of the first requirements for colonization by a new organism is an ability to adhere to a host surface. Many bacteria have surface structures (*pili* or *fimbriae*) that bind to lectins and other receptors on host epithelial cells. These interactions are often very specific. For example, glycolipid found on renal epithelia act as receptors for *E. coli* that may lead to colonization and subsequent pyelonephritis. Viruses and fungi can use similar mechanisms. For example, human immunodeficiency virus (HIV) has a membrane glycoprotein that binds to CD4, a surface antigen found on human helper T cells. This binding permits attachment, followed by penetration and infection. In all cases, subsequent to adherence, the organism must cope with the host microenvironment to establish colonization or infection.

### Determinants of Pathogenicity

Pathogenicity or virulence is what allows a colonizing (either indigenous or pathogenic) organism to become dangerous. Unfortunately, pathogenicity *in vivo* is exceedingly complex and only just beginning to be understood. Increasingly it is recognized that many bacteria that are ordinarily not regarded as pathogenic in fact are capable of producing infection and disease, particularly in circumstances in which host defense mechanisms are less than intact. Thus, the distinctions between a pathogen and a nonpathogen, or between virulent and avirulent organisms, has become somewhat blurred. Almost all microorganisms that are human parasites potentially may cause infection and therefore can be considered potentially pathogenic when host defense mechanisms are impaired. Clearly there is a continuum of disease-producing capability. Nevertheless, it is common practice to use the terms *pathogen* or *nonpathogen*, or *virulent* or *avirulent*, to indicate the *relative* capacities of parasites to cause

disease. At least three factors are important in characterizing an organism's virulence: (1) ability to grow in the host environment, (2) ability to fight initial and ongoing host defense mechanisms, and (3) ability to damage or destroy the host. These topics are discussed in greater detail in the review article by Smith.

An organism's growth rate is a vital determinant of pathogenicity. Other things being equal, a rapidly multiplying organism can harm the host more effectively than a slow-growing one. Studies of bacterial growth *in vivo* often involve comparison of wild-type organisms to temperature-sensitive or nutrient-sensitive mutants that theoretically cannot multiply *in vivo*. Using ratios of the quantities of these organisms following inoculation, one can estimate doubling times. Growth requirements are multifactorial but studies show that nutritional conditions are often rate limiting. Oxygen tension and iron limitation are two factors that have been studied. Since specific nutrient availability varies from site to site within a host, organisms may show predilection for specific sites. Also important is selection and phenotypic variation—microbes often show extraordinary ability to adapt to averse circumstances. For example, *Neisseria gonorrhoeae* can express different pilin proteins in human hosts when compared to *in vitro* cultures, presumably because of adaptational changes required for better adherence. Of prime clinical importance today are organisms that adapt to antibiotics present in the environment by acquiring episomes that code for antibiotic-inactivating enzymes, or by simple selection of antimicrobial agent–resistant clones that then spread from patient to patient. Of interest, nutrient depletion may play a significant role in bacterial survival in abscesses. Most antimicrobials require active organism growth to kill the microbe. In an (nutrient depleted) abscess, microbes are typically quiescent, making antimicrobials less active than expected, which is one reason that most abscesses cannot be cured by antibiotic treatment alone.

Some organisms are able to survive not just by growing rapidly but by resisting host defenses. For example, certain gram-negative bacteria have thick capsules that resist phagocytosis. Others can resist the bactericidal activity of complement, allowing them to survive in the blood. Some bacteria avoid destruction by creating (or selecting) protected environments like abscesses with oxygen tension or acidity unfavorable to host defenses. Other defenses to be overcome include constant epithelial cell turnover or constant unidirectional fluid flow through host conduits such as the ureter or urethra.

Organisms can harm the host by producing toxins (e.g., anthrax, pseudomembranous colitis from *Clostridium difficile*), by damaging tissues (e.g., gangrene from *C. perfringens*), or by compromising vital physiologic functions of the host (e.g., pneumonia impairing oxygen exchange, meningitis causing increased intracranial pressure, and AIDS causing immune suppression). Specific mechanisms of host damage by pathogenic organisms are discussed in other chapters.

## Interactions with Commensal Flora

Even more complex than pathogenicity is the concept of interaction between a host's commensal flora and new colonizers or invading organisms. A list of mechanisms is given in Table 2–1. Many of the important protective mechanisms are direct effects of indigenous flora. Bacteriocins are protein antibiotics made by viridans group streptococci (normally found in the oropharynx) that impede colonization by more potentially pathogenic organisms such as *Streptococcus pneumoniae*, *S. pyogenes*, and gram-negative bacilli. Bacterial interference is another form of protection and is the process where prior attachment by one species inhibits colonization by another, presumably due to a limited number of binding sites. Metabolic end products of indigenous flora may be toxic to potential

pathogens, particularly in the gastrointestinal tract. For example, some strains of enterococci have been shown to inhibit the growth of *C. difficile*.

Specific interactions will be described in later sections of this chapter corresponding to the particular body sites in which they occur.

## Selective Antimicrobial Agent Modulation

One important method of taking advantage of bacterial interaction merits a separate heading: selective antimicrobial modulation. Sepsis is a fairly common and sometimes devastating complication of the granulocytopenia that follows treatment for malignant diseases. Infection usually results from *Pseudomonas aeruginosa*, *Escherichia coli* and other Enterobacteriaceae, *Staphylococcus aureus*, and *Candida albicans*. Infecting strains of these organisms are often resistant to multiple antimicrobial agents, making treatment even more difficult. Methods of prevention historically have included laminar-airflow rooms (wherein air and airborne contaminants are cleansed and continually flowing away from the patient), total isolation, and intensive broad-spectrum antimicrobial treatment once infection develops that is intended to treat any and all potential pathogens.

In 1972, van der Waaij characterized the concept of "colonization resistance." As few as $10^1$–$10^2$ *E. coli* cells could colonize a germ-free animal, whereas $10^7$ were needed to colonize a normal animal. Subsequent experiments showed that animals with suppressed aerobic flora but normal anaerobic flora were almost as resistant to colonization as the conventional animal—$10^6$ organisms were needed to colonize with *E. coli*. Thus, indigenous anaerobes, which rarely caused infections themselves, seemed to confer resistance to colonization by the more virulent aerobic bacteria (and yeasts). Antibiotic regimens were then created that were selective against likely pathogenic aerobic organisms, sparing the protective anaerobes.

This developing approach to prevention of infection is called selective antimicrobial modulation. It can afford good protection for granulocytopenic patients without the cost and psychologic trauma of total isolation and may reduce serious infections originating from gut organisms. However, as with any use of antibiotics, organisms with natural (intrinsic) or acquired resistance to the antimicrobial regimen may be selected out from the

---

**TABLE 2–1. MECHANISMS BY WHICH INDIGENOUS MICROORGANISMS INHIBIT POTENTIAL PATHOGENS***

**DIRECT EFFECTS**
Production of bacteriocin
Production of toxic metabolic end products
Induction of low oxidation-reduction potential
Degradation of toxins
Depletion of essential nutrients
Suppression of adherence
Inhibition of translocation

**INDIRECT EFFECTS**
Enhancement of antibody production
Stimulation of phagocyte production
Stimulation of clearance mechanisms
Augmentation of interferon production
Deconjugation of bile acid

*From Mackowiak, P. A. The normal microbial flora. *N. Engl. J. Med.* **307**:83, 1982. With permission. Adapted from Savage, D. C. Colonization by and survival of pathogenic bacteria on mucosal surfaces. In: Britton, G., and Marshall, K. C., eds. *Adsorption of Microorganisms to Surfaces.* New York: John Wiley & Sons, 1980.

**TABLE 2–2.    MICROORGANISMS FOUND ON THE SKIN**

| MICROORGANISM | RANGE OF PREVALENCE (%) |
| --- | --- |
| *Staphylococcus epidermidis* | 85–100 |
| *S. aureus* | 10–15 |
| *Streptococcus pyogenes* (group A) | 0–4 |
| *Propionibacterium acnes* (anaerobic diphtheroids) | 45–100 |
| Corynebacteria (aerobic diphtheroids) | 55 |
| *Candida* sp. | Common |
| *Clostridium perfringens* (especially lower extremities) | 40–60 |
| Enterobacteriaceae | Uncommon |
| *Acinetobacter calcoaceticus* | 25 |
| *Moraxella* sp. | 5–15 |
| *Mycobacterium* sp. | Rare |

remaining host flora, overgrow, and then cause infections themselves that can be even more difficult to treat.

# INDIGENOUS FLORA BY ANATOMIC REGION

## Skin

Due to its external location, the skin is constantly bathed in many kinds of environmental microorganisms throughout life, no matter how one tries to avoid this exposure. Table 2–2 lists most of the common indigenous skin flora. Some species live on the surface epithelial layer and are easily wiped off. Others live in deeper layers of the epidermis, or in hair follicles and sweat glands. Deep glands are protected from the external atmosphere and provide an anaerobic environment where bacteria such as *Propionibacterium acnes* (anaerobic diphtheroids) may thrive. Some areas of the skin may be thicker, warmer, oilier, or drier than other areas, providing a variety of microenvironments favorable to different species. For example, *Clostridium perfringens* is localized to the perineum and thighs, whereas *Staphylococcus aureus* favors the nose, perianal region, and axillae.

Skin flora often present as laboratory contaminants. *Staphylococcus epidermidis* is a hardy, gram-positive coccus that is found nearly everywhere on the skin. Even with good skin disinfection, this organism is occasionally isolated from blood cultures. Since *S. epidermidis* is potentially a cause of bacteremia and endocarditis, one must interpret cultures positive for this organism with caution. *Propionibacterium* species, and aerobic diphtheroids (*Corynebacterium* species) can cause similar problems.

The skin flora provides an example of beneficial bacterial interaction. Many indigenous gram-positive organisms enzymatically digest the lipids produced by sebaceous glands. The resultant compounds can have antifungal and even antibacterial activity, particularly against gram-negative organisms. Unfortunately, these breakdown products may have unpleasant odors, especially where they are concentrated in areas such as underarms. Commercial deodorants work in part by suppressing gram-positive bacteria. The result is a shift in the normal flora, specifically, to an overgrowth of gram-negative bacteria.

### Nose and Nasopharynx

A list of indigenous nasopharyngeal organisms is given in Table 2–3. The outermost portion of the nasopharynx and the external nares contain much the same flora as the skin. Staphylococci, including *Staphylococcus aureus*, especially favor the anterior surfaces of the inside of the nares. Aerobic diphtheroids, or corynebacteria, a group of rarely pathogenic gram-positive bacilli, are also present in abundance.

Flora from the posterior nasopharynx is not as well characterized due to the difficulty of culturing the area. One may find anaerobes, viridans streptococci, *Streptococcus pneumoniae*, *Haemophilus influenzae*, and even *Neisseria meningitidis*. These last three organisms are usually thought of as pathogenic, but indigenous (colonizing) strains are mostly nonencapsulated and nonvirulent.

### Oropharynx

As a routine throat culture will demonstrate, there is quite a large variety of microorganisms populating the oropharynx. A representative list is provided in Table 2–4. Staphylococci are present in abundance, as well as alpha-hemolytic streptococci (so

TABLE 2–3.  MICROORGANISMS FOUND IN THE NASOPHARYNX

| MICROORGANISM | RANGE OF PREVALENCE (%) |
|---|---|
| *Staphylococcus aureus* | 20–85 |
| *S. epidermidis* | 90 |
| Corynebacteria (aerobic diphtheroids) | 5–80 |
| *Streptococcus pneumoniae* | 0–17 |
| *S. pyogenes* (group A) | 10 |
| Viridans streptococci | 95 |
| *Moraxella catarrhalis* | 12 |
| *Haemophilus influenzae* and *H. parainfluenzae* | 35–65 |
| *Neisseria meningitidis* | 0–10 |
| Enterobacteriaceae | Uncommon |

named because they show partial "green" hemolysis on sheep blood agar plates). Most of these are classified under the name "viridans group streptococci" that includes *S. mitis, S. mutans, S. milleri, S. sanguis,* and *S. salivarius.* Diphtheroids and treponemes are also present. *Actinomyces species,* which are really anaerobic gram-positive bacteria, can be isolated from the tonsils. Like the nasopharynx, avirulent strains of *S. pneumoniae* and *H. influenzae* can be found, along with *Branhamella (Moraxella) catarrhalis,* a penicillin-resistant, neisseria-like organism that occasionally causes pneumonia and sinusitis.

Research has shown that the indigenous oropharyngeal flora can protect the host from colonization by group A beta-hemolytic streptococci (*Streptococcus pyogenes*), the agent of "strep throat," rheumatic fever, bacteremia, and nephritis. Clinically, *S. salivarius,* an indigenous streptococcus, was isolated more often in children who were not colonized by *S. pyogenes.* Subsequently, *in vitro* studies showed that growth of *S. pyogenes* was inhibited by cell-free filtrates of *S. salivarius.* The inhibition was reversed by pantothenic acid. Further investigation showed that *S. salivarius* produced a substance that interfered with the use of pantothenate by *S. pyogenes.* The indigenous flora also protects against *N. meningitidis, S. aureus, Mycobacterium tuberculosis,* and *Legionella pneumophila.*

It is well known that seriously ill patients experience a shift of their oropharyngeal flora toward gram-negative bacilli, which can then lead to nosocomial pneumonia. Alterations in bacterial adhesins may play a role. Additionally, many ill, hospitalized patients are given antimicrobial agents that eliminate the normal oropharyngeal flora, creating a void easily filled by the aggressive, drug-resistant gram-negative bacilli found in hospitals.

### Mouth

The mouth provides many different kinds of surfaces for indigenous flora. The gums and buccal mucosa provide epithelial attachment sites for streptococci. Gingival crevices

TABLE 2–4.  MICROORGANISMS FOUND IN THE OROPHARYNX

| MICROORGANISM | RANGE OF PREVALENCE (%) |
|---|---|
| *Staphylococcus aureus* | 35–40 |
| *S. epidermidis* | 30–70 |
| Corynebacteria (aerobic diphtheroids) | 50–90 |
| *Streptococcus pyogenes* (group A) | 0–9 |
| *S. pneumoniae* | 0–50 |
| Viridans streptococci | 75–100 |
| *Moraxella catarrhalis* | 10–97 |
| *Neisseria meningitidis* | 0–15 |
| *Haemophilus influenzae* and *H. parainfluenzae* | 20–35 |
| Enterobacteriaceae | Uncommon |
| *Acinetobacter calcoaceticus* | 5–30 |
| Anaerobic streptococci | Common |
| *Bacteroides fragilis* | Common |
| *Prevotella melaninogenica* | Common |
| *P. oralis* | Common |
| *Fusobacterium* sp. | Common |

**TABLE 2–5.   MICROORGANISMS FOUND IN THE MOUTH INCLUDING SALIVA AND TOOTH SURFACES**

| MICROORGANISM | RANGE OF PREVALENCE (%) |
|---|---|
| *Staphylococcus epidermidis* | 75–100 |
| *S. aureus* | 10–35 |
| Viridans streptococci | 100 |
| Peptostreptococci | Common |
| *Streptococcus pneumoniae* | 25 |
| Lactobacilli | 95 |
| *Actinomyces israelii* | Common |
| Enterobacteriaceae | 65 |
| *Eikenella corrodens* | 0–5 |
| *Bacteroides fragilis* | Common |
| *Prevotella melaninogenica* | Common |
| *P. oralis* | Common |
| *Fusobacterium nucleatum* | 15–90 |
| *Mycobacterium* sp. | 0–3 |
| *Candida albicans* | 6–50 |
| *Treponema denticola* and *T. refringens* | Common |

and spaces between teeth provide protective environments for anaerobes. Carious teeth provide additional microenvironments.

Streptococci are the most important indigenous flora in the mouth (Table 2–5). The streptococci (e.g., *Streptococcus mutans*), combined with inadequate dental hygiene, promote the production of plaque (see Chapter 9). Teeth coated with plaque have a lower redox potential that favors the growth of indigenous anaerobic bacteria such as *Prevotella melaninogenica*, *Prevotella oralis*, and peptostreptococci. Cavities are soon formed, further improving the microenvironment for these organisms, and a vicious circle is created leading to infection and more tooth destruction.

Indigenous flora, particularly in the presence of advanced dental disease, can be a source of extraoral infections. Contaminated saliva may be aspirated, causing pneumonia or lung abscess. Dental caries may lead to abscess of the jaw from another indigenous microbe, *Actinomyces israelii*. Tooth extraction and other dental manipulation that causes bleeding can result in transitory bacteremia, and occasionally endocarditis develops from this event in patients with prior cardiac valve disease. Happily, correction of dental problems removes the protected colonization sites along with many of the consequences.

## Stomach

The acid pH of the normal stomach prevents growth of most microorganisms and quickly kills ingested bacteria. In certain clinical situations, though, gastric sterility may be compromised. Illnesses or medication that can raise gastric pH may result in colonization of the stomach. These include gastric malignancy, pernicious anemia, intestinal reflux, rapid gastric emptying syndromes, excessive antacid intake, or ingestion of histamine ($H_2$) blockers. Also, some organisms such as mycobacteria have chemically inert waxy cell walls that may be more resistant to acid exposure and can survive transit through the stomach. When microorganisms are present in the stomach, they usually mirror the oropharyngeal flora plus ingested (food) microbes.

## Small Intestine

The indigenous flora of the small bowel varies from proximal to distal regions. The proximal small bowel is protected by the stomach, which acts as a gatekeeper by killing most organisms before they reach the duodenum. The duodenal mucosa itself is exposed to the acid pH during the gastric emptying phase, providing further protection. Nevertheless, patients with abnormal physiology, including the syndromes mentioned above, may be colonized with organisms including *Enterococcus faecalis*, lactobacilli, or diphtheroids. Diverticula, or blind outpouchings of the bowel, can provide additional isolated, protected environments for colonizing bacteria to grow.

The ileum shows various species of colonic organisms such as anaerobes and Enterobacteriaceae. Interestingly, *Candida albicans* is found in the small intestine of 40% of the population. Although carriage is asymptomatic in healthy patients, systemic candidiasis may result from this intestinal colonization during immunosuppression and neutropenia.

Like the stomach, the biliary system is normally sterile due to the local harsh chemical environment. Only a few organisms can survive, including *Salmonella* species, *E. faecalis*, *C. perfringens*, and *Bacteroides fragilis*. Hepatobiliary reflux (reverse flow), due to obstruction with subsequent inoculation of the gallbladder and bile ducts, may result in colonization and serious infection (acute cholecystitis).

## Large Intestine

The large intestine is a veritable storehouse for bacteria. At $10^{12}$ organisms per gram of fecal material, the large intestine has the highest density of bacteria in the body. Bacteria constitute most of the dry weight of feces. Studies have shown that the bulk of fecal bacteria consists of anaerobes that often outnumber facultative aerobes (including Enterobacteriaceae) by a factor of at least 300:1. One analysis of the stool using serial dilutions plus thorough culturing isolated 113 different species. Table 2–6 contains the results of this study. This listing contains organisms often isolated from sites of infection, as well as many that rarely, if ever, cause infection.

Most of the colonic flora are clinically benign when they remain intraluminal. Only the facultative aerobes and a small fraction of the anaerobes can cause problems. For example *Bacteroides fragilis* represents only a tiny percentage of the normal flora but a disproportionately large fraction of isolates from anaerobic cultures of infected sites. Capsular virulence factors may explain the difference, but much is still unknown. Of the facultative aerobes, *Escherichia coli* causes a disproportionately high number of infections, especially urinary tract and postsurgical infectious complications. Certain colonic organisms when present in a clinical setting of sepsis can offer clues to associated diagnoses. *Streptococcus bovis* or *Clostridium septicum* isolated from a blood culture may indicate a search for an occult colonic malignancy is needed.

Like the oropharynx, indigenous flora can help prevent colonization and infection by exogenous organisms like *Vibrio cholerae*, *Shigella* species and *Salmonella* species. The mechanisms have been described earlier and include bacteriocin production and bacterial interference or competition. Short-chain fatty acids produced by anaerobes are toxic and inhibitory for *Shigella* species, *Pseudomonas aeruginosa*, and *Klebsiella pneumoniae*. Specific IgA can prevent attachment of *V. cholerae*. Of course, bowel motility with continuous peristalsis can prevent colonizing organisms from gaining a foothold. Also, indigenous flora can be altered by exogenous factors such as immunosuppression or antibiotic therapy, as well as by ingestion of specific bacteria associated with infection (e.g., salmonella or *C. difficile*). As a result, there may be overgrowth of *Candida albicans* or infection by salmonella or *C. difficile*, leading to diarrhea (see Case Histories).

## Genitourinary Tract

Most of the genitourinary tract in both sexes is sterile. This includes the kidneys, ureters, bladder, and proximal urethra. The ure-

**TABLE 2–6.   RANK AND FREQUENCY OF BACTERIAL SPECIES IN FECAL FLORA\***

| RANK | PERCENTAGE | ORGANISM(S) |
|---|---|---|
| 1 | 12 | *Bacteroides vulgatus* |
| 2 | 7 | *Fusobacterium* sp. |
| 3 | 6.5 | *Bacteroides adolescentia* |
| 4 | 6 | *Eubacterium aerofaciens* |
| 5 | 6 | *Peptostreptococcus productus* II |
| 6 | 4.5 | *Bacteroides thetaiotaomicron* |
| 7 | 3.6 | *Eubacterium eligens* |
| 8 | 3.3 | *Peptostreptococcus productus* I |
| 9 | 3.2 | *Eubacterium biforme* |
| 10 | 2.5 | *Eubacterium aerofaciens* III |
| 11 | 2.3 | *Bacteroides distasonis* |
| 28 | 0.7 | *Bacteroides ovatus* |
| 29 | 0.6 | *Bacteroides fragilis* |
| 59–75 | 0.13 | *Enterococcus faecalis* |
| 76–113 | 0.06 | *Escherichia coli*, *Klebsiella pneumoniae*, and 37 other bacterial species |

\*Adapted from Moore, W. E. C., and Holdeman, L. V. The human fecal flora of 20 Japanese-Hawaiians. *Appl. Microbiol. 27*: 916, 1974. With permission.

thral meatus and distal urethral segment are often contaminated (colonized) with skin flora. The short female urethra and proximity to the anal orifice helps explain the increased frequency of urinary tract infections resulting from this colonization in women.

In contrast, the lower female genital tract is rich in microorganisms (Table 2–7). Most prevalent and important are the lactobacilli. Present at birth and throughout the fertile years, lactobacilli are sensitive to the physiologic changes of the cervical and vaginal epithelium resulting from hormonal stimuli. The greatest number of lactobacilli can be cultured during the proliferative endometrial phase (the first 2 weeks following menses). Lactobacilli make lactic acid, resulting in a pH of the vagina and cervical os in a healthy female ranging from 4.4–4.6. Other organisms commonly growing at this pH include enterococci, *C. albicans*, and anaerobes such as *C. perfringens*.

Bacterial interactions abound in the genitourinary area. The acid pH created by the lactobacilli has many physiologic effects. It prevents overgrowth of gram-negative bacilli, and inhibitory substances can also inhibit colonization by *Neisseria gonorrhoeae*. Inhibitory lactobacilli are isolated from a smaller percentage of women with gonorrhea than from women without gonorrhea. Acid production from lactobacilli also helps activate sperm. Exogenous influences can disrupt the normal flora and lead to disease. Oral contraceptives change the usual hormonal cycles, thus altering the population of lactobacilli. The vaginal pH may rise, leading to overgrowth of *C. albicans* ("moniliasis"). Anaerobes, particularly *C. perfringens*, are present in the cervicovaginal canal and may be an important source of infection following trauma or surgery (see Case Histories).

## SUMMARY

From this chapter, it is evident that the human body is populated by an immense variety of microbial tenants. For the most part they are harmless or beneficial commensals, but by various mechanisms that are only beginning to be understood, they interact with each other, with the host, and with potential invading organisms. They are sometimes beneficial in terms of protecting us from outside pathogens but at times can be harmful, overgrowing and damaging their host. Further examples of host–microbe interactions are described in other chapters.

## CASE HISTORIES

### CASE HISTORY 1

A 58-year-old man presented at an outpatient clinic with fever, chills, malaise, and a cough productive of thick greenish sputum. A chest x-ray showed consolidation of the left lower lobe. He was diagnosed with pneumococcal pneumonia, admitted to the hospital, and because of a penicillin allergy and past intolerance to erythromycin was started on clindamycin. The respiratory symptoms cleared but 5 days later the patient developed severe diarrhea persistent for 72 h. The stool was cultured for the cause of this nosocomial diarrhea.

### TABLE 2–7.    MICROORGANISMS FOUND IN THE FEMALE GENITAL TRACT

| MICROORGANISM | RANGE OF PREVALENCE (%) |
|---|---|
| *Lactobacillus acidophilus* | 50–75 |
| *Bacteroides* sp. | 60–80 |
| *Clostridium* sp. | 15–30 |
| *Peptostreptococcus* sp. | 30–40 |
| *Bifidobacterium* sp. | 10 |
| *Eubacterium* sp. | 5 |
| Corynebacteria (aerobic diphtheroids) | 45–75 |
| *Staphylococcus aureus* | 5–15 |
| *S. epidermidis* | 35–80 |
| *Enterococci (group D streptococcus)* | 30–80 |
| Group B streptococci (*S. agalactiae*) | 5–20 |
| Enterobacteriaceae | 18–40 |
| *Acinetobacter* sp. | 5–15 |
| *Candida albicans* | 30–50 |
| *Trichomonas vaginalis* (protozoa) | 10–25 |
| Herpes simplex virus | Common |

The laboratory recovered *Clostridium difficile* with virtual absence of normal flora, and a simultaneous diarrheal specimen was positive for *C. difficile* toxin B.

In this case a shift in the normal flora incorporating a new organism, *C. difficile*, was due to an exogenous influence (antibiotics). *C. difficile* is nosocomially acquired in many institutions and the risk of colonization with this potential pathogen is about 8% per week in the hospital. Taking antibiotics inhibits portions of the normal colonic flora, thereby permitting toxigenic strains of *C. difficile* to become established and, in the right setting, cause severe diarrhea.

## CASE HISTORY 2

A 27-year-old woman presents with fever, knee pain, and lower abdominal pain. Her history reveals that in the past 4 years she has had one previous live birth and one induced abortion. During an office visit 1 month earlier, she had indicated to her physician that she might be pregnant. This was confirmed and at the time she indicated she could not afford to raise another child. She was informed that Medicaid no longer paid for abortions. One week ago she traveled to Mexico, where an induced abortion was obtained. Now she is hospitalized with fever and tachycardia. Her uterus is markedly tender and was not easily examined because of abdominal guarding. Blood cultures are done and *C. perfringens* is isolated. An emergent hysterectomy was performed, but she continued to deteriorate and died from renal and cardiac failure. *C. perfringens* was also isolated from the removed endometrial tissue.

This case illustrates that a fatal infection can occur due to contamination of the uterus by an indigenous vaginal organism (*C. perfringens*) during an abortion procedure. Clostridia can easily proliferate in necrotic tissue, and once established, the infection causes increasing necrosis often associated with bacteremia. The accompanying toxin production and hemolysis causes organ failure at distant sites that may culminate in death of the patient.

## REFERENCES

### Books

Murray, P. R., Baron, E. J., Pfaller, M. A., Tenover, F. C., and Yolken, R. H., eds. *Manual of Clinical Microbiology.*
6th ed. Washington, DC: American Society for Microbiology, 1995.
Skinner, F. A., and Carr, J. G., eds. *The Normal Microbial Flora of Man.* London: Academic Press, 1974.
Savage, D. C. Survival on mucosal epithelia, epithelial penetrations and growth in tissues of pathogenic bacteria. In: Smith, H., and Pearce, J. H., eds. *Microbial Pathogenicity in Man and Animals.* New York: Cambridge University Press, 1972.

### Review Articles

Mackowiak, P. A. The normal microbial flora. *N. Engl. J. Med. 307*:83–93, 1982.
Smith, H. Pathogenicity and the microbe in vivo. *J. Gen. Microbiol. 136*:377–393, 1990.

### Original Articles

Crow, C. C., Sanders, W. E., and Longley, S. Bacterial interference II. Role of the normal throat flora in prevention of colonization by group A *Streptococcus. J. Infect. Dis. 128*:527–532, 1973.
Gorbach, S. L. Intestinal microflora. *Gastroenterology 60*: 1110–1129, 1971.
Mackowiak, P. Microbial synergism in human infections. *N. Engl. J. Med. 298*:21–26, 1978 and *298*:83–87, 1978.
Mason, C., Nelson, S., and Summer, W. Bacterial colonization: Pathogenesis and clinical significance. *Immunol. Allergy Clin. North Am. 13*:93, 1993.
Noble, W. C. Skin microbiology: Coming of age. *J. Med. Microbiol. 17*:1–12, 1984.
Nord, C. E., Kager, L., and Heimdahl, A. Impact of antimicrobial agents on the gastrointestinal microflora and the risk of infections. *Am. J. Med. 76*(5A):99–106, 1984.
Roszak, D. B., and Colwell, R. R. Survival strategies of bacteria in the natural environment. *Microbiol. Rev. 51*: 365–379, 1987.
Sanders, C. C., and Sanders, W. E. Enocin: An antibiotic produced by *Streptococcus salivarius* that may contribute to protection against infections due to group A streptococci. *J. Infect. Dis. 146*:683–690, 1982.
Summanen, P. Recent taxonomic changes for anaerobic gram-positive and selected gram-negative organisms. *Clin. Infect. Dis. 16*(Suppl. 4):S168, 1993.
van der Waaij, D., Berghuis, J. M., and Lekkerkirk, J. E. Colonization resistance of the digestive tract of mice during systemic antibiotic treatment. *J. Hyg. (Cambridge) 70*:605–610, 1972.

# 3

# THE IMMUNE SYSTEM AND MICROBE-INDUCED AUTOREACTIVE HOST RESPONSES AND AUTOIMMUNE DISEASE

STEPHEN D. MILLER, Ph.D. and CARL WALTENBAUGH, Ph.D.

## THE IMMUNE SYSTEM: WHO NEEDS IT?

The vast majority of microorganisms that contact either the skin or the mucosal membranes do not enter the tissues of the body. Those relatively few microbes that do enter the body are usually quickly eliminated. These barriers to infection are collectively defined as a biologic system that is called the immune system. Host defenses against microbial infection can be divided into two general categories, the innate immune system and the adaptive immune system. Innate immune defenses are always present and are very important in maintaining a first line of defense to infection. Innate host defenses do not require a previous encounter with an infectious organism for maximal response, yet these responses are very rapid and occur within hours or minutes of exposure to the infectious organism. As important as the innate immune system is, this first line of defense is only good until breached. Compromise by cut, abrasion, insect bite, puncture wound, hypodermic needle, or alteration in pH allows opportunistic infection by pathologic organisms. The adaptive immune system rises to meet these threats. Substances or organisms that provoke adaptive immune responses are collectively known as immunogens or antigens. The adaptive immune system tailors its responses to an invading organism. Initial adaptive immune responses are slow, taking a week or more to develop, but most importantly they are specific for the invading organism. Once exposed to an immunogen or microbial threat, the adaptive immune system alters the qualitative and quantitative nature of subsequent responses to the same threat or stimulus. In other words, the immune system remembers. Two hallmarks of the adaptive immune system are specificity and memory. Often the same cells (e.g., macrophages) play critical roles in both innate and adaptive immune responses.

## Innate Immune System

External natural defenses are the body's first line of defense against infection and include mechanical, chemical, and biologic barriers that lie external to the basement membrane of the integument. The skin and the mucous membranes of the respiratory tract, gastrointestinal tract, among others, provide barriers to infection. The skin is the largest "organ" of the body, weighing 5 kg in adults, and its keratinized epithelium presents an impervious mechanical barrier to most microorganisms. Only when this barrier is breached by abrasion or puncture or by a breakdown of the integrity of the epidermis may organisms enter. Microbial entrance to the body is usually through the "wet" or mucous membranes such as the upper respiratory tract as by rhinoviruses or through the intestinal tract by enteroviruses and bacteria such as salmonella. Hairs and cilia in the nasal and respiratory tract serve to filter and sweep out microbes and other foreign particles. These defenses can be easily impaired. For example, cigarette smoke diminishes the ability of cilia to beat in a coordinated rhythmic fashion, and the bronchial epithelium of heavy smokers is no longer ciliated, leaving the individual with diminished capacity for self-cleansing of the respiratory tract. The strong, periodic flushing of the urinary system with urine helps prevent microbes from advancing up the urethra to infect the bladder and kidneys. The mucous membranes of the respiratory and gastrointestinal tract, as well as tears and saliva, help to trap and/or wash away microbial and other external materials. Natural chemical defenses include glands in the skin that secrete a variety of substances, such as fatty acids, giving the skin its pH of about 5.5, which inhibits microbial growth. Likewise, the basic or acidic pH levels in different parts of the body, (e.g., the gastrointestinal tract), inhibit the growth of certain microbial organisms. Biologic natural defenses include a population of harmless, "residential" symbiotic microbes on the surface of the skin, in the oral cavity, in the gut, and so forth, that are important because, by colonizing these areas, they inhibit the colonization of potentially harmful organisms.

For most individuals, the vast majority of microbes are excluded from the tissues. Occasionally, microorganisms cross the skin's basement membrane, and additional innate natural defenses are mobilized. These are categorized as either cell-mediated or humoral (fluid) mechanisms. Phagocytic cells (e.g., monocytes and polymorphonuclear leukocytes) actively ingest microbes and secrete antimicrobial toxins. These represent some of the most primitive cellular defenses in that phagocytic cells are found in all vertebrate animals as well as in many invertebrates. Some invertebrates have soluble molecules (agglutinins) in their sera and tissue fluids that cause the clumping of microbes. In vertebrates, a series of serum proteins comprise the complement system, including the alternative pathway of complement, and are capable of nonspecifically initiating damage to microbial invaders. Complement molecules by their attachment to microorganisms may enhance phagocytosis, a process known as opsonization, or binding of complement may lead directly to the cytolysis of the invading microorganism. Complement proteins also interact with antibodies (in the adaptive immune system) to help inflict more specifically targeted damage. In addition, a number of cytokines, or molecular protein messages secreted by cells, such as the interferons (alpha, beta, gamma), tumor necrosis factor-alpha, and so forth are responsible for limiting the spread and growth of microorganisms and facilitate their destruction.

The reticuloendothelial or mononuclear phagocytic system is the collective term for a variety of cells including monocytes, alveolar and other macrophages, Kupffer cells in the liver, and so forth. These cells are involved in the clearance of particulate and soluble substances from the circulation, tissue fluids, and organs. Mononuclear phagocytes and neutrophils provide defense against microbial infection generally by phagocytosis and proteolytic digestion of the engulfed microbial particles. Opsonins such as complement and immunoglobulin that bind to microbes are, in turn, bound by receptors (e.g., for the third component of complement [C3] and for the Fc portion of the immunoglobulin molecule) on the surfaces of these cells. The macrophage advances pseudopodia over the opsonized portion of the microbe, and the microbe is internalized into a phagocytic vacuole that fuses with lysosomal vacuoles in the cytoplasm. Fusion of the granule contents of lysosomal vesicles with the phagosomal vacuole results in the enzymatic destruction of the microorganism. Particle ingestion by phagocytes may occur over a very wide pH range and is accompanied by increased glucose oxidation.

Although many microorganisms are easily destroyed by this mechanism, certain pathogens, such as *Listeria, Salmonella, Mycobacterium, Chlamydia, Rickettsia, Trypanosoma,* and *Legionella pneumophila* have evolved the means to parasitize macrophages and to survive and replicate within them.

Natural killer (NK) cells are an important group of lymphocytes found both in the peripheral blood and ubiquitously in the organs and tissues of the body. While their exact function remains somewhat of a mystery, NK cells appear to play a vital role in the regulation of microbial infection and in the regulation and differentiation of hemopoietic and lymphoid cells. Their direct cytolytic activity, as their name implies, is important in the destruction of microorganisms, either by direct lysis of microorganisms or through the destruction of infected cells. Although regulation of microbial infection may be their primary function, NK cells also appear to be important in antitumor resistance.

## Adaptive Immune System

### Specialized Cells of the Adaptive Immune System and Their Products

Leukocytes, cells of the adaptive immune system, traverse the entire body via the circulatory system. Accumulations of white blood cells in tissues (spleen, thymus, lymph nodes, Peyer's patches, and appendix) together with leukocytes found in the circulation constitute the organs and tissues of the adaptive immune system. Each leukocyte has its own specific tasks to perform. Five types of leukocytes compose the adaptive immune system, and these can be divided into two general categories based upon morphology. Lymphocytes and monocytes are the two types of agranular leukocytes, those without overt cytoplasmic granules, and are thus classified as mononuclear cells. Granular leukocytes, or granulocytes, have multilobed nuclei and are classified upon the staining characteristics of their cytoplasmic granules as eosinophils, basophils, and neutrophils (or polymorphonuclear leukocytes).

**Lymphocytes.** Lymphocytes are the "workhorses" of the immune system. Generally, all lymphocytes look alike both by light and electron microscopy. Histologists often classify lymphocytes according to size: small (4–7 $\mu$m), medium (7–11 $\mu$m), and large (11–15 $\mu$m). Stimulated lymphocytes often transform into large lymphoblastic cells (up to 30 $\mu$m). Although morphologically similar, lymphocytes may differ widely in function. Immunologists further classify lymphocytes based upon embryologic function and by distinguishing molecules expressed on the cell surface.

B lymphocytes, or B cells, are responsible for the production of immunoglobulins and antibodies. In birds, a blind cloacal sac called the bursa of Fabricius serves as the indoctrination site for these precursors of antibody secreting (plasma) cells. Mammals do not have this organ, but the bone marrow appears to serve as the equivalent differentiation site. The term B cell is a mnemonic for the bursal or bone marrow origin of these cells, which normally comprise 5–20% of all peripheral blood lymphocytes. Cell-surface molecules are used to characterize lymphocyte subsets. All B cells express immunoglobulin both on their cell surface and within the cytoplasm. Immature or pre-B cells express cytoplasmic but not cell surface immunoglobulin. Cells that secrete immunoglobulin are termed plasma cells. Moreover, B cells are antigen-specific; that is, a single B cell produces immunoglobulin of only one antibody specificity recognizing a single antigenic determinant or epitope. B cells also express receptors for the third component of complement (C3R) on their surface. Complement is a collective term for those serum proteins that act in concert to lyse cells when the appropriate antibody is bound to the surface of a cell; these complement proteins comprise the classical complement pathway. C3, the third component of complement, binds to antigen-antibody complexes, and the C3R serves to concentrate antigen–antibody complexes at the B-cell surface. B-cells also express surface receptors for the Fc portion of the immunoglobulin molecule (FcR). Conformational changes in the Fc portion of the immunoglobulin molecule occur when antibody binds to antigen; the FcR can then bind this antigen–antibody complex. The FcR thus appears to concentrate antigen at the surface of the B cell. Major histocompatibility complex (MHC) class II molecules are also expressed on the surfaces of B lymphocytes.

Thymic-derived lymphocytes or T cells originate embryologically in the bone marrow as prothymocytes and migrate via the circulation to the thymus. Lymphocytes within the thymus (thymocytes) are indoctrinated by mechanisms that are just now becoming understood to develop the ability to distinguish self from non-self (foreign) antigens. This is discussed further later in this chapter. Fully mature T cells exit from the thymus and populate peripheral lymphoid organs and tissues. Collectively, T cells display a number of diverse functions; they regulate the immune response, they mediate immune responses, and they are responsible for effector function. T cells display distinguishing surface molecules. T cells, like B cells, have the ability to recognize epitopes specifically, through a cell-surface antigen-specific receptor (the T-cell receptor [TcR]). The TcRs expressed by a single cell all have identical antigenic specificity. This means that there is a distinct TcR for each antigenic epitope recognized. Since there are estimated to be between $10^7$ and $10^9$ potential epitopes, there must be nearly this number of distinct T cells. In addition to the TcR, T cells express a molecular complex known as CD3 (for cluster of differentiation) that associates on the cell surface with the TcR and is responsible for signal transduction. In addition, accessory molecules known as CD4 and CD8 are found on the surfaces of T lymphocytes; they are important to the function of the TcR and give us an indication as to the function of the cell. T cells comprise 60–70% of all peripheral blood lymphocytes.

B cells (5–20%) and T cells (60–70%) do not account for all the peripheral blood lymphocytes. Lymphocytes that are immunoglobulin-negative and do not bear CD3 markers are termed null cells. Included in this group are NK cells and the cells responsible for antibody-dependent cell-mediated cytotoxicity (ADCC) and lymphokine-activated killer (LAK) cell function.

**Monocytic Cells.** Monocytes and the reticuloendothelial or mononuclear phagocytic system are involved in the clearance of particulate and soluble substances from the circulation, tissue fluids, and organs as discussed above for the innate immune system. Distinguishing surface characteristics of these cells include FcR and C3R expression as well as the expression of MHC class II molecules. These cells play a critical role in the development of the adaptive immune response. Monocytes or macrophages *phagocytose* (e.g., engulf foreign particles, dead cells), *process* (enzymatically degrade this matter), and *present* the processed antigen on the cell surface in association with MHC class II molecules. Immunologists collectively term these cells antigen-presenting cells (APCs), and this function is called antigen presentation.

EOSINOPHILS. Eosinophilis are easily recognized in peripheral blood smears by their eosin-staining cytoplasmic granules and segmented nuclei. Eosinophils are able to phagocytose antigen–antibody complexes and microorganisms, although less efficiently than other cell types. Their ability to release toxic substances against nonphagocytosable surfaces probably accounts for their ability to kill certain metazoan parasites, such as *Trypanosoma cruzi*. The release of cationic substances from the eosinophil granules causes a certain amount of collateral damage to the surrounding tissues and is probably responsible for damage seen at the site of inflammation

BASOPHILS. Basophils both synthesize and store in their granules histamine, proteoglycans, and proteases. Granules are stained metachromatically with basic dyes. Surface receptors (Fc$_\varepsilon$RI) bind immunoglobulin E (IgE) with high affinity. Binding of multivalent antigen to this surface IgE causes the cells to degranulate and secrete mediators responsible for an immediate hypersensitivity reaction. Basophils (the circulating form) and mast cells (the tissue form) are sparsely distributed.

POLYMORPHONUCLEAR CELLS OR NEUTROPHILS. are the most numerous peripheral leukocytes, accounting for 60–70% of all circulating leukocytes. These are the classic cells of acute inflammation and are found at sites within hours of tissue injury. These cells can ingest and kill invading microorganisms using reactive oxygen compounds and microbicidal proteins stored in their granules. The importance of this defense is well illustrated by patients with profound neutropenia or neutrophil dysfunction, who often present with overwhelming infections.

## Initiation of Adaptive Immune Responses

The immune response is initiated after foreign antigen is processed by the antigen-presenting cells and peptides derived from that antigen are presented on the cell surface in a complex that includes MHC class II molecules (Fig. 3–1). This antigenic peptide–MHC II complex is recognized by the alpha-beta TcR on CD4+ T cells. The alpha-beta TcR is physically associated with the CD3 complex that is expressed on the surface of all mature T cells and is necessary for membrane expression of the alpha-beta heterodimer critical for trans-

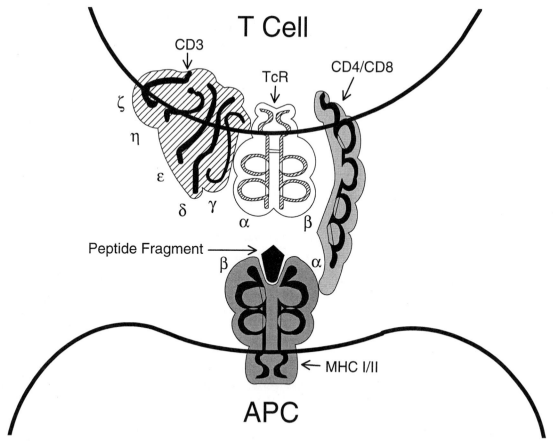

**FIGURE 3–1.** Structure of the $\alpha\beta$ TcR complexed to peptide and MHC. The T cell $\alpha\beta$ receptor has a combining site for peptide-MHC. The processed peptide fragment is bound in the groove of an MHC class I or II molecule on the surface of an antigen presenting cell (APC). Other molecules involved in T cell recognition and activation, the $\gamma$, $\delta$, $\varepsilon$, $\eta$, and $\xi$ chains of the CD3 molecule and the CD4/CD8 accessory molecules are shown.

ducing signals required for T-cell activation. Histocompatibility between the antigen-presenting cell and the CD4+ T cell is necessary for activation to occur.

B and T lymphocytes each bear receptors (surface immunoglobulin molecules and T-cell receptors, respectively) that confer the ability to discern fine antigenic differences. Although of distinctly separate lineages, the basic tenet for both B and T cells is that each cell expresses antigen receptors of only *one specificity*. It is estimated that these receptors enable our immune systems to recognize a very large number (between $10^7$ and $10^9$) of potential antigenic determinants or epitopes. This also means that there must be a separate T and/or B cell for each epitope recognized. The diversity of the immunoglobulin molecules that serve as B-cell receptors results from somatic recombination of hundreds of variable (V) gene segments, dozens of diver-sity (D) gene segments, and several joining (J) gene segments. Binding of soluble antigen to surface immunoglobulin on a B lymphocyte, in conjunction with T-cell help, results in B-cell clonal expansion and eventually the secretion of antibody molecules. Activation of T cells differs in that soluble antigen must be processed and immunogenic peptides presented to the T cell on the cell surface of antigen-processing cells in conjunction with MHC molecules, as described above. In addition to T-cell receptor occupancy, T-cell activation requires the delivery of appropriate costimulatory signals mediated in part by the CD28/B7-mediated pathway. The alpha-beta TcR complex is composed of a 40- to 50-kD acidic alpha-glycoprotein covalently linked to a 40- to 45-kD basic beta-glycoprotein; they are noncovalently associated at the cell surface with the CD3 complex, which is itself composed of five protein chains. The TcR alpha- and beta-glycoproteins are transmembrane and contain extracellular variable and constant domains analogous to immunoglobulins, as well as a connecting segment, a transmembrane segment, and a short intracytoplasmic tail. The antigenic diversity of the TcR is generated by the combination of approximately 30 V-beta, two diversity (D), and 12 J-beta gene segments, and in the alpha chain by approximately 100 V-alpha and 50 J-alpha segments.

Most adaptive immune responses are T-cell dependent; that is, they are regulated by T cells and involve multiple cell–cell interactions. Two types of CD4-bearing helper T ($T_H$) cells, termed $T_H1$ and $T_H2$, defined both by their lymphokine secretion patterns and by their functions, are responsible for regulation of most adaptive immune response and are represented diagramatically in Figure 3–1. $T_H1$ cells produce interleukin-2 (IL-2), interferon-gamma (IFN-gamma) and lymphotoxin (TNF-beta) and appear to be important in helping cell-mediated immune responses. $T_H2$ cells produce IL-4, IL-5, IL-6, and IL-10 and appear to be responsible for the development of most humoral immunity. In addition to their stimulatory effects, at least several of these $T_H1$- or $T_H2$-produced cytokines are cross-inhibitory. For example, IFN-gamma, an important stimulator of cell-mediated delayed hypersensitivity (DTH) responses, is a potent inhibitor of $T_H2$ function. Conversely, IL-10, produced by $T_H2$ cells, acts upon APCs and inhibits IFN-gamma production and other cytokine synthesis by $T_H1$ cells. IFN-gamma and IL-10 appear to play important cross-inhibitory roles in the course of immune responses to infectious organisms. Moreover, infectious organisms by their route of infection and/or the cytokines they induce may alter the $T_H1$-$T_H2$ balance and thus alter the course of the immune response.

### Cell-Mediated Immunity

Cell-mediated immune responses are directed by T cells and involve direct cell-to-cell contact by T cells or macrophages to cause the death of invasive organisms. Microorganisms are engulfed by macrophages (phagocytosis), enzymatically degraded (processed), and displayed on the surface of APCs in association with MHC class II molecules (presentation). Certain infectious organisms induce, by mechanisms that are not fully understood, macrophages to produce interleukin-12 (IL-12), a cytokine that appears necessary for the development of cell-mediated immune responses. A CD4 T cell specific for the particular antigenic peptide is stimulated as described above to further differentiate into a $T_H1$ T cell. Stimulated $T_H1$ cells produce a variety of cytokines including IL-2 and IFN-gamma. IFN-gamma is critical for the recruitment and activation of macrophages that cause the cellular infiltration characteristic of DTH responses. Although IFN-gamma is necessary for the development of DTH responses, it inhibits the development of $T_H2$-controlled responses.

Cytotoxic T lymphocytes (CTLs) function in the cell-mediated immune response. For years immunologists believed that CD4-bearing lymphocytes ($T_H1$) helped CD8-bearing CTLs kill cells expressing antigens in association with MHC class I cell surface molecules. Since all nucleated cells in the body express MHC class I, CTLs are very efficient at clearing (i.e., killing) cells that are the repositories for intracellular infectious agents such as viruses. Recently, however, this view has been revised. Genetically manipulated mice, unable to make CD8 lymphocytes ($beta_2$-microglobulin knockouts), are not overtly susceptible to viral infection, and are able to produce CD4-bearing CTLs. Conversely, mice that lack CD4 lymphocytes (CD4 knockouts), develop CD8 CTL responses that do not differ from non-genetically manipulated individuals. This indicates that CD4+, $T_H1$ help is not absolutely necessary for the development of CD8-mediated CTL responses.

### Humoral Immunity

With the recognition of the universality of microorganisms about 100 years ago, a new paradox arose, the normal resistance of animals to microbial infection. Immunology was born about the same time when a general method of immunization against infectious disease was demonstrated. Related to this was the observation that blood, held outside the body, resisted putrefaction much longer than other body tissues. Freshly drawn blood would kill at least some types of bacteria. Gradually the idea of special agents in the blood, adapted to defend the body against bacterial invasion, gave "birth" to a new class of humors, specific antibodies. In more contemporary terms, humoral immunity refers to antibody production in response to an antigenic stimulus.

Microorganisms that do not induce macrophages to produce IL-12 are engulfed by macrophages (phagocytosis), enzymatically degraded (processed), and displayed on the surface of APCs in association with MHC class II molecules (presentation). The development of a humoral immune response is outlined in Figure 3–2. IL-12 appears to be inhibitory to the development of $T_H2$ cells; when IL-12 is not present or in very low concentration, a humoral immune response develops. $T_H2$ cells produce a variety of cytokines including IL-4, IL-5, IL-6, and IL-10. Both IL-4 and IL-10, while helpful in the development and maturation of B cells into plasma (antibody-secreting) cells, are inhibitory to the development of cell-mediated ($T_H1$-mediated) immune responses.

B cells are the only cells destined to become antibody-secreting or plasma cells. Multipotential stem cells give rise to the progenitors of all blood cells, including cells of the B-cell lineage. Committed progenitor cells proceed through a number of discernible steps. Early B-cell precursors undergo $VDJ_H$ immunoglobulin gene rearrangement. Large cells that express cytoplasmic but not surface immunoglobulin class M (IgM) are termed pre-B cells, and newly formed B cells express both cytoplasmic *and* surface IgM. Mature B cells express both IgM and IgD on their cell surfaces. At this stage, however, B cells may be considered developmentally arrested and require activation to become antibody-secreting cells. Cell surface immunoglobulin serves as the antigen receptor on B cells. The physical binding of either soluble or particulate antigen (e.g., microorganisms) to B-cell antigen receptors is necessary but not sufficient for the activation of B cells to become antibody-secreting cells. $T_H2$ cells provide the second necessary cytokine signals for B-cell activation. Both molecular and biochemical changes occur as a consequence of this activation. Immunoglobulin secreted by plasma cells differs in both quantity and quality from that ex-

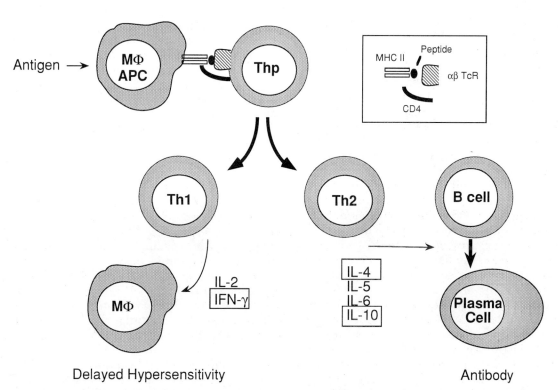

**FIGURE 3–2.** Diagrammatic structure of the alpha-beta TcR complexed to antigen plus MHC. The T-cell alpha-beta receptor has a combining site for antigen-MHC. The antigenic peptide (represented by the *black pentagon*) is bound by an MHC molecule on the surface of an antigen-presenting cell in a groove created by two alpha helices (*circles*) and a beta-pleated sheet (*platform*). Other molecules involved in T-cell recognition and activation, the gamma, delta, and epsilon chains of CD3, and the "accessory" or "co-stimulatory" molecules, CD4 and CD8, are shown. (From Blackman, M., Kappler, J., and Marrack, P. The role of the T-cell receptor in positive and negative selection of developing T-cells. *Science 248:*1335, 1990. With permission.)

pressed on the surfaces of B cells. The membrane-anchoring domain of immunoglobulin is not present in the secreted form of immunoglobulin. Also, activated B and plasma cells switch the constant portion of their immunoglobulin heavy chains, a process known as isotype or class switching by deleting portions of the cell's genomic DNA. (For a more detailed discussion of these molecular and biochemical processes, please refer to the texts by Abbas et al., or Janeway and Travers cited at the end of this chapter.) As the humoral immune response "matures," antibodies of IgG, IgA, and/or IgE isotypes become prevalent in the serum and/or in the tissue fluids.

## Progression of Adaptive Immune Responses

A paradox of the immune system is that an individual has all of his/her antigen-specific *precommitted* T and B cells shortly after birth and prior to encounter with antigen. There are an estimated $10^7$–$10^9$ epitopes recognized separately by T and B lymphocytes, yet the human body contains "only" $10^9$–$10^{10}$ lymphocytes. Thus, a few epitope-specific T lymphocytes must interact with an equally small number of T (for a $T_H1$ response) or B (for a $T_H2$ response) cells. The immune system answers this paradox by clonally expanding the number of antigen-specific T and/or B cells (antigen-specific proliferative responses) upon activation, and this accounts for much of the lag phase seen in the development of a primary immune response. This clonal expansion has a twofold effect: (1) to increase the number of antigen-specific T cells and thereby increase the likelihood of an encounter with an effector cell (such as an antigen-specific B cell); and (2) a second later encounter with antigen does not require the same initial lag time, since the same degree of clonal expansion of lymphocytes is not required. Therefore, a secondary immune response is characterized by a shorter lag phase, a more rapid and prolonged level of immune response and, in the case of a humoral immune response, the production of large amounts of antibodies of the IgG, IgA, and/or IgE isotypes. This secondary immune response and the rapidity with which it occurs are the hallmarks of immunologic memory.

## IMMUNITY GONE AWRY: MICROBE-INDUCED AUTOREACTIVE HOST RESPONSES AND AUTOIMMUNE DISEASE

The tools of modern cellular and molecular biology have enabled the recent advancement in our knowledge of how host immune responses can be directed against constituents of our own tissues or cells, the process known as "autoimmunity." It has been recognized for decades that autoimmune responses are often preceded by or associated with certain microbial infections. However, the precise relationship between those cellular and/or humoral immune responses and the pathogenesis of self-tissue damage has been difficult to establish. For example, the existence of a tissue-reactive autoantibody in certain pathologic conditions does not confirm a causal relationship between the disease and the presence of the self-reactive antibody. In fact, the autoantibody response may be an "epiphenomenon," secondary but unrelated to the disease pathology.

There are, however, a number of examples of microbe-induced immune responses that are central to disease pathogenesis. The primary examples are the development of acute rheumatic fever following group A streptococcal upper respiratory tract infection, acute poststreptococcal glomerulonephritis following skin or throat infection (see Chapter 7), acute encephalomyelitis in humans receiving certain viral vaccines, and the so-called reactive arthropathies that occur in selected individuals recovering from acute gastrointestinal infection caused by *Salmonella*, *Shigella*, *Yersinia*, or other agents.

The precise mechanisms by which the majority of autoimmune diseases arise remains unclear; however, there are multiple theories to explain the origin of autoreactivity. The simplest explanation is a spontaneous loss of self-tolerance due to unknown mechanisms (see below). Several alternate hypotheses related to microbe-induced, self-directed responses have recently been proposed. First, certain autoimmune phenomena may result from the presentation of self determinants that are normally sequestered from the immune system, either as a result of trauma or secondary to infection-induced, chronic inflammatory tissue damage. This phenomenon has been termed "*epitope spreading*" and has been shown to play a role in the chronic pathology of several experimental autoimmune diseases. Alternatively, the "*molecular mimicry*" hypothesis maintains that certain antibody or T-cell–mediated autoimmune diseases arise as a result of cross-reactive immune responses, wherein a response to a microbe-encoded antigenic determinant cross-reacts with a determinant(s) on a self-antigen. This is exemplified by the induction of antibodies against the M protein of *Streptococcus pyogenes*, which cross-react with a cardiac myocyte cell membrane protein (see Chapter 7). Lastly, it has been proposed that self-reactive responses may be activated via the action of bacterial or viral superantigens that can activate T-cell subsets in a polyclonal manner.

### Self–Non-self Recognition

The immune system is highly efficient in its ability to mobilize responses to an extraordinarily diverse range of foreign (i.e., *non–self-*) antigenic stimuli by the mechanisms described above. By contrast, under normal circumstances, the host's *self* antigenic determinants are in large part ignored by the immune system. This ability to selectively avoid developing immune responses against self-epitopes is found even in primitive forms of life, suggesting that there is parallel acquisition of both immune responsiveness and selective self-nonresponsiveness. Clarifying the mechanisms by which self-tolerance is induced and maintained is crucial for the understanding of the pathogenesis and treatment of autoimmune disease.

The interaction of the TcR alpha-beta–CD3 complex with foreign processed antigen and MHC leads to activation of the TcR alpha-beta–CD4+ lymphocytes. The most critical determinant of whether an immune response will occur is conferred by the TcR alpha-beta-heterodimer that recognizes the complex of processed foreign peptide and MHC molecule on appropriate APCs. It is presumed that T cells with specificity for self-antigens are negatively selected (either deleted or inactivated) during thymic maturation of immature T cells. The resultant failure of T cells to recognize self-antigens is termed *tolerance.*

### Tolerance

At least three mechanisms have been proposed to explain how tolerance, or nonresponsiveness, to self-antigens develops. These

include: (1) *clonal deletion*—the clonal elimination of autoreactive T-cell clones early in thymic development; (2) *clonal anergy*—the functional inactivation of autoreactive T-cell clones either during thymic development or in the periphery; and (3) active *suppression* of autoreactive T-cell clones. Until recently, it has been difficult to determine the relative contributions of these three mechanisms to the maintenance of self-tolerance. However, recent advances including: (1) the construction of transgenic mice that express specific T-cell receptors; (2) the demonstration that some TcR beta-chain variable domains preferentially confer reactivity to specific self or to foreign antigens; and (3) the use of monoclonal antibodies to identify T cells that bear TcRs for a specific antigen have helped clarified this picture. These studies have supported a role for both thymic clonal deletion and peripheral anergy in the induction and maintenance of self-tolerance. T-cell precursors bearing high-affinity autoreactive TcRs are negatively selected (i.e., deleted) during early thymus development. In addition, self-reactivity against organ-specific antigens not expressed at high levels or inefficiently presented in the thymus is mediated by the induction of peripheral anergy. It is believed that presentation of self-peptides by "nonprofessional" tissue-resident APCs lacking appropriate co-stimulatory molecules leads to the functional inactivation of those autoreactive T cells, which may escape thymic deletion. At present, there is little evidence for a major role for suppressor T cells in maintaining self-tolerance.

Tolerance to non–self-antigens also occurs, but appears to be of less clinical relevance, except as to its desirability in transplant recipients. Mechanisms of induction of tolerance to non–self-antigens are varied and complex, and they are beyond the scope of this chapter.

### Autoreactive Responses in Humans

In general, humans remain tolerant of self-antigens, a fact that contributes to the healthy state. However, a number of pathologic conditions are characterized by the development of autoimmunity, or the failure of self-tolerance. In general, autoimmune *responses* are thought to be rather common, whereas the occurrence of autoimmune *disease* is relatively rare. That is, the quality and magnitude of the autoimmune mechanisms triggered may determine whether clinically apparent disease develops. The development of disease is dependent upon the antigenic properties of the inducing autoantigen, the mode of antigen presentation, the genetic make-up of the host, and the accessibility of the target antigen to immune effector mechanisms.

Clinical autoimmune disorders result from a variety of effector pathways, humoral and/or T-cell–mediated, that may result in cell dysfunction, damage, or death. Effector mechanisms include $T_H1$ cell-directed mononuclear cell inflammatory processes that in many respects are identical to classic DTH-mediated tissue damage. Autoreactive $T_H1$ cells produce proinflammatory chemokines and cytokines, such as macrophage inflammatory protein (MIP) –1 alpha, IFN-gamma, and lymphotoxin (i.e., TNF-beta), which promote the chemoattraction and activation of mononuclear inflammatory cells to sites of autoantigen presentation. Activated mononuclear cells then mediate bystander tissue destruction via enhanced release of proteolytic enzymes, cytotoxic cytokines, oxygen radicals, nitric oxide, and increased phagocytic capacity. Autoimmune diseases in which $T_H1$-directed responses play a major pathologic process include multiple sclerosis, insulin-dependent diabetes mellitus (IDDM), rheumatoid arthritis, autoimmune orchitis, Hashimoto's thyroiditis, and many other organ-specific autoimmune responses.

Autoreactive $T_H2$ clones facilitate proliferation and differentiation of autoreactive B-cell clones producing autoantibodies, which can participate in complement-mediated cell damage, immune complex-mediated injury, or ADCC. Autoantibodies can also blockade or down-regulate the expression of cell receptors (e.g., in myasthenia gravis), or act as false transmitters (e.g., in Graves' disease). Other examples of antibody-mediated autoimmune disorders include the group of classic systemic autoimmune diseases—systemic lupus erythematosus (SLE), rheumatoid arthritis, scleroderma, Sjögren's syndrome, dermatomyositis, and mixed connective tissue disease (MCTD). These disorders are characterized by spontaneous production of autoantibodies that react with cellular proteins and/or nucleic acids. It has recently been established that each of these disorders is characterized by its own distinctive set of autoantibodies. SLE is associated with several autoantibodies including anti-DNA (both single-stranded and native double-stranded DNA), anti-Sm (complexes of small nuclear RNAs and proteins that are

important for splicing of precursor mRNA), and anti-PCNA (proliferating cell nuclear antigen, involved in DNA replication and repair). In scleroderma, autoantibodies to centromere proteins involved in cell mitosis and spindle function are common, as is anti-Scl-70 (DNA topoisomerase I). Careful study of the patterns of autoantibodies in various disorders suggests that the immunogens *in vivo* may be subcellular particles in structurally distinct cellular compartments, rather than individual proteins. Certain autoantibodies are directed against autoepitopes that are critical for certain cellular functions (e.g., catalytic sites of enzymes). In fact, these autoantibodies are being utilized to study the molecular structure of intracellular molecules and to clarify their biologic function.

Autoantibodies serve as convenient markers for diagnosing autoimmune diseases. Although an autoantibody may not be involved directly in disease pathogenesis, it may offer important clues as to the nature of disease-relevant T-cell autoantigens/epitopes and/or the events involved in initiation of the autoimmune disease. For the most part, the role of specific exogenous factors in triggering or exacerbating autoimmune responses remains unclear. Certain chemical agents, such as mercuric chloride in mice and rats and the drug procainamide in humans, clearly initiate autoantibody formation. Physical alteration of self-antigens, for example, by tissue injury, has also been proposed as a possible mechanism by which an autoimmune response might be triggered. The role of infectious agents is relatively clear in a few disorders (see below), but in many other autoimmune diseases their role is clearly speculative.

## Microbe-Induced Autoreactive Responses

As outlined previously, there are several proposed mechanisms by which microbes might trigger autoreactive immune responses leading to development of autoimmune clinical disorders. In some circumstances, infectious agents may induce in host tissues expression of an altered or neoepitope that is not present on uninfected tissue, nor on the infecting agent. Coxsackie B virus–induced myocarditis/myocardiopathy in mice is associated with an early acute phase directly related to viral infection and a later phase mediated by a T-cell autoimmune response directed against a new epitope on myocardial fibers and unrelated to viral antigen. Alternatively, chronic $T_H1$-mediated inflammatory responses against microbial agents which have the ability to persist in particular target organs or tissues can lead to the release of normally sequestered antigens and, in a secondary fashion, result in the priming of self-reactive immune responses. It has recently been demonstrated that *epitope spreading* plays a major role in the *chronic* T-cell–mediated pathogenesis of both autoimmune (experimental autoimmune encephalomyelitis [EAE]) and Theiler's virus-induced demyelinating diseases in the SJL/J mouse. Thus, autoimmune responses against a non–cross-reactive, immunodominant epitope on proteolipid protein, the major protein component of central nervous system (CNS) myelin, are demonstrable following chronic CNS demyelination initiated by specific $T_H1$ cells targeting a CNS-persistent virus. In addition, epitope spreading has been described in the T-cell–mediated destruction of pancreatic beta cells that occurs spontaneously in the non–obese diabetic (NOD) mouse.

A particularly striking association between microbial infection and suspected autoimmune disease is evident in the so-called *reactive arthropathies* (including Reiter's syndrome) and in ankylosing spondylitis. Reactive arthropathy is of acute onset and occurs 2–6 weeks after a preceding gastrointestinal or genitourinary tract infection has subsided. The disease is episodic and primarily involves peripheral joints. The implicated infectious agents include *Shigella, Salmonella, Yersinia, Campylobacter, Clostridium,* and *Chlamydia* species. These illnesses are considered to be reactive rather than infective because no viable organisms are detectable in the inflammatory sites, and antibiotic therapy is completely ineffective. However, recent studies have reported the persistence of bacterial DNA in synovial cells from patients with reactive arthritis, but not from controls.

There is a strong association between these arthropathies and expression of the HLA-B27 haplotype, particularly in Caucasians. For example, approximately 90% of patients with ankylosing spondylitis, about 80% of those with Reiter's syndrome, and 60–80% of those with reactive arthropathies are B27-positive. This contrasts with about 6–8% B27-positivity in the general Caucasian population. Several hypotheses have been proposed to explain how HLA-B27 and the bacteria noted above might interact to induce reactive arthropathy.

One is that HLA-B27 is important in the presentation of bacterial antigens in the form of peptides to putative disease-associated T cells. However, it has not been definitively established that reactive arthropathies are T-cell mediated, nor have disease-inducing bacterial peptides been identified. A second hypothesis is that HLA-B27 molecules serve as cell-surface receptors for certain factors elaborated only by arthritis-inducing organisms, and that the genes encoding these factors are on plasmids and become integrated into the host cell genome. Few experimental data support this idea.

Another hypothesis to explain the pathogenesis of reactive arthropathies involves *molecular mimicry.* The mimicry hypothesis suggests that cross-reactive antigens exist between HLA-B27 or HLA-B27 complexed to particular processed host peptides and components or products of the disease-triggering bacteria, so that a B27-restricted response to bacterial determinants initiates the disease. The structure of HLA-B27 molecules, like other HLA class I cell-surface glycoproteins, includes a polymorphic heavy chain and a noncovalently associated light-chain peptide, beta$_2$-microglobulin. The HLA class I (HLA-A, B, and C alleles) genes have an exon-intron structure, and the exons encode a leader peptide and three extracellular domains (alpha$_1$, alpha$_2$, alpha$_3$), as well as transmembrane and cytoplasmic portions. Polymorphisms among the class I alleles reflect amino acid substitutions mainly in the N-terminal alpha$_1$- and alpha$_2$-domains. Six HLA-B27 alleles have been defined by isoelectric-focusing gel electrophoretic differences, and they differ by 1–4 amino acid substitutions in eight variable positions in the alpha$_1$- and alpha$_2$-domains. X-ray crystallographic studies of HLA class I molecules indicate that the alpha$_2$- and beta$_2$-microglobulin domains have tertiary structures resembling immunoglobulin constant domains and that the alpha$_1$- and alpha$_2$-domains form a platform of eight beta strands topped by two alpha helices, with a long groove between the helices. The polymorphic residues of HLA class I molecules such as B27 tend to be clustered in this groove and are the sites at which peptide antigens are bound and serve as the TcR recognition site. All eight of the B27 variable positions point into this groove and thus appear functionally important.

Monoclonal antibodies have been used for the evaluation of possible cross-reactivity or mimicry between HLA antigens and bacterial determinants. A monoclonal antibody raised against *Yersinia enterocolitica* that also reacted specifically with HLA-B27 has been described, as have HLA-B27–directed monoclonal antibodies that cross-react with a 16-kD component of a strain of *Y. enterocolitica* and two strains of *Klebsiella pneumoniae*, or with a 20-kD molecule on a strain of *Shigella flexneri*. Cross-reactivity between B27 and a 19-kD component of *Y. pseudotuberculosis* has also been reported. Other investigations have reported monoclonal anti-B27 antibodies that react with 23-kD and 36-kD envelope components in strains of *Shigella flexneri, S. sonnei, Salmonella typhimurium, K. pneumoniae,* and *Escherichia coli.*

Utilizing a somewhat different approach, other investigators have compared the amino acid sequence of HLA-B27 with a computer bank of known protein sequences in order to identify a bacterial protein with close sequence homology. The most homologous were six consecutive amino acids shared by B27 (residues 72–77 in the hypervariable region) and *K. pneumoniae* nitrogenase (residues 188–193). Antibodies raised against the B27 peptide reacted not only with the peptide used for immunization, but also with peptides from *Klebsiella* nitrogenase containing the six consecutive amino acids. Peptides with single amino acid substitutions demonstrate substantially less cross-reactivity. Thus, amino acid homology between HLA-B27 and *Klebsiella* nitrogenase results in immunologic cross-reactivity. Sera from HLA-B27–positive patients with Reiter's syndrome or ankylosing spondylitis frequently react to these peptides, whereas sera from B27-positive normals do not. Therefore, it may be possible that many patients with these disorders have antibodies against self–HLA-B27 that are induced during an infection with *Klebsiella*. Sections of articular tissue from B27-positive patients with ankylosing spondylitis showed strong reactivity of the cells of the synovial lining and vascular endothelium with antibodies raised against peptides derived from B27 or from nitrogenase; this was not found in control articular tissues. These studies support the hypothesis that ankylosing spondylitis patients express the epitope shared by HLA-B27 and *Klebsiella* nitrogenase, such that it is accessible to a cross-reactive immune response. Thus, a possible sequence of events related to this molecular mimicry is as follows: *K. pneumoniae* infection or colonization induces an immune response that also recognizes self-B27–specific antigens; the shared antigen has enhanced expression in articular tissues, and the result is an autoimmune disorder such as ankylosing spondylitis or Reiter's syndrome.

Another classic instance of molecular mimicry in an antibody-mediated autoimmune disease relates to group A streptococcal M proteins and myosin, a relationship that may contribute to the pathogenesis of the carditis of acute rheumatic fever (see Chapter 7). Although several cross-reactive systems between streptococcal and mammalian antigens have been described, the best characterized system is that involving myosin. Sera from patients with acute rheumatic fever or chronic rheumatic heart disease contain elevated levels of antimyosin antibodies that cross-react with M protein, especially M types 1, 5, 6, and 19. Pepsin treatment of M protein leads to removal of its amino-terminal half (referred to as Pep M protein), and the epitope cross-reactive with myosin was localized to this Pep M protein. Using synthetic-overlapping peptides that encompass the entire sequence of the Pep M5 molecule, the Pep M5 epitope recognized by human and murine cross-reactive antibodies was localized to a 14-amino acid sequence in the carboxy region of Pep M5, and a pentameric sequence (positions 184–188) was found to be essential for inhibiting the cross-reactive antibodies.

Similar instances of molecular mimicry have been investigated that involve homologies between other important mammalian proteins, such as alpha-gliadin, insulin, and acetylcholine receptor, and a variety of microbial proteins. Mimicry between a major surface glycoprotein of *Streptococcus mutans* (an oral streptococcus) and human IgG heavy chains has recently been demonstrated. Thus, numerous examples of cross-reactivity between antimicrobial antibodies and self-determinants have been described that may contribute to antibody-mediated tissue injury.

Mimicry at the T-cell level is less well documented in association with T-cell–mediated autoimmune disorders. However, recent studies both in the T-cell–mediated NOD mouse model of spontaneous IDDM and in human IDDM patients have demonstrated T-cell cross-reactivity between coxsackievirus P2-C protein and an epitope (amino acids 247–279) on glutamate decarboxylase (GAD65), a pancreatic beta-cell–specific enzyme. This interesting finding may indicate that molecular mimicry at the T-cell level contributes to the pathogenesis of human IDDM. It is likely that multiple mechanisms of induction of anti–self-responses (e.g., molecular mimicry and epitope spreading), acting either alone or in concert, are operative in different autoimmune diseases. Considerable additional study is required to elucidate the significance of these and other instances of cross-reactivity between host and microbial antigens and their ultimate relationship to autoimmune disorders.

## CASE HISTORY

### CASE HISTORY 1

In 1985, contaminated dairy milk led to the largest outbreak of acute salmonellosis in the United States, with over 16,000 well-documented cases occurring in the greater Chicago area alone. Following resolution of their acute gastrointestinal illnesses, a number of individuals developed additional symptoms. A 45-year-old woman complained of the onset of acute right-knee swelling, pain, and tenderness 6 weeks after her acute salmonellosis that had been characterized by 3 days of fever, diarrhea, and vomiting. The knee complaints regressed after 1 week, but recurred 2 months later. Physical examination was negative except for swelling, redness, and tenderness of the right knee. At that time, laboratory investigation yielded an erythrocyte sedimentation rate of 60 mm/h (Westergren method), WBC = 14,000/mm$^3$, HLA-B27 was positive, rheumatoid factor and antinuclear antibody were negative, and stool culture was negative. Treatment with nonsteroidal anti-inflammatory agents was instituted with prompt response. Three months later, another episode of arthritis of the right knee necessitated additional therapy.

This is a typical example of reactive arthritis in a B27-positive individual following acute salmonellosis.

## REFERENCES

### Books

Abbas, A., Lichtman, A. H., and Pober, J. S. *Cellular and Molecular Immunology*, 2nd edition. Philadelphia: W. B. Saunders Co., 1992.
Dupont, B., ed. *Immunology of HLA*. Vol. I and Vol. II. New York: Springer-Verlag, 1989.

Janeway, C. A., Jr., and Travers, P. *Immunobiology: The Immune System in Health and Disease*. New York: Garland Publishing, Inc., 1994.
Rose, N. R., and MacKay, I. R., eds. *The Autoimmune Diseases*. New York: Academic Press, 1985.
Schumacher, H. R., Jr., Klippel, J. H., and Robinson, D. R., eds. *Primer on Rheumatic Diseases*. Atlanta, GA: Arthritis Foundation, 1988.

### Review Articles

Blackman, M., Kappler, J., and Marrack, P. The role of the T-cell receptor in positive and negative selection of developing T-cells. *Science 248*:1335–1341, 1990.
Marrack, P., and Kappler, J. The T-cell receptor. *Science 238*:1073–1079, 1987.
Miller, S. D., and Karpus, W. J. The immunopathogenesis and regulation of T-cell mediated demyelinating diseases. *Immunol. Today 15*:356–361, 1994.
Miller, S. D., McRae, B. L., and Vanderlugt, C. L., et al. Evolution of the T-cell repertoire during the course of experimental immune-mediated demyelinating diseases. *Immunol. Rev., 144*:225–244, 1995.
Rose, N. R. Pathogenic mechanisms in autoimmune diseases. *Clin. Immunol. Immunopathol. 53*:S7–16, 1989.
Schattner, A., and Rager-Zisman, B. Virus-induced autoimmunity. *Rev. Infect. Dis. 12*:204–222, 1990.
Sinha, A. A., Lopez, T., and McDevitt, H. O. Autoimmune diseases: The failure of self-tolerance. *Science 248*:1380–1388, 1990.
Tan, E. M. Antinuclear antibodies: Diagnostic markers for autoimmune diseases and probes for cell biology. *Adv. Immunol. 44*:93–151, 1989.
Tan, E. M. Interactions between autoimmunity and molecular and cell biology. *J. Clin. Invest. 84*:1–6, 1989.
Yu, D. T. Y., Choo, S. Y., and Schaak, T. Molecular mimicry in HLA-B27-related arthritis. *Ann. Intern. Med. 111*:581–591, 1989.
Zauderer, M. Origin and significance of autoreactive T-cells. *Adv. Immunol. 45*:417–433, 1989.

### Original Articles

Atkinson, M. A., Bowman, M. A., Campbell, L., et al. Cellular immunity to a determinant common to glutamate decarboxylase and coxsackie virus in insulin-dependent diabetes. *J. Clin. Invest. 94*:2125–2129, 1994.
Bjorkman, P. J., Sapier, M. A., Samraouri, B., et al. Structure of the human class I histocompatibility antigen, HLA-A2. *Nature 329*:506–512, 1987.
Bjorkman, P. J., Sapier, M. A., Samraouri, B., et al. The foreign antigen binding site and T-cell recognition regions of class I histocompatibility antigens. *Nature 329*:512–518, 1987.
Chen, J.-H., Kono, D. H., Young, A., et al. A *Yersinia pseudotuberculosis* protein which cross-reacts with HLA-B27. *J. Immunol. 139*:3003–3011, 1987.
Cunningham, M. W., McCormack, J. M., Fenderson, P. G., et al. Human and murine antibodies cross-reactive with streptococcal M protein and myosin recognize the sequence Gln-Lys-Ser-Lys-Gln in M protein. *J. Immunol. 143*:2677–2683, 1989.
MacDonald, H. R. Mechanisms of immunological tolerance. *Science 246*:982, 1989.

Morel, P. A., Erlich, H. A., and Fathman, C. G. A new look at the shared epitope hypothesis. *Am. J. Med. 85* (Suppl. 6A):20–22, 1988.

Oldstone, M. B. A. Molecular mimicry: Immunologic cross-reactivity between dissimilar proteins (microbial and self) that share common epitopes can lead to autoimmunity. *Cell 50*:819–820, 1987.

Schlosstein, L., Terasaki, P., Bluestone, R., et al. High association of HLA antigen B27 with ankylosing spondylitis. *N. Engl. J. Med. 288*:704–706, 1973.

Tian, J., Lehmann, P. V., and Kaufman, D. L. T-cell cross-reactivity between coxsackievirus and glutamate decarboxylase is associated with a murine diabetes susceptibility allele. *J. Exp. Med. 180*:1979–1984, 1994.

# 4

# BACTERIA–HOST INTERACTIONS

JOHN R. WARREN, M.D.

A *parasite* is a life form that lives on or in another life form, the *host*. *Infection* is parasitism of the host by a microorganism, and *bacterial infection* parasitism of the host by bacteria. When parasitism by bacteria results in host injury, the expression of host injury is known as *bacterial disease*. Bacterial disease is due to *pathogenic* (disease-producing) properties intrinsic to bacteria. *Virulence* is the degree of pathogenicity of a bacterial parasite for a host. Different bacteria vary widely in their virulence. Some species of bacteria are highly virulent and cause disease in normal hosts, whereas others are weakly virulent and produce disease only in hosts with deficient defenses against bacterial invasion.

Pathogenic properties of bacteria include the ability to produce toxic proteins (*exotoxins*), which directly injure host cells; cell-wall molecules (*adhesins*) and structures (*fimbriae*), which strongly enhance attachment of bacteria to mucosal surfaces as a prelude to invasion; and surface *capsules*, which enable bacteria to elude phagocytic cells and thereby cause disease by proliferation within the extracellular spaces of tissue (*extracellular bacterial parasites*). Another important group of bacterial organisms causes disease by infection and growth inside tissue macrophages (*facultative intracellular parasites*) because of the ability of the parasites to elude enzymic and oxygen-mediated killing mechanisms of intracellular phagolysosomes.

The human host has developed both natural and acquired mechanisms of defense to protect itself from pathogenic bacteria. Natural mechanisms operate at external cutaneous and internal mucosal surfaces of the human organism and serve to impede both attachment and invasion of bacteria and their exotoxins. Once bacterial invasion occurs, natural tissue mechanisms are available that impede growth and spread of bacteria, including oxygenation of tissue by arterial blood (which prevents tissue infection by *obligately anaerobic bacteria*) and *complement activation* (which results in lysis of unencapsulated bacteria). Infection successfully stopped by these mechanisms will not cause disease, since host injury is minimal. However, with virulent bacteria, invasion and spread provoke an inflammatory response which within hours produces efflux into infected tissue of blood *polymorphonuclear neutrophils*, and exudation of plasma proteins (including *complement* and *kininogen*) in an attempt to contain infection. Almost invariably, this inflammatory response becomes manifest as disease with heat, redness, and pain of infected tissue, as well as systemic reactions of *fever* and peripheral blood *neutrophilic leukocytosis*. If infection is fulminant or persistent, the inflammatory response itself can be injurious to the host, with local tissue necrosis and hypotensive shock due to systemic actions of inflammatory cytokines on the vascular endothelium. Injury due to persistent inflammation is a prominent feature of disease caused by facultative intracellular bacteria, in which the *chronic granulomatous inflammatory* response produced by intracellular bacteria results in tissue necrosis.

In the absence of specific immunity, polymorphonuclear neutrophils are unable to efficiently ingest and kill virulent encapsulated extracellular bacteria. Humoral immunity provides *opsonizing antibody*, which "coats" extracellular bacteria and thereby makes them "palatable" to neutrophils for ingestion and killing. Likewise, in a host without specific immunity, tissue macrophages infected by facultative intracellular parasites cannot inhibit growth of the parasites. However, immune activation of T lymphocytes generates release by the T cells of *cytokines*, which directly activate tissue macrophages for killing of the parasites.

Bacterial disease results from a dynamic interplay between pathogenic properties of bacteria that promote host invasion on the one hand and mechanisms by which the host protects itself against bacterial invasion and disease on the other hand. Diagnosis and treatment of bacterial disease require a thorough understanding of bacterial and host factors responsible for this dynamic interaction, which is the focus of this chapter.

## DEGREE OF BACTERIAL PARASITISM

Diseases caused by bacteria can be classified according to the degree of bacterial parasitism of the human host. The degree of host parasitism in bacterial disease varies over a wide spectrum, and includes the following: absence of true parasitism characteristic of the food-poisoning syndromes caused by *enterotoxins* ingested with contaminated food; overgrowth of normal bacterial microflora by toxin-producing bacteria with local actions of toxin on mucosal surfaces; superficial infection of mucosal surfaces or devitalized wound tissue by toxigenic bacteria with systemic absorption of toxin; invasion of bacteria across epithelial surfaces of the host, with dissemination to and proliferation of bacteria within the extracellular interstitium of tissue (extracellular parasites); and the most intimate form of host parasitism, growth of the bacterial parasite within macrophages of host tissue (facultative intracellular parasites).

### Bacterial Exotoxins

A number of bacteria produce disease by the synthesis and secretion of protein exotoxins. *Diphtheria* is the prototype for disease produced by bacterial exotoxin. Diphtheria begins as a superficial infection of the pharynx by strains of *Corynebacterium diphtheriae* lysogenized by a bacteriophage, *prophage-beta*, which possesses the structural $tox^+$ gene for the diphtheria toxin molecule. Toxin secreted by diphtheria bacilli is absorbed systemically from the pharyngeal site of infection and binds to cells of target organs to cause disease. The heart is highly sensitive to the toxic actions of diphtheria, with cardiac failure the leading cause of death. The myocarditis of diphtheria is sterile (no diphtheria bacilli can be recovered by culture) and is caused by direct action of the diphtheria toxin molecule on cardiac myocytes. A primary target of diphtheria toxin is elongation factor 2 (EF-2), the eukaryotic protein factor required for translocation of polypeptidyl-transfer RNA to accept amino acids from aminoacyl-transfer RNA in ribosomal protein chain elongation. A peptide fragment (fragment A) of the diphtheria toxin molecule is internalized by host cells (Fig. 4–1), where it acts as an enzyme to catalyze the transfer of ADP-ribose from cytosolic nicotinamide adenine dinucleotide to EF-2, with formation of ADP-ribose–EF-2. ADP-ribose–EF-2 is inactive as a translocase, and profound inhibition of ribosomal protein synthesis develops within minutes in heart muscle cells. One molecule of diphtheria toxin can kill a single cell by repeated cycles of ADP-ribosylation of EF-2. *Tetanus* is another exotoxin disease in which, like diphtheria,

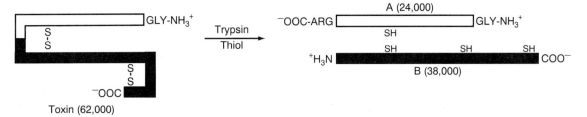

Toxin (62,000)

**FIGURE 4–1.** Diphtheria toxin. Diphtheria toxin is secreted by *Corynebacterium diphtheriae* as a single-chain protein, which is nicked (cleaved) in its closed disulfide loop by protease to form two fragments, A and B, held together by a disulfide bond. Fragment B binds to membrane receptors of host target cells and following reduction of the disulfide bond fragment A is internalized by target cells. Fragment A causes toxic suppression of ribosomal protein synthesis in target cells by inactivation of elongation factor-2. (From Pappenheimer, A. M., and Gill, D. M. Diphtheria. Science *182*:353–358, 1973. Copyright 1973 American Association for the Advancement of Science. With Permission.)

there is limited host parasitism by the bacterial organism that produces toxin. Contamination of devitalized tissue by spores of *Clostridium tetani* results in growth of tetanus bacilli in the anaerobic depths of penetrating (puncture) wounds with production of toxin. Tetanus toxin produced locally in a wound migrates in peripheral nerve fibers by retrograde intraaxonal transport to the anterior horns of the spinal column, where it localizes in presynaptic membranes of *inhibitory afferent fibers*. Tetanus toxin blocks the release of inhibitory neurotransmitters and results in sustained motor stimulation of voluntary muscles with generalized muscle spasm.

Toxin-induced disease frequently occurs upon the ingestion of food contaminated by enterotoxins produced by *Staphylococcus aureus*, *Bacillus cereus*, or *Clostridium perfringens*. Nausea and vomiting develop a few hours after ingestion of enterotoxin, and when prolonged or severe the loss of fluid leads to prostration, dehydration, and hypotension. However, recovery is usually complete within 24 h. There is no true host parasitism, and the food-poisoning syndrome is due entirely to enterotoxins absorbed from contaminated food. *Botulinum toxin* produced by *Clostridium botulinum* can also contaminate food. When absorbed from ingested food, this neurotoxin localizes at cholinergic neuromuscular junctions and blocks the presynaptic release of acetylcholine. A state of flaccid paralysis develops, which initially affects voluntary muscles supplied by the cranial nerves causing double vision and difficulty in speaking and swallowing, followed by paralysis of muscles of the trunk and extremities. *Botulism* can result in death, most often by ventilatory insufficiency.

Diarrheal illness follows colonization and overgrowth of the normal colonic bacterial flora by toxin-producing bacteria. Diarrhea often complicates treatment with broad-spectrum antibiotics, related to antibiotic suppression of the normal colonic flora and overgrowth by enterotoxin-producing *Clostridium difficile*. Hemorrhagic diarrhea is produced by *verotoxin* secreted by strains of *Escherichia coli* O157:H7, which heavily colonize the large intestinal flora following ingestion of rare or undercooked ground beef contaminated with *E. coli* O157:H7. Systemic absorption of verotoxin from the colon can produce the hemolytic-uremic syndrome (HUS), with thrombocytopenia, hemolytic anemia, and acute renal failure, especially in children younger than 5 years of age. Voluminous watery diarrhea is produced by the attachment of *Vibrio cholerae* to the small intestinal mucosa, with secretion by the cholera bacilli of an enterotoxin that acts locally on intestinal mucosal cells to increase their cyclic adenosine monophosphate (cAMP) content. The increase in cAMP inhibits active absorption of $Na^+$ and stimulates active secretion of $Cl^-$ by the small intestinal mucosa, resulting in an outpouring of isotonic fluid into the intestinal lumen and watery diarrhea.

## Extracellular Parasites

The extracellular bacteria actively invade subcutaneous tissue, submucosal tissue, and tissue of deep organs to produce disease. These microorganisms strongly adhere to host cutaneous and mucosal surfaces by bacterial cell-wall structures known as *adhesins* and can penetrate the epithelium of these surfaces, especially mucosal surfaces, to invade underlying tissue. Penetration of tissue lymphatics can lead to widespread dissemination of the parasite with secondary infection of single or multiple organs. Infection of the pharyngeal mucosa by *Neisseria meningitidis* with bacteremic dissemination of meningococci to the meninges of the brain and development of *meningococcal meningitis* is an important clinical example. Extracellular parasites adherent to a mucosal surface can also invade laterally to reach and infect organs whose drainage depends on structures lined by the mucosal surface. Ascending urinary tract infection by *Escherichia coli* with development of *pyelonephritis* reflects this mechanism. Also, extracellular bacteria adherent to the pharyngeal mucosa can be aspirated into deep airspaces of the lung, especially in debilitated hospital patients, and invade alveolar spaces through walls of bronchioles, causing bacterial pneumonia.

Regardless of the route of infection, disease is produced by rapid multiplication of these organisms in the extracellular spaces of tissue. The doubling time of extracellular bacterial growth is short (an hour or so), and millions of organisms rapidly establish residence at sites of tissue infection. The extracellular bacteria possess surface structures, especially polysaccharide capsules, which block their ingestion by neutrophils. However, if phagocytosis of extracellular bacteria occurs, they are highly susceptible to microbial killing mechanisms that operate within the phagolysosomes of neutrophils. Consequently, the neutrophilic inflammatory response is an important line of defense against host invasion by extracellular bacterial parasites. The clinical signs of extracellular bacterial disease directly reflect the neutrophilic inflammatory response, including elevated body temperature; increased numbers of peripheral blood neutrophils; presence of neutrophils in body secretions such as sputum and urine; swelling, redness, and heat of infected tissue; and development of infiltrates on x-ray. If infection becomes persistent, tissue will be injured by the neutrophilic inflammation, with necrosis and abscess formation.

### Facultative Intracellular Parasites

The facultative intracellular bacterial parasites are capable of proliferation outside human cells, and their extracellular growth contributes to the transmission of bacteria from infected to uninfected individuals (disease caused by facultative bacteria is communicable), increase of microbial mass in infected tissue, and spread of organisms within the infected host. However, facultative intracellular parasites cause disease by growth of the organisms inside cells of the host, most frequently tissue macrophages. Facultative intracellular parasites are resistant to killing by polymorphonuclear neutrophils, and killing can be accomplished only by *activated macrophages*. A prominent feature of infection by facultative intracellular parasites is the development of a cell-mediated immunologic reaction that is responsible for the manifestations of disease and the destruction of infected tissue. Tuberculosis is an important example of disease produced by a facultative intracellular parasite, in this instance *Mycobacterium tuberculosis* (see Chapter 13).

## PROPERTIES OF PATHOGENIC BACTERIA

### Bacterial Adherence

Adherence of bacteria to a host surface is the first step in bacterial invasion. The surfaces of bacterial prokaryotic cells and host eukaryotic cells are negatively charged, and charge repulsion tends to repel bacteria from host cells. However, surfaces of pathogenic bacteria display surface protein ligands called *adhesins*, which bind in a stereochemically specific manner with *complementary receptor molecules* in the plasma membranes of host cells. This binding is best envisioned at the molecular level as a lock-and-key mechanism analogous to antigen–antibody and enzyme–substrate interactions. Adhesin-receptor binding bridges the gap between bacterium and host cell, overcoming the forces of charge repulsion. In addition, the constant flow of secretions across mucosal surfaces combined with continuous desquamation of epithelial cells from these surfaces (see discussion below) would, in the absence of strong adhesin-receptor binding, quickly dislodge bacteria from mucosal surfaces before invasion into submucosal tissue could occur.

Adhesin proteins of gram-negative bacteria are located at the tips of delicate filamentous structures known as *fimbriae* or *pili*, which cover the bacterial surface. Three major types of fimbriae have been identified for the gram-negative organism *Escherichia coli*. *Type 1* fimbriae contain adhesin protein that binds to mannose-containing receptors of lower urinary tract cells and are strongly associated with invasive infection of the urinary bladder (*bacterial cystitis*). Adhesive protein of *type P* fimbriae of *E. coli* binds to galactose-galactose determinants (P blood group glycolipid) in membranes of uroepithelial cells. Organisms with type P fimbriae are prevalent in ascending infection of the kidneys causing *pyelonephritis*, including clinically severe forms of pyelonephritis in which the patient becomes bacteremic (*urosepsis*). *Type S* fimbriae contain adhesin protein that specifically binds to sialic acid of host cell membrane galactosides and are associated with the pathogenesis of meningitis and bacteremia in infants. Adhesins for other pathogenic strains of gram-negative bacteria are present in the fimbriae of *Neisseria gonorrhoeae*, which bind to receptor glycolipids of urogenital tract cells containing lactosylceramide and gangliotriaosylceramide, and of *Shigella flexneri*, which bind to fucose/glucose determinants of colonic epithelial cell receptors.

Surfaces of gram-positive bacteria are covered by a fine irregular fuzz, or *fibrillae*. Fibrillae of the streptococci are composed of *lipoteichoic acid*, which is a polyglycerol phosphate containing saturated and unsaturated long-chain fatty acids esterified to the glycerol moiety. Part of the lipoteichoic acid is situated deep in the streptococcal cell wall, but a significant fraction is secreted onto the streptococcal cell surface with fatty acid chains freely extending above the surface. Because of its hydrophobicity, lipoteichoic acid avidly binds to the adhesive host glycoprotein *fibronectin* present on the surface of pharyngeal mucosal cells. The oropharynx is normally colonized by the viridans streptococci, a heterogeneous group of streptococci which demonstrate alpha-hemolysis (green hemolysis) on sheep blood agar. Fibronectin does not bind well to gram-negative bacteria, suggesting that a function of this host adhesive protein is to fix gram-positive rather than gram-negative cells to host surfaces. Hospitalized, debilitated, or aged individuals develop heavy pharyngeal colonization by gram-negative bacteria, which predisposes to aspiration pneumonia. An increase in salivary proteases that occurs in these individuals digests cell-bound fibronectin, and thereby increases the adherence of gram-negative bacteria to pharyngeal epithelial cells.

The invasive gram-positive organism *Streptococcus pyogenes* (group A streptococcus) contains *M protein* complexed with its cell surface lipoteichoic acid. M protein is strongly associated with the virulence of *S. pyogenes*, and serves as an adhesin for the binding of these streptococci to epithelial cells in producing *acute pharyngitis* (see Chapter 7). Adhesins associated with other gram-positive bacterial diseases include glucan-binding protein for *Streptococcus mutans*, which causes tooth decay (*caries*), and N-acetyl-D-glucosamine–binding protein present in *Streptococcus agalactiae* (group B streptococcus) (neonatal meningitis and bacteremia).

## Antiphagocytic Capsules

Most extracellular bacteria that cause disease are encapsulated. Capsules block the attachment of bacteria to neutrophils for phagocytosis in the absence of specific anticapsular antibody. Most bacterial capsules are polysaccharide in composition. The hydrophilic and acidic nature of capsular polysaccharide impedes contact of bacteria with the hydrophobic, negatively charged membranes of host neutrophils. In addition, capsules block complement-activating structures in the underlying cell wall of bacteria, such as endotoxin of gram-negative bacteria. As a consequence, encapsulated strains of bacteria do not efficiently fix complement in the absence of antibody. As will be discussed below, complement activation is a key event for the phagocytosis and killing of bacteria by polymorphonuclear neutrophils. Capsules can also mask bacterial surface structures that are antigenic and prevent an effective host immune response. Some important examples of capsules associated with bacterial virulence include the 83 different polysaccharide capsules of *Streptococcus pneumoniae;* the polyribitol phosphate capsule of *Haemophilus influenzae* type b; the group A, B, C, Y, and W-135 polysaccharide capsules of *Neisseria meningitidis;* the K1 polysaccharide capsule of *Escherichia coli;* and the capsular type III polysaccharide of group B streptococcus (*Streptococcus agalactiae*).

## Intracellular Parasitism of Phagocytes

Facultative intracellular parasites evade both oxidative and nonoxidative killing inside cells, primarily macrophages. Nonoxidative killing of bacteria results from the acidity of phagolysosomes (pH~4.5) as well as from the acidic activation of lysosomal proteases and lipases. Oxidative killing in macrophages is caused by production within phagolysosomes of oxygen radicals, especially · OH and · NO. One group of intracellular bacterial parasites is able to physically escape the phagosome and live in the cytosol, away from the killing activity of the phagolysosomes. An important example is *Listeria monocytogenes*, a cause of neonatal meningitis and bacteremia, which leaves the phagosome and multiplies within the cytosolic compartment of macrophages. *L. monocytogenes* produces a hemolytic factor, *listeriolysin O*, which allows the organism to escape the phagosome by lysing its membrane. A second group of intracellular bacteria inhibits the fusion of phagosomes with lysosomes. *Legionella pneumophila*, the bacterial cause of Legionnaires' disease, actively multiplies within the phagosome of infected macrophages by inhibiting fusion (and thus acidification) of the phagosomes with lysosomes. *Mycobacterium tuberculosis* also resides within the phagosomes of infected macrophages and inhibits fusion of phagosomes with acidic lysosomes by sulfolipids and other inhibitory substances of the mycobacteria. Yet a third mechanism of intracellular bacterial parasitism is seen with *Salmonella* species, which are resistant to the acidic and oxidative environment of macrophage phagolysosomes and can actively replicate within the phagolysosomes.

## MECHANISMS OF HOST DEFENSE AGAINST BACTERIA

Mechanical, chemical, and microbiologic mechanisms exist in the normal host that in-

hibit the attachment and invasion of cutaneous and mucosal surfaces by bacterial pathogens. When successful, these *primary mechanisms* prevent bacterial infection. However, with virulent microorganisms and/or a compromised host, bacteria can breach these natural barriers to invade and cause infection. Within hours, infection provokes the vascular and cellular events of *inflammation*. Inflammatory responses develop in infected tissue, and constitute *secondary mechanisms* of host defense to contain the spread of infection (Fig. 4–2). Immunologic responses develop in a few days to several weeks, the time required depending on the type of individual pathogen and the immunocompetence of the infected host. The essential purpose of immunologic responses is to amplify the intensity and efficiency of inflammatory responses, thus serving as *tertiary mechanisms* for the eradication of infection from the host.

### Surface Barriers to Infection

#### *Skin*

The skin is a natural mechanical and chemical barrier to invasion by bacteria. The heavily keratinized superficial layer of skin epidermis and its many layers of tightly adherent squa-

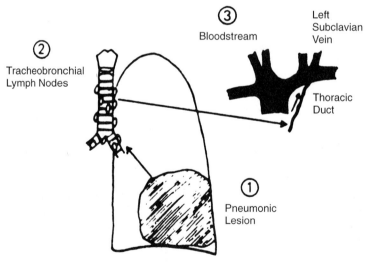

**FIGURE 4–2.** The pneumonic lesion. Invasion of bronchioles and alveoli by bacteria provokes a neutrophilic inflammatory response in which polymorphonuclear neutrophils fill the alveolar spaces. This inflammatory response gives infected lung a solid texture (consolidation), and the consolidated region constitutes the pneumonic lesion. If infection is not contained within the pneumonic lesion by the inflammatory response, bacteria will invade draining lymphatics and spread to tracheobronchial lymph nodes, and from the lymph nodes enter the blood circulation via the thoracic duct to cause a bloodstream infection (bacteremia). The development of bacteremia in pneumonia indicates inadequate secondary inflammatory and tertiary immunologic defenses of the host and is associated with a substantial increase in mortality. (From Wood, W. B., Jr. Studies on the cellular immunology of acute bacterial infections. *The Harvey Lectures.* New York: Academic Press, 1951–1952: 72–98. With permission.)

mous epithelial cells constitute a thick mechanical barrier to bacterial invasion. Epithelial cells of the skin are continuously dividing cells, and constant sloughing of superficial cells serves to remove bacterial pathogens attached to cutaneous surfaces. The acidity of unsaturated fatty acids present in sebaceous gland secretions (skin pH~5.5) readily inactivates bacteria other than skin commensals, providing a chemical decontamination mechanism. Breaks in the skin, such as traumatic or surgical wounds, breach this natural barrier and offer a route of bacterial invasion for pathogens such as *Staphylococcus aureus* and the gram-negative rods. In addition, placement of intravascular catheters in the peripheral and central circulation facilitates host invasion by bacteria that are normal skin commensals. An intravascular catheter is a foreign body that creates a skin wound while offering a solid surface along which bacteria can invade through the catheter tunnel in subcutaneous tissue, to enter the blood circulation. Bacteremia acquired from an infected intravascular catheter is most frequently due to the coagulase-negative staphylococci, especially *Staphylococcus epidermidis*, normally present in skin flora.

### Respiratory Tract

The thin, nonkeratinized mucosal epithelium of the respiratory tract is more easily penetrated by bacteria than the thick, keratinized epidermis of skin. Natural defense of the respiratory tract depends on clearance of inhaled particles containing bacteria by aerodynamic filtration, mucociliary mechanisms, and coughing. Hairs within the nostrils filter out large particles from incoming air, which is then subjected to turbulence as it flows across the turbinate bones. Particles larger than 10 $\mu$m are deposited by this turbulent flow on the nasal mucosa lining the turbinates, and are swept by the mucociliary lining (see below) to the back of the throat and swallowed. Air leaving the nasal cavities sharply changes direction as it recurves through the posterior pharynx, and particles about 10 $\mu$m in size impact on the mucosal lining of the posterior pharyngeal wall to be swallowed. Particles less than 10 $\mu$m in diameter are likely to reach the bronchial tree. The mucociliary lining of the bronchial tree consists of ciliated epithelial cells, goblet cells, and submucosal mucous glands. A film of mucus is secreted onto the surfaces of the ciliated epithelial cells by goblet cells and mucous glands. This mucus film is propelled upward in the bronchial tree by beating cilia of the epithelial cells. Repetitive bifurcation of the bronchial tree slows the velocity of inhaled air, and particles between 3 and 10 $\mu$m in size settle onto the upward moving mucus film, to be transported to the posterior pharynx. Mucus in the posterior pharnyx is removed by coughing or is swallowed. Coughing expels particle-laden mucus and air from the respiratory tract, and swallowing brings bacteria enmeshed in mucus into contact with the acid pH of gastric secretions, which is bactericidal for many pathogens.

Particles less than 5 $\mu$m in diameter are likely to reach the alveolar spaces due to their small size. The major natural defense against these particles is phagocytosis by alveolar macrophages. Alveolar macrophages are well suited to this task, demonstrating a phagocytic capacity for bacteria comparable to that of neutrophils.

Normally the lungs are sterile, since bacteria inhaled in particles are efficiently removed by mucociliary clearance, coughing, and swallowing, or are destroyed and removed by alveolar macrophages. However, several mechanisms operate either singly or in combination that allow bacteria to infect the lung. Injury to the ciliated epithelium of the bronchial tree by viral infection (especially influenza virus), cigarette smoking and atmospheric pollutants, accumulation of excessive and abnormally viscid mucus secretions as in cystic fibrosis or chronic bronchitis, or the genetic *immotile cilia syndrome* in which cilia of the respiratory epithelium are immobile due to defects in organization of microtubules suppresses normal clearance by the mucociliary blanket. Suppression of the cough reflex typically occurs with debilitated hospital patients, who as a consequence aspirate oropharyngeal secretions heavily contaminated with bacteria, especially gram-negative bacteria, into the deep airspaces of the lung. Pulmonary edema that develops as a complication of a variety of cardiovascular, renal, hepatic, and malignant diseases provides a favorable growth medium for invasive bacteria in the bronchiolar and alveolar spaces. Finally, because of their small size, inhaled respiratory droplet nuclei (1–5 $\mu$m in diameter) containing tuberculosis bacilli provide ready access of the bacilli to alveolar macrophages. This bacillus is a facultative intracellular parasite (see above), which in the nonimmune host readily infects alveolar macrophages.

## Alimentary Tract

Gastrointestinal secretions greatly assist the elimination of bacteria from the alimentary tract by promoting the flow of luminal contents through the mouth, stomach, and intestine. Saliva is constantly swallowed and cleanses the mouth of food particles and sloughed epithelial cells with attached bacteria. Large volumes of mucus secretions bathe surfaces of the stomach and intestine, where glycoproteins in the mucus block attachment of bacteria to the gastric and intestinal epithelium. Unattached bacteria in the mucus secretions are swept away by peristalsis, and in the normal host their multiplication in the intestine is balanced by their passage to the exterior. The acidity of gastric secretions (pH < 4) is a formidable barrier to the many bacteria and bacterial exotoxins that are acid sensitive.

The importance of secretions is apparent in a number of conditions that increase host susceptibility to intestinal bacterial infection. Stasis of intestinal secretions is caused by obstruction of colonic diverticuli or the appendix. Increased intraluminal pressure within these obstructed structures combined with bacterial overgrowth of the stagnant secretions causes *purulent diverticulitis* or *appendicitis*. Complications include perforation with development of pericolonic or periappendiceal abscesses, or even generalized peritonitis. The importance of the gastric barrier as a protective mechanism is clearly seen with the enteric pathogens *Salmonella* or enterotoxin-producing *Vibrio cholerae*. Individuals with hypochlorhydria or achlorhydria secondary to either gastric resection or atrophic gastritis demonstrate an increased susceptibility to salmonellosis or cholera. In addition, studies with volunteers have shown that concomitant ingestion of sodium bicarbonate solution with *Salmonella typhi* or *Vibrio cholerae* greatly decreases disease-producing doses of these microorganisms. However, some bacteria such as the tubercle bacilli are highly resistant to the bactericidal action of gastric acid and gain ready access to the intestine. Intestinal tuberculosis is caused by tubercle bacilli from lung lesions that are coughed into the posterior pharynx and then swallowed.

## Urinary Tract

Complete emptying of the bladder by micturition (urination) is of central importance for natural resistance of the urinary tract to infection. Urine is normally sterile, since frequent micturition effectively removes bacteria by dilution with fresh ureteric urine. Also, normal urine is acidic (pH<6), and an acid pH effectively inhibits the growth of potential urinary tract pathogens, especially *Escherichia coli*. Obstructive conditions of the lower urinary tract such as benign prostatic hyperplasia or urethral stricture result in the presence of residual urine in the bladder following micturition. Residual urine inevitably becomes infected with bacteria, and this is frequently followed by invasive bacterial infection of the bladder wall (*bacterial cystitis*). Ascending infection of the kidneys (*bacterial pyelonephritis*) can develop from regurgitation of bladder urine into the ureters and renal pelves due to incompetence of the vesicoureteral valves, atony of smooth muscle in pregnancy combined with ureteral obstruction by the enlarged gravid uterus, or ureteral obstruction by stones or pelvic tumor. The common denominator in all of these infections is obstruction to normal urine outflow.

The male urethra is about 20 cm in length and is distant from the anus, the source of intestinal bacteria for urinary tract infection. Thus, the male urethra has a high degree of natural resistance to infection. In contrast, the much shorter female urethra (~5 cm long) is dangerously close to the anus. Furthermore, distention of the short female urethra during micturition produces turbulent flow in which the peripheral part of the urine stream is reversed, and intestinal bacteria that colonize the urethral meatus are carried into the bladder. Urinary tract infections are much more common in women than men, especially young females. Urinary tract infection becomes prevalent in men only during the late adult years with the development of obstructive prostatic enlargement.

## Conjunctivae

As seen with mucosal surfaces of the respiratory, gastrointestinal, and urinary tracts, flow of secretions (in this instance tears) provides natural resistance to infection of the conjunctivae. Tears wash bacteria-containing particles into tear ducts, which drain into the nasal cavities. Tears also contain a high concentration of the basic protein *lysozyme*, which lyses some gram-positive bacteria by enzymically degrading their rigid peptidoglycan layer. Trauma or irritation by a foreign body (such as a contact lens) accompanied by direct mechanical inoculation of bacteria (especially *Pseudomonas aeruginosa*) is often responsible for conjunctival infection.

## Endogenous Microbiota

An important component of surface defense against bacterial pathogens is the presence of commensal microorganisms that normally colonize these surfaces (*the endogenous microbiota*), especially the mucosal epithelium of the pharynx, large intestine, and vagina (see Chapter 2). Commensalism is a form of host–parasite interaction in which the parasite (commensal) lives on a surface of the host and is beneficial to the parasite but not harmful to the host. Commensals block host surface attachment sites used by invasive bacteria and produce acid metabolites toxic to pathogens. The pharynx is normally colonized by the viridans streptococci, which are of low virulence and whose presence inhibits colonization by more virulent gram-negative bacteria (see discussion above). The colonic endogenous microbiota consists predominantly of obligately anaerobic bacteria, especially *Bacteroides*, which are present in enormous numbers, approximately $10^{12}$ organisms per gram of feces. The anaerobic commensals suppress colonization of the colon by pathogens such as *Salmonella* that are not normally present in the intestine. Also, predominant species of the anaerobic microflora inhibit overgrowth of the colon by bacterial species normally present in small numbers. Treatment with broad-spectrum antibiotics reduces the numbers of predominant commensals, often with overgrowth of the colon by *Clostridium difficile* normally present in low numbers. Toxin-producing strains of *C. difficile* cause a necrotizing colitis with abdominal pain and diarrhea. Finally, the acid pH (pH~5) of the vagina in women during reproductive life provides a natural barrier against invasion by bacterial pathogens, especially *Neisseria gonorrhoeae*. The acid pH is due to the endogenous vaginal microbiota. Lactobacilli normally colonize the vagina and metabolize glycogen produced by the vaginal epithelium under the action of estrogen. Glycogen metabolism by lactobacilli produces large amounts of lactic acid giving an acid pH.

## Tissue Barriers to Invasion

### Arterial Oxygenation

The obligate anaerobic bacteria grow in the absence but not presence of oxygen. The toxicity of oxygen for anaerobic bacteria is due, at least in part, to absence of enzymes that degrade oxygen radicals produced by bacterial oxygen metabolism (see Chapter 27). Tissue oxygenation is a primary host defense against tissue infection by the anaerobes, and tissue oxygenation is maintained by arterial blood flow. When blood supply is impaired by arterial occlusion or tissue is destroyed by trauma, infection, or tumor, anaerobic conditions within the infarcted or necrotic tissue favor the growth of obligately anaerobic bacteria.

### Complement Activation

The *complement system* (Table 4–1) consists of serum proteins which, when activated, generate a *membrane attack complex* (MAC) capable of lysing unencapsulated bacteria. Unencapsulated bacteria are killed by lysis when added to serum that contains complement but lacks specific antibody to the organisms. Such unencapsulated bacteria are referred to as *serum sensitive*, and are generally avirulent for humans. Since killing of serum-sensitive organisms occurs in the absence of antibody, their lack of invasiveness for host tissue

### TABLE 4–1.  ACTIVATED COMPLEMENT FACTORS*

| Factors | Activity | Function in Bacterial Infection |
|---|---|---|
| C3b, C3bi[†] | Bacterial opsonins | Increase phagocytosis of bacteria by neutrophils |
| C3a, C5a[‡] | Vascular permeability factors | Increase exudation of antibody and complement |
| C5a | Chemotaxin | Increased numbers of neutrophils |
| C56789 | Membrane attack complex | Lysis of unencapsulated bacteria and fastidious gram-negative species[§] |

*The complement system is a cascade of reactions. The *classic pathway* is initiated when antibody–antigen complexes activate the first component of complement (C1). Activated C1 acts on C4 and C2 as a protease to produce *C3 convertase*, which cleaves C3 to C3a and C3b. The *alternate pathway* is initiated when C3b interacts with bacterial cell-wall components (endotoxin, teichoic acid) in the presence of plasma *properdin* proteins. Stimulation of the alternate pathway occurs in the absence of antibody to bacterial antigen. Activation of the remaining components of complement follows the same sequence (C5 → C9) in the classic and alternate pathways.

[†]C3bi is the stable product of C3b.

[‡]C3a and C5a are anaphylatoxins that increase vascular permeability by stimulation of histamine release by mast cells and basophils. Histamine acts directly on venules to increase vascular permeability.

[§]The fastidious bacteria include *Neisseria gonorrhoeae*, *N. meningitidis*, and *Haemophilus influenzae*.

is most likely due to their complement sensitivity.

## Inflammatory Mechanisms

### Neutrophilic Inflammation

The polymorphonuclear neutrophil is a postmitotic, terminally differentiated white blood cell that has a multilobed nucleus (two to five lobes) and cytoplasm rich in highly specialized lysosomal granules. Neutrophils fully mature in the bone marrow (Fig. 4–3), from which they are released into the blood circulation to find their way into the extravascular spaces of infected tissue. The normal bone marrow has a large reserve of neutrophils, and approximately $10^{11}$ neutrophils are released each day. The peripheral blood white cell count in normal adults is $4.5–11.0 \times 10^3/\mu L$, with an average of 56% (range, 45–67%) of the white cells constituted by neutrophils. In bacterial infection, *especially infection by extracellular bacteria*, there is an increase in the release of neutrophils from the bone marrow, causing an elevated peripheral blood white cell count (*neutrophilic leukocytosis*) (Fig. 4–3). Newly released neutrophils circulate for only a few hours before they migrate from blood

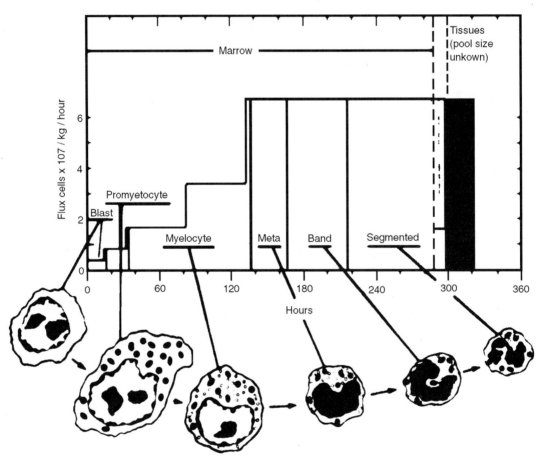

**FIGURE 4–3.** Maturation of polymorphonuclear neutrophils in the bone marrow. The average times required for proliferative (blast cells → myelocytes) and nonproliferative phases of differentiation (metamyelocytes → mature segmented neutrophils) are indicated on the abscissa, and the number of cells fluxing into and out of each maturation phase on the ordinate. The bone marrow reserve of mature neutrophils is frequently depleted in severe infections with the release of immature forms into the circulation, especially band forms. Also, the proliferative nature of promyelocyte and myelocyte differentiation explains the sensitivity of bone marrow neutrophil maturation to cytotoxic irradiation and drugs. Cytotoxic agents often cause profound decrease in the numbers of circulating neutrophils (*neutropenia*), resulting in increased susceptibility to bacterial infection. (From Bainton, D. F. In: Weissmann, G., ed., *The Cell Biology of Inflammation.* Elsevier/North-Holland, 1980:1–25. With permission.)

vessels into extracellular sites of tissue infection. Neutrophils are *phagocytic cells* that readily ingest particles as large as bacteria. Neutrophils are so highly phagocytic that they are considered one of two types of "professional phagocyte" produced in the bone marrow, the other being the monocytes-macrophages. Extracellular bacteria ingested by neutrophils are contained within a membrane-enclosed cytoplasmic vacuole known as a *phagosome.* Bacteria-containing phagosomes fuse with the specialized lysosomes of neutrophils, and active oxygen species produced within the phagolysosomes kill the ingested bacteria. Neutrophils that are actively killing bacteria produce large amounts of $H_2O_2$ in their phagolysosomes by the reactions:

$$2O_2 + NADPH \rightarrow 2O_2^- \cdot + NADP^+ + H^+$$
$$O_2^- \cdot + O_2^- \cdot + 2H^+ \rightarrow O_2 + H_2O_2$$

The first reaction produces superoxide anion ($O_2^- \cdot$) by the catalytic action of the *NADPH oxidase system,* a transmembrane multicomponent structure of enzymic and electron-transport proteins. Superoxide radicals are unstable, and at the acid pH of phagolysosomes undergo spontaneous collisional dismutation, producing $H_2O_2$. Both $O_2^- \cdot$ and $H_2O_2$ have bactericidal activity, but many bacteria produce enzymes that degrade these activated oxygen species, especially catalase, which converts $H_2O_2$ to $H_2O$ and $O_2$. Oxygen radicals highly active in bacterial killing are produced by the *myeloperoxidase system* and the Fenton reaction, both of which use $H_2O_2$ as a substrate (Table 4–2).

Early in the neutrophilic inflammatory response, an increased flow of blood to infected tissue is accompanied by marked increase in the permeability of blood vessels (especially venules) for plasma proteins. Exudation of plasma protein from blood vessels results in high concentrations of complement proteins

in the extravascular spaces of infected tissue. Complement coats the surfaces of extracellular bacteria and becomes activated by bacterial cell-wall components to form the peptide fragments C3b and C3bi (Table 4–1). Coating of bacterial cells by plasma proteins is known as *opsonization,* and the complement fragments C3b and C3bi (Table 4–1) as *opsonins.* Plasma membranes of polymorphonuclear neutrophils contain specific receptors (CR1, CR2, and CR3) for C3b and C3bi, which avidly bind these complement fragments on bacterial surfaces, thereby promoting phagocytosis of the bacteria by neutrophils. Activation of complement in the absence of antibody to bacteria does not utilize the initial complement components C1, C4, and C2, and is referred to as the *alternate pathway* of complement activation (Table 4–1). *The alternate pathway enables the infected host to opsonize bacteria for neutrophil phagocytosis in the absence of a specific immune response.* Complement activation also produces factors that increase the permeability of blood vessels (C3a, C5a) and exudation of plasma proteins. In addition, C5a attracts increasing numbers of neutrophils to sites of infection, since C5a is a *chemotaxin* for neutrophils (Table 4–1). Complement fragments act with vasoactive amines, other peptides, oxidized fatty acids, and lipids to amplify the neutrophilic inflammatory response as *chemical mediators of inflammation* (Table 4–3).

### Chronic Mononuclear and Granulomatous Inflammation

Unlike extracellular bacterial parasites, the facultative intracellular bacterial parasites are *not* susceptible to the killing activity of polymorphonuclear neutrophils. Indeed, the primary pathogenic determinant of the facultative parasite is its ability to grow within host cells, especially macrophages. *Without immunity there is not an effective inflammatory response*

---

**TABLE 4–2.    OXYGEN RADICALS ACTIVE IN THE KILLING OF BACTERIA BY NEUTROPHILS\***

| RADICAL | PRODUCTION | KILLING |
|---|---|---|
| Hypochlorous ($HOCl \cdot$) and hypoiodous ($HOI \cdot$) acid | $H_2O_2$ and halide ion ($Cl^-$, $I^-$) bind to myeloperoxidase with formation of acid radicals | Halogenation and amino acid decarboxylation of bacterial cell walls |
| Hydroxyl ($\cdot OH$) | $H_2O_2$ reduced by ferrous iron ($Fe^{2+}$) to $\cdot OH$ radical (Fenton reaction)[†] | Lipid peroxidation of bacterial cell walls and membranes |

\*Bacterial killing occurs within the phagolysosomes of neutrophils formed by the fusion of bacteria-containing phagosomes with azurophilic granules, highly specialized lysosomes that contain the enzyme myeloperoxidase.

[†]The reduction of $H_2O_2$ results in the oxidation of $Fe^{2+}$ to $Fe^{3+}$ ion. Superoxide anions ($O_2^- \cdot$) produced by phagolysosomal membranes of activated neutrophils in turn reduce $Fe^{3+}$ ion to $Fe^{2+}$ ion, allowing the continued production of $\cdot OH$ radical.

**TABLE 4–3.   CHEMICAL MEDIATORS OF INFLAMMATION\***

| MEDIATOR | ACTIVITY | PRODUCTION |
|---|---|---|
| Histamine | Vasodilatation, increased vascular permeability | Secretion by mast cells, basophils, and platelets |
| Serotonin (5-hydroxytryptamine) | Vasodilatation, increased vascular permeability | Secretion by platelets |
| Bradykinin | Vasodilatation, increased vascular permeability | Activation of plasma Hageman factor (factor XII) and kinin system[†] |
| Leukotrienes (LT) | Neutrophil chemotaxis (LT type $B_4$), increased vascular permeability (LT types $C_4$, $D_4$, $E_4$) | Synthesis by inflammatory cell membranes (neutrophils, macrophages) |
| Prostaglandin (PG) | Vasodilatation, fever (PG type $E_2$)[‡] | Synthesis by inflammatory cell membranes (neutrophils, macrophages) |
| Platelet activating factor (PAF) | Vasodilatation, neutrophil chemotaxis[§] | Synthesis by inflammatory (neutrophils, macrophages) cell and endothelial cell membranes |

\*Activity of complement factors C3a and C5a as chemical mediators of inflammation is described in Table 4–1.

[†]The plasma kinin system is a cascade of reactions starting with factor XIIa (a = activated), which acts as a protease on plasma prekallikrein to produce kallikrein, which in turn acts as a protease on plasma high-molecular-weight kininogen to produce bradykinin. Factor XIIa is produced by surface activation of factor XII upon contact of factor XII with vascular basement membrane, collagen, or elastin in injured tissue. The kinin system thus represents an important nonimmune mechanism for the generation of inflammatory mediators.

[‡]Fever production results from prostaglandin synthesis in the thermoregulatory centers of the hypothalamus. Hypothalamic prostaglandin synthesis is stimulated by the cytokines interleukin-1 and tumor necrosis factor-alpha.

[§]PAF acts on mast cells to stimulate histamine release, and also acts directly on vascular endothelial cells and neutrophils.

*to contain facultative intracellular parasites,* and the parasite widely disseminates to infect different organ systems. With the eventual occurrence of cell-mediated immunity, a *chronic mononuclear cell inflammatory response* develops in which infected tissue becomes heavily infiltrated with macrophages and lymphocytes. Macrophages in this response mature from blood monocytes (Fig. 4–4) that emigrate into areas of mononuclear cell inflammation. Under the influence of lymphokines produced by T lymphocytes present in the inflammatory cell infiltrate (see below), macrophages become activated for the killing of intracellular parasites. The activated macrophages become enlarged and epithelium-like in appearance, and are referred to as *epithelioid cells* (Fig. 4–4). Senescent epithelioid cells fuse to form giant cells with many nuclei arranged on the periphery (*Langhans-type giant cell*) or diffusely through the cell (*foreign body-type giant cell*). Frequently, tissue infiltrates of epithelioid cells, giant cells, and lymphocytes become organized into focal aggregates known as *granulomas. Granulomatous* inflammation is a hallmark of infectious disease caused by the facultative intracellular bacteria.

### Immunologic Mechanisms

#### Humoral Immunity

Circulating IgM and IgG antibodies function as antitoxins and opsonins in humoral immunity toward bacterial exotoxins and extracellular bacteria. The initial immune response with first exposure of the host to a microbial exotoxin or extracellular bacteria is formation of IgM antibodies, large pentameric molecules (MW~800,000 D) whose Fab region has a relatively low affinity of binding to epitopes of exotoxin molecules or bacterial cells. The increased vascular permeability at tissue sites of neutrophilic inflammation results in the localization of IgM antibody at these sites. Within approximately 10 days, IgG antibodies appear that have a relatively high affinity of binding to the same bacterial epitopes. The production of IgG antibodies exceeds and outlasts IgM antibodies, and long-term humoral immunity to exotoxins and extracellular bacteria depends on IgG antibodies.

Immunity to diphtheria is the prototype for humoral immunity to bacterial exotoxins. The diphtheria toxin molecule consists of two protein chains, A and B, held together by a single disulfide bond (Fig. 4–1). The A chain contains the toxic catalytic site for the ADP-ribosylation of EF-2, and the B chain binding sites for the attachment of diphtheria toxin to host target cells. Immunity to diphtheria is provided by the ability of humoral antibody to combine with cell attachment sites on the B chain, thereby blocking the binding of diphtheria toxin to host target cells. Before neu-

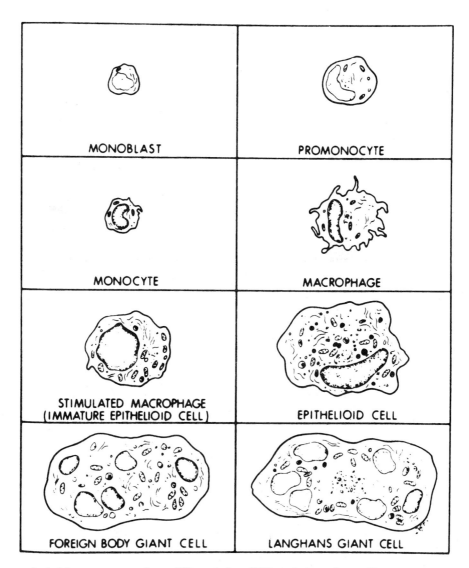

**FIGURE 4–4.** Monocyte-macrophage differentiation. Differentiation of monoblasts to monocytes occurs in the bone marrow. Monocytes released into the circulation enter tissue within 1 day to become tissue macrophages. With further stimulation by cytokines, especially interferon-gamma, macrophages undergo further differentiation into states activated for the killing of intracellular bacterial parasites. Senescent macrophages undergo membrane fusion to form multinucleate giant cells, which are especially prominent in granulomas. (From Adams, D. O. The granulomatous inflammatory response. A review. *Am. J. Pathol. 84*:164, 1976. With permission.)

tralizing antibody can be produced in individuals without previous exposure to diphtheria toxin or toxoid, significant amounts of diphtheria toxin will be internalized by host target cells, especially heart muscle cells. Only individuals previously immunized with diphtheria toxoid, treated with high levels of neutralizing diphtheria antitoxin, or made immune by a previous infection with toxin-producing *Corynebacterium diphtheriae* will be effectively protected. The importance of diphtheria toxoid

immunization is dramatically illustrated by the current outbreak of diphtheria in the New Independent States (NIS) of the former Soviet Union (Fig. 4–5).

The opsonic activity of humoral antibodies greatly increases clearance of encapsulated extracellular bacteria in infected tissue by neutrophilic inflammation. Antigen-binding sites of the Fab region of IgG attach to bacterial capsular epitopes, and concomitantly the Fc region of IgG binds to Fc receptors

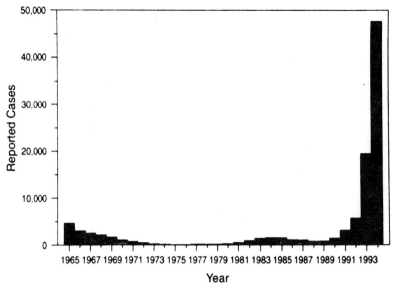

*Data for 1994 are provisional.

Source: World Health Organization.

**FIGURE 4–5.** Reported number of diphtheria cases in the New Independent States (NIS) of the former Soviet Union. This epidemic of diphtheria began in 1990 in the Russian Federation and spread to Ukraine in 1991 and to 12 of the 13 remaining NIS during 1993–1994. Although reasons for the epidemic are not fully understood, inadequate vaccination with diphtheria toxoid resulted in large numbers of susceptible children and adults. The high clinical effectiveness of diphtheria toxoid in preventing diphtheria was confirmed in this epidemic when toxoid was appropriately used for vaccination. (From Centers for Disease Control, *MMWR 44*(10):177–181, March 17, 1995. With permission.)

(FcγR) in neutrophil membranes. Also, when bound to bacterial surfaces, IgG and IgM activate the classic complement pathway by interaction of the Fc portion of IgG and IgM with C1 (Table 4–1). Classic pathway activation generates high concentrations of C3b and C3bi on bacterial surfaces, which bind to the specific complement receptors of neutrophil membranes. IgG-mediated and IgG/IgM plus complement-mediated phagocytosis by neutrophils is critical for recovery from infectious diseases caused by encapsulated extracellular bacteria. Extracellular bacterial infection frequently occurs when antibody production is suppressed by treatment of malignant disease by cytotoxic drugs and irradiation, genetic or acquired immunodeficiency disease, or hematologic malignancy.

Secretory IgA antibody does not function as an opsonin. However, its abundance on mucous surfaces of the respiratory, alimentary, and genitourinary tracts serves to block the binding of bacterial adhesins to epithelial cell receptors at these portals of entry for infection. Thus, IgA immunity prevents invasive infection by inhibiting attachment of pathogenic bacteria to mucous membranes.

### Cell-Mediated Immunity

Macrophage activation is the central event in cell-mediated immunity to facultative intracellular parasites. These parasites are resistant to killing by polymorphonuclear neutrophils, monocytes, and quiescent (nonactivated) tissue macrophages. Furthermore, disease caused by facultative intracellular parasites is characterized by infection of macrophages. Infected macrophages display parasitic antigen on the macrophage membrane in association with *class II major histocompatibility complex* (MHC) molecules. The membrane *T-cell receptor* (TcR) complex of T lymphocytes specifically binds to parasitic antigen, and membrane *CD4 molecules* of helper T lymphocytes concomitantly bind to the macrophage class II MHC molecules. This "focused" interaction of helper T cells with infected macrophages induces secretion by T cells of the cytokine *interferon-gamma* (IFN-gamma), which acts locally in tissue (*paracrine effect*) to activate infected macrophages for killing of intracellular parasites. A specific subset of antigen-sensitive helper T cells, $T_H1$ cells, releases IFN-gamma as well as the cytokine *interleukin-2* (*IL-2*), which acts as an *autocrine factor* to promote the proliferative expansion of antigen-sensitive helper T-cell populations. Evidence has accumulated that the cytokine *interleukin-12* (*IL-12*) produced by macrophages stimulates the differentiation of CD4+ T lymphocytes to $T_H1$ cells. The importance of CD4+ T lymphocytes for cell-mediated immunity in the recovery from diseases caused by facultative intracellular bacteria is clearly demonstrated by their prevalence in the acquired immunodeficiency syndrome (AIDS), in which CD4+ cells are destroyed by human immunodeficiency virus type 1 (HIV-1) infection.

Cells infected with intracellular parasites can also activate *cytotoxic T lymphocytes*, a population of T cells that uses lymphocyte membrane *CD8 molecules* for recognition of microbial antigen complexed with *MHC type* I *molecules* of infected cells. Cytotoxic T lymphocytes directly kill infected cells by lysis. Although previously thought to occur only in cell-mediated immunity toward obligate intracellular parasites, especially viruses, recent evidence indicates that cytotoxic T cells may contribute to immunity in facultative intracellular bacterial disease as well (see Chapter 13).

## TISSUE INJURY IN BACTERIAL DISEASE

### Direct Injury

Many pathogenic bacteria release enzymes that directly damage tissue, especially the extracellular connective tissue matrix and blood vessels, thereby promoting the local spread of bacteria through tissue and systemically in the blood circulation. Invasive streptococci produce *hyaluronidase*, which degrades hyaluronic acid of the connective tissue matrix, with rapid spread of streptococcal infection through tissue, especially a rapidly spreading and diffuse infection of the soft tissues of the skin known as *cellulitis*. Particulary virulent strains of group A streptococcus ("flesh-eating bacteria") produce large amounts of protease and cause a necrotizing cellulitis that extensively undermines surrounding tissue. *Clostridium perfringens* infections are associated with gangrenous necrosis of traumatized tissue contaminated with clostridial spores, which germinate to form vegetative bacilli in the anaerobic regions of traumatized tissue. *C. perfringens* bacilli release collagenase and hyaluronidase which degrade extracellular matrix proteins, as well as phospholipases which act on host cell membranes of muscle cells causing *myonecrosis*, membranes of the endothelium of blood vessels producing hemorrhagic necrosis of tissue, and red cell membranes causing a hemolytic anemia. The gram-negative pathogen *Pseudomonas aeruginosa* produces the exoenzyme *elastase*, which degrades and damages the elastin of blood vessel walls.

### Inflammatory Injury

The inflammatory response to bacterial infection, whether neutrophilic, chronic mononuclear, or granulomatous, can itself result in injury of tissue. Three mechanisms operate separately and together to cause inflammatory tissue injury. First, neutrophils and macrophages release lysosomal neutral proteases into tissue by active secretion (exocytosis), passive regurgitation through incompletely sealed phagolysosomes, and (especially with short-lived neutrophils) passive release from necrotic inflammatory cells. These neutral proteases can degrade collagen and elastin of the extracellular connective tissue matrix, the basement membrane of blood vessels, and cartilage. Second, external membrane surfaces of activated neutrophils and macrophages release oxygen radicals ($O_2^-$ · and · OH) that injure host parenchymal and stromal cells primarily by lipid peroxidation. Third, the cytokine *tumor necrosis factor-alpha* (*TNF-alpha*) secreted by activated macrophages (and to a lesser extent by neutrophils) has toxic actions on host tissue cells.

Antiprotease and antioxidant mechanisms exist to protect infected tissue against inflammatory injury. The serum antiprotease *alpha$_1$-antitrypsin* neutralizes neutrophil lysosomal elastase at sites of inflammation. Interestingly, radicals released by inflammatory cells can oxidatively inactivate alpha$_1$-antitrypsin and thereby promote tissue injury by inflammatory cell proteases. The serum iron-transport protein *transferrin* binds the ferric form of iron and removes iron as a catalyst for the Fenton reaction. The serum copper-transport protein *ceruloplasmin* has ferroxidase activity, which converts ferrous to ferric iron for binding and removal by transferrin.

Intracellular mechanisms are also available

to protect host cells against the oxidant stress of inflammatory responses. The cytosolic enzyme *superoxide dismutase* rapidly converts $O_2^- \cdot$ to $H_2O_2$ at the neutral pH of cytosol, and $H_2O_2$ in turn is decomposed to harmless $O_2$ and $H_2O$ by the enzyme *catalase*. Also, the cytosolic *glutathione peroxidase* system (glutathione is a tripeptide of glutamic acid, cysteine, and glycine) inactivates $H_2O_2$ by the reactions:

$$2GSH + H_2O_2 \rightarrow GSSG + 2H_2O$$

$$GSSG + NADPH \rightarrow 2GSH + NADP^+$$

in which GSH is reduced glutathione, GSSG is oxidized glutathione, and $NADP^+$ is nicotinamide adenine dinucleotide phosphate. Thus, the reduced forms of the cytosolic cofactors glutathione and $NADP^+$ provide potent antioxidant mechanisms for the protection of host cells in inflamed tissue. If infection is promptly contained by the inflammatory response, within a day or so, these protective mechanisms are effective, and little or no residual tissue injury is caused by the infection. However, when infection is persistent and inflammation becomes chronic (weeks, months, or years), these protective mechanisms are unable to cope with ever-increasing numbers of inflammatory cells entering the infected tissue, and inflammatory injury of tissue inevitably results. An important pathologic manifestation of inflammatory injury observed with extracellular bacteria is *liquefaction necrosis* of infected tissue, with the production of *pus* (a semifluid mixture of necrotic inflammatory and tissue debris) and *abscesses* (focal collections of pus in an organ or confined space of the body). *Ulcers* can also develop in which sloughing of inflamed necrotic tissue produces excavations of mucosal and cutaneous surfaces. The inflammatory response towards facultative intracellular bacteria can also be complicated by tissue liquefaction and ulceration, but *caseation necrosis* is much more common, in which necrotic tissue has the appearance of friable, cheesy material.

## SYSTEMIC REACTIONS IN BACTERIAL DISEASE

Activation of macrophage function is an important feature of bacterial disease. Macrophage processing of microbial antigen occurs during infection with both extracellular and facultative intracellular bacteria. In gram-negative bacterial disease, endotoxin of the gram-negative cell wall stimulates macrophages directly (see Chapter 32). Also, parasitism of macrophages by facultative intracellular bacteria stimulates the production of IFN-gamma, which activates macrophage function. Two cytokines with systemic effects in the host are released by activated macrophages, *interleukin-1* (*IL-1*) and TNF-alpha. The toxic action of TNF-alpha on host cells of infected tissue has already been discussed. Systemically, both IL-1 and TNF-alpha cause fever by direct stimulation of prostaglandin synthesis in the thermoregulatory center of the hypothalamus (Table 4–3), neutrophilic leukocytosis by acceleration of the bone marrow release of neutrophils, and increase in the serum levels of acute-phase proteins (including alpha$_1$-antitrypsin and complement) by stimulation of their synthesis. These systemic effects are host protective. Fever enhances immune responsiveness in infection. The benefit to the infected host of increased availability of neutrophils, serum antiproteases, and complement is clear. However, IL-1 and TNF-alpha can also act systemically on the vascular endothelium to induce widespread vasodilation accompanied by marked increased in vascular permeability to plasma (see discussion in Chapter 32). The resultant reduction in the effective circulating volume of blood results in hypoperfusion of tissue and shock. The mortality of bacterial infection is substantially increased when complicated by the development of shock.

## CASE HISTORIES

### CASE HISTORY 1

A 68-year-old man experiences increasing fatigue, shortness of breath, and anorexia during the summer and autumn months. In early January, he develops severe chills and fever, accompanied by chest pain on his right side and a cough productive of abundant yellow mucoid sputum containing flecks of blood. His niece brings him to the emergency department, where physical examination reveals a man in severe respiratory distress, breathing 28 times per minute, and with a heart rate of 110/min. His right hemithorax shows limited expansion on inspiration, dullness to percussion, and bronchial breath sounds. A chest x-ray reveals numerous patchy infiltrates in the right middle and lower lobes of lung. His laboratory results include a white blood cell count of $18.4 \times 10^3/\mu L$ (reference range = $4.5$–$11.0 \times 10^3$) with 60% segmented neutrophils (reference range =

45–67%) and 25% band forms (reference range = 0–11%), a hemoglobin of 6.0 g/dL (reference range = 12.6–17.4), and a total serum protein of 13.0 g/dL (reference range = 6.0–7.8) with an albumin of 2.2 g/dL (reference range = 3.2–4.6). Microscopic examination of a sputum Gram's stain shows numerous polymorphonuclear neutrophils and a pure population of gram-positive lancet-shaped diplococci morphologically consistent with *Streptococcus pneumoniae*. He is admitted to the hospital, where three sets of blood cultures are sent to the laboratory, treatment with parenteral penicillin is initiated, and he is transfused with 3 units of packed red blood cells. Over the next few days his respiratory status improves dramatically. The microbiology laboratory reports that his sputum and blood cultures are positive for *Streptococcus pneumoniae*, which is susceptible to penicillin (minimal inhibitory concentration = 0.03 μg/mL).

Because of abnormally high total serum protein accompanied by a decrease in serum albumin concentration noted at admission, a serum protein profile is ordered. Quantitative measurement of serum immunoglobulins reveals a marked elevation of his IgG level to 9600 mg/dL (reference range = 650–1600) and suppression of IgM level to 20 mg/dL (50–300) and IgA to 40 mg/dL (40–350). Serum protein electrophoresis shows a restricted protein band in the gamma-globulin region, which immunofixation electrophoresis demonstrates to be a monoclonal IgG immunoglobulin. Because of these serum protein abnormalities, bone marrow aspiration and biopsy are performed. Microscopic examination of the bone marrow reveals many large, pleomorphic plasma cells that constitute approximately 45% of the cells in his marrow. Consequently chemotherapy with cytotoxic drugs is implemented.

## CASE 1 Discussion

Multiple myeloma is a malignant neoplasm of plasma cells in which the clonal expansion of malignant plasma cells suppresses the polyclonal production of immunoglobulin by normal plasma cells needed by the host to respond to invasion by encapsulated bacteria. This is particularly evident with *S. pneumoniae*, a prevalent pathogen in individuals with multiple myeloma. A primary IgM response is necessary to opsonize encapsulated *Streptococcus pneumoniae* efficiently for phagocytosis and killing by polymorphonuclear neutrophils early in the course of infection. Despite an apparently adequate response of polymorphonuclear neutrophils as shown by purulent sputum and neutrophilic leukocytosis, marked suppression of IgM due to multiple myeloma resulted in the acute development of pneumococcal pneumonia in this elderly man. His case clearly demonstrates the critical role of immunologic responses in amplifying the intensity and efficiency of inflammatory responses in eradicating infection. It is important to note that the increasing worldwide incidence of penicillin resistance among *S. pneumoniae* requires laboratory testing of susceptibility to penicillin for all invasive infections with this microorganism.

## CASE HISTORY 2

A 48-year-old man with a long history of alcohol-induced cirrhosis injures his right lower leg in a fall, in which superficial abrasions disrupt the skin in several different areas. The abrasions are heavily contaminated by soil and water during the fall. He removes the soil by holding the leg abrasions under tap water for several minutes. Over the next several days, large and coalescent blisters (bullae) develop in the skin around his leg abrasions, and the abrasions weep slightly turbid, serous fluid. He develops chills, and by the time he enters the hospital the skin blisters have extended along the inner aspect of his left thigh. He is febrile with a blood pressure of 90/60 mm Hg, and three sets of blood cultures are submitted to the laboratory. In addition, fluid is aspirated from several skin blisters, which on visual examination appears turbid. Gram's stain examination of the blister fluid reveals numerous polymorphonuclear neutrophils and gram-negative rods. He is treated with intravenous fluid, as well as parenteral piperacillin and gentamicin. Within 3 days the microbiology laboratory reports that the blister fluid and blood cultures are positive for growth of *Aeromonas hydrophila*, which is resistant to ampicillin but susceptible to the cephalosporins, extended-spectrum penicillins (including piperacillin), and aminoglycosides (including gentamicin).

## CASE 2 Discussion

*Aeromonas hydrophila* is a gram-negative bacillus that is ubiquitous in the environment, including soil and water (both fresh and salt water). An important portal of entry for this microorganism is offered by breaks in the integrity of skin, such as trauma during swimming, or in accidents where skin breaks are contaminated by soil and/or water. This case demonstrates that superficial abrasions with exposure of underlying dermis can be sufficient to compromise the ability of skin to function as a primary defense mechanism against bacterial invasion. An important underlying factor which promoted the development of bacteremia in this man was cirrhosis, in which clearance of bacteria from the blood by hepatic phagocytic Kupffer cells is lost due to shunting of blood around the liver.

## REFERENCES

**Book**

Mims, C. A., Dimmock, N. J., Nash, A., and Stephen, J. *Mims' Pathogenesis of Infectious Disease*. New York: Academic Press, 1995.

## Review Articles

Burman, L. A., Norrby, R., and Trollfors, B. Invasive pneumococcal infections: Incidence, predisposing factors, and prognosis. *Rev. Infect. Dis.* 7:133–142, 1985.

Busse, W. W. Pathogenesis and sequelae of respiratory infections. *Rev. Infect. Dis.* 13:S477–S485, 1991.

Cossart, P., and Mengaud, J. *Listeria monocytogenes*—a model system for the molecular study of intracellular parasites. *Mol. Biol. Med.* 6:463–474, 1989.

Gibbons, R. J. Bacterial attachment to host tissues. In: Gorbach, S. L., Bartlett, J. G., and Blacklow, N. R., eds. *Infectious Diseases.* Philadelphia: W.B. Saunders Co., 1992:7–17.

Goldmann, D. A., and Pier, G. B. Pathogenesis of infections related to intravascular catheterization. *Clin. Microbiol. Rev.* 6:176–192, 1993.

Guerrant, R. L., Hughes, J. M., Lima, N. L., and Crane, J. Diarrhea in developed and developing countries: Magnitude, special settings, and etiologies. *Rev. Infect. Dis.* 12:S41–S50, 1990.

Janda, J. M., Guthertz, L. S., Kokka, R. P., and Shimada, T. *Aeromonas* species in septicemia: Laboratory characteristics and clinical observations. *Clin. Infect. Dis.* 19:77–83, 1994.

Johnson, J. R. Virulence factors in *Escherichia coli* urinary tract infection. *Clin. Microbiol. Rev.* 4:80–128, 1991.

Knoop, F. L., Owens, M., and Crocker, I. C. *Clostridium difficile:* Clinical disease and diagnosis. *Clin. Microbiol. Rev.* 6:251–265, 1993.

Marrie, T. J. Community-acquired pneumonia. *Clin. Infect. Dis.* 18:501–515, 1994.

Musher, D. M. Infections caused by *Streptococcus pneumoniae:* Clinical spectrum, pathogenesis, immunity, and treatment. *Clin. Infect. Dis.* 14:801–809, 1992.

Petri, W. A., Jr., and Mann, B. J. Microbial adherence. In: Mandell, G. L., Bennett, J. E., and Dolin, R., eds. *Principles and Practice of Infectious Diseases.* New York: Churchill Livingstone, 1995:11–19.

Raoult, D., and Brouqui, P. Intracellular location of microorganisms. In: Raoult, D., ed. *Antimicrobial Agents and Intracellular Pathogens.* Boca Raton: CRC Press, 1993:39–61.

Rupp, M. E., and Archer, G. L. Coagulase-negative staphylococci: Pathogens associated with medical progress. *Clin. Infect. Dis.* 19:231–245, 1994.

Scheld, W. M., and Mandell, G. L. Nosocomial pneumonia: Pathogenesis and recent advances in diagnosis and therapy. *Rev. Infect. Dis.* 13:S743–S751, 1991.

Stamm, W. E., Hooton, T. M., Johnson, J. R., et al. Urinary tract infections: From pathogenesis to treatment. *J. Infect. Dis.* 159:400–406, 1989.

Tarr, P. I. *Escherichia coli* 0157:H7: Clinical, diagnostic and epidemiological aspects of human infection. *Clin. Infect. Dis.* 20:1–10, 1995.

# 5

# VIRUS–HOST INTERACTIONS

BETSY C. HEROLD, M.D. and PATRICIA G. SPEAR, Ph.D.

The past few decades have been characterized by intense activity in the field of virology. Many previously unrecognized viral pathogens have been discovered. Previously unrecognized viral diseases, such as the acquired immunodeficiency syndrome (AIDS), have also been identified. The decade has seen the development of new techniques, especially in molecular biology, which serve as tools for diagnosis as well as for unraveling the mysteries of viral pathogenesis. There have been advances in the development of antiviral therapies and immunization strategies. Viruses, however, remain a major cause of human disease and continue to challenge scientists and clinicians.

Viruses are obligate intracellular parasites. They differ in fundamental ways, however, from bacterial, fungal, and protozoan intracellular parasites. Viruses are inert in their extracellular forms but have the capacity to invade cells. In the intracellular environment, the nucleic acid component of the virus is released to redirect the biosynthetic activities of the cell toward production of progeny virus particles. The virus contributes the genetic instructions for this process, such as genetic information for the viral enzymes, regulatory proteins, and structural proteins needed for its replication, but otherwise must use the host cell machinery for its replication.

Every step of viral replication from entry into the cell, to the expression of viral genes, to the egress of progeny virus requires functional interactions between viral and cell proteins and nucleic acids. This means that a particular virus is suited for (has evolved for) replication in some cell types and species but not in others. Even if a cell is not permissive for viral replication (because it lacks one or more components required for that replication), the virus may still be able to invade the cell and, through the expression of a subset of viral genes, alter the properties of the cell. For example, the virus may induce cell proliferation under conditions that would normally not be conducive to cell proliferation.

Virus-induced pathology in the intact animal or human depends on the effects of the virus on each cell type it can invade and on the immune responses provoked by viral antigens. Infected cells may be killed by the virus, especially if the cells are permissive for viral replication. Infected cells may also be killed by induced cytotoxic responses of the host directed against the virus-infected cells. Finally, infected cells may survive and evade the immune response. Rarely are the cells permissive for viral replication in this latter situation. More often, the cells are latently infected; that is, a subset of viral genes are expressed but virus is not produced. Latently infected cells can be important in pathogenesis because they harbor a reservoir of virus that is not eliminated on recovery from disease and that can later be reactivated to cause a recurrence of disease. Finally, by inducing cells to proliferate in the absence of the normal signals for cell proliferation, as mentioned above, viruses can be one of the multiple factors that contribute to the induction of cancer.

Following a brief discussion of virus structure and classification, we focus first on describing various kinds of virus–cell interactions, and considering the consequences to the virus and the cell. Viral pathogenesis in the intact host is then addressed, with discussion of the factors that influence host resistance and susceptibility to viral disease.

## VIRUS STRUCTURE AND CLASSIFICATION

Viruses are composed of nucleic acid, a capsid or protein coat and, in some instances, an outer membranous envelope. Viruses are quite small (10–300 nm) and cannot be visualized with the light microscope, making rapid clinical diagnosis difficult. With the advent of electron microscopy in the 1940s, viral particles could be visualized. Electron microscopy has since played a major role in studies of the etiology of viral disease, in diagnosis, and in the delineation of viral structure. Most recently, x-ray crystallography and electron microscopic analyses combined with computer-assisted image reconstructions have enabled researchers to produce very detailed images of virus particles, also called *virions* (Fig. 5–1).

Virus classification depends on properties of the viral genome and of the particle in which it is packaged. The differentiating properties of the viral genome include the nature of the nucleic acid (DNA or RNA), the number of strands to the nucleic acid (single- or double-), its shape (linear or circular), and size of the genome. Most DNA viruses associated with human disease have genomes of double-stranded DNA. RNA viruses are usually single-stranded, except for reoviruses, which have a double-stranded RNA genome. For single-stranded RNA viruses, the genome may be either positive sense (the same polarity as messenger RNA [mRNA]), negative sense (antipolar to the mRNA), or rarely, ambisense (part of the genome has the same polarity as mRNA and the rest is antipolar). The sizes of viral genomes and numbers of genes

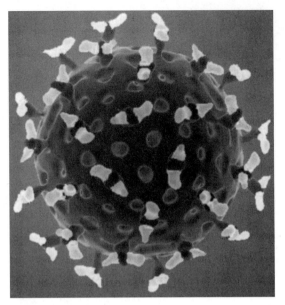

**FIGURE   5–1.** Three-dimensional structure of a rotavirus–Fab complex reconstructed by computer analysis from multiple electron-microscopic images of frozen, hydrated specimens. The virus particle has a diameter of 76 nm. The icosahedral surface of the virion is perforated by 132 aqueous channels. Sixty spikes, which are dimers of the viral protein VP4, extend from this surface. Two Fab fragments from a neutralizing monoclonal antibody against VP4 are shown (in lighter tone) at the distal end of each spike. (Photograph courtesy of B. V. V. Prasad, Baylor College of Medicine, Houston, TX; reprinted by permission from Prasad, B. V. V., Burns, J. W., Marietta, E., Estes, M. K., and Chiu, W. Localization of VP4 neutralization sites in rotavirus by three-dimensional cryoelectron microscopy. *Nature 343*:476–479; copyright © 1990 Macmillan Magazines Limited.)

encoded range from about 2 kilobases (kb) (one or two genes) to about 300 kb (100–200 genes).

The differentiating properties of the virus particle include the size, morphology, and symmetry of the protein coat, or capsid, and the presence or absence of a membranous envelope as an outer coat (Fig. 5–2). The viral genome can be coated with proteins in a helical array (especially for single-stranded RNA viruses) or surrounded by an icosahedral protein shell. The arrangement of the capsid proteins in the helical nucleocapsid or in the icosahedral shell is characteristic for each distinct family of viruses. Some viruses also possess a viral envelope composed of a lipid bilayer and various proteins or glycoproteins specified by the virus. These viruses acquire their envelopes by budding through a virus-modified patch of host cell membrane. Thus, the envelope is composed of host cell lipids and viral membrane proteins and may con-

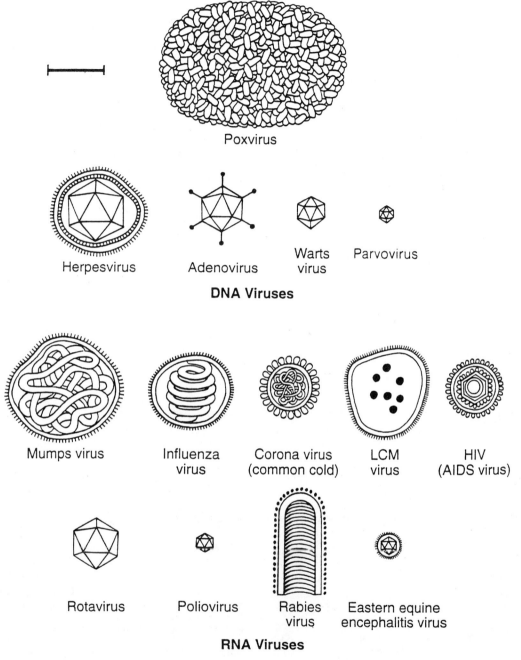

Poxvirus

Herpesvirus    Adenovirus    Warts virus    Parvovirus

**DNA Viruses**

Mumps virus    Influenza virus    Corona virus (common cold)    LCM virus    HIV (AIDS virus)

Rotavirus    Poliovirus    Rabies virus    Eastern equine encephalitis virus

**RNA Viruses**

**FIGURE 5–2.** Differences in virion morphology exhibited by members of different virus families. The genomes of some viruses are enclosed within icosahedral protein shells, whereas those of others (particularly single-stranded RNA viruses) are associated with proteins to form a helical nucleoprotein complex. A biologic membrane composed of lipids and viral proteins and glycoproteins forms the outer surface for some, but not all, viruses. (From Fields, B. N. Biology of viruses. In: Schaechter, M., Medoff, G., Eisenstein, B. I., eds. *Mechanisms of Microbial Disease.* 2nd ed. Baltimore: Williams & Wilkins, 1993:386. With permission.)

tain small amounts of host membrane proteins in addition. The structural proteins and envelope (if present) of the virus particle serve at least two roles. They protect the viral genome from degradation in the extracellular environment and provide the vehicle required to dock with and invade a cell. The outer surface of the virus particle, whether this is the protein capsid or the viral envelope, mediates attachment of the virus to a host cell, initiating the process that leads to penetration of the viral genome into the cell.

## VIRUS–CELL INTERACTIONS

Viral infection of an animal or human being requires the invasion of individual cells at the portal of entry and replication of virus in at least some of these cells. Virus may then spread to cells in other tissues. If an infected cell has all the factors required for viral replication, a productive infection occurs. Otherwise, an abortive or latent infection occurs. These nonproductive infections can also have profound effects on the individual cell and on the natural history of the disease. Following a discussion of viral entry into cells, the various kinds of productive and nonproductive infections are described.

### Entry of Virus into a Cell

Specific attachment or adsorption of a virion to a cell precedes virus penetration into the cell and is mediated by binding of a viral protein (antireceptor) to a cell-surface receptor. Recently, receptors for several clinically important viruses have been identified, including the CD4 molecule for the human immunodeficiency virus (HIV), the CR2 complement receptor for Epstein-Barr virus (EBV), ICAM-1 for rhinoviruses, and heparan sulfate proteoglycans for herpes simplex virus (HSV).

It is coming to be recognized that presence of a cell-surface receptor appropriate for the attachment of virus may be necessary but not sufficient to allow penetration of the virus into the cell. A possible explanation is that penetration may require specific molecular interactions between the virion surface and the cell membrane, in addition to the interaction required for attachment of the virus to the cell. For example, adenovirus binds to unknown cell surface receptors via the fiber protein extending from each vertex of the virion. It was shown recently that entry of cell-bound adenovirus depends on interactions of the

vertex base protein (penton) with specific members of the family of integrin proteins (cell-surface adhesion molecules).

There are fundamental differences in the way enveloped and nonenveloped viruses penetrate into cells. For enveloped viruses, penetration results when the virion envelope fuses with a cell membrane (Fig. 5–3). The virion envelope may fuse directly with the cell plasma membrane, following attachment of the virus to the cell surface (Fig. 5–3A). Alternatively, the virion envelope may fuse with an endosome membrane, after the entire virion has been taken into the cell by receptor-mediated endocytosis (Fig. 5–3B). For nonenveloped viruses, the virion is either translocated across the plasma membrane or translocated across an endosome membrane following endocytosis. The pathway of entry is characteristic for each virus and may also be influenced by the host cell.

### Viral Replication

The stages in a viral replicative cycle (following adsorption and penetration of virus)

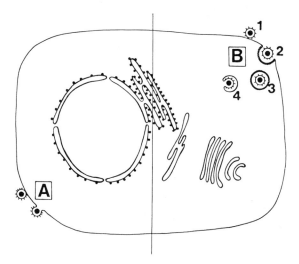

**FIGURE 5–3.** Pathways by which enveloped viruses can enter cells to initiate infection. The virion–cell fusion required to release the nucleocapsid into the cytoplasm may occur at the plasma membrane (*A*) or with the membrane of an endosome (*B*), depending upon the virus. The temporal sequence of events in the endocytic pathway (*B*) is thought to be similar to that defined for receptor-mediated endocytosis of other ligands. These events include attachment of virus to the cell surface (1), lateral movement to a clathrin-coated pit (2), ingestion by the cell in a coated vesicle (3), transition of the vesicle from coated to uncoated (endosome), and fusion of the virion with the membrane of the endosome (4). (From Spear, P. G. Virus-induced cell fusion. In: Sowers, A. E., ed. *Cell Fusion.* New York: Plenum Publishing Corporation, 1987: 6. With permission.)

include uncoating of the viral genome, viral gene expression, replication of the viral genome, assembly of progeny virus, and egress of the progeny virus from the infected cell.

Penetration of virus into a cell is accompanied by and followed by disassembly of the virus particle and release of the viral genome. The viral genome is then translocated to the compartment of the cell where viral gene expression can occur (either the nucleus or cytoplasm, depending on the virus). The strategies for expressing the genetic information encoded in each viral genome are different for each virus family. Figures 5–4 and 5–5 outline the strategies of gene expression and replication for the major families of viruses that cause human disease.

A few general observations are pertinent. First, DNA viruses can use cell RNA polymerases for transcribing their genes and cell DNA polymerases for replicating their genomes. DNA viruses, however, always encode their own regulatory proteins needed to direct transcription and replication to the viral genome. Many DNA viruses also encode their own DNA polymerases and some of the other enzymes and factors required for replication of the genome.

Second, RNA viruses must encode their own RNA polymerases because there appear to be no cell enzymes capable of transcribing genetic information from RNA to RNA or replicating RNA using RNA as a template, at least not for viral RNA genomes. These viral RNA polymerases (often called *transcriptases/replicases*) are usually highly specific for the homologous RNA viral genome. In cases where the input parental RNA genome is not of positive polarity and therefore cannot serve as mRNA, a viral transcriptase must be packaged with the viral genome in the virion. This is to permit production of mRNA, using the parental genome as template, as soon as the virus penetrates into the cell.

Third, retroviruses and hepadnaviruses (hepatitis B virus) both encode reverse transcriptases (RTs) which are packaged in virions and are required for replication of the genome. Their strategies for use of the RTs (which transcribe RNA to produce a double-stranded DNA copy) are quite different, however, as outlined in Figure 5–4.

Fourth, a common strategy for the production of functional viral proteins is synthesis of viral polyproteins, followed by proteolytic cleavage of the polyproteins to yield the individual viral proteins. This strategy is especially important for RNA viruses, including retroviruses. The proteases required are usually encoded by the virus. The proteolytic cleavages may accompany, and may be required for, dynamic processes such as replication of the viral genome or assembly of progeny virus particles.

Assembly of progeny virions takes place in the cell compartment where replication of the viral genome occurred. Most RNA viruses are assembled in the cell cytoplasm, whereas most DNA viruses are assembled in the cell nucleus. For enveloped viruses, the final step in assembly is acquisition of the envelope by budding of the nucleocapsid through a patch of cell membrane modified to contain viral membrane proteins and glycoproteins. This envelopment can occur at the inner nuclear membrane, endoplasmic reticulum, Golgi apparatus, or the plasma membrane, depending on the virus (Fig. 5–6).

For an enveloped virus that acquires its envelope from the plasma membrane, the final step in assembly releases the virus from the cell. For other enveloped viruses, an exocytic process is required to transport the virions from cisternae of the endoplasmic reticulum or Golgi apparatus to the outside of the cell. For nonenveloped viruses, the progeny virus must escape from the nuclear or cytoplasmic compartment of the cell. It has been thought that this escape might depend upon lysis of the cell. More recent evidence suggests, however, that specific mechanisms may exist for the secretion or extrusion of nonenveloped virions. In general, the mechanisms governing the egress of viruses from infected cells are not well understood.

Death of the infected cell is the usual, but not invariant, consequence of viral replication. The precise mechanisms by which viruses kill cells are poorly understood. Many viruses produce specific inhibitors of cell macromolecular syntheses, presumably to provide a selective advantage for viral gene expression. For example, poliovirus produces a protease that inactivates a cap-binding protein required for the translation of capped cell mRNAs but not for the uncapped viral mRNA. Virus-induced inhibition of cell protein synthesis can render cells sensitive to host cytokines that induce cell death by apoptosis. Viruses that can replicate without killing the host cell include retroviruses.

Many of the stages of each viral replicative cycle can be exploited in the development of antiviral drugs. Most of the antiviral drugs

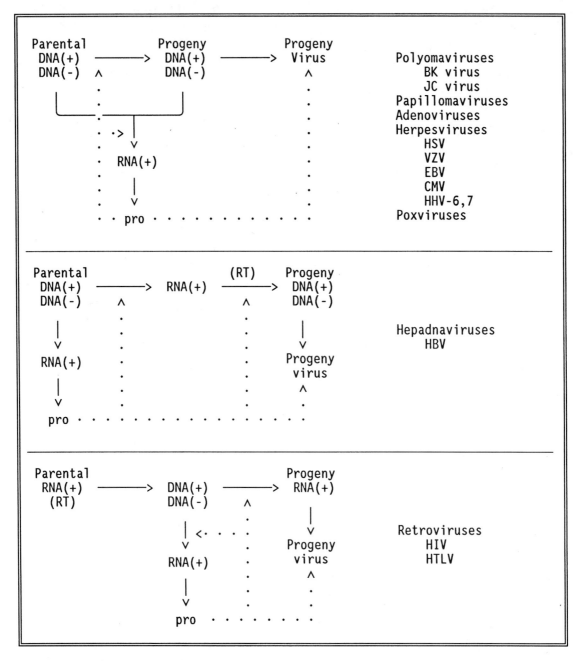

**FIGURE 5–4.** Strategies for gene expression and viral replication by selected DNA viruses and retroviruses. For all the DNA viruses listed in *A*, except poxviruses, the viral DNA is transported to the cell nucleus where it is transcribed into mRNA (RNA(+)) by cell RNA polymerase. The mRNA goes to the cell cytoplasm where it is translated into protein (pro). Viral proteins regulate transcription of the viral genome, participate in replication of the viral genome, and package the progeny viral genomes into virions, as indicated by the *dotted lines*. Adenoviruses and herpesviruses encode their own DNA polymerases, whereas polyomaviruses and papillomaviruses use the cell DNA polymerase. Poxviruses replicate entirely in the cell cytoplasm. These viruses encode all the enzymes required for transcription and replication of the viral genome. A viral RNA polymerase packaged in the virion mediates initial transcription of the viral genome. For hepadnaviruses (*B*), the viral genome is also transported to the cell nucleus where it is transcribed by cell RNA polymerase. Some of the transcripts produced serve as mRNA. A special full-length transcript is packaged into immature virus particles, along with a viral reverse transcriptase (RT). During the final stages of virion morphogenesis, the packaged RNA is transcribed into double-stranded DNA (the RNA is degraded subsequent to the reverse transcription; some nicks and gaps remain in the DNA). Viral proteins regulate transcription of the viral genome, mediate reverse transcription, and package the viral genome. For retroviruses (*C*), the viral RNA genome is introduced into cells along with an RT that was also packaged in the virion. This RT immediately transcribes the viral RNA genome into a double-stranded DNA, which is

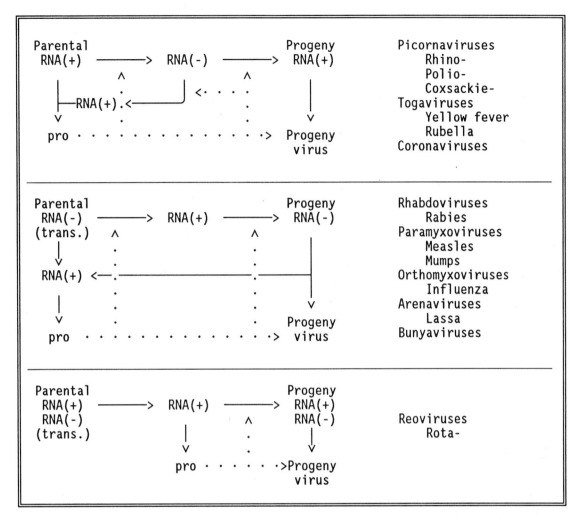

**FIGURE 5–5.** Strategies for gene expression and viral replication by selected RNA viruses. The RNA genomes of the viruses listed in *A* serve as mRNA immediately on entry into the cell cytoplasm. Newly synthesized viral proteins serve as transcriptase–replicase, first to transcribe the viral genome to produce a negative-polarity template. This template is then transcribed to produce positive-polarity RNA. Some of the RNA(+) serves as mRNA to make more viral proteins, including the virion proteins, and the remaining RNA(+) is packaged into virions. The RNA genomes of the viruses listed in *B* are of negative polarity and are introduced into cells along with a viral transcriptase (trans.). This transcriptase immediately transcribes the viral genome to produce mRNAs that are translated to produce viral proteins. These proteins include a replicase that transcribes the viral genome to yield a positive-polarity copy and then transcribes this copy to yield progeny viral genomes. Reoviruses (*C*) have segmented genomes of double-stranded RNA. On entry into a cell, the virion is converted to a protein core containing the RNA genome and a viral transcriptase. The transcriptase transcribes the RNA genome to yield mRNA, which is released from the core and translated to produce viral proteins. These proteins include a replicase that produces double-stranded RNA segments from each mRNA. These segments are packaged into progeny virions.

then integrated into the cell genome. A viral integrase catalyzes this integration. Cell RNA polymerase transcribes the integrated viral DNA (proviral DNA). Differential splicing of the transcripts yields several mRNAs needed for the production of the viral proteins. Full-length transcripts can be packaged into virions along with RT. Viral proteins regulate transcription and splicing, mediate reverse transcription and integration, and package progeny RNA into virions.

currently in use block viral genome replication. For example, acyclovir inhibits herpesvirus (HSV and varicella-zoster virus [VZV]) DNA replication. This drug, an analog of guanidine, is highly selective against herpesviruses and relatively nontoxic because herpesvirus thymidine kinases can phosphorylate acyclovir (phosphorylation is required for its inhibitory activity) much more efficiently than host cell kinases. Azidothymidine (AZT) specifically inhibits HIV reverse transcriptase and can therefore inhibit the initiation of HIV infection in previously uninfected cells. Unfortunately, viral mutants that are resistant to AZT arise at high frequency, limiting the usefulness of the drug during the course of treating a patient. A new generation of anti-HIV drugs targets the viral protease (essential for production of functional viral proteins), and several are currently being tested in clinical trials.

## Latent and Persistent Infections

A nonproductive infection results when a virus invades a cell that does not possess all the factors required for virus replication. The replicative cycle can be blocked at whatever stage requires the missing cell factor or factors. If the block occurs early in the replicative cycle, the parental viral genome may gradually be lost or diluted out by cell division. If the block occurs late in the replicative cycle, the cell may be killed but without releasing any progeny infectious virus.

Certain viruses, particularly DNA viruses, have evolved mechanisms for the long-term maintenance of viral genomes in cells that are nonpermissive for viral replication. This usually requires the controlled expression of a particular subset of viral genes and repression of most other viral genes, along with controlled replication of the viral genome in concert with the replication of cell DNA. If the latent infection is established in a nondividing quiescent cell (resting B lymphocyte for EBV) or in a postmitotic cell (neuron for HSV), then the requirement for viral gene expression may be minimized because viral genome replication would not be required. This maintenance of viral genomes in nonpermissive cells is analogous to lysogeny of bacteria by bacteriophage and, in eukaryotic systems, is called a *latent infection*. In latently infected cells, maintenance of viral genomes depends on cell viability, whereas in productively infected cells virus replication is usually incompatible with cell survival. Latent infection ap-

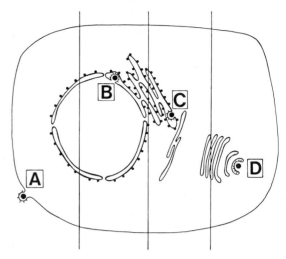

**FIGURE 5–6.** Envelopment of nucleocapsids by modified patches of cell membrane during the final stages of virion morphogenesis. Members of different virus families characteristically acquire their envelopes by budding through the plasma membrane (*A*), the inner nuclear membrane (*B*), membrane of the endoplasmic reticulum (*C*), or the Golgi apparatus (*D*). (From Spear, P. G. Virus-induced cell fusion. In: Sowers, A. E., ed. *Cell Fusion*. New York: Plenum Publishing Corporation, 1987:5. With permission.)

pears to be an alternative to productive infection, and not just an aborted productive infection. Under appropriate conditions, however, latently infected cells can be induced to produce virus, which means that the state of the cell governs whether latent or productive infection occurs.

Latent infections are central to the pathogenesis of certain virus infections, such as members of the herpesvirus family. Molecular details of the virus–cell interaction in latency are best understood for EBV, principally because latently infected B lymphocytes can be cultured and studied *in vitro*. EBV maintains a few copies of its genome, as circular episomes, in latently infected cells. It does so by expressing a viral protein that binds to an origin of DNA replication in the viral genome, thereby directing cell DNA polymerase to replicate the genome in a controlled fashion during each S phase of the cell cycle. If the latently infected B cell is induced to produce virus, then viral DNA polymerase is expressed and catalyzes the exponential replication of viral genomes, using a different origin of DNA replication. Latently infected B lymphocytes can be isolated from EBV-positive individuals long after primary infection with this virus, whether or not the infection was symptomatic.

Retroviruses present a special case with regard to latency. These viruses have evolved the enzymatic machinery required to produce a double-stranded DNA copy of the RNA genome and then to integrate this DNA (called *proviral DNA*) into the cell genome. As described in Figure 5–4, this integration of proviral DNA is required for viral replication. Viral replication depends upon transcription of the integrated proviral DNA by cell RNA polymerase to produce progeny RNA genomes. Perhaps because maintenance of the template required for production of viral genomes depends upon cell viability, retrovirus replication usually does not result in cell death and is compatible with cell proliferation. Moreover, integration of proviral DNA ensures that an infected cell and its daughter cells are permanently altered genetically and can rarely if ever be "cured" of the infection. Whether cells carrying proviral DNA will be productively or latently infected depends upon whether the appropriate cell factors are present for transcribing the proviral DNA and for producing virus particles. Theoretically, cells can remain latently infected with a retrovirus for a long time and then begin to produce virus only when the cell is stimulated by external events to produce the factors required for virus production. This possibility has been invoked to explain the variable, but often very long, incubation period of AIDS. On the other hand, it is now appreciated that HIV replication and virus-induced loss of T cells occur at much higher rates during the incubation period than previously thought.

Most RNA viruses do not transcribe their genetic information into DNA and do not have any known mechanisms for establishing latent infections of the kinds just described. Persistent, chronic infections with RNA viruses and at least one DNA virus (hepatitis B virus) do occur, however, both *in vivo* and, in some instances, in cultured cells. In persistently infected populations of cultured cells, virus replication and spread of infection may occur at reduced rates and levels so that cell proliferation can outpace cell death resulting from cytotoxic effects of the virus. Some of the factors that enable the establishment of persistent, chronic infections include the generation of defective viruses and the induction of interferon, both of which can modulate the replication of wild-type virus. Certain RNA viruses have the capacity to persist for long periods in individuals who have recovered from the primary disease and then perhaps to

cause a different kind of secondary disease. For example, long after recovery from measles, a condition called subacute sclerosing panencephalitis (SSPE) may occur. SSPE is due to the abortive replication of persistent measles virus in cells of the central nervous system.

## Virus-Induced Proliferation of Cells

Many DNA viruses encode proteins that can stimulate cell division or other cell processes. An important role of these proteins is to induce the production of cell enzymes and other factors required for viral DNA replication. If these viral stimulatory proteins, sometimes called *viral oncogenes,* are expressed in the absence of other viral proteins, the cells may be immortalized (converted from cells that can divide only a finite number of times to cells that can divide indefinitely) or may even be transformed from normal to malignant. A number of DNA viruses (including polyomaviruses and adenoviruses) can cause tumors in animals other than the natural host. Abortive infection of nonpermissive cells allows the viral oncogenes to be expressed in the absence of viral replication (illegitimate recombination between the viral genome and the cell genome is required to alter permanently the genotype and phenotype of the transformed cells).

Some DNA viruses can induce the proliferation of latently infected cells. The subsets of viral genes expressed under these conditions are those encoding proteins that induce cell division and that ensure replication of the viral genome in concert with the cell genome. Virus-induced cell proliferation is an important aspect of pathogenesis in diseases caused by viruses such as papillomaviruses and EBV.

Papillomaviruses can induce the proliferation of latently infected cells in the basal layers of epidermis, resulting in a benign tumor or wart. When the cells in the basal layer move toward the outer surface and differentiate, viral replication is activated. EBV induces the proliferation of latently infected B lymphocytes, immortalizing the cells and enabling them to proliferate indefinitely in the absence of the antigenic stimulus usually required. Practical use is made of this phenomenon to isolate permanent cell lines from individuals for genetic studies or for use of the cells as autologous antigen-presenting cells in *in vitro* assays of immune function.

The cells that are induced to proliferate in

response to virus infection express viral antigens and are usually highly immunogenic. The normal immune system, once primed for attack, can readily contain or eliminate these latently infected, proliferating cells. The consequences of deficiencies in this immunity are discussed below. For EBV, and perhaps for other DNA viruses, there may be two kinds of latent infection—one in which cell proliferation is induced and another in which it is not. Latent infection in which cell proliferation is induced can explain the *in vitro* results observed and certain aspects of the pathology of infectious mononucleosis (this self-limiting lymphoproliferative disease appears to be due to the virus-induced proliferation of B lymphocytes and to the even more pronounced proliferation of T lymphocytes in response to the latently infected B cells) (see Chapter 8). Latently infected cells that do not express the viral genes required for cell proliferation may not be very immunogenic (due in part to the more limited expression of viral genes) and could persist for long periods in the infected individual. This kind of latent infection could explain the long-term persistence of EBV in the lymphocytes of asymptomatic individuals.

## VIRUS–HOST INTERACTIONS

Specific properties of each virus direct the kinds of diseases it can cause. These properties are determined by the genetic content of the virus, the evolution of which is influenced by interactions of the virus with its natural host. Severity of disease and specific pathologic features of disease are governed not only by properties of the virus but also by the response of the host to virus infection. The response of the host is determined by immune status and genetic polymorphisms that can result in variations among human beings in innate resistance to a particular infectious agent and/or in ability to react to infection with that agent by the activation or induction of various protective cells and products. The remainder of this chapter addresses these issues, emphasizing the interplay between virus and host that governs the outcome of infection.

### Determinants of Viral Pathology

The signs, symptoms, and pathology of disease caused by a particular virus depend in part on the virus–cell interactions that govern the portal of entry, the rate of viral replication and spread, the route of spread of infection, and the target organs or tissues. The nature of the disease is also dependent on the vigor and nature of the host response, in part because the induced protective responses can contribute to the pathology of disease as well as to the containment of virus spread and the reduction in severity of disease.

Some of these points can be illustrated by comparison of the different diseases caused by two viruses, influenza virus and VZV, both of which use the respiratory tract as portal of entry. Both viruses can infect cells in the respiratory epithelium. Influenza virus replication remains largely localized to the respiratory epithelial cells, however, whereas VZV replication occurs also in other cells and tissues. Influenza virus replication can be accompanied by extensive destruction of the respiratory epithelium, due to viral cytotoxicity and to induced host responses directed against the infected cells. The systemic symptoms of disease (malaise, headache, myalgia, cachexia), as well as localized respiratory symptoms, can be accounted for in large part by the action of cytokines and monokines released from cells of the immune system that respond to the localized infection. On the other hand, VZV usually causes less pathologic change in the respiratory tract but is able to infect leukocytes attracted to the primary sites of infection, resulting in viremia and the spread of virus infection to the skin and mucosal surfaces and to the nervous system. VZV can replicate in localized patches of cutaneous or mucocutaneous epithelium, causing the characteristic chicken pox. VZV also infects cells of the peripheral nervous system to establish latent infections. The entry of VZV into nerve cells is either via the circulatory system or via neural routes. Whereas influenza virus is eliminated from the host during recovery from disease, VZV is not eliminated because of the ability of the virus to establish latent infections. At variable times after recovery from chicken pox (or after a primary infection that causes no apparent disease), the latent virus can be activated, by unidentified stimuli, to cause shingles or zoster. In zoster, virus replication probably begins in cells of the peripheral nerves, accounting for the severe pain that can result, and then spreads via axons to the skin, causing the characteristic zoster lesions, which have a dermatomal distribution.

The cellular and molecular determinants of the differences in disease caused by influenza and VZV are not yet understood. Although the initial binding of both viruses to cells is via receptors that are widely distributed on many cell types (sialic acid for influenza virus and probably glycosaminoglycan chains for VZV), other viral and cell factors required for viral entry or replication must account for the fact that influenza virus usually fails to infect leukocytes or cells of the nervous system, whereas VZV can infect both.

The different evolutionary histories and properties of influenza virus and VZV determine the differences in basic features of disease as commonly manifested. However, variations in the host response can influence the nature of disease. For example, individuals who can mount vigorous protective responses to the initial stages of influenza virus or VZV infection may experience only mild respiratory symptoms with either virus (with possibly the only difference in consequences being that the VZV-infected person is then at risk for subsequent zoster). On the other hand, immunodeficient individuals usually respond differently to infection by these two viruses. In the case of influenza virus, immunodeficiency does not generally result in widespread dissemination of viral infection and replication. Severe pneumonia may occur and may be lethal, especially if there is a secondary bacterial pneumonia. In the case of VZV, widespread dissemination of viral infection and replication can occur, affecting several organ systems including the central nervous system and resulting in death or permanent neurologic damage.

In addition to the constitutional or genetic differences among individuals that influence their ability to mount induced protective responses, there may also be genetic differences among individuals that influence innate susceptibility to a particular virus. For example, a particular virus may require for cell entry a cell surface receptor that is polymorphic in human beings (encoded by a gene that has multiple forms or alleles). This virus may be able to use some forms of the polymorphic receptor for entry more efficiently than others, making the cells of some individuals more susceptible than those of others. Because innate susceptibility or resistance to viral disease is influenced by multiple genetic loci of the host, identifying the most important determinants has been difficult even for inbred strains of animals. In some cases, however, one genetic determinant may be dominant. For example, some inbred strains of mice are resistant to infection by mouse hepatitis virus (a coronavirus) because their cells lack the correct form of the cell surface receptor required for viral entry. Also, mice, which are normally resistant to human poliovirus infection, can be rendered susceptible by introducing the gene for the human poliovirus receptor into the cells of the mice (as in transgenic mice).

Certain hereditary defects of humans result in extreme susceptibility to disease caused by a particular virus. One is an X-linked defect that manifests itself when the individual is exposed to EBV. As many as 75% of people with this X-linked defect (Duncan's syndrome) develop fatal lymphoproliferative disease as a result of EBV infection. Another genetic defect results in the condition called epidermodysplasia verruciformis, in which the individual suffers throughout life from multiple, disseminated warts caused by papillomaviruses. Apparently, resistance to the development of warts and ability to resolve the warts are greatly impaired. The genetic mutations responsible for these diseases have not yet been identified, and it is not clear whether the mutations alter innate susceptibility to disease or the ability to induce the appropriate protective responses.

## Host Responses to Viral Infection and Viral Defenses

The severity of viral disease is quite variable in animal or human populations. As indicated above, the consequences of virus infection for the individual may include no clinically evident disease, mild or severe (even fatal) acute disease, or chronic or persistent disease. The outcome depends not only on the viral and host factors discussed in the preceding section but also on the efficacy of various induced host responses to the virus and the ability of the virus to escape the consequences of these responses. The induced host responses include *antigen-independent* protective responses that are triggered by alterations in virus-infected cells, cell injury and stress, etc., and *antigen-specific* immune responses, such as the production of antibodies and cytotoxic T cells. Both types of responses are important in prevention or moderation of disease after virus infection. Their importance is highlighted by the fact that certain of the most successful viral pathogens have evolved mechanisms to either prevent or blunt these protective responses.

## Antigen-Independent Protective Responses

These responses include the production of interferons (IFNs), activation of natural killer (NK) cells, activation of macrophages to produce proinflammatory cytokines such as interleukin 1 (IL-1) and tumor necrosis factor-alpha (TNF-alpha), and activation of complement components. These antigen-independent responses are the earliest line of defense against virus infection, and in an individual without preexisting immunity to a virus, the only line of defense against disease until antigen-specific responses can be mounted.

An IFN was first described in 1957 when Issacs and Lindenmann found that chick chorioallantoic membranes infected with influenza virus or heat-inactivated influenza virus produced a soluble factor capable of protecting other cells from viral infection. Normal cells do not usually produce IFNs but can be induced to do so by various stimuli, including virus infection, double-stranded RNA (often produced in virus-infected cells), and the induction of immune responses. IFNs do not have direct antiviral activity, but induce cells to produce various factors that interfere with viral infection and replication. This induction requires the binding of an IFN to a specific cell surface receptor. Therefore, IFNs are relatively species-specific because they have evolved to recognize receptors expressed on cells of the homologous species. The effects of IFNs are not virus-specific inasmuch as most viruses are susceptible to the antiviral activities induced.

IFNs are a family of proteins encoded by three distinct subfamilies of genes. The multiple forms of IFN-alpha are expressed, principally by leukocytes, as the products of about 15 different nonallelic genes. Different forms of IFN-beta are encoded by at least two nonallelic genes and are expressed principally in fibroblasts. Finally, there appears to be only one genetic locus for IFN-gamma, which is produced by activated T lymphocytes.

The multiple mechanisms by which IFNs exert their antiviral effects have not all been defined. Two of the cell products known to be induced by IFNs could act to inhibit viral protein synthesis, provided double-stranded RNA is present. One of these products is a protein kinase that, when activated by double-stranded RNA, phosphorylates and inactivates a factor required for the initiation of protein synthesis. The other is a synthetase of 2,5-oligoA (an unusual polyadenylic acid); the synthetase is activated by double-stranded RNA to produce 2,5-oligoA, which in turn activates a latent RNase capable of degrading mRNA. Whatever the mode of action of IFNs, their physiologic importance (not necessarily for antiviral activity alone) is underscored by the number of genes encoding the various forms. The importance of antiviral effects of the IFNs is evident from findings that anti-IFN antibodies, capable of neutralizing IFN activity, can greatly increase the severity of viral disease in experimental animals. In addition to interfering with viral replication, the various forms of IFN have a plethora of other activities, including modulation of cell growth and differentiation, enhancement of the expression of histocompatibility antigens (which can potentiate antigen recognition), and enhancement of NK cell activity.

NK cells are large granular cytotoxic lymphoid cells that are distinguishable from other lymphoid cells such as T cells that bear the characteristic CD4 and/or CD8 markers and B cells that bear antibody receptors. When activated by the IFNs produced early in a virus infection, NK cells have the capacity to kill "abnormal" target cells, including virus-infected cells (and tumor cells). It is not clear how the target cells are recognized as abnormal by the NK cells. Recent evidence suggests that down-regulation of class I major histocompatibility (MHC) antigen expression may render cells more sensitive to NK cell cytotoxicity. Many viruses are able to mediate this down-regulation of MHC class I antigen expression, as discussed below. The effect could be to render the virus-infected cells more resistant to killing by antigen-specific cytotoxic T cells but more sensitive to killing by NK cells.

In certain experimental systems, NK cells have been shown to contribute to resistance to viral infection. For example, depletion of NK cells by administration of appropriate antibodies or by the use of beige (mutant) mice, which have impaired NK cell cytolytic activity, increases the susceptibility of mice to infection by murine cytomegalovirus. The clinical importance of NK cells in host defense against viral infections is reflected in the increased frequency and severity of viral infections in patients with selective deficiencies of this cell type.

Cells of the macrophage/monocyte lineage are also activated by virus infection through the action of IFNs and perhaps other products of infected cells in the throes of stress responses. As a result, the macrophages produce proinflammatory cytokines such as IL-1 and TNF-alpha. These cytokines bind to cell surface receptors expressed on a variety of cell types and have multiple effects. Principal activities are chemoattraction and activation of neutrophils and induction of the expression of cell adhesion molecules that enable leukocytes to move from blood vessels into the affected tissues. In addition, IL-1 and TNF-alpha have antiviral activity. Through IFN-like activity or synergy with an IFN, they can render cells nonpermissive for viral replication. Also, TNF can kill infected cells by inducing an apoptotic (cytolytic) response.

The term complement refers to a set of serum proteins that can be activated to engage in a cascade of proteolytic reactions, resulting in the release of anaphylatoxins, chemoattractants for phagocytic cells, and in the assembly of membrane attack complexes that can cause cell lysis or virus neutralization (see Chapter 3). Although complement activation can be triggered by antigen–antibody complexes (principally via the classic pathway of complement activation), there are also antigen-independent mechanisms of activation (via alternative pathways). In ways that are not completely understood, viruses and infected cells can trigger complement activation, even in the absence of antiviral antibodies, resulting in neutralization of virus or in killing of virus-infected cells.

### Antigen-Specific Immune Responses

The immune response to viruses, as to other antigens, results in the production of antibodies, cytotoxic T cells, delayed-type hypersensitivity (DTH) T cells, and so forth. The antibodies can neutralize viral infectivity, either by blocking the adsorption of virus to cells or by blocking the penetration of virus into cells. Antibodies (with the participation of complement or cells that mediate antibody-dependent cell cytotoxicity) and cytotoxic T cells can kill virus-infected cells, thereby limiting the production of progeny virus and the spread of infection. T cells mediating DTH can direct the attack of activated macrophages to virus-infected cells.

Both antibodies and T cells are important effectors of antigen-specific responses against viruses. Circulating antibodies persist longer after vaccination or recovery from disease than do virus-specific T cells and are useful as markers of immunity. In an immune individual, persisting antibodies probably play a key role in limiting the numbers of cells infected by a subsequent exposure to virus and in aborting the spread of infection so that clinical disease does not occur. Persisting antibodies, which can promote the processing of viral antigens for presentation to T cells, probably also aid in boosting immunity through activation of all arms of the antigen-specific response. During primary exposure to a virus and secondary exposures that result in disease, however, the antigen-independent responses described above and the antigen-specific cell-mediated responses may be more important than antibodies in limiting the spread of virus infection and reducing the severity of disease. Containment of virus infection depends in large part on killing virus-infected cells before they can produce progeny virus for dissemination.

During the primary response to an infectious agent, various factors, mostly not yet identified, influence the nature of the cytokine response, which in turn can influence whether the antigen-specific response is shifted toward cell-mediated responses ($T_H1$) or antibody-mediated ($T_H2$) responses (see Chapter 3). One of the key regulatory cytokines is IL-12, which is produced by monocytes, macrophages, neutrophils, dendritic cells, and B cells. IL-12 can activate NK cells and also stimulate helper T cells to shift toward the $T_H1$ or cell-mediated type of response. In this type of response, the T cells are induced to produce INF-gamma and to help other T cells express cytolytic activity. Another cytokine, IL-4, shifts the helper T-cell response toward the $T_H2$ type of response or the production of antibodies. The activities of IL-12 have been shown to be very important for protection from certain helminths and intracellular bacteria and protozoa. These activities of IL-12 (activation of NK cells and promotion of cell-mediated responses and the production of IFN-gamma) are probably also important for infections with most viruses. It has been shown, for example, that low doses of exogenously added IL-12 are very effective in limiting disease caused by murine cytomegalovirus in mice.

The devastating consequences of viral infections in immunocompromised individuals demonstrate the importance of the immune response in the normal virus–host interaction. Interestingly, patients with agammaglobulinemia can respond adequately, if not optimally, to many viral infections, with the exception of enterovirus infections. This is consistent with the ideas presented above, that antibodies are not as important as cell-mediated immunity for the control of many viral diseases (except for those caused by enteroviruses).

The immune response is, to some extent, a double-edged sword in many viral diseases. Some antiviral antibodies may actually enhance the spread of infection. These include antibodies that can bind to virions without neutralizing their infectivity. These antibodies can block the binding of neutralizing antibodies or can facilitate the infection of cells that are devoid of virus receptors but express Fc receptors. In addition, some of the pathology observed in viral infections can be due principally to immune effector mechanisms. This immunopathology may be of negligible consequence or it may be the major cause of distress, particularly in chronic viral diseases. For example, the liver damage associated with hepatitis B virus is due primarily to immune responses to the persistently infected cells. The virus itself may not cause much cytopathology (see Chapter 19).

Another aspect of the interaction between viruses and the immune system is crucial to pathogenicity. A number of viruses can infect cells of the immune system and thus modify the activities of these cells. HIV is the most prominent example. As a consequence of infecting CD4+ T lymphocytes and macrophages, HIV impairs the immune system to the extent that opportunistic infections invariably occur and result in fatal disease (see Chapter 23). EBV induces the proliferation of B lymphocytes, thereby abrogating the normal controls of B-cell function and proliferation. A number of viruses, most notably measles virus, can suppress certain aspects of the immune system, by mechanisms that are not yet understood. This immunosuppression can explain, for example, the association of measles virus infection with the reactivation of tuberculosis.

### Viral Defenses

Viruses have evolved a variety of mechanisms for foiling both the antigen-independent and antigen-specific protective responses of the host. The most interesting and numerous defense activities are associated with products of the larger DNA viruses, probably because these viruses have sufficient genetic material so that a number of genes can be reserved for activities not strictly required for viral replication.

Several different strategies have evolved to protect viruses against IFNs. Adenoviruses and EBV produce large quantities of low-molecular-weight RNAs that interfere with the double-stranded RNA-dependent activation of the IFN-induced protein kinase that can block protein synthesis. Poxviruses and retroviruses encode other products that inhibit the antiviral activity of IFN-alpha and IFN-beta. Poxviruses also express secreted molecules that can serve as receptors for interferon-gamma. These receptor decoys inhibit the action of IFN-gamma by competing with human cell-associated receptors for the binding of IFN. Influenza virus induces a cellular inhibitor of IFNs.

Viral defenses against cytokines rely on receptor decoys, inhibition of proteases required for cytokine processing, inhibition of downstream effects of cytokines, and expression of viral cytokines that can regulate induced responses. Members of the poxvirus family produce at least two different soluble secreted molecules that can act as receptors for IL-1 and TNF-alpha, respectively. When these cytokines are bound to the secreted viral receptor decoys, they are unavailable for binding to receptors on the surfaces of human cells, which is a requirement for their activity. Members of the poxvirus family also produce a protease inhibitor that prevents the cleavage of pro–IL-1 to yield the biologically active cytokine. An important effect of TNF-alpha and perhaps other cytokines is to induce apoptosis of virus-infected cells. Normal uninfected cells are able to produce proteins that counteract the apoptotic signal generated by the binding of TNF-alpha to its receptor whereas, it is thought, virus-infected cells generally cannot produce these protective cell proteins due to redirection of macromolecular synthesis to viral proteins. Some viruses, notably members of the adenovirus, herpesvirus, and poxvirus families, express their own proteins that protect the infected cell from apoptosis. EBV influences cytokine effects by a completely different mechanism. This virus encodes a homologue of IL-10. Like the human version of IL-10, the EBV cytokine inhibits the synthesis of TNF-alpha and IFN-gamma by macrophages and $T_H1$ cells and tends to shift the immune response toward the $T_H2$ type.

Both herpesviruses and poxviruses encode proteins that interfere with complement activation. Herpes simplex virus expresses a glycoprotein that binds C3b and accelerates its decay, thus down-modulating both the classic and alternative pathways of complement activation. Poxviruses and another herpesvirus (*H. saimiri*) encode C4-binding proteins that can block the classic pathway of activation. Herpesviruses also express Fc receptors that can bind the Fc domains of IgG, thereby blocking various effector functions mediated by the Fc region including complement activation.

Several mechanisms have evolved to protect virus-infected cells from killing by cytotoxic T cells, through interference with the presentation of antigen by class I MHC antigens. Adenoviruses can inhibit the transcription of genes for MHC class I heavy chains and also express a glycoprotein that sequesters MHC class I molecules in the endoplasmic reticulum. Murine cytomegalovirus also blocks the transport of peptide-loaded MHC class I molecules out of the endoplasmic reticulum. Human cytomegalovirus encodes a homologue of MHC class I heavy chains that competes with cell heavy chains for interaction with beta$_2$-microglobulin, thus inhibiting assembly of functional antigen-presenting complexes. In addition, herpes simplex virus encodes a protein that binds to the transporter associated with antigen processing, preventing peptide translocation into the endoplasmic reticulum.

Finally, genetic variations resulting in altered antigenic structures of viral proteins can be a powerful defense against the host immune response. Some viruses such as VZV exhibit little antigenic variability. Recovery from primary disease usually confers life-long immunity to superinfection (although reactivation of virus to cause zoster occurs). Other viruses exhibit sufficient antigenic variability such that development of immunity to one antigenic type does not confer immunity to other types. There are many serotypes of rhinovirus circulating simultaneously in human populations, which explains in part why an individual can suffer from rhinovirus colds repeatedly. Influenza virus also exhibits antigenic variation but in a sequential fashion, such that one type replaces another in human populations, as immunity to the earlier type becomes established (see Chapter 12). Replication of HIV is associated with an extremely high mutation rate. In individual patients, new antigenic variants arise that can be resistant to preexisting neutralizing antibodies. Mutations in the viral targets of antiviral drugs (reverse transcriptase, for example) also occur, and some of these mutations can confer resistance to the antiviral drugs.

### Immunity to Viral Disease

Despite the viral defenses against host protective responses, recovery from infection is usually a consequence of developing immunity, and specific immune responses can be exploited to prevent viral disease. Vaccination is an effective means of preventing certain viral diseases despite our ignorance of the particular antigens and effector mechanisms that provide the protection. The diseases for which effective vaccines are currently available are, for the most part, those caused by viruses that are antigenically stable and in which recovery from primary infection is accompanied by the development of long-lasting immunity to disease. In general, the vaccines currently in use are either live attenuated viruses that cause asymptomatic infection or inactivated whole viruses that include most or all viral antigens (see Chapter 40).

There are risks associated with the use of live attenuated or killed whole viral vaccines, including the possibility that the live vaccine virus could induce a latent infection with consequences that might not be evident for many years. In addition, the dominant epitopes for viruses that exhibit antigenic variation are often the most variable epitopes, so that vaccination with the whole virus induces variant-specific, but not cross-reactive, immunity. Given that it is now technically feasible to produce genetically engineered subunit vaccines, considerable attention is being focused on identifying for particular viruses the few antigens and epitopes, among many, that can induce effective cross-reactive immunity. Because T cells as well as B cells must be able to respond to the vaccine and because T cells recognize peptide fragments that can associate with MHC antigens, considerable attention must also be focused on determining how to formulate and administer the vaccine so that the antigens are processed and presented properly to T cells and B cells.

### Viruses and Cancer

Several viruses are probably cofactors in the causation of human cancers, including papillomaviruses, EBV, human T-cell lymphotropic virus (HTLV), and hepatitis B virus (HBV). Establishing a causal role for these viruses in cancer is complicated by the relatively low incidence of cancer compared with incidence of virus infection, the long interval between virus infection and detection of the cancer, and the occasional appearance of similar cancers in the absence of virus infection.

The first three of the viruses mentioned above, and possibly the fourth, share the ability to induce the proliferation of infected cells under certain conditions. Papillomaviruses and EBV can stimulate the proliferation of latently infected cells, whereas productively infected cells are probably killed as a consequence of viral replication. For HTLV, virus-induced proliferation of cells may occur either in productively or latently infected cells. This virus-induced cell proliferation is not synonymous with malignant transformation, but possibly predisposes the dividing cells to mutations caused by carcinogens that act during DNA replication. In any event, the development of one of the cancers associated with these viruses probably depends upon multiple contributory factors, which may usually but not always include virus infection.

Certain of the many serologic types of papillomavirus appear to have a causative role in cancers of the urogenital tract, particularly cervical carcinoma. DNAs of types 16 or 18 are found in most of the cervical carcinomas screened. Expression of viral gene products known to be involved in inducing cell proliferation and immortalization is also regularly detected in the cancer cells.

EBV has been associated with Burkitt's lymphoma and with a nasopharyngeal carcinoma that occurs predominantly in people of Chinese extraction. More is known about the genetic basis for the lymphoma than the carcinoma. A chromosomal translocation that brings the c-*myc* oncogene under the control of the immunoglobulin locus is invariably found in cells of Burkitt's lymphoma. The possibility exists that this chromosomal translocation occurs more readily in B lymphocytes that have been stimulated to divide by EBV gene products, but the translocation and Burkitt's lymphoma can also occur in the absence of EBV infection. The EBV-positive Burkitt's lymphoma cells do not express the EBV proteins required to induce cell division in normal B lymphocytes. This implies that the translocation is the key event in the malignant transformation. Possibly cancer cells that express these EBV proteins are eliminated by the immune system inasmuch as B lymphocytes that express these proteins are highly immunogenic.

EBV can cause fatal lymphoproliferative disease or lymphoma in immunodeficient individuals. In early stages, the proliferating B cells may be polyclonal, suggesting that nonmalignant immortalized B cells may simply be dividing continually, as they would in cell culture, without the usual constraints supplied by the immune system. In the later stages of disease, one or a few clones of proliferating B cells may predominate, suggesting that these clones have acquired mutations conferring a selective advantage for proliferation.

Just as EBV can immortalize B lymphocytes *in vitro*, HTLV-1 can immortalize T lymphocytes *in vitro*. Human infections with HTLV-1 are largely asymptomatic, indicating that the normal immune system can control the proliferation of the HTLV-1 infected cells *in vivo*. A small percentage (about 1%) of infected individuals eventually become ill with the malignant disease called adult T-cell leukemia. A dominant clone of HTLV-1–infected, malignant cells is present in most cases, indicating that the malignant transformation required a genetic event, as yet unidentified, subsequent to HTLV-1 infection.

The evidence that HBV has a role in hepatocellular carcinoma is largely based on epidemiologic studies. The incidence of this type of carcinoma is highest in populations where HBV infection is most prevalent. Integrated hepatitis B virus DNA and viral gene products have been detected in cancer cells. The molecular linkage between HBV infection and the carcinoma is not understood, however.

## SUMMARY

The consequences of virus–host interactions are determined by the multiple kinds of virus–cell interactions that can occur and by the protective host responses provoked by virus infection and the expression of viral antigens. As the molecular details of the virus–cell interactions and the immune responses are revealed, new approaches to preventing and curing viral diseases will also be revealed. This is a time of accelerating progress in this area of medical research.

## CASE HISTORY

### CASE HISTORY 1

A 5-year-old female with a history of acute lymphocytic leukemia presents with low-grade fever, abdominal pain, and jaundice. She has received intravenous gammaglobulin therapy in the past year. Her immunizations, including hepatitis B vaccine, are complete. On physical examination her temperature is 38°C, and the exam is remarkable for scleral icterus and a tender liver palpable 3 cm below the right costal margin. The remainder of the examination is normal. Laboratory tests showed alanine aminotransferase (SGPT) of 240 units/L, aspartate aminotransferase (SGOT) of 350 units/L, and total bilirubin of 5.0 mg/dL. Serologic studies show IgG-HAV–negative, IgM-HAV–negative, HBsAg–negative, anti-HBs–positive, anti-HBc–negative, anti-HBe-negative, and anti-HCV–positive by recombinant immunoblot assays (RIBA).

### CASE 1 Discussion

This is most likely a case of acute hepatitis C infection; the patient's anti-HBs antibody reflects hepatitis B viral vaccination. This patient probably contracted the hepatitis C virus from contaminated intravenous gammaglobulin. In 1994 the Centers for Disease Control received reports on acute HCV infection in recipients of specific lots of an intravenous immunoglobulin product. The product was removed from the market. Since May 1994, the manufacturing process for all immunoglobulin products now includes a solvent-detergent treatment designed to inactivate viruses. These products no longer pose any risk for HCV transmission to recipients. The liver damage associated with HCV infection is primarily a result of the host immune response to the virus, not a direct cytopathic effect of viral infection. Unfortunately, chronic hepatitis develops in more than 60% of persons infected with HCV. This child's liver disease has persisted for more than 6 months and she has entered a study protocol to evaluate the response to alpha-interferon.

## REFERENCES

### Books

Fields, B. N., and Knipe, D. M., eds. *Fields' Virology.* 2nd ed. New York: Raven Press, 1990.

### Reviews

Biron, C. A. Cytokines in the generation of immune responses to, and resolution of, virus infection. *Curr. Opin. Immunol. 6*:530, 1994.

Brutkiewicz, R. R., and Welsh, R. M. Major histocompatibility complex class I antigens and the control of viral infections by natural killer cells. *J. Virol. 69*:3967, 1995.

Dubin, G., Fishman, N. O., Eisenberg, R. J., Cohen, G. H., and Friedman, H. M. The role of herpes simplex virus glycoproteins in immune evasion. *Curr. Top. Microbiol. Immunol. 179*:111, 1992.

Gooding, L. R. Virus proteins that counteract host immune defenses. *Cell 71*:5, 1992.

Gooding, L. R. Regulation of TNF-mediated cell death and inflammation by human adenoviruses. *Infect. Agents Dis. 3*:106, 1994.

Hall, S. S. IL-12 at the crossroads. *Science 268*:1432, 1995.

Pickup, D. J. Poxviral modifiers of cytokine responses to infection. *Infect. Agents Dis. 3*:116, 1994.

Weinberg, R. A. Oncogenes, anti-oncogenes, and the molecular bases of multistep carcinogenesis. *Cancer Res. 49*:3713, 1989.

Weismann, C., and Weber, H. The interferon genes. *Prog. Nucleic Acid Res. Mol. Biol. 33*:251, 1986.

### Primary Publications

Coffin, J. M. HIV population dynamics in vivo: Implications for genetic variation, pathogenesis, and therapy. *Science 267*:483, 1995.

Dalgelish, A. G., Beverly, P. C. L., Clapham, P. R., et al. The CD4 (T4) antigen is an essential component of the receptor for the AIDS retrovirus. *Nature 312*:763, 1985.

Fingeroth, J. D., Weiss, J. J., Tedder, T. F., et al. Epstein-Barr virus receptor of human B lymphocytes is the C3d receptor CR2. *Proc. Natl. Acad. Sci. USA 81*:4510, 1984.

Gregory, C. D., Rowe, M., and Rickinson, A. B. Different Epstein-Barr virus-B cell interactions in phenotypically distinct clones of a Burkitt's lymphoma cell line. *J. Gen. Virol. 71*:1481, 1990.

Hill, A., Jugovic, P., York, I., et al. Herpes simplex virus turns off the TAP to evade host immunity. *Nature 375*:411, 1995.

Issacs, A., and Lindenmann, J. Virus interference: I. The interferon. *Proc. R. Soc. Lond. 147*:258, 1957.

Mendelsohn, C., Wimmer, E., and Racaniello, V. Cellular receptor for poliovirus: Molecular cloning, nucleotide sequence, and expression of a new member of the immunoglobulin superfamily. *Cell 56*:855, 1989.

Schrier, P. I., Bernards, R., Vaessen, R. T. M. J., et al. Expression of class I major histocompatibility antigens switched off by highly oncogenic adenovirus 12 in transformed rat cells. *Nature 305*:771, 1983.

Webster, R. G., Laver, W. G., Air, G. M., et al. Molecular mechanisms of variation in influenza viruses. *Nature 296*:115, 1982.

Weis, W., Brown, J., Cusack, S., et al. Structure of the influenza virus hemagglutinin complexes with its receptor, sialic acid. *Nature 333*:426, 1988.

# 6

# TEMPERATURE REGULATION, THE PATHOGENESIS OF FEVER, AND THE APPROACH TO THE FEBRILE PATIENT

A TODD DAVIS, M.D. and JOHN P. PHAIR, M.D.

Fever, or an elevated body temperature, is the hallmark of infection; however, patients seriously ill with infection can be afebrile or have lower than normal temperature. In addition, there are many causes of fever other than infection. This chapter briefly reviews regulation of body temperature, the pathogenesis of fever, and an approach to the febrile adult and pediatric patient.

## REGULATION OF BODY TEMPERATURE

Body temperature in humans is the net result of heat production by metabolic processes and/or muscle activity and heat loss by conduction, evaporation (sweating), and radiation. The ambient temperature activates compensatory mechanisms leading to a steady-state temperature over a broad range (13°–60°C in dry air for adults). This results in a range of normal adult body temperatures between 36° and 37.3°C. Most individuals have a diurnal rhythm, with the temperature being lowest in the morning hours at the end of sleep and highest in the late afternoon.

Like most other physiologic processes, thermoregulation is developmentally influenced.

For example, the newborn infant has a relatively low metabolic rate and a large surface area–to-mass ratio. In addition, the newborn has relatively little subcutaneous fat, particularly over the head. Accordingly, low heat production, coupled with poor insulation and a large surface area from which to conduct and radiate heat, may explain why a significant minority of infected newborns are either normothermic or hypothermic. Conversely, fever is much more commonly present during infection in 3-month-olds. The typical 3-month-old has developed a thicker layer of subcutaneous fat, has increased the metabolic rate by 50%, and has a somewhat lower surface area–to-mass ratio than a newborn.

The thermoregulatory center is located in the anterior hypothalamus. There are apparently heat-sensitive temperature centers in the preoptic region of the anterior hypothalamus and in the skin. The hypothalamus serves to integrate all the afferent messages from all the temperature centers. If the body temperature is higher than the "set point temperature" in the hypothalamus, the sympathetic centers in the hypothalamus are inhibited. This results in increased blood flow to the skin through dilated blood vessels, the net result increasing the rate of heat transfer eightfold. Sweating will also be initiated, which dissipates heat at ten times the resting metabolic rate.

Conversely, if the thermoregulatory set point is higher than the core body temperature, vasoconstriction occurs by activation of the sympathetic centers in the hypothalamus. Heat production increases by 10–15%, and most importantly, shivering occurs, which increases total body production of heat four to five times over the resting metabolic state.

## FEVER

An elevation of body temperature occurs in a number of physiologic and pathophysiologic settings. As mentioned above, exercise can raise the body temperature. Long-distance runners at the finish of a race can record temperatures of 38°–38.5°C. Heat stroke is a pathologic and dangerous elevation of body temperature that can be the consequence of such exercise and of dehydration due to inadequate fluid intake or to the failure, due to disease or debility, of the heat-dissipation mechanisms in conditions of extremely high ambient temperature. Malignant hyperthermia is a rare hereditary disease occurring in association with general anesthesia. It appears to result from an inappropriate release of calcium from muscles upon exposure to an anesthetic agent and is accompanied by muscle rigidity, rhabdomyolysis, and acidosis. Another uncommon cause of excessive elevation of body temperature (≥41°C) is associated with antipsychotic drugs, such as haloperidol, phenothiazines, and thioxanthenes. This condition, known as neuroleptic malignant syndrome, is characterized by fever, muscular rigidity, autonomic dysfunction, and changes in mental status. This syndrome results from blockage of central dopamine receptors, which leads to uncontrolled muscular contractions in association with peripheral vasoconstriction. Thus, heat is generated that cannot be dissipated.

All of these conditions are instances of elevated body temperature, but not fevers. Fevers are the result of conditions that produce alteration in the thermoregulatory center through the effects of cytokines produced by macrophages.

The majority of fevers, however, are the result of conditions that produce alteration in the thermoregulatory center through the effects of cytokines produced by macrophages.

Beeson in the 1940s performed experiments demonstrating that stimulated phagocytic cells release a factor(s) that produces fevers in rabbits.

It is now established that the cytokines (interleukin-1–beta [IL-1–beta], interleukin-6, tumor necrosis factor-alpha and interferons-beta and -gamma) act independently as endogenous pyrogens. They apparently exert their influence by passing through the fenestrated capillaries in the organum vasculosum. At least part, if not the entire effect, is mediated by the local production of prostaglandin $E_2$. Seemingly, increased concentrations of prostaglandin $E_2$ activate the thermoregulatory cold-sensitive neurons in the preoptic area of the hypothalamus and decrease the firing of warm-sensitive neurons, thereby raising the thermostatic set point.

IL-1 has a wide variety of effects in addition to inducing hypothalamic up-regulation of body temperature (Fig. 6–1). It can stimulate hepatic production of acute-phase reactants such as fibrinogen. Elevated fibrinogen levels are the primary cause of more rapid than normal erythrocyte aggregation and sedimentation, which explains the elevated sedimentation rate seen in patients with infectious or inflammatory diseases. Other serum proteins, such as C-reactive protein, also increase in concentrations. The source of this increased protein production by the liver are amino acids derived from muscle breakdown or proteolysis, which is mediated by IL-1. Low serum iron and serum zinc and elevated serum copper levels also appear to be induced by IL-1 and/or other cytokines released by stimulated or phagocytosing mononuclear cells. Finally,

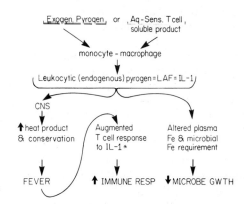

**FIGURE 6–1.** Pathways of endogenous pyrogen production with resulting fever and associated effects on host immune responses and iron metabolism.

leukocytosis, the other characteristic manifestation of infection, occurs as a consequence of release of IL-1 and other cytokines. In addition to mediating these characteristics of inflammation, IL-1 up-regulates the immune system. An elevated body temperature is associated with a more efficient response by thymic-derived lymphocytes (T cells), which play a central role in the induction of the immune response.

With the accumulated understanding of the augmented inflammatory and immune responses associated with fever, the febrile response has been viewed as conferring an advantage to the host. The primary cell defending the host against bacteria, the polymorphonuclear leukocyte, is released from the marrow and is more adherent to endothelial cells, thus enhancing diapedesis into tissue. Some viruses are very temperature-sensitive, surviving and replicating at 37°C, but not at 39°C. Lowered serum iron is thought to provide a less favorable milieu for iron-dependent bacteria. The augmented T-cell function may facilitate the specific immune response to microbial invasion. While the beneficial effect of elevated temperature in infected cold-blooded animals has been amply documented, this has not been demonstrated definitively in individual humans. Lowering the fever associated with influenza, chickenpox, and rhinovirus infections with acetaminophen prolongs viral shedding. Elderly patients with bacteremia who do not mount a fever have a poorer prognosis than similarly aged individuals who develop a febrile response. However, this latter finding may reflect the association of debility, poor prognosis, and failure to respond with the normal inflammatory response, rather than a poorer prognosis because of the muted febrile response.

Furthermore, there is a physiologic cost associated with the febrile response. Heart rate increases, possibly straining a damaged heart. Skeletal muscle proteolysis results in negative nitrogen balance, which persists for prolonged periods following resolution of the fever.

Thus, the balance of the advantageous and deleterious effects of fever are as yet unresolved. There are undoubtedly both positive and negative effects in the individual patient, the overall effect depending upon the balance of the two. Some have argued that the effects of fever on human disease should be viewed from a population perspective rather than from an individual perspective. This argument suggests that in an otherwise productive, intact member of society in his/her productive years, the production of inflammatory cytokines causing fever may be salubrious, whereas in the no-longer-productive senescent individual, the adverse consequences of the inflammatory response with fever may lead to death, thus benefitting those who remain alive. This argument, if valid, would apply more to pre–20th century civilization than to the soon-to-be 21st century.

## Approach to the Febrile Adult

The basic approach to the febrile adult should focus upon establishing the cause of the fever and then instituting appropriate therapy. Treatment of the temperature elevation itself is generally unnecessary except in special situations; for example, the patient who cannot tolerate tachycardia, the child who has seizures, or the elderly patient who becomes disoriented with fever. Salicylates or nonsteroidal antiinflammatory agents are generally quite adequate to control fever, but they have the adverse effects of inhibiting platelet aggregation, thus inhibiting clotting, and producing gastric irritation, erosions, and often bleeding. With extreme temperatures above 40°C, as in patients with heat stroke or malignant hyperthermia, cooling blankets are used to help control fever.

Except for malaria, the pattern of the fever curve provides little information about the etiology of the underlying condition. It has been suggested that fevers secondary to drug hypersensitivity are continuously elevated, whereas those associated with an abscess resemble a picket fence. However, most patients with drug fever demonstrate a diurnal variation in temperature with a return to the normal range in the morning, and many infected patients are constantly febrile.

The diagnosis of the cause of fever in most patients can be established by obtaining a thorough history and performing an adequate physical examination. Basic and necessary laboratory studies include a complete blood count with differential count; examination of the urine; chest x-ray; and culture of appropriate specimens including blood, urine, or sputum. These studies usually suggest whether or not the fever is due to infection or to some other cause.

Fevers that persist without explanation for several weeks despite such an evaluation are termed *fevers of unknown origin* (FUOs). They represent one of the most challenging problems for a diagnostician. In general, FUOs are the result of common diseases presenting in an uncommon manner or uncommon conditions presenting typically (Table 6–1). When approaching a patient with FUO, the physician must devise a diagnostic plan that can distinguish between a disease that is generalized, such as miliary (disseminated) tuberculosis, endocarditis, or noninfectious conditions such as sarcoidosis or neoplastic, lymphoproliferative disease, and a localized process such as an abscess or other occult infection or tumor. The patient's history should be reevaluated, specifically to search for potential exposure to unusual infections. Examples of such exposure include travel to areas of endemic infection, exposure to certain wild animals through hunting, to pets, to drugs, or possible distant exposure to persons with tuberculosis. The physical examination bears repeating on several occasions, emphasizing a search for the changing murmur of endocarditis, the bony tenderness of chronic osteomyelitis, or right upper quadrant tenderness associated with a liver abscess or cryptogenic cholecystitis. Potential exposure to fungal infections, as might occur for individuals who explore caves, work with soil, or who have traveled for the first time to the Ohio/Mississippi Valley or the Southwest, warrants serologic assays for fungal antibody.

Cryptogenic localized infections commonly overlooked include abscessed teeth, pyelonephritis (occasionally), hepatic abscess, or pelvic tuberculosis. A diagnostic procedure that is often useful is examination and culture of the bone marrow in the presence of unexplained neutropenia, anemia, or thrombocytopenia. Specific diseases readily identified by bone marrow culture include disseminated histoplasmosis and other fungal infections, tuberculosis, typhoid, or brucellosis. Com-

puted tomography (CT) and ultrasonography can be extremely helpful in searching for localized infections or tumors. The recent introduction of scans using [111] indium-labeled polymorphonuclear leukocytes can aid in the discovery of localized abscesses. Laparoscopy and peritoneoscopy in persons with pelvic or abdominal symptoms, in combination with the new radiologic techniques, have obviated almost entirely the use of diagnostic laparotomy in the management of FUOs. Finally, there are increasingly useful serologic tests that can screen for and ultimately identify antibodies found in specific collagen vascular diseases, such as systemic lupus erythematosus or mixed connective tissue disease. This group of conditions represents a large proportion of diseases reported in all series of adult patients with unexplained fever.

Other specific laboratory studies that can be useful include seeking polymorphonuclear leukocytes in the stool, which can be the earliest sign of inflammatory bowel disease, especially in patients with atypical abdominal complaints. Abnormalities of the serum concentrations of hepatic enzymes may indicate that a liver biopsy is in order. Histologic examination and culture of liver tissue can be extremely helpful, often diagnosing miliary tuberculosis, sarcoidosis, or granulomatous hepatitis. In the presence of normal liver enzyme levels the yield from liver biopsy is disappointing.

Occult neoplasms are almost as common as occult localized or disseminated infections as a cause of prolonged fever. In addition to non-Hodgkin's and Hodgkin's lymphoma, renal cell carcinoma is a common cause of fever. Therefore, radiologic or ultrasound examination of the kidney is often part of the evaluation of these patients. The availability of CT

## TABLE 6–1. CATEGORIES OF FEVER OF UNKNOWN ORIGIN*

| Diagnostic Categories | Petersdorf & Beeson 1961 Series (n = 100)[†] (%) | Jacoby & Swartz 1973 Series (n = 128) (%) | Larson et al. 1982 Series (n = 105) (%) |
|---|---|---|---|
| Infection | 36 | 40 | 30 |
| Neoplastic disease | 19 | 20 | 31 |
| Connective tissue diseases | 15 | 15 | 9 |
| Granulomatous and miscellaneous diseases | 23 | 15 | 18 |
| Undiagnosed | 7 | 10 | 13 |

*Adapted from Petersdorf, R. G., and Beeson, P. B., *Medicine* 40:1, 1961; Jacoby, G. A., and Swartz, M. N., *N. Engl. J. Med.* 289: 1407, 1973; and Larson, E. B., Featherstone, H. J., and Petersdorf, R. G., *Medicine* 61:269, 1982. With permission.
[†]Number of patients indicated within brackets.

and gallium scans allows for examination of the retroperitoneum and can define enlarged lymph nodes suggesting lymphoproliferative disease.

The evaluation of a patient with an unexplained fever is always easier in the absence of previous antimicrobial therapy. In general, therapeutic trials of antibiotics are not useful in this situation unless there is strong evidence of abacteremic ("culture-negative") endocarditis or occult tuberculosis. Finally, it must be recognized that the most well-organized and thorough evaluation can fail to establish the cause of the fever. Reappraisal at a later time sometimes is successful but, more than occasionally, fever disappears and is never explained or, less happily, the underlying disease is diagnosed only at autopsy.

### The Febrile Child

Fever is not always a presenting sign in children with infections. Neonates (<28 days of age) may be seriously ill with an acute or chronic infection and yet be afebrile. In infants and older children, there is no clear correlation between the height of the fever and the seriousness of the infection. Among neonates, two general classifications of infections occur: congenital or perinatally acquired infections, such as TORCH infections (Table 6–2); and acute bacterial sepsis and meningitis.

## ACUTE CHILDHOOD INFECTIONS

After birth, the neonate's immune system continues to mature slowly, a fact that modifies the presentation and severity of many illnesses compared with that of the older child and adult who have fully intact immune systems. For example, only about 60% of neonates respond with fever during an episode of meningitis or bacterial sepsis. The other 40% are either afebrile or hypothermic. Although irritability and lethargy may be seen in almost all children with bacterial meningitis, systemic symptoms such as respiratory distress, apnea, and jaundice are found uniquely in meningitic neonates as opposed to older children (Table 6–3).

Newborn infants are at particular risk, for a short time, for some viral pathogens. If the mother develops varicella (chickenpox) from 4 days before delivery to 48 h afterward, her child is at particular risk to develop serious and potentially fatal varicella. However, if the mother develops chickenpox more than 5 days before delivery, her offspring is at little risk. The immunologic factors underscoring these phenomena are currently unknown but include transplacental passage of IgG to varicella virus. Some coxsackievirus B or echovirus infections that may be asymptomatic or cause only mild constitutional symptoms in the mother may result in devastating encephalitis and myocarditis (coxsackievirus) or hepatitis (echovirus) in the newborn.

Some viral illnesses during the neonatal period and early infancy present with fever, some irritability or lethargy, but no abnormal physical findings. In those circumstances, the careful physician must simply assure himself or herself that no serious, treatable pyogenic infection is being overlooked. When doubt

TABLE 6–2.   CLINICAL MANIFESTATIONS OF GENERALIZED CONGENITAL (TORCH) INFECTIONS*

|  | RUBELLA | CYTOMEGALOVIRUS | TOXOPLASMOSIS | HERPES SIMPLEX | TREPONEMA PALLIDUM |
|---|---|---|---|---|---|
| Hepatosplenomegaly | + | + | + | + | + |
| Jaundice | + | + | + | + | + |
| Petechiae | + | + | + | + | + |
| Meningoencephalitis | + | + | + | + | + |
| Chorioretinitis | ++ | + | ++ | + | + |
| Microcephaly | − | ++ | + | + | − |
| Hydrocephalus | + | − | ++ | − | − |
| Intracranial calcifications | − | ++ | ++ | − | − |
| Myocarditis | + | − | + | + | − |
| Bone lesions | ++ | − | + | − | ++ |

*From Remington, J. S., and Klein, J. O., eds., *Infectious Diseases of the Fetus and Newborn*. Philadelphia: W. B. Saunders Co., 1995. With permission.
   (−) Absent or rare.
   (+) Occurs regularly in infected infants.
   (++) Somewhat characteristic for a given kind of infection.

**TABLE 6–3.    COMPARISON OF SYMPTOMS IN NEONATES WITH BACTERIAL INFECTIONS AND METABOLIC OR CENTRAL NERVOUS SYSTEM DISORDERS**

| | IRRITABILITY | LETHARGY | POOR FEEDING OR VOMITING | HIGH-PITCHED CRY | TREMORS | CONVULSIONS | CYANOSIS |
|---|---|---|---|---|---|---|---|
| Sepsis | + + | + + | + + | + | + | + | + + |
| Meningitis | + + | + + + | + + + | + + | + | + + | + |
| Hypoglycemia* | + + | + + | + + | + + | + + + | + + | + + |
| Hypocalcemia* | + + | + + | + + | + + | + + + | + + | + |
| CNS abnormalities | + + | + + | + + | + + | + | + + | + |

| | RESPIRATORY DISTRESS | APNEA | JAUNDICE | FEVER |
|---|---|---|---|---|
| Sepsis | + + | + + | + + | + + + |
| Meningitis | + + | + + | + + | + + + |
| Hypoglycemia* | + | + + | + | + |
| Hypocalcemia* | + | + + | + | + |
| CNS abnormalities | + | + | + | + |

*The majority of infants with these conditions are asymptomatic. When symptoms occur, tremulousness is most frequent.
(+) Incidence 0–10%.
(++) Incidence 11–50%.
(+++) Incidence 51–100%.

exists, a broad-spectrum antibiotic should be begun and continued until a variety of cultures are negative.

On the other hand, some viral illnesses are milder in infants than in adults. For example, poliomyelitis occurring early in infancy (defined as <2 years of age) rarely results in permanent paralysis. In populations with poor hygiene and sanitation, contact with the virus early in life, when the risk of paralysis is low, confers life-long immunity. Hepatitis A in children younger than 2 years of age presents either with vague constitutional symptoms or gastrointestinal complaints such as vomiting and diarrhea. Jaundice rarely occurs. By age 5 or 6, jaundice much more frequently accompanies this infection. The changes in the maturing immune system that underlie these varying responses to infection are not well understood.

In the child older than 3 months with sudden onset of fever, the diagnosis is usually evident from the associated symptoms. Thus, those viruses causing upper respiratory infections usually present with cough and/or coryza. Stridor and/or wheezing occasionally occur. In later childhood, the child is able to complain about a sore throat. An erythematous pharynx or exudative tonsillitis points to the diagnosis. Gastrointestinal disease, exanthems with febrile diseases, and enanthems are all readily diagnosed. Urinary tract infections, particularly in young children, do not have any characteristic clinical findings. Indeed, some children with urinary tract infec-

tions present only with fever, while some may have gastrointestinal symptoms as well. Because of the nonspecific nature of the symptoms of urinary tract infections in early childhood, it is important to obtain a urine specimen, particularly in girls, when a source of fever is not readily apparent.

There are a few acute pediatric infectious diseases that present subtly and for which a diagnosis is rarely made unless the possibility of their occurrence is considered. Two important examples of such diseases are retropharyngeal abscess and suppurative pericarditis. Other diseases must be diagnosed rapidly because they are life-threatening or they may cause long-term disability if not treated promptly. Included among these are bacterial meningitis, tuberculous meningitis, herpes encephalitis, epiglottitis, and septic arthritis of the hip.

## FEVER OF UNKNOWN ORIGIN IN CHILDREN

Like adults, children occasionally present with fever of unknown origin. FUO is considered when a fever has been present for 2–3 weeks without any apparent cause. Happily, most of these fevers resolve in time without a diagnosis being established. Nonetheless, a careful search for an etiology is imperative, beginning by considering five large categories of disease entities: infectious diseases, neoplasia, inflammatory bowel disease, rheumatologic conditions, and other entities.

With this conceptual framework, a careful history sometimes points to a diagnosis. Useful clues include recent foreign travel; exposure to psittacine birds (psittacosis); ingestion of imported cheeses (listeriosis, brucellosis); close contacts with someone with a chronic cough (tuberculosis); abdominal pain and diarrhea (inflammatory bowel disease); and fleeting macular rashes with fever, swelling or redness of the joints, or morning stiffness (juvenile rheumatoid arthritis).

If history and physical examination fail to yield a diagnosis, then a number of imaging studies should be undertaken to exclude occult neoplasms or infections. Useful tests include a chest radiograph, bone nuclear scintigraphy, abdominal CT scan, and gallium scintigraphy. If these tests are normal, a bone marrow examination should be considered for histologic review and culture for bacterial and fungal pathogens.

Diagnosing the child with a fever of unknown origin remains one of the most challenging intellectual exercises in medicine despite the increased diagnostic tools now available. The answer, however, usually yields to clinical insight.

## CASE HISTORIES

### CASE HISTORY 1

A 4-day-old infant was born 36 h after the premature rupture of membranes and weighed 2000 g. The child had fed normally until the fourth day of life, when he vomited an early morning feeding. The child was difficult to arouse 4 h later, suckled poorly, and took only a half ounce of formula. Four hours later, when the child was still lethargic and feeding poorly, a physician was summoned. The child was afebrile, but was noted to have somewhat elevated respiratory rate, with slight flaring of the alae nasi and slight retractions of the intercostal spaces; he also appeared "jittery." He suckled poorly and demonstrated no Moro reflex.

### CASE 1 DISCUSSION

Sepsis, hypoglycemia, and hypocalcemia were included in the differential diagnosis. Specimens of blood, cerebrospinal fluid (CSF), and urine were obtained. Blood glucose and calcium were normal. CSF glucose and protein were within normal limits. Only five white blood cells (all monocular) were present in the CSF, all mononuclear, and Gram's stain was negative. Antibiotics were administered empirically because of the progressive nature of the clinical signs and symptoms. However, over the next 48 h, respiratory distress worsened and apnea developed, which necessitated mechanical ventilation. The child continued to be lethargic and irritable, with jaundice and hepatomegaly noted 24 h after the institution of antibiotic treatment. The child died from *Escherichia coli* sepsis 2 days after the institution of antibiotic therapy.

This case illustrates several principles in the care of newborns. First, the presentation of severe illness is often subtle but rapidly progressive. In this child, the first noted abnormality occurred on the fourth day of life. He very likely acquired *E. coli* during passage through the birth canal, with a number of days elapsing for invasion by the bacteria and multiplication in the bloodstream. The onset of the illness was nondescript, vomiting at early morning feeding, 4 h later sucking poorly and being somewhat lethargic. Eight hours after the onset of symptoms, the nurses were convinced that the child was ill and summoned a physician. This 8- to 12-h interval between the first observation of subtle symptoms and the unequivocal evidence of illness is quite common.

The child manifested no signs or symptoms specific to a particular site of infection. Rather, the child showed constitutional symptoms (i.e., an elevated respiratory rate, flaring of the alae nasi, both changes designed to maximize flow of oxygen to his lungs). In addition, he was showing some signs of neurologic disturbance, having an absent Moro reflex.

Sepsis, meningitis, hypoglycemia, hypocalcemia, and a central nervous system hemorrhage all can present with similar signs and symptoms. Therefore, the physician included all of these in the differential diagnosis and appropriate laboratory tests were obtained. The CSF glucose, protein, and cell count were all within normal limits. Accordingly, there was no evidence at that time that the child had meningitis. Although this child never went on to develop meningitis, the initial spinal tap data indicated that there was no evidence of meningitis *at that time*. Occasionally, CSF parameters can be entirely normal very early in the course of meningitis.

Despite the institution of antibiotic therapy and supportive therapy, such as mechanical ventilation, the child had progressive illness. In many respects, septic neonates act as if they have been poisoned metabolically.

Most neonatal *E. coli* infections are caused by a strain with a capsule designated K1. In contrast, children with meningomyelocele who become infected with *E. coli* usually have a non-K1 strain. The K1 capsular strains are much more virulent than non-K1 strains. For example, in one study a number of years ago, approximately one third of all children with K1 *E. coli* infections died, whereas none with non-K1 infections died. This pattern of strain difference within a species is seen repeatedly in clinical medicine.

## CASE HISTORY 2

Mr. and Mrs. Jones both developed hepatitis A within 1 week of each other. While they were perplexed about how they acquired hepatitis A, they assumed they were simply unlucky, since they ate at restaurants quite frequently and speculated that it was their misfortune to have a hepatitic cook contaminate their food. However, when they learned that the parents of Vicky Smith also had hepatitis, they began to wonder. Vicky attended the same day-care center as their child, Trudy. Could there be a connection through their daughter?

The Jones' expressed their concern to the director of the day-care center, who in turn notified the public health authorities.

## CASE 2 DISCUSSION

The public health department sent a young epidemiologist to investigate the possible role of the day-care center in the illness in the adults. The epidemiologist found that 2 months prior to the Jones' illness, a child had been ill with gastroenteritis and was absent for a week. There was no other case of vomiting and diarrhea in the day-care center until 2 weeks later. Over the ensuing 2 weeks, half of the children in the day-care center had been ill, with vomiting and diarrhea for various periods of time, including Trudy Jones and Vicky Smith.

Upon questioning parents of day-care attendees, the epidemiologist found two additional families in which the mothers had developed hepatitis. In both cases, their children were 17 and 18 months of age, respectively, and still in diapers.

Blood specimens were obtained from all children in the day-care center. Eighty percent of those who had a history of gastroenteritis in the preceding 3 months had antibodies to hepatitis A. Conversely, only 10% of those without symptoms had antibodies to hepatitis A. None of the children had ever been noted to be jaundiced. For unknown reasons, jaundice rarely accompanies hepatitis A in children less than 24 months.

With these data in hand, the public health authorities concluded that a case of hepatitis A had been introduced into the nursery. Because all of the children were less than 2 years old and were in diapers, massive contamination in the day-care center led to other children becoming sick and then serving as a reservoir for spread of infection among their parents.

The outbreak was terminated by emphasizing hygienic procedures in the day-care center, and more importantly, by administering immune serum globulin to all children who had not been ill and to the healthy parents of children in the day-care center.

## CASE HISTORY 3

A 38-year-old housewife in previous good health developed fever (as high as 103°F [39.5°C]), frontal headache, intense generalized muscular aching, and an intermittent nonproductive cough on January 4. She took to bed and over the next 5 days slowly improved as her symptoms were treated. On January 9 (the sixth day of illness) she suddenly experienced severe right-sided pleuritic chest pain, sharp rise in fever to 104°F (40°C), marked increase in cough, and increasing breathlessness. A few hours later in the emergency room, she appeared acutely ill, tachypneic, and cyanotic and was noted to be coughing up traces of purulent sputum.

Physical examination revealed a temperature of 103.8°F (39.9°C); pulse, 110/min; blood pressure, 90/60; and respirations, 32/min. The nail beds were dusky; the skin reflected dehydration. Coarse inspiratory rales and impaired resonance were noted over the lower right lateral-posterior chest.

Laboratory data: Hemoglobin, 14.5 g/dL; white blood count, 16,000/mm$^3$ with 82% segmented neutrophils. Urinalysis was within normal limits. Sputum smear showed many polymorphonuclear leukocytes and many gram-positive cocci with occasional gram-positive rods and rare gram-negative coccobacilli. Chest roentgenogram revealed a nondescript density in the right lower lung. Arterial blood gases were $PO_2$ 43 mm Hg, $PCO_2$ 13 mm Hg, and pH 7.48.

## CASE 3 DISCUSSION

The type of initial illness and its occurring in the winter season point to influenza. The abrupt departure from an otherwise uneventful convalescence strongly suggests complicating secondary bacterial pneumonia, namely, preceding respiratory infection, purulent sputum, pleuritic chest pain, and leukocytosis. The sputum smear is consistent with pneumococcal or staphylococcal infection. Staphylococci and pneumococci are among the most common causes of bacterial pneumonia complicating influenza. Nafcillin, a semisynthetic and penicillinase-resistant derivative of penicillin, was administered, since a beta-lactamase (penicillinase) — producing strain of staphylococcus could be present. This particular semisynthetic penicillinase-resistant antimicrobial agent is highly effective against the pneumococcus and against penicillin-resistant as well as penicillin-susceptible staphylococci. Therapy is initiated only after sputum has been collected and cultured and two blood cultures drawn in rapid succession from two separate venipuncture sites have been secured.

During the next 3 days, the patient showed gradual clinical improvement, even though there was an increase in the right lung infiltrate based on physical findings and chest roentgenograms. Sputum culture revealed a heavy growth of *Staphylococcus aureus*, resistant to penicillin. Blood cultures were sterile. Serologic tests using paired sera showed a greater than fourfold antibody rise against influenza virus, "Asian" A2 strain. On the fourth hospital day, defervescence occurred, with improvement in the chest physical examination.

## CASE HISTORY 4

A 46-year-old female with a diagnosis of systemic lupus erythematosus established 6 months previously entered the hospital on February 15, with a 3-day history of shaking chills and fever spiking to 105°F (41°C) in association with attempts to decrease her daily prednisone dose from 60 to 20 mg/day. She appeared chronically ill and was weak and anorexic.

Physical examination revealed a temperature of 102°F (38.8°C); pulse, 100/min; blood pressure, 110/70; and respirations, 28/min. The patient had pale mucous membranes, a scaly erythematous maculopapular rash over both cheeks and the bridge of her nose, and patchy bitemporal alopecia. The remainder of the examination was within normal limits.

Laboratory data: hemoglobin, .10.5 g/dL; leukocyte count, 4700/mm³ with normal differential. Urinalysis revealed 2+ proteinuria and a normal sediment. One of four blood cultures taken during the first 2 days of hospitalization was reported positive for a gram-positive coccus, tentatively identified as *Staphylococcus epidermidis*. Urine cultures were negative. Chest roentgenogram was within normal limits.

On the third hospital day, the patient's temperature approached 105°F (41°C) and she showed signs of clinical deterioration.

## CASE 4 DISCUSSION

This patient was known to have a primary disease, systemic lupus erythematosus, associated with defective immunity. This fact, plus her corticosteroid therapy, should alert the physician to an increased likelihood of infection. There is no evidence of an infectious process to explain the single blood culture yielding a common microorganism constituting part of the normal flora of the skin. Therefore, the isolated microorganism is considered a contaminant. For these reasons, no antimicrobial therapy is prescribed, even though a strong plea to "cover the patient" with an antimicrobial agent was made by the house staff. The patient's prednisone dosage was increased on the premise that the fever and chills were due to increased activity of the autoimmune disease process in the face of decreased prednisone therapy.

The patient became afebrile, and marked clinical improvement occurred after the daily dose of prednisone was increased to 60 mg for 3 days. Two additional blood cultures taken during this period were sterile.

Another reason for withholding antimicrobial therapy in this patient is the propensity for antimicrobial drugs to alter the normal bacterial flora of the host. In an already debilitated host receiving an antiinflammatory drug such as prednisone, microbial "opportunists" may induce serious pneumonia or invade the bloodstream to cause systemic infection involving many different organ systems; that is, life-threatening "superinfections." The occurrence of superinfection is an important reason for not prescribing antimicrobial therapy unless clear evidence exists for doing so.

# REFERENCES

### Books

Feigin, R. D., and Cherry, J. D. *Textbook of Pediatric Infectious Diseases.* Vols. I and II. 3rd ed. Philadelphia: W. B. Saunders Co., 1992.

Remington, J. S., and Klein, J. O. *Infectious Diseases of the Fetus and Newborn Infant.* 4th ed. Philadelphia: W. B. Saunders Co., 1995.

Stiehm, E. R. *Immunologic Disorders in Infants and Children.* 4th ed. Philadelphia: W. B. Saunders Co., 1995.

### Review Articles

Jaffe, D., and Davis, A. T. The febrile child. In: Schwartz, M. W., Charney, E. B., Curry, T. A., and Ludwig, S., eds. *Principles and Practice of Clinical Pediatrics.* Chicago: Year Book Medical Publications, Inc., 1987:394.

Kasper, D. L. Bacterial capsule—old dogmas and new tricks. *J. Infect. Dis.* 153:407, 1986.

Mackowiak, P. A. Fever: Blessing or curse? A unifying hypothesis. *Ann. Intern. Med.* 120(12):1037–1040, 1994.

Moltz, H. Fever: Causes and consequences. *Neurosci. Biobehav. Rev.* 17(3):237–269, 1993.

Saper, C. B., and Breder, D. C. The neurologic basis of fever. *N. Engl. J. Med.* 330(26):1880–1886, 1994.

Schmidt, K. D., and Chan, C. W. Thermoregulation and fever in normal persons and in those with spinal cord injuries. *Mayo Clin. Proc.* 67:469–475, 1992.

Wilson, C. B., Penix, L., Weaver, W. M., et al. Ontogeny of T lymphocyte function in the neonate. *Am. J. Reprod. Immunol.* 28(3–4):132–135, 1992.

### Original Articles

Albrecht, P., Ennis, F. A., Saltzman, E. J., et al. Persistence of maternal antibody in infants beyond 12 months: Mechanism of measles vaccine failure. *J. Pediatr.* 91:715, 1977.

Allsop, P., and Twigley, A. J. The neuroleptic malignant syndrome. Case report with a review of the literature. *Anesthesia* 42:49, 1987.

Atkins, E., and Bodel, P. Clinical fever: Its history, manifestations and pathogenesis. *Fed. Proc.* 38:57, 1979.

Azaz, Y., Fleming, P. J., Levine, M., et al. The relationship between environmental temperature, metabolic rate, sleep rate, and evaporative water loss in infants from birth to three months. *Pediatr. Res.* 32(4):417–423, 1992.

Bodel, P. Spontaneous pyrogen production by mouse histiocytic and myelomonocytic tumor cell lines in vitro. *J. Exp. Med.* 147:1503, 1978.

Cluff, L. E., and Johnson, J. E., III. Drug fever. *Prog. Allergy* 8:149, 1964.

Corey, L., Stone, E. F., Whitley, R. J., et al. Difference between herpes simplex virus type 1 and type 2 neonatal encephalitis in neurological outcome. *Lancet 1*: 1, 1988.

Cornblath, M., Joassin, G., Weisskopf, B., et al. Hypoglycemia in the newborn. *Pediatr. Clin. North Am. 13*:905, 1966.

Dinarello, C. A., Cannon, G. G., Wolff, S. M., et al. Tumor necrosis factor (cachectin) is an endogenous pyrogen and induces production of interleukin-1. *J. Exp. Med. 163*:1433, 1986.

Horstmann, D. M. Poliomyelitis—severity and type of disease in different age groups. *Ann. N. Y. Acad. Sci. 61*:946, 1955.

Miller, E., Cradock-Watson, J. E., and Ridehalgh, M. K. S. Outcome in newborn babies given anti–varicella-zoster immunoglobulin after perinatal maternal infection with varicella-zoster virus. *Lancet 2*:371, 1989.

Musher, D. M., Fainstein, V., Young, E. J., et al. Fever patterns: Their lack of clinical significance. *Arch. Intern. Med. 139*:1225, 1979.

Petersdorf, R. G. Fever of unknown origin. *Ann. Intern. Med. 70*:864, 1969.

Roberton, N. R. C., and Smith, M. A. Early neonatal hypocalcemia. *Arch. Dis. Child. 50*:604, 1975.

# II  UPPER RESPIRATORY TRACT INFECTION AND SEQUELAE

## 7

# BACTERIAL INFECTIONS OF THE UPPER RESPIRATORY TRACT

STANFORD T. SHULMAN, M.D.

Upper respiratory tract infections (URIs) are among the leading reasons people of all ages in the United States seek medical attention. URIs account for considerable morbidity and have very substantial economic consequences for society. Several years ago it was estimated that more than 27 million office visits occur annually in the United States for sore throat complaints, and innumerable days are lost from school and work as a result of these infections. In certain circumstances,

URIs have potentially life-threatening consequences (e.g., streptococcal pharyngitis and acute rheumatic fever), and some URIs are themselves life-threatening (e.g., diphtheria).

Infections of the upper respiratory tract include acute inflammatory processes involving the nose, paranasal sinuses, middle ear cavity, the oropharynx and tonsils, peritonsillar or retropharyngeal tissues, and the laryngeal–epiglottic region. Many URIs involve overlapping anatomic regions. However, it is impor-

## TABLE 7–1. SIMPLIFIED STREPTOCOCCAL CLASSIFICATION SCHEME AND ASSOCIATED CLINICAL CONDITIONS

BETA-HEMOLYTIC STREPTOCOCI (COMPLETE HEMOLYSIS)

　　Group A (*S. pyogenes*): streptococcal pharyngitis, impetigo, toxic shock-like syndrome, invasive infections; acute rheumatic fever, acute glomerulonephritis (see text)

　　Group B (*S. agalactiae*): neonatal and peripartum infections (see Chapter 26)

　　Group C (*S. equisimilis* and four others): pyogenic infections, probably pharyngitis

　　Group G: probably pharyngitis

ALPHA-HEMOLYTIC STREPTOCOCI (INCOMPLETE HEMOLYSIS)

　　*S. pneumoniae* (pneumococcus): pyogenic infections including pneumonia, meningitis, septicemia (see Chapter 11)

　　Viridans streptococci (*S. mutans* and many others): endocarditis, dental caries, dental infections (see Chapters 9 and 33)

GAMMA-HEMOLYTIC STREPTOCOCI (NO HEMOLYSIS)

　　Anaerobic and microaerophilic streptococci(Peptostreptococcus): brain, liver abscesses

　　Group D streptococci*

　　　　Enterococci (*Enterococcus faecalis, E. faecium, E. durans*): endocarditis, urinary infections (see Chapters 15 and 33)

　　　　Nonenterococci (*S. bovis, S. equinus*): endocarditis

---

*Enterococcal strains are occasionally alpha- or even beta-hemolytic, and some nonenterococcal group D organisms may be alpha-hemolytic. Hemolysis here refers to hemolysis of sheep RBC in agar.

---

tant that physicians identify the primary sites of pathology in order to conclude accurately which are the most likely etiologic agents. There may be therapeutic implications to identifying the site of infection; for example, inflammation of the epiglottis (epiglottitis) in a child is virtually always due to *Haemophilus influenzae* type b, and laryngotracheobronchitis is almost always viral in etiology.

Considerable misinformation exists regarding infections of the upper respiratory tract, resulting in several important practical problems: (1) the large majority of URIs are viral in origin and do not respond to antibiotic therapy—a fact that is frequently ignored, resulting in many patients receiving unnecessary and costly treatment with antibiotics; (2) it is often forgotten that "strep throat," acute pharyngitis/tonsillitis caused by group A streptococci (*S. pyogenes*), is the most important upper respiratory infection and should be treated with appropriate antibiotics to prevent its complications; and (3) physicians often overlook the fact that it is impossible to differentiate reliably between viral and strep-

tococcal pharyngitis/tonsillitis on clinical grounds alone. Accurate differentiation requires a simple diagnostic test, such as a throat culture or a rapid antigen detection test, in order to avoid unnecessary overtreatment with antibiotics of the majority who have nonstreptococcal disease.

A simplified classification schema for clinically important streptococci (Table 7–1) is based primarily upon their typical hemolytic activity on sheep blood agar and upon the antigenic reactions of their cell-wall carbohydrates, as developed by Lancefield (see below).

## ANATOMY OF THE UPPER RESPIRATORY TRACT

Consideration of the anatomy of the upper respiratory tract leads to appreciation for the highly organized and extensive lymphoid structures of the region and their intimate relationship with the oral, nasal, and pharyngeal cavities. The great German anatomist, Wilhelm Waldeyer (1836–1921), described what is now known as *Waldeyer's ring*, the circular band of lymphoid tissue that guards the entrance to the respiratory and gastrointestinal tracts. Anteriorly, this ring is composed of submucosal lymphoid tissues of the posterior part of the tongue; laterally, of the palatine tonsils, peritonsillar lymphatics, and adenoids adjacent to the pharyngeal orifices of the eustachian tubes; and posteriorly, of the submucosal lymphoid tissue of the posterior pharyngeal wall. Additionally, the ring has a rich network of lymphatics and regional cervical lymph nodes. These lymphoid structures often react to infection in proximate regions (hyperplasia, hypertrophy), generally contributing to control of the infection but occasionally resulting in symptoms. An example of such a symptom is the swollen, tender anterior cervical nodes most typically associated with acute streptococcal pharyngitis.

Anatomically, the upper respiratory tract may be envisioned as a passageway from the lips and nose to the trachea and bronchi, with a number of mucosally lined, narrow side passages that lead to somewhat larger mucosally lined cavities that are normally filled with air. These cavities (the middle ear, mastoid antrum and air cells, and paranasal sinuses) normally communicate with the oropharynx and nasopharynx. Obstruction of connecting passages, such as the eustachian tube or sinus ostia, contributes significantly to development of infection within these cavities. The intimate relationship among various lymphoid tissues, the mucosal surface, and the orifices of the communicating structures is remarkable and contributes to disease manifestations.

## Normal Flora

The mucosal surfaces of the nose, mouth, and the remainder of the upper respiratory tract are normally colonized by a complex variety of bacterial species. The fascinating situation that exists in the oral cavity is outlined in Chapter 2. Under normal circumstances, the middle ear cavity and the paranasal sinuses are sterile. The pharynx, larynx, and trachea are colonized by anaerobic cocci and bacilli, as well as by aerobes, including *Streptococcus pneumoniae*, alpha-hemolytic streptococci, *Haemophilus influenzae*, neisseria, and coagulase-negative staphylococci. The character of the organisms that normally colonize these mucosae is important when examining and understanding organisms isolated in cultures of these sites, including bronchoscopic specimens, from ill individuals.

The normal flora appear to confer a certain degree of protection against infectious diseases originating at the mucosal surface. This protection manifests itself by providing *nonspecific* stimulation of the immune system, by providing *specific* immunization that leads to protection against pathogens with cross-reactive antigens, and by hampering colonization by other organisms through complex competitive mechanisms (collectively termed *bacterial interference*, or colonization resistance). The importance of the normal flora is readily apparent from studies of germ-free animals, which show deficient development of the immune system and excessive susceptibility to overwhelming infection.

Normal flora demonstrate a remarkable tropism for specific locations (e.g., the regions of the mouth). Certain species of alpha-hemolytic streptococci characteristically colonize the anterior portion of the tongue, whereas other viridans species typically colonize the posterior portion, the gingivae, or the buccal mucosa. The precise determinants for these characteristic niches in the complex ecology of the oral cavity, for example, remain poorly defined but must depend at least in part upon specific mucosal receptors and binding molecules on the surface of microbes and epithelial surfaces.

## PHARYNGITIS/TONSILLITIS

The most important bacterial cause of pharyngitis and tonsillitis is group A beta-hemolytic streptococci (*S. pyogenes*). The importance of this agent is due to its extreme frequency as a cause of pharyngotonsillar infection (with a great deal of associated morbidity), to its relatively infrequent complicating purulent infections (e.g., cervical lymphadenitis, sinusitis), and to its very important nonpurulent sequelae (acute rheumatic fever and acute glomerulonephritis) (Table 7–2). Because acute rheumatic fever and resultant rheumatic heart disease are major illnesses that are, for the most part, preventable by prompt diagnosis and treatment of acute streptococcal pharyngitis, clinical strategies for treating patients with acute pharyngitis focus on streptococcal pharyngitis in particular. In addition, invasive infections with *S. pyogenes* with severe features including necrotizing fasciitis or streptococcal toxic shock–like syndrome, have highlighted the importance of this agent.

In 1868, Theodor Billroth coined the term *streptococcus* from the Greek (*streptos* = chain, *kokkos* = berry) for chain-forming cocci isolated from infected wounds. Ferdinand Widal in 1889 considered streptococci from all clinical sources to belong to a single species, *S. pyogenes*, and to be the primary cause of "septic sore throat" as well as of other illnesses. By 1923, A. R. Felty and A. B. Hodges had established sporadic acute pharyngitis as a specific entity related to beta-hemolytic streptococci.

## Group A Streptococci

These organisms, all now classified as *S. pyogenes*, are characterized by the presence of a specific cell-wall carbohydrate, A carbohydrate, first defined serologically by Rebecca Lancefield around 1930 (see Table 7–1). The Lancefield serogrouping scheme distinguishes streptococcal groups on the basis of cell-wall carbohydrate antigenicity. Within group A streptococci, different cell-wall protein antigens (termed M, T, and R proteins) allow distinction of more than 80 serotypes. Although the group-specific cell-wall carbohydrate does not appear to be a virulence factor, M proteins are important determinants of virulence because of their antiphagocytic properties. M proteins stimulate the development of long-lasting opsonic type-specific antibody, which then overcomes the antiphago-

**TABLE 7–2. BIOLOGIC DIFFERENCES BETWEEN POSTSTREPTOCOCCAL GLOMERULONEPHRITIS AND RHEUMATIC FEVER**

| BIOLOGIC FEATURE | ACUTE GLOMERULONEPHRITIS | ACUTE RHEUMATIC FEVER |
| --- | --- | --- |
| Preceding infection | Pharyngeal or skin | Pharyngeal only |
| Geographic distribution | Uniform, more in tropics | More in developing countries |
| Age | Any age | Rare <4 yr, >30 yr |
| Sex incidence | Males predominate | Equal |
| Attack rate after streptococcal infection | Variable (to 28%) | Constant; pharyngeal strains only |
| Second attacks | Rare; may occur after skin infections | Common; prevent with prophylaxis |
| Average latent period between infection and first attack | Pharyngeal: 10 days Skin; 3 weeks | 18 days |
| Latent period between infection and later attack | Shortened as compared with first attack | Same as latent period of first attack |
| Relation of degree of ASO* increase to incidence of first attacks | No relation | Incidence proportional to degree of ASO increase |
| Serum complement and C3 levels | Decreased | Increased |
| M types of initiating group A hemolytic streptococcus | Pharyngeal: 1, 2, 3, 4, 12, 15 Skin: 49, 52, 55, 59, 60, 61 | Any pharyngeal type, particularly 1, 3, 5, 6, 18. Skin strains are *not* rheumatogenic |

*Antistreptolysin O titer.

cytic effect of a specific M protein, leading to protection against strains that express that M protein (but not most other M proteins).

### Growth

Group A streptococci grow optimally at 34°–37°C and have complex nutritional requirements. Media containing brain and heart extracts, peptone, and glucose are most often utilized, frequently supplemented with whole blood. Solid media usually employ sheep blood for optimal growth and for visualization of the characteristic beta, or complete, hemolysis adjacent to areas of bacterial growth. *S. pyogenes* is homofermentative, producing mainly L-lactic acid from glucose, and is catalase-negative. The organisms are nonmotile and are facultative, growing well under aerobic and anaerobic conditions.

### Identification

Group A streptococci grow readily on standard laboratory media, forming discrete pinpoint colonies. On sheep blood agar they usually produce a large zone of beta (clear) hemolysis around each colony. Group A streptococcus (GAS) hemolytic activity relates to the extracellular elaboration of two hemolysins, typically an oxygen-labile immunogenic protein, streptolysin O; and an oxygen-stable, nonimmunogenic protein, streptolysin S. He-

molysis on the surface of a blood agar plate is due primarily to streptolysin S, whereas subsurface hemolysis is due to streptolysin S and streptolysin O. Antibody responses to streptolysin O are important clinically (see below). Gram's stains show gram-positive cocci in short-to-medium chains, and group A may be differentiated from other streptococci by several methods, based generally on demonstrating the presence of cell-wall A carbohydrate. These methods include agglutination of latex particles coated with anti–A carbohydrate antibody, reaction of acid-extracted or enzymatically extracted cell-wall carbohydrate with specific antisera in a capillary precipitin test, or counterimmunoelectrophoresis (CIE). A frequently employed presumptive test for group A streptococci is the determination of sensitivity to the antibiotic bacitracin, to which about 95% of group A organisms (but only 5–10% of beta streptococci of other groups) are sensitive. Bacitracin impairs peptidoglycan synthesis and alters the membrane permeability of GAS.

### Morphology

These gram-positive cocci are approximately 0.8 $\mu$m in diameter and grow in chains, particularly in purulent exudates. The organisms are composed of an outer capsule, a complex cell wall with attached fimbriae, a cytoplasmic membrane, a nucleus, ribosomes, and cytoplasmic granules (Fig. 7–1). The capsule, composed of hyaluronic acid, polymerized glucuronic acid, and N-acetylglucosamine, is more apparent early in growth; the later production of hyaluronidase removes the capsule. Infected individuals frequently respond with antihyaluronidase antibodies following GAS infection. The capsule may play an antiphagocytic role. The fimbriae that project from the cell wall are composed, in part, of the M, T, and R proteins. The cell wall is a rigid structure that maintains the shape and osmotic integrity of the cell but is permeable to nutrients. Enzymatic degradation of the cell wall leads to osmotic lysis of the streptococcal cell unless it is maintained in a hyperosmolar environment. Streptococcal cell-wall structure is complex, composed of a peptidoglycan; intercalated A carbohydrate (a polymer of rhamnose and terminal N-acetylglucosamine residues); lipoteichoic acid (LTA); and the M, T, and R proteins. The proteins, carbohydrate, and lipoteichoic acid extend outward to form the fimbriae. Enzymes located at or adjacent to the cell membrane at the base of the cell wall are responsible for synthesis of the cell-wall components and are the penicillin-binding proteins.

The M proteins are among the most important components of GAS organisms because they are key virulence factors. Their antiphagocytic activity relates primarily to their ability to block alternative complement pathway activation. In experimental animals, increased quantity of M protein correlates with enhanced virulence, whereas anti-M protein is protective against GAS organisms of the homologous M type. Infection in man leads to the production of anti-M antibody, which is protective and long-lived. Subsequent GAS infections may occur but only with organisms that possess different M proteins. The structure of a number of M proteins has been characterized very thoroughly and homologies to mammalian myosin have been found. Peptide sequences from conserved domains of several M proteins are under evaluation as possible vaccines. T proteins are trypsin-resistant antigens generally associated with specific M proteins. Like M proteins, T proteins are useful in serologically typing organisms—for epidemiologic purposes, for example. However, T proteins appear to be unrelated to virulence, and antibody to T protein is not protective. Similarly, the R proteins, which share some sequence homology with M proteins, are unrelated to virulence or to protection. Another group of GAS surface structures are the serum opacity reaction (SOR) proteins, which possess lipoproteinase activity. These proteins correlate closely with M types and are utilized for typing purposes and for epidemiologic studies. In addition, certain surface proteins of GAS that nonspecifically bind the Fc end of immunoglobulin molecules have been recognized. LTAs, which are phosphate-diesterglycerol compounds found in many grampositive bacterial cell walls, are covalently bound to cell-membrane lipids. In streptococci, LTA extends to the cell surface and serves as the major ligand for attachment of

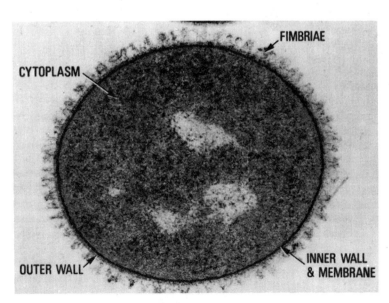

**FIGURE 7–1.** Cross-section of a group A streptococcus cell, type 23. Filamentous fimbriae are attached to the opaque outer cell wall. The inner wall is electron-dense. The thin protoplast membrane is forced against the inner surface of the wall by the internal osmotic pressure of the cell and is not clearly visible. In several places, a separation between the wall and membrane may be seen ($\times$ 126,500). (Courtesy of Dr. Roger Cole, National Institute of Allergy and Infectious Diseases, National Institutes of Health.)

GAS to epithelial cell surfaces. LTA also functions in cation exchange reactions. The GAS cell-wall peptidoglycan is a rigid cross-linked polymer of N-acetylglucosamine—an N-acetylmuramic acid covalently bound to peptide bridges. Peptidoglycan is immunogenic, but its role in virulence and immunity is poorly defined. Peptidoglycan also possesses potent adjuvant, pyrogenic, and mitogenic activity. Interference with peptidoglycan synthesis is the major mechanism by which penicillins are bactericidal for GAS, which are universally sensitive to penicillin activity. The cell membrane of GAS is 60–70% protein and the remainder is composed of phosphatidyl lipids. The membrane serves as a permeability barrier and is rich in enzyme systems with synthetic and oxidative functions.

A variety of bacteriophages are commonly present within GAS, and it has become apparent that they encode for a number of extracellular products including erythrogenic (or pyrogenic) exotoxins A, B, and C, and streptolysin S, as well as antibiotic resistance. Erythrogenic toxin A is most likely responsible for the classic skin rash of scarlet fever and is encoded by a temperate phage.

Reports of severe GAS infections caused by strains that elaborate erythrogenic exotoxin A, a toxin that has otherwise been rarely observed in strains of GAS isolated in recent years, have generated considerable interest. Clinically, these illnesses resemble toxic shock syndrome, and it is noteworthy that streptococcal exotoxin A is similar in many respects to staphylococcal TSST-1, the mediator of toxic shock syndrome. GAS also produces several bacteriocins, small proteins of approximately 8000 d that kill a variety of other bacterial species and thus may be important in initiation or persistence of mucosal colonization or infection by GAS.

### Extracellular Products

In addition to the previously mentioned hemolysins (streptolysins O and S), GAS elaborates a wide variety of extracellular substances, most with enzymatic activity not toxic to mammalian or bacterial cells. These include hyaluronidase, which may facilitate tissue invasion by GAS; desoxyribonucleases A, B, C, and D, which are immunologically distinct and two of which possess RNAse activity as well; streptokinases, which activate the plasmin–plasminogen fibrinolytic system; nicotinamide adenine dinucleotidase (NADase); and others. The phage-related erythrogenic toxins noted above are pyrogenic, they enhance endotoxic shock, and they are neutralized by specific antibody. The latter is the basis of the classic Dick test to demonstrate the presence or absence of immunity to scarlet fever. A C5a peptidase that cleaves and inactivates the chemotactic complement activation product C5a is produced by GAS and has been shown to delay accumulation of polymorphonuclear neutrophils (PMNs) at foci of streptococcal infection.

### Clinical Features of Streptococcal Pharyngitis/Tonsillitis

Streptococcal pharyngitis/tonsillitis is an exceptionally common clinical condition. Of the estimated more than 27 million visits to physicians each year in the United States for sore throat complaints, only approximately 15–20% represent GAS pharyngitis/tonsillitis, but this amounts to a very substantial number of cases. Most importantly, streptococcal pharyngitis/tonsillitis is the only common cause of pharyngitis that warrants antibiotic therapy because untreated GAS infection can lead to the development of acute rheumatic fever and chronic rheumatic heart disease.

Streptococcal pharyngitis is most typically an acute infection of school-aged children, although it may occur at any age. These patients manifest the relatively sudden onset of sore throat, fever, dysphagia, and tender anterior cervical lymph nodes. Rhinorrhea, cough, coryza, and hoarseness are absent. Examination reveals tonsillopharyngeal erythema, frequently with whitish exudates composed of fibrin, bacteria, white blood cells, and debris; petechiae may be present on the soft palate, and tender anterior cervical adenitis is characteristic. Younger children with streptococcal infection typically manifest coryza, excoriated nares, general adenopathy, and a more chronic course. In contrast, in older children and young adults, abdominal pain and headache are frequently prominent symptoms, and tonsillopharyngeal exudates are more constant. *Scarlet fever* is a GAS pharyngeal infection with an accompanying erythematous rash; it reflects an acute streptococcal infection caused by a lysogenized strain of GAS (i.e., one that carries a phage encoding for the toxin causing the rash).

Unfortunately, the clinical features of streptococcal infection are quite variable and overlap with the signs and symptoms of other forms of pharyngitis. Thus, clinical assessment must be supplemented by laboratory testing to obtain an accurate diagnosis—either throat culture or rapid GAS antigen detection test (see below).

The primary importance of accurately identifying and promptly treating acute streptococcal pharyngitis is that untreated or inadequately treated patients are particularly likely to develop acute rheumatic fever (see below).

### Epidemiologic Features

Streptococcal pharyngitis occurs primarily in endemic form; that is, sporadic cases, rather than in the epidemics prevalent prior to World War II in the United States. Foodborne epidemics or outbreaks in military populations are occasionally encountered, but streptococcal pharyngitis is most often endemic. Although it was once thought that streptococcal pharyngitis and acute rheumatic fever were diseases primarily of temperate climes, it is now apparent that they are worldwide in distribution. It has been suggested that urbanization of developing tropical countries has contributed to increases in acute rheumatic fever. The striking seasonality of acute streptococcal pharyngitis has been documented, particularly in temperate regions. Late winter and early spring peaks (January–April) with summer nadirs (July–August) are highly typical. Factors contributing to this cycle include the increased contact between children once they reach school age and the possible effect of intercurrent viral respiratory pathogens upon microbial flora–epithelial cell relationships and upon host immunologic factors. Age is also an important epidemiologic characteristic of streptococcal pharyngitis. Children between 5 and 10 years old experience the highest rates of infection; substantially lower frequencies occur in children 3 years old and younger and in those over 10 years old. Some researchers have observed a secondary peak at approximately 12 years of age and at 18–20 years (related to military recruits). The role of tonsillectomy in preventing streptococcal pharyngitis is controversial, with conflicting data in the literature. In general, removal of the tonsillar lymphoid tissue is not warranted on the basis of frequent episodes of streptococcal pharyngitis alone.

GAS organisms are transmitted primarily by direct contact with large droplets or respiratory secretions rather than by air-borne spread or contamination of inanimate objects (fomites). Thus, spread within family groups or classrooms is common. Contagiousness ap-

pears maximal during the acute stage of illness and during the first 2 weeks after acquisition of the organism. Antibiotic therapy with an appropriate agent, especially penicillin, is associated with prompt suppression of contagiousness; children can therefore return to school after 24 h of therapy. Individuals who are chronically colonized in the pharynx with GAS (streptococcal carriers) pose little transmission risk. Spread of GAS infection and the frequency of poststreptococcal complications are clearly facilitated by crowded living conditions.

### Diagnosis

The following is a profile of the classic patient with acute streptococcal pharyngitis: a 5- to 10-year-old child with sudden onset of fever, sore throat, and perhaps headache, nausea, malaise, and abdominal pain, whose examination shows moderate to severe tonsillopharyngeal erythema, tonsillar hypertrophy and exudates, palatal petechiae, and hypertrophied tongue papillae, with tender and enlarged anterior cervical nodes. When this classic picture is present, the clinician can expect a high degree of diagnostic precision based on clinical criteria alone. Unfortunately, however, most patients with acute streptococcal pharyngitis do not manifest this picture, but rather present with only some of these typical signs and symptoms. Thus, the clinician must rely upon laboratory studies for accurate diagnosis. This conclusion is confirmed by experience with scoring systems that attempt to differentiate those infected with GAS from those not infected. These systems ascribe point values to epidemiologic features (age, season), symptoms (sore throat, headache, absence of cough), signs (abnormal pharynx or cervical nodes, fever), and laboratory findings (leukocytosis). Even the best such scoring system is unable to predict the presence or absence of GAS with sufficient accuracy to eliminate the need for adjunctive laboratory tests. However, it is possible to identify a subgroup of patients (at least 20–30%) with an extremely low probability of streptococcal pharyngitis, particularly those with rhinorrhea and cough who appear to have viral infections. For the remaining 70%, the clinical impression must be confirmed by laboratory studies. Serum streptococcal antibody levels are *not* useful for diagnosis of acute streptococcal pharyngitis because demonstration of a significant increase (fourfold or greater) in antibody titer over 2–4 weeks is necessary—a procedure that is clearly impractical. In addition, there is evidence that prompt antibiotic therapy can abort the antibody responses following GAS infection.

The standard, time-tested, and most reliable method for diagnosing streptococcal pharyngitis is the performance of the throat culture. This entails obtaining a swab of the posterior pharyngeal and tonsillar region and streaking it on a plate containing sheep blood agar, a method in widespread practice in the United States since about 1960. This practice was pioneered by Burtis Breese and Frank Disney, Rochester, N.Y. pediatricians, who began to use this technique around 1953. After 18–24 h of incubation at 37°C, beta-hemolytic streptococci appear as small colonies surrounded by large zones of beta or complete hemolysis. Differentiation of group A from other serogroups of beta streptococci can be made on a presumptive basis by finding inhibition of growth of subcultured organisms using discs impregnated with the antimicrobial agent *bacitracin*. About 95% of bacitracin-sensitive (i.e., growth-inhibited) beta streptococci are group A organisms, whereas 99% of bacitracin-resistant beta streptococci belong to other serogroups and are collectively referred to as non–group A beta streptococci, lacking the potential to lead to acute rheumatic fever. The blood agar plate is streaked from the site of initial application of the throat swab using a sterile wire loop. The procedure should include an agar stab to enable subsurface growth. The stab frequently enhances the beta hemolysis related to streptolysin O (oxygen-labile) production.

The throat culture is the standard against which other diagnostic tests for streptococcal pharyngitis are compared, even though it is associated with only approximately 90% accuracy. Culture is limited because it cannot distinguish reliably between patients with active streptococcal infection and those who are chronic pharyngeal carriers of GAS but who may have a coincidental acute viral pharyngitis. The former patients tend to have heavier growth of GAS on the culture plate than the latter group, but sufficient overlap in the intensity of growth exists to render this distinction unreliable.

In the past 5 years, a large number of rapid diagnostic tests that detect GAS antigen have been developed and marketed. A patient's throat swab is first subjected to a brief extraction step (usually with nitrous acid) to release cell-wall A carbohydrate from GAS organisms, followed by an immune reaction employing anti–A carbohydrate antibody. This reaction is made readily detectable—a color change or agglutination is used to distinguish between specimens that are positive and negative for GAS. Results are generally available in 10–30 min. The marketed tests vary considerably in their *sensitivity* (the fraction of culture positives that are positive by the rapid test) and their *specificity* (the fraction of rapid test positives that are culture-positive), when compared with simultaneous culture results. High specificity (i.e., few false-positives) but varying and frequently inadequate sensitivity (i.e., too many false-negatives) are usually seen. Thus, a positive test is usually valid and may serve as the basis for initiating treatment, but a negative test is less reliable and should be backed up by a culture. Rapid tests are also incapable of distinguishing between GAS carriage and active infection. They serve as a useful adjunct to the clinician but should not completely displace the throat culture in routine clinical practice until their sensitivity improves.

### Treatment

Acute streptococcal pharyngitis/tonsillitis is generally a self-limited illness. Over a period of days, symptoms spontaneously subside in the large majority of instances. A small minority of untreated patients develop suppurative complications (e.g., cervical adenitis, peritonsillar abscess) or nonsuppurative complications (e.g., acute glomerulonephritis, acute rheumatic fever). The primary reason that streptococcal pharyngitis should be identified and treated is *to prevent acute rheumatic fever and resultant rheumatic heart disease.*

Despite almost five decades of penicillin use to treat streptococcal pharyngitis, group A streptococci have not developed resistance to penicillin; not a single penicillin-resistant strain has been found. Thus, penicillin remains the drug of choice given either orally for 10 days or as a single parenteral injection of a depot preparation (benzathine penicillin). Oral regimens have the practical problem of relying upon patient compliance for the entire 10 days, whereas parenteral penicillin is painful and may be associated with higher rates of significant allergic reactions. Individuals known or suspected to be allergic to penicillin should be treated with alternative, non–beta-lactam agents, such as erythromycin or clindamycin. Even though streptococcal pharyngitis is self-limited, antibiotic treatment is associated with somewhat accelerated clearing of fever and other signs and symptoms of streptococcal pharyngitis. In contrast to its response to penicillin, GAS resistance to erythromycin is well documented and reflects, in general, the frequency of usage of the agent in a particular population. For example, in Japan and Finland, where erythromycin has been used very freely, as many as 62% and 24% of GAS isolates, respectively, have been found to be erythromycin-resistant. Antibiotics that cannot be recommended for treatment of streptococcal pharyngitis include sulfa drugs (which are useful for *prevention* but not for *treatment*), trimethoprim-sulfamethoxazole, tetracyclines, and chloramphenicol.

## Purulent Complications of Streptococcal Pharyngitis

Prior to the availability of antibiotics, purulent streptococcal complications were very common and greatly feared, having substantial associated mortality (Table 7–3). In the antibiotic era, purulent infections that represent direct extension of GAS from the pharynx to adjacent structures are much less common, but they still occur. These infections include (1) *peritonsillar abscess* (''quinsy''): presenting as fever, dysphagia, and referred ear pain, with asymmetry of the tonsils and a bulge in the peritonsillar area; (2) *retropharyngeal abscess*: presenting as fever, dysphagia, drooling, stridor, and extension to the neck, with a bulging mass in the posterior pharyngeal wall; (3) suppurative *cervical lymphadenitis*: presenting as tender swollen cervical nodes that may become fluctuant, representing lymphangitic spread from the tonsils; and (4) otitis media, sinusitis, and mastoiditis, all more commonly due to bacteria other than GAS but occasionally complicating streptococcal pharyngitis. Therapy of these purulent complications of course includes an antibiotic effective against GAS. Peritonsillar and retropharyngeal abscesses require surgical drainage;

### TABLE 7–3.    COMPLICATIONS OF GROUP A STREPTOCOCCAL PHARYNGITIS

Purulent
  Cervical adenitis, sinusitis, otitis media
  Peritonsillar and retropharyngeal abscess
  Sepsis, metastatic infection
  Streptococcal toxic shock–like syndrome (rare)

Nonpurulent
  Acute rheumatic fever
  Acute glomerulonephritis

### TABLE 7–4.    DIAGNOSTIC CRITERIA: STREPTOCOCCAL TOXIC SHOCK SYNDROME*

I. Isolation of *S. pyogenes* from
  A. A normally sterile site (e.g., blood, CSF)
  B. A nonsterile site (e.g., throat, sputum, vagina)
II. Clinical features
  A. Hypotension: systolic BP $\leq$90 mm Hg (adults) or less than fifth percentile for children
                AND
  B. At least two of the following:
  1. Renal impairment
  2. Coagulopathy (e.g., thrombocytopenia, low fibrinogen)
  3. Liver involvement (e.g., aminotransferase or bilirubin elevation)
  4. Adult respiratory distress syndrome (ARDS)
  5. Generalized macular red rash
  6. Soft tissue necrosis (e.g., necrotizing fasciitis)
Defininte case = IA and IIA and IIB
Probable case = IB and IIA and IIB

*Adapted from JAMA *269*:390–391, 1993. With permission.

each may present early as a cellulitis that has not yet walled off to form an abscess. Drainage is not helpful until an abscess has developed. Cervical adenitis may resolve with antibiotic therapy alone or may suppurate and require drainage.

Streptococcal toxic shock syndrome (STSS) is the term now used to describe the occurrence of shock and multiorgan dysfunction associated with severe group A streptococcal infection. Invasive infections like necrotizing fasciitis are often present. A skin rather than pharyngeal or other mucosal portal of entry is usual. The diagnostic criteria for STSS are presented in Table 7–4.

## Nonpurulent (or Nonsuppurative) Complications of Streptococcal Pharyngitis

### Acute Rheumatic Fever

Acute rheumatic fever (ARF) is a major medical disorder that occurs in selected individuals following untreated upper respiratory tract infection with GAS. This systemic inflammatory illness involves connective tissue and produces *carditis* (which may lead to heart disease that is frequently permanent or at least long-standing), joint inflammation (*arthritis* or arthralgia, with transient involvement only), and neurologic involvement (*chorea,* transient only). From 1925 to 1950, rheumatic fever and resultant rheumatic heart (valvular) disease (RHD) was the leading cause of death in American children and adolescents 5–19 years of age and the leading cause of heart disease in those younger than 40. Although suspected as being related to streptococcal infection in the late 19th century, ARF was unequivocally linked to recent GAS pharyngitis around 1930, following Lancefield's identification of the cell-wall A carbohydrate that distinguishes GAS and following Todd's subsequent development of the antistreptolysin O serologic test that enabled documentation of recent GAS infection. A steady decline in the frequency of ARF and RHD and in mortality from these illnesses clearly had begun as early as 1900 or 1910, antedating Lancefield's work, the institution of effective control measures, and the development of antibiotic and corticosteroid therapy. The occurrence of ARF and RHD decreased markedly during the 1960s and particularly during the 1970s and early 1980s. Recent generations of U.S. medical students and house officers had been trained without encountering patients with ARF. In 1985, the Jones Memorial Lecture to the American Heart Association was entitled "The Virtual Disappearance of Rheumatic Fever in the United States," and the American Heart Association sponsored a symposium entitled "Management of Pharyngitis in an Era of Declining Incidence of Rheumatic Fever" (see Shulman in reference list). In addition to convincing evidence of a decline in the *incidence* of ARF in the United States, the *severity* of ARF had also decreased substantially even before penicillin or corticosteroids had become available.

The striking decline in ARF and RHD in the first half of this century was due, in large measure, to improved living conditions with less crowding and improved nutrition and sanitation. However, it is difficult to ascribe the more striking fall in ARF since 1950 to such nonspecific societal improvements. Thus, other possible explanations were sought for the near-disappearance of ARF by 1985 in the United States. One hypothesis was that there might have been a sharp decline in the frequency of acute streptococcal pharyngitis in children, but no data support this prospect. Some suggested that a decline in incidence of some other disorder like measles or rubella, resulting from successful vaccine programs, might have contributed by the elimination of some necessary cofactor, but even fewer data support this hypothesis. Close analysis of patterns of access to health care suggests that this is at least an important contributing factor to the observed decline in ARF. In Baltimore, for example, the incidence

of ARF in the inner city during the 1960s declined only in those populations living in proximity to comprehensive care clinics and not in those residing in areas not served by such clinics. This suggests that accurate diagnosis and timely treatment of streptococcal pharyngitis contributed in a major way to the decline.

The epidemiologic picture changed around 1985–1986 when a completely unexpected substantial resurgence in ARF was noted in several areas of the United States, most dramatically in the intermountain region near Salt Lake City, but also in Pittsburgh, Columbus, and Akron, and several other locales. This resurgence lasted 2–3 years, and ARF appears to have resumed its earlier decline. Although ARF had traditionally been an illness with greatest incidence in the lowest socioeconomic groups of our society, the outbreaks in the 1980s appeared to be focused on white, suburban, middle-class children. That this resurgence was not a nationwide phenomenon was suggested by survey data that fail to demonstrate an overall increase in ARF nationally but rather indicate focality of the outbreaks. Of great interest is the observation that highly mucoid, heavily encapsulated strains of GAS were recovered on throat culture of family members, random community sources, and occasionally from ARF patients themselves in Salt Lake City, Akron, and several other areas during this resurgence of ARF. Unfortunately, the precise relationship between these mucoidal isolates, which represent several different M types (even within a single geographic area), and the increase in ARF is unclear. The application of the tools of modern molecular biology to study these GAS isolates may provide important insights into the pathogenesis of this major medical disease.

ARF characteristically demonstrates its peak incidence in children 5–12 years of age, being relatively rare under the age of 4 years and in adulthood. This parallels the age distribution of streptococcal pharyngitis. However, chronic rheumatic heart disease that represents the residua of earlier ARF is important in adults and accounts for a sizable fraction of those who require placement of prosthetic heart valves. ARF is characterized by a propensity to recur after subsequent GAS infections (see below). Table 7–2 contrasts certain features of ARF with those of acute poststreptococcal nephritis.

**Clinical Features.** A single diagnostic test for ARF does not exist, prompting T. Duckett

Jones in 1944 to develop what have since become known as the Jones criteria for the diagnosis of ARF. The subsequently modified and revised Jones criteria stand as the worldwide standard for diagnosis of first attacks of ARF (Table 7–5). These criteria are divided into five major criteria, several minor (or less specific) criteria, and an absolute requirement for evidence of a recent GAS infection, either by positive throat culture or rapid antigen test or by serologic demonstration of elevated or rising antibody titer to a GAS antigen. The diagnosis of ARF requires the combination of at least one major criterion and two minors, or two majors, plus evidence of recent GAS infection. The Jones criteria were designed specifically to decrease the overdiagnosis of ARF and to set some minimum requirements for diagnosis; not all patients who meet the Jones criteria necessarily have ARF. Individualized assessment is mandatory.

CARDITIS. The most important manifestation of ARF is cardiac inflammation, since this leads to the only long-term sequelae of an episode (or an "attack") of ARF. Carditis is present in approximately 50% of ARF patients, manifested as tachycardia and murmurs of mitral and/or aortic valve insufficiency. Involvement of endocardium (valves), myocardium (myocarditis), or pericardium (pericarditis, effusion) may occur, with valvular involvement invariably present. Myocarditis or pericarditis without valvular involvement is rarely, if ever, related to ARF. Echocardiographic evidence of mitral insufficiency that is not apparent by auscultation does not fulfill the Jones criterion for carditis. When all three cardiac layers are involved, the term *pancar-*

*ditis* is used, referring to a very serious, even life-threatening, acute disease. Clinical symptoms associated with acute rheumatic carditis include dyspnea (and other features of congestive heart failure) and chest pain. Following ARF with carditis, patients are frequently left with chronic mitral and/or aortic valve insufficiency that may lessen in severity with time or may alternatively evolve to the development of stenotic valvular lesions, generally over at least 5–10 years. Recurrent episodes of ARF are frequently associated with increasingly severe rheumatic heart disease. Pathologically, the hallmark of rheumatic carditis is the Aschoff body, a perivascular aggregation of large cells with polymorphous nuclei and basophilic cytoplasm rosetting around an avascular core of fibrinoid necrosis. The Aschoff body is of uncertain origin and can probably be seen in other cardiac disorders, but it remains most characteristic of rheumatic carditis.

ARTHRITIS. The most common major manifestation of ARF is migratory polyarthritis, seen in about 75% of attacks. Typically, this involves the large joints, particularly the knees, ankles, wrists, and elbows, and rarely affects smaller joints. The involved joints are usually exquisitely tender, with even the friction of a bedsheet inducing pain; redness, heat, and swelling are also usually present. The degree of patient discomfort frequently seems disproportionate to the objective findings. Most characteristic is the migratory nature of the arthritis, so that without therapy an involved joint becomes normal within 1–5 days while other previously uninvolved joint(s) become inflamed. Untreated patients manifest an average of six involved joints over

**TABLE 7–5. JONES CRITERIA (1992 REVISION) FOR GUIDANCE IN THE DIAGNOSIS OF ACUTE RHEUMATIC FEVER**

| MAJOR MANIFESTATIONS | MINOR MANIFESTATIONS |
|---|---|
| Carditis | *Clinical* |
| Polyarthritis | Fever |
| Chorea | Arthralgia |
| Erythema marginatum | |
| Subcutaneous nodules | |
| | *Laboratory* |
| | Acute-phase reaction |
| | (erythrocyte sedimentation |
| | rate, C-reactive protein) |
| | Prolonged PR interval |
| *Additional Criteria* | |
| Supporting evidence of preceding streptococcal infection | |
| (increased ASO or other streptococcal antibodies), or | |
| Positive throat culture for group A streptococci | |

1–2 weeks. Also highly characteristic is the dramatic response of the arthritis of ARF to even small doses of salicylate, a feature well known to clinicians of 100 years ago. There appears to be somewhat of an inverse relationship between the severity of arthritis and the incidence of cardiac involvement in ARF. The migratory arthritis of ARF does not lead to chronic or deforming joint disease.

CHOREA. Sydenham's chorea (or St. Vitus dance) occurs in about 10% of ARF patients, manifesting as uncoordination, choreoathetoid movements, emotional lability, poor school performance, and facial grimacing. Symptoms are frequently exacerbated by stress. Sydenham's chorea usually develops weeks to months after the other manifestations of ARF; that is, the latent period between acute streptococcal infection and onset of chorea is substantially longer than the approximately 3 weeks between GAS infection and the other major manifestations of ARF. Even though chorea may last several months, it is not associated with persistent neurologic findings.

SUBCUTANEOUS NODULES. These are seen only rarely in ARF and are firm nodules approximately 1 cm in diameter palpable along extensor surfaces of tendons near bony prominences. Most patients with this finding have prominent rheumatic heart disease.

ERYTHEMA MARGINATUM. This is also a rare manifestation of ARF, a macular nonpruritic erythematous rash with irregular margins and clear center. The rash is evanescent, exacerbated by warming as with a warm wash cloth, and appears on the trunk and extremities but not on the face.

MINOR MANIFESTATIONS OF ACUTE RHEUMATIC FEVER. These features of ARF are more nonspecific than the major manifestations discussed above. They are divided into clinical manifestations (i.e., fever and arthralgia) and laboratory manifestations (i.e., prolonged PR interval on ECG, and presence of acute-phase reactants, such as elevated sedimentation rate or C-reactive protein). Arthralgia can be used as a minor criterion only if arthritis is not used as a major.

EVIDENCE OF RECENT GROUP A STREPTOCOCCAL INFECTION. This is an absolute requisite in addition to the major and minor Jones criteria. Approximately 20% of ARF patients harbor GAS on throat culture at the time of presentation; the other 80% are culture-negative, presumably after spontaneous clearing of their earlier pharyngeal infection.

Therefore, alternative evidence of recent GAS infection must be sought, usually in the form of serum antibody against streptococcal products or antigens; for example, antistreptolysin O, anti-DNase B, antihyaluronidase, or anti–A carbohydrate. A single antibody test will be positive in about 80% of patients with ARF; therefore, when ARF is suspected clinically, it may be necessary to obtain several streptococcal antibody assays to establish the diagnosis of ARF. An exception to the requirement for recent GAS evidence can be made in patients with Sydenham's chorea as their sole major manifestation, because the long latency between GAS infection and onset of chorea may allow decline of antistreptococcal titers to near-baseline levels

**Recurrences.** One of the most characteristic features of ARF is its propensity to recur in the same individual with subsequent acute GAS infections, as emphasized almost 100 years ago by Sir William Osler. Recurrences tend to mimic the first attack in clinical manifestations, but there is a cumulatively increasing frequency (and severity) of cardiac disease as the number of recurrences increases. This is the basis for the recommendations for long-term antibiotic prophylaxis to prevent GAS infections and thus to prevent recurrences of ARF in individuals who have had at least one attack.

**Pathogenesis of Acute Rheumatic Fever.** The evidence that ARF is directly related to GAS infection can be summarized as follows:

1. One half to two thirds of ARF patients give a clear history of a recent upper respiratory illness, usually sore throat, and 20% still harbor GAS in the pharynx.

2. Streptococcal antibody tests provide serologic confirmation of recent GAS infection in those with or without such clinical evidence.

3. Titers of antistreptococcal antibodies are higher in ARF patients than in those following uncomplicated GAS infection.

4. The age distribution of ARF parallels that of acute streptococcal pharyngitis.

5. Antibiotic therapy for acute streptococcal pharyngitis that is instituted within 9 days of the onset of symptoms appears highly effective in preventing ARF.

6. Long-term, continuous prophylactic administration of antibiotics is highly effective in preventing recurrent episodes of ARF in susceptible individuals.

The precise mechanism(s) by which GAS infection of the upper respiratory tract leads to ARF remains unclear despite many decades of intense investigation. The concept of the "susceptible host" with genetically determined susceptibility has become accepted even though the precise determinants of susceptibility have been difficult to define. In some, but not all, patient populations it appears that the presence of a specific HLA-D locus marker correlates with susceptibility to ARF (i.e., DR4 in those of European ancestry, DR2 in those of African ancestry). Family clustering of ARF supports a genetic predisposition, and a specific B-lymphocyte surface antigen may be more common in rheumatic individuals. That only up to 3% of individuals with untreated streptococcal pharyngitis in epidemic circumstances, and a much lower percentage in endemic circumstances, go on to develop ARF also suggests that a host susceptibility factor is operative.

The proposed pathogenetic mechanisms that lead to the clinical manifestations that we recognize as ARF fall into three general categories: (1) persistent streptococcal infection; (2) reaction to a toxic streptococcal product or component; and (3) an aberrant immune response to group A streptococci. Essentially no evidence supports persistent GAS infection within affected tissues, as highlighted by the failure of massive amounts of penicillin to alter ARF. A direct toxic effect of one of the many extracellular products elaborated by GAS, including streptolysin O (which is directly toxic to myocardial cells in tissue culture), seems unlikely because of the latent period between acute streptococcal pharyngitis and onset of ARF.

By far, most attention has focused upon an immune-mediated pathogenesis of ARF. The following support the hypothesis that ARF is an immune-mediated disorder: (1) the striking clinical similarity of ARF to certain diseases that clearly have an immune pathogenesis; (2) the approximately 3 week latent period between acute streptococcal pharyngitis and the onset of ARF; (3) the antigenicity of many streptococcal products and constituents; and (4) the extensive immunologic cross-reactivity that exists between GAS constituents and human tissues (Table 7–6). The cross-reactivity existing between streptococcal cell membrane and cardiac sarcolemma and subsarcolemma, or between group A carbohydrate and cardiac valvular glycoprotein, suggests the possibility that GAS triggers an immune response that is misdirected against cross-reactive host "self" antigens, resulting in tissue damage that manifests clinically as ARF. In addition, serum heart-reactive antibodies can be demonstrated in patients with acute rheumatic carditis, and antineuronal antibodies are found in sera from those with chorea. However, a central role in pathogenesis of ARF for any specific immune reaction has been difficult to prove, and the precise pathogenetic mechanisms are still unclear. The absence of an animal model for ARF has significantly hampered pathogenetic studies.

Central to pathogenetic considerations, of course, is the group A streptococcus. Although it had long been thought that all GAS strains were equally capable of triggering the events that lead to ARF, more recent evidence (primarily epidemiologic) suggests that a relatively limited number of M types are usually linked to ARF. These have been considered to be *rheumatogenic* strains, but it is not known what confers rheumatogenicity. As noted above, the recent resurgence of ARF in selected areas of the United States has been associated with heavily encapsulated (mucoid) GAS strains of several serotypes that earlier had been implicated in epidemics of ARF. Further analysis of such strains and identification of a "rheumatogenic factor" will be necessary to further our understanding of this disorder.

Although its full significance has not yet

### TABLE 7–6. CROSS-REACTIVITY BETWEEN GROUP A STREPTOCOCCI AND HUMAN TISSUES

| Cross-Reactive Streptococcal Constituent | Human Tissue Component |
|---|---|
| M protein | Human tropomyosin and myosin |
| Cell membrane | Sarcolemma and subsarcolemma |
| M protein | Sarcolemma and subsarcolemma |
| Group A carbohydrate | Heart valve glycoprotein |
| Cell membrane | Neurons of caudate and subthalamic nuclei |
| Hyaluronic acid | Connective tissue protein–polysaccharide complex |

been clarified, a fascinating relationship between the structure of certain streptococcal M proteins and human myosin has been described. Antibodies reactive against M protein types 5 and 6, for example, cross-react with myosin and suggest a possible role in pathogenesis of acute rheumatic fever. The epitope responsible for this cross-reactivity has been localized to a specific short amino acid sequence of M protein. Additional studies of this epitope are necessary to clarify its possible involvement in pathogenesis of ARF.

### Treatment

ACUTE EPISODES. *Acute* episodes of ARF are treated with *antiinflammatory drugs, antibiotics,* and *cardiac drugs* when needed. Antiinflammatory therapy comprises aspirin (50–100 mg/kg/day in four doses) for those without carditis or with mild carditis, or corticosteroids (prednisone at 2 mg/kg/day in four doses) for those with significant cardiomegaly or congestive failure. Joint symptoms resolve dramatically. Although acute cardiac manifestations resolve promptly with steroids, there is no evidence that the ultimate incidence of residual chronic rheumatic valvular dysfunction is reduced by the use of steroids. When steroids are used, they are withdrawn gradually after 2–4 weeks, with salicylates phased in during the prednisone taper. All patients with ARF should receive oral penicillin or erythromycin or an injection of depot penicillin to achieve at least 10 days of therapy to ensure eradication of any residual GAS. Cardiac medications such as diuretics and digoxin should be used as necessary in patients with congestive failure.

CHRONIC THERAPY. After the acute illness has subsided, *chronic therapy* for rheumatic fever includes long-term administration of prophylactic antistreptococcal antibiotics to prevent further episodes. Acceptable secondary prophylaxis regimens include intramuscular injections of benzathine penicillin ($1.2 \times 10^6$ units for those over 60 lb, $0.6 \times 10^6$ units for those under 60 lb) every 3–4 weeks, or oral penicillin (250 mg) twice daily or oral sulfadiazine (500 mg) twice daily. The oral regimens are slightly less effective than the parenteral regimen, and they rely upon patient compliance but are more convenient. Benzathine penicillin is painful but does not require daily patient cooperation. The duration of rheumatic fever prophylaxis is somewhat controversial but should be maintained for at least 5 years from the last attack or until age 21 years, or, in the case of those with significant residual cardiac disease, perhaps for life. Clearly the greatest risk of recurrent ARF is in the first 5 years after an attack and in those with increased exposure to those with GAS upper respiratory infection (school teachers, parents of young children, etc.).

### Acute Poststreptococcal Glomerulonephritis

The other nonsuppurative complication of GAS infection is acute glomerulonephritis (AGN), described by Richard Bright in 1836. This important renal disorder contrasts with ARF in many respects. Examination of the epidemiologic, pathogenetic, and biologic differences between these illnesses should yield insights into our understanding of these diseases (Table 7–2).

The most striking epidemiologic differences between AGN and ARF relate to the fact that AGN develops following *either pharyngeal or skin infection* with GAS, whereas ARF occurs only following upper respiratory infection, never after streptococcal skin infection. The explanation for this is not at all clear. AGN is quite common in very young children, generally related to preceding streptococcal pyoderma or impetigo. These skin infections are most common in the warmer months, related to streptococcal superinfection of insect bites or sites of minor trauma. Males predominate in patients with AGN, perhaps because of their increased frequency of minor trauma. Second episodes of AGN are unusual.

The M types of GAS frequently associated with AGN are limited in number and represent the so-called nephritogenic types (particularly types M1, M2, M3, M4, M12, and M15, in addition to higher numbered pyoderma types like M49, M52, M55, M59, M60, and M61). Even within a given nephritogenic M type, only certain strains of the nephritogenic types seem to be capable of initiating AGN.

**Clinical Features.** AGN is typically characterized by the sudden onset of edema, hematuria, and decreased urination. Hypertension, azotemia, hematuria, and proteinuria also occur. Although a large number of infectious agents, including group C streptococci, other bacteria, and some viruses, can lead to development of acute glomerulonephritis, GAS is the most common. There is usually evidence of previous pyoderma or streptococcal pharyngitis. The latent period between GAS pharyngeal infection and onset of AGN is approximately 10 days, in contrast to a longer

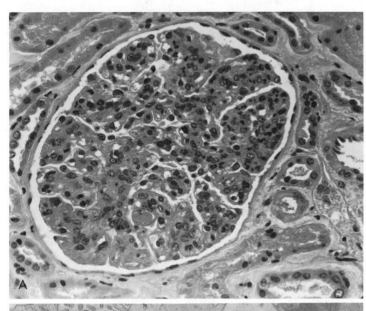

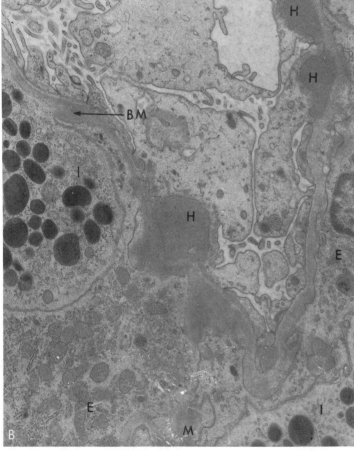

**FIGURE 7–2.** Poststreptococcal acute diffuse glomerulonephritis. *A,* Proliferation and exudation in biopsy obtained 30 days after onset. Hematoxylin and eosin stain. *B,* Characteristic electron-dense subepithelial "humps." BM, basement membrane; E, endothelial cell; H, hump (immune deposit); I, inflammatory cell; M, basement membrane–like material (in mesangium). Electron microscopy (× 12,000). (Both from Jennings, R. B., and Earle, D. P. In: Becker, E. L., ed. *Structural Basis of Renal Diseases.* New York: Harper & Row, 1968. With permission.) *Illustration continued on opposite page*

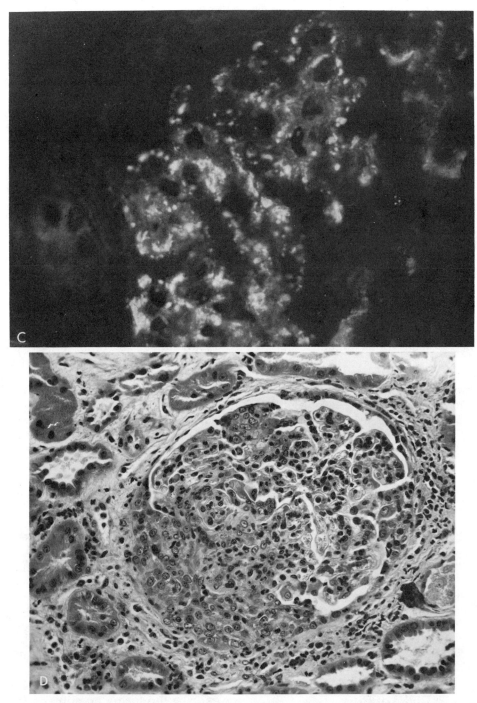

**FIGURE 7–2.** *Continued C,* Characteristic deposition of IgG in a granular pattern along the glomerular capillary basement membrane. Immunofluorescent anti-IgG stain. (Courtesy of Dr. Elizabeth V. Potter.) *D,* Crescent formation characteristic of severe acute glomerulonephritis. Hematoxylin and eosin stain. (From Jennings, R. B., and Earle, D. P. In: Becker, E. L., ed. *Structural Basis of Renal Diseases.* New York: Harper & Row, 1968. With permission.)

latent period of up to 6 weeks (usually 3 weeks) following streptococcal skin infection or pyoderma. AGN is generally a self-limited illness in children, only rarely leading to chronic renal disease. By contrast, in adults, up to 20% of episodes of AGN result in chronic renal disease, sometimes leading to renal insufficiency in 10–30 years.

Serologic or culture evidence of recent or active GAS infection usually confirms the diagnosis of AGN in acute hypocomplementemic nephritis with hypertension and azotemia.

**Pathogenesis.** AGN appears to be a classic immune-mediated disorder and is usually associated with profoundly depressed serum complement levels (total complement, C3, properdin). Proliferative or exudative glomerular changes with diffuse involvement of virtually all glomeruli are characteristic (Fig. 7–2). Crescent formation may occur. Immunofluorescence studies demonstrate fine granular staining for IgG, C3, and C1q, and electron microscopy shows subepithelial humps of electron-dense material in capillary walls. Among the candidate streptococcal antigens that may lead to this immune-complex nephritis is a 45-kD streptokinase termed nephritis strain—associated protein (NSAP); endostreptosin, an antigen derived from cytoplasm and cell membrane of nephritogenic GAS; and a streptococcal protease.

**Therapy.** Penicillin or erythromycin therapy is given to eradicate streptococci, and diuretics and antihypertensive agents are used as necessary. AGN tends to be a self-limited disorder, particularly in children, and immunosuppressive therapy is not warranted.

**Prophylaxis.** Effective prevention of AGN by prompt treatment of acute streptococcal infections is not clearly documented, in contrast to ARF; indeed, most evidence suggests that it is not possible to prevent AGN effectively. Since recurrent attacks of AGN are quite rare (in direct contrast to ARF), long-term prophylactic antibiotics as used in ARF are not warranted or recommended.

## DIPHTHERIA

A very important and now very rare acute bacterial infection of the upper respiratory tract in the United States is diphtheria—the result of extracellular toxin production by toxigenic strains of *Corynebacterium diphtheriae*. This illness was described as a distinct entity by Pierre Brettonneau in 1821, who recognized its contagious nature. Around 1883, Theodor Klebs and Friederich Löffler observed the causative agent in smears of diphtheritic membranes, isolated the organism on artificial media, and produced fatal infection in guinea pigs. In 1923, a safe and effective vaccine composed of formalin-treated toxin was introduced by Gaston Ramon.

*Corynebacterium diphtheriae* is also known as the Klebs-Löffler bacillus, and is a gram-positive, nonmotile, nonsporulating, pleomorphic gram-negative rod that sometimes has a club-shaped appearance. Media containing tellurite are best for recovery of *C. diphtheriae* because they inhibit other flora. Colonies may be rough or smooth in appearance, frequently classified as gravis, mitis, or intermedius. Toxin production does not correlate with colonial morphology and is present in strains of *C. diphtheriae* that are lysogenic for a prophage or phage encoding for diphtheria toxin. Toxin production *in vitro* is inversely related to the inorganic iron content of the medium.

Epidemiologically, diphtheria occurs worldwide, particularly in areas where immunization with diphtheria toxoid is not near-universal. An explosive epidemic of diphtheria in the former Soviet Union has affected about 100,000 individuals since 1991, with almost 50,000 reported cases in 1994. Fatality rates range from 3–23%. In the United States only very small numbers of cases have been reported yearly (Fig. 7–3), primarily in unimmunized patients. Transmission is most efficient in crowded circumstances and occurs by droplets during coughing or sneezing by a carrier or a person with disease. Fomites appear unimportant. *C. diphtheriae* infection of skin may occur in the unimmunized, who thereby may be predisposed to respiratory colonization and infection.

The pathogenesis of diphtheria begins with *C. diphtheriae* mucosal colonization of the nose or mouth, with toxin elaboration by lysogenized strains occurring after an incubation period of several days. Tissue necrosis and local inflammation occurs in areas of colonization, eventually producing an adherent gray-black pharyngeal membrane that includes fibrin, blood, inflammatory cells, and epithelial cells and that bleeds on attempts to remove it. The membrane and underlying edema may compromise the airway, and the membrane may extend into the major bronchi. Toxin is absorbed through the damaged mucosa and car-

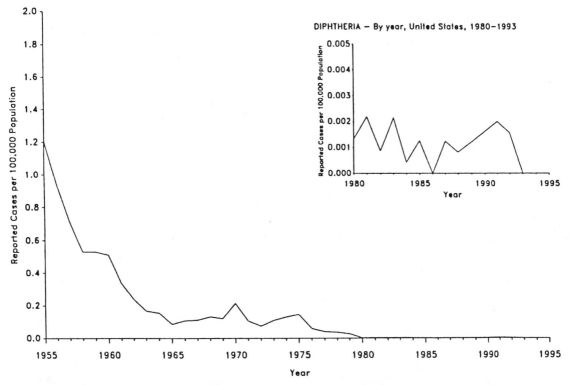

**Figure 7–3,** Diphtheria—by year, United States, 1955–1993. (Data from Centers for Disease Control. *MMWR 42*(53):27, 1994.

ried to distant sites. Fragment B of the 63-kD polypeptide toxin binds to receptors on the cell membrane, and the smaller fragment A then enters the cell, interfering with protein synthesis by enzymatically inactivating elongation factor 2 by ADP ribosylation. Diphtheria toxin has particular tropism for cardiac, neural, and renal cells. Antitoxin is effective in neutralizing circulating diphtheria toxin, but is ineffective once toxin is fixed to the cell membrane. Clinical manifestations appear some time after tissue fixation of toxin, with myocarditis appearing 10–14 days and peripheral neuritis 3–7 weeks after onset of disease.

### Clinical Features

The result of the interaction between *C. diphtheriae* and the human host is determined by the virulence of the specific organism (i.e., its ability to adhere, to multiply, and to elaborate toxin) and by the immune status of the host (whether or not serum antitoxin is present). Immune individuals may become colonized but not ill with *C. diphtheriae* and serve as reservoirs of infection.

Diphtheria develops after an incubation pe-

riod of 1–5 days and is conveniently classified by the anatomic location of the affected membrane (nasal, tonsillar, pharyngeal, laryngeal or laryngotracheal, and nonrespiratory). Tonsillar and pharyngeal diphtheria is characterized by the insidious onset of anorexia, malaise, low-grade fever, and sore throat. A membrane of varying extent forms within 1–2 days, depending upon the host's immune status, covering the tonsils and pharyngeal walls and extending inferiorly to the larynx and trachea. Cervical adenopathy varies but may be associated with edema of the soft tissues of the neck, producing a "bull-neck" appearance. In milder cases the membrane sloughs after 7–10 days and recovery ensues. However, severe cases are associated with increasing toxemia followed by prostration, tachycardia, stupor, coma, and death within 6–10 days. Palatal paralysis is the most common manifestation of diphtheritic neuritis, associated with difficulty swallowing. Ocular palsies and diaphragmatic palsy may be seen. Severe diphtheria is also associated with diphtheritic myocarditis and with arrhythmias, congestive failure, and ECG changes.

## Diagnosis

Because of its potential severity, diphtheria must be suspected on clinical grounds and therapy not withheld pending confirmation. Accurate confirmation of diphtheria requires isolation of *C. diphtheriae* on tellurite media from material from beneath the membrane. Recovered diphtheria organisms should be tested for toxin production, usually by inoculation of guinea pigs.

Other laboratory tests are of little value. ST and T wave changes on ECG may be present in patients with myocarditis. The classic test of the immune status of a patient is the Schick test, in which a small amount of diphtheria toxin is injected intracutaneously inducing, in the absence of antitoxin, a local inflammatory response. A toxoid control is necessary because some persons are sensitized to the toxin.

## Treatment

The best treatment of diphtheria, of course, is prevention by appropriate immunization (see Chapter 40). Once diphtheria is suspected, aggressive therapy to neutralize free toxin with antitoxin and to eradicate *C. diphtheriae* with antibiotics is essential. Equine antitoxin must be given intravenously in a single large dose (40,000–120,000 units) to neutralize all free toxin and to attempt to avoid reaction to the horse serum (see Chapter 40). Prior sensitivity to horse serum should be assessed with a test dose of 0.1 mL of 1:1000 dilution intracutaneously or into the conjunctiva; if positive, careful desensitization is necessary. In addition to antitoxin, penicillin or erythromycin is administered for about 7 days. Diphtheria immunization is given following recovery, since at least 50% fail to develop immunity after natural infection.

## OTHER BACTERIAL CAUSES OF PHARYNGITIS

### *Arcanobacterium haemolyticum*

This organism (formerly *Corynebacterium haemolyticum*) causes a scarlet fever–like illness with acute pharyngitis and a scarlatinal rash, particularly in teenagers and young adults. The peak age appears to be 15–20 years. Although well described in Scandinavia and Britain, this has been little studied in the United States. These patients fail to respond to penicillin therapy but have dramatic clinical responses to erythromycin. Clinical features exhibited by patients from whom *A. haemolyticum* has been recovered include tonsillitis or pharyngitis, and about 50% have an associated scarlatinal rash appearing several days after the onset of pharyngeal symptoms. Recovery of *A. haemolyticum* was 80-fold more common in those who were symptomatic than in normal, age-matched individuals.

### *Neisseria gonorrhoeae*

Acute pharyngitis due to this agent is the result of oral–genital sexual contact and presents as an ulcerative, exudative tonsillopharyngitis. Culture on selective media for recovery of gonococci is necessary to establish the diagnosis. Therapy with penicillin or ceftriaxone resolves this infection.

## OTITIS MEDIA

Infection of the middle ear is extremely common in children, one associated with high morbidity but very low mortality. It has been shown by prospective cohort studies that by the age of 3 years two thirds of American children have experienced at least one episode of otitis media (OM), and one third of children have had three or more episodes. OM is the most frequent illness diagnosed and the most frequent reason for physician visits by children except for well-baby and well-child care. Middle ear effusion persists for weeks to months after an episode of acute OM: 40% still are present at 1 month and 10% at 3 months. Because conductive hearing impairment accompanies middle ear effusion and because many patients develop chronic effusions or chronic infections of the middle ear cavity and adjacent structures, OM is an extremely important disorder, particularly in childhood.

## Anatomy and Physiology

Under normal circumstances the mucosa-lined middle ear cavity communicates with the nasopharynx via the mucosa-lined eustachian tube. The eustachian tube serves three functions: (1) to *ventilate* the middle ear cavity (i.e., equilibrate air pressure, replenish oxygen); (2) to facilitate *clearance* of secretions produced in the middle ear cavity; and (3) to *protect* the middle ear cavity from reflux of nasopharyngeal secretions. Under normal circumstances, the eustachian tube is functionally collapsed at rest but opens intermittently during swallowing by contraction of the ten-sor veli palatini muscle. Eustachian tube dysfunction can take the form of obstruction or of abnormal patency and is crucial to the pathogenesis of OM. Most simply, obstruction of the eustachian tube tends to prevent drainage of secretions, whereas excessive patency facilitates aspiration of pharyngeal organisms into the normally sterile middle ear cavity. Both circumstances predispose to acute OM. In young children, the eustachian tube is more susceptible to functional obstruction because its cartilaginous support is less than in older children and adults. In addition, the tube is very short in infants and young children and enters the pharynx at a less acute angle than in adults, making aspiration of nasopharyngeal flora much easier. In effect, the dysfunction associated with a short floppy eustachian tube appears to account in large part for the frequency of OM in this population. Nasal allergy also contributes to the development of OM, presumably by leading to mucosal swelling that extends to the eustachian tube, where it can compromise the lumen.

## Bacteriology

The microbiology of acute OM has been defined by middle ear fluid cultures obtained by tympanocentesis (needle aspiration through the tympanic membrane). Viruses and mycoplasmas are rarely recovered from middle ear fluid, but bacteria that are among the normal flora of the upper respiratory tract are very commonly isolated, particularly *Streptococcus pneumoniae* and *Haemophilus influenzae*. *S.pneumoniae* is the most important cause of OM at all ages, recovered from about 33% of middle ear aspirates in acute OM. *H. influenzae* is recovered from about 20% of aspirates, with 90% of those isolates nontypable (nonencapsulated) and only 10% representing type b strains (see Chapter 21). *Moraxella* (formerly *Branhamella*) *catarrhalis* (6–10%), *Staphylococcus aureus* (2%), GAS (2%), and mixed isolates (6%) represent the remainder of isolates. Approximately 30% of aspirates fail to yield pathogens; it has been shown that excellent anaerobic culturing technique decreases this category somewhat. Of importance is the observation that increasingly the isolates of *H. influenzae* and *M. catarrhalis* (as well as *S. aureus*) are beta-lactamase producers and therefore resistant to penicillin and ampicillin. Additionally, strains of *S. pneumoniae* with decreased sensitivity to penicillin are being isolated with increasing frequency. This of

course has therapeutic implications. Chronic suppurative OM is associated with infection with organisms that are more difficult to eradicate, including *Pseudomonas aeruginosa*, *Proteus mirabilis*, and *S. aureus*.

## Therapy

Decongestant and antihistaminic medications are of little or no value in treating acute OM. Antibiotic therapy with agents effective against the common pathogens clearly speeds resolution of symptoms and hastens clearance of middle ear effusions. Common choices include amoxicillin, cefaclor, erythromycin-sulfadiazine, and trimethoprim-sulfamethoxazole. In most circumstances, middle ear aspiration is not performed to determine the etiologic agent, but is generally used for patients who are treatment failures or compromised hosts for whom it is most important to establish a specific etiology because of the possibility of unusual pathogens.

Persistent middle ear effusion predisposes patients to recurrent acute episodes of OM. In addition, persistent effusion or infection leads to hearing impairment, usually conductive but occasionally sensorineural as well. Protracted hearing impairment in young children is thought to be associated with impaired speech development. Other untoward sequelae include perforation of the tympanic membrane, tympanosclerosis, adhesive fibrotic changes of the tympanic membrane with fixation of ossicles, chronic suppurative OM with chronic drainage through a perforated tympanic membrane, cholesteatoma formation within the middle ear, mastoiditis (see below), labyrinthitis representing spread of infection into the inner ear, facial nerve paralysis, and (rarely) suppurative intracranial complications (e.g., epidural or subdural empyema, brain abscess, meningitis). Mastoiditis is caused by the same organisms that cause OM; indeed, the mastoid air cells are directly contiguous to the middle ear cavity. Extension of infection from mastoids to contiguous intracranial areas occurs occasionally.

## SINUSITIS

Infection of the paranasal sinuses bears many similarities to infection of the middle ear cavity. The normal physiology of the sinuses depends upon: (1) patency of the ostia; (2) function of the ciliary apparatus; and (3) the quality of the mucosal secretions. Ostial obstruction or ciliary dysfunction predisposes to infection of the normally sterile paranasal sinuses. Sinus development varies: ethmoidal and maxillary sinuses are patent at birth, sphenoidal sinuses begin to develop at about 2 years of age, and frontal sinuses are usually very small until 5 or 6 years of age. Full sinus development may not be complete until about 20 years of age.

Obstruction of the ostial-meatal complex of the sinuses is facilitated by the small diameter of the ostia: maxillary sinus ostia are about 2.5 mm in diameter and ethmoidal air cell ostia are only 1–2 mm in diameter. Factors that predispose to sinus ostial obstruction include those related to mucosal swelling, including viral infection, allergy, immotile cilia, chemical irritation by medications (rhinitis medicamentosa), barotrauma (diving), and facial trauma. In addition, nasal polyps, foreign bodies, tumors, deviated nasal septum, and congenital choanal atresia may each lead to mechanical ostial obstruction. The most important of these factors that create mucosal swelling are clearly allergies and viral URIs. Sinusitis is an extremely common disorder, frequently subclinical and self-limited, but often requiring medical attention.

## Microbiology

The paranasal sinuses are normally sterile. When acute sinusitis develops, the responsible bacterial organisms are the same that cause acute otitis media; that is, *H. influenzae* (nontypable) and *S. pneumoniae* most often, with lower frequencies of *M. catarrhalis*, *Staphylococcus aureus*, and *Streptococcus pyogenes*. In older children and adults, penicillin-sensitive anaerobes such as *Peptostreptococcus*, *Peptococcus*, and *Bacteroides* are recovered as well. Chronic sinusitis is characterized by a similar distribution of pathogens, with more anaerobes and gram-negative bacilli.

## Clinical Features

The clinical features of sinusitis are somewhat age-dependent, and the physician's challenge is to distinguish simple upper respiratory tract infection or allergy from secondary bacterial infection of the sinuses. Only the patients with secondary infection will benefit from antibiotic therapy. Young children most commonly manifest persistent rhinorrhea (serous or purulent), frequently with a daytime cough that is worse at night. Children rarely demonstrate sinus tenderness, but periorbital edema may be seen, as well as postnasal drain-

age and foul-smelling breath. In older children and adults, headache and dental and facial pain, with evidence of sinus tenderness to palpation, are more common complaints. Transillumination of the sinuses with a bright light may be a useful adjunctive test for diagnosing maxillary or ethmoidal sinusitis, particularly in older children and adults. Sinusitis is a clinical diagnosis based upon signs and symptoms. Imaging studies that may support the diagnosis of sinusitis include computed tomography or radiographs that show air–fluid levels, complete opacification, or substantial mucosal thickening of the sinuses, and possibly ultrasound studies of the sinus region. Nasopharyngeal and throat culture results do *not* correlate with the organisms within sinuses, and they thus should not be relied upon.

## Treatment

The goals of antimicrobial therapy of acute sinusitis are to achieve clinical improvement and sterilization of sinus secretions, and to prevent chronic sinusitis as well as the intracranial and orbital complications of sinusitis. Based upon the spectrum of organisms isolated from infected sinuses, one can predict that antibiotics such as amoxicillin, ampicillin with clavulanate, cefaclor or other expanded spectrum cephalosporin, or trimethoprim-sulfamethoxazole would be appropriate. Parenteral cephalosporins such as cefuroxime, or ampicillin with sulbactam may be useful in hospitalized patients. Local or systemic administration of vasoconstrictive agents may contribute to reopening the sinus ostia, thereby improving the drainage of secretions. Occasionally, surgical drainage is necessary in a particularly ill patient with acute or chronic sinusitis or the patient with intracranial spread of infection from the sinuses.

## CASE HISTORIES

### CASE HISTORY 1

A 23-year-old school teacher (sixth grade) saw her physician in early March because of a persistent sore throat and low-grade fever of approximately 3 days' duration. When her symptoms first began she had taken an oral tetracycline preparation that a neighbor had given to her. Physical examination revealed several discrete white to yellow-gray patches of exudate over both tonsillar areas. Marked point tenderness at the angle of the right jaw coincided with enlarged palpable submandibular cervical lymph nodes.

A throat culture was obtained, and the patient was told that if she had streptococci in her throat culture she would be notified and should then start penicillin therapy. Forty hours after this visit, the patient was contacted by telephone and told that a heavy growth of group A beta-hemolytic streptococcus was identified by culture. Although she reported that fever had subsided and that her sore throat was improved, she was strongly urged to take a full 10-day course of penicillin. A follow-up throat culture taken 10 days after starting therapy failed to reveal beta-hemolytic streptococci.

## Case 1 Discussion

Several points about this case are worth emphasizing. First, the patient is an elementary school teacher and thus is almost constantly exposed to young children of an age (5–14 years) most prone to harbor group A streptococci in their respiratory tracts. Second, the time of year when her illness developed coincides with the peak occurrence of streptococcal pharyngitis. Third, close questioning is often necessary to elicit a history of self-medication. In some instances, this may be very important. For example, it may help explain delay in isolating a microorganism by culture. Note that the neighbor had some of her oral tetracycline preparation "left over," evidence that patients frequently do not consume all of an oral medication for the full course. Fourth, note that tetracycline, which is ineffective against group A streptococci, did not prevent heavy growth of the organism. Fifth, although the physician found clinical manifestations consistent with streptococcal disease of the oropharynx, the exudative process was minimal and the pharynx was not "beefy red," as is frequently the case. Perhaps the best indicator of streptococcal disease in this patient was the marked tenderness over the enlarged cervical lymph nodes beneath the right jaw. Sixth, note that when streptococci were isolated, the patient was instructed to take the eradicative 10-day course of penicillin, even though clinical features had begun to resolve spontaneously. Eradicative therapy was effective, as shown by the follow-up throat culture. Posttreatment cultures are not usually obtained.

## Case History 2

A 10-year-old boy was seen by an intern at 6 P.M. on July 2 in an emergency clinic because of fever of several hours' duration, headache, and sore throat. Oral temperature was 102.4°F (39°C). The posterior pharynx was intensely erythematous; the tonsils were swollen, red, and partially covered with a skim milk–like exudate. The remainder of the physical examination was normal. A throat culture was obtained. Aspirin, fluids, and bed rest were recommended as supportive therapy and he was instructed to return the next day.

On July 3, he appeared to be less acutely ill, temperature was 101.6°F (38.7°C) and the tonsillar exudate was thicker, resembling cottage cheese in consistency. The original throat culture was reported to be free of beta-hemolytic streptococcal colonies. A second throat swab was negative by a rapid antigen test for group A streptococci. In addition, throat and rectal swabs for viral culture and an acute-phase serum for baseline serologic studies were obtained.

The boy improved rapidly and felt well by July 6, and he returned to his normal activities. A convalescent-phase serum was obtained 3 weeks later. The laboratory studies revealed the following: viral cultures—throat, adenovirus type 3; rectum, no virus isolated. Serologic studies:

| | ANTIBODY TITER OF SERA COLLECTED | |
|---|---|---|
| ANTIGEN | *July 3* | *July 24* |
| Streptolysin O | 1:100 | 1:100 |
| Adenovirus (group-soluble antigen | <1:4 | 1:16 |
| Heterophil | <1:56 | <1:56 |

## Case 2 Discussion

The illness in this 10-year-old boy erroneously could have been considered to be streptococcal. The harried clinic staff could have simply given the patient a "shot of penicillin." However, the intern recognized that summer is not when group A streptococcal respiratory infection is prevalent and that a virus was more likely responsible for this illness. Therefore, symptomatic measures were employed. The validity of this approach was verified by failure of two throat swabs to yield group A streptococci. Note that the cooperative parents did not demand that an antimicrobial agent be given and brought the patient back for follow-up.

Further retrospective evidence that this infection was not streptococcal was provided by the lack of a rise in antistreptolysin O titer. Isolation of type 3 adenovirus from the throat and a diagnostic, greater than fourfold rise in antibody to adenovirus group antigens proved that this patient had an acute adenovirus infection. Such special laboratory procedures are not often available or warranted but provided instructive data in this instance.

Note that the emergency clinic staff was aware that infectious mononucleosis can simulate streptococcal pharyngitis, as evidenced by their request for a heterophil titer (see Chapter 8).

## Case History 3

A 10-year-old boy developed fever and sore throat in April. His physician diagnosed streptococcal pharyngitis, confirmed by a positive rapid GAS antigen-detection test, and prescribed 10 days of oral penicillin. The patient rapidly improved, discontinued his medication after 3 days, and was well until 3 weeks after the onset of sore throat when he developed fever to 103°F and exquisite pain in the left knee. At this time the knee was mildly red and swollen but very painful to touch, he was unable to bear weight, and a loud apical systolic murmur radiating to the axilla was noted. He was hospitalized and confined to bed rest without medication. By the next morning, the left knee was much improved but the right wrist was very painful and slightly swollen. He was mildly tachypneic, quite tachycardic (pulse 140/min), and the liver was palpable 3 cm below the right costal margin. Laboratory studies indicated 1+ cardiomegaly on chest x-ray, WBC of 18,000/mm³ with 70% PMNs, 10% bands, 15% lymphocytes, ESR = 60 mm/h (uncorrected), throat culture negative for *Streptococcus pyogenes*, prolonged PR interval, and antistreptolysin O titer = 1:1600. Echocardiogram showed a small pericardial effusion, mild left ventricular dilatation, and moderate mitral regurgitation. Therapy with prednisone, penicillin, digitalis, and diuretics was instituted. The patient was markedly improved by the next day from both the arthritic and cardiac perspectives. Prednisone was tapered over the next 2 weeks, and aspirin was instituted. When seen 6 months later, the patient had persistent evidence of mild mitral regurgitation without congestive failure. He was receiving monthly injections of benzathine penicillin prophylaxis and had been instructed regarding the importance of endocarditis prophylaxis. Five years later, no evidence of residual cardiac disease was detectable. He had been highly compliant with his monthly prophylaxis.

## Case 3 Discussion

The failure to receive 10 days' treatment for acute streptococcal pharyngitis placed this child at risk for acute rheumatic fever (ARF). His clinical illness fulfilled the modified Jones criteria (Table 7–5) with two major and three minor (fever, acute-phase reactants, prolonged PR interval) criteria and evidence of previous streptococcal infection. The migratory nature of the arthritis is striking. Prompt suppression of the acute manifestations by antiinflammatory therapy (begun only after the diagnosis was established) is typical. Corticosteroids were chosen because of the evidence for congestive heart failure. This case demonstrates that in some patients healing of their cardiac lesions occurs if they are protected from recurrent attacks of ARF and from infective endocarditis.

## Case History 4

A 17-year-old high school student with no prior known renal disease developed sore throat and fever of 103°F on November 18, lasting 3 days. On November 28, he developed hematuria, puffy eyelids, and swollen ankles. A physician noted an in-flamed pharynx, enlarged and reddened tonsils, and palpable cervical lymph nodes, as well as pitting edema of his feet and pretibial areas and blood pressure of 165/105 mm Hg. Urine contained 4+ protein, 20–30 erythrocytes and 25–30 leukocytes per high-powered field, some hyaline and granular casts, and one erythrocyte cast. The physician admitted the patient to a hospital where he was given bed rest and 10 days of oral penicillin. Throat culture revealed 4+ group A streptococci, antistreptolysin O titer was 1:500 (elevated), C3 level was 53 mg/dL (normal, 110–160), and serum creatinine was 2.5 mg/dL (normal, <1.5 mg/dL).

## Case 4 Discussion

This teenager presents with typical postpharyngeal acute poststreptococcal glomerulonephritis. Oliguria and hypertension persist up to 1–2 months, and the disease process resolves spontaneously. Younger patients rarely develop chronic renal disease, but adults may develop evidence of progressive glomerulonephritis.

# REFERENCES

**Books**

Bluestone, C. D., and Klein, J. O. *Otitis Media in Infants and Children.* 2nd ed. Philadelphia: W. B. Saunders Co., 1994.

Breese, B. B., and Hall, C. B., eds. *Beta-Hemolytic Streptococcal Disease.* Boston: Houghton-Mifflin, 1978.

Shulman, S. T., ed. *Pharyngitis: Management in an Era of Declining Rheumatic Fever.* New York: Praeger, 1984.

Taranta, A., and Markowitz, M. *Rheumatic Fever,* 2nd ed. New York: Kluwer, 1990.

Wannamaker, L. W., and Matsen, J. M., eds. *Streptococci and Streptococcal Diseases: Recognition, Understanding, and Management.* New York: Academic Press, 1972.

**Review Articles**

Ayoub, E. M., and Kaplan, E. L. Host-parasite interaction in the pathogenesis of rheumatic fever. *J. Rheumatol.* 18(Suppl.30):6–11, 1991.

Bluestone, C. D. Management of otitis media in infants and children: Current role of old and new antimicrobial agents. *Pediatr. Infect. Dis. J.* 7:S129–136, 1988.

Gordis, L. The virtual disappearance of rheumatic fever in the United States. *Circulation* 72:1155–1162, 1985.

Stollerman, G. H. Rheumatogenic group A streptococci and the return of rheumatic fever. *Adv. Intern. Med.* 35:1, 1990.

Taubert, K., Rowley, A. H., and Shulman, S. T. Seven-year national survey of Kawasaki disease and acute rheumatic fever. *Pediatr. Infect. Dis. J.* 13:704–708, 1994.

**Articles**

Banck, G., and Nyman, M. Tonsillitis and rash associated with *Corynebacterium haemolyticum. J. Infect. Dis.* 154:1037–1040, 1986.

Bisno, A. L., Shulman, S. T., and Dajani, A. S. The rise and fall (and rise?) of rheumatic fever. *JAMA 259*:728–729, 1988.

Breese, B. B. A simple scorecard for the tentative diagnosis of streptococcal pharyngitis. *Am. J. Dis. Child. 131*:514–517, 1977.

Committee on Rheumatic Fever, Endocarditis, and Kawasaki Disease of the Council on Cardiovascular Disease in the Young. The American Heart Association. Prevention of rheumatic fever. *Pediatr. Infect. Dis. J. 8*: 263–266, 1989.

Committee on Rheumatic Fever, Endocarditis, and Kawasaki Disease of the Council on Cardiovascular Disease in the Young. The American Heart Association. Jones Criteria, 1992 Update. Guidelines for the diagnosis of rheumatic fever. *JAMA 268*:2069–2073, 1992.

Cunningham, M. W., McCormack, J. M., Fenderson, P. G., et al. Human and murine antibodies cross-reactive with streptococcal M proteins and myosin recognize the sequence Gln-Lys-Ser-Lys-Gln in M protein. *J. Immunol. 143*:2677–2683, 1989.

Lancefield, R. C. A microprecipitin-technic for classifying hemolytic streptococci. *Proc. Soc. Exp. Biol. Med. 38*:473 –478, 1938.

Massell, B. F., Chute, C. G., Walker, A. M., et al. Penicillin and the marked decrease in morbidity and mortality from rheumatic fever in the United States. *N. Engl. J. Med. 318*:280–286, 1988.

Potter, E. V., Lipschultz, S. A., Abidh, S., et al. Twelve to 17 year follow-up of patients with post-streptococcal acute glomerulonephritis in Trinidad. *N. Engl. J. Med. 307*:725–729, 1982.

Stevens, D. L., Tanner, M. H., Winship, J., et al. Severe group A streptococcal infections associated with a toxic shock-like syndrome and scarlet fever toxin A. *N. Engl. J. Med. 321*:1–7, 1989.

Veasy, L. G., Wiedmeier, S. E., Orsmond, G. S., et al. Resurgence of acute rheumatic fever in the intermountain area of the United States. *N. Engl. J. Med. 316*:421–427, 1986.

# 8

# VIRAL INFECTIONS OF THE UPPER RESPIRATORY TRACT, INFECTIOUS MONONUCLEOSIS, AND THE CHRONIC FATIGUE SYNDROME

BEN Z. KATZ, M.D.

In Chapter 12, viral infections of the lower respiratory tract are discussed. Some of the viral agents discussed in that chapter (e.g., influenza, parainfluenza, and respiratory syncytial virus) also cause upper respiratory tract disease, usually in concert with disease elsewhere in the respiratory tree. In this chapter, viral agents whose pathology is limited to the upper respiratory tract are delineated, followed by descriptions of infectious mononucleosis and the chronic fatigue syndrome.

## THE COMMON COLD

Colds are among the most frequently occurring illnesses worldwide. Typically, children in the United States average three to eight colds per year, while adults experience half that number. Ten percent of pediatricians' office visits are due to colds.

Colds are most frequent in the winter months, although cold temperature per se does not cause or increase susceptibility to colds; generally, it is thought that the crowded condition of schoolrooms, day-care centers, and offices during the winter promotes transmission. School-aged children serve as the chief reservoir of cold viruses; as new viruses capable of causing colds are introduced into the classroom, spread occurs. Students then bring the viruses home to their family members, who then spread them to the community. Smokers do not have more colds per year than nonsmokers, but their colds are more severe, probably because the preexisting mucociliary damage caused by smoke exacerbates the tissue injury caused by the offending virus.

Rhinoviruses (*rhin* is Greek for nose) account for about one third of all colds. They are members of the Picornaviridae (small RNA virus) family. Rhinoviruses contain a single-stranded, positive-sense RNA genome surrounded by an icosahedral protein capsid.

The virus has the ability to survive for considerable periods of time on fomites.

Coronaviruses are responsible for about 15% of colds. They are positive-stranded RNA viruses that grow poorly in tissue culture and are not as easily spread as rhinoviruses.

Adenoviruses and myxoviruses (which are discussed in Chapter 12) each cause about 5% of colds. No organism is recovered from about 30% of patients with colds; nevertheless, it is assumed that the majority of these colds are also viral in origin.

In general, cold viruses are transmitted mainly via people's hands (fomites); small- and large-particle aerosols (see Chapter 12) play a more minor role in transmission. Cold viruses usually gain access to the respiratory tract via self-inoculation or inhalation into the respiratory epithelium of the nasal mucosa; occasionally inoculation via the conjunctiva can occur. Following virus acquisition, local replication of the virus in the respiratory tract occurs, eventually resulting in increased amounts of nasal secretions that are thicker than usual.

Symptoms (nasal stuffiness, sore throat, sneezing) begin 2–3 days following infection. There is abrupt onset of watery nasal discharge, nasal stuffiness, and modest irritation of the throat. Brisk rhinorrhea persists for 2–4 days and then gradually subsides. Nasal discharge initially is thin (mucoid and acellular) but becomes thicker as virus replicates, causing inflammatory cells and detached epithelial cells to accumulate in the secretions. Colds are generally afebrile infections; at most, low-grade fevers (temperature elevations of about 1°F) are seen. Viral shedding is maximal 2–7 days following infection. Viremia is uncommon; the sinuses, however, may be involved. Local interferon is produced, and this presumably plays a role in controlling infection. Serum and especially secretory antibody are produced and may play a role in limiting infection as well. The role of cell-mediated immunity in the pathogenesis of colds (if any) is unknown.

Physical findings are usually limited to hyperemia and edema of the nasal and pharyngeal mucosa. The skin around the nares can become red and swollen, particularly when rhinorrhea is intense. Physical examination should focus on ruling out diseases more serious than a simple cold, especially if the patient complains of unusual (e.g., facial pain, earache) or unusually severe (e.g., high fever or severe pharyngitis) symptoms. Marked pharyngeal injection or exudate, pseudomembrane formation, palatal petechiae or vesicles in the oropharynx shift consideration to streptococcal pharyngitis, diphtheria, mononucleosis, or coxsackie or adenoviral infection, respectively. The nasal turbinates should be inspected for polyps, which may suggest allergic rhinitis or cystic fibrosis, and for foreign bodies in children. Adults and adolescents should be questioned about cocaine use; patients who smoke should be reminded that smokers have more severe colds. Secondary bacterial infection of the middle ear and sinuses occasionally occurs; otoscopic examination of the tympanic membranes and physical and radiographic examination of the sinuses are appropriate when patients complain of headache, sinus tenderness, or purulent nasal discharge.

Laboratory work-up is generally not necessary. Culture or serologic confirmation of the causative viral agent has no effect on management and is not cost-effective. One exception is the patient with acute oropharyngitis who requires an antigen screen and/or culture for group A beta-hemolytic streptococcal (*Streptococcus pyogenes*) infection, as discussed in Chapter 7.

Management of the typical cold is symptomatic. Antibiotics are unwarranted unless bacterial superinfection has occurred. Sympathomimetic amines (e.g., phenylephrine and pseudoephedrine) produce vascular constriction and thus decrease mucus production. Decongestants may also be used, but rebound vasodilatation can occur. Antihistamines may reduce sneezing; in addition, most antihistamines have a sedative effect, which may be beneficial at nighttime but can interfere with daytime activities. Cough can usually be controlled with dextromethorphan, a nonnarcotic cough suppressant. Analgesics such as aspirin or acetaminophen are useful for patients with headache or constitutional symptoms.

Practical measures that can interrupt the transmission of cold viruses include fluids to prevent drying and inspissation of mucus, the covering of sneezes and coughs (preferably with a tissue or handkerchief), and frequent handwashing. The latter two measures will prevent hand-to-hand, hand-fomite-hand, and large-droplet transmission of cold viruses.

## ACUTE VIRAL OROPHARYNGITIS

Pharyngitis is a common feature of the common cold, influenza, respiratory syncytial virus infection, and infectious mononucleosis. In acute oropharyngitis, however, inflammation of the mucosa of the mouth or throat is the patient's dominant complaint.

In school-aged children, group A streptococcus is the single most common cause of acute pharyngitis (see Chapter 7). In children under 6, viral causes predominate. In general, viral pharyngitis (except for mononucleosis) is not severe and is not associated with cervical lymphadenopathy; symptoms are nonspecific and consist of sore throat, fever, hoarseness, cough, rhinitis, conjunctivitis, and otitis media. The four acute viral pharyngitites discussed in this section comprise distinct syndromes linked to specific viral agents, and are easily recognized clinically.

### Acute Herpetic Gingivostomatitis

Most cases of acute herpetic gingivostomatitis are due to herpes simplex virus serotype 1 (HSV-1). HSV-1 (oral herpes) is an endemic virus that infects 75% of the population by age 5. Humans are the only natural reservoir, so all new infections are the result of person-to-person spread. Transmission is usually via saliva (generally from someone with lesions) either through kissing or the sharing of secretions that occurs between children at play. HSV is a double-stranded DNA virus with a fragile lipid envelope, so viability on fomites is limited. Cells of the skin or mucous membranes have receptors for the viral membrane glycoprotein D, and thus they serve as the portal of viral entry. Following a brief (several day) incubation period, acute replication of HSV-1 leads to viral nuclear inclusions, the fusion of adjacent infected cells to produce multinucleated giant cells, and vesicles. Classically, one sees grouped vesicles on an erythematous base (Fig. 8–1). Other symptoms that may be seen with primary infection include fever, lymphadenopathy, malaise, myalgias, inability to eat, and irritability. Because of friction, vesicles in the oropharynx rupture, leading to ulcer formation; the absence of vesicles in mouth lesions occasionally makes the diagnosis of a herpes infection of the mouth difficult. Mucosal ulcers generally heal without scarring unless they become secondarily infected.

Immunocompetent individuals develop an antibody response to HSV-1 within days and generate cytotoxic T lymphocytes capable of destroying cells infected with HSV-1 within 2–3 weeks of infection. Many cases of primary oral herpes are asymptomatic or mild, lacking conspicuous vesicles or ulcers; seroconversion is thus the only means for verifying the herpetic etiology in such cases. Some individuals,

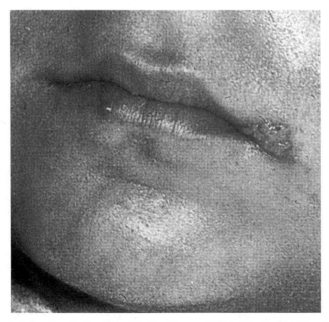

**FIGURE 8–1.** Acute herpetic gingivostomatitis "cold sore." Note the grouped vesicles on the (erythematous) base at the corner of the mouth. (From Simon, C. and Janner, M. *Atlas of Pediatric Diseases with Differential Diagnosis.* 2nd ed. Stuttgart: F. K. Schattauer, 1990. With permission.)

on the other hand, including those with impaired cell-mediated immunity, may experience a protracted infection with severe, painful, ulcerative stomatitis accompanied by fever and anterior cervical lymphadenopathy.

All herpes viruses can exist in a latent state following acute infection. Periodically, the virus may reactivate and cause recurrent infection, which is generally milder than primary disease; for oral herpes the lesions of reactivation infection are on the outer lip and are often referred to as "fever blisters" or "cold sores" (Fig. 8–1). The site of latency of HSV-1 is the trigeminal ganglion, which becomes infected during the primary episode. Only a minority of individuals experience clinically obvious episodic reactivation. Compared to genital HSV-2 infection, reactivation of oral herpes is milder and occurs one-sixth as often. Reactivation infections are worse in patients with eczema and can be triggered by local stimuli such as injury or sunlight exposure, or systemic conditions such as emotional stress, menstruation, coincident infection, or fevers. No conspicuous defects in cell-mediated immunity can be identified in the majority of HSV-1 seropositive individuals who experience recurrent lesions. The frequency of recurrence is unpredictable; recurrences generally become less severe with time. Acyclovir is active against HSV but is generally not indicated in the immunocompetent host.

In contrast, patients with impaired cell-mediated immunity are at risk for severe mucocutaneous ulceration and dissemination of the virus into the lower respiratory tract and elsewhere from either primary or recurrent herpetic infections. Oral or intravenous acyclovir is generally indicated in this setting.

Specific laboratory diagnosis is usually not necessary. However, herpes simplex viruses grow very rapidly in tissue culture; overnight growth is not unusual. Vesicle fluid and, preferably, the base of a freshly unroofed vesicle, vigorously swabbed, are the best sources of live virus. The earlier in the illness the specimen is obtained, and the faster it is placed in transport medium and brought to the viral diagnostic laboratory, the more likely one is to grow the virus.

## Adenoviral Pharyngoconjunctival Fever

Several adenovirus serotypes can infect the upper respiratory tract. As mentioned previously and as discussed in Chapter 12, adenoviruses can cause simple colds and pneumonia. In addition, adenoviruses cause a unique triad of fever, pharyngitis, and conjunctivitis, appropriately termed acute pharyngoconjunctival fever.

Acute pharyngoconjunctival fever can occur sporadically or in community-wide outbreaks; in the latter situation it usually occurs in the summer and is generally centered around swimming pools or other fomites. Several nosocomial outbreaks have also been traced to the contaminated hands of health care workers; this is probably related to the ability of the virus to survive for at least brief periods of time on fomites (see Chapter 12). It appears that the conjunctivae need to be inoculated directly for pharyngoconjunctival fever to develop.

Young children are most likely to be affected. The incubation period is 2–4 days. Lymphoid hyperplasia with prominent tonsillar and cervical lymph node enlargement and enlargement of the adenoids occurs as well; in fact, adenovirus was first isolated from adenoidal tissue, whence its name.

Laboratory confirmation of the diagnosis of pharyngoconjunctival fever is rarely necessary. Adenoviruses grow in the standard tissue culture systems used in virology laboratories. Direct antigen detection and serologic tests are also available.

## Herpangina and Hand-Foot-and-Mouth Syndrome

Enterovirus infections are common in warm weather months. The enteroviruses are single-stranded RNA viruses that include the polioviruses, coxsackieviruses, and echoviruses. These viruses often produce both upper and lower respiratory tract infections, often accompanied by a rash or meningitis. Many other organisms can produce similar syndromes. However, two distinctive enteroviral upper respiratory tract syndromes have been described: herpangina and hand-foot-and-mouth syndrome.

Herpangina (*anchone* means constricting in Greek) is an acute-onset febrile illness with characteristic, discrete vesicular lesions distributed on the *posterior* portion of the oropharynx: the posterior buccal, tonsillar, lingual, and pharyngeal mucosal surfaces. As is true for herpetic gingivostomatitis (in the *anterior* oropharynx), these vesicles can convert to open ulcers due to mechanical forces in the mouth. Fever can be as high as 104°F, and sore throat pain may be so intense that swallowing is difficult. Other symptoms can include headache and backache. Coxsackie A enteroviruses are the most frequently associated with herpangina, but coxsackie B and echoviruses can also produce this syndrome.

Hand-foot-and-mouth syndrome is generally linked to coxsackie A16 and also has fever and vesicles as prominent features of illness; other enteroviruses can cause this syndrome as well. Painful oral lesions follow the onset of fever. These lesions begin as vesicles and subsequently erode into ulcers. In contrast to herpangina, hand-foot-and-mouth oral vesicles are distributed *anteriorly* in the oropharynx; on the buccal and gingival mucosa and on the tongue. As its name implies, patients develop vesicles on the hands and feet as well as in the mouth; vesicles can also be found elsewhere on the body in a minority of cases.

Both herpangina and hand-foot-and-mouth syndrome are self-limited, usually resolving within a week. Laboratory diagnosis is rarely necessary. Viral culture of the pharynx, vesicle fluid, or the vesicular base often yields a pathogen when culture confirmation is sought. Serologic testing is of limited value.

## INFECTIOUS MONONUCLEOSIS

Infectious mononucleosis (IM) is a clinical entity usually caused by primary infection with Epstein-Barr virus (EBV). Other common etiologies include cytomegalovirus and toxoplasmosis (see below). Acute pharyngotonsillitis is a very prominent feature; generally the most severe cases of pharyngitis are seen with IM and *Streptococcus pyogenes*. IM also commonly involves the lymph nodes, spleen, liver, and peripheral blood; rarely, the lungs, kidney, skin, myocardium, and central nervous system are involved.

EBV, like HSV, is a ubiquitous double-stranded DNA herpesvirus that exists in both a latent and lytic form and is spread via secretions, usually saliva. Initial EBV infection usually occurs in young children. In developing countries and areas of developed countries with crowding or suboptimal sanitation, EBV seropositivity rates of almost 100% are common by age 5. Primary EBV infection is usually asymptomatic or clinically nonspecific in young children; thus, IM is uncommon in this age group.

In the upper socioeconomic groups of affluent societies, up to 50% of individuals entering adolescence escape infection with EBV. However, since the virus is shed sporadically in saliva by all seropositive individuals, seronegative adolescents and young adults may encounter EBV. It is these older individuals who then often develop IM. EBV is occasionally transmitted via blood transfusion. By age 30, EBV seroprevalence approaches 100% in all social strata of all countries.

After a 30- to 50-day incubation period, about one half of adolescents and young adults primarily infected with EBV develop IM. It may be because many of the clinical manifestations of IM are due to the body's immune response to the virus that IM is usually not seen in young children who lack robust immune responses.

Infection is often heralded by 3–5 days of mild headache, malaise, and fatigue. This is typically followed by fever, lymphadenopathy, and sore throat. The disease in children is generally mild; in adults it is more severe and has a more protracted course. Recurrences have only rarely been reported.

The temperature usually rises to 103°F and gradually falls over a variable period of time, averaging 6 days. In a severe case it is not unusual for temperatures to hover between 104° and 105°F and to persist for several weeks. Younger children are more likely to be afebrile or to have only minimal temperature elevation.

Generalized lymphadenopathy is a hallmark of IM. Shortly after the onset of illness, the lymph nodes rapidly enlarge. Any chain may become enlarged, but the cervical group is the one most commonly involved. The nodes are usually single, firm, tender, 2–4 cm in diameter, and not matted. Massive mediastinal and hilar lymph node enlargement leading to respiratory embarrassment is sometimes seen. Mesenteric lymphadenitis frequently has been confused with acute appendicitis. Lymph node enlargement gradually subsides over a period of days to weeks, depending on the severity and extent of involvement.

Sore throat is one of the cardinal symptoms of IM. The tonsils are usually enlarged, reddened and, in more than 50% of patients covered with an exudate. Petechiae appear on the palate between the 5th and 17th days of illness in up to 25% of IM patients. Six to 20 lesions are usually seen, grouped for the most part at the juncture of the hard and soft palate; they usually become brownish in color within 2 days and then fade.

Between the second and third weeks of illness moderate enlargement of the spleen occurs in approximately 50% of cases. In rare instances, splenic enlargement may be followed by trauma-induced or (less commonly) spontaneous splenic rupture that may lead to hemorrhage, shock, or death. Once splenomegaly is appreciated, repeated splenic examinations should be discouraged.

The triad of lymphadenopathy, splenomegaly, and exudative pharyngitis in a febrile patient is typical but not pathognomonic of infectious mononucleosis. Other less common manifestations of primary EBV infection include hepatitis, rash, and pneumonia as well as immunologic, cardiac, and hematologic complications. Characteristically, a rash is seen in patients with IM treated with ampicillin or related antibiotics.

### Pathogenesis

EBV enters the oropharynx in saliva and replicates in oropharyngeal mucosal cells, producing lytic destruction of pharyngeal epithelium and resulting in severe pharyngitis. EBV is lymphotropic, attaching to the C3d (complement) receptor on the cytoplasmic membrane of mature B cells. It is in the lymphoid tissue of the oropharynx that B cells are infected. Binding of EBV to B lymphocytes activates cellular signals that trigger a polyclonal proliferative response, resulting in worsening pharyngitis, lymphadenopathy, and hepatosplenomegaly. The disease resolves when reactive and EBV-specific cytotoxic T cells, natural killer (NK) cells, and neutralizing antibodies against EBV develop.

### Laboratory Findings and Diagnosis

**Hematologic Profile.** The white blood cell count is variable during the first week of IM. An absolute increase in the number of *atypical lymphocytes* in the second week of illness is a characteristic finding. The atypical lymphocytes are generally not EBV-infected B cells, but T cells reactive to the infected B cells. They are larger than normal lymphocytes with basophilic, vacuolated cytoplasm and in-

dented nuclei. Atypical lymphocytes are not specific for infectious mononucleosis. However, in infectious mononucleosis, there are usually more than 10% atypical cells in the peripheral smear. In young children, atypical lymphocytosis is seen less often.

**Heterophil Antibodies.** Heterophil antibodies were the first serologic markers described (by Paul and Bunnell) in association with IM. A heterophil antibody test is the most commonly used test to diagnose IM. Most sera of patients with infectious mononucleosis cause sheep red blood cells to agglutinate after they have been absorbed with guinea pig kidney antigens but not after absorption with beef red blood cells. The reverse is occasionally true of sera from uninfected individuals (see Table 8–1). The heterophil antibody responsible for this differential absorption in IM is principally of the IgM class, appears during the first and second weeks of illness, and disappears gradually over 6 months. Young children under 4 with acute EBV infection are likely to be heterophil antibody–negative.

Heterophil antibodies are not specific for IM. However, a differential heterophil antibody response in the appropriate clinical setting is virtually pathognomonic for acute IM. Rapid heterophil slide tests (e.g., the monospot test) have been developed as diagnostic tests for IM. The advantages of these tests include a low incidence of false positive-reactions, a high degree of specificity, and rapidity and ease of performance. These rapid tests are a valuable diagnostic aid in clinical practice.

**Antibody Titers to Specific EBV Antigens (see Fig. 8–2).** The first antibodies generated during the course of primary EBV infection are against the viral capsid antigen (VCA) complex of EBV. Generally, both IgM and IgG anti-VCA antibodies are measured. The IgM antibodies are transient; the IgG antibodies persist for life.

Later in the course of primary EBV infection, antibodies against the early antigen (EA)

### TABLE 8–1.   HETEROPHIL ANTIBODY REACTIONS IN NORMAL AND IM* SERA

| | AUGGLUTINATION OF SHEEP RED BLOOD CELLS AFTER ABSORPTION WITH | |
| --- | --- | --- |
| IN THE PRESENCE OF | *Guinea Pig Kidney Cells* | *Beef Red Blood Cells* |
| Some normal human sera | − | + |
| Most IM* sera | + | − |

*IM = Infectious mononucleosis.

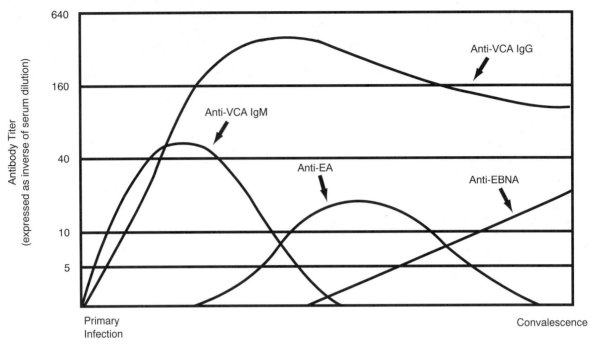

**FIGURE 8–2.** Idealized antibody responses to primary EBV infection. A titer of less than 1:5 is considered negative.

complex are generated. (These antigens are produced by the virus prior to EBV DNA replication.) EA antibodies are present transiently, usually disappearing after 6 months; however, low levels of antibody against the EA complex may be detectable in healthy individuals for years after acute IM.

Antibody against the EBV nuclear antigen (EBNA) complex appears more slowly, taking from 1–6 months to become detectable. (The EBNA complex consists of neoantigens produced in the nucleus of all EBV-infected B cells.) In contrast to the kinetics of the antibody responses against VCA and EA, antibodies to EBNA *rise* during convalescence and then level off. All late convalescent sera from healthy individuals contain modest antibody titers against EBNA.

Because of the differing kinetics of the different EBV antibody responses, one can often diagnose EBV infection based on a single serum sample. Thus, the presence of antibodies against VCA and the absence of antibodies to EBNA is diagnostic of a *primary* EBV infection. Acute illness may also be diagnosed if IgM antibody to VCA is present, but this assay is difficult to perform and may yield false-positive reactions if rheumatoid factor is present in the blood. An unusually high antibody response to VCA or EA in the presence of antibodies against EBNA may be a sign of secondary or *reactivated* EBV infection. Modest titers to both VCA and EBNA are characteristic of past disease (see Table 8–2).

**Autoantibodies.** Autoantibodies, which may or may not cause symptoms, are occasionally produced during IM. For example, one may see antinuclear antibodies and rheuma-

**TABLE 8–2.    TYPICAL SEROLOGIC PROFILES OF PRIMARY AND CONVALESCENT EBV INFECTION**

| TYPE OF INFECTION | SEROLOGIC PROFILES(S): PRESENCE OF |
|---|---|
| Primary | IgM−VCA<br>or<br>IgG−VCA ± EA + no antibody against EBNA |
| Convalescent | IgG−VCA + EBNA ± EA |

toid factor; these usually produce no clinical sequelae. In contrast, antiplatelet antibodies have been associated with thrombocytopenia, and production of anti-I, anti-i, and anti-HLA class I antibodies may be associated with severe hemolytic disease. Hypogammaglobulinemia or isolated IgA deficiency may also be seen.

**Detection of the Virus.** EBV does not grow in standard viral culture systems. The presence of biologically active virus can be assayed by means of the virus' ability to immortalize cultured B lymphocytes from an EBV-seronegative individual. This so-called immortalization assay is time consuming (6–8 weeks) and requires specialized tissue-culture facilities. Viral genomic material can be found in lymphoid tissue and occasionally in the peripheral blood if there is a high level of leukoviremia (e.g., in acute IM or in the immunosuppressed). The most specific method for demonstrating EBV DNA or RNA in pathologic material is nucleic acid hybridization.

### Treatment

Infectious mononucleosis is a self-limited disease; treatment is chiefly supportive. Bed rest is indicated in the acute stage of disease. Aspirin and saline gargles usually control the pain or discomfort caused by the enlarged lymph nodes and pharyngitis. In severe cases, codeine or meperidine may be required.

Short courses of corticosteroid therapy may have a beneficial effect. In many instances, symptoms referable to the throat and enlarged lymph nodes improve within 24 h on steroids. Nevertheless, many experts are reluctant to use steroids for what is ultimately a self-limited disease because the long-term effects of such intervention on the normal immune response to EBV are unknown and because of rare reports of neurologic complications following steroid use. Nevertheless, steroids should be considered for treatment of severe cases of IM such as those characterized by respiratory embarrassment or symptomatic hematologic complications.

Contact sports should be avoided until the patients are fully recovered. In patients with splenomegaly, contact sports should be avoided until the spleen has returned to its normal size; this usually takes 2–6 months.

Acyclovir acts on the lytic (but not the latent) phase of EBV replication. When given parenterally to patients with acute IM, acyclovir reduces the level of oropharyngeal viral replication; however, after cessation of treatment, replication returns to previously high levels. There is little or no reduction in the number of EBV-infected B cells in the peripheral circulation and little effect on the clinical course of acute IM. High-dose oral acyclovir is ineffective clinically as well. Therefore, acyclovir is not recommended for routine therapy of acute IM.

Individuals who have impaired cell-mediated immunity may experience especially severe primary or reactivated EBV infection or suffer from an uncontrolled, malignant lymphoproliferative disorder. Patients with the *X-linked lymphoproliferative syndrome* (Duncan's syndrome) have a genetically defective (probably NK cell) immune response to EBV infection. Severe or fatal infectious mononucleosis is seen in two thirds of these patients, and profound, secondary hypogammaglobulinemia or B-cell lymphoma occurs in the remainder. *Organ transplant recipients* treated with immunosuppressive agents (especially antithymocyte globulin and cyclosporine) may develop EBV-associated B-cell lymphoproliferative diseases, including lymphomas. *Human immunodeficiency virus (HIV) infection* is linked to several EBV-associated diseases including oral "hairy" leukoplakia, lymphoid interstitial pneumonitis, and malignant lymphoma. There is also a strong association between EBV and nasopharyngeal carcinoma. Ironically, the role played by EBV in African *Burkitt's lymphoma*, in which the virus was first discovered, is unclear. Acyclovir is often given to immunosuppressed patients with documented or suspected EBV infection, although its efficacy in these situations is debatable.

### Mononucleosis Syndromes

EBV is the most common cause of infectious mononucleosis (50–90% of cases); the virus is responsible for all cases of heterophil-positive IM and about one third of heterophil-negative IM. The other two thirds of the patients with heterophil-negative IM lack VCA IgM antibody and have an illness due to some other agent. Primary cytomegalovirus (CMV) infection, particularly when acquired after childhood, can produce an illness with pharyngitis, lymphadenopathy, and fever that follows a clinical course very similar to EBV-induced IM, although the atypical lymphocytosis is usually less dramatic. CMV can be isolated from urine during the acute illness, and serum contains IgG CMV-specific antibody. A rapid urine "shell vial" culture assay is now widely available. In total, CMV causes 3–8% of cases of IM.

Primary symptomatic infection with *Toxoplasma gondii* causes 1–3% of cases of IM. Toxoplasma infection can be acquired from contact with infected cats or from the ingestion of improperly cooked meat, particularly lamb or pork. Following ingestion, the organism invades the blood, proliferates and disseminates, and produces fever and lymphadenopathy. Hepatitis and atypical lymphocytosis are uncommon. Acute toxoplasmosis can be diagnosed by demonstrating specific IgM antibody or a significant rise in IgG antibody against the organism.

Human herpesvirus 6 (HHV-6) is a recently characterized member of the herpes virus family that, like EBV, is lymphotropic. HHV-6 causes roseola infantum, a common childhood exanthem, and some cases of nonspecific childhood febrile illnesses or febrile seizures. Evaluation of patients with mononucleosis syndromes but without serologic evidence of acute EBV, CMV, or toxoplasma infection reveals that approximately one third have demonstrable IgM antibody specific for HHV-6. In most cases, a 1- to 3-week-long febrile illness with mild pharyngitis, cervical adenopathy, lymphocytosis, with atypical lymphocytes and abnormal liver function studies is seen.

Acute infection with *human immunodeficiency virus type 1 (HIV-1)* is associated with symptoms about half of the time; the disease seen is often described as either "flu-like" or "mononucleosis-like." This illness usually occurs 3–8 weeks following acquisition of HIV. Standard enzyme-linked immunosorbent assay (ELISA) HIV serology may be negative at this early phase of illness. HIV antigen can be detected in serum, however, and antibody is invariably detected upon repeat testing 2–3 months later. This acute infection usually lasts a maximum of 1–4 weeks.

The first step in the laboratory evaluation of a patient with a mononucleosis syndrome is a heterophil antibody. If the heterophil test is negative, EBV-VCA, urine for CMV, and toxoplasmosis IgM titers are the tests of choice. Serologic testing for HHV-6 is not widely available. Antigen and antibody assays for acute HIV infection are appropriate for patients at risk.

A minority of mononucleosis cases have no etiologic agent identified. Since lymphoma can have features that resemble mononucleosis early in the course of disease, adenopathy that persists for more than a few weeks, especially if associated with anemia, weight loss, or abnormalities on chest radiography, should be considered for excisional biopsy.

## CHRONIC FATIGUE SYNDROME

In the past decade considerable attention has been given in both the medical and lay press to a chronic clinical entity known by a variety of names (e.g., neurasthenia, fibromyalgia, "sick building syndrome") over the past half-century, characterized principally by disabling, persistent fatigue. Fever, pharyngitis, tender lymphadenopathy, arthralgias, and myalgias are frequent accompanying complaints. The clinical signs and symptoms of this illness suggest an infectious etiology, and several reports in the mid-1980s implicated EBV, either as a chronically persistent primary infection, or as a reactivated infection, since afflicted patients had modestly elevated EBV antibody titers. Upon further study, however, no consistent relationship with EBV or any other pathogen (e.g., brucella, influenza, retroviruses, enteroviruses, HHV-6, CMV, *Borrelia burgdorferi*, or toxoplasma) has been found. The disease is now termed *chronic fatigue syndrome* (CFS). A screening evaluation to rule out malignancy; autoimmune disease; and endocrinologic, neuromuscular, or psychiatric disorders is often necessary.

Immunologic evaluations of CFS patients have shown aberrations (e.g., NK cell dysfunction). There is a high incidence of depressive symptoms in these patients; whether the immunologic aberrations cause the depression or *vice versa* is unclear. However, after an initial set of screening tests (e.g., chest x-ray, complete blood count, tuberculin skin test, urinalysis, erythrocyte sedimentation rate), continued laboratory studies are usually unnecessary and only reinforce the idea that the patient is seriously ill. Supportive counseling, caring follow-up, and perhaps antidepressive medication are all that is recommended for CFS at this time, as there is no proven, effective specific therapy. The prognosis of CFS in adolescents is much better than that in adults, in that most adolescents are significantly improved within 1 or 2 years.

## CASE HISTORIES

### CASE HISTORY 1

A 19-year-old college sophomore was seen at the student health clinic in early October complaining of malaise and fever. She stated that 3 days earlier, she became aware of a marked reduction in her level of activity. Later that day she felt more tired and had so much difficulty remaining alert that she had to return to her dorm room for a nap. Upon awakening, after reading for a little less than an hour, she went back to sleep. The following morning she had little appetite and was weary and inattentive despite three cups of coffee. By evening a mild sore throat developed. She was 100.8°F, orally. She took Tylenol and cough drops. Over the next 2 days she remained feverish and sleepy.

She had a boyfriend. She had no ill contacts. She grew up on a farm in Idaho and was the oldest in a family of six. She experienced the usual childhood illnesses and was up-to-date on her immunizations, including a second measles vaccine. She had had several "strep throats" but never had "mono." She had no chronic medical problems and was taking no medications. She occasionally had wine with dinner or smoked a "joint" but vigorously denied other drug use.

Physical examination demonstrated a young woman who appeared tired and listless. Oral temperature was 100.6°F; the rest of her vital signs were normal. Inspection of the oropharynx showed modest enlargement of the tonsils with hyperemia; there were no petechiae, vesicles, ulcerations, or exudates. There was moderate, nontender cervical lymphadenopathy, with the largest detectable lymph node measuring about 2.0 cm in diameter. Lungs were clear to auscultation. Cardiac exam was normal. Abdomen was soft and nontender; there was no hepatomegaly or splenomegaly.

The health service physician believed that she was suffering from IM and obtained a complete blood count and heterophil antibody titers (a "monospot"). The white blood cell count was 12,500/mm³ with 45% neutrophils and 45% lymphocytes; there were 2% atypical lymphocytes. Hemoglobin was 13.6 g/dL, platelets 310,000/mm³. Monospot was negative. A throat swab for a rapid test for *Streptococcus pyogenes* was negative; a culture was sent.

The patient was asked to call the health service office the next day for the results of the throat culture, at which time antibiotics would be prescribed if *S. pyogenes* was isolated. She was instructed to rest, maintain a good fluid intake, and take acetaminophen for temperature elevations above 101°F. The next day, the throat culture grew only normal upper respiratory tract flora. The patient returned to the health service still complaining of fatigue and low-grade fever. Physical examination was unchanged. An additional blood sample was obtained for a mononucleosis serologic profile, which included tests for IgM and IgG antibodies against EBV, CMV, and toxoplasma. Urine for CMV by the rapid "shell vial" technique was also ordered. Instructions for supportive care were repeated. When the patient returned 5 days later, she stated that she had begun to feel better: she

was less sleepy, her throat was better, and her appetite was nearly normal. At this time, the following serologic results were available:

EBV VCA IgG 1:160, IgM negative, EBNA 1:40.
CMV IgG and IgM 1:40; rapid urine "shell vial" assay was positive.
Toxoplasma IgG and IgM negative.

## CASE 1 Discussion

The presence of low titers of EBV VCA IgG, modest anti-EBNA titers, and the absence of EBV VCA IgM indicated past but not current EBV infection. She had no history of "mono," so she probably had had an asymptomatic EBV infection during childhood. Lack of IgM antibody against toxoplasma ruled out that potential etiology. Primary CMV infection was verified by the presence of IgM antibody specific for CMV and the presence of CMV in the patient's urine. She was told that she had probably been infected with CMV several weeks earlier, most likely via the salivary route. Since she was experiencing her primary CMV infection as an adult, a mononucleosis syndrome was not unusual. She was advised that her illness was self-limited and that no complications or sequelae were expected. Her boyfriend never became ill; he had serologic evidence only of old CMV disease and may have been the source of her primary infection during a time when he shed CMV asymptomatically.

## CASE HISTORY 2

A previously healthy pathology resident arrived in the emergency room complaining of eye pain. Two days earlier he noticed an irritating sensation that felt like a foreign body in his left eye, which rapidly progressed to constant, severe pain accompanied by diffuse conjunctival hyperemia and excessive tearing. The pain was sufficiently severe that he had difficultly sleeping. The discomfort was intensified by bright light. He never actually saw a foreign body in his eye, however. Use of topical over-the-counter eyedrops produced no relief. He was married and had two preschool-aged children who were healthy. He had no significant family history.

On physical examination, the patient had a low-grade fever (100.4°F). The rest of his vital signs were normal. Ocular examination showed that the left eye was diffusely injected with a small amount of thin, yellow discharge. Throat was mildly injected and there was a palpable left preauricular lymph node. The rest of the examination was normal.

A culture and Gram's stain of the discharge were obtained. Gram's strain revealed a few neutrophils and no organisms. The patient was given Gantrisin (sulfisoxazole) eye drops. The patient was scheduled for ophthalmology clinic the next day. The working diagnosis was conjunctivitis, and the patient was instructed to wash his hands frequently to minimize the likelihood of spread.

The bacterial culture of the eye discharge yielded only a few colonies of *Staphylococcus epidermidis*, which was felt to be normal flora. In the ophthalmology clinic, a specimen for virus culture was obtained. The patient was again sent home. After 48 h, one of the cultured monolayer cell lines stained positive with fluorescein-conjugated antibody to adenovirus group antigen. Two days later, the fibroblast monolayer in that tissue culture tube showed cytopathic changes consistent with adenovirus growth.

Two days later the conjunctivitis was moderately improved. However, sore throat worsened and fever persisted. Upon further questioning it was revealed that 2 days before the onset of symptoms, the resident performed an autopsy on an elderly patient who had died with a fulminant, poorly characterized pneumonia. He wore no eye protection during the autopsy and recalled that while dissecting the lungs, something splashed into his eye. Adenovirus was subsequently cultured from the autopsied lung.

One week later, the patient's conjunctivitis, pharyngitis, and fever had resolved. The ophthalmologist concluded that the pathology resident suffered from pharyngoconjunctival fever that began following accidental inoculation of his conjunctiva; subsequently the virus spread via the nasolacrimal duct, causing the characteristic syndrome.

## REFERENCES

### Books

Feigin, R. D., and Cherry, J. D., eds. *Textbook of Pediatric Infectious Diseases.* 3rd ed. Philadelphia: W. B. Saunders Co., 1992.

Fitzpatrick, T. B., Eisen A. Z., Wolff, K., Freedberg, I. M., and Austen, K. F., eds. *Dermatology in General Medicine.* 3rd ed. New York: McGraw-Hill, 1987.

Mandell, G. L., Bennett, J. E., and Dolin, R., eds. *Principles and Practice of Infectious Diseases.* 4th ed. New York: Churchill Livingstone Co., 1995.

Schlossberg, D., ed. *Infectious Mononucleosis.* New York: Springer-Verlag, 1983.

### Articles and Chapters

Buchwald, D., Sullivan, J. L., and Komaroff, A. L. Frequency of "chronic active Epstein-Barr virus infection" in a general medical practice. *JAMA* 257:2303–2307, 1987.

Carter, B. D., Edwards, J. F., Kronenberger, W. G., Michalczyk, L., and Marshall, G. C. Case control study of chronic fatigue in pediatric patients. *Pediatrics* 95:179–86, 1995.

D'Alessio, D. J., Meschievitz, C. K., Peterson, J. A., et al. Short-duration exposure and the transmission of rhinoviral colds. *J. Infect. Dis.* 150:189–194, 1984.

D'Angelo, L., Hierholzer, J. C., Keenlyside, R. A., et al. Pharyngoconjunctival fever caused by adenovirus type 4: Report of a swimming pool-related outbreak with recovery of virus from pool water. *J. Infect. Dis. 140:* 42–46, 1979.

Edwards, K. M., Thompson, J., Paolini, J., et al. Adenovirus infections in young children. *Pediatrics* 76:420–424, 1985.

Forbes, B. A. Acquisition of cytomegalovirus infection: An update. *Clin. Microbiol. Rev. 2:*204–216, 1989.

Fukuda, K., Straus, S. E., Hickie, I., et al. The chronic fatigue syndrome. *Ann. Intern. Med. 121:*953–959, 1994.

Hall, C. B., Long, C. E., Schnabel, K. C., et al. Human herpesvirus-6 infection in children. *N. Engl. J. Med. 331:*432–438, 1994.

Hendley, J. O., and Gwaltney, J. M., Jr. Mechanisms of transmission of rhinovirus infections. *Epidemiol. Rev. 10:*242–258, 1988.

Holmes, G. P., Kaplan, J. E., Gantz, N. M., et al. Chronic fatigue syndrome: A working case definition. *Ann. Intern. Med. 108:*397–399, 1988.

Horwitz, C. A., Henle, W., Henle, G., et al. Long-term serological follow-up of patients for Epstein-Barr virus after recovery from infectious mononucleosis. *J. Infect. Dis. 151:*1150–1153, 1985.

Huovinen, P., Lahtonen, R., Ziegler, T., et al. Pharyngitis in adults: The presence and coexistence of viruses and bacterial organisms. *Ann. Intern. Med. 110:*612–616,1989.

Kesler, H. A., Blaauw, B., Spear, J., et al. Diagnosis of human immunodeficiency virus infection in seronegative homosexuals presenting with an acute viral syndrome. *JAMA* 258:1196–1199, 1987.

Katz, B. Z. Epstein-Barr virus. In: Long, S. S., Prober, C. G., and Dickering, C. K., eds. *The Principles and Practice of Pediatric Infectious Diseases.* New York: Churchill Livingstone Co. (in press).

Kirov, S. M., Marsden, K. A., and Wongwanich, S. Seroepidemiological study of infectious mononucleosis in older patients. *J. Clin. Microbiol. 27:*356–358, 1989.

Knight, P. J., Mulne, A. F., and Vassy, L. E. When is lymph node biopsy indicated in children with enlarged peripheral nodes? *Pediatrics 69:*391–396, 1982.

Levandowski, R. A., and Rubenis, M. Nosocomial conjunctivitis caused by adenovirus Type 4. *J. Infect. Dis. 143:*28–31, 1981.

Naclerio, R. M., Proud, D., Kagey-Sobotka, A., et al. Is histamine responsible for the symptoms of rhinovirus colds? A look at the inflammatory mediators following infection. *Pediatr. Infect. Dis.* 7:218–222, 1988.

Okuno, T., Takahashi, K., Balachandra, K., et al. Seroepidemiology of human herpesvirus 6 infection in normal children and adults. *J. Clin. Microbiol. 27:*651–653, 1989.

Pacini, D. L., Collier, A. M., and Henderson, F. W. Adenovirus infections and respiratory illness in children in group day care. *J. Infect. Dis. 156:*920–927, 1987.

Slap, G. B., Brooks, J. S. J., and Schwarz, S. When to perform biopsies of enlarged peripheral lymph nodes in young patients. *JAMA* 252:1321–1326, 1984.

Steeper, T. A., Horwitz, C. A., Ablashi, D. V., et al. The spectrum of clinical and laboratory findings due to human herpesvirus 6 (HHV-6) in patients with mononucleosislike illnesses not due to EBV or CMV. *Am. J. Clin. Pathol. 93:*776–783, 1990.

Steeper, T. A., Horwitz, C. A., Hanson, M., et al. Heterophil-negative mononucleosis-like illnesses with atypical lympcytosis in patients undergoing seroconversions to the human immunodeficiency virus. *Am. J. Clin. Pathol. 89:*169–174, 1988.

Straus, S. E., Dale, J. K., Tobi, M., et al. Acyclovir treatment of the chronic fatigue syndrome: Lack of efficacy in a placebo-controlled trial. *N. Engl. J. Med. 319*: 1692–1698, 1988.

Sumaya, C. V., and Ench, Y. Epstein-Barr virus mononucleosis in children. II. Heterophil antibodies and viral specific responses. *Pediatrics 75*:1011–1019, 1985.

Szilagyi, P. G. Viruses and the common cold. *Pediatr. Virol. 5*(3):1–4, 1990.

Tindall, B., Barker, S., Donovan, B., et al. Characterization of the acute clinical illness associated with human immunodeficiency virus infection. *Arch. Intern. Med. 148*:945–949, 1988.

Turner, B. R., Hendley, J. O., and Gwaltney, J. M., Jr. Shedding of infected ciliated epithelial cells in rhinovirus colds. *J. Infect. Dis. 145*:849–853, 1982.

Yungbluth, M. Infectious mononucleosis and viral infections of the upper respiratory tract. In: Shulman, S. T., Phair, J. P., and Sommers, H. M., eds. *The Biologic and Clinical Basis of Infectious Diseases*, 4th ed. Philadelphia: W. B. Saunders Co., 1992.

# 9

# DENTAL INFECTIONS AND OTHER DISEASES OF THE ORAL CAVITY

JAMES L. DUNCAN, D.D.S., Ph.D.

The most common infections of the oral cavity are dental caries and periodontal disease, afflictions that are almost ubiquitous in civilized populations. Caries is a microbial attack that occurs directly on the teeth, whereas periodontal disease involves the supporting structures of the teeth.

Both diseases occur in an area of the body characterized by the presence of a complex indigenous microbial flora as well as dynamic host defense mechanisms. The situation is complex because the mouth is frequently exposed to environmental extremes with respect to temperature, pH, viscosity and osmolarity, and chemical composition of the materials taken in. Furthermore, a considerable number of saprophytic organisms enter each day, via food, water, and other substances. Despite these continuous assaults from without, the types of organisms constituting the indigenous microbial flora of the oral cavity gener-

ally remain relatively constant, varying, however, with the presence or absence of teeth, in certain oral diseases, and after the administration of certain drugs, such as antibiotics.

A variety of microbial ecosystems can be found in the oral cavity; for example, the composition of the microbial flora found in a deep periodontal pocket differs from that found in superficial dental plaque or on the buccal mucosa. Local environmental factors, such as pH, oxidation–reduction potential, and availability of appropriate nutrients, account in part for the types of organisms found. An additional characteristic that is important in microbial colonization of both hard and soft oral tissues is that of selective adherence of microorganisms. Organisms can persistently colonize the oral cavity only if they are able to attach to host tissues, and there is abundant evidence that certain oral microorganisms selectively colonize particular tissue surfaces. Most of the organisms that initially adsorb to oral surfaces are thought to desorb subsequently, and only a small proportion of the initially adherent organisms become firmly bound and result in persistent colonization. The adsorption and desorption processes occur continuously, and the number of microorganisms present in the saliva (up to $10^9$ organisms per milliliter) is a reflection of the organisms that have become dislodged.

### Host Defense Mechanisms

Despite the presence of large numbers of organisms in intimate contact with the mucosa, and not infrequent traumatic incidents that occur in the oral cavity, acute infections of the oral tissues are relatively uncommon. This is undoubtedly a reflection of the host defense mechanisms that operate in the mouth.

Mechanical defense processes remove enormous numbers of microorganisms from the oral cavity. These include the flow of saliva, desquamation of the oral mucosa; and the motion of the lips, cheeks, and tongue. The latter process helps cleanse some of the surfaces of the teeth and moves the saliva, desquamated epithelial cells, and microorganisms to the back of the mouth where they are swallowed. Dental caries most frequently develop in areas that are inaccessible to these cleansing effects.

In addition to its physical properties, saliva contains a number of substances that contribute to the host's defenses. These include lysozyme, lactoferrin, and lactoperoxidase, as well as salivary glycoproteins that may aggregate certain microorganisms and prevent their attachment to the teeth and oral mucosa. The predominant immunoglobulin present in saliva is secretory immunoglobulin A (IgA), produced by the major salivary glands and the numerous minor salivary glands present throughout the oral mucosa. Salivary IgA antibody is thought to contribute to immunity in the oral cavity primarily by interfering with the adherence of microorganisms to oral tissues. This effect, which can be readily demonstrated in *in vitro* models of bacterial adherence, is the basis of some of the vaccines against dental caries that have been tested in experimental animals. An additional source of immune elements in the oral cavity is the gingival sulcus. The fluid that seeps into the sulcus from the gingival tissues contains IgG, IgA, and IgM immunoglobulins; comple-

ment and other serum proteins; and phagocytic cells, primarily segmented neutrophils. All these components are thought to contribute to normal host defense mechanisms within the gingival tissues and in the gingival sulcus.

## DENTAL CARIES

### General Considerations

Dental caries attacks the hardest, most calcified tissues of the body, the enamel and dentin of the teeth, and is characterized by an initial demineralization of the inorganic material of these structures, followed by the destruction of their organic components. The demineralization of the calcified components of enamel and dentin is due to lactic acid produced by the fermentation of dietary carbohydrates by bacteria found in the oral cavity.

Once initiated, caries progresses into the enamel layer of the tooth, and eventually advances to the dentoenamel junction, where the infection spreads laterally to involve large numbers of dentinal tubules. The lesion progresses through the dentin by decalcification of the inorganic components and proteolysis of the organic matrix of the tissue. Microorganisms are readily apparent in the dentinal tubules. Dentin is a vital tissue, and in response to the insult and irritation of the advancing lesion, the dentinal tubules may become sealed off by calcification, and additional layers of dentin may be produced. Without treatment, however, the lesion often progresses to the dental pulp.

### Role of Diet and Tooth Morphology in Caries

For caries to occur, appropriate microorganisms, fermentable carbohydrates in the diet, and susceptible sites on the teeth all must be present. The importance of dietary fermentable carbohydrates in the development of dental caries is supported by a large number of epidemiologic and laboratory studies. An increase in the consumption of sugar, especially sucrose, results in an increase in the incidence of caries. In addition to making up a large percentage of the carbohydrates consumed in the United States, sucrose can be uniquely metabolized by certain oral streptococci to form glucose polymers that contribute to the structure of dental plaque.

Caries does not attack the teeth in a uniform manner; rather, there appear to be certain regions on the teeth that are more vulnerable than others. The occlusal surfaces are most frequently affected, and caries that occurs here is described as *pit and fissure caries* because the process is thought to be initiated as a result of the trapping of food debris and microorganisms in the pits and fissures that are characteristic of these surfaces. Caries also occurs at certain sites on the smooth surfaces of the teeth. *Smooth surface caries* is seen primarily on the interproximal surfaces of the teeth near the point at which they contact the adjacent teeth. Caries in this region is related to the formation of dental plaque, which holds microorganisms and their metabolic end products in close contact with the tooth enamel. Smooth surface caries is also found at the cervical region of the teeth, where the gingiva contacts the enamel. *Root surface caries* may develop in elderly people when a portion of the root may be exposed due to receding periodontal tissues. Carious lesions are not seen frequently on other smooth surface areas of the teeth that are more readily cleansed by the movement of lips, cheeks, and tongue and by the flow of saliva. Some teeth are more susceptible to caries than are others. When caries is present, the first and second molars are almost always affected. Caries is seen infrequently on cuspids and mandibular incisors.

## Dental Plaque

Plaque is an aggregation of bacteria, extracellular bacterial products, and certain salivary constituents that adheres firmly to the surface of the teeth (Fig. 9–1). It is of primary importance in the development of caries, especially of the smooth surface variety. The accumulation of plaque allows continual contact between acidogenic microorganisms and the enamel surface, where the localized production of lactic acid initiates the destruction of the hydroxyapatite structure of the enamel. Bacteria make up about two thirds of the bulk of dental plaque, and the number of organisms may be as high as $10^{10}$–$10^{11}$ bacteria per gram wet weight of plaque. Intercellular material of bacterial or salivary origin makes up the plaque matrix.

Studies of plaque formation show that there is an initial adsorption of salivary glycoproteins to the enamel surface, forming a thin, amorphous film called the *acquired pellicle*. Certain oral microorganisms, including streptococci and actinomycetes, selectively adsorb to this material; other bacteria may spe-

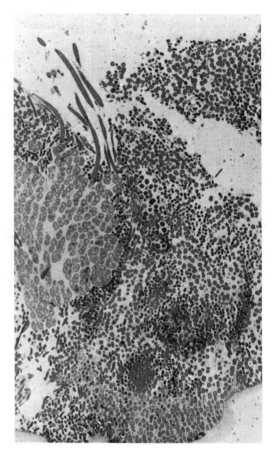

**FIGURE 9–1.** Electron micrograph of a thin section from dental plaque. The microbial flora is seen to consist primarily of cocci, although a few rods and filamentous forms are also present ($\times$ 1900). (From Lai, C-H., Listgarten, M. A., and Rosan, B. Immunoelectron microscopic identification and localization of *Streptococcus sanguis* with peroxidase-labeled antibody: Localization of *Streptococcus sanguis* in intact dental plaque. *Infect. Immun. 11*:200, 1975. With permission.)

cifically adhere to previously bound bacteria. Within a few hours, microcolonies and aggregates of bacteria can be observed. As the organisms multiply, some produce extracellular polysaccharide polymers, glucans and fructans, which are products of sucrose metabolism. The microcolonies eventually coalesce to form a continuous mass of bacteria and polysaccharides on the tooth enamel.

Plaque is a heterogeneous material, and the microbial flora and composition of the matrix differs considerably, depending on the age of the plaque, its location in the mouth, and even the site on an individual tooth from which it is taken. Plaque overlying carious lesions differs from plaque obtained from noncarious areas of the same tooth. Cariogenic plaque contains high levels of *Streptococcus mutans* compared with noncariogenic plaque.

## Bacteriology of Dental Caries

The critical role of microorganisms in dental caries was demonstrated unequivocally in experiments with germ-free rats during the 1950s. Such animals developed no caries even when they were maintained on a cariogenic diet; upon implantation of streptococci, however, dental caries appeared. Animal model studies as well as clinical and epidemiologic investigations over the past three decades all point to one organism as being of primary importance in the initiation of dental caries: *Streptococcus mutans.*

### *Streptococcus mutans*

Over the past 30 years, a voluminous literature dealing with *S. mutans* and its role in caries has accumulated. The organism was first isolated from human carious lesions in 1924 by J. K. Clarke, who suggested that the ability of *S. mutans* to adhere to the surface of teeth was of great importance. Unfortunately, the organism was forgotten for four decades, only to be rediscovered in the 1960s. Organisms that are now included in the mutans streptococcus group are separated into eight antigenic serotypes (a–h) and seven species: *S. mutans* (serotypes c, e, f); *S. sobrinus*

(d, g); *S. cricetus* (a); *S. rattus* (b); *S. ferus* (c); *S. macacae* (c); and *S. downei* (h). The most important member of this group in human dental caries is *S. mutans,* serotype c. There is a strong positive correlation between the presence and numbers of *S. mutans* in plaque and the development of caries.

Several unusual physiologic properties of this organism may contribute to its virulence. First, *S. mutans* produces glucosyltransferase enzymes, which synthesize polymers of glucose, known as glucans, from sucrose. The glucosyltransferase enzymes are associated with the bacterial cell surface and produce both water-soluble and water-insoluble glucans. The sticky, water-insoluble glucan molecules synthesized by *S. mutans* are thought to contribute to plaque development (Fig. 9–2) and microbial colonization of the smooth surfaces of the teeth. Second, *S. mutans* produces higher levels of lactic acid than other organisms commonly found in plaque and remains metabolically active at low pH. Third, *S. mutans* stores large amounts of intracellular polysaccharides that may be used as reserve energy sources when dietary carbohydrates are not present.

## Treatment and Prevention

Because the reparative ability of enamel and dentin is minimal, the treatment of caries

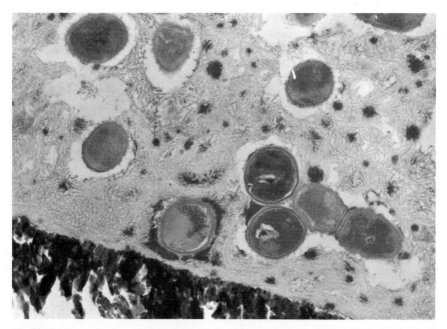

**FIGURE 9–2.** Electron micrograph of sectioned *Streptococcus mutans* cells attached to extracted human enamel, after growth in a 5% sucrose medium. The microorganisms are enmeshed in an extensive fibrillar matrix of extracellular polysaccharide. (Courtesy of Dr. N. Tinanoff.)

requires that all the affected tissues be removed. The affected tooth structure is then replaced by one of several types of inert filling materials.

A number of effective, low-cost procedures are available to prevent the disease. Many of these are based on the use of fluorides, either systemically in public water supplies or in topical applications of fluoride in toothpastes, or in gels applied in the dental office. In addition, the use of inert polymers to seal pits and fissures is very effective in preventing caries on occlusal surfaces of the teeth.

The prevalence of dental caries has dramatically declined in the United States and other industrialized countries over the past 20–30 years. Surveys carried out in 1987 indicated that 50% of U.S. children between the ages of 5 and 17 years had no decay in their permanent teeth. Although this decline has been attributed to the increasing availability of fluoride in water and processed foods and in topical applications, large reductions have also occurred in unfluoridated areas in several countries. The reasons for this substantial reduction in tooth decay, which cannot apparently be attributed to fluoridation, are unknown.

## INFECTIONS OF THE DENTAL PULP AND PERIAPICAL TISSUES

The dental pulp is a loose connective tissue lined at its periphery by a layer of odontoblasts, specialized cells that are responsible for the formation of dentin. With the exception of the foramen at the apex of the roots of the teeth, the pulp is completely enclosed by dentin, on top of which lies cementum or enamel (Fig. 9–3). Although these calcified structures protect the pulp, they are unyielding and therefore indirectly contribute to the pressure, pain, and tissue necrosis that may be associated with an inflammatory response in the pulp.

The healthy, vital pulp of an intact tooth is nearly always free of microorganisms. There are several routes by which bacteria can infect the dental pulp, but by far the most important is the extension of caries through the enamel and dentin into the pulp chamber. When bacteria break through into the pulp chamber, an acute inflammatory response is elicited at the exposure site. The infectious process may then spread so that the entire pulp becomes acutely inflamed, with partial or total necrosis

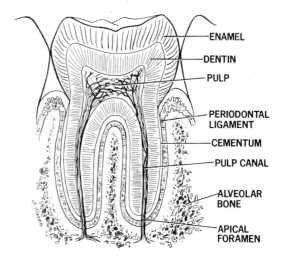

**FIGURE 9–3.** Diagrammatic representation of a mandibular molar, illustrating the tooth structures and periodontal tissues.

of the pulp tissue. The inability of the pulp to tolerate edema and the lack of significant collateral blood circulation severely limit the ability of the pulp to cope with bacterial invasion and tissue necrosis.

The determination of whether the pathologic condition of the pulp is reversible is based on clinical findings. A frank, carious exposure of the pulp requires that the pulp tissue be removed and the pulp chamber and root canals filled with an inert material.

As might be expected, the microorganisms that can be cultured from infected, necrotic pulps consist of bacteria that are commonly found in the oral cavity. In virtually all cases, these are mixed infections and include alpha-hemolytic (viridans) and nonhemolytic streptococci as well as a number of strict anaerobic organisms. The latter organisms include *Porphyromonas endodontalis*, *P. gingivalis* and *Prevotella intermedius* (all of which produce black-pigmented colonies on blood agar), and *Peptostreptococcus* species.

The inflammatory and degenerative processes that occur in the infected pulp may extend through the apical foramen into the surrounding bone of the periapical region. The involvement of the periapical tissues may take several forms. *Chronic apical periodontitis* can be a relatively asymptomatic condition characterized by the presence of a radiolucent area in the periapical region of a nonvital tooth (Fig. 9–4). Histologically, the lesion may appear as a granuloma, chronic abscess, or cyst. *Acute apical periodontitis* is characterized by an acute inflammatory response with abscess forma-

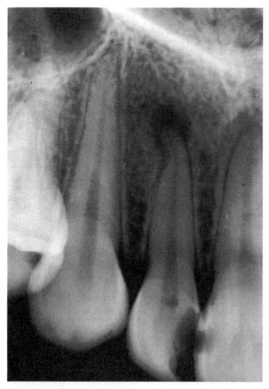

**FIGURE 9–4.** Dental radiograph showing a pathologic lesion at the apex of a maxillary lateral incisor. A large carious lesion is present in the crown of the tooth. (Courtesy of Dr. E. Stephen Smith.)

olar bone and the cervical regions of the teeth; *periodontal ligament,* composed of collagen fibers that are attached to the cementum of the tooth and are inserted into the gingiva, alveolar bone, and cementum of the adjacent teeth; *cementum,* the calcified bone-like structure that covers the dentin of the roots of the teeth; and *alveolar bone,* ridges of maxillary and mandibular bone into which the roots of the teeth are embedded. Although acute infections of the periodontium occur, the disease that is most common and of greatest concern is a chronic inflammatory condition known as periodontal disease.

Periodontal disease involves the gingival sulcus (or crevice) and surrounding tissues (Fig. 9–5); the sulcus and marginal gingiva are unusual because of the unique interface between the humoral and secretory immune systems in this region. The tissues are bathed in crevicular fluid, which contains cellular and soluble humoral immune elements, as well as saliva, which contains secretory IgA and other antimicrobial substances.

Several forms of periodontal disease are recognized: *Gingivitis* is seen as an inflammation of the more superficial soft tissues of the periodontium and is characterized by the red,

tion. Swelling is often present, pain may be severe, and the tooth is extremely sensitive to percussion and palpation. The microbial flora isolated from periapical lesions is very similar to that found in necrotic dental pulp tissue.

Apical abscesses may occasionally penetrate the cortical plate of the maxillary or mandibular bone and drain via a fistula into the oral cavity or to the face. On rare occasions, the infection may extend into fascial spaces of the head and neck. The rapid spread of infection, most frequently into submaxillary and parapharyngeal spaces, with attendant airway obstruction, often makes such an extension a life-threatening situation.

## PERIODONTAL DISEASE

### General Considerations

Diseases of the periodontium affect those tissues that support and anchor the teeth (Figs. 9–3 and 9–5). These include the *gingiva,* the coral-pink-colored mucous membrane that covers and is attached to the alve-

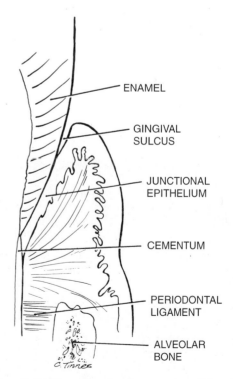

**FIGURE 9–5.** Diagrammatic representation of the gingival sulcus region.

ENAMEL

GINGIVAL SULCUS

JUNCTIONAL EPITHELIUM

CEMENTUM

PERIODONTAL LIGAMENT

ALVEOLAR BONE

inflamed appearance of the gingiva and the loss of the normal contour of the gingival margins. Gingivitis may remain as a stable, chronic condition for many months or years without further affecting the function of the other periodontal tissues. Chronic gingivitis may lead to the migration of the junctional epithelium toward the apex of the tooth, deepening the gingival sulcus. *Acute necrotizing ulcerative gingivitis* is an acute form of gingivitis seen primarily in young adults. Epidemiologic studies suggest that emotional stress, fatigue, malnutrition, and neglected oral hygiene are contributing elements to the disease. Acute necrotizing ulcerative gingivitis is characterized by pain and bleeding with necrosis and erosion of the gingival papillae between the teeth (Fig. 9–6). In many cases, a grayish pseudomembrane covers the margins of the affected gingiva.

The most serious form of periodontal disease, seen primarily in adults, is one in which the inflammatory process involves not only the gingiva but also the periodontal ligament and alveolar bone. In this condition, known as *adult periodontitis,* the apical migration of the junctional epithelium seen in chronic gingivitis is exaggerated, resulting in the formation of a *periodontal pocket* between the cementum and the surrounding tissues. These pockets allow a greater accumulation of debris, plaque, and calculus in the area. The periodontal ligament is eventually destroyed, and resorption of alveolar bone is seen (Fig. 9–7), resulting in increased mobility and eventual loss of the affected teeth. Periodontitis in adults has traditionally been thought to be a slow but continuous process. However, more recent data suggest that the progression of the disease may be discontinuous, with episodic and relatively brief bursts of tissue destruction at a given site, followed by longer periods of remission and repair. *Localized juvenile periodontitis* is an uncommon form of periodontal disease found primarily in young people, which affects permanent molars and incisors. The disease is characterized by reduced numbers of bacteria (compared with those observed in adult periodontitis), minimal plaque formation, and less severe inflammation.

Periodontal disease is said to be a widespread and common affliction, but this statement is a reflection of the common occurrence of gingivitis. Serious, advanced periodontitis is much less frequently seen. Several epidemiologic factors appear to be correlated with risk of periodontal disease, the most important being age and oral hygiene. With increasing age, there is anincrease in the number of individuals affected. Microbial plaque, lying in close proximity to the gingival tissues, is thought to be an important factor in the initiation of gingivitis.

## Microorganisms as Initiating or Contributing Factors in Periodontal Disease

A considerable amount of evidence indicates that oral microorganisms play a role in the initiation of gingivitis and in the more destructive forms of periodontal disease. Clinicians have long noted the direct relationship between the microbial plaque burden in the cervical regions of the teeth and the presence

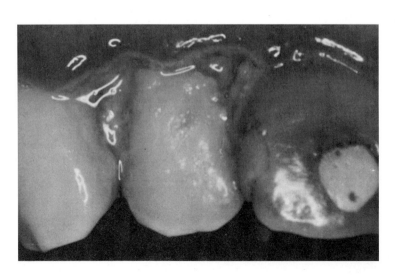

**FIGURE 9–6.** Acute necrotizing ulcerative gingivitis. The interdental papillae have eroded, and a grayish pseudomembrane is present on the marginal gingiva. (Courtesy of Dr. E. Stephen Smith.)

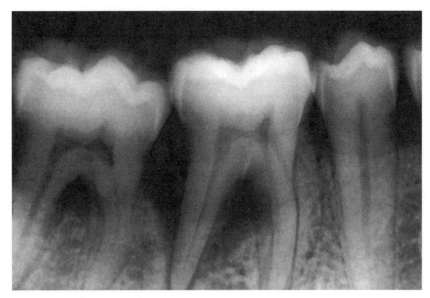

**FIGURE 9–7** Advanced periodontitis. Extensive loss of alveolar bone around the first and second molars can be seen. (Courtesy of Dr. E. Stephen Smith.)

and severity of gingivitis, and that gingival inflammation can be reduced or eliminated by procedures that remove the plaque and by antibiotics and other antimicrobial agents. In addition, several microorganisms isolated from the human oral cavity have been shown to produce periodontal disease in experimental animals.

### Gingivitis

The flora that can be isolated from the normal gingival sulcus region is complex, consisting of gram-positive species, primarily *Streptococcus* and *Actinomyces,* as well as some gram-negative species, including *Veillonella.* As gingivitis develops over a period of days or weeks, there is an increase in the number of organisms present, seen primarily as an increase in the numbers of gram-positive filamentous *Actinomyces* species (Table 9–1). With time, there is an increase in the number of certain gram-negative organisms in the gingival sulcus, including *Porphyromonas* and *Fusobacterium.* Spirochetes are also present. The complexity of the flora found in the gingival sulcus is illustrated by a study of experimental gingivitis in four subjects, from whom 166 bacterial species and subspecies were isolated. The flora became more diverse as gingivitis developed, and sequential colonization by certain species was observed.

### Acute Necrotizing Ulcerative Gingivitis

The microbial flora associated with this acute form of gingivitis is characterized by increased numbers of spirochetes, which appear to invade the gingival tissues. These spirochetes include *Treponema denticola, Borrelia gingivalis,* and others that bear antigens similar to those of *T. pallidum.* Gram-negative anaer-

**TABLE 9–1.  MICROBIAL FLORA OF THE GINGIVAL SULCUS**

| CONDITION | CHARACTERISTIC FEATURES OF THE MICROBIAL FLORA |
|---|---|
| Normal | Complex flora, with *Streptococcus, Actinomyces,* and *Veillonella* present in greatest numbers. |
| Gingivitis | Increased numbers of microorganisms, especially gram-positive, filamentous actinomycetes. Some gram-negative organisms (*Porphyromonas, Fusobacterium*) may increase in number. |
| Advanced periodontitis | Predominantly gram-negative rods, including *Porphyromonas, Prevotella, Bacteroides, Fusobacterium, Campylobacter, Eikenella, Capnocytophaga,* and *Actinobacillus.* Other organisms include *Treponema* and *Peptostreptococcus.* |

obes, including *Prevotella intermedius* and *Fusobacterium* species are also present.

### Adult periodontitis

As much as 75% of the bacterial population found in the gingival sulcus region in periodontitis consists of gram-negative organisms, many of which are obligate anaerobes (Table 9–1). Various organisms, including *Porphyromonas, Prevotella, Bacteroides, Fusobacterium, Campylobacter,* and *Actinobacillus,* have been isolated from periodontal pockets. Recent studies have emphasized the possible role in periodontitis of the black-pigmented, asaccharolytic organism, *Porphyromonas gingivalis.* This gram-negative anaerobe produces several proteases that may contribute to the tissue damage seen in periodontitis. Spirochetes, including *Treponema denticola,* are also present in greatly increased numbers. These organisms localize on the outer surface of the plaque in intimate contact with the epithelium of the gingival sulcus.

### Localized juvenile periodontitis

The organism thought to be of primary importance in localized juvenile periodontitis is *Actinobacillus actinomycetemcomitans,* a facultative, gram-negative coccobacillus. This organism is invariably present in relatively high numbers in the disease, and it is known to produce several substances, including leukotoxin and endotoxin, that may contribute to pathologic processes.

### Mechanisms of Tissue Destruction in Periodontal Disease

#### Microbial Products

Histologic studies have demonstrated that in most cases of periodontal disease the bacteria usually remain confined to the periodontal pocket and seldom are found in large numbers in the underlying connective tissues. For this reason, the possibility that microbial products penetrate the permeable junctional epithelium and act directly or indirectly to initiate or contribute to the tissue destruction seen in periodontal disease has been investigated.

A number of studies suggest a role for endotoxin in producing tissue damage in periodontal disease. The amount of endotoxin found in crevicular fluid correlates with the severity of periodontal inflammation, and endotoxin preparations from cultures of the gram-negative bacteria that dominate the microbial flora in periodontitis have been shown to be highly destructive to gingival tissues. Endotoxin is known to induce the production of inflammatory cytokines by mononuclear cells, and one such product, interleukin-1 (IL-1), is known to stimulate bone resorption in organ cultures. Endotoxin is also known to enhance the ability of macrophages to produce oxygen radicals and to release collagenase.

A number of organisms associated with periodontal disease, including *P. gingivalis, B. forsythus,* and *T. denticola,* produce several trypsin-like proteolytic enzymes, and in some cases, collagenase. Although these enzymes are undoubtedly important in the nutrition and metabolism of these organisms, they may also contribute to the destruction of periodontal tissues. Other bacterial products such as the metabolic end products $H_2S$ and butyrate, or cell wall peptidoglycan, may also stimulate destructive events in the periodontium.

#### Destructive Immune Mechanisms

The immune response in periodontal disease is complex; in addition to providing protection, it also undoubtedly contributes to the destruction of periodontal tissues. Interest in the possibility that immune elements might contribute to the tissue destruction seen in periodontitis was initially aroused by the demonstration that peripheral blood leukocytes from patients with periodontal disease underwent proliferative responses and produced cytokines after incubation with dental plaque bacteria, whereas leukocytes from normal individuals were unresponsive. The histopathologic changes in periodontal disease, including infiltration of increased numbers of macrophages, lymphocytes, and plasma cells into the affected tissues, are compatible with a role for immune elements in the disease. For example, IL-1, a cytokine secreted primarily by macrophages that plays an important role in immunologic and inflammatory reactions, stimulates prostaglandin and collagenase release from connective tissue and induces bone resorption as measured by $Ca^{2+}$ release from organ cultures of fetal rat bones. Significant levels of IL-1 activity have been detected in gingival crevicular fluid obtained from patients with periodontitis, and peripheral blood mononuclear cells can be stimulated by antigens present in dental plaque to produce IL-1 (originally described as osteoclast-activating factor). Other cytokines, including tumor necrosis factor and lymphotoxin, may contribute to bone resorption.

The protective and/or destructive role of antibody in periodontal disease is uncertain. B lymphocytes and plasma cells increase and predominate in the periodontium in advanced disease; immunoglobulin-containing cells, primarily of the IgG isotype, are present; and IgG antibody, some of which is thought to be locally produced, is present in the periodontal tissues. In addition to this localized response, serum levels of IgG to *P. gingivalis* and other organisms that are associated with periodontitis may be elevated. A destructive role for antibody in the pathogenesis of periodontal disease is entirely speculative, but could include complement fixation with the release of chemotactic factors, antibody-dependent cytotoxicity, and opsonization of tissue-associated antigens.

## OTHER ORAL INFECTIONS

A large number of bacterial, mycotic, and viral infections may produce oral manifestations. The reader should consult an oral pathology textbook for a complete description of those lesions. The diseases described here are among the more important primary infections of the oral tissues.

### Candidiasis

Oral candidiasis, or *thrush*, is the most common fungal infection of the mouth. *Candida albicans* is an opportunistic organism, normally found in the oral cavity, whose numbers are thought to be held in check by other members of the oral flora and by host defense mechanisms. Overgrowth of the organism is seen primarily in newborn infants, diabetics, or persons who have immunodeficiencies; candidiasis is uncommon in healthy adults who have not received broad-spectrum antibiotics or corticosteroids. Oral and esophageal candidiasis is one of the most frequent opportunistic infections seen in patients with the acquired immunodeficiency syndrome (AIDS).

Infection is characterized by the presence of white plaques or patches on the buccal mucosa, tongue, palate, and other mucous membrane surfaces. These lesions, which consist of masses of mycelial and yeast forms, may remain as discrete areas or coalesce to form a continuous white to gray pseudomembrane. Parts of the pseudomembrane may be stripped from the underlying tissue, revealing a red, bleeding surface. Chronic forms of candidiasis are also present in the oral cavity. These include denture stomatitis, a chronic infection of the mucosa underlying dentures in some individuals.

### Herpes Simplex

The most important viral disease affecting the oral mucosa is infection by herpes simplex virus type 1 (HSV-1). Primary HSV-1 infections most commonly occur in the mouth, usually in children between the ages of 6 months and 6 years. The majority of primary infections are thought to be subclinical, but in many children a severe gingivostomatitis with high fever occurs, characterized by the appearance of vesicles that progress to form ulcers.

An important property of HSV is its tendency to persist in a latent state in nerve tissues, particularly sensory ganglia, and to cause localized recurrent infections, despite the presence of circulating neutralizing antibodies. Recurrent infections are often associated with certain stimuli, such as sunlight, menstruation, fatigue, and emotional stress, which are thought to trigger viral replication, resulting in clinical disease. It is estimated that up to one third of the population has recurrent episodes, the majority suffering more than one attack each year; many persons develop one or more recurrent lesions each month. Labial herpes infections, known as cold sores or fever blisters, are the most common form of the recurrent disease; usually the outer third of the lower or upper lip is affected. A prodromal period, characterized by a burning or tingling sensation, precedes vesicle formation at the site. The vesicles rupture, leaving a shallow ulcer, which becomes covered with a brownish crust, and the lesions heal within 7–10 days after their appearance.

Transmission of HSV-1 to patients from the hands of dental personnel with herpetic whitlow (a soft-tissue herpetic infection of the finger pulp) has been documented.

### Actinomycosis

Several species of *Actinomyces* are found in the oral cavity, where they are associated with dental plaque and carious lesions, the gingival sulcus, and periodontal pockets. Actinomycosis in the cervicofacial region is a chronic granulomatous infection characterized by firm, nodular swelling and persistent, draining sinus tracts. *A. israelii* is usually the causative organism, although other reports have also implicated *A. naeslundii*. There frequently appears to be a relationship between actino-mycosis and previous trauma to the area, such as a blow to the teeth, fractures, or dental extractions. These events presumably allow the organisms to penetrate into the soft tissues or bone under anaerobic conditions and facilitate establishment of chronic infection.

### Venereal Infections of the Oral Cavity

It has long been known that syphilitic lesions can occur in and around the oral cavity. Chancres of the lip are the most common extragenital primary lesions, but they may also be found on the tongue, palate, and other oral tissues. In the secondary stage of syphilis, grayish white mucous patches may be found in the oral cavity, usually on the tongue or buccal mucosa, and the gumma of tertiary syphilis may involve the tongue or palate.

The frequency with which gonococci can be isolated from the oropharynx has only recently been appreciated. Data from a number of studies now suggest that the pharynx may be an important reservoir of *Neisseria gonorrhoeae*. Discrete lesions within the oral cavity thought to be due to gonococcal infection have rarely been described.

Venereal transmission of HSV-2 has been reported to cause oral lesions or asymptomatic infections of the oral cavity.

## DISEASES BEARING A SPECIAL RELATIONSHIP TO THE ORAL CAVITY

Certain diseases, although they are not considered to be oral infections, are especially important in the practice of dentistry. They are significant from the standpoints of the increased risk of disease for dentists or the role of dental health personnel in the transmission of disease.

### Hepatitis B

The increased risk of hepatitis B in dentists, particularly in oral surgeons, has been well documented over the past three decades. Of additional concern is the possibility that a dentist who has contracted hepatitis B may transmit the disease to patients. At least nine outbreaks of hepatitis B traceable to dentists or oral surgeons have been reported in the United States since 1974. In each outbreak, the implicated dentist was seropositive for HBsAg and did not use gloves during dental or surgical procedures.

The nature of dental practice offers a variety of means for the transmission of hepatitis B virus (see Chapter 19). The dentist's hands are almost constantly in contact with the patient's saliva and frequently with the patient's blood. The presence of viral antigens in the blood of infected individuals is well known, but HBsAg is also known to be present in the saliva of a high proportion of persons who have acute hepatitis B or who are chronic HbsAg carriers.

There are widely recommended and easily available measures to protect dentists (and all health care workers) against hepatitis B and to prevent transmission of the virus from dentist to patient. These include vaccination with the safe and effective recombinant hepatitis B vaccine and the routine use of gloves when treating patients.

### Acquired Immunodeficiency Syndrome

Manifestations of AIDS are seen in the oral cavity of a significant number of AIDS patients, and indeed, oral lesions may be the first clinical expression of human immunodeficiency virus (HIV) infection (see Chapter 23). Oral tumors may be present in up to half of the patients with Kaposi's sarcoma, and in some patients the mouth is the only site involved. Oral/esophageal candidiasis is the most common oral infection, present in 70% of AIDS patients in some studies. Other oral changes include a white hyperplasia of the epithelium, termed *hairy leukoplakia*, and recurrent herpetic lesions. In addition, changes in the periodontal tissues are present in many patients; these changes are seen as a generalized gingivitis and rapidly progressive periodontitis characterized by gingival recession and rapid and extensive alveolar bone loss.

The AIDS public health crisis has important implications for the practice of dentistry, especially in the area of infection control and in the diagnosis and management of oral infections and pathologic lesions related to the syndrome. It is estimated that more than 1 million people in the United States are infected with HIV, and dental professionals are likely to be exposed to some persons infected with HIV before those persons know they have been infected or become ill. Recommended infection control precautions require that blood, saliva, and crevicular fluid from all patients be regarded as infective; gloves should be used for contact with oral mucous membranes of all patients, and surgical masks and protective eyewear should be worn during dental procedures in which splashing or spattering of blood, saliva, or gingival fluids is likely.

## Infective Endocarditis

Infective endocarditis is a disease of considerable importance in the practice of dentistry. Large numbers of viridans (alpha-hemolytic) streptococci colonize the oral cavity, and alpha-hemolytic streptococci are the most frequent cause of endocarditis. Furthermore, many dental procedures, especially extractions and manipulation of periodontal tissues, virtually always result in transient bacteremia of alpha-hemolytic streptococci or other organisms. The transitory bacteremia may have unfortunate consequences for individuals with rheumatic heart disease or congenital heart defects or for those who have prosthetic heart valves. The blood-borne organisms may lodge on and colonize damaged heart valves or other parts of the endocardium, initiating an episode of endocarditis (see Chapter 33). In some endocarditis episodes, the patient is found to have a history of recent dental work, even though a causal relationship may be difficult to establish.

Although the prophylactic administration of antibiotics at the time of oral surgery to prevent infective endocarditis is a widely accepted procedure, the effectiveness of antibiotic prophylaxis in preventing bacterial endocarditis remains unproved. A number of factors influence the establishment of intravascular infection and the efficacy of prophylactic antibiotics. The management of cardiac patients at risk must be influenced by the American Heart Association recommendations for the prevention of bacterial endocarditis and include consultation with the patient's physician.

## REFERENCES

### Books

Genco, R. J., ed. *Molecular Pathogenesis of Periodontal Disease.* Washington, D.C.: American Society for Microbiology, 1994.

Grant, D. A., Stern, I. B., and Listgarten, M. A. *Periodontics.* 6th ed. St. Louis: C. V. Mosby Co., 1988.

Marsh, P., and Martin, M. *Oral Microbiology.* 3rd ed. London: Chapman and Hall, 1992.

Nisengard, R. J., and Newman, M. G. *Oral Microbiology and Immunology.* 2nd ed. Philadelphia: W. B. Saunders Co., 1994.

Schluger, S., Yuodelis, R. A., Page, R. C., et al. *Periodontal Disease.* 2nd ed. Philadelphia: Lea & Febiger, 1990.

Seltzer, S., and Bender, I. B. *The Dental Pulp.* 3rd ed. Philadelphia: J. B. Lippincott Co., 1984.

Shafer, W. G., Hine, M. K., and Levy, B. M. *A Textbook of Oral Pathology.* 4th ed. Philadelphia: W. B. Saunders Co., 1983.

Slots, J., and Taubman, M. A. *Contemporary Oral Microbiology and Immunology.* St. Louis: Mosby—Year Book, Inc., 1992.

Topazian, R. G., and Goldberg, M. H. *Oral and Maxillofacial Infections.* 3rd ed. Philadelphia: W. B. Saunders Co., 1994.

### Review Articles

Corey, L., and Spear, P. G. Infections with herpes simplex viruses. *N. Engl. J. Med. 314*:686, 1986.

Cottone, J. A. Recent developments in hepatitis: New virus, vaccine, and dosage recommendations. *JADA 120*: 501, 1990.

Coykendall, A. L. Classification and identification of the viridans streptococci. *Clin. Microbiol. Rev. 2*:315, 1989.

Cutler, C. W., Kalmar, J. R., and Genco, C. A. Pathogenic strategies of the oral anaerobe, *Porphyromonas gingivalis. Trends Microbiol. 3*:45, 1995.

Diesendorf, M. The mystery of declining tooth decay. *Nature 322*:125, 1986.

Farber, P. A., and Seltzer, S. Endodontic microbiology. I. Etiology. *J. Endodont. 14*:363, 1988.

Hirsch, R. S., and Clarke, N. Infection and periodontal disease. *Rev. Infect. Dis. 11*:707, 1989.

Johnson, B. D., and Engel, D. Acute necrotizing ulcerative gingivitis. A review of diagnosis, etiology and treatment. *J. Periodontol. 57*:141, 1986.

Kolenbrander, P. Intergeneric coaggregation among human oral bacteria and ecology of dental plaque. *Annu. Rev. Microbiol. 42*:627, 1988.

Loesche, W. J. Role of *Streptococcus mutans* in human dental decay. *Microbiol. Rev. 50*:353, 1986.

Loesche, W. J. Bacterial mediators in periodontal disease. *Clin. Infect. Dis. 16*(Suppl. 4):S203, 1993.

Mayrand, D., and Holt, S. C. Biology of asaccharolytic black-pigmented *Bacteroides* species. *Microbiol. Rev. 52*: 134, 1988.

Robinson, P. Periodontal diseases and HIV infection. *J. Clin. Periodontol. 19*:609, 1992.

Shah, H. N., and Gharbia, S. Ecophysiology and taxonomy of *Bacteroides* and related taxa. *Clin. Infect. Dis. 16* (Suppl. 4):S160, 1993.

Shaw, J. H. Causes and control of dental caries. *N. Engl. J. Med. 317*:996, 1987.

Tanner, A., and Stillman, N. Oral and dental infections with anaerobic bacteria: Clinical features, predominant pathogens, and treatment. *Clin. Infect. Dis. 16*(Suppl. 4):S304, 1993.

Williams, R. C. Periodontal disease. *N. Engl. J. Med. 322*: 373, 1990.

### Original Articles

Dajani A. S., Bisno A. S., Chung K. J., et al. Prevention of bacterial endocarditis. *JAMA 264*:2919–2922, 1990.

Dewhirst, F. E., Stashenko, P., Mole, J. E., et al. Purification and partial sequence of human osteoclast-activating factor: Identity with interleukin 1B. *J. Immunol. 135*:2562, 1985.

Holt, S. C., Ebersole, J., Felton, J., et al. Implantation

of *Bacteroides gingivalis* in nonhuman primates initiates progression of periodontitis. *Science 239*:55, 1988.

Imamura, T., Pike, R. N., Potempa, J., and Travis, J. Pathogenesis of periodontitis: A major arginine-specific cysteine proteinase from *Porphyromonas gingivalis* induces vascular permeability enhancement through activation of the kallikrein/kinin pathway. *J. Clin. Invest. 94*:361, 1994.

Kabashima, H., Maeda, K., Iwamoto, Y., et al. Partial characterization of an interleukin-1-like factor in human gingival crevicular fluid from patients with chronic inflammatory periodontal disease. *Infect. Immunol. 58*:2621, 1990.

Klein, R., Harris, C., Small, C., et al. Oral candidiasis in high risk patients as the initial manifestation of the acquired immunodeficiency syndrome. *N. Engl. J. Med. 311*:354, 1984.

Klein, R. S., Phelan, J. A., Freeman, K., et al. Low occupational risk of human immunodeficiency virus infection among dental professionals. *N. Engl. J. Med. 318*: 86, 1988.

Manzella, J. P., McConville, J. H., Valenti, W., et al. An outbreak of herpes simplex virus type 1 gingivostomatitis in a dental hygiene practice. *JAMA 252*:2019, 1984.

Riviere, G. R., Wagoner, M. A., Baker-Zander, S. A., et al. Identification of spirochetes related to *Treponema pallidum* in necrotizing ulcerative gingivitis and chronic periodontitis. *N. Engl. J. Med. 325*:539, 1991.

Winkler, J., Murray, P., Grassi, M., et al. Diagnosis and management of HIV-associated periodontal lesions. *JADA 119*:25S, 1989.

# III    LOWER RESPIRATORY TRACT INFECTION

# 10

## INFECTIONS OF THE LOWER RESPIRATORY TRACT: GENERAL CONSIDERATIONS

JOHN P. PHAIR, M.D.

**PATHOGENESIS OF LOWER RESPIRATORY TRACT INFECTION**

**ETIOLOGY**

**SPECIFIC SYNDROMES**

**PREVENTION**

**CASE HISTORY**

**REFERENCES**

The lower respiratory tract is vulnerable to infection by a wide variety of microorganisms because it is one of the organ systems that communicate directly with the environment. Its physiologic function, the exchange of gases, can result in exposure to bacteria, fungi, viruses, and other potentially pathogenic agents. In addition, the entire blood supply must pass through the pulmonary capillary bed, and bloodstream infections can produce secondary infection in the lower respiratory tract. The lower respiratory tract, comprising the bronchial tree, the pulmonary parenchyma, and the pleura, can be the locus of infection that presents as similar or quite distinct symptom complexes with a variety of physical findings.

Infections of the lower respiratory tract represent a constantly increasing cause of morbidity and mortality. This is in part a consequence of smoking; it is estimated that 30% of both men and women in the United States smoke. Smoking predisposes to a breakdown in upper airway and bronchial defense mechanisms necessary to protect the lungs and results ultimately in chronic obstructive lung disease. Chronic obstructive lung disease in turn is associated with infection, significant levels of disability, neoplastic disease, and death. It is estimated that chronic respiratory disease, including asthma, represents the fifth leading cause of death in the United States. In addition, pneumonias and related lower respiratory tract infections acquired during hospitalizations are an increasing and extremely difficult problem. Patients with severe, debilitating medical and surgical illness are extremely vulnerable to pulmonary infections and much of the therapeutic intervention for such patients leads to an increased risk of lower respiratory tract infections. This problem is discussed more fully in Chapter 25.

The patient with lower respiratory tract infection usually presents with signs and symptoms referable to the chest. Fever and cough are the two most prominent complaints. With involvement of the pleura, chest pain is also present. Physical examination provides evidence of lung involvement, inflammation of bronchi, or the presence of pleural fluid. The cornerstones of diagnosis are chest radiography (x-ray) and microscopic examination and culture of expectorated sputum or pleural fluid if available.

The chest x-ray can demonstrate consolidation of a lobe or lobule of the lung representing fluid-filled alveoli. With consolidation an "air bronchogram," air-filled bronchi surrounded by fluid-filled alveoli, can be seen on a chest film. Absence of an air bronchogram suggests collapse of a lung segment or atelectasis. Diffuse interstitial processes, if chronic, usually represent inflammatory or granulomatous involvement of the alveolar septa or, if acute, edema due to heart failure or fluid overload. In these circumstances, pleural disease with effusions is usually found at the base of the lung and, if not loculated, moves when the patient is repositioned. An air–fluid level with a pleural effusion can result from a bronchopleural fistula. In the lung, an air–fluid level is seen in conjunction with a partially fluid-filled emphysematous cyst or a lung abscess. The latter is usually thick-walled, whereas the former is thin-walled. The physician must evaluate the history, physical examination, and the chest radiograph to determine if the patient's complaints are related to upper (Chapters 7 and 8) or to lower respiratory tract disease. If lower tract disease is the most likely cause of the patient's complaints, infection must be distinguished from other causes of bronchial, lung, or pleural disease (Table 10–1). Pulmonary embolism, hemorrhage, lung tumors, congestive heart failure, hypersensitivity pneumonitis, or vasculitis can present with pulmonary symptoms, fever, and an abnormal chest film. An elevated white cell count in the peripheral blood can be helpful for diagnosis, as is careful examination of expectorated sputum. However, invasive procedures, such as bronchoscopy

with lavage, transbronchial biopsy, and/or open lung biopsy, may ultimately be required to determine the cause of lower respiratory tract disease.

## PATHOGENESIS OF LOWER RESPIRATORY TRACT INFECTION

The great majority of lower respiratory tract infections are the consequence of inhalation or aspiration of microorganisms. The upper airway is designed to warm, humidify, and screen inspired air to reduce the number of organisms or other foreign aerosolized particles reaching the bronchi. The nasal turbinates, mucus, and nasal hairs serve to trap such inhaled particles. Those organisms that traverse the nasal passages and reach the trachea are screened again by the cilia and mucous of this major airway. The cilia serve to carry particles trapped in mucus up to the pharynx (the so-called mucociliary elevator), thus providing a second barrier to colonization of the lower bronchial tree or alveoli, which in normal individuals remains sterile. Immunoglobulins, especially IgA, are contained in the mucus and provide another defense against microbial invasion.

The majority of organisms that produce lower respiratory infection first colonize the nasal and pharyngeal epithelium. Colonization is the result of an interaction of a surface molecule on the microorganism, an adhesin, interacting with a receptor on cells of the nasopharyngeal mucous membrane. In the healthy person, normal flora of the nasopharynx has an advantage in this ecology. As an example, in normal individuals, gargling of aerobic enteric organisms does not result in prolonged colonization of the pharynx. Cultures obtained 60 min after such exposure grow the usual flora of the oropharynx.

Certain pathogenic bacteria, such as *Streptococcus pneumoniae*, *Haemophilus influenzae*, and *Neisseria* species, however, can colonize the nasopharynx, and colonization rates with these organisms rise in the colder months of the year. In the setting of an intercurrent viral upper respiratory infection the defense mechanisms discussed above (normal ciliary function, for example) are altered, and inhalation of these organisms into the lower respiratory tract occurs, setting the stage for infection of the alveoli.

Other pathologic situations that favor colonization of the oropharynx with organisms

---

**TABLE 10–1.   DIFFERENTIAL DIAGNOSIS OF LOWER RESPIRATORY TRACT INFECTION**

Pulmonary tumor, primary or metastatic
Pulmonary embolism
Pulmonary hemorrhage
Congestive heart failure
Hypersensitivity pneumonitis
Vasculitis

associated with bronchitis and pneumonia include acute and chronic alcoholism and severe intercurrent illness. Alcohol ingestion, in addition to being associated with colonization of the upper airway by aerobic gram-negative bacilli, leads through its central nervous system effects to a diminished gag reflex and poor tracheobronchial ciliary function, thus altering important defenses of the respiratory tract. The pathogenic bacteria that colonize the upper airway in this situation gain access to the respiratory tract and produce pneumonia. Alcoholism is also associated with nausea and vomiting that, when coupled with loss of the gag reflex, can lead to aspiration either of the oropharyngeal flora or stomach contents. When vomitus is aspirated, a chemical pneumonitis is produced that increases the susceptibility of the pulmonary parenchyma to bacterial infection.

Severe illness also is associated with changes in the surface secretions of the oropharynx that favor colonization by organisms capable of producing bronchial or pulmonary infections. For reasons that are not clear, severe illness is associated with an increase in salivary protease activity, a reduction of mucosal fibronectin, and augmentation of the ability of gram-negative bacilli to colonize these surfaces. Immobilization due to debility also favors aspiration of organisms of the upper airway into the lower respiratory tract. In critically ill patients, antacids or $H_2$ blockers are used to prevent gastric ulceration (stress ulcers), resulting in a rise in stomach pH. The stomach, which is normally sterile, then can be colonized with bacteria. These bacteria are capable of retrograde colonization of the pharynx and, subsequently, causing pneumonia.

Specific intravascular infections lead to metastatic infection in the lungs. An example are the multiple foci of pneumonitis that occur in endocarditis involving the tricuspid and pulmonary valves (see Chapter 33). Vegetations break off from the valves as septic pulmonary emboli, lodge in the pulmonary capillaries, and serve as foci for phlebitis and pneumonitis. Pelvic infections with anaerobic organisms such as *Bacteroides* species also cause thrombophlebitis and septic pulmonary emboli—infections seen most frequently as a complication of parturition or septic abortion.

Finally, inhalation of irritant gases, such as cigarette smoke, alters the bronchial epithelium, leading to a loss of the cilia-bearing columnar epithelial cells and ultimately to chronic inflammation, with or without microbial infection of the bronchi. Acute bronchitis, in contrast, can occur as a direct result of viral or bacterial infection independent of such irritant effects. Structural damage to bronchi due to chronic infection can produce saccular pockets in the bronchial wall, collecting mucous secretions that commonly become infected with oropharyngeal bacteria. This condition, known as *bronchiectasis*, results in further destruction of the bronchial tree. A common condition underlying severe bronchiectasis is cystic fibrosis, an autosomal recessive disorder associated with mucus plugging of bronchi, chronic infection, and destruction of the integrity of the bronchial wall. The usual cause of infection of the pleural space is direct extension of infection from the lungs. Purulent infection of the pleural space is a closed space infection similar to an abscess and is termed *empyema*.

## ETIOLOGY

Any microorganism, given the appropriate circumstances and host factors, can cause lower respiratory tract infection. However, among bacteria, the common causes of lower respiratory tract infection in normal adults include *Streptococcus pneumoniae*, *Mycoplasma pneumoniae*, and *Legionella* species—the usual causes of community-acquired pneumonia. Group A streptococcus (*S. pyogenes*) causes outbreaks of pneumonia in such closed populations as recruit camps and boarding schools. *Staphylococcus aureus* and *Haemophilus influenzae* are uncommon causes of pneumonia in adults except in association with influenza epidemics. Lung infections with these organisms are more commonly seen in children. Children also commonly develop pneumococcal and mycoplasmal pulmonary infections. Among compromised hospitalized patients, *S. aureus* and aerobic gram-negative bacilli including *Legionella* are common causes of pneumonia (see Chapter 25). Aspiration pneumonia is usually due to the aerobic and particularly the anaerobic oropharyngeal flora. Mycobacterial infections are primarily lower respiratory tract infections and are discussed in Chapter 13.

Most of the deep mycoses, such as histoplasmosis, blastomycosis, coccidioidomycosis, and cryptococcosis, begin as lower respiratory tract infections following inhalation of the infecting form of these fungi. A more complete description of these infections is found in Chapter 14.

Viral infection is probably the most common cause of acute bronchitis and pneumonia in adults and children. It can be caused by any of the "respiratory viruses," including adenovirus, influenza, parainfluenza, and respiratory syncytial virus, as well as the enteroviruses. Coxsackievirus is the cause of epidemic pleurodynia, a form of pleuritis which, as its name implies, occurs in outbreaks (see Chapter 12).

## SPECIFIC SYNDROMES

There are a variety of specific clinical syndromes due to infection of the lower respiratory tract (Table 10–2). *Pneumonia*, the most common lower respiratory tract infection, is discussed in Chapter 11 (community-acquired) and Chapter 25 (nosocomial pneumonia).

*Acute bronchitis* is usually a self-limited infection of the bronchial tree due to viral infection. Similar symptoms can be seen with infection due to *Mycoplasma pneumoniae*. Patients usually seek medical attention because of a persistent cough that can be paroxysmal. Often the cough is nonproductive, but puru-

lent sputum may be expectorated even when the infection is due to viral infection. Patients complain of difficulty sleeping because of the cough and of tightness or discomfort in the anterior chest. Fever is not always present, but when it occurs it is usually low grade. Patients note chills but not rigors. Acute bronchitis is often preceded by an upper respiratory tract infection. The physical examination generally reveals normal breath sounds upon auscultation of the chest, but occasionally wheezes and rhonchi are present. Therapy can be aimed at controlling symptoms, unless it is suspected that the infection is due to *M. pneumoniae*. Usually, mycoplasmal infections occur in outbreaks within a geographic locale, and in interepidemic years the most common cause of acute bronchitis is viral infections, which should not be treated with antibiotics.

*Chronic bronchitis* represents a condition of chronic inflammation of the bronchi most commonly due to prolonged cigarette smoking. Smoking the equivalent of 20 cigarettes per day for 20 years (20 pack-years) is associated with changes in the bronchi that predispose to chronic bronchitis and that are often found in association with emphysema. An increase in the prevalence of chronic bronchitis and emphysema is found in persons who are heterozygotic for alpha$_1$-antitrypsin deficiency, even with minimal smoking. The diagnosis of chronic bronchitis is made on the basis of the history of 3 consecutive months of productive cough, 2 years in a row. Acute exacerbations of chronic bronchitis occur secondary to intercurrent viral or bacterial infection. Such exacerbations are associated with either increased sputum production or a marked reduction in sputum produced by cough. Usually, the patient seeks medical attention because of increasing shortness of breath. An emphysematous chest (hyperexpanded) with low diaphragms and diminished breath sounds is a common finding upon physical examination. The body temperature and white cell count usually are not elevated, and the chest x-ray commonly does not reveal pulmonary infiltrates. Evaluation of arterial blood gases reveals respiratory acidosis or compensated respiratory acidosis in severely ill patients with hypoxemia. Management usually includes antibiotics effective against *S. pneumoniae* and *H. influenzae*, such as ampicillin or trimethoprim-sulfamethoxazole. The chronic treatment for such patients includes cessation of smoking, bronchial hygiene, and in some patients prolonged antibiotic therapy.

**TABLE 10–2.   LOWER RESPIRATORY TRACT INFECTION**

| INFECTION | ETIOLOGY |
| --- | --- |
| Bronchitis | |
|   Acute | Respiratory viruses |
| | *Mycoplasma pneumoniae* |
|   Chronic | Respiratory viruses |
| | *Streptococcus pneumoniae* |
| | *Haemophilus influenzae* |
| Pneumonia | |
|   Community-acquired | Respiratory viruses |
| | *Streptococcus pneumoniae* |
| | *Legionella pneumophila* |
| | *Mycoplasma pneumoniae* |
| | *Chlamydin pneumoniae* |
|   Hospital-acquired | Aerobic gram-negative bacilli |
| | *Staphylococcus aureus* |
| | *Chlamydin pneumoniae* |
|   Aspiration/necrotizing | Oropharyngeal flora (anaerobic/aerobic organisms) |
| Lung abscess | Oropharyngeal flora |
| Bronchiectasis | Oropharyngeal flora |
| | *Pseudomonas aeruginosa* |
| | Aerobic/anaerobic bacteria |
| Empyema | Group A streptococcus |
| | *Streptococcus pneumoniae* |
| | *Staphylococcus aureus* |

Antibiotics are often administered prophylactically in the winter months when respiratory infections occur with increased frequency.

*Pneumonia* following aspiration of vomitus, a foreign object, or oropharyngeal flora commonly results in a necrotizing process with destruction of pulmonary tissue and production of a lung abscess. Patients with a lung abscess complain of fever, foul-smelling, often fetid sputum, and chest discomfort. There is commonly a history of alcoholism, seizures, impaired swallowing or cough mechanisms, loss of consciousness, or aspiration of a foreign object; for example, symptoms develop following inhalation of food. Organisms isolated by invasive techniques such as transtracheal aspiration include both aerobic and anaerobic flora of the oropharynx. The fusobacterium and other anaerobic microbial species are the cause of the fetid odor of the breath and sputum. Physical examination often reveals an area of consolidation. Amphoric breath sounds (blowing across the top of a bottle) sometimes can be heard if the abscess cavity communicates with a bronchus. The peripheral white count is elevated and the chest x-ray reveals a fluid-filled, or partially filled, thick-walled cavity. Treatment is dependent upon drainage, which is achieved by bronchoscopy or by having the patient practice postural drainage (chest physical therapy). Postural drainage is accomplished with the patient lying across the bed with the arms upon a chair, placing the head lower than the thorax. Coughing, aided by chest percussion, usually results in expectoration of large amounts of sputum. Antibiotic therapy has greatly reduced the morbidity due to lung abscess and has largely eliminated the need for surgical drainage. The agents of choice must be active against the oropharyngeal flora. Penicillin G, ampicillin, first-generation cephalosporins, and clindamycin are all effective against this infection.

*Bronchiectasis* can be managed in much the same fashion as a lung abscess. Stimulation of coughing to drain infected secretions and institution of similar antibiotics usually control acute exacerbations. Prolonged antibiotic therapy with the agents listed above can lead to superinfection with antibiotic-resistant gram-negative bacilli, such as *Pseudomonas aeruginosa*, which require treatment with an enhanced-spectrum penicillin or cephalosporin in combination with an aminoglycoside. These agents must be given parenterally. In general, lung abscess and bronchiectasis require a minimum of 2 weeks of parenteral antibiotic therapy. Follow-up oral antibiotic therapy of a lung abscess is usually continued until there is evidence of a substantial decrease in size of the cavity on chest x-ray.

*Empyema,* or infection of the pleural cavity, is usually the result of extension of an underlying pneumonia to the pleural space. Although empyema can occur with any form of bacterial pneumonia, it is seen in a minority of cases of infection due to *S. pneumoniae.* In contrast, 50% of pneumonias due to group A streptococcus are complicated by empyema. This is presumably due to the multiplicity of enzymes produced by *Streptococcus pyogenes* that interfere with the inflammatory barriers that usually localize infection (see Chapter 7).

*Necrotizing pneumonia* following aspiration also is associated with empyema due to destruction of lung tissue and spread of infection to the pleural cavity. Pulmonary infections with actinomyces are also commonly complicated by empyema because of the predilection of infection with this organism to cross tissue barriers. Empyema can be suspected from physical findings compatible with the presence of fluid between the lung and outer chest wall. Breath sounds are distant and there is flatness or lack of resonance with percussion of the thorax of the affected side. Unless the infection is loculated, a chest x-ray will demonstrate pleural fluid that changes in position with the patient lying on the involved side. The diagnosis is established by needle aspiration of the empyema fluid, which can be viscous and contains many leukocytes, a high concentration of protein, and a low concentration of glucose. The concentration of the enzyme lactic dehydrogenase is much higher than in serum. A Gram's stain often can suggest the etiologic agent(s), but cultures provide the definitive evidence of the cause of the underlying pneumonia as well as the empyema. Treatment generally requires placement of a chest tube with suction to ensure drainage, and appropriate antibiotic therapy. The choice of antibiotics is dictated by the identity of the isolated organism(s) and the results of antibiotic susceptibility tests. Tube drainage is continued as long as fluid is draining. Antibiotic therapy is continued usually until the chest tube is removed or for a minimum of 3 weeks. A complication of empyema due to necrotizing pneumonia is the development of a bronchopleural fistula. In the preantibiotic era undrained empyema could dissect through the chest wall and drain spontaneously, producing empyema necessitans.

## PREVENTION

Prevention of lower respiratory tract disease represents a major challenge to the medical profession. The single most important step is cessation of smoking. Additionally, reduction in excessive use of alcohol decreases the prevalence of bacterial pneumonias, aspiration pneumonia, and lung abscess. Recently, it has been suggested that administration of non-absorbable antibiotics by mouth, to prevent colonization of the stomach when gastric acidity is reduced, will prevent hospital-acquired pneumonia. Finally, as discussed in Chapter 40, immunization to prevent influenza and pneumonia due to *Streptococcus pneumoniae* and *Haemophilus influenzae* in selected groups of the population can further reduce the prevalence of lower respiratory tract infections.

## CASE HISTORY

### CASE HISTORY 1

A 52-year-old man with a long history of alcohol abuse and a 50 pack-year smoking habit is admitted with fever and cough productive of foul-smelling sputum. These symptoms have been present for 3 weeks following an alcoholic binge during which the patient lost consciousness. He had become anorectic, lost 5 lb, and noted a dull discomfort in his right chest. He had fetid halitosis, a temperature of 102°F, and was in moderate distress, with 20 respirations per minute. His thorax expanded normally with inspiration, and breathing was not associated with pain. The right and left hemithoraces were equally resonant to percussion, but auscultation revealed crackles over the right posterior chest. Breath sounds were accentuated in this area. His white blood cell count was 12,200/mm³, with 70% neutrophils and 10% band forms. Gram's stain of the sputum revealed many neutrophils, gram-negative bacilli and coccobacilli, and gram-positive cocci. Forty-eight hours later, the laboratory reported the presence of "normal oropharyngeal flora" in the sputum culture. The chest x-ray demonstrated a thick-walled cavity in the upper segment of the right lower lobe with an air–fluid level surrounded by an infiltrate. The diagnosis of lung abscess was made, and therapy was initiated with intravenous penicillin G, $1 \times 10^6$ units every 4 h. Bronchial hygiene was established with postural drainage and chest percussion. This was productive of large amounts of sputum. Within 3 days the sputum no longer had a fetid odor and

the daily temperature elevation was lower. In view of this response, penicillin V, 500 mg by mouth every 6 h, was substituted for intravenous penicillin G. After 10 days the patient was eating well, had gained 3 lb, and was afebrile. A repeat x-ray showed clearing of the infiltrate and a decrease in the size of the cavity. Sputum cytology did not demonstrate any malignant cells. The patient, after counseling, agreed to join Alcoholics Anonymous and to attempt to give up smoking. He was discharged with a prescription for penicillin V with instructions to return to the pulmonary clinic in 2 weeks.

### CASE 1 DISCUSSION

This is the typical presentation of a lung abscess that commonly develops following aspiration of vomitus during an alcoholic binge. The infection is polymicrobial, reflecting the aerobic and anaerobic oropharyngeal bacteria. Therefore, the culture of sputum does not grow a specific pulmonary pathogen such as Klebsiella or *S. pneumoniae*. The bacteria constituting the oropharyngeal flora are generally susceptible to penicillin. Occasionally, infection with the beta-lactamase–producing *Bacteroides fragilis* occurs, requiring treatment with clindamycin or cefoxitin. Establishing drainage of the abscess is necessary and usually can be accomplished adequately by postural drainage. Surgical intervention is therefore not usually required.

Once the inflammatory response is decreased, it is necessary in adults to determine if the abscess has developed in the necrotic center of a lung tumor. Cytologic examination of cells in the sputum can be helpful, as is the continued response to therapy. If repeat x-rays do not demonstrate improvement in the abscess, bronchoscopy is required to rule out the presence of bronchial carcinoma, especially in smokers. Prolonged antibiotic therapy for 4–6 weeks is advocated for treatment of lung abscess. Thus, it is important to provide for appropriate follow-up during convalescence after hospital discharge.

## REFERENCES

**Books**

Niederman, M. S., Sarosi, G., and Glassroth, J., ed. *Respiratory Infections: A Scientific Basis for Management.* Philadelphia: W. B. Saunders Co., 1994.

**Articles**

Bartlett, J., Gorbach, S., and Finegold, S. The bacteriology of aspiration pneumonia. *Am. J. Med. 56:*202–207, 1974.
Bartlett, J., Gorbach, S., Tally, F., et al. Bacteriology and treatment of primary lung abscess. *Am. Rev. Respir. Dis. 109:*510–524, 1974.

DePaso, W. J. Aspiration pneumonia. *Clin. Chest Med. 12*: 269–284, 1991.

Gleeson, K., and Reynolds, H. Y. Life threatening pneumonia. *Clin. Chest Med. 15*:581–602, 1994.

Lebowitz, M., and Burrows, B. The relationship of acute respiratory illness history to the prevalence and incidence of obstructive lung disorders. *Am. J. Epidemiol. 105*:544–554, 1977.

Levison, M., Mangura, C., Larber, B., et al. Clindamycin compared with penicillin for the treatment of anaerobic lung abscess. *Ann. Intern. Med. 98*:466–471, 1983.

Monto, A., and Ross, H. The Tecumseh study of respiratory illness. X relation of acute infection to smoking, lung function and chronic symptoms. *Am. J. Epidemiol. 107*:57–64, 1978.

Tablan, O. C., Anderson, L. J., et al. Guideline for prevention of nosocomial pneumonia. *Am. J. Infect. Control 22*:247–292, 1994.

Thorsteinsson, S., Musher, D., and Fagan, T. The diagnostic value of sputum culture in acute pneumonia. *JAMA 233*:894–895, 1975.

Wood, D. Role of fibronectin in the pathogenesis of gram-negative bacillary pneumonia. *Rev. Infect. Dis. 9*: S386–390, 1987.

# 11

# COMMUNITY-ACQUIRED BACTERIAL PNEUMONIA

JOHN P. PHAIR, M.D.

Before the antibiotic era, bacterial pneumonia was a leading cause of morbidity and mortality in the United States, and it remains an important form of infection that is difficult to manage. Antibiotic treatment, however, has greatly altered the clinical approach to this disease. A wide variety of bacteria cause infection of the lungs both in previously healthy individuals and in those with underlying debilitating disease. This chapter discusses the causes of community-acquired pneumonia and their differing clinical presentations and management. Bacterial pneumonia can involve an entire single lobe, multiple lobes, lobular segments, or can present as bronchopneumonia, defined as a patchy involvement of one or several lobes. It can develop explosively or have a more indolent onset. Multiple complications can arise due to either hematogenous or contiguous spread of the infecting organism. The frequency of such complications differs with the infecting organism.

## DIAGNOSIS AND DIFFERENTIAL DIAGNOSIS

Bacterial pneumonia should be suspected in patients whose signs of infection include chills, fever, and symptoms referable to the lower respiratory tract. An elevated peripheral neutrophil count with early forms of neutrophils is common, although neutropenia can also be found, especially in patients with bacteremic pneumonia. A chest x-ray should demonstrate pulmonary infiltrates (Figs. 11–1 and 11–2); however, early in the course of the infection or in dehydrated patients, the x-ray can be misleading. Although this constellation of findings is helpful in suggesting infection in the lungs, it does not establish the etiology of the pneumonia. The causative organism can be identified definitively only by isolation from cultures of sputum, pleural fluid (if available), or blood. Thoracentesis should be performed if pleural fluid is present, and a minimum of two blood cultures should be obtained from every patient in whom bacterial pneumonia is suspected. In some forms of pulmonary infection, such as that due to *Mycoplasma pneumoniae* or *Legionella*, serology can be extremely helpful but only in retrospect (Table 11–1).

It is important to collect sputum in an appropriate manner because bacteremia or pleural involvement does not occur in every patient. Culture of sputum obtained following a deep cough can establish the etiology of the infection. A Gram's stain of sputum is extremely useful in determining whether or not the specimen represents secretions from the

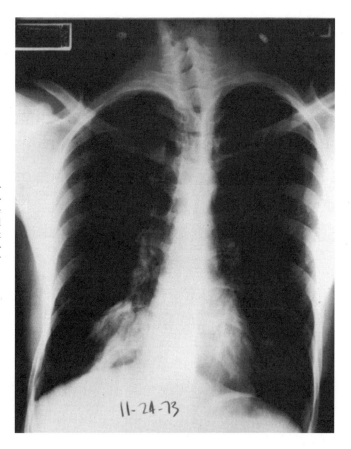

**FIGURE 11–1.** Posteroanterior chest roentgenogram of the patient discussed in Case History 1. Note the fairly well-defined density in the lower right lung field. Without the right lateral roentgenographic projection (see Fig. 11–2), it would be impossible to know whether the pneumonic infiltrate occupies the right middle or right lower lobe of the lung.

site of infection or merely expectorated saliva. Culture of improperly collected sputum can be misleading about the cause of the infection. Expectorated sputum in bacterial pneumonia should contain more than 25 neutrophils and not more than 10 epithelial cells per high-powered field. If a good specimen is obtained and a predominant organism is present, a skilled microscopist can provide a tentative etiologic diagnosis from the Gram's stain. Some patients cannot produce sputum spontaneously. For these patients, an appropriate sputum specimen can be induced using inhaled nebulized steam and gentle chest percussion. Children under the age of 7 or 8 rarely are capable of producing adequate sputum specimens. Invasive techniques such as transtracheal aspiration by needle, in which sterile saline is instilled and then aspirated, were utilized in the recent past to overcome difficulties in obtaining a high-quality sputum sample. This technique is now used less frequently as it is associated with bleeding and other complications. Bronchoscopy with bronchial lavage and brushings or transbronchial biopsy is now utilized more frequently

in specific situations and can be extremely useful in determining etiology.

It is important to recognize that not all patients with fever, respiratory symptoms, and a pulmonary infiltrate have pneumonia. Other common causes of these signs and symptoms include pulmonary embolism (with or without infarction), primary or metastatic lung tumors, or, less commonly, pulmonary hemorrhage, among many other conditions. Thus, the physician is required to decide if the pulmonary symptoms are due to infection, and, if so, to establish a bacteriologic cause. At this point a decision regarding empiric antibiotic therapy is necessary. Once culture results are available, antibiotic treatment should be modified to use the safest, most conveniently administered, and least expensive effective agent.

## ETIOLOGY

Of the bacterial causes of community-acquired pneumonia, *Streptococcus pneumoniae*, *Haemophilus influenzae*, and *Klebsiella pneumoniae* have been well recognized for many years.

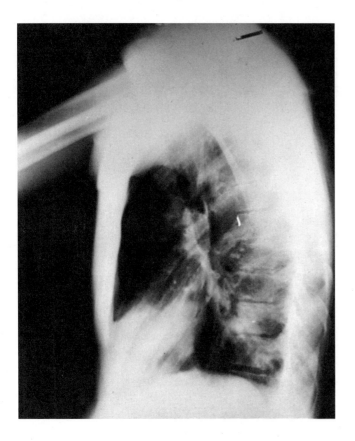

**FIGURE 11–2.** Right lateral chest roentgenogram of the patient discussed in Case History 1. Although difficult to discern because of the cardiac shadow, the density noted in the right lung (Fig. 11–1) appears to be within the middle lobe and also the lower lobe of the right lung. The "stringy" densities confined to the hilar region are not uncommon in patients with bronchial asthma.

They are extracellular pathogens that are killed by phagocytic cells, neutrophils, and macrophages. *Staphylococcus aureus* and group A streptococcus are also extracellular pathogens but, in contrast to the three organisms listed above, are less frequent causes of pneumonia. Legionella, mycoplasma, and moraxella are more recently identified causes of pulmonary infections and raise specific issues relevant to diagnosis and treatment. The three most common bacterial causes of community-acquired pneumonia in adults are *Streptococcus pneumoniae, Mycoplasma pneumoniae, Chlamydia pneumoniae,* and *Legionella pneumophila* (Table 11–2). In children, *Haemophilus influenzae, S. pneumoniae,* and *Staphylococcus*

**TABLE 11–1. DIFFERENTIAL DIAGNOSTIC FEATURES OF BACTERIAL VS. NONBACTERIAL PNEUMONIA**

| FEATURE | PNEUMOCOCCAL LOBAR PNEUMONIA | VIRAL–MYCOPLASMAL PNEUMONIA |
|---------|------------------------------|------------------------------|
| Onset | Sudden | Gradual |
| Rigors | Single chill | "Chilliness" |
| Facies | "Toxic" | Well |
| Cough | Productive | Paroxysmal; nonproductive |
| Sputum | Purulent (bloody) | Mucoid |
| Herpes labialis | Frequent | Rare |
| Temperature | 103°–104°F | <103°F |
| Pleurisy | Frequent | Rare |
| Consolidation | Frequent | Rare |
| Gram's stain (sputum) | Neutrophils; cocci | Mononuclear cells; mixed flora |
| White blood cell and differential count | >15,000/mm³ Immature neutrophils | >15,000/mm³ Normal |
| Chest roentgenogram | Defined density | Nondefined infiltrate |

**TABLE 11–2.   ETIOLOGIC CATEGORIES OF INFECTIOUS PNEUMONIA AMONG HOSPITALIZED PATIENTS AT YALE–NEW HAVEN MEDICAL CENTER***

| MICROBIAL AGENT ISOLATED | JULY 1969– JAN. 1972 | | JULY 1979– JAN. 1982 | |
|---|---|---|---|---|
| | Percentage | | Percentage[†] | |
| *Streptococcus pneumoniae* | 46.0 | | 21.0 | |
| *Staphylococcus* sp. | 6.8 | | 3.4 | |
| *Haemophilus influenzae* | 3.8 | | 3.2 | |
| *Klebsiella* sp. | 1.8 | | 3.0 | |
| Other bacteria | 9.5 | | 22.0 | |
|   Total bacteria | | 67.9 | | 52.6 |
| *Mycoplasma pneumoniae* | 5.6 | | 3.4 | |
| Fungi (*Candida* and others) | <7.2 | | 13.2 | |
| Influenza | 1.0 | | 3.4 | |
| Cytomegalovirus | 0 | | 1.5 | |
| "Unspecified virus(es)" | 16.5 | | 28.0 | |
|   Total viruses | | 17.5 | | 32.9 |
| Miscellaneous agents | 2.1 | | 4.4 | |
|   Total patient records reviewed | | 935 | | 1175 |

*Adapted from Fick, R. B. Jr., and Reynolds, H. Y. Changing spectrum of pneumonia—news media creation or clinical reality? *Am. J. Med. 74*:1, 1983. With permission. Etiologic categories modified by the author of this chapter as follows: "Other bacteria" includes other streptococci, *Pseudomonas aeruginosa*, *Legionella pneumophilia*, and *Mycobacterium tuberculosis*; "miscellaneous agents" includes *Pneumocystis carinii*, *Chlamydia* sp., and parasitic microorganisms.

[†]Cumulative total percentage exceeds 100% because more than one agent was isolated in some patients.

*aureus* are also seen frequently, but legionella infection is very uncommon.

## SPECIFIC FORMS OF PNEUMONIA

### Pneumococcal Pneumonia

*Streptococcus pneumoniae* are gram-positive diplococci that require an enriched medium for growth *in vitro*. On blood agar plates colonies produce alpha, or green, hemolysis. When heavily encapsulated, the colonies appear mucoid. These organisms are facultative anaerobes that often are difficult to maintain in culture because of autolysis produced by an endogenous enzyme, muramyl-L-alanine amidase. This enzyme, activated by a variety of stimuli including bile, is the basis of the bile solubility of these organisms, and distinguishes them from other alpha-hemolytic streptococci. *S. pneumoniae* is sensitive to optochin, and this characteristic is used to identify the organism when isolated in culture.

The serologic reactions of the capsular polysaccharide identify more than 80 separate serotypes of *S. pneumoniae*. The amount of capsular polysaccharide produced by an organism correlates roughly with virulence within a specific serotype. Thus, a type 3 *S. pneumoniae* with a large capsule is, in general, more virulent than a type 3 pneumococcus with less capsular polysaccharide. Normally, humans are resistant to pneumococci, which

is a part of the normal nasopharyngeal flora. Those *S. pneumoniae* that bind well to respiratory epithelial cells appear to be more pathogenic than those that are less firmly bound. With aspiration or inhalation into the lower respiratory tract, in the absence of antibody specific for the capsular polysaccharide, the organism replicates and edema and neutrophils fill the alveoli. The mechanism of alveolar cell injury that leads to the inflammatory response is not clearly delineated. The capsule inhibits phagocytosis by neutrophils. In the presence of opsonins (specific antibody or complement), ingestion and killing of the organism by phagocytes is rapid. In the absence of antibiotic therapy, recovery is associated with production of specific antibody. Without therapy, the infection can spread via the lymphatics to the hilar nodes and contiguous organs as well as hematogenously producing metastatic infection.

Pneumonia due to *S. pneumoniae* is the most common form of bacterial lung infection requiring hospitalization. It can occur in any age group and on a background of good health as well as in the presence of an underlying disease. In the colder months of the year, the "respiratory season," an increased number of normal individuals carry *S. pneumoniae* asymptomatically in the pharynx. Humans thus constitute the most important reservoir of this microorganism. Aspiration of *S. pneumoniae*, or the pneumococcus, into the lower respiratory tract is enhanced by a preceding viral upper respiratory illness that interferes with the normal upper respiratory tract defense mechanisms (see Chapter 8). In addition, alcohol ingestion increases the risk of developing pneumococcal pneumonia.

Classically, this infection has a sudden onset, heralded by a single severe rigor, and followed by a precipitous increase in body temperature and cough productive of rusty sputum. The patient usually is dyspneic and often complains of pleuritic chest pain. Examination of the chest reveals evidence of consolidation of a lobe, including limited expansion of the thorax on the affected side, increased tactile fremitus, dullness to percussion, bronchial breath sounds, and rales. Not uncommonly, the physical signs of consolidation are absent, especially if the patient is seen early in the course of the infection. Furthermore, the classic history of the acute illness can be absent or greatly altered. For example, elderly individuals complain only of fever and shortness of breath and often are unable to produce sputum.

The laboratory usually provides adjunctive evidence of infection. The peripheral white count typically is elevated, and there are many young forms of neutrophils seen on smear, the so-called shift to the left. Acutely, arterial blood gases often reveal marked hypoxemia. The arterial oxygen can be disproportionately low in relation to the actual amount of lung involvement, reflecting marked shunting of blood within the pulmonary vasculature.

In the untreated patient, the temperature continues to remain high for 7–10 days. The "crisis" at the end of this period is marked by a rapid rise in fever to levels of 105°F and is associated with the appearance of detectable levels of serum antibody to the capsular polysaccharide of the infecting pneumococcus. Once the peak of the fever is reached, the temperature drops precipitously to normal or below. The crisis is sometimes associated with cardiopulmonary collapse but more often heralds the beginning of convalescence. Appropriate antibiotic therapy, with penicillin G or erythromycin, in the majority of young healthy individuals infected with a susceptible organism is associated with rapid defervescence. In older or debilitated patients, in contrast, the temperature often falls more slowly, requiring 5–7 days to reach normal levels. Complications that were prevalent in the preantibiotic era include empyema, pericarditis, pyogenic arthritis, endocarditis, and meningitis. Empyema and pericarditis are due to direct extension of the infection to the contiguous structure; the remaining complications represent metastatic infection following bacteremia. Antibiotic therapy has greatly reduced the prevalence of these complications except in patients who delay seeking medical attention or who have a defect in host defenses such as hypogammaglobulinemia. The initial response to antibiotic therapy can be followed by recrudescence of fever. This can be due to development of one of the complications of pneumococcal pneumonia noted above, or it can represent a hypersensitivity reaction to the antibiotic used in treatment. Less commonly, the development of a sterile nonpurulent pleural effusion, in reaction to the underlying pneumonia, is the cause of the new fever. Drug fevers can mimic fevers seen with infection. The temperature may rise daily so that the fever curve resembles a picket fence. In other patients drug fever results in a constant temperature elevation marked by a dampened diurnal variation. This hypersensitivity reaction responds within 2–3 days to cessation of administration of the antibiotic. Drug fevers often occur without rash, eosinophilia, or other common manifestations of an allergic response.

The mortality rate for this form of pneumonia remains at 15–20% despite the availability of curative antibiotic therapy. Approximately one in five patients with pneumococcal pneumonia has positive blood cultures before initiation of treatment. Bacteremia, involvement of multiple lobes, advanced age, and metastatic infection all independently worsen the prognosis. Splenectomized individuals are also at great risk of developing fulminant infection with circulatory collapse and disseminated intravascular coagulation as a consequence of bacteremic pneumococcal infections (see Chapter 24).

The polysaccharide capsule of *S. pneumoniae* inhibits phagocytosis of the organism by neutrophils. Antibody to the capsule serves as an opsonin and is protective. Immunization designed to induce specific antibody to capsular polysaccharide was shown to reduce the frequency of pneumococcal infection before the antibiotic era. With the widespread availability of penicillin G and other effective agents, further development of vaccines was discontinued after World War II. The realization that bacteremic pneumococcal infection continued to be associated with high mortality renewed interest in developing a means of preventing this often-lethal form of pneumonia. Although there are more than 80 serotypes, a limited number account for the majority of bacteremic pneumonias. Therefore, a vaccine containing the polysaccharides of the 23 serotypes most commonly associated with bacteremia has been developed for use in "high-risk" individuals, including those with immune deficiencies, postsplenectomy patients, individuals with chronic cardiac and pulmonary disease, and the elderly. Controversy about the usefulness of the vaccine has continued since its introduction to clinical use (see Felice in the references for a complete discussion of this issue).

Although antibiotic resistance of *S. pneumoniae* has been recognized for almost 30 years, penicillin-resistant organisms had not posed a serious clinical problem until recently. The mechanism of resistance lies in an altered affinity of the penicillin-binding proteins (PBPs) for penicillins. PBPs are enzymes responsible for synthesis of the cell wall of the organism. An intermediate and high level of penicillin resistance have been described. Penicillin-susceptible pneumococci usually are inhibited by penicillin concentrations less than 0.02 $\mu$g/mL, those with intermediate susceptibility require 0.1 to 1.0 $\mu$g/mL, and resistant pneumococci require concentrations of at least 2.0 $\mu$g/mL to inhibit growth. The prevalence of organisms with this high level of resistance varies but has been reported to be near 40% in Spain and higher in Eastern Europe and South Africa. In the United States high-level resistance has been localized to specific geographic regions. These organisms generally are also resistant to other commonly used orally administered antibiotics and require therapy with vancomycin. The rising prevalence of these highly penicillin-resistant *S. pneumoniae* are further justification for use of the pneumococcal vaccine.

## Legionella Pneumonia

In August 1976, a pneumonic illness with a high fatality rate occurred among men and women who attended a state American Legion convention in Philadelphia. The majority of affected individuals had stayed at a single hotel and became ill within 2–3 days after returning home. Treatment with penicillins or cephalosporin antibiotics was not associated with improvement. Many of the individuals, in addition to pneumonia, were noted to have diarrhea, renal and hepatic dysfunction, or change in mental status.

The isolate associated with the outbreak in Philadelphia was initially identified by methods used for isolation of rickettsia, inoculation of embryonated eggs. It was later grown on artificial media containing a higher concentration of cysteine than is present in commonly used media. In addition, ferric pyrophosphate stimulates growth but is not necessary for primary recovery of the organism. Following isolation, the organisms can be identified by immunofluorescent stains. Six serotypes of the organism *Legionella pneumophila* have been identified; type 1 caused the outbreak in Philadelphia. Closely related organisms, *L. bozemanii* and *L. micdadei*, also have been isolated from patients with similar forms of pneumonia. *L. micdadei* is unique in that it does not produce a beta-lactamase and appears to be associated most commonly with infection in compromised hosts. With identification of the etiologic organism, stored specimens from previous outbreaks of unexplained febrile illnesses revealed that this aerobic gram-negative bacillus had been the cause not only of pneumonia but also of a febrile illness that was short in duration and less lethal. This latter illness was termed Pontiac fever. With the isolation of *Legionella*, an assay for antibody to the bacteria and a simplified culture technique were developed. It is now apparent that *Legionella* species are a relatively common cause of pneumonia in adults, accounting for a significant proportion of the hospitalizations resulting from pulmonary infection. Serologic surveys have documented that approximately 5% of the population has antibody to these organisms.

The pneumonic form is by far the most common manifestation of this infection, and it occurs both in outbreaks and episodically. Individuals with chronic bronchitis or emphysema, cardiac disease, or immunodeficiencies are clearly more susceptible to this infection and have the highest morbidity and mortality. The organism is water-borne and can live in hot water systems as well as in air-conditioning ducts. This finding explains the outbreaks localized to a single building such as hotel or hospital. The organism, however, is ubiquitous and has been isolated from shower heads in homes and from the banks of rivers.

Legionella infections generally present with rigors, fever, and respiratory symptoms, but the onset is somewhat less explosive than pneumonia due to *S. pneumoniae*. The cough is often nonproductive and, in contradistinction to other forms of bacterial pneumonia,

Gram's stains of sputum reveal mononuclear cells rather than neutrophils. A paucity of microorganisms is found in smears of sputum. A high peripheral white count is generally present. If there is renal and hepatic involvement, elevation of serum creatinine, blood urea nitrogen, and hepatic enzymes are noted. Hyponatremia and hypophosphatemia suggest this form of pneumonia. The findings on chest x-ray can vary. The pneumonia can be lobar, but more commonly presents as a bronchopneumonia involving multiple lobes with or without a pleural effusion. The infection can also produce cavitary disease.

Diagnosis of legionella pneumonia requires a high degree of suspicion by the physician. The clinical presentation, although generally different from that of pneumonia due to S. pneumoniae and Mycoplasma pneumoniae, can mimic these infections completely. Acutely, the diagnosis is suggested by a serum antibody titer, using an indirect immunofluorescent technique, of greater than 1:64. If the titer is greater than 1:256 the diagnosis can be made more confidently. A fourfold rise or fall in antibody titer over a 4- to 6-week period is diagnostic of infection with a species of Legionella.

The antibiotics shown to be effective are the macrolides, fluoroquinolones, and rifampin. Erythromycin has been the most widely used form of therapy, and it is generally administered intravenously, 1 g every 6 h. The penicillins and cephalosporins are ineffective because these organisms, except for L. micdadei, produce a beta-lactamase that renders them resistant to beta-lactam agents.

### Mycoplasmal Pneumonia

Pulmonary infection due to Mycoplasma pneumoniae is most commonly diagnosed in young adults and older children. In the late 1930s, an atypical form of lung infection that differed from classic "pneumococcal pneumonia" was first described. During World War II the clinical features of the illness were delineated and the association of serum antibodies that aggregated erythrocytes in the cold and agglutinins for the MG streptococcus were noted. Eaton produced pneumonia in rats and hamsters with filtered sputum obtained from infected patients and documented that serum from convalescent patients protected the animals. In the 1950s, Liu identified the "Eaton agent" on bronchial epithelium of chick embryos using immunofluorescent techniques. Chanock and co-workers in the early 1960s proved that this agent caused "atypical pneumonia" and successfully cultured the organisms on artificial media.

M. pneumoniae requires supplemental enriched media for in vitro replication. It is slow-growing and has the typical properties of a mycoplasma. It is a small prokaryotic organism, bounded by a cell membrane and lacking a cell wall. Mycoplasma are the smallest free-living organisms, distinct from viruses in that they can be grown on cell-free media. They grow under both aerobic and anaerobic conditions. The inability of this organism to synthesize a cell wall renders it resistant to antibiotics that inhibit cell-wall synthesis, such as penicillins, cephalosporins, and vancomycin. Macrolides, tetracyclines, and fluroquinolone antibiotics that inhibit protein synthesis or DNA gyrase activity provide effective therapy.

Glycolipids in the cell membrane of M. pneumoniae induce both specific antibody and nonspecific antibody responses. Thus, a positive serologic test for syphilis sometimes develops following infection with this organism. A specific mycoplasmal lipid sequence apparently interacts with the erythrocyte antigens I and i, and presumably this is the basis for the induction of the cold hemagglutinin antibody—the cold agglutinins. Occasionally, high titers of the cold hemagglutinin are associated with hemolysis.

The infection is documented in susceptible populations in the temperate climates throughout the year. Thus, in the warmer months pneumonia due to M. pneumoniae increases relative to the decreasing prevalence of Streptococcus pneumoniae infection. When epidemics occur, mycoplasma infection can account for 15–20% of pneumonic illness in a community. However, the infection is usually mild and accounts for a small number of hospitalized patients even in epidemic periods. Upper respiratory infection with the organism is common in children under 5 years of age; pulmonary infection occurs most commonly in school-aged children and young adults. It is common to obtain a history of upper respiratory infections spreading through children in the family of an adult patient with this form of pneumonia for weeks before the pulmonary infection occurred. Attack rates are estimated to be very high once one member of a family or a closed population, such as boarding school students or military recruits, is infected.

Respiratory secretions contain M. pneumoniae for a week before the onset of clinical symptoms, but the concentration is highest at the time of onset of disease. The organism can then be detected in respiratory secretions for weeks after convalescence. The organism attaches to respiratory epithelium through the interaction of a membrane protein termed P1 and a cell-surface receptor. It is thought that oxidants produced by *M. pneumoniae* damage cells. It also has been postulated that clinical symptoms are the result of the immunologic response by the host to the organism. Immunologically mediated pathology could account for more disease occurring in older children and young adults who had been immunized by exposure to the organism early in life and for the relatively infrequent pneumonias due to this organism occurring in immunocompromised patients. The characteristic cellular infiltrate induced by infection consists of lymphocytes and plasma cells. Patient recovery from infection is associated with detection of specific IgG and IgA antibody in respiratory secretions. Thus, the immune response may be involved in production of clinical manifestations as well as in recovery.

Mycoplasmal pneumonia is generally mild, with fever and cough being the prominent signs. The disease begins slowly with nonspecific symptoms such as headache, malaise, and fever. Symptoms increase over the course of a few days before a nonproductive cough is noted that is often associated with substernal discomfort. Symptoms of an upper respiratory infection can be present. Rigors are not reported commonly by patients, and fever can range from low grade to 40°C. Examination of the chest can reveal wheezing, rhonchi, or rales, or can be negative. A minority of patients have myringitis and some patients complain of muscle tenderness and joint discomfort. Gastrointestinal symptoms include anorexia, nausea, and vomiting.

The chest x-ray usually demonstrates bronchopneumonia, which can involve multiple lobes, and a small pleural effusion is present in a quarter of the patients. The white blood cell count is often normal but can be moderately elevated. Few young neutrophilic forms are seen in the differential smears in contrast to results for pneumonococcal pneumonia. Sputum smears reveal phagocytic cells but usually contain mixed pharyngeal flora. The diagnosis is supported by the finding of cold agglutinins in serum usually within a week of the onset of the illness. The cold agglutinin is an IgM antibody directed against the I antigen on the red cell surface and can

be detected at the bedside by cooling anticoagulated blood obtained from the patient to 4°C and observing red cell aggregation. When the antibody is present in very high concentrations, erythrocytic aggregation can be seen at room temperature. A rise in specific complement-fixing antibodies to the organism late in the infection establishes the diagnosis.

The pneumonic form of mycoplasmal infection is generally self-limited but on rare occasion can be fatal. The course is shortened by treatment with erythromycin or tetracycline therapy for 7 days, if initiated early in the infection. Complications include meningitis, encephalitis, pericarditis, myocarditis, and erythema multiforme or its more severe form, Stevens-Johnson syndrome. Patients with sickle cell anemia develop severe illness with mycoplasmal pneumonia, marked by a brisk leukocytosis and pleural effusions. Other causes of atypical pneumonia that resemble that caused by *M. pneumoniae* include psittacosis, Q fever, and infections with *Chlamydia pneumoniae* as well as with *Legionella*. Treatment with tetracycline is effective for pulmonary infection with these agents, but erythromycin more effectively treats Legionnaire's disease, a more common infection. Moreover, tetracycline should not be used in children under 8 years of age, as it stains the developing permanent teeth.

### Pneumonia Caused by *Haemophilus influenzae*

*Haemophilus influenzae* type b is a common cause of lower respiratory infection in children; but its most dramatic manifestations are epiglottitis or meningitis (see Chapter 21). In adults serious infection with this small gram-negative coccobacillus is less frequent. In common with *Streptococcus pneumoniae*, *H. influenzae* type b is encapsulated by polysaccharide which inhibits phagocytosis by neutrophils in the absence of opsonic antibody.

Exposure in childhood to *H. influenzae* type b is thought to result in immunity and the lessened frequency of infection due to this encapsulated serotype in adults. In addition, cross-reactivity of the capsular polysaccharide with some pneumococcal types and with the *Escherichia coli* K1 antigen has been documented. Six antigenic types of capsular polysaccharide of *H. influenzae* have been distinguished: types a through f. Type b is by far the most frequent cause of serious infection. The role of unencapsulated (nontypable) *H. influenzae* in disease is less clearly defined.

Such organisms, as well as the encapsulated strains, are found in the normal pharyngeal flora. Frequent isolation of these bacteria from sputum specimens in patients with chronic bronchitis has led to the use of antibiotics to prevent and treat acute exacerbations of bronchitis. The role of *H. influenzae* in the pathogenesis of these acute episodes, however, remains problematic.

The pathogenesis of pulmonary infection due to *H. influenzae* is similar to pneumonia produced by the pneumococci. The organism, residing in the upper airway, reaches the lower respiratory tract when the normal defense mechanisms are altered, usually by a viral infection or alcohol ingestion. If the organism is encapsulated, phagocytosis by alveolar macrophages and neutrophils is inhibited. Bacterial replication occurs, followed by an inflammatory reaction and symptoms of pneumonia. In adults the onset is less dramatic than that of classic pneumococcal pneumonia, but severe dyspnea, cough, and fever are prominent features of the clinical picture. Lobar pneumonia is less frequently seen with *H. influenzae* than in pulmonary infection due to *S. pneumoniae*. The chest x-ray often demonstrates diffuse bronchopneumonia involving multiple lobes. In children, *H. influenzae* pneumonitis is frequently associated with bacteremia, but it is unclear whether the bacteremia is a primary or secondary event.

Treatment with ampicillin was previously effective. However, an increasing percentage of encapsulated and unencapsulated (nontypable) strains now produce beta-lactamase and are resistant to ampicillin and to first-generation cephalosporins. The extended-spectrum second- and third-generation cephalosporins are the empiric treatment of choice for serious infection due to *H. influenzae*. If the laboratory demonstrates lack of beta-lactamase production by the clinical isolate, ampicillin can be substituted. The availability of an effective vaccine for *H. influenzae* type b has greatly reduced serious infections due to this organism in children (see Chapter 40).

### Klebsiella Pneumonia

Pneumonia due to the aerobic gram-negative bacilli of the *Klebsiella* species is an uncommon cause of community-acquired pneumonia. Pulmonary infection with the low-numbered serotypes of these organisms was formerly called Friedländer's pneumonia. These organisms were first isolated in the late 19th century by Karl Friedländer, a clinician and microbiologist. The low-numbered serotypes are encapsulated by a polysaccharide capsule that is antiphagocytic and, therefore, a virulence factor.

The pneumonic form of infection with *Klebsiella* is most common among alcoholics and debilitated or elderly patients. The clinical onset is sudden, but a rigor is not a component of the classic picture. Fever and leukocytosis are usually present, but, as in many severe infections due to gram-negative bacilli, hypothermia and neutropenia may occur and are associated with a poor prognosis. The sputum produced by patients with klebsiella pneumonia is usually thick and tenacious. The chest x-ray can reveal either lobar or lobular infiltrates. Often with lobar involvement the volume of the affected lobe is expanded, marked by a convex bowing of the interlobar fissure. It is not uncommon to find cavity formation as a consequence of this necrotizing infection. The Gram's stains of the sputum should demonstrate neutrophils in abundance and many short, thick, gram-negative bacilli. Failure to recognize this form of pneumonia and to begin appropriate treatment can result in rapid death. In the preantibiotic era mortality rates reached 80%.

At the present time the most effective antibiotics used to treat klebsiella pneumonia are the extended-spectrum second- and third-generation cephalosporins. Many isolates are now resistant to the first-generation cephalosporins, cephalothin, and cefazolin. It has been suggested that the addition of an aminoglycoside such as gentamicin enhances survival of these patients. However, except for patients with neutropenia due to cytotoxic therapy or a hematologic malignancy, there is little information to indicate that the addition of these potentially toxic agents is beneficial.

### Staphylococcal Pneumonia

Pulmonary infection due to *Staphylococcus aureus* is a rare form of pneumonia except in immunocompromised patients and occasionally in infants and children. The pneumonia is generally a diffuse bronchopneumonitis that complicates a preceding viral upper respiratory infection and is especially common during community outbreaks of influenza. The clinical onset generally differs from that of pneumococcal infection in that staphylococcal pulmonary infections are insidious; chills are uncommon, but fever is high and the patient appears septic. Sputum can be purulent and is classically described as salmon-pink. However, in many patients, it is blood-tinged, and in some sputum production is scant, especially early in the course of the infection. If sputum is available, grape-like clusters of staphylococci are easily demonstrated by Gram's stain. As the disease progresses the chest radiograph often demonstrates multiple, small-cavitary lesions or abscesses or one or two large abscess cavities with air–fluid levels. Complications include spread of the infection to the pleura (empyema) or pericardium, and (with bacteremia) infection of cardiac valves (endocarditis), bone, kidneys, or meninges. Before the availability of effective antibiotic therapy, the prognosis was extremely poor, with mortality reaching 80–90% in some series. More recently, mortality is in the range of 5–10%.

Antibiotics of choice for treatment of severe staphylococcal infections are the penicillinase-resistant penicillins. At present the most commonly used forms of these antibiotics are nafcillin or oxacillin. The great majority (90%) of community-acquired, as well as hospital-acquired, *S. aureus* pneumonia are penicillin-resistant. An increasing number of these organisms are also methicillin-resistant (MRSA). The increased prevalence of MRSA infections is well documented in such epidemiologically restricted populations as intravenous drug users, but they are increasing in prevalence throughout society. Therefore, monitoring of the susceptibility pattern of *S. aureus* isolates, both hospital-acquired and community-acquired, is necessary. The antibiotic used to treat MRSA infection is vancomycin.

Endocarditis of the tricuspid and pulmonary valves due to *S. aureus* is diagnosed frequently among intravenous drug users and is seen in individuals with left-to-right shunts resulting from congenital cardiac disease. Septic emboli from these infected valves typically lodge in the pulmonary capillary bed and produce multiple scattered areas of bronchopneumonia. This is probably the most common form of hematogenously acquired pulmonary infection.

## Group A Streptococcal Pneumonia

Pneumonia is an uncommon form of infection due to this organism; however, it can be an especially virulent clinical illness. Most often, pneumonia due to group A streptococcus occurs, epidemically, in closed populations following an outbreak of a viral upper respiratory infection. However, sporadic cases are seen. The details of the microbiology and pathogenic potential of this organism are presented in Chapter 7.

The pathogenesis of pneumonia due to this organism is similar to that for *Streptococcus pneumoniae*. Following alteration in the normal host defenses of the upper airway, often as a consequence of viral infection, the organism reaches the lower respiratory tract. The onset of signs and symptoms is explosive, and the patient is usually extremely toxic. The extracellular products that contribute to the virulence of this organism influence the clinical picture of pulmonary infection. The pneumonia spreads rapidly and empyema is documented in up to 50% of cases. Management requires early recognition and institution of therapy with penicillin. Mortality due to group A streptococcal pneumonia is low unless treatment is delayed.

## Pneumonia Caused by *Moraxella catarrhalis*

Although sinusitis and otitis media are the most common infections associated with *Moraxella catarrhalis* (formerly named *Branhamella catarrhalis*), bronchopulmonary infections have been reported with increasing frequency over the past decade. However, respiratory tract infections are most definitively documented in patients with a significant compromise of host defenses. In patients who are the recipients of organ grafts, *M. catarrhalis* pneumonitis can develop rapidly, be associated with moderate to severe toxicity, but respond rapidly to appropriate antimicrobial therapy. Beta-lactamase production has been increasingly documented in clinical isolates. Therefore, ampicillin, which had been universally effective, can no longer be used empirically. A broad-spectrum cephalosporin or the combination of a beta-lactamase inhibitor such as clavulanic acid plus ampicillin are the agents to be used when this organism is suspected.

The pathogenesis of pneumonia due to this member of the normal oropharyngeal flora closely mimics that of *Haemophilus influenzae* or *Streptococcus pneumoniae*—that is, aspiration from the usual locus of colonization, failure or absence of defense mechanisms, bacterial replication, and an inflammatory response in the alveoli.

## Pneumonia Due to Chlamydia Species

Two species of this specialized bacterium cause pulmonary infection. *Chlamydia psittacci* is a rare cause of pneumonia in the United States. The organism causes ornithosis and is acquired most commonly following exposure to chronically infected psittacine birds. Although uncommon, the pneumonia produced by this organism is usually bilateral and found in the lower lobes. Other manifestations include diarrhea, myalgia, and headache. Patients have chills, high fever, temperature-pulse disassociation, and truncal skin lesions (Horder spots), which are pink papules that blanch with application of pressure. Mortality approaches 40%.

More common is a milder form of respiratory infection due to the totally unrelated *Chlamydia pneumoniae* that apparently is a strictly human pathogen. First isolated in 1965 in Taiwan and later in association with an acute respiratory infection, the organism was initially called the TWAR agent. Serologic studies in Washington, Nova Scotia, and Finland have demonstrated that *Chlamydia pneumoniae* can be responsible for up to 10% of community-acquired pneumonic infections in a given year. The prevalence of antibody increases with age, being relatively low in children. The majority of infections are mild, causing fever, nonproductive cough, and pharyngitis. This symptom complex is followed by bronchitis and pneumonia in some patients. Infection in elderly patients, especially those with underlying disease, is more severe. The chest x-ray generally demonstrates a single infiltrate. Diagnosis can be established only by increase in antibody titer. Treatment with tetracycline is more effective than erythromycin for infection with either chlamydia species.

*Chlamydia trachomatis*, a venereal pathogen, is the most common cause of afebrile pneumonia in young infants. About 20–50% of infants born vaginally to mothers who harbor this organism in their genital tracts develop conjunctivitis 1–3 weeks after birth unless ophthalmic prophylaxis with erythromycin is given. About half of the infected infants develop afebrile pneumonitis. Affected infants present with a staccato cough and tachypnea without fever; rales may be present and infiltrates are apparent on chest x-ray. Chlamydiae are present in conjunctival and nasopharyngeal secretions, and cytoplasmic inclusions are often present in these secretions. Chlamydial pneumonitis is frequently associated with mild peripheral eosinophilia and hyperimmunoglobulinemia. Erythromycin given orally for 14 days is effective in this infection.

## CASE HISTORIES

### CASE HISTORY 1

A 30-year-old lawyer was seen in the emergency room for fever, cough, and pain in the right side of the chest with breathing. He had been well until 7 days before when he had caught a "cold," which he thought was improving. Two nights before coming to the hospital he had "partied" with friends and become intoxicated. The day before he noted a severe chill, followed by fever, chest pain, and cough productive of yellow sputum.

Physical examination revealed a young man in moderate respiratory distress. He was febrile (39°C), breathing 20 times per minute, and had a tachycardia of 110/min. His blood pressure was 120/80. The positive physical findings were limited to a "fever blister" on his lower lip, limited expansion of the right thorax on inspiration, dullness to percussion over the right posterior lung fields, and bronchial breath sounds.

The white count was 12,000/mm$^3$ with an increase in young neutrophils (30%), and the chest x-ray revealed right lower and middle lobe pneumonitis. Gram's stain of expectorated sputum revealed neutrophils and gram-positive, lancet-shaped diplococci. One sputum culture and two blood cultures were obtained.

The patient was hospitalized and penicillin G (600,000 units) was administered intravenously. This was followed in 4 h by procaine penicillin (600,000 units) given intramuscularly. The procaine penicillin was then given every 12 h for the next 48 h. At that point the patient was afebrile and felt subjectively much better. The sputum culture grew *Streptococcus pneumoniae*, but the blood cultures were sterile. With the clinical improvement the therapy was changed to 500 mg penicillin V by mouth every 6 h. He continued to improve and was discharged on the fourth hospital day to continue the oral penicillin for 3 more days at home. He was seen by his physician a week following discharge and requested to return to work because he felt well.

### CASE 1 DISCUSSION

This is a typical presentation of pneumonia due to *Streptococcus pneumoniae*. The lower respiratory signs and symptoms developed on the background of an upper respiratory infection and acute alcohol ingestion and were associated with an exacerbation of herpes simplex infection. The initial sign was a rigor. In this healthy young man the response to penicillin therapy was rapid. The organism's usual extreme susceptibility to penicillin allows for low parenteral and low oral doses of penicillin to be used in therapy. Early discharge was possible because the absence of documented bacteremia reduces the risk of arthritis, meningitis, or endocarditis, which can complicate bloodstream infection. A follow-up chest x-ray would continue to demonstrate a pulmonary infiltrate, because x-ray findings commonly lag behind clinical improvement by several weeks.

## CASE HISTORY 2

A 50-year-old air-conditioner repairman was admitted to the hospital with pneumonia. He had noted onset of chills, fever, and cough 3 days before admission. At admission he was somewhat confused but able to give a complete history. He stated that he had diarrhea for the past 2 days, as well as the respiratory symptoms. He was a heavy smoker but did not drink alcohol. He was febrile (39.5°C), breathing 25 times per minute, had a tachycardia of 120/minute, and his blood pressure was 90/60. Rales were heard over the left posterior lung fields, and a chest x-ray confirmed the presence of pneumonitis in the left lower lobe. He could not produce sputum. The white count was elevated (13,500/mm$^3$), and there was a shift to the left. Serum chemistries revealed elevated levels of transaminase, bilirubin, blood urea nitrogen, and creatinine. The serum sodium value was below normal. Two blood cultures were obtained.

Therapy was initiated with erythromycin, 1 g intravenously every 6 h, as empiric therapy for a community-acquired pneumonia. The history of diarrhea, liver function, and renal abnormalities on a background of good health suggested to a consultant the possibility of Legionnaire's pneumonia. Serologic studies for antibody to *Legionella* and *Mycoplasma* were obtained on the second hospital day. By the fourth hospital day, although the patient remained febrile, he was clear mentally and subjectively improved. The blood cultures were sterile, but the titer of antibody to *Legionella* type 2 was 1:64. There were no antibodies to *Mycoplasma*. Therapy was continued with erythromycin. By day 7 he was afebrile, and asking to go home. The abnormal serum chemistries had improved. He was discharged to continue erythromycin (500 mg orally) every 6 h for 7 additional days.

## CASE 2 DISCUSSION

The presence of mental status changes, diarrhea, and abnormalities in renal and liver function in association with pneumonia alerted the physician to the possibility of infection with *Legionella pneumophila*. The patient's occupation exposed him to potentially contaminated aerosols in air-conditioning ducts. The antibody titer of 1:64 was suggestive but not diagnostic of this infection. Approximately 5% of the population has antibody to this organism. The diagnosis could be proved by obtaining a convalescent sera and demonstrating a significant ($\geq$ fourfold) rise or fall in the antibody titer.

The three most common causes of community-acquired pneumonia in adults can be treated effectively with erythromycin.

*Legionella* and *Mycoplasma* are resistant to such beta-lactam antibiotics as penicillin, but *Streptococcus pneumoniae* is susceptible to both penicillin and erythromycin.

## REFERENCES

### Books

Heffron, R. *Pneumonia.* Cambridge, MA: Harvard University Press, 1979.

Neiderman, M. S., Sarose, G. A., and Glassroth, J., eds. *Respiratory Infections.* Philadelphia: W. B. Saunders, Co., 1994.

### Articles

Austrian, R. Pneumococcal infection and pneumococcal vaccine. *N. Engl. J. Med.* 297:938–939, 1977.

Austrian, R., and Gold, J. Pneumococcal bacteremia with especial reference to bacteremic pneumococcal pneumonia. *Ann. Intern. Med.* 60:759–776, 1964.

Busk, M., Rosenow, E., and Wilson, W. Invasive procedure in the diagnosis of pneumonia. *J. Infect. Dis. 155*: 855–861, 1988.

Carpenter, J. Klebsiella pulmonary infections: Occurrence at one medical center and review. *Rev. Infect. Dis.* 12:672–682, 1990.

Fedson, D. S. Pneumococcal vaccination in the prevention of community-acquired pneumonia. *Semin. Respir. Infect.* 8:285–293, 1993.

Fekety, R., Caldwell, J., Gump, D., et al. Bacteria, virus, and mycoplasma in acute pneumonia in adults. *Am. Rev. Respir. Dis.* 104:499–507, 1971.

Finegold, S. M. Aspiration pneumonia. *Rev. Infect. Dis.* 13(Suppl. 9):S737–742, 1991.

Fraser, D., Tsai, T., Ornstein, W., et al. Legionnaire's disease. Description of an epidemic of pneumonia. *N. Engl. J. Med.* 297:1189–1197, 1977.

Gaydos, C. A., et al. Diagnosis of *Chlamydia pneumoniae* infection in patients with community-acquired pneumonia by PCR. *Clin. Infect. Dis.* 19:157–160, 1994.

Gopal, V., and Bisno, A. Fulminant pneumococcal infection in "normal" asplenic hosts. *Arch. Intern. Med. 137*: 1526–1530, 1977.

Grayston, J., Alexander, E., Kenny, G., et al. *Mycoplasma pneumoniae* infections. Clinical and epidemiologic studies. *JAMA 191*:369–374, 1965.

Grayston, J. T. *Chlamydia pneumoniae* (TWAR) infections in children. *Pediatr. Infect. Dis. J.* 13:675–684, 1994.

Hahn, H., and Beaty, H. Transtracheal aspiration in the evaluation of patients with pneumonia. *Ann. Intern. Med.* 72:183–187, 1970.

Johnston, R. B., Jr. Pathogenesis of pneumococcal pneumonia. *Rev. Infect. Dis.* 13(Suppl. 6):S509–517, 1991.

Klagman, K. P. Pneumococcal resistance to antibiotics. *Clin. Microbiol. Rev.* 3(7):196, 1990.

Lim, I., Shaw, D. R., Stanley, D. P., et al. A prospective hospital study of the etiology of community-acquired pneumonia. *Med. J. Aust.* 151:87–91, 1989.

Luby, J. P. Southwestern Internal Medicine Conference: Pneumonia in adults due to mycoplasma, chlamydia and virus. *Am. J. Med. Sci.* 294:45–64, 1987.

Marrie, T. J. Bacteraemic pneumococcal pneumonia. *J. Infect.* 24:247–255, 1992.

Stout, J., Yu, V., Vickers, R., et al. Ubiquitous *Legionella pneumophila* in the water supply of a hospital with endemic Legionnaire's disease. *N. Engl. J. Med. 306:* 466–468, 1982.

Stover D., Zaman, M., Hajdu, S., et al. Bronchoalveolar lavage in the diagnosis of diffuse pulmonary infiltrates in the immunocompromised host. *Ann. Intern. Med. 101:*1–7, 1984.

Tillotson, J., and Lerner, A. Pneumonias caused by gram-negative bacilli. *Medicine 45:*65–76, 1966.

Wallace, R., and Musher, D. In honor of Dr. Sarah Branham a star is born: The realization of *Branhamella catarrhalis* as a respiratory pathogen. *Chest 90:*447–450, 1986.

Wallace, R., Musher, D., and Morton, R. *Haemophilus influenzae* pneumonia in adults. *Am. J. Med. 64:*87–93, 1978.

Warshauer, D., Goldstein, E., Akers, T., et al. Effect of influenza viral infection on the ingestion and killing of bacteria by alveolar macrophages. *Am. Rev. Respir. Dis. 115:*269–277, 1977.

# 12

# VIRAL INFECTIONS OF THE LOWER RESPIRATORY TRACT

BEN Z. KATZ, M. D. and RICHARD B. THOMSON, JR., Ph.D.

Viral lower respiratory tract infections are frequent occurrences worldwide. The majority of these infections occur in otherwise healthy individuals and are community acquired. Infections are usually acute in onset, last less than 1–2 weeks, and resolve without sequelae. Because of respiratory compromise, patients with viral infections of the lower respiratory tract tend to be sicker than patients with upper respiratory tract infection, and thus are more likely to seek medical attention.

This chapter deals with lower respiratory tract infections, defined as infection below the level of the epiglottis, including the glottis and trachea and extending downward through the bronchial tree, alveoli, and into the parenchymal portion of the lung. These infections are subdivided into several syndromes, based principally on the anatomic structure(s) involved clinically and radiographically. Fortuitously, each of these syndromes is caused primarily by a single family of viruses. Thus, this chapter discusses each syndrome along with its major viral etiologic agent: influenza and influenza virus, croup (acute laryngotracheobronchitis) and parainfluenza virus, bronchiolitis and respiratory syncytial virus, viral pneumonia and adenovirus.

The tracheobronchial mucosa is a dense layer of ciliated columnar cells and mucin-secreting goblet cells. The mucosa changes abruptly at the level of the alveolus to a flattened, attenuated, gas-permeable epithelial monolayer similar to the endothelium of capillaries. In the nose, mouth, pharynx, and larynx, ciliated cells are intermixed with stratified squamous epithelium; however, in the lower respiratory tract the ciliated cells represent a continuous, homogeneous mucosal surface. The ciliated columnar epithelial cells are rich in surface receptors that bind viruses. Thus, respiratory viruses can be expected to infect a wide range of epithelial cells in both the upper and lower respiratory tracts. Anatomic factors as well as the modifying influence of the host immune response often dictate at what site in the respiratory tract clinical symptoms will be most pronounced following infection with a particular virus.

## INFLUENZA

Influenza is an acute, febrile respiratory illness that is caused exclusively by influenza virus types A or B. Although both of these viruses can also produce nondescript upper respiratory infections that clinically resemble ordinary upper respiratory tract infections, influenza (''the flu'') is a specific syndrome with a distinctive clinical presentation and epidemiologic pattern.

### Virology of Influenza Viruses

Influenza viruses are single-stranded, negative-sense RNA viruses. They are the only members of the Orthomyxoviridae family, and all have the same structural and morphologic features (Fig. 12–1). Influenza virus may be either spherical or elongated and has a lipid bilayer envelope that encircles the helical nucleocapsid. The influenza virus envelope is acquired from the host cell's cytoplasmic membrane as the newly assembled viral nucleocapsid exits the cell by budding. Two glycoprotein virally encoded antigens, hemagglutinin (HA) and neuraminidase (NA), are located in this lipid envelope. These two proteins play an essential role in pathogenesis and laboratory diagnosis, as will be discussed. The HA antigen is embedded by its hydrophobic end into the lipid bilayer of the viral envelope; its hydrophilic end projects above the viral surface and functions as the ligand for attachment of the virion to receptors on the ciliated columnar epithelial cells of the respiratory tract. HA also can bind to guinea pig, chicken, and human erythrocytes (a fortuitous observation that led to its name and aids in laboratory diagnosis). The infectious cycle of influenza begins when HA anchors the virus to respiratory epithelium, initiating fusion of the viral envelope with the cytoplasmic membrane of the host cell so that the nucleocapsid can be released into the cytosol. HA is also the inciting antigen against which neutralizing antibodies develop.

The NA antigen is an enzyme that hydrolyzes the glycosidic linkage of sialic acid to glycoprotein. Its contribution to the pathogenesis of influenza is not entirely clear; it may be needed for the envelopment and final release of mature virions from the infected cell. Like HA, NA spikes are anchored in the virion envelope and project above the viral surface. Matrix proteins on the inner surface of the lipid bilayer are responsible for type specificity (A or B).

The influenza virus genome is organized into eight separate helical segments of RNA, each of which encodes one to three proteins. The segmented genome allows for genetic reassortment, resulting in major antigenic change (*antigenic shift*), which has implications for the epidemiology, pathophysiology, treatment, and prevention of influenza. Genetic reassortment occurs because human influenza A viruses are able to infect many animal species, including birds and pigs. Coinfection of an animal cell with both human and animal influenza strains results in random assortment of the genome segments, creating hybrid viruses. Human progeny viri-

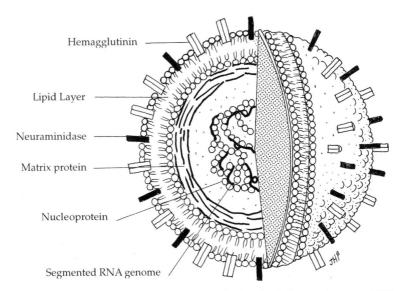

**FIGURE 12–1.** Diagram of influenza virus virion. The single-stranded, negative-sense RNA genome is divided into eight segments. The lipid bilayer envelope contains separate neuraminidase and hemagglutinin glycoprotein antigens. Matrix proteins are responsible for type specificity (A or B).

ons, encoding antigenically novel HA or NA antigens, lead to influenza strains to which the population has no or inadequate immunity (Fig. 12–2). Antigenic shift results in influenza pandemics every 9–39 years. In two pandemics (1957 and 1968), novel viruses were most likely generated by human strains that captured exogenous RNA from avian influenza viruses. The more dramatic the HA and NA antigenic alterations produced, the more susceptible the general population to infection, and the more severe the ensuing influenza outbreak. The pandemics of 1957 and 1968 began in The People's Republic of China and spread to the rest of Asia, Australia, Europe, and the Americas (Table 12–1).

A specific influenza virus strain can also have minor antigenic change resulting from mutation of the viral genome—so called *an-*

### TABLE 12–1.  INFLUENZA A PANDEMICS RESULTING FROM ANTIGENIC SHIFT*

| YEAR OF ORIGIN | SUBTYPE |
| --- | --- |
| 1918 | H1N1 |
| 1957 | H2N2 |
| 1968 | H3N2 |
| 1977 | H1N1 |

*Pandemics resulting from the introduction of novel influenza subtypes through genome reassortment.

*tigenic drift*. Antigenic drift is a consequence of (generally four) random point mutations in the RNA genome. RNA viruses, in general, do not have an efficient replication repair mechanism, giving rise to relatively frequent mutations. Fortunately, the immunologic characteristics of the virus usually remain

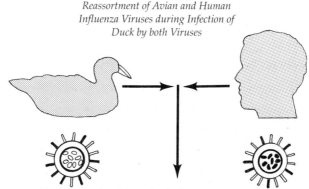

*Reassortment of Avian and Human Influenza Viruses during Infection of Duck by both Viruses*

*Reassortant virus Maintains Pathogenieity in Humans and Represents an Antigenically Novel Influenza subtype*

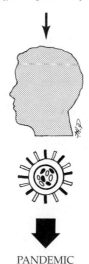

PANDEMIC

**FIGURE 12–2.** Postulated antigenic shift resulting from genome reassortment between human and duck influenza A viruses. Note that genome segments from different viruses are highlighted with light and dark shades.

**TABLE 12–2. H3N2 INFLUENZA A EPIDEMICS RESULTING FROM ANTIGENIC DRIFT BETWEEN 1968 AND 1986\***

| |
|---|
| A/Hong Kong/68 |
| A/England/72 |
| A/Port Chalmers/73 |
| A/Victoria/75 |
| A/Texas/77 |
| A/Bangkok/79 |
| A/Philippines/82 |
| A/Mississippi/85 |
| A/Leningrad/86 |

*Epidemics result from mutation of HA and NA genes.

fairly stable following such drift and thus annual wintertime influenza outbreaks due to these "new" strains are contained at relatively low levels and at most develop into regional epidemics, not worldwide pandemics (Table 12–2).

To date, three major hemagglutinin (HA 1–3) and two major neuraminidase (NA 1, 2) subtypes resulting from antigenic shift have been identified. Antigenic drift, resulting from mutation, dictates that precise identification of influenza A strains also include the geographic site and year in which the virus was first identified. As a result, human influenza A viruses are classified by the virus type (A or B), HA subtype (1–3), NA subtype (1, 2), and geographic site and year discovered (e.g., influenza A/Hong Kong/68/H3N2).

Influenza B undergoes antigenic drift but not antigenic shift. Major antigenic variation (shift) does not occur, apparently, because human strains of influenza B do not coinfect other animals. Minor antigenic changes (drift) occur as a result of random mutations, giving rise to low rates of infection year to year.

During an epidemic season, one influenza strain typically predominates, but two or more additional strains can often be isolated from a minority of the infected population. Careful surveillance to identify prevalent strains and emerging mutants or reassortant viruses is needed to ensure that annual vaccine formulations include appropriate antigens for the upcoming season (see below).

## Pathogenesis

Influenza is spread easily from person to person. Respiratory tract secretions are rich in influenza virus during acute illness, and virus is incorporated into small-particle aerosol droplets by sneezing, coughing, and talking. The fragile lipid envelope and glycoprotein HA spikes make viral survival on inanimate objects very short, but low humidity and low ambient temperature can prolong survival on these surfaces.

Initially, virus is introduced into the respiratory tract by aerosol inhalation. It attaches via its HA envelope antigen to a ciliated columnar epithelial cell, becomes internalized within the host cell, and promptly begins its replicative cycle. New virions are released in less than 24 h. The infection then spreads to nearby cells on the respiratory mucosal surface.

The incubation period for influenza is 1–3 days, after which time enough virus has accumulated to produce symptoms. Up to 70% of nonimmune individuals develop classic influenza following primary infection. The diagnosis of influenza should be reserved for those patients who have a systemic febrile illness with lower respiratory tract signs. Severe upper airway illness, even if caused by influenza virus, should not be labeled as "the flu."

As with most viral infections, recovery from acute influenza requires an adequate cell-mediated immune response. CD4 lymphocytes exposed to viral antigen initiate clonal expansion of specific cytotoxic CD8 lymphocytes that recognize and destroy host cells that contain influenza virus. Because of these CD4 and CD8 responses, lymphocytic, rather than neutrophilic, infiltrates characterize influenza infection pathologically. The lymphocytic process promptly and efficiently terminates viral replication but also temporarily accelerates cytonecrosis of respiratory tract epithelium. The newly regenerated replacement epithelium has a metaplastic appearance (see Fig. 12–3).

Influenza virus antigens also stimulate a humoral B-lymphocyte response with the production of specific IgM, IgG, and IgA antibodies. IgM antibody is detected approximately 1 week after the onset of influenza and persists for 2–3 months. IgG antibody follows shortly thereafter and can persist for years. Secretory IgA antibody appears in nasal secretions in parallel with the development of humoral IgG but generally cannot be detected after 3–6 months. Protection against reinfection is correlated with adequate concentrations of both serum and secretory antibody. Neutralizing antibody directed against HA antigen stereotactically interferes with its binding to cells of the respiratory tract and thus prevents viral attachment and infection. Antibody against NA modifies existing viral infection, possibly

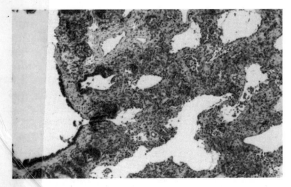

**FIGURE 12–3.** Fatal influenza A virus pneumonia in a 26-year-old woman. Bronchiolar mucosa has been destroyed and replaced by metaplastic epithelium (*arrow*). Alveolar walls are distorted and thickened by edema and dense lymphocytic infiltrate. Hematoxylin and eosin stain, × 25.

by interfering with the release of newly replicated virus from host cells. High levels of serum antibody against HA and NA protect against reinfection; low antibody concentrations moderate the severity of illness.

## Epidemiology

Influenza outbreaks occur annually during cold weather months in temperate climates; in the tropics influenza can occur year-round. The clustering of cases within a 1- to 2-month epidemic is a characteristic feature of influenza, as is the increase in the death rate from primary viral pneumonia and bacterial superinfection during these epidemics.

There have been 19 epidemics of influenza in the United States between 1957 and 1986. Each epidemic caused greater than 10,000 deaths, mainly in those over 65 years of age. The cause of death in these individuals is usually either pneumonia (primary viral or secondary bacterial) or an exacerbation of chronic cardiopulmonary disease.

## Clinical Illness

The systemic features of influenza are abrupt in onset and include fever (up to 104°F), chills, headache, myalgias, lumbosacral backache, nonproductive cough, rhinorrhea, sore throat, and profound weakness. Headache and muscle aches are conspicuous complaints and their intensity parallels the height of fever. Fever usually lasts 2–4 days. Dry cough, sore throat, and rhinorrhea are less intense at the outset, but become more prominent as the fever subsides. Necrosis of infected respiratory epithelial cells is marked, and respiratory complaints likely reflect this

damage. Viral shedding, and hence infectivity, is roughly proportional to the severity of pharyngitis, cough, and coryza.

Physical findings are nonspecific. Physical examination is more valuable for ruling out other serious lower respiratory tract diseases than for confirming a diagnosis of influenza. The pharyngeal mucosa is hyperemic but without exudate, and enlargement of tonsillar and anterior cervical lymph nodes is limited. The conjunctivae are somewhat inflamed and there is often a clear nasal discharge, but rhinorrhea is less than with the common cold. Cough is nonproductive and often accompanied by substernal discomfort; pleural rubs are uncommon and the lung fields are clear to auscultation. Despite headache, myalgia, and lower back pain, objective neurologic and musculoskeletal findings are lacking. Exhaustion is often the most pronounced early feature of influenza, and this is generally the symptom that resolves most slowly, usually taking about a week. Although acute influenza can be quite debilitating, recovery within 1–2 weeks is the rule and is uneventful in the majority of cases.

Although physicians are often consulted regarding influenza in adults, especially the elderly, children may also be infected, and there are several differences between influenza in adults and children. For example, children often experience more sustained fever and shed virus for longer periods of time than adults. Influenza more easily provokes asthma and febrile seizures in children than in adults. Reye's syndrome, a rare complication of influenza consisting of sudden hepatocyte steatosis with mitochondrial damage and encephalopathy, has been linked with the use of salicylate antipyretics (aspirin) in children. Reye's syndrome is rare now that salicylate use in small children with influenza (and chickenpox) has been widely discouraged.

The two most common complications of influenza are primary viral pneumonia and secondary bacterial pneumonia. Viral pneumonia occurs in less than 1% of cases, but mortality is high. Primary influenza virus pneumonia generally occurs in patients with underlying heart disease, particularly rheumatic mitral stenosis, but sporadic cases in otherwise healthy individuals are occasionally reported. Healthy pregnant women have an unexplainable but well-recognized higher risk for influenzal pneumonia. Primary viral pneumonia usually presents after a few days of

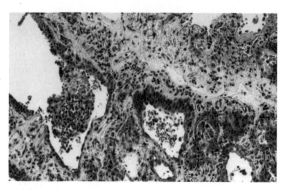

**FIGURE 12–4.** Acute influenza in a 34-year-old man. Note necrotic epithelial debris in bronchial lumen (*arrow*) and lymphocytic inflammatory infiltrate (*double arrow*). Hematoxylin and eosin stain, × 40.

illness. Extensive cellular damage is seen throughout the tracheobronchial mucosa, the distal bronchioles, and the alveolar epithelium. An acute interstitial pneumonitis and severe hypoxia then develops. Despite intensive supportive care, mortality rates as high as 30% are seen. Figure 12–4 shows the histopathologic features of primary influenzal pneumonia.

Secondary bacterial pneumonia is thought to develop when epithelial damage in the tracheobronchial tree disrupts mucociliary clearance. In addition, neutrophil chemotaxis is impaired. Both defects result in decreased clearance of bacteria aspirated into the lower respiratory tract. Patients who develop secondary infection are often elderly and/or have underlying lung disease, hypertension, or ischemic or valvular heart disease. A biphasic pattern of illness is typical; the acute illness appears to resolve, but then fever recurs accompanied by a *productive* cough with purulent sputum (see Fig. 12–5). Chest x-ray often reveals a lobar pneumonia. In some cases viral and bacterial pneumonia develop simultaneously. *Streptococcus pneumoniae, Staphylococcus aureus,* and *Haemophilus influenzae* are the usual secondary bacterial pathogens; if promptly treated with antibiotics most patients respond favorably. Other serious but, fortunately, rare complications of acute influenza include encephalitis, transverse myelitis, myositis with rhabdomyolysis, pericarditis, and myocarditis.

## Diagnosis

The diagnosis of influenza is usually apparent (especially during an epidemic) from its characteristic clinical picture of acute lower respiratory tract infection without evidence of pneumonia and prominent systemic symptoms such as myalgia and fatigue. When laboratory confirmation of the clinical diagnosis is required, there are both cell culture and rapid non–culture-dependent diagnostic tests

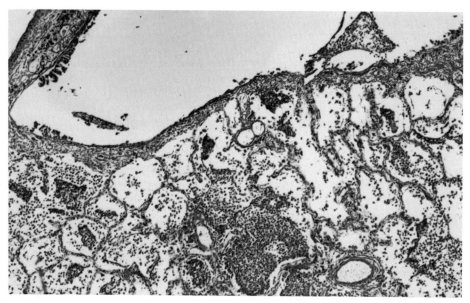

**FIGURE 12–5.** Fatal secondary bacterial bronchopneumonia following influenza. Bronchial epithelium shows focal metaplastic change from prior influenzal damage. Alveolar walls are normal, but alveolar spaces are consolidated with neutrophils and fibrin from acute bacterial infection (*arrows*). Hematoxylin and eosin stain, × 40.

available. Cell culture entails inoculating respiratory secretions into a susceptible cell line. Influenza A and B grow readily in primary monkey kidney cell cultures. Virus is abundant in respiratory secretions during the first few days of illness. Optimal specimens include secretions aspirated from the nasopharynx, bronchoalveolar lavage fluid collected during bronchoscopy, sputum which contains tracheobronchial cells, and secretions collected by vigorous pharyngeal swabbing. Specimens need to be placed in viral transport medium (VTM), which is a broth that contains antibiotics to inhibit contaminating upper respiratory bacterial flora and protein to help stabilize viruses present. Although immediate inoculation of cell culture is optimal, specimens in VTM can be refrigerated up to 24 h before inoculation. Conventional cell culture detects morphologic changes in virally infected cells, referred to as cytopathic effect (CPE). In general, CPE is detected within 4–7 days. Influenza-infected cell cultures can be detected in 2–3 days by performing a hemadsorption test. Guinea pig red blood cells, added to the cell culture, attach (hemadsorb) to infected cells because of the presence of HA glycoproteins in the host cell membrane. If the centrifugation-enhanced shell vial cell culture technique is used, influenza virus can be identified in 1–2 days. The shell vial method identifies viral antigen, produced early during the course of cell culture infection, by fluorescent antibody staining. Viral growth in conventional or shell viral cell culture is required for subtyping.

These same respiratory specimens can be used with rapid, non–culture-dependent diagnostic tests, utilizing type-specific (influenza A or B) monoclonal antibodies in a fluorescent antibody staining or enzyme immunoassay format. Direct, non–culture-dependent tests for influenza are less sensitive than cell culture–based tests but are more rapid. Serologic diagnosis of influenza has considerable value for the epidemiologic investigation of outbreaks; in individual cases, however, results are usually not positive until convalescence, when a fourfold rise in antibody titer has developed, and are not very helpful.

## Treatment and Prevention

Inactivated vaccines are able to prevent infection or lessen the severity of disease; the benefit in high-risk patients (see below) is considerable. Influenza vaccine is reformulated yearly based on the strains that circulated in the Far East the previous year. Since antigenic shift is an unlikely event from year to year, the vaccine usually provides adequate protection. Typically the vaccine includes three antigenic types. In recent years, two influenza A types and a single B type have been combined in a trivalent vaccine. The vaccine is administered in early fall (in temperate climates in the Northern Hemisphere) so that protective antibody levels are achieved before the predictable winter outbreaks. Two doses of vaccine 1 month apart are necessary the first time a child (<9 years) receives influenza vaccine; however, only one dose is necessary in adults. Component ("split") vaccines are used in children younger than 13 years; children younger than 3 years receive half the adult dose of vaccine.

Serious side effects of vaccination are rare. Local irritation is common. Transient fever is seen in less than 5% of inoculees. During 1976, a national immunization program to prevent an anticipated swine influenza epidemic was linked to cases of Guillain-Barré syndrome (GBS); the associated mortality rate among those with GBS was 5%. There has been no subsequent association of influenza vaccine with GBS, and there have been no other recorded deaths linked to flu vaccination; however, because the number of vaccinations administered in 1976 was so much greater than normal, one cannot rule out rare side effects not seen on a yearly basis, when standard amounts of vaccine are administered only to high-risk patients.

Influenza vaccination is indicated in those individuals at risk of high morbidity following infection, such as the elderly (those over 65 or in nursing homes) and patients with underlying health problems such as hemodynamically significant cardiovascular disease, pulmonary disease (asthma, bronchopulmonary dysplasia), diabetes, renal disease, hemoglobinopathies (especially sickle cell anemia); and in immunocompromised patients such as those with collagen vascular disease, malignancy, and human immunodeficiency virus (HIV) infection. Immunocompromised patients may have a reduced antibody response. It is also recommended that health care workers (physicians, nurses, and allied personnel) in hospitals, clinics, and chronic care facilities be immunized to prevent the spread of influenza to their patients and to ensure continued efficient delivery of medical care in the event of an influenza outbreak. The only absolute contraindication to vaccination is hypersensitivity to chicken eggs, since immunizing virus strains are propagated in this medium.

Amantadine hydrochloride can prevent or ameliorate disease caused by influenza A if given early in the course of infection. The drug interferes with uncoating of the viral nucleocapsid within infected cells. Unvaccinated or recently vaccinated high-risk individuals, household contacts of index cases, and health care workers may benefit from prophylactic administration of amantadine during periods of high influenza activity. Side effects of amantadine are largely confined to the gastrointestinal tract and central nervous system, and consist mainly of insomnia, dizziness, anorexia, and nausea. Side effects occur in up to 15% of patients given amantadine, mainly those with underlying renal or neurologic disease and the elderly; side effects are reversible once the drug is discontinued. Rimantadine, an analog of amantadine, has recently been licensed for prophylaxis of influenza A disease in children and adults and has an overall lower risk of side effects than amantadine (6–10%). Use of both amantadine and rimantadine has provoked the emergence of resistant influenza A virus strains (related to mutations of the matrix proteins), especially in children (probably because they shed larger amounts of virus than adults and thus have a higher chance of producing mutations that lead to resistance); the effect these resistant strains may have on the epidemiology and management of influenza is still unclear.

In most individuals management of uncomplicated, acute influenza need only be sup-
portive. Rest is often recommended, since most patients are exhausted for the first few days of illness. Adequate hydration can usually be maintained without the use of intravenous fluids. Acetaminophen is used to treat fever and myalgias; *salicylates are contraindicated in children with influenza* because of the risk of Reye's syndrome. Antibiotics are reserved for cases of secondary bacterial superinfection of the lower respiratory tract.

Influenza virus is highly contagious; virus is spread by the respiratory route (via inhalation of aerosols) as well as by direct inoculation from animate or inanimate objects. Therefore, respiratory isolation of patients with influenza is mandatory in hospitals and nursing homes as is strict handwashing following patient contact.

## CROUP: ACUTE LARYNGOTRACHEOBRONCHITIS

Croup is the term used to describe several clinical illnesses with varying degrees of inflammation involving the larynx (resulting in hoarseness), trachea (producing stridor), and bronchi (characterized by cough). The relative degree of involvement of each of these anatomic regions in croup varies considerably, but generally there is some involvement of all three areas.

Croup is usually associated with infection with parainfluenza virus; it must be distinguished, however, from epiglottitis (usually due to *Haemophilus influenzae* type b) and bacterial tracheitis (usually due to *Staphylococcus aureus*) (Table 12–3). Other causes of airway

**TABLE 12–3.   MAJOR INFECTIOUS CAUSES OF CHILDHOOD UPPER RESPIRATORY OBSTRUCTION**

|  | ACUTE SUPRA(EPI)GLOTTIS | ACUTE LARYNGOTRACHEOBRONCHITIS (CROUP) | BACTERIAL TRACHEITIS |
|---|---|---|---|
| Usual etiology | *Haemophilus influenzae* type b | Parainfluenza virus | *Staphylococcus aureus* |
| Usual age | >3 yr | <3 yr | 6 mo–3 yr |
| Onset | Acute | Gradual, nocturnal | Gradual |
| Natural history | Progressive | Usually not progressive | Progressive |
| Appearance | Toxic | Usually not toxic | Toxic |
| Physical examination | Red, edematous epiglottis | Stridor | Purulent secretions |
| Chest x-ray | Lateral neck: increased size of epiglottis and aryepiglottic folds | Chest: subglottic inflammation and narrowing | Chest: subglottic inflammation |
| Treatment | Antibiotics, intubation | Supportive usually | Antibiotics, intubation |

obstruction (e.g., foreign body, diphtheria, or peritonsillar and retropharyngeal abscesses) should also be considered.

### Virology of Parainfluenza Viruses

The parainfluenza viruses include four serotypes (1–4) of enveloped paramyxoviruses that contain a negative-sense, single-stranded, nonsegmented RNA genome and, like influenza virus, possess neuraminidase- and hemagglutinin-containing glycoproteins. They differ from influenza viruses in that they do not undergo much antigenic variation. Nevertheless, parainfluenza viruses can reinfect previously infected individuals with high efficiency. Parainfluenza viruses can also cause pharyngitis, upper respiratory tract infection, bronchitis, and pneumonitis. Parainfluenza 4 is much less common and generally causes only mild upper respiratory tract symptoms.

### Pathogenesis

The majority of cases of croup are caused by parainfluenza virus type 1. Other etiologies include parainfluenza virus types 2 and 3, influenza virus, and respiratory syncytial virus; less commonly, adenovirus, rhinovirus, and measles virus are implicated.

In croup, inflammation is thought to begin in the larynx and then extend to the trachea and bronchi. Thick secretions are produced that can lead to atelectasis and mucus plugging, which in turn lead to increased respiratory effort and hypoxia. The inspiratory stridor and cough characteristic of croup ("croupy cough") probably result from laryngeal irritation and accumulated secretions.

Immunity to parainfluenza infection is only transient. Nevertheless, repeat infections in older children and adults are milder than those seen in infancy and childhood.

### Epidemiology

Croup is characteristically seen in young children: the peak incidence is at 2 years of age; about 75% of cases are younger than 3; and boys outnumber girls 2:1. As with most respiratory illnesses, croup peaks in the late fall–early winter, but cases can be seen year-round.

### Clinical Illness

Illness typically begins at night with the upper respiratory tract symptoms of coryza, nasal irritation, hoarseness, sore throat, cough, and fever. Shortly thereafter, signs of upper airway obstruction gradually develop, including the classic "croupy" cough that sounds like a barking seal. Respirations then become increasingly stridorous. Symptoms usually begin to resolve after a few days but may progress to respiratory obstruction, with retractions, tachypnea, tachycardia, fatigue, restlessness, and anxiety. Duration of illness is typically 7–10 days.

### Diagnosis

Specific diagnosis can be established by virus isolation in cell culture (using a primary monkey kidney cell line) or by serologic testing that demonstrates at least a fourfold increase in antibody titer between paired acute and convalescent sera. Rapid diagnosis can be achieved using centrifugation-enhanced shell vial cell culture (see "Influenza" above) or by demonstrating parainfluenza antigen directly in respiratory tract secretions that contain epithelial cells by fluorescent antibody staining.

### Treatment and Prevention

No specific therapy or prophylaxis exists. Treatment is supportive, including minimal disturbance, hydration, and mist therapy. Racemic epinephrine can be used to decrease the obstruction, but rebound can occur. The use of steroids is controversial. Rarely do these patients require intubation.

Transmission occurs by inhalation of aerosol as well as by direct inoculation from animate and inanimate objects, as is true for influenza. Therefore, respiratory isolation and strict handwashing are mandatory for containing infection.

## BRONCHIOLITIS

Bronchiolitis is a common form of acute viral infection of the lower respiratory tract that occurs principally in children under 2 years of age. Respiratory syncytial virus (RSV) is responsible for 50–90% of cases of acute bronchiolitis; other causes of bronchiolitis include parainfluenza virus types 1 and 3, adenovirus, rhinovirus, influenza virus, measles viruses, and *Mycoplasma pneumoniae*.

### Virology of Respiratory Syncytial Virus

RSV is a paramyxovirus. As with other paramyxoviruses, RSV has a negative-sense, single stranded non-segmented RNA genome. However, unlike other paramyxoviruses, RSV does not contain hemagglutinin or neuraminidase antigens. RSV contains a fusion protein (the F glycoprotein), which helps the virus enter infected respiratory tract cells and mediates fusion with neighboring host cells, forming syncytia (thus giving the virus its name). The lack of a segmented genome or HA and NA proteins means that the antigenic composition of RSV remains relatively stable year to year.

### Pathogenesis

RSV adheres to ciliated columnar epithelial cells throughout the respiratory tract probably via the F glycoprotein. Consequently, viral replication, cytonecrosis, edema, and inflammation occur along the entire respiratory epithelial surface, causing upper and lower respiratory tract symptoms. The most severe pathology is found in the distal airways. Inflammation of the small bronchi and bronchioles leads to luminal narrowing, and as necrotic debris accumulates, plugs of sloughed epithelial and inflammatory cells block the smallest airways (see Fig. 12–6). This inflammation produces dramatic obstruction in very young children, whose small airways readily occlude. The negative intrathoracic pressure created during inspiration allows air to flow through a partially obstructed bronchiole, but air becomes trapped in the alveolar spaces as the cross-sectional area of the bronchiole decreases with the positive pressure of expiration. Hyperinflation results, and eventually ventilation and oxygenation may be impaired leading to dyspnea, air hunger, and intense respiratory effort. Hypoxia leads to restlessness, tachycardia, and tachypnea, and as the added work of ventilation becomes fatiguing, carbon dioxide is retained.

The cellular immune response in RSV-induced bronchiolitis is primarily lymphocytic. A specific CD8 (cytotoxic) T-lymphocyte response is initiated, which peaks at approximately the fifth day of illness and is critical for the containment and elimination of the virus. The humoral (antibody) immune response to RSV follows. IgM is expressed after a few days and disappears within a few weeks. Specific IgG and IgA antibodies appear by the second week and wane within a few months. There is some evidence that the severity of symptoms in subsequent infections may be greater in patients who have high concentrations of RSV-specific IgE or other RSV-specific antibodies; this would account for the fact that (1) the worst RSV bronchiolitis is seen in infants 2–5 months of age when maternal antibody is present and (2) that in some vaccine trials, vaccinees developed worse disease following natural infection than unvaccinated controls.

### Epidemiology

Outbreaks of bronchiolitis are 2–5 months in length, from early winter to early spring, as with most respiratory infections. They generally begin on the West Coast of the United States and move east and are worst in urban areas. When RSV is in a community, other respiratory viruses tend to disappear. As with influenza, the reservoir of respiratory paramyxoviruses between epidemics is not obvious. Humans are the only known host; presumably low levels of infection persist in the community.

Bronchiolitis is most common between 2 and 5 months of age. In the second year of life the incidence drops by at least one half; after the second year of life the incidence of bronchiolitis is negligible.

RSV bronchiolitis appears more virulent than bronchiolitis due to other pathogens. Nearly all primary infections occur in the first year of life and are symptomatic; symptomatic reinfection in early childhood is also common. Adult RSV infections can also be clinically apparent and range from diseases as trivial as a mild cold to an illness as severe as influenza or pneumonia.

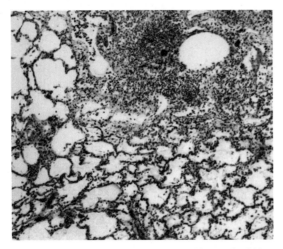

**FIGURE 12–6.** RSV bronchiolitis in an 18-month-old boy. There is acute necrotizing inflammation of terminal bronchiole (*arrows*) with minimal focal extension into surrounding alveoli. Hematoxylin and eosin stain, × 25.

### Clinical Illness

The incubation period for RSV bronchiolitis is 3–4 days. There then follows a nonspecific upper respiratory tract prodrome of rhinorrhea, low-grade fever, decreased appetite, and cough. Wheezing is heard on physical examination, which may also reveal coryza, pharyngeal hyperemia, low-grade fever, and otitis media. Mild cases regress spontaneously within 5 days.

Children at *high risk* for developing severe bronchiolitis include those with underlying heart, lung, or renal disease; prematures; and those with compromised immune function. Mortality is rare and usually linked to complicating pneumonias. Other rare complications include meningitis, myocarditis, heart block, and rash.

In severe cases, cough and wheezing progress and the child becomes dyspneic. Hyperexpansion of the chest occurs with intercostal and subcostal retractions. Tachypnea may be seen with hypoxemia and apnea. Cyanosis and elevated $Pco_2$ are seen only in the most severely affected infants with life-threatening bronchiolitis.

Chest x-ray may be normal or reveal air trapping, peribronchial thickening, interstitial pneumonia, atelectasis, or segmental consolidation resembling lobar pneumonia. A complete blood count (CBC) shows only a modest elevation of the white blood cell count (WBC) with or without a left shift. The intensity of wheezing and retractions does not accurately predict the $Po_2$. Serum electrolytes reflect accompanying dehydration (if any).

## Diagnosis

As with influenza and croup, diagnosis is usually made clinically but can be confirmed by virus isolation or rapid RSV antigen detection. The best material to send for testing is that which is aspirated from the nasopharynx during routine suctioning. A useful technique is to cut the entire suction catheter with sterile scissors and send it in a sterile container to the clinical virology laboratory.

Rapid RSV antigen assays are sensitive and specific and can be completed in less than 4 h. Respiratory tract secretions can be assayed for antigen by fluorescent antibody staining or enzyme immunoassay methodologies. Viral culture takes 3–7 days. RSV, unfortunately, is the slowest growing and most fastidious of the pediatric respiratory viral pathogens. Serologic diagnosis provides little meaningful clinical information.

## Treatment and Prevention

Children sick enough to require hospitalization are usually hypoxic and therefore require supplemental humidified oxygen. Intubation and mechanical ventilation are only rarely needed. Nebulized racemic epinephrine and bronchodilators have been shown to be beneficial in some studies; their use, however, along with that of steroids, remains controversial. Intravenous rehydration is often needed; care must be taken, however, not to overhydrate the patient. Antibiotics are not appropriate unless there is serious concern about a secondary bacterial pneumonia or otitis media.

Ribavirin, a guanosine analog, has broad antiviral activity, including activity against RSV. When administered as a small-particle aerosol, ribavirin reaches the distal airways and inhibits RSV replication, thereby potentially minimizing further tissue damage and ameliorating the severity of disease. Oxygenation is significantly improved and the duration of viral shedding is reduced. However, the clinical usefulness of the drug and whether it should be used in intubated subjects is controversial. Ribavirin cannot replace supportive measures in the treatment of RSV-associated bronchiolitis; nevertheless, its use should be considered in high-risk patients. Ribavirin is expensive (at least $3000 per course in 1995). Although ribavirin is teratogenic in several animal model studies, aerosol therapy has not been linked to any damage in either patients, health care workers, or their offspring. Levels of the drug in the blood are barely detectable in patients following aerosol therapy and are undetectable in workers caring for the patients. Hyperimmune globulin was licensed in early 1996 as a prophylactic modality in high-risk patients.

As was true for influenza and parainfluenza viruses, RSV is spread from person to person, principally via the respiratory (air-borne) route as well as directly by contaminated hands. RSV is highly contagious, even in the hospital setting. Vigorous hand-washing practices can substantially limit nosocomial transmission of this virus by health care workers. Unfortunately, gowns and gloves are often necessary just to encourage or remind health care workers (mainly physicians) to wash their hands. Goggles further decrease spread in hospitals, especially when used by nurses and respiratory therapists. Cohorting of babies with similar respiratory tract infections due to the same agent in the same room is reasonable.

## PNEUMONIA

In general, viruses cause at least 50% of cases of pneumonia. In contrast to bacterial pneumonias, viral pneumonias are generally less acute and are associated with *nonproductive* coughs, *low-grade* fevers, and myalgias. Infiltrates on chest x-ray are generally patchy, although lobar infiltrates can occur. Pleural effusions are infrequently seen.

Pneumonia can complicate the course of viral infections of the lower respiratory tract in either adults or children. This is especially well appreciated in influenza A pandemics but can also be seen with RSV and parainfluenza infections. For example, in cases of croup or bronchiolitis, extension of virus into the adjacent alveolar epithelium is not an infrequent complication. Secondary bacterial infection can occur as well.

One viral agent of pneumonia not previously discussed in this chapter is adenovirus. Adenoviruses, although an infrequent cause of pneumonia, result in the most severe viral pneumonias seen in previously healthy patients.

Adenovirus is a double-stranded, nonenveloped, icosahedral-shaped DNA virus that is commonly recognized as a cause of conjunctivitis and/or pharyngitis. However, it also produces severe pneumonia in young children (generally 3–18 months of age) and adults, especially in military recruits, where crowded living in barracks appears to be the major risk factor. Adenoviruses are divided into 42 serotypes. Serotypes 3, 4, 7, 14, and 21 are responsible for most pneumonias. Because they are nonenveloped, adenoviruses can survive for at least brief periods of time on environmental surfaces.

As with most of the other viral pathogens, a specific diagnosis of adenoviral pneumonia can be made by viral culture, antigen detection, or serology. There is no specific therapy. Because of the limited number of serotypes that cause pneumonia, a vaccine was developed by the military to prevent infection in soldiers. Isolation procedures, similar to those described for influenza virus infection, should be used when a patient with adenoviral pneumonia is admitted to the hospital.

## CASE HISTORIES

### Case History 1

A 70-year-old man was examined in the emergency department (ED) in January because of a worsening nonproductive cough, fever, weakness, fatigue, and decreased appetite of 3 days' duration. His past medical history included a recent diagnosis of Waldenström's macroglobulinemia for which he received three cycles of chemotherapy. He had no known sick contacts. The most recent 7-day cycle finished 1 day prior to his ED visit. The patient's WBC count was $1.0 \times 10^3 \mu L$, with a differential of 79% segmented neutrophils, 11% band neutrophils, 6% lymphocytes, 2% monocytes, and 2% eosinophils. A chest x-ray showed a patchy, right-sided lung infiltrate.

1. What viral etiologies should be included in the differential diagnosis?
2. What laboratory diagnostic test(s) would rapidly identify a virus causing this pneumonia?
3. Is it necessary to identify a viral etiology for this hospital admission?
4. Are antiviral agents available for treatment of adult viral pneumonias?
5. What prophylaxis should this patient have been given prior to chemotherapy?

### Case 1 Discussion

This immunocompromised patient may have bacterial or viral pneumonia. January is the usual time for respiratory viruses to cause morbidity in the community. In addition to influenza virus, a neutropenic adult may have disease caused by adenovirus, respiratory syncytial virus and, less frequently, parainfluenza virus. Two rapid fluorescent antibody stains, using monoclonal antibodies specific for influenza A and B, were performed on smears prepared from nasopharyngeal aspirates. Numerous influenza A infected cells were identified. In addition, cell culture confirmed the identity of the isolate and provided the state public health laboratory with virus for subtyping. Subtyping of select strains is important to detect antigenic shift and drift, which impact the composition of future vaccines. Once admitted to the hospital the patient requires a private room or cohorting with other patients with influenza virus. The antiviral agent amantadine hydrochloride may decrease the severity of influenza A (not influenza B) disease if administered early in the course of illness. Influenza vaccine is recommended for the elderly, even those who are healthy but especially if underlying disease exists.

### Case History 2

A 9-month-old Black girl presents to the emergency room in January with fever, cough, and rapid respirations. She was well until 1 week earlier, when she developed rhinorrhea and cough. One day prior to being seen, she developed increased cough, anorexia, fever to 102°F rectally, and rapid breathing. Several family members have had rhinorrhea, cough, and temperatures of 100.5°F rectally.

Physical examination showed an infant in moderate respiratory distress. Vital signs were: temperature, 101°F rectally; pulse, 140/min; respiration, 46/min; blood pressure, 90/50. Clear nasal discharge was present. Tympanic membranes were normal. Neck was supple, without adenopathy. Moderate subcostal and intercostal retractions and mild nasal flaring were present. Fine expiratory wheezes were heard bilaterally, and the expiratory phase was prolonged. No stridor was present. The cardiac exam was normal. The liver was palpated 3 cm below the right costal margin and the spleen 2 cm below the left costal margin.

Chest x-ray showed hyperinflated lungs with flat diaphragms and increased perihilar markings throughout both lung fields. CBC showed WBC = 14,000/mm$^3$ with 25% PMNs, 5% bands, 60% lymphocytes, 5% eosinophils, and 5% monocytes; hemoglobin was 11 g/dL and hematocrit 36%. SGPT was 23 (normal, <40).

After observing that she was comfortably able to suck on a bottle, the child was discharged to home with a cool mist humidifier to be seen again in 2 days.

1. What epidemiologic clues are useful in this history?
2. What are the likely etiologic agents?
3. What organ systems are affected in this child?
4. What do the lab findings suggest?
5. What additional diagnostic test(s) might be useful?
6. What therapy may be available to treat this problem?

## CASE 2 DISCUSSION

Viral respiratory illness is suggested because the child is presenting in the winter, has only a low-grade fever, and has prominent rhinorrhea and contacts with cold symptoms (e.g., clear nasal discharge).

The child manifests mild respiratory distress with some tachypnea, nasal flaring, retractions, and wheezing. These symptoms are typical of bronchiolitis, a viral illness usually caused by RSV. The apparent hepatosplenomegaly is probably the result of air-trapping and depressed diaphragms; SGPT was normal. The baby takes the bottle well; thus, her respiratory distress is not so severe that it interferes with feeding.

Chest x-ray showed air-trapping and perihilar streaking but no infiltrates; this is typical of bronchiolitis. The CBC has a normal WBC count with a lymphocytic predominance, most consistent with a viral illness. Additional laboratory tests that would be helpful include a rapid RSV antigen detection test on upper respiratory tract secretions. Intravenous ribavirin may be used for RSV infection in seriously ill children or in those at high risk for developing severe disease, such as those with preexisting lung disease or congenital heart disease. The child should be seen again in 1–2 days

for follow-up to assess whether the respiratory distress has worsened and whether there is evidence of a bacterial superinfection.

## REFERENCES

### Books

Feigin, R. R., and Cherry, J. D., eds. *Textbook of Pediatric Infectious Diseases*. 3rd ed. Vol. II. Philadelphia: W. B. Saunders Co., 1992.

Fields, B. N., et al., eds. *Virology*. 2nd ed. New York: Raven Press, 1990.

Kilbourne, E. D. *Influenza*. New York: Plenum Medical Book Co., 1987.

Mandell, G. L., Bennett, J. E., and Dolin, R. eds. *Principles and Practice of Infectious Diseases*. 4th ed. New York: Churchill Livingstone Co., 1995.

Stuart-Harris, C. H., Schild, G. C., and Oxford, J. S. *Influenza: The Viruses and the Disease*. 2nd ed. London: Edward Arnold, 1985.

### Articles and Chapters

Centers for Disease Control. Prevention and control of influenzae, Part I, Vaccines. *MMWR 43*(RR-9):1–13, 1994.

Douglas, R. G., Jr. Prophylaxis and treatment of influenza. *N. Engl. J. Med. 322*:443–450, 1990.

Englund J. A., Sullivan, C. J., Jordan, M. C., et al. Respiratory syncytial virus infection in immunocompromised adults. *Ann. Intern. Med. 109*:203–208, 1988.

Gala, C. L., Hall, C. B., Schnabel, K. C., et al. The use of eye-nose goggles to control nosocomial respiratory syncytial virus infection. *JAMA 256*:2706–2708, 1986.

Glezen, W. P., and Couch, R. B. Interpandemic influenza in the Houston area, 1974–76. *N. Engl. J. Med. 298*: 587–592, 1978.

Hall, C. B., et al. Respiratory syncytial virus infection in children with compromised immune function. *N. Engl. J. Med. 315*:77–81, 1986.

Hall, C. B., McBride, J. T., Walsh, E. E., et al. Aerosolized ribavirin treatment of infants with respiratory syncytial viral infection: A randomized double-blind study. *N. Engl. J. Med. 308*:1443–1447, 1983.

Hayden, F. G., Belshe, R. B., Clover, R. D., et al. Emergence and apparent transmission of rimantadine-resistant influenza A virus in families. *N. Engl. J. Med. 321*: 1696–1702, 1989.

Hierholzer, J. C. Adenoviruses in the immunocompromised host. *Clin. Microbiol. Rev. 5*:262–274, 1992.

Komshian, S. V., Chandrasekar, P. H., and Levine, D. P. Adenovirus pneumonia in healthy adults. *Heart Lung 16*:146–150, 1987.

LaVia, W. V., et al. Respiratory syncytial virus puzzle: Clinical features, pathophysiology, and prevention. *J. Pediatr. 121*:503–510, 1992.

Leclair, J. M., Freeman, J., Sullivan, B. F., et al. Prevention of nosocomial respiratory syncytial virus infections through compliance with glove and gown isolation precautions. *N. Engl. J. Med. 317*:329–334, 1987.

MacDonald, N. E., Breese Hall, C., Suffin, S. C., et al. Respiratory syncytial viral infection in infants with congenital heart disease. *N. Engl. J. Med. 307*:397–400, 1982.

Meert, K. L., et al. Aerosolized ribavirin in mechanically

ventilated children with respiratory syncytial viruslower respiratory tract disease: A prospective, double-blind, randomized trial. *Crit. Care Med.* 22:566–572, 1994.

Shaw, M. W., Arden, N. H., and Maassab, H. F. New aspects of influenza virus. *Clin. Microbiol. Rev.* 5:74–92, 1992.

Steinhauser, D. A., et al. Receptor binding and cell entry by influenza viruses. *Semin. Virolo.* 3:91–100, 1992.

Stretton, M., and Newth, C. J. Croup and epiglottitis: The critical early diagnosis. *J. Respir. Dis.* 11:1087–1100, 1990.

Vainionpaa, R., and Hyypia, T. Biology of parainfluenza viruses. *Clin. Microbiol. Rev.* 7:265–275, 1994.

Welliver, R. C. Detection, pathogenesis, and therapy of respiratory syncytial virus infections. *Clin. Microbiol. Rev.* 1:27–39, 1988.

# 13
# MYCOBACTERIAL INFECTIONS

JOHN R. WARREN, M.D.

Tuberculosis is an infectious disease of humans caused by the microorganism *Mycobacterium tuberculosis*. Most individuals infected with *M. tuberculosis* do not develop the disease tuberculosis. However, when it does occur, tuberculosis is marked by chronicity with tissue necrosis due to delayed-type hypersensitivity. Mycobacterial species other than *M. tuberculosis*, including the "atypical" mycobacteria and the causative agent of leprosy, also produce human disease. Diagnosis and effective treatment depend on awareness of the wide spectrum of mycobacterial disease.

## TUBERCULOSIS

### Microbiology

The *Mycobacterium tuberculosis* complex of organisms consists of five species: *M. tuberculosis*, *M. bovis*, *M. africanum*, *M. ulcerans*, and *M. microti*. In the past, *M. bovis* was a frequent cause of human tuberculosis, usually acquired by the ingestion of milk contaminated with *M. bovis*. However, with eradication of *M. bovis*

mastitis in dairy herds and the pasteurization of milk, tuberculosis due to *M. bovis* has been largely eliminated. *M. africanum* is a rare cause of human tuberculosis in Africa. *M. ulcerans*, the causative agent of necrotizing cutaneous ulceration in Africa and Australia, grows only at cooler skin temperatures (30°–31°C). *M. microti* is an animal pathogen.

*Mycobacterium tuberculosis* is the cause of human tuberculosis in the United States and other developed countries. *M. tuberculosis* is a facultative intracellular parasite that produces disease by growth within macrophages. *M. tuberculosis* can also proliferate extracellularly in infected tissue, and is able to grow *in vitro* in cell-free culture systems. Humans are the natural reservoir of *M. tuberculosis*, but the organism is highly virulent for the guinea pig, which has served as an experimental model for the pathogenesis of tuberculosis. *M. tuberculosis* is an obligate aerobe whose growth is favored by 5–10% $CO_2$ tension, and is inhibited by acid pH below 6.5 and long-chain fatty acids. Optimal growth of tubercle bacilli occurs at temperatures of 35°–37°C, consistent with their ability to infect internal organs, es-

**157**

pecially the lungs. This microorganism is a non–spore-forming, nonmotile bacillus measuring approximately 0.4 × 4.0 μm, whose cell wall has a very high content of lipid. Lipid constitutes 25–60% of the organism's dry weight, as compared with 0.5% for gram-positive bacteria and 3.0% for gram-negative bacteria. This accounts for the acid-fast staining by mycobacteria. Tubercle bacilli grow very slowly: their doubling time is 12–20 h, as compared with less than 1 h for most other bacterial pathogens.

No exotoxins, endotoxins, or tissue-necrotizing enzymes have been discovered for *M. tuberculosis*. However, an array of glycolipids and peptides have been implicated in the virulence and hypersensitivity of tuberculous infection. *Cord factor* is a glycolipid that causes virulent strains of *M. tuberculosis* to grow as ropes, bundles, or serpentine cords in liquid media. Cord factor can be extracted from tubercle bacilli with organic solvents, and when extracted the bacilli become avirulent. However, the exact role of cord factor in the pathogenesis of tuberculosis is presently unknown. Tubercle bacilli ingested by macrophages in the nonimmune host reside in phagosomes that seldom provoke lysosomal fusion. Consequently, multiplication of tubercle bacilli is unimpeded within macrophages until immunity develops. The mycobacterial *sulfatides*, polyanionic trehalose glycolipids associated with virulence of *M. tuberculosis*, are readily taken up by lysosomes, and modify lysosomal membranes so that lysosome fusion with phagosomes is inhibited. A primary component of host responses to infection with *M. tuberculosis* is the development of delayed-type hypersensitivity against *tuberculin antigens*, products that are released or secreted by tubercle bacilli during intracellular growth in macrophages. Several constituents of the mycobacterial cell wall, especially *muramyl dipeptide* and a glycolipid *wax D*, enhance tuberculin hypersensitivity.

## Pulmonary Tuberculosis

Pulmonary tuberculosis is a disease that results from infection of the lung with an *M. tuberculosis* complex organism—in the United States almost always *M. tuberculosis* itself. Pulmonary infection is due to inhalation of *droplet nuclei*, small (1–5 μm) particles containing a few (one to three) tubercle bacilli. Coughing, sneezing, or talking by an individual with respiratory tract disease due to *M. tuberculosis* produces aerosols of respiratory secretions, which rapidly dry, forming droplet nuclei.

Droplet nuclei remain suspended in the air until inhaled, after which they reach deep alveolar spaces of the lung because of their small size. Respiratory aerosols that fall to surfaces (floors, tables) or inanimate objects, such as bedding or clothing (fomites), become associated with particles of dust or lint before they dry. The association with dust or lint increases particle size (>5 μm), and these *secondary aerosols* are not highly infectious, since they can be efficiently cleared by the mucociliary apparatus of the respiratory tract. Consequently, the tuberculosis patient is the primary source for transmission of tubercle bacilli, and environmental surfaces and fomites are not important. Although tuberculosis is not highly contagious, in overcrowded or substandard living conditions 25–50% of persons with close and sustained contact with individuals whose sputum smears are microscopically positive for tubercle bacilli will become infected. To prevent transmission of *M. tuberculosis*, an individual with tuberculosis should be placed in respiratory isolation until effective drug therapy has been implemented and three consecutive sputum smears microscopically negative for tubercle bacilli have been obtained on different days.

A total of 5–15% of individuals infected with *M. tuberculosis* develop active tuberculosis. The likelihood of active disease varies with age and is greatest in infants, young adults, and persons older than age 60 years. Individual groups at increased risk for tuberculosis include the homeless, inmates of correctional facilities, migrant farm workers, recent immigrants to the United States, and nursing home elderly. Poor nutrition, silicosis, cancer (especially bronchogenic carcinoma), diabetes mellitus, human immunodeficiency virus (HIV) infection, and treatment with immunosuppressive corticosteroids or cytotoxic drugs increase susceptibility to tuberculosis. The number of tuberculosis cases declined steadily until the mid-1980s (Fig. 13–1), when that trend reversed. The number of new tuberculosis cases reported in the United States increased from 9.3/100,000 population in 1985 to 10.5/100,000 population in 1992, a 12.9% increase. If the decline in tuberculosis from 1980 through 1984 had continued through 1992, there would have been approximately 51,700 fewer cases during 1985–1992 than were actually reported. The resurgence in tuberculosis primarily involves individuals infected with HIV-1. Infection with HIV-1 is currently the strongest predictor for the de-

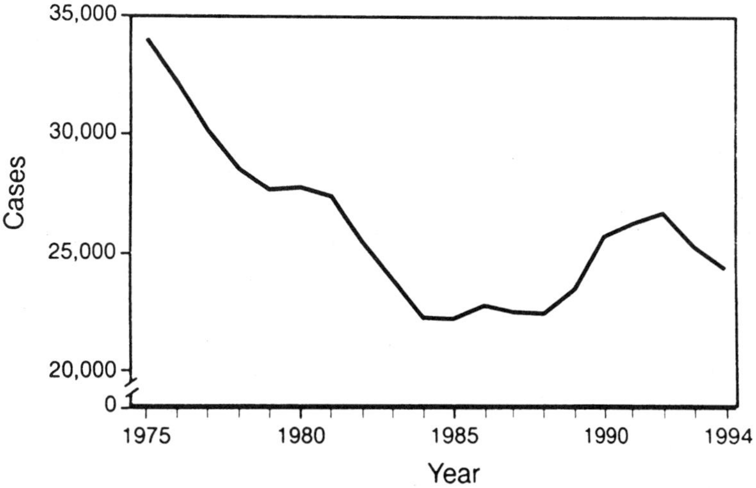

**FIGURE 13–1.** The annual number of tuberculosis cases in the United States for the period 1975–1994. (From Centers for Disease Control. *MMWR 44*(20):387–395, May 26, 1995. With permission.)

velopment of tuberculosis in the United States. The largest increases in tuberculosis have occurred among African-Americans and Hispanics aged 25–44 years, the age group where excess acquired immunodeficiency syndrome (AIDS) occurs. A substantial decrease in the number of tuberculosis cases was observed from 1992–1994 (Fig. 13–1), perhaps reflecting the effectiveness of prevention and control measures implemented during the alarming increase in this disease during 1989–1993.

### Primary Tuberculosis

*Primary tuberculosis* occurs in individuals who have no immunity to *M. tuberculosis*. Inhaled tubercle bacilli in droplet nuclei reach the alveoli, where they are ingested by alveolar macrophages. Since immunity is absent, tubercle bacilli multiply logarithmically within nonactivated alveolar macrophages. Also, tubercle bacilli escape via draining lymphatics and establish separate foci of infection in ipsilateral hilar lymph nodes of the lung. From the hilar lymph nodes, bacilli spread via the thoracic duct into the circulation and seed multiple organs, including the bone marrow, liver, spleen, kidneys, meninges, and (of particular importance in the development of chronic pulmonary tuberculosis) the posterior regions of the apices of the upper lung lobes and superior segments of the lower lobes. This bacillemic phase of infection is clinically silent. However, within 2–6 weeks the infected host develops *cellular hypersensitivity* to tubercle bacilli, which evokes a granu-

lomatous inflammatory response at sites of tissue infection. Granulomas are produced consisting of focal aggregates of macrophages, Langhans' giant cells, lymphocytes, and granulation tissue (fibroblasts and capillaries) (Fig. 13–2), which are referred to as *tubercles*. Granulomas in the lower lobes of lung and hilar lymph nodes enlarge and undergo central *caseation necrosis* (Fig. 13–3). Caseation necrosis is a manifestation of hypersensitivity to mycobacterial antigen. In caseation necrosis, dead tissue consists of gray to white granular debris that has the appearance of friable, cheesy material (hence the term *caseous*). Concomitant with hypersensitivity, *cell-mediated immunity* is expressed by differentiation of macrophages to *epithelioid cells* —enlarged and activated macrophages that assume the morphologic appearance of epithelial cells (Fig. 13–2). Activated macrophages are able to suppress the proliferation of phagocytosed tubercle bacilli, and infection is contained. Also, cytotoxic T lymphocytes are generated, which attack and release tubercle bacilli from quiescent (unactivated) macrophages, with subsequent uptake of the released bacilli by activated macrophages.

The development of hypersensitivity and immunity occurs during primary infection, which for most individuals is subclinical. The only evidence that infection has taken place is the development of cutaneous delayed hypersensitivity to tuberculin protein. Healing of tissue granulomas occurs by fibrosis. The fibrotic granulomas often calcify to produce

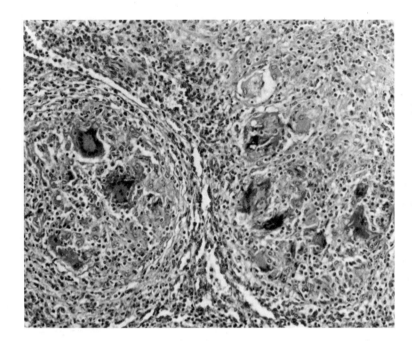

**FIGURE 13-2.** Tuberculous granulomas (tubercles). Two granulomas are shown, each consisting of a compact collection of large activated macrophages (epithelioid cells), multinucleated giant cells, and small dark lymphocytes. (From Warren, J. R., Scarpelli, D. G., Reddy, J. K., and Kanwar, Y. S. *Essentials of General Pathology.* New York: Macmillan Publishing Company, 1987. With permission.)

the *Ghon complex,* a complex of calcified pulmonary and hilar node granulomas.

Progressive primary tuberculosis, when it occurs, is observed most frequently in infants and in adults with AIDS. Roentgenograms in primary tuberculosis frequently show dense infiltrates in a lower or midlung field, accompanied by large, occasionally massive hilar or mediastinal lymphadenopathy. Fever and lassitude may be present, and hilar or mediastinal lymphadenitis may compress a bronchus, causing a brassy cough. The bacillemic phase may result in life-threatening miliary–meningeal tuberculosis.

### Chronic Pulmonary Tuberculosis

*Chronic pulmonary (reactivation) tuberculosis* occurs in individuals who have some degree of immunity to *M. tuberculosis.* The bacillemic phase of primary infection results in dissemination of tubercle bacilli to the posterior apical regions of the upper lung lobes or the superior segments of the lower lobes. The subsequent development of cell-mediated immunity contains but does not eradicate tubercle bacilli, and cavitary disease can develop in these pulmonary regions a short time after the bacillemic phase of primary infection, or (more commonly) after a long latent period. Viable tubercle bacilli persist for years within the "healed" fibrocalcific granulomas of primary infection, and there is always the potential for activation of these lesions with

development of clinical disease. Chronic pulmonary tuberculosis most often occurs in the posterior regions of the lung apex because of the relatively high oxygen tension and low lymphatic drainage in these regions. HIV infection, advanced age, diabetes mellitus, cancer, and immunosuppression for any reason, including that resulting from corticosteroids, can lower cell-mediated immunity sufficiently to cause reactivation of latent organisms and development of chronic pulmonary tuberculosis. Because of hypersensitivity, large areas of caseous necrosis are surrounded by a granulomatous rim of epithelioid cells and Langhans' giant cells (Fig. 13–3).

Accumulation of large concentrations of mycobacterial antigen results in severe hypersensitivity, and caseous centers of tubercles become liquefied. Liquefaction necrosis is one of the most harmful host responses in tuberculosis. The liquefied caseum is an excellent culture medium for tubercle bacilli, which multiply extracellularly and attain large numbers. Erosion of liquefied caseum into a bronchus results in drainage of necrotic material into the bronchial tree and cavitation of the lung. Cavity formation is the pivotal event in chronic pulmonary reactivation tuberculosis, since tubercle bacilli proliferate to enormous numbers in the ambient $O_2$ tension of air, and bronchial drainage of necrotic material establishes new exudative foci of infection within the lung (*bronchogenic spread*). Pulmonary and

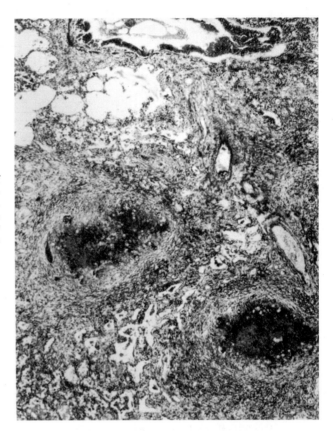

**FIGURE 13-3.** Caseating granulomas. Two areas of caseous necrosis are present in the central region of tuberculous granulomas (lower half of the field). (From Warren, J. R., Scarpelli, D. G., Reddy, J. K., and Kanwar, Y. S. *Essentials of General Pathology.* New York: Macmillan Publishing Company, 1987. With permission.)

systemic signs and symptoms are often pronounced, with hectic fever, productive cough, night sweats, weight loss, dyspnea, and even hemoptysis. Cell-mediated immunity in conjunction with appropriate drug treatment slows the progression of pulmonary tuberculosis, and healing of cavities ensues with fibrosis and dystrophic calcification. Apical calcified lesions present on chest roentgenogram in the region of the clavicle are referred to as *Simon's foci.*

### Extrapulmonary Tuberculosis

As described previously, lymphohematogenous spread of tubercle bacilli occurs during primary infection of individuals who have no tuberculous immunity. This phase is most often (but not always) transient, since acquisition of cell-mediated immunity usually prevents disease, but it creates a situation in which most organs are seeded with tubercle bacilli. Extrapulmonary tuberculosis in adults generally results from later development of a predisposing condition, including immunosuppressive treatment (particularly the use of steroids), HIV infection, or chronic illness (es-

pecially renal failure, connective tissue disease, and diabetes mellitus), which causes reactivation of a latent tuberculous focus.

### Disseminated (Miliary) Tuberculosis

Disseminated tuberculosis involves two or more noncontiguous tuberculous sites, and/or the presence of *Mycobacterium tuberculosis* in the blood (*mycobacteremia*). The pathologic lesions in disseminated tuberculosis range from tiny caseous granulomas that resemble millet seeds—hence the term *miliary tuberculosis*—to larger granulomatous nodules. Disseminated tuberculosis occurs in young children under 3 years of age, and in adults especially over the age of 65 years with the immunosuppression of cancer, alcoholism, malnutrition, or chronic hemodialysis, and in AIDS. The presenting symptoms of miliary tuberculosis are nonspecific and evolve over several weeks, with fever, anorexia, sweats, and weight loss. Although less common, headache is an ominous sign indicating meningeal involvement. Abnormal laboratory findings are also nonspecific, and a mild anemia, elevated erythrocyte sedimentation rate (ESR), hyponatremia, and polyclonal gammopathy are typically present. In most patients, the discovery of a miliary or reticulonodular infiltrate on chest roentgenogram raises the suspicion of miliary tuberculosis. Despite its atypical presentation, prompt diagnosis and treatment of disseminated tuberculosis are critical, since untreated disseminated tuberculosis is almost uniformly fatal within 1 year.

### Isolated Organ Tuberculosis

*Isolated organ tuberculosis* is an extrapulmonary disease caused by hematogenous seeding of a particular organ system, especially the central nervous system (CNS), pericardium, genitourinary tract, and peripheral lymph nodes. Frequently an asymptomatic latent period (sometimes years) follows the hematogenous seeding of extrapulmonary organs.

**Tuberculous Meningitis.** This disease most often results from rupture of a tubercle into the subarachnoid space, with development of granulomatous meningitis at the base of the brain. Low-grade fever, headache, and altered mental state in a patient with clinical evidence of tuberculosis—especially miliary lesions on a chest roentgenogram—suggest tuberculous meningitis. Meningeal inflammation can result in fibrous encasement of cerebral arteries with accompanying ischemia and infarction of dependent brain tissue, or obstruction of basilar cisterns and ventricular foramina leading to hydrocephalus.

**Tuberculous Pericarditis.** Tuberculous pericarditis most often results from rupture of a hilar or mediastinal caseous lymph node into the pericardial space. The pericardial effusion may or may not be accompanied by signs of infection (fever, pericardial pain). Fibrous organization of a caseous effusion can progress to pericardial constriction and cardiac failure.

**Renal Tuberculosis.** Renal tuberculosis originates from a primary lung focus with lymphohematogenous spread and bilateral cortical seeding of the kidneys. This disease reflects extension of cortical foci of infection to the medulla, where the hypertonic environment inhibits cell-mediated immunity. This form of extrapulmonary tuberculosis has an especially long latent period, generally greater than 5 years. Tuberculous bacilluria causes cystitis, and local urinary symptoms and signs, including dysuria with hematuria and pyuria, are frequent. The scarring of chronic renal tuberculosis may lead to obstructive uropathy.

**Tuberculous Lymphadenitis.** This is the most common form of extrapulmonary tuberculosis, accounting for about one third of cases of predominantly extrapulmonary disease. Mostly occurring in otherwise healthy individuals, tuberculous lymphadenitis initially appears as rapidly enlarging, firm lymph nodes, which later undergo caseation necrosis, may soften and become matted, and form draining fistulae. Approximately 70% of tuberculous lymphadenitis is cervical in location.

Other forms of isolated organ tuberculosis include skeletal tuberculosis of the spine (*Pott's disease*), granulomatous hepatitis, tuberculous peritonitis, and pleural tuberculosis.

## Cell-Mediated Immunity and Hypersensitivity

Macrophages from experimental animals immunized with tubercle bacilli greatly inhibit the intracellular proliferation of tubercle bacilli. The increased microbicidal activity of macrophages during infection with facultative intracellular parasites is referred to as *macrophage activation*. A number of important facts have emerged in studies on macrophage activation in mycobacterial disease. First, once established, macrophage activation is nonspecific, and enhanced bactericidal activity is directed not only toward the inducing mycobacterial species, but also against unrelated facultative intracellular bacteria. Second, induction of macrophage activation depends upon specific interaction between immune lymphocytes and the infecting organism. Lymphokines, peptides that act as intercellular signals between lymphoid cells, are secreted by specific lymphocytes upon contact with homologous mycobacterial antigen, and the lymphokines activate macrophages for intracellular killing. The lymphokine *interferon-gamma* (IFN-gamma) plays the major role in activating macrophages for inhibition of mycobacterial growth. Third, macrophage activation is under the control of T lymphocytes. Antibody against thymocytes or T cells ablates the ability of splenic lymphocytes to activate macrophages, and mice deficient in T lymphocytes develop persistent mycobacterial infections. Fourth, mycobacterial antigen is processed by macrophages and is displayed on the macrophage membrane in association with class II histocompatibility antigens. T lymphocytes become specifically sensitized by contact with mycobacterial antigen and, upon later exposure to mycobacterial antigen and the same class II antigens, release the inflammatory lymphokines responsible for macrophage activation.

Lymphocytes and macrophages exist side by side in granulomas, where macrophages become highly activated by local T-cell secretion of IFN-gamma. T cells also secrete *macrophage chemotactic factor* (MCF), which attracts macrophages to local sites of infection, and *migration inhibitory factor* (MIF), which holds macrophages at sites of infection. Consequently, macrophages are present within granulomas in large numbers. *Tumor necrosis factor-alpha* (TNF-alpha) released from macrophages in granulomas supports the development of large epithelioid cells in granulomas and mycobacterial elimination. These macrophage recruitment and activation mechanisms within granulomas are of critical importance, since the mere presence of activated macrophages without granuloma formation is insufficient to control mycobacterial infection.

### Role of T Cells in Immunity

In recent years, a great deal has been discovered concerning the roles of T-lymphocyte subsets in the cell-mediated immunity of tuberculosis. Quiescent CD4+ helper/inducer T cells are activated by mycobacterial antigen displayed on macrophage membranes with histocompatible class II antigen. Helper T-cell activation is supported by interleukin-1 (IL-1) produced by the macrophage. The activated CD4+ cell, in turn, produces interleukin-2 (IL-2) and expresses large numbers of IL-2 receptors on its membrane. Consequently, IL-2 acts as an autocrine factor, producing clonal expansion of the immunologically specific CD4+ lymphocytes, which secrete IFN-gamma, MIF, and MCF. Recently, a role has become apparent for CD8+ cytotoxic T lymphocytes in the cell-mediated immunity of tuberculosis. Depletion of CD8+ cells in mice renders them more susceptible to infection with *M. tuberculosis*, and cloned CD8+ cell lines obtained from mice immunized with tubercle bacilli can destroy infected macrophages. A model for cell-mediated immunity in tuberculosis has emerged, in which both macrophage activation and macrophage lysis provide potent mechanisms for host defense (Fig. 13–4). Cytotoxic T lymphocytes destroy nonactivated macrophages infected with and unable to suppress the intracellular proliferation of *M. tuberculosis*. Lysis of nonactivated macrophages results in the release of their content of bacilli into extracellular tissue spaces, where the organisms are ingested and killed by activated macrophages.

### Cell-Mediated Damage

Tissue injury (caseation necrosis, liquefaction) occurs in tuberculous lesions when tu-

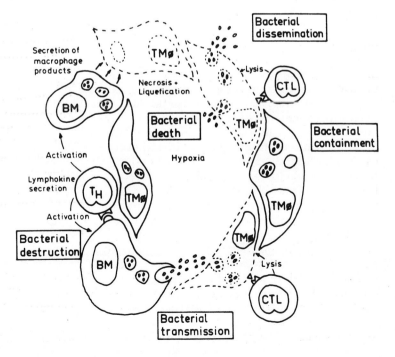

FIGURE 13–4. A proposed model for T-lymphocyte–macrophage interactions in a tuberculous granuloma. BM, unactivated macrophage (blood-borne monocyte); T$_H$, CD4+ helper T cell; TM$\phi$, activated tissue macrophage; CTL, CD8+ cytolytic T cell. (From Kaufmann, S. H. E. In vitro analysis of the cellular mechanisms involved in immunity to tuberculosis. *Rev. Infect. Dis. 11*:S448, 1989. With permission.)

berculin protein antigens reach high local concentrations. This injury reflects cell-mediated damage due to lymphocytes and macrophages mobilized in the immune response to the tuberculin antigens. Cellular immunity is usually sufficient to suppress the proliferation of tubercle bacilli, and caseation necrosis is limited to focal areas such as the upper lung lobes. However, if cellular immunity is depressed, bacillary proliferation produces a high concentration of tuberculoprotein, and extensive tissue destruction results from hypersensitivity to tuberculoprotein. Caseation necrosis and liquefaction result from the release by activated macrophages of hydrolytic enzymes, reactive $O_2$ intermediates, and TNF-alpha. In addition, activated macrophages secrete procoagulant factors, which cause thrombosis of local blood vessels and ischemia. Destruction of host tissue also occurs through lysis of tissue macrophages by CD8+ T lymphocytes.

## Cutaneous Tuberculin Reaction

Many years ago, Robert Koch recognized the hypersensitivity response induced by infecting guinea pigs with *M. tuberculosis*. Subcutaneous infection by tubercle bacilli in a nonimmune guinea pig caused a persistently infected ulcer that failed to heal. In contrast, secondary infection by tubercle bacilli at another subcutaneous site in the infected animal elicited brisk formation of an indurated lesion, which ulcerated and then healed rapidly. In subsequent work, Koch demonstrated that a crude extract of a boiled culture of tubercle bacilli (*old tuberculin*) produced a similar secondary response when injected into an infected animal. The tuberculin hypersensitivity of infected individuals was initially thought to be of potential therapeutic usefulness. It was soon recognized, however, that the tuberculous patient is inordinately sensitive to tuberculin, and that hypersensitivity (allergy) can be deleterious in the presence of high tuberculin concentration. However, cutaneous tuberculin hypersensitivity is very important for the clinical diagnosis of tuberculous infection. Products prepared from old tuberculin by fractionation with trichloroacetic acid, ammonium sulfate, and alcohol are designated *purified protein derivative* (PPD) of tuberculin. In reality PPD consists of a heterogeneous mixture of mycobacterial cell-wall proteins and polysaccharides. A single lot of PPD (designated PPD-S) has been adopted as the biologic standard by which all clinical PPD prep-

arations are standardized. A 5-TU (tuberculin unit) dose of PPD is equivalent to 0.0001 mg of PPD-S in 0.1 mL of solution. Extensive clinical studies have demonstrated that 90% of individuals with at least 10 mm of induration 2–3 days following an intracutaneous 5-TU dose of PPD are infected with *M. tuberculosis*, and that essentially 100% of individuals with a 20-mm reaction are infected. The persistence of cutaneous tuberculin hypersensitivity requires the continued presence of tubercle bacilli, although in many individuals the bacilli are present in small numbers and in a slowly replicating, slowly metabolizing form without clinical disease. Histologically, the cutaneous indurated lesion of tuberculin hypersensitivity consists primarily of infiltrates of mononuclear cells in the superficial and deep dermis, and fibrin deposition in the interstitium. The induration is due mostly to fibrin.

A positive *tuberculin reaction* is generally defined as induration 10 mm or greater 2–3 days following intracutaneous injection of a PPD dose equivalent to 5 TU (*intermediate-strength PPD*). In certain situations (contact investigations, HIV-infected persons, presence of upper lobe fibrotic lesion on chest x-ray), the threshold for a positive test is lowered to 5 mm to enhance the sensitivity of the test. A positive tuberculin reaction indicates probable clinical or subclinical infection by *M. tuberculosis*. However, both false-positive and false-negative reactions occur. False-positive reactions can be due to infection with nontuberculous mycobacteria, especially *M. kansasii*, or vaccination with bacille Calmette-Guérin (BCG) (an attenuated strain of *Mycobacterium bovis*) within the previous 15 years. *False-negative reactions* (anergy) can occur in patients with active tuberculosis, but most of these patients become tuberculin-positive when their illness begins to resolve with antituberculosis chemotherapy. Cutaneous hypersensitivity to tuberculin in infected patients can also be lost due to suppression of cellular immunity by viral infections, lymphoreticular malignancies, AIDS, and corticosteroid therapy. Thus, the absence of a positive tuberculin test does not necessarily mean the absence of tuberculous infection.

## Chemotherapy of Tuberculosis

Effective chemotherapy for tuberculosis is based on two fundamental principles. First, spontaneous genetic resistance is present in populations of tubercle bacilli not previously exposed to the primary antituberculous

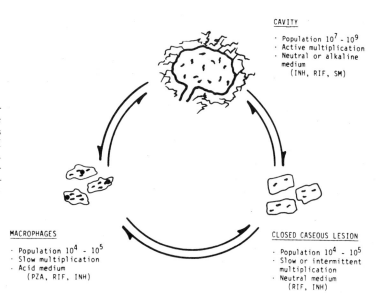

CAVITY
· Population $10^7$ - $10^9$
· Active multiplication
· Neutral or alkaline
  medium
  (INH, RIF, SM)

MACROPHAGES
· Population $10^4$ - $10^5$
· Slow multiplication
· Acid medium
  (PZA, RIF, INH)

CLOSED CASEOUS LESION
· Population $10^4$ - $10^5$
· Slow or intermittent
  multiplication
· Neutral medium
  (RIF, INH)

**FIGURE 13–5.** Three populations of tubercle bacilli in tuberculosis. Drugs active against each population are indicated as INH (isoniazid), RIF (rifampin), SM (streptomycin), and PZA (pyrazinamide). (From Dutt, A. K., and Stead, W. W. Present chemotherapy for tuberculosis. *J. Infect. Dis. 146:*698, 1982. With permission.)

drugs. The frequency of genetic drug-resistant mutants is estimated at 1 in $10^5$ tubercle bacilli for streptomycin, 1 in $10^6$ for isoniazid (INH) and ethambutol, and 1 in $10^8$ bacilli for rifampin. Second, tubercle bacilli in the infected patient exist as three different bacterial populations: extracellularly in cavitary lesions and closed caseous lesions, and intracellularly in macrophages (Fig. 13–5). *M. tuberculosis* is an obligate aerobe, and rapidly proliferates to large numbers ($10^7$–$10^9$ organisms) in the high oxygen tension of open cavities. However, in closed caseous lesions and within macrophages, where oxygen tension is reduced, only low numbers ($10^4$–$10^5$) of slowly growing, metabolically inert tubercle bacilli are present. Based on these principles, a combination of bactericidal drugs rather than a single drug is necessary in the chemotherapy of active disease where large numbers of tubercle bacilli are present, to prevent overgrowth by drug-resistant bacteria (Fig. 13–6). In addition, it is necessary to use drugs that are bactericidal not only for extracellular tubercle bacilli in cavities but for slowly growing bacilli in closed caseous lesions and in macrophages. These slowly metabolizing organisms are selectively killed by the drugs rifampin and INH. Rifampin and INH are also bactericidal against rapidly proliferating tubercle bacilli in cavitary lesions. Combination chemotherapy that includes rifampin and INH for a prolonged period (9 months) is sufficient to eliminate both rapidly growing cavitary organisms and slow-growing bacilli in noncavitary

lesions. Most patients on an effective combination regimen convert to negative sputum cultures within 2 months, and relapse is infrequent.

### Primary Drug Resistance

*Primary drug resistance* refers to the presence of a predominantly drug-resistant population of tubercle bacilli in a previously untreated patient. The occurrence of primary drug resistance reflects person-to-person transmission of drug-resistant strains. The prevalence of drug-resistant strains, in turn, reflects the degree of supervision of patients on antituberculous medication. In the United States, where supervision is generally good, the prevalence of primary drug-resistant infection is approximately 9%. However, some areas in the United States, notably Southern California, south Texas, and New York City, show a substantially higher prevalence of primary drug resistance. In Southeast Asia, where antituberculosis drugs can be obtained without physician supervision, the prevalence of primary drug resistance is about 50%.

### Secondary Drug Resistance

*Secondary drug resistance* is the emergence of a drug-resistant strain during antituberculous chemotherapy and among persons previously treated with such drugs. Secondary drug resistance occurs in a patient who fails to complete a full course of chemotherapy after initial improvement during early therapy and

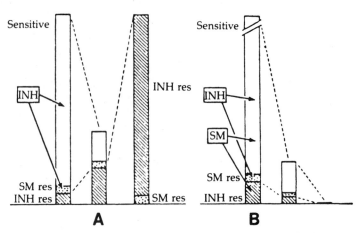

**FIGURE 13–6.** Emergence of drug-resistant bacteria in tuberculosis treated with a single drug. In panel *A*, the patient is treated only with isoniazid (INH). In active tuberculosis with $10^7$–$10^9$ bacilli, INH-resistant mutants present at a frequency of $10^6$ emerge, and soon constitute the majority of organisms. In panel *B*, the patient is treated with both INH and streptomycin (SM). Streptomycin suppresses the INH-resistant mutants, and INH suppresses the streptomycin-resistant mutants. Consequently, neither drug-resistant mutant can overgrow, and the combination drug therapy is successful where single drug therapy fails. (From Crofton, J. Some principles in the chemotherapy of bacterial infections. *Br. Med. J.* 2:209, 1969. With permission.)

then suffers a relapse with a drug-resistant strain. Such patients provide a source of infection for uninfected individuals, and the occurrence of secondary drug resistance promotes a high prevalence of primary drug resistance.

### Tuberculosis Chemotherapy

Rifampin, INH, streptomycin, pyrazinamide, and ethambutol are considered "first-line" drugs in tuberculosis therapy. Streptomycin is active only against extracellular bacilli, whereas pyrazinamide has specific bactericidal activity against organisms in the acidic environment of phagosomes in macrophages. Ethambutol is not a bactericidal drug, but penetrates both the extracellular and intracellular environments of lesions and deters emergence of resistant mutants. The addition of pyrazinamide to INH and rifampin for the first 2 months of therapy allows targeting of each of the three bacterial subpopulations (Fig. 13–5). A combination of pyrazinamide plus streptomycin or ethambutol, together with INH and rifampin, is indicated for patients with suspected or proven single-drug-resistant infection. In infections with multiple drug resistance, "second-line" drugs (ethionamide, cycloserine, capreomycin, kanamycin) or alternative agents (rifabutin, amikacin, ciprofloxacin, ofloxacin) should be used. The use of combination chemotherapy to kill both extracellular and intracellular tubercle bacilli

is also required for extrapulmonary (miliary, isolated organ) tuberculosis.

Chemoprophylaxis with INH deserves special mention. Converting a skin test from negative to positive reactivity, especially in individuals who are close contacts of patients with active tuberculosis, mandates 1 year of INH chemoprophylaxis to prevent tuberculosis years later. Also, individuals with upper lobe fibrotic lesions of the lung and a positive tuberculin test, and younger individuals (<35 years of age) with positive tuberculin reactivity but without documented conversion, should have 1 year of INH prophylaxis. Contacts of INH-resistant cases of tuberculosis will not benefit from INH prophylaxis. Such contacts should be treated with rifampin, unless the contact strain is resistant to both INH and rifampin. In the latter situation, the drug susceptibility of the source case must be considered in the design of chemoprophylaxis with other drugs, including pyrazinamide, ethambutol, streptomycin and other aminoglycosides, and fluoroquinolones.

Chemoprophylaxis is a misnomer, since the real intent is therapy of subclinical but active *M. tuberculosis* infection. Small numbers of tubercle bacilli are present in subclinical infection and thus use of a single drug is effective. In older individuals (>35 years) with a positive skin test but without documented conversion, contact with active cases, HIV infection, fibrotic pulmonary lesions, or other circumstances known to increase the risk of progressive tuberculosis, INH prophylaxis is not recommended because of the risk of INH hepatotoxicity in older age groups.

The single most important principle in controlling the spread of tuberculosis in communities and hospitals is prompt initiation and maintenance of effective combination antituberculosis chemotherapy to render patients with active disease noninfectious. *Directly observed therapy* (DOT) is a highly effective component of tuberculosis control programs, in which the health care worker directly observes administration of medications to patients. The other public health imperative is to reduce the reservoir of individuals latently infected with *M. tuberculosis* by PPD skin testing and chemoprophylaxis.

## NONTUBERCULOUS MYCOBACTERIAL DISEASE

### Overview

Mycobacteria other than *M. tuberculosis* (MOTT) are an important cause of human disease, including chronic pulmonary infection, lymphadenitis, skin and soft tissue infection, and disseminated mycobacteremia. Prior to their identification with species names, MOTT organisms were designated by early investigators as the "atypical" mycobacteria. This historic designation is no longer appropriate but remains widely used. MOTT organisms differ from *M. tuberculosis* in a number of important respects. First, MOTT species are ubiquitous in the environment, found in water, soil, and house dust. Most infections with MOTT are acquired from a natural reservoir. Person-to-person transmission of disease, if it occurs, is exceptional. In contrast, there is no natural reservoir of *M. tuberculosis*, and the spread of tuberculosis is by direct contact with infectious cases. Second, the human pathogenicity of MOTT varies greatly for different species, whereas *M. tuberculosis* is an obligate pathogen for humans. Third, MOTT organisms are commonly recovered in cultures of human secretions and fluids as contaminants, MOTT may colonize individuals as saprophytes without causing invasive disease, or MOTT may cause true invasive disease. This differs sharply from *M. tuberculosis*, which when recovered in culture is *always* considered a pathogen. Because of the ubiquity and variable pathogenic potential of MOTT, it is necessary to understand the disease-produc-

ing spectrum of the various MOTT species and carefully consider the evidence for clinical disease in individual patients (presence of infiltrates on chest roentgenogram, enlarged lymph nodes, nonhealing wounds, skin abscesses or ulcers, or constitutional signs). Multiple isolates of the same MOTT organism and absence of other potential pathogens suggest disease due to the MOTT organism.

### Runyon Classification Method

The Runyon method for the classification of MOTT is based on pigmentation and growth rate. The *photochromogens* (Runyon group I) produce bright yellow to orange beta-carotene pigment when exposed to visible light, but are unpigmented when grown in the dark. The *scotochromogens* (Runyon group II) are pigmented in the dark, usually a deep yellow to orange, and the pigmentation darkens with prolonged exposure to light. The *nonphotochromogens* (Runyon group III) are unpigmented or light yellow and are not affected by light. *Rapid growers* (Runyon group IV) are unpigmented species that produce colonies in less than 7 days when isolated by subculture. The Runyon classification provides clinically relevant information when MOTT species are initially examined in patient cultures. Also, the major Runyon groupings provide a highly useful conceptual framework for understanding MOTT disease. However, definitive diagnosis of MOTT disease requires complete microbiologic identification of isolates to the species level.

Those MOTT species responsible for the majority of human disease are discussed individually in the following sections.

### *Photochromogens (Runyon Group I)*

*Mycobacterium kansasii* is a photochromogenic acid-fast bacillus that characteristically produces chronic granulomatous pulmonary disease in older-aged white men with underlying chronic obstructive pulmonary disease. Chest roentgenograms typically show involvement of an upper lobe with one or more cavities. Most strains are susceptible to rifampin and slightly resistant to INH. Prolonged combination chemotherapy with rifampin, INH, and ethambutol (the latter to suppress emergence of rifampin and INH resistance) is generally adequate. Disseminated disease with *M. kansasii* has been observed in AIDS. *M. marinum* is a photochromogen that has an optimal growth temperature of 31°–32°C, and which grows poorly if at all at 37°C. Infection with

*M. marinum* is confined to superficial cutaneous tissue, and is characteristically acquired from skin trauma while in contact with contaminated nonchlorinated fresh or salt water. Small skin papules develop within 2–8 weeks, often with progression to a verrucous or ulcerated lesion. Cutaneous lesions frequently resolve spontaneously, but persistent infection requires surgical excision or chemotherapy. Most strains of *M. marinum* are INH resistant, but are susceptible to combination therapy with rifampin and ethambutol.

### Scotochromogens (Runyon Group II)

The vast majority of scotochromogenic mycobacteria do not produce human disease. They are ubiquitous organisms that frequently contaminate specimens or colonize patients. Consequently, it is important to recognize *M. scrofulaceum*, *M. szulgai*, and *M. xenopi*, because these scotochromogenic species can produce disease. *M. scrofulaceum* is associated with cervical granulomatous lymphadenitis (scrofula) in children (most often in those 1–5 years old), which is unilateral and typically submandibular in location. Surgical excision of involved nodes is almost always curative; some patients are treated medically, often with clarithromycin. *M. szulgai* is an unusual scotochromogen in that it is scotochromogenic when grown at 37°C but photochromogenic at 25°C. Although clinical isolates of *M. szulgai* are infrequent, most are associated with disease. The predominant form of disease is chronic cavitary pulmonary infection in middle-aged men. *M. xenopi* is recognized by its optimal growth at 41°–42°C and an ability to produce pulmonary disease in immunosuppressed individuals. *M. gordonae* is a common saprophytic scotochromogen that rarely produces human disease, but is often recovered in culture as a contaminant.

### Nonphotochromogens (Runyon Group III)

The *Mycobacterium avium* complex (MAC) organisms (*M. avium* and *M. intracellulare*) are the nonphotochromogens most frequently associated with human disease. Four forms of disease due to MAC infection are commonly seen:

1. Chronic cavitary pulmonary disease occurs, typically in a middle-aged white man with preexisting lung disease, including chronic obstructive pulmonary disease, bronchiectasis, and silicosis. Clinical presentation of MAC pulmonary disease resembles tuberculosis, with a sputum-producing cough, fatigue, weight loss, fever, night sweats, and occasionally hemoptysis.

2. Chronic fibronodular disease with or without cavitation is caused by MAC especially in elderly white women, with cough and progressive respiratory symptoms over years.

3. MAC may cause cervical lymphadenitis in children and sometimes in adults, indistinguishable from adenitis due to *M. scrofulaceum*.

4. Disseminated MAC infection occurs in immunocompromised states, especially due to adrenocorticosteroid therapy or HIV infection.

Most immunocompromised patients with disseminated MAC infection present with fever, weight loss and, in many AIDS patients, gastrointestinal symptoms, including abdominal pain and diarrhea. In patients with gastrointestinal disease, aggregates of foamy macrophages are present in the small intestinal mucosa, which resemble those in Whipple's disease but (unlike in Whipple's disease) contain numerous intracellular acid-fast bacilli. The heavy mycobacterial load has led to the proposal that the gastrointestinal tract is the portal of entry for MAC in AIDS patients with a gastrointestinal syndrome. MAC is an environmental organism that can colonize individuals without causing disease. Thus, a diagnosis of MAC disease should be made only after repeated isolation of MAC in culture from a patient with signs and symptoms consistent with MAC disease. Chemotherapy of MAC disease is difficult because of resistance to the first-line antimycobacterial drugs among clinical strains. The newer macrolide antibiotics clarithromycin and azithromycin have been found to alleviate symptoms and reduce the mycobacterial load in disseminated MAC disease. Although there is yet no consensus, clarithromycin or azithromycin combined with ethambutol and/or rifabutin (a rifampin derivative) holds promise. However, no combination of antimycobacterial drugs eradicates MAC infection in AIDS patients, and restoration of immune capacity is the only hope for these patients. An unusual nonphotochromogen has recently been discovered, *Mycobacterium genavense*, which causes disseminated infection identical to MAC, but which unlike MAC will not grow on solid media. Extended incubation of a blood specimen in broth culture is required to detect the organism. Another unusual nonphotochromogen, *Mycobacterium haemophilum*, causes multiple skin nodules in transplant (renal, bone marrow) and AIDS patients that can ulcerate and progress to draining fistulae. *M. haemophilum* grows optimally at the cooler temperatures of skin (20°–30°C), and is unique among the mycobacteria in its growth requirement for iron (ferric ammonium citrate, hemoglobin).

### Rapid Growers (Runyon Group IV)

The human pathogens in this group are *M. fortuitum* and *M. chelonei. M. fortuitum* and *M. chelonei* are environmental organisms present in water, soil, and dust, and most human infections are due to accidental inoculation of skin and soft tissue during surgery or with trauma. Median sternotomy in cardiovascular surgery, augmentation mammoplasty, peritoneal dialysis, hemodialysis, surgical insertion of a percutaneous catheter, and arthroplasty have been implicated in postsurgical infections. Patients present with failure of the wound to heal. Cutaneous infections due to trauma can resemble pyogenic infection with suppuration or may progress to chronic ulceration with sinus tract formation. Like other mycobacteria, treatment for *M. fortuitum* and *M. chelonei* infection is best done with a combination of drugs to avoid emergence of resistance. Unlike most other mycobacteria, however, these rapid growers are susceptible to drugs generally used in the therapy of infection due to facultative bacteria. The aminoglycosides are most active therapeutically, especially amikacin (preferably combined with cefoxitin, doxycycline, ciprofloxacin, or rifampin).

### Leprosy

Leprosy is a chronic infection of the skin, mucous membranes, and peripheral nerves by *M. leprae* (Hansen's bacillus). *M. leprae* is an acid-fast bacillus that grows very slowly. When injected into the footpads of mice, its doubling time is 11–13 days. It is an obligate pathogen for humans, and transmission of the bacillus is by direct and prolonged contact with individuals shedding large numbers of bacilli from open skin lesions or in nasal mucus. The leprosy bacillus does not grow in cell-free culture systems and can be detected only by acid-fast staining of infected tissue. The incidence of leprosy in the United States is increasing as a result of increased immigration from areas of the world where leprosy is common, especially India, Vietnam, Laos, and the Phillipines.

### Tuberculoid Leprosy

The clinical spectrum of leprosy reflects the degree of cell-mediated immunity toward the leprosy bacillus. At one extreme of the spectrum, tuberculoid granulomas form in the skin and peripheral nerves of patients with T-lymphocyte responsiveness to *M. leprae.* This form of leprosy is designated *polar tuberculoid leprosy.* Only rare bacilli are present in the granulomas, and the tuberculoid form is not contagious. The tuberculoid granulomas result in raised erythematous plaques of the skin with flattened pale (healed) centers. These areas are *anesthetic* due to involvement of cutaneous nerve fibers by the granulomatous inflammatory response.

### Lepromatous Leprosy

At the opposite extreme of the spectrum are patients who lack T-lymphocyte reactivity to leprosy bacilli, and who have huge numbers of acid-fast bacilli within macrophages (*lepra cells*). There is no granulomatous inflammatory response, but instead nodular or diffuse aggregates of foamy macrophages appear in the skin, mucous membranes, and peripheral nerves. This form of leprosy is designated *polar lepromatous leprosy.* These aggregates are distributed bilaterally and symmetrically as erythematous nodular lesions of the skin, which often coalesce to impart diffuse thickening of the facial skin (*leonine facies*). In severe disease, perforation of the nasal septum and destruction of nasal cartilages can occur. Lepromatous skin and mucous membrane lesions contain large numbers of bacilli, and the lepromatous form is contagious. Because of lack of host resistance, lepromatous leprosy is more extensive and more difficult to cure.

Forms intermediate between tuberculoid and lepromatous leprosy are variable in their tissue reactions and bacillary load, and there is a clinically silent phase that can last for many years during which the bacilli slowly proliferate and disseminate.

### Diagnosis

As in tuberculosis, cutaneous hypersensitivity develops in leprosy. *Lepromin* is a crude preparation of bacillary antigens obtained from lepromatous nodules, which can be used as a skin-test antigen to gauge the intensity of delayed-type hypersensitivity in individual patients. Positive reactions are biphasic, consisting of transient induration at 48 h, followed by progressive nodule formation that is maximal at 3–4 weeks, sometimes with ulceration. Histologically, these nodules consist of tuberculoid inflammation. A positive lepromin test is typical in tuberculoid leprosy, but the lepromatous patient is anergic (nonreactive) to lepromin. However, patients with lepromatous leprosy characteristically have a polyclonal gammopathy with antibodies to *M. leprae*. These antibodies are not protective, but rather are deleterious, since immune complex formation often leads to an Arthus-type vasculitis and *erythema nodosum leprosum* (ENL). ENL is associated with painful necrosis of skin nodules, fever, arthralgias, and sometimes even glomerulonephritis. ENL can be fatal.

### Treatment

Infection with *M. leprae* tends to be persistent, especially in lepromatous leprosy, and prolonged chemotherapy is necessary to control and, it is hoped, eradicate the leprosy bacilli. Dapsone (4,4'-diaminodiphenylsulfone [DDS]) is the mainstay of therapy and is usually combined with clofazimine (a lipophilic drug that selectively concentrates in infected macrophages) and rifampin to suppress emergence of DDS resistance.

## LABORATORY DIAGNOSIS OF MYCOBACTERIAL INFECTION

Although mycobacteria may infect almost any tissue or organ, they most frequently infect the lungs, urogenital tract, gastrointestinal tract, meninges, and blood. Pulmonary secretions are present in expectorated sputum, aerosol-induced sputum, gastric lavage (due to swallowing), and bronchoscopy washings. Voided urine specimens are useful for the laboratory diagnosis of urogenital infections and disseminated disease. The shedding of mycobacteria into the respiratory or urogenital tracts is irregular. Thus, a minimum of three early-morning sputum, gastric lavage, or urine specimens should be collected on three separate days. Fecal specimens are submitted for evaluation of enteric disease and blood specimens for disseminated disease, especially with MAC infection in AIDS patients.

Pulmonary, urogenital, and fecal specimens are contaminated by bacterial commensals (normal flora), and consequently the recovery of mycobacteria requires both decontamination and concentration. The "gold standard" for bacterial decontamination is brief treatment (15–20 min) of specimens with 2% NaOH solution containing N-acetyl-L-cysteine (NALC). NALC acts as a mucolytic agent, thereby releasing mycobacteria trapped in mucin strands for detection by acid-fast stain and culture. Following decontamination, hypotonic phosphate buffer is added to terminate NaOH decontamination and also to lower the specific gravity of the specimen. The high cell-wall lipid content of mycobacteria renders them buoyant during centrifugation. Thus, the specific gravity of the specimen must be low in order to concentrate mycobacteria by centrifugation. The specimen is subjected to centrifugation, and mycobacteria are concentrated in a pellet, which is retrieved for acid-fast staining and culture.

Specimens obtained from normally sterile sources (blood; cerebrospinal, pleural, peritoneal, or joint fluid; and tissue) do not require decontamination, and can be either processed directly by acid-fast staining and culture or first concentrated by centrifugation.

The laboratory detection and evaluation of mycobacteria are accomplished by (1) acid-fast staining; (2) growth in culture; and (3) species identification by nucleic acid hybridization, growth properties, pigmentation, and biochemical phenotype. Although other procedures have been found useful, especially the analysis of cell-wall long-chain fatty acids by gas–liquid chromatography, they have yet to achieve general use in clinical mycobacteriology laboratories. Once isolated, the antimicrobial drug susceptibility of a mycobacterium must be carefully determined under strictly defined conditions.

### Acid-Fast Staining

The *mycosides* are mycolic acid–containing glycolipids and glycolipid–peptide complexes, which imbue mycobacteria with *acid fastness*. To perform a *Ziehl-Neelsen acid-fast stain*, a smear is briefly heated to obtain deep penetration of carbolfuchsin into mycobacterial cell walls. In the *Kinyoun stain*, a higher carbolfuchsin concentration is utilized so that heating is not necessary. When the red dye fuchsin is combined with phenol (carbolic acid) as a mordant to intensify dye binding, the bound fuchsin resists decolorization with acid-alcohol solution (acid fastness). Avid binding of fuchsin to cell-wall mycolic acid forms a barrier that traps fuchsin inside the mycobacterial cell. Tubercle bacilli stained with carbolfuchsin appear as red, irregularly beaded, slim rods in oil immersion microscopy. Other mycobacteria stain similarly, but there are some notable variations. *M. kansasii* is strongly acid-fast with long rods that are banded, and MAC organisms appear as pleomorphic coccobacillary acid-fast forms. Rapid growers are acid-fast by carbolfuchsin staining, but unlike other mycobacteria (which do not stain with crystal violet of the Gram's stain), *M. chelonei* and *M. fortuitum* appear as gram-positive diphtheroids by Gram's stain. More sensitive fluorochrome stains are now available, in which fluorescent dyes (auramine O–rhodamine) bind in acid-fast fashion to cell-wall mycolic acid. Mycobacteria display a characteristic bright yellow to golden color by fluorescent microscopy. One limitation is failure of most rapid growers to stain with fluorochromes. Thus, negative fluorochrome stains should be confirmed by a carbolfuchsin stain, with specimens obtained from body sites where infection with rapid growers characteristically occurs (surgical wounds, percutaneous catheters, traumatic cutaneous lesions).

Acid-fast stains can detect mycobacteria in specimens concentrated by centrifugation when present in numbers of 10,000 bacilli per milliliter or more. Patients with open cavitary disease shed large numbers of mycobacteria, and acid-fast smears of sputum are highly sensitive for detection of disease in such individuals. However, in patients with less advanced disease in which cavitation has not occurred, positive smears are less frequent. When the optimal three to five early-morning sputum specimens are obtained for patients with pulmonary tuberculosis, 60–80% of them will have at least one positive acid-fast smear. Tuberculous meningitis is particularly difficult to detect by acid-fast smear and culture, since there may be very few organisms in the cerebrospinal fluid (CSF). A minimum of 4 mL of CSF is recommended for recovery of mycobacteria, prolonged centrifugation must be performed to concentrate bacilli in a pellet for acid-fast staining and culture, and several CSF specimens should be submitted for an individual patient.

## Growth and Species Identification in Culture

The most commonly used medium for the culture of mycobacteria is the *Löwenstein-Jensen* (LJ) *medium*, which is a solid, egg-based, heat-inspissated medium containing the inhibitory agent malachite green to prevent overgrowth by normal bacterial flora. Also, defined *Middlebrook media* are available, in both liquid (7H9) and transparent (7H10, 7H11) agar-based forms. They contain salts, vitamins, oleic acid, albumin, catalase, glycerol, and dextrose to support mycobacterial growth. The 7H11 medium can be made selective for the growth of mycobacteria by the addition of antibiotics that suppress overgrowth by normal bacterial flora. In a significant improvement, $^{14}C$-labeled palmitic acid has been incorporated into Middlebrook 7H9 broth as a metabolic substrate for mycobacteria (BACTEC 12B broth, Becton Dickinson). When present, mycobacteria convert $^{14}C$-palmitic acid in BACTEC 12B broth to $^{14}CO_2$, and the accumulation of $^{14}CO_2$ gas allows rapid detection of the mycobacteria (*radiometric culture systems*). Standard laboratory practice dictates use of at least two of the three different media (LJ, 7H10 or 7H11, radiometric broth) for clinical specimens. In general, growth of *M. tuberculosis* complex and MOTT organisms is initially detected in 1–3 weeks in radiometric broth, and after somewhat longer times with the solid media. Following appearance in culture, it is necessary to determine whether an isolate is a member of the *M. tuberculosis* complex or a MOTT organism. The identification of mycobacteria by biochemical reactions requires several weeks to months. A much more rapid way to accomplish identification is by use of acridinium-ester–labeled DNA probes (AccuProbe, Gen-Probe Inc.) that are specific for unique rRNA genes of *Mycobacterium tuberculosis* complex, MAC, and *Mycobacterium kansasii*. These gene probes can provide an identification of organisms growing in culture within 2 h. Not infrequently, MOTT organisms other than *M. kansasii* and MAC must be characterized by pigmentation, growth rate, and species identification by a variety of biochemical tests. The identification of the same species of MOTT organism in multiple cultures, the occurrence of a lesion or disease consistent with the MOTT species identified, and absence in culture of another organism that could be responsible for the lesion or disease is strong evidence of disease caused by the MOTT species.

## Nucleic Acid Amplification

Chromosomal DNA or ribosomal RNA of *M. tuberculosis* complex can be readily and directly detected in patient specimens by am-

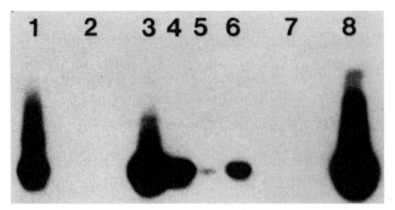

**FIGURE 13–7.** Direct detection of *M. tuberculosis* in clinical specimens by polymerase chain reaction (PCR) assay. A 336-bp repetitive element in the *M. tuberculosis* genome was amplified by PCR and the amplified product then hybridized to a $^{32}$P-labeled nucleic acid probe for visualization by autoradiography after purification by agarose gel electrophoresis. DNA directly isolated from CSF of a patient with tuberculous meningitis (lane 1), lung biopsy tissue from pulmonary tuberculosis (lane 3), and pleural fluid from tuberculous effusions (lanes 4 through 6) were strongly positive for presence of *M. tuberculosis* DNA. CSF from a patient with pneumococcal meningitis (lane 2) and pleural fluid from a patient with a malignant effusion (lane 7) were negative. Lane 8 is an *M. tuberculosis* chromosomal DNA–positive control. (From DeWit, D., Steyn, L., Shoemaker, S., and Sogin, M. Direct detection of *Mycobacterium tuberculosis* in clinical specimens by DNA amplification. *J. Clin. Microbiol. 28:* 2437, 1990. With permission.)

plification using the polymerase chain reaction (PCR) or reverse transcriptase (RT) assay. PCR assay is sensitive to fewer than ten tubercle bacilli and can rapidly and directly detect tubercle bacilli in a variety of clinical specimens (Fig. 13–7). Although still in its infancy, nucleic acid amplification is powerful and specific, and likely will assume an important role in the laboratory diagnosis of mycobacterial disease.

## Drug Susceptibility Testing

If more than 1% of bacilli in a strain of *M. tuberculosis* isolated from a patient are resistant to a drug, that drug is unlikely to be effective in therapy. Consequently, drug susceptibility assays have been established for *M. tuberculosis* that quantitatively measure whether fewer or more than 1% of organisms in an isolate are drug resistant. These assays are performed with the drug incorporated into transparent Middlebrook agar or broth (Fig. 13–8), and are referred to as proportion susceptibility assays. The proportion susceptibility assay is also clinically useful for measurement of rifampin susceptibility with *M. kansasii*, but has poor predictive power for other MOTT species. Microbroth measurement of minimal inhibitory concentrations is useful to assess the activity of amikacin, cefoxitin, and ciprofloxacin in infection caused by the rapid growers, *M. fortuitum* and *M. chelonei*.

## CASE HISTORIES

### CASE HISTORY 1

A 62-year-old, barrel-chested white male complained of increasing shortness of breath and fever. He was a heavy cigarette smoker, and his shortness of breath was attributed to chronic obstructive pulmonary disease. However, the dyspnea had considerably worsened in the preceding 3 weeks. Physical examination revealed a temperature of 100°F, pulse rate of 90/min, respiration of 24/min, and a blood pressure of 110/80 mm Hg. Chest roentgenogram revealed small, scattered pneumonic infiltrates in both upper lobes, accompanied by several small cavities. Sputum Gram's stain performed the first hospital day showed numerous neutrophils (>25 per low-power field), only occasional oropharyngeal epithelial cells (less than ten), and scattered gram-positive cocci and a few gram-negative cocci and rods. Routine bacterial culture of the sputum showed a mixed flora of alpha-hemolytic streptococci, coagulase-negative staphylococci, diphtheroids, and *Haemophilus* species. Three sets of blood cultures submitted the first day were negative after 1 week's incubation. Because of the appearance of the chest roentgenogram, three early-morning sputum specimens obtained on three different days were submitted for auramine O–rhodamine acid-fast stain and mycobacterial culture. The first two sputum specimens were negative by acid-fast stain, but the third specimen revealed golden-colored acid-fast bacilli present in small numbers (ten bacilli per entire smear). Thus, the patient was placed in respiratory

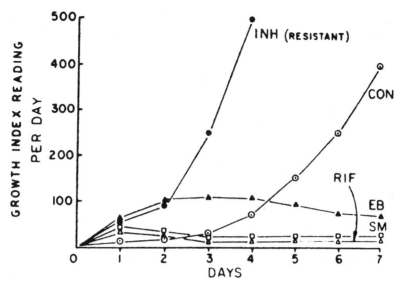

**FIGURE 13–8.** A 1% threshold as determinant of drug resistance for *M. tuberculosis*. Growth of *M. tuberculosis* in drug-containing BACTEC 12B radiometric broths is directly compared with growth in control broth in which the inoculum of organisms is only 1/100th that used for drug-containing broths. As can be seen, growth in isoniazid (INH)-containing broth is greater than growth in the control broth, indicating more than 1% of organisms are resistant to INH. Hence, this isolate is considered INH-resistant. In contrast, growth in the presence of rifampin (RIF), streptomycin (SM), and ethambutol (EB) is less than in the control broth, indicating that fewer than 1% of the organisms are resistant to these drugs. Therefore, this isolate is considered susceptible to RIF, SM, and EB. (From Siddiqui, S. H., Libonati, J. P., and Middlebrook, G. Evaluation of a rapid radiometric method for drug susceptibility testing of *Mycobacterium tuberculosis*. *J. Clin. Microbiol. 13*:908, 1981. With permission.)

isolation to prevent possible transmission of acid-fast bacilli to other individuals, and combined therapy was instituted with rifampin, INH, and ethambutol. Within 5 days of inoculation of radiometric BACTEC 12B broth with the acid-fast–positive sputum, a positive growth index (GI) was recorded (GI >10), and by the next day the GI value exceeded 100. After confirmation by Kinyoun stain that organisms growing in the radiometric broth were acid-fast bacilli, the broth was concentrated by centrifugation. Organisms in the pellet tested by gene probe were positive for *M. kansasii* but negative for *M. tuberculosis* complex and MAC. Since communicability of infection was no longer a possibility, the patient was released from respiratory isolation. Within 6 weeks, agar susceptibility testing had been completed that demonstrated rifampin susceptibility of the isolate. By this time, however, the patient had been discharged from the hospital on therapy with rifampin, INH, and ethambutol, and was doing well at home.

## CASE 1 DISCUSSION

*Mycobacterium kansasii* produces pulmonary disease that closely resembles tuberculosis with chronic granulomatous cavitary disease of the upper lobes of lung. However, unlike *M. tuberculosis*, there is no risk for acquisition by health care workers or other patients of *M. kansasii* infection from

individuals with *M. kansasii* disease, and thus respiratory isolation is not necessary. Pulmonary disease due to *M. kansasii* occurs primarily in the southern region of the United States from Texas to Florida, and the middle west extending up the Mississippi River valley to Illinois. Laboratory testing of rifampin susceptibility is necessary for clinical isolates of *M. kansasii*, as this drug has excellent activity against the organism. Disease due to rifampin-susceptible strains will respond well to combined therapy with rifampin, INH, and ethambutol, with almost 100% of sputum cultures converting to negative after 6 months of therapy. Alternative drugs are necessary with rifampin-resistant *M. kansasii*, including clarithromycin, sulfamethoxazole, or ciprofloxacin. Pyrizinamide lacks activity against any of the nontuberculous mycobacteria, and has no role in the treatment of disease due to *M. kansasii*.

## CASE HISTORY 2

A 36-year old woman developed fever, chronic cough, night sweats, and a 20-lb weight loss over a period of several weeks. A few days before admission she experienced acute shortness of breath and left-sided pleuritic chest pain. The patient was placed in respiratory isolation on admission to the hospital. Chest x-ray revealed a large left pleural effusion, and computed tomography (CT) scan of the chest demonstrated a few small infiltrates in the left upper lung lobe in addition to the pleural effusion. The initial diagnosis was community-acquired pneumonia, and treatment with erythromycin was initiated. Upon interview she described a several-year habit of intravenous heroin use, and occasional use of cocaine. She gave informed consent for serologic testing for HIV-1 infection, which was positive both by enzyme immunoassay (EIA) and Western blot. Several early-morning sputum specimens were negative by auramine stain for acid-fast bacilli, but skin testing with intermediate strength PPD produced a 12-mm area of redness and induration within 48 h. According to the patient, a tuberculin skin test performed several years earlier had been read as negative by her physician. Thus, even though the acid-fast stain of sputum had been negative, tuberculosis chemotherapy was implemented with rifampin, INH, pyrazinamide, and ethambutol. In addition, a tissue biopsy of left lung pleura for histology and culture was performed, and pleural effusion was obtained by thoracentesis of the left chest for acid-fast smear and mycobacterial culture. A diagnosis of granulomatous pleuritis was reported for the pleural biopsy, but the biopsy was negative on acid-fast stain as was the pleural effusion. The patient was discharged from the hospital, but arrangements were made for a public health nurse to visit her home three times weekly to directly supervise administration of tuberculosis medications. Two weeks later, acid-fast bacilli were reported as growing in BACTEC 12B broth inoculated with pleural biopsy tissue and thoracentesis fluid. A few days later the organisms were identified as *Mycobacterium tuberculosis* complex by gene probe testing. Drug susceptibility testing of the *M. tuberculosis* revealed full susceptibility to rifampin, INH, ethambutol, and streptomycin. During a routine clinic visit several months later, no pleural effusion was observed on chest x-ray and her lungs were described as "now basically clear." After 8 weeks of culture, her sputum specimens were negative for growth of acid-fast bacilli.

## Case 2 Discussion

The laboratory diagnosis of pleural tuberculosis can be difficult. Delayed hypersensitivity plays a major role in the development of tuberculous pleuritis, and relatively few mycobacteria are present. Acid-fast smears of pleural effusion are frequently negative, and culture is often delayed in showing growth of acid-fast bacilli or is negative. Multiple biopsy of parietal pleura with histology and culture is the most sensitive procedure to obtain a specific diagnosis. Diagnosis of tuberculous pleuritis is important, since if not treated the pleural effusion will resolve only to be followed in several years by active pulmonary parenchymal tuberculosis. The strong association of tuberculosis with HIV-1 disease is well established, and the presentation of tuberculosis in HIV-1 patients is often

atypical with disseminated or isolated organ tuberculosis (including tuberculous pleuritis). This reflects the occurrence of exogenous primary infection with *M. tuberculosis* as well as reactivation tuberculosis with dissemination in AIDS patients. Physicians should "think TB" when any patient has chronic cough and fever, especially in the setting of immunosuppression, even if radiographic findings are not typical of tuberculosis, and acid-fast smears of respiratory or other specimens are consistently negative. Prompt respiratory isolation and empiric tuberculosis chemotherapy are clinically appropriate. Isolation of *M. tuberculosis* in culture with drug susceptibility testing of the isolate remains the foundation for long-term treatment of such patients, especially with emergence of INH- and/or rifampin-resistant strains of *M. tuberculosis* for AIDS patients.

## Case History 3

A 44-year-old man developed fever, malaise, shortness of breath, intractable diarrhea, and rectal pain. His HIV-1 serology (EIA and Western blot) had become positive the previous year. Chest x-ray demonstrated diffuse bilateral pulmonary inflitrates, and arterial blood gas measurement revealed him to be markedly hypoxic. Sputum production was induced by inhalation of aerosolized saline. Direct fluorescent antibody (DFA) stain of the induced sputum was positive for cysts of *Pneumocystis carinii*. However, auramine stain was negative for acid-fast bacilli, methenamine silver stain was negative for yeast and hyphal forms (although confirming the presence of *Pneumocystis carinii* cysts), and Gram's stain was negative for bacteria. He was treated with intravenous trimethoprim-sulfamethoxazole with resolution of shortness of breath and pulmonary infiltrates within a few days. However, diarrhea persisted as did fever and malaise. Thus, a specimen of diarrheal stool was sent for acid-fast smear and culture. Within a few hours the laboratory reported presence of large numbers of acid-fast bacilli in his stool. In response to this information, treatment with clarithromycin, rifabutin, and ethambutol was implemented, and blood was submitted to the laboratory for mycobacterial culture. Three weeks later the stool and blood cultures were reported as positive for MAC organisms. By this time the patient's fever had resolved, and he desribed himself as feeling "much better."

## Case 3 Discussion

The frequent occurrence of diarrhea due to MAC in AIDS patients implicates the gastrointestinal tract as a major portal of entry for this organism. Thus, MAC joins *Salmonella* and *Listeria monocytogenes* as facultative intracellular parasites that invade the host from the gut, most likely via parasite-infected monocytes/macrophages traverse the gut mucosa. Dissemination of MAC is best demonstrated by recovery of the organism in blood culture. This case demonstrates the multiple infections that can occur in AIDS patients at any given time, and the need for comprehensive microbiologic evaluation of these patients to identify a treatable infectious etiology. It is now appreciated that drug treatment of disseminated MAC infection in AIDS significantly reduces morbidity.

# REFERENCES

## Books

Bloom, B. R., ed. *Tuberculosis. Pathogenesis, Protection, and Control*. Washington, D. C.: American Society for Microbiology Press, 1994.

Frideman, L. N., ed. *Tuberculosis. Current Concepts and Treatment*. Boca Raton: CRC Press, 1994.

Schlossberg, D., ed. *Tuberculosis*. 3rd ed. New York: Springer-Verlag, 1994.

## Review Articles

Ellner, J. J., Hinman, A. R., Dooley, S. W., et al. Tuberculosis symposium: Emerging problems and promise. *J. Infect. Dis. 168*:537–551, 1993.

Centers for Disease Control. Guidelines for preventing the transmission of *Mycobacterium tuberculosis* in health-care facilities. *MMWR 43*:1–132, 1994.

Inderlied, C. B., and Salfinger, M. Antimicrobial agents and susceptibility tests: Mycobacteria. In: Murray, P. R., Baron, E. J., Pfaller, M. A., Tenover, F. C., and Yolken, R. H., eds. *Manual of Clinical Microbiology*. 6th ed. Washington, D. C.: American Society for Microbiology Press, 1995:1385–1404.

Jacobs, R. F. Multiple-drug resistant tuberculosis. *Clin. Infect. Dis. 19*:1–10, 1994.

Kim, J. H., Langston, A. A., and Gallis, H. A. Miliary tuberculosis: Epidemiology, clinical manifestations, diagnosis, and outcome. *Rev. Infect. Dis. 12*:583–590, 1990.

Lockwood, D. N. J. and McAdam, K. P. W. Leprosy. In: Gorbach, S. L., Bartlett, J. G., and Blacklow, N. P. eds. *Infectious Diseases*. Philadelphia: W. B. Saunders Co., 1992:1256–1266.

Menzies, D., Fanning, A., Yuan, L., and Fitzgerald, M. Tuberculosis among health care workers. *N. Eng. J. Med. 332*:92–98, 1995.

Sepkowitz, K. A. AIDS, tuberculosis, and the health care worker. *Clin. Infect. Dis. 20*:232–242, 1995.

Tenover, F. C., Crawford, J. T., Huebner, R. E., et al. The resurgence of tuberculosis: Is your laboratory ready? *J. Clin. Microbiol. 31*:767–770, 1993.

Woods, G. L., and Washington, J. A. II. Mycobacteria other than *Mycobacterium tuberculosis:* Review of microbiologic and clinical aspects. *Rev. Infect. Dis. 9*:275–291, 1987.

Woods, G. L. Disease due to the *Mycobacterium avium* complex in patients infected with human immunodeficiency virus: Diagnosis and susceptibility testing. *Clin. Infect. Dis. 18*:S227–S232, 1994.

## Original Articles

Alland, D., Kalkut, G. E., Moss, A. R., et al. Transmission of tuberculosis in New York City. An analysis by DNA fingerprinting and coventional epidemiologic methods. *N. Eng. J. Med. 330*:1710–1716, 1994.

Flesch, I., and Kaufmann, S. H. E. Mycobacterial growth inhibition by interferon-γ activated bone marrow macrophages and differential susceptibility among strains of *Mycobacterium tuberculosis. J. Immunol. 138*:4408–4413, 1987.

Kindler, V., Sappino, A. P., Grau, G. E., et al. The inducing role of tumor necrosis factor in the development of bactericidal granulomas during BCG infection. *Cell 56*:731–740, 1989.

Miller, N., Hernandez, S. G., and Cleary, T. G. Evaluation of Gen-Probe amplified *Mycobacterium tuberculosis* direct test and PCR for direct detection of *Mycobacterium tuberculosis* in clinical specimens. *J. Clin. Microbiol. 32*:393–397, 1994.

Pezzia, W., Raleigh, J. W., Bailey, M. L., et al. Treatment of pulmonary disease due to *Mycobacterium kansasii*: Recent experience with rifampin. *Rev. Infect. Dis. 3*:1035–1039, 1981.

Reisner, B. S., Gatson, A. M., and Woods, G. L. Use of Gen-Probe AccuProbes to identify *Mycobacterium avium* complex, *Mycobacterium tuberculosis* complex, *Mycobacterium kansasii*, and *Mycobacterium gordonae* directly from BACTEC TB broth cultures. *J. Clin. Microbiol. 32*:2995–2998, 1994.

Small, P. M., Shafer, R. W., Hopewell, P. C. et al. Exogenous reinfection with multidrug-resistant *Mycobacterium tuberculosis* in patients with advanced HIV infection. *N. Engl. J. Med. 328*:1137–1144, 1993.

Wallace, R. J., Jr., Dunbar, D., Brown, B. A., et al. Rifampin-resistant *Mycobacterium kansasii*. *Clin. Infect. Dis. 18*:736–743, 1994.

# 14
# FUNGAL INFECTIONS

GARY A. NOSKIN, M.D. and JOHN P. PHAIR, M.D.

Infections due to various fungi are common and may be classified as either endemic or opportunistic. In the case of endemic mycoses, the risk of infection results from living in a geographic area that is the natural habitat of that organism. The most common endemic mycoses in North America are due to *Histoplasmosis capsulatum*, *Blastomyces dermatitidis*, and *Coccidioides immitis*. Infection with these fungi is acquired by inhalation of conidia. Although the endemic mycoses are significant causes of morbidity, it is the opportunistic fungi that are increasing in incidence and are associated with a high mortality in immunocompromised hosts (see Chapter 24). This chapter reviews the epidemiology, microbiology, pathology, and clinical manifestations of the most common endemic mycoses as well as the opportunistic fungal infections. While the distinction between endemic and opportunistic fungi is for convenience of presentation, it should be realized that some organisms, such as *Cryptococcus neoformans*, can infect both healthy individuals and immunocompromised hosts.

The pathogenic fungi can be classified as yeasts, which are spherical organisms that reproduce by budding, or molds, which have hyphae that branch, elongate, and release infective spores or conidia. Many of the fungi that cause deep infections are dimorphic; that is, they exist as yeast forms in tissue and mold forms in the environment.

Diagnosis of systemic fungal infections can be difficult and usually requires biopsy of involved tissue to demonstrate invasion by fungal elements. Fungal cultures of ordinarily sterile sites can aid in the diagnosis, but may not distinguish colonization from infection. For example, blood cultures which are the mainstay of diagnosis of bloodstream infections are only positive in about 50% of patients with disseminated fungemia proved at autopsy. On the other hand, fungal cultures can also lead to false-positive results. In one study, only 10% of patients with a positive sputum culture for *Aspergillus fumigatus* had documented invasive aspergillosis. These factors have led to considerable interest in improving the laboratory diagnosis of fungal infections, primarily those infecting immunocompromised hosts. Serologic tests can be useful in the diagnosis of histoplasmosis, coccidioidomycosis, and cryptococcosis, but are of limited value in the diagnosis of blastomycosis, candidiasis, or aspergillosis. Recently, assays of urine or blood for histoplasma antigen have been developed to facilitate the diagnosis of

**TABLE 14–1.   RISK FACTORS FOR FUNGAL INFECTIONS**

Underlying host defects
Neutropenia
T-cell dysfunction
B-cell dysfunction
AIDS
Diabetes mellitus
Cytotoxic chemotherapy
High-dose corticosteroids
Broad-spectrum antibiotics
Prosthetic devices
Central venous catheters
Indwelling bladder catheterization
Solid organ or bone marrow transplantation
Severe burns

disseminated histoplasmosis. Culture for *Coccidioides immitis* and *Histoplasma capsulatum* should be performed only in laboratories specially equipped to perform these isolation techniques, as laboratory personnel can be infected by the mold form of these organisms.

In general, the host defense mechanisms that control these infections involve the phagocytic cells, polymorphonuclear leukocytes, monocytes, and macrophages. In some instances, serum opsonins appear to augment phagocytosis, but for the endemic mycoses, cell-mediated responses appear to be the primary host defense mechanism.

There is no evidence for the existence of exotoxins in pathogenic fungi; however, several fungal endotoxins have been described. *Candida albicans* produces several cell-wall glycoproteins such as proteinase, phospholipase A, and lysophospholipase that facilitate tissue invasion. *Aspergillus fumigatus* produces fumigatoxin, which leads to hemorrhage and tissue necrosis and phthioic acid, which stimulates granuloma formation.

Mycotic infections generally result from exposure to environmental sources of the infecting organisms or activation of endogenous flora secondary to other diseases or therapy for these illnesses (Table 14–1). Except for candidal infections and superficial mycoses, there is no evidence of person-to-person spread.

## HISTOPLASMOSIS

*H. capsulatum* is an organism ubiquitous in certain areas of North, Central, and South America (Fig. 14–1). In the United States, most cases occur in the Ohio and Mississippi river valleys. In 1905, Samuel Darling first noted and named the organism following identification from autopsy tissue obtained in Panama. It was not until World War II that the widespread nature of this infection in endemic areas was appreciated. Culture of soil in endemic areas contaminated by bat excrement is usually positive, and localized outbreaks have occurred when such sites have been disturbed by construction. Bats, although carriers of the fungus, do not become infected or ill.

### Pathology

Infection occurs following the inhalation of spores released from hyphae, with the spores then germinating within tissue. Within days, the yeast form of the fungus can be demonstrated in pulmonary macrophages. In the previously uninfected host, intracellular proliferation occurs. The mononuclear phagocytes containing the yeast can be found in regional nodes, and throughout the reticuloendothelial system within 2 weeks. This primary infection leads to an immune response, inflammation, and necrosis at the site of mononuclear cell accumulation. With the onset of the immune response, the macrophages are activated and kill the intracellular yeast. Ultimately, the areas of caseous necrosis calcify; however, viable organisms can be recovered from such lesions long after the initial infection. In individuals with impaired T-cell immunity, infection is not controlled and these individuals are prone to dissemination.

Most individuals exposed to this fungus are asymptomatic or develop nonspecific constitutional symptoms that are self-limited. In fact, symptomatic disease occurs in only 1% of all patients and is most commonly characterized by fever, cough, chest pain, and fatigue. Although patients usually recover uneventfully, fatigue and weakness may persist for months. Infection is extremely common in endemic areas, with 80% of persons growing up in the Ohio Valley having evidence of prior infection by age 18 years. Rarely, the acute infection can be severe enough to produce life-threatening illness. In young children, the primary infection can be associated with evidence of dissemination including hepatic and splenic involvement. In normal adults, hepatosplenomegaly is uncommon, but evidence of dissemination can be documented. Cutaneous manifestations, such as erythema nodosum or erythema multiforme, are associated with the immune response to the fungus.

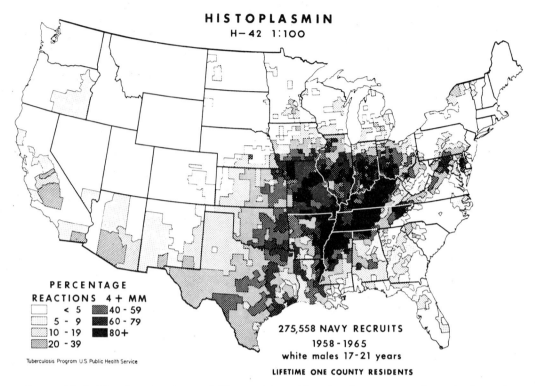

**FIGURE 14–1.** Map shows incidence of skin reactivity to histoplasmin among naval recruits. In southern Kentucky, middle Tennessee, and other areas, the incidence of skin reactivity is as high as 90–95%. (From Edwards, L. B., Acquaviva, F. A., Livesay, V. T., et al. An atlas of sensitivity of tuberculin, PPD-B, and histoplasmosis in the United States. *Am. Rev. Respir. Dis. 99.*1, 1969. With permission.)

Involvement of the pericardium, pleura, or mediastinal nodes or development of mediastinal fibrosis can complicate acute infection. The most serious complication, however, is uncontrolled dissemination, which is fatal if untreated. Clinically recognized disseminated histoplasmosis occurs in 1 in 2000 exposed individuals, invariably in those with impaired host immunity. Most patients develop prolonged fever, weight loss, hepatosplenomegaly, skin lesions, adrenal insufficiency, pancytopenia, and abnormalities of hepatic function. This syndrome is well recognized in human immunodeficiency virus (HIV)–infected patients residing in endemic areas.

The majority of individuals have no radiographic evidence of histoplasmosis; however, approximately, 25% have calcified hilar adenopathy. In patients exposed to a large inoculum, multiple small, round calcifications can be observed on chest x-ray.

## Diagnosis

The diagnosis of histoplasmosis must be suspected clinically in order to be established. A fourfold or greater rise in the titer of complement-fixing antibody to *H. capsulatum* is generally considered diagnostic. Biopsy and culture of bone marrow or liver also can lead to the diagnosis. Culture of blood using lysis centrifugation is often positive in patients with disseminated disease. Careful examination by an experienced observer of a Wright's stain of peripheral blood is positive in almost all patients with disseminated infection and about half of those with subacute disease. Recently, histoplasma antigen detection from blood or urine has been useful in diagnosing disseminated histoplasmosis, especially in acquired immunodeficiency syndrome (AIDS) patients, and is particularly useful to monitor therapy. Antigen levels fall with successful treatment and tend to increase with relapse. Skin testing with histoplasmin elicits a positive response several weeks after exposure to the organism. Although not useful for diagnosis, skin testing is helpful in establishing the epidemiology of this infection.

## Treatment

Therapy is generally unnecessary for acute histoplasmosis in the normal host. However, immunocompromised patients or those with disseminated or chronic pulmonary histoplasmosis should be treated. Amphotericin B is fungicidal against *H. capsulatum* and remains the treatment of choice for patients with moderate to severe infections. The optimal duration of therapy is unknown; however, patients should receive 0.5–0.7 mg/kg daily for at least 7–14 days. If clinical improvement occurs, then treatment can be changed to ketoconazole or itraconazole; otherwise, amphotericin B should be continued until 2.0 g is administered (for adults). The adult dosage of itraconazole is 200 mg twice daily and for ketoconazole 400 mg daily. For chronic pulmonary histoplasmosis, treatment should continue for at least 12 months because of the high relapse rate. For immunocompetent patients with disseminated histoplasmosis, 6 months of antifungal therapy is appropriate. In AIDS patients, however, following induction, treatment should be continued indefinitely. Fluconazole is less active than ketoconazole or itraconazole against *H. capsulatum*

and its role in treatment of histoplasmosis requires additional investigation.

## BLASTOMYCOSIS

*Blastomyces dermatitidis* also is endemic in the central United States; however, this disease extends farther into the northern Midwest than does histoplasmosis (Fig. 14–2). Thus, in Chicago and Wisconsin, blastomycosis is more common than histoplasmosis. The disease was originally described in Chicago by Thomas C. Gilchrist, who ultimately isolated the organism and proved that it was a fungus. At room temperature it grows as a mold with terminal conidia—the infectious form of the fungus. At 37°C, however, the fungus grows as a yeast and in tissue is seen to bud with a characteristic broad base ("broad-based buds = blastomycosis").

Cases of endemic or sporadic blastomycosis account for the majority of infections, but a few epidemics have been reported primarily

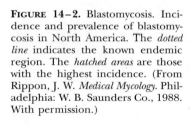

**FIGURE 14–2.** Blastomycosis. Incidence and prevalence of blastomycosis in North America. The *dotted line* indicates the known endemic region. The *hatched areas* are those with the highest incidence. (From Rippon, J. W. *Medical Mycology.* Philadelphia: W. B. Saunders Co., 1988. With permission.)

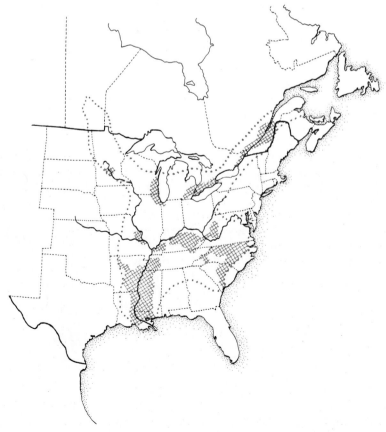

from Wisconsin and Minnesota. Infection generally occurs in individuals with significant outdoor exposure, especially in wooded areas. Although *B. dermatitidis* causes disease following inhalation of spores from soil or decaying vegetation, the organism has not been isolated consistently from soil samples.

### Pathology

As with histoplasmosis, the primary site of infection by blastomycosis is the lung following inhalation of the conidia. The fungus is then cleared by alveolar macrophages that kill the conidia, explaining why some persons do not develop infection despite significant exposure. At body temperature, those conidia that are not killed convert to yeast forms that trigger an inflammatory response resulting in the formation of noncaseating granulomas. As this transformation occurs, the fungus can disseminate.

The inflammatory response involves polymorphonuclear phagocytes as well as mononuclear phagocytes. These phagocytic cells are capable of inhibiting replication of ingested organisms. This pyogranulomatous tissue response is unique to blastomycosis. In animal models, intracellular inhibition of proliferation is associated with previously induced cell-mediated immune responses. Cytokines, such as interferon and other lymphokines, have been shown to augment this cellular activity. Specific antibody can be detected, but because of difficulties in obtaining purified antigens, assays are difficult to interpret. Cross-reactivity with other fungal antigens is common.

It is assumed that the majority of acute pulmonary cases of blastomycosis are self-limited, as many patients have recovered without antifungal therapy during large outbreaks. Individuals who seek medical attention generally have chronic disseminated disease. With a careful medical history, a long period of illness often can be documented. The organism can produce multisystem involvement, although cutaneous lesions are the most common manifestation. The skin lesions of blastomycosis may be mistaken clinically and histologically for squamous cell carcinoma necessitating a fungal stain for diagnosis.

Like histoplasmosis, the clinical manifestations of blastomycosis are nonspecific. Patients generally complain of fever, weight loss, and fatigue. An important historic clue is an individual who works outside or is frequently

exposed to wooded areas (e.g., hunters). The most common presentation of pulmonary blastomycosis is a pulmonary infiltrate or mass lesion (Fig. 14–3). Bone, joint, genitourinary, and meningeal involvement can occur. In disseminated disease, lesions can occur in virtually every organ and in severe cases may lead

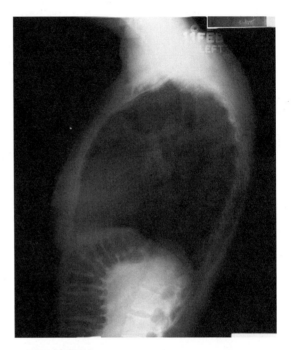

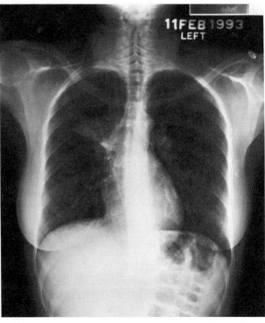

**FIGURE 14–3.** Posteroanterior and lateral chest radiograph of a woman from Chicago that demonstrates a right paratracheal infiltrate. Cultures obtained at bronchoscopy revealed *Blastomyces dermatitidis*.

to adult respiratory distress syndrome (ARDS). The classic clinical triad of blastomycosis is pulmonary, skin, and bone lesions.

There is no difference in the clinical manifestations of blastomycosis between immunocompromised patients and those with normal host defenses. Interestingly, unlike other endemic mycoses, blastomycosis has not been reported to be a significant pathogen in HIV-infected persons.

### Diagnosis

The diagnosis of blastomycosis is made by identification of the characteristic budding yeast in tissue or by isolating the organism from secretions. Unlike other fungi, *B. dermatitidis* is easy to detect in both smears and cultures. Cytologic examination of sputum, bronchial lavage fluid, pleural fluid, or pus can reveal the yeast forms and suggest the diagnosis.

Serologic tests such as complement fixation and immunodiffusion are not reliable for the diagnosis of blastomycosis but are useful for epidemiologic studies. Complement-fixing antibody to *B. dermatitidis* cross-reacts with *H. capsulatum* and other fungal antigens. Immunodiffusion appears to be the most useful serologic test; however, the sensitivity is only 70–80%. Until antigen testing is available for *B. dermatitidis*, the diagnosis of blastomycosis will require identification of the organism in tissue or culture.

### Treatment

Because blastomycosis may be a self-limiting infection, therapy is reserved for patients with disseminated disease or those who progress without treatment. Amphotericin B is the treatment of choice for blastomycosis, with a cure rate over 90% when a total of 2.0 g is administered to adults. Of the oral antifungal agents, itraconazole and ketoconazole have the greatest activity against *B. dermatitidis*. For patients with mild to moderate infection, therapy with one of these agents for 6 months is reasonable. Limited trials with fluconazole have to date been disappointing. Comparative studies evaluating the various antifungal agents are needed before definitive recommendations can be made with regard to optimal therapy. However, for patients with severe infection, ARDS, central nervous system (CNS) involvement, or who fail oral therapy, amphotericin B remains the treatment of choice.

## COCCIDIOIDOMYCOSIS

Coccidioidomycosis is an endemic mycosis found in the southwestern United States, northern Mexico, Central America, and central South America (Fig. 14–4). Recently, there has been a marked increase in coccidioidomycosis in California and Brazil. These areas are characterized by high temperatures in the summer and mild winters. *Coccidioides immitis*, the etiologic agent, is a soil fungus that is found as a mold. Coccidioidomycosis can cause disease in people of all ethnic groups and regardless of immune status. However, immunocompromised patients and African-Americans have a poorer prognosis. Cases are generally sporadic, but local epidemics can occur, especially when the soil is disturbed, as the spores can be blown many miles by high winds.

Arthroconidia, barrel-shaped hyphae of the mold form, break up, become air-borne, and are inhaled. In pulmonary tissue they swell and develop a thick-walled structure termed a *spherule*. The spherule contains endospores that are released to form new spherules. As with histoplasmosis and blastomycosis, inhalation and pulmonary infection account for the majority of cases of coccidioidomycosis, also known as "valley fever" because of its prominence in the San Joaquin Valley of California. Infection can also occur from direct inoculation, especially in the laboratory. Person-to-person spread does not occur except in rare circumstances.

### Pathology

In tissue, the spherules induce a granulomatous reaction resulting in caseous necrosis. Yeast cells, macrophages, and neutrophils can be demonstrated at loci of infection. In the presence of ruptured spherules, neutrophils predominate but the spherules and endospores are resistant to both phagocytosis and killing by these cells. Activated macrophages are capable of killing the organisms following ingestion, and thus the lymphocyte-macrophage–mediated response is central to control of this infection. Patients with defective cell-mediated immunity such as those with HIV infection, hematologic malignancies, and on immunosuppresive medications are at increased risk of infection.

### Diagnosis

Like the other endemic mycoses, the majority of coccidioidal infections are asympto-

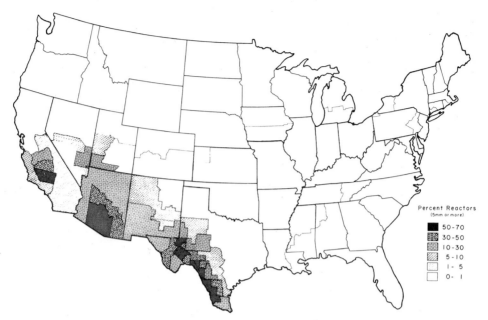

**FIGURE 14–4.** Geographic distribution of frequency of coccidioidin reactors among 48,676 young adults. *Coccidioides immitis* is known to exist in areas of high incidence. A low incidence of positive reactions occurs in areas where histoplasmosis is endemic. A low incidence of positive cutaneous reactions to coccidioidin also may be observed in certain other geographic regions, such as the Mississippi River and Ohio River areas, in which histoplasmosis is endemic, because of antigenic cross-reactivity between coccidioidin and histoplasmin skin-test reagents. (From Edwards, P. Q., and Palmer, C. E. Prevalence of sensitivity to coccidioidin, with special reference to specific and nonspecific reactions to coccidioidin and to histoplasmin. *Dis. Chest 31*:35, 1957. With permission.)

matic. Only 40% of infected persons develop symptomatic disease characterized by productive cough; chest pain; and constitutional complaints of fever, night sweats, and fatigue. As with other fungal infections, erythema nodosum and erythema multiforme can occur. Erythema nodosum occurs most frequently in young women and is associated with a good prognosis. A chest radiograph may be normal or demonstrate pneumonia with or without pleural involvement. The hilar nodes are often enlarged. Approximately 5–10% of infected individuals develop a cavity or a residual nodule, and very few progress to severe pneumonia or chronic pulmonary disease. Potentially life-threatening dissemination occurs in fewer than 1%, this being a more common finding in men, persons of non-European descent, and pregnant women. Immunocompromised individuals, especially those with HIV infection or an organ transplant, are at high risk for disseminated coccidioidomycosis. Chronic pulmonary coccidioidomycosis can resemble chronic cavitary histoplasmosis, tuberculosis, or bronchiectasis, and occasionally leads to development of a bronchopleural fistula.

Primary pulmonary infection with dissemination can lead to involvement of joints, bones, skin, and meninges. Meningitis is the most lethal complication if unrecognized or untreated. Early diagnosis is the essential element in successful treatment of this complication. Analysis of the cerebrospinal fluid (CSF) shows typical findings of low glucose, elevated protein, and a moderate mononuclear cell pleocytosis. Culture and tests for antibody in CSF, which is positive in 70% of cases, establishes the diagnosis, which should be suspected in an individual with meningitis of unknown etiology who has been in an endemic area in the recent past.

Direct examination of tissue, pus, or respiratory secretions can allow for direct visualization of the organism. In the case of disseminated disease, the fungus is commonly identified by bone marrow or liver biopsy. If coccidioidomycosis is suspected, the microbiology laboratory should be notified because this organism represents a biohazard to laboratory personnel. Unlike the blastomycosis, serologic testing is helpful in the diagnosis and management of patients with coccidioidomycosis. Serum IgM antibody to *C. immitis* can be detected usually within 21 days of infection by precipitin or latex agglutination reactions. Complement-fixing IgG antibody develops later and persists for a longer time. Elevated levels of this antibody persist in disseminated disease, and serum titers continue to rise in the absence of effective treatment. Titers greater than 1:16 are suggestive of disseminated disease. While serologic tests are important clinically, they must be interpreted with caution because of cross-reactivity with *B. dermatitidis* and *H. capsulatum.*

Delayed type hypersensitivity skin testing using coccidioidal antigens is useful for epidemiologic purposes. Most individuals develop a positive skin test within 3 weeks of infection. Patients who do not respond to skin testing are more likely to have disseminated disease and generally respond poorly to therapy. The antigen utilized most frequently for skin testing is *coccidioidin,* which is derived from the mycelial phase. *Spherulin,* a filtrate of the spherule or endospore phase, is more reactive and may lead to more false-positive results by stimulating antibody responses.

### Treatment

Most infections with *C. immitis* are self-limited and do not require treatment. The "gold standard" therapy for coccidioidomycosis is amphotericin B, which is reserved for patients with severe primary infection or disseminated disease. Patients with persistent symptoms, rising antibody titers, and anergy should receive therapy. Chronic cavitary disease usually requires surgical resection. For patients with meningitis, amphotericin B should be administered intravenously as well as intrathecally. The optimal therapy for coccidioidomycosis is unknown; however, adult patients should receive at least 30 mg/kg of amphotericin B.

Ketoconazole has been shown to have activity against *C. immitis,* and in open trials using this agent it was found to be efficacious, but relapse rates were high. Initial clinical trials with fluconazole and itraconazole have been encouraging. An advantage of fluconazole is that it penetrates the blood-brain barrier and may be useful in the treatment of meningitis. The possibility that liposomal or lipid complex forms of amphotericin B will allow higher doses to be administered safely is currently under investigation.

### SPOROTRICHOSIS

Sporotrichosis is generally a cutaneous fungal infection that results from infection with *Sporothrix schenckii.* This soil fungus produces multiple nodules along the lymphatics in the skin and subcutaneous tissue. Extracutaneous sporotrichosis is rare and often indicates that the patient is immunocompromised. The organism is found in soil, on tree bark, shrubs, and plants. Although *S. schenckii* has a worldwide distribution, most infections occur in temperate and tropical zones.

### Pathology

*S. schenckii* is a dimorphic fungus that grows as a mold at room temperature and as a yeast at 37°C. This organism is easy to identify in the laboratory by its conidiophores, which form a cluster resembling a daisy or palm tree. Infection occurs most commonly following puncture by thorns or plant fragments, which result in inoculation of the subcutaneous tissue. The initial reddish purple nodules characteristic of sporotrichosis appear 1–10 weeks after exposure. The lesion is a granuloma consisting of histiocytes and giant cells, surrounded by lymphocytes and plasma cells. Although the organism spreads via the lymphatic system, hematogenous dissemination is rare.

### Diagnosis

This infection should be suspected in a patient presenting with multiple cutaneous nodules in a lymphatic distribution who has frequent outdoor exposure, such as agricultural workers or gardeners. Demonstration of *S. schenckii* in tissue or culture is necessary for definitive diagnosis of infection. Serologic tests are also of value for confirmation if cultures are negative. The lesions of sporotrichosis are highly suggestive of infection with this organism, but must be distinguished from tuberculosis, tularemia, syphilis, and other cutaneous fungal infections. Extracutaneous infection is uncommon, but may involve bone and joints. Pulmonary disease and evidence of other organ involvement is unusual. Rarely, spread of infection to the meninges has been reported in immunocompromised hosts.

### Treatment

The cutaneous form of sporotrichosis responds to therapy with a saturated solution of oral potassium iodide plus local heat. The mechanism of action of iodide against this yeast is not known because this agent has no *in vitro* activity against the organism. For extracutaneous infection, amphotericin B is the treatment of choice. Of the oral antifungal agents, results with ketoconazole have been disappointing, but preliminary studies show that itraconazole may have a role for patients without CNS involvement.

## CRYPTOCOCCOSIS

In contrast to the previously described fungal infections, cryptococcosis is not associated with a specific geographic locality and can be viewed as both an endemic and opportunistic infection. *Cryptococcus neoformans*, the causative organism, has a worldwide distribution and is associated with pigeon and other bird feces. Skin testing indicates that exposure followed by an immune response to the fungus is common. Most of the infections that result from exposure to this organism occur in immunocompromised individuals. Currently, HIV-infected persons represent the largest group of individuals with cryptococcosis. In the United States, this infection occurs in 5–7% of HIV-infected patients and in up to 30% in Africa. In contrast to the normal host, 90% of AIDS patients infected with *C. neoformans* develop meningitis. This fungus is acquired via inhalation and person-to-person transmission has not been documented.

### Pathology

*C. neoformans* is a yeast surrounded by a polysaccharide capsule that effectively interferes with phagocytosis by neutrophils or macrophages. The organism is killed efficiently by neutrophils and macrophages that have been activated by T-cell–derived cytokines, and many patients who develop cryptococcosis have demonstrable defects in cell-mediated immunity. In addition, specific antibody is induced by infection and in combination with complement aids the cellular response to infection. The polysaccharide capsule and the cell wall of the fungus directly activate the alternative complement pathway.

Presumably, cryptococci are inhaled, and the lungs are the primary site of infection. The primary infection is generally asymptomatic; however, an occasional patient presents with a primary respiratory illness. This presentation has been more common in patients with AIDS than in other patient groups. When the organism escapes from the respiratory tract, the next most common site is the central nervous system. It is unclear why this fungus has such a propensity for the meninges, but if untreated, cryptococcal meningitis is uniformly fatal. Other extrapulmonary foci of infection that result from dissemination include prostate, skin, bones, retina, and myocardium.

### Diagnosis

Individuals predisposed to develop cryptococcosis include diabetics, patients receiving corticosteroids, those with hematologic malignancies, or severe immunosuppression secondary to HIV infection or transplantation. However, prior to the "AIDS era" approximately half of the diagnosed cases occurred in individuals with no known defect in immunity or predisposing condition. Currently, the great majority of patients diagnosed with cryptococcal meningitis in the United States are HIV infected. The most serious complication of infection with this fungus is meningitis, which can be difficult to recognize. Clinically, patients may complain of headache, nausea/vomiting, mental status changes, loss of vision, and focal neurologic findings. The major site of infection is the meninges at the base of the brain. The cranial nerves are commonly involved, and diplopia due to involvement of the sixth cranial nerve may be the only sign of CNS disease. Patients may have low-grade fever, but often are afebrile. More than half of patients have no meningeal signs. Occasionally, a cryptococcoma, or large granuloma in the brain, produces focal neurologic findings, but the physical examination is usually not helpful unless cranial nerve abnormalities are present (Fig. 14–5).

To establish the diagnosis requires a high degree of suspicion and a lumbar puncture. The CSF classically demonstrates low glucose and high protein concentrations plus a mononuclear pleocytosis; however, the CSF may be normal. Characteristically, cryptococcal organisms can be demonstrated by an India ink stain of the CSF. More recently, the use of cryptococcal latex agglutination has been shown to be more sensitive than the India ink stain. Because infection with *C. neoformans* is a basilar meningitis, CSF fungal cultures may be negative. CSF cultures obtained from the cisterna magna by a cisternal tap produce a higher yield. Adverse prognostic findings include a high titer of cryptococcal antigen in CSF or blood (>1:1024), hypoglycorrhachia, and a poor inflammatory response. Serum titers of cryptococcal antigen can be very high. False-positive reactions occur in the presence of serum antiglobulins (rheumatoid factors),

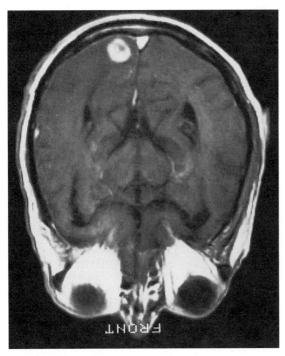

**FIGURE 14–5.** Magnetic resonance imaging (MRI) of the brain with gadolinium in a man complaining of worsening headache and ataxia. MRI reveals a solitary, enhancing lesion in the posterior fossa. Because of concerns about possible malignancy, the lesion was resected. Histologic exam demonstrated many encapsulated yeast forms consistent with *Cryptococcus neoformans*. The patient responded to a course of amphotericin B.

and the cryptococcal antigen detection assay must be accompanied by appropriate controls to prevent misinterpretation on this basis.

### Treatment

The treatment of cryptococcosis has changed considerably over the past few years primarily due to the presence or absence of concurrent HIV infection. For patients without AIDS, treatment of cryptococcal disease remains intravenous amphotericin B 0.3 mg/kg/day in combination with oral 5-flucytosine, 150 mg/kg/day in divided doses. The combination of amphotericin B plus 5-flucytosine is synergistic against cryptococci, but may be poorly tolerated because of the bone marrow suppressive effects of 5-flucytosine. Because 5-flucytosine has such a narrow therapeutic window, levels must be monitored closely. Alternatively, if amphotericin B is used alone, the dose should be increased to 0.5–0.8 mg/kg/day. The total duration of therapy is 6 weeks if the CSF becomes sterile within the first several weeks of therapy. If cultures of the CSF remain persistently positive, then therapy

should be prolonged. Renal function and electrolytes must be carefully monitored while patients are receiving amphotericin B. Because of rapid development of resistance, 5-flucytosine should not be used alone.

It usually is not possible to cure patients with AIDS of cryptococcal meningitis; therefore, following induction therapy life-long maintenance therapy is required. For induction therapy both amphotericin B and fluconazole have been evaluated. Because of early deaths in fluconazole-treated patients, initial therapy should include amphotericin B 0.5–0.8 mg/kg/day until the patient demonstrates symptomatic improvement (usually 2 weeks). If the patient is responding amphotericin B can be changed to fluconazole 400 mg daily in adults for 8–10 weeks followed by life-long maintenance with fluconazole 200 mg daily. If the initial response is slow or the patient remains seriously ill, then amphotericin B should be continued for a total dose of 2.5 g in adults. In AIDS patients with mild disease, treatment with fluconazole alone has yielded favorable results. Itraconazole is not as effective as fluconazole for cryptococcal meningitis. Liposomal preparations of amphotericin B are currently being evaluated for the treatment of this infection.

## CANDIDIASIS

*Candida* species have emerged as important pathogens causing a wide array of infections, primarily in immunocompromised hosts. These yeasts reproduce by budding and are commonly isolated from soil, inanimate objects, the gastrointestinal tract, and the female genital tract. In disease states, these organisms can be isolated from skin, urine, blood, and CSF. Recent data suggest that during the 1980s there was a fivefold increase in candidemia. Furthermore, in some university teaching hospitals, *Candida* species are the most common cause of bloodstream infection. This emphasizes the changing epidemiology of bloodstream infections in the United States and underscores the importance of *Candida* as a significant pathogen.

Presumably, most individuals become colonized with *Candida* during passage through the vagina at birth. Although confirmation is difficult, approximately 80% of healthy individuals over 1 year of age exhibit cell-mediated delayed hypersensitivity skin-test reactions to candidal antigens. Ultimately, the majority of clinical infections result from failure or suppression of normal defense mechanisms.

## Pathology

There are hundreds of *Candida* species, although only a few of them are human pathogens. The most commonly identified species that result in clinical disease are: *C. albicans, Torulopsis (Candida) glabrata, C. krusei, C. lusitaniae, C. parapsilosis,* and *C. tropicalis.* Although *C. albicans* and *C. tropicalis* are the most frequent causes of infection, the epidemiology appears to be changing. The host defenses against infection with these organisms are altered by diseases such as diabetes mellitus; infection with HIV; cancer; or therapy with antibiotics, corticosteroids, immunosuppressive medications, or neutropenia. The overall incidence of candidal infections has increased in parallel with the increased use of antimicrobial agents, corticosteroids, and central venous access devices. The most common cause of candidal infection is the use of broad-spectrum antibiotics, which suppress the normal bacterial flora of the oropharynx, lower gastrointestinal tract, and vagina and result in proliferation of the yeast. Oropharyngeal (thrush) or vaginal overgrowth is the most common form of infection; however, fungemia is becoming increasingly recognized. The mechanism(s) by which *Candida* enter the bloodstream is unknown, but the gastrointestinal tract is the most likely portal of entry. The combination of intestinal surgery or trauma, broad-spectrum antibiotics, and central venous catheters is associated with an increased incidence of fungemia. Other conditions that predispose to candidemia include injection drug use, indwelling bladder catheters, burns, prolonged hospitalization, organ transplantation, and hyperalimentation. In short, the increasing incidence of candidemia is the result of improved medical technology.

Use of medications that reduce the number of polymorphonuclear leukocytes or alter their function, such as corticosteroids, also favors infection with *Candida* species. Breaks in the natural protective barrier of the skin due to maceration or catheters predispose to colonization, tissue invasion, and fungemia in some cases. Finally, alteration in the lymphocyte-macrophage–mediated immune function leads to mucosal or skin infection with *Candida* species.

## Diagnosis

The most common clinical manifestation of candidal overgrowth is oropharyngeal infection, or thrush. This is usually recognizable by creamy white patches that can be scraped from mucosal surfaces. The finding of thrush in nondiabetic patients not receiving antibiotics or corticosteroids should increase the clinician's suspicion for immune dysfunction. In cases in which the diagnosis is uncertain, the lesions can be scraped and examined with potassium hydroxide or cultured. Thrush can also present as atrophic lesions of the tongue and buccal membranes, and under dentures. Patients receiving antibiotics or inhaled corticosteroids, those with cancer or HIV infection, and normal young infants or those with congenital T-cell defects all have an increased incidence of thrush. In HIV-infected patients, early lesions may be subtle, manifested only by angular cheilosis or mucosal erythema. Since candida are part of the normal oral flora, the isolation of this organism from sputum, especially in patients with pneumonia, presents a diagnostic challenge. To establish the diagnosis of candidal pneumonitis, documentation of pulmonary tissue invasion is necessary. This requires a transthoracic needle biopsy, bronchoscopy with transbronchial biopsy, or an open lung biopsy. Other extremely common infections that occur with the use of antibiotics are candidal vaginitis and infection or colonization of the bladder in association with use of a Foley catheter. *Torulopsis glabrata* urinary tract infection may complicate diabetes mellitus, and in some patients lead to pyelonephritis and occasionally perinephric abscesses.

Candidal involvement of the esophagus results in painful swallowing (odynophagia) and the sensation of food "sticking" substernally. Candida esophagitis occurs in neutropenic or immunodeficient patients and establishes the diagnosis of AIDS in an HIV-infected patient. In the neutropenic patient, involvement of the upper or lower gastrointestinal tract is well recognized as leading to fungemia and metastatic infection in bones and joints, heart valves, renal parenchyma, eyes, and meninges, and to multiple small abscesses of the liver and spleen. This latter complication represents an increasingly prevalent problem in patients receiving intensive chemotherapy who have prolonged periods of neutropenia and have received antibiotic therapy for febrile illnesses.

Candidal endocarditis occurs in injection drug users, patients with prosthetic heart valves, and those with prolonged central venous catheters. It represents the most common form of fungal endocarditis and presents a major problem with respect to therapy. Without surgical intervention, the mortality associated with fungal endocarditis is about 99%. Therefore, resection of the infected valve in combination with amphotericin B is generally required for cure.

One of the more recently recognized manifestations of candidemia is endophthalmitis. Examination of the fundi reveals cotton-ball–like lesions (cotton-wool spots) in the choroid and retina. Endophthalmitis may be the first indication that a patient is fungemic, and it can be sight-threatening. Because of the classic funduscopic appearance, a retinal examination is essential for any patient with documented or suspected fungemia.

In order to improve the recovery of fungi from blood, cultures should be performed by the lysis-centrifugation technique. This method increases the likelihood for a positive culture and diminishes the time necessary for growth. Approximately half of patients with disseminated candidiasis at autopsy have not had a positive blood culture prior to death. In addition, the mortality in patients with documented fungemia is high and approaches 80% for neutropenic patients with multiple positive cultures. Therefore, because of limitations in diagnosis, empiric antifungal therapy is often necessary for immunosuppressed patients with multiple risk factors.

Chronic disseminated candidiasis (formerly hepatosplenic candidiasis) is being recognized with increasing frequency in patients with hematologic malignancies. Interestingly, this infection often manifests itself following the resolution of neutropenia and is characterized by fever, hepatosplenomegaly, and abnormal liver function tests. The diagnosis can be identified by computed tomography (CT) showing multiple small lesions in the liver and spleen and confirmed by biopsy.

## Treatment

Treatment of patients with candidal infections is still evolving. Management of superficial infections generally involves the use of topical agents such as nystatin or clotrimazole; however, ketoconazole and fluconazole can be used for refractory cases. For candidal esophagitis or cystitis, fluconazole can be given orally or intravenously depending on the severity of the infection. In immunocompromised patients with candidemia or other systemic infections, amphotericin B remains the treatment of choice. However, recent data suggest that, for patients without neutropenia, the response rate with fluconazole is comparable to amphotericin B. In patients who initially respond to amphotericin B or are intolerant of this agent, fluconazole is a reasonable alternative. While the optimal duration of therapy is unknown for patients with fungemia, a minimum of 500 mg of amphotericin B should be administered to adults. Liposomal and lipid complex preparations of amphotericin B are currently under investigation for treatment of disseminated candidal infections. The widespread use of fluconazole for treatment of fungal infections has been associated with development of resistant *Candida* species.

## ASPERGILLOSIS

Species of *Aspergillus* are ubiquitous in our environment and are responsible for a wide array of diseases in humans. The spectrum of illness due to these organisms ranges from benign colonization of the paranasal sinuses to life-threatening invasion of the lungs in immunocompromised hosts. Additionally, hypersensitivity to the conidia of *Aspergillus* species may lead to allergic alveolitis, or allergic bronchopulmonary aspergillosis (ABPA). Invasive aspergillosis has become an increasingly important infection leading to significant morbidity and mortality in patients undergoing organ transplantation, receiving cytotoxic chemotherapy for hematologic malignancies, or infected with HIV. The two species most commonly associated with human disease are *A. fumigatus* and *A. flavus*.

### Pathology

Complement enhances the ingestion or killing of *Aspergillus* conidia by neutrophils and monocytes. Antibody is induced upon exposure, but whether or not the humoral response contributes to protection is unclear. Invasion of tissue by this organism can lead to hemorrhage and necrosis. *A. fumigatus* has a propensity to invade blood vessels, which contributes to tissue necrosis and hematogenous dissemination. Although the pathogenesis of aspergillosis is not completely understood, the presence of phthioic acid in fungal cells has been shown to facilitate experimental infection. Furthermore, *Aspergillus* species produce extracellular enzymes such as proteases and peptidases that contribute to tissue invasion. Acutely infarcted areas surrounded by necrotizing abscesses are highly suggestive of aspergillosis. Identification of this fungus is based on recognizing wide-based, septated hyphae that branch at acute angles in histologic sections. Despite the tendency for angioinvasive disease, pathogenic aspergilli are rarely cultured from blood.

### Diagnosis

Three major syndromes can be attributed to *A. fumigatus.* ABPA results from colonization of the respiratory tract with the organism which then releases antigenic substances leading to allergic manifestations. Secondly, *Aspergillus* can colonize pulmonary cavities that develop following tuberculosis, histoplasmosis, or sarcoidosis leading to aspergillomas or fungal balls. Finally, in profoundly immunocompromised hosts, *Aspergillus* can cause invasion of the lung parenchyma leading to invasive aspergillosis.

ABPA is associated with elevated levels of specific IgG and IgE and with eosinophilia, recurrent wheezing, bronchial plugging, and ultimately bronchiectasis, but rarely with invasion of lung tissue. The immune response to the fungus or to products produced by the organism is presumed responsible for the pathogenic process.

Aspergillomas are usually asymptomatic; signs and symptoms are generally those of the underlying disease. Hemoptysis can occur but is usually not due to tissue or vascular invasion by the fungus.

The most serious form of aspergillosis is invasive disease of the lung, occurring in immunosuppressed patients, especially those with neutropenia. This illness is progressive and is associated with fever, a rapidly enlarging lesion on chest x-ray, invasion of blood vessels, and spread to the pleura with chest pain. With involvement of the pulmonary vasculature, hemoptysis and hematogenous spread to other organs are common. Despite profound immunosuppression, infection with *Aspergillus* is relatively uncommon in HIV-infected individuals, although the incidence may be increasing. In AIDS patients, two forms of aspergillosis have been described— an invasive form in which cough and fever predominate and a bronchial obstructing form characterized by dyspnea, cough, and chest pain. Children with chronic granulo-matous disease also are highly susceptible to invasive aspergillosis. In this setting the disease is more indolent, but contiguous spread to pleura and vertebral bodies and hematogenous dissemination can occur.

### Treatment

Therapy for disease due to *Aspergillus* is dependent on the host and clinical syndrome. ABPA is a noninvasive process that is treated with corticosteroids. Systemic prednisone is superior to inhaled steroids, and antifungal therapy is of no benefit. Aspergillomas have a variable course that range from benign to rapidly progressive. If the fungus ball remains stable in size and does not impair the patient's functional capacity, close observation is reasonable. However, if the lesion grows or impinges on the bronchi, then surgical resection is the preferred treatment. Invasive aspergillosis is difficult to treat and is associated with an overall mortality of approximately 80%. Outcome is more favorable in solid organ transplantation recipients than in patients with leukemia or following bone marrow transplantation.

Standard antifungal therapy for invasive aspergillosis is amphotericin B. Despite widespread use of this agent the most appropriate dose and duration of therapy are unknown. The addition of 5-flucytosine or rifampin has been suggested by some investigators. Oral itraconazole occasionally is an effective alternative for patients who cannot tolerate amphotericin B. Finally, new preparations of amphotericin B that allow for the delivery of high concentrations to tissue without the toxicity are being investigated.

## MUCORMYCOSIS

Fungi of the order Mucorales are opportunistic pathogens that result in rhinocerebral and pulmonary infection. These organisms include *Rhizopus, Mucor,* and *Absidia* species; infections due to these fungi are referred to as mucormycosis. Like *Aspergillus* species, these molds are ubiquitous in the environment and can lead to life-threatening infections in immunocompromised patients. These organisms are typically found on decaying organic material, but have also been isolated from nonsterile adhesive tape. The high prevalence of these fungi in the environment results in universal exposure, but disease is limited to individuals with severe immunocompromise, diabetes mellitus, or trauma.

## Pathology

The spores of these fungi are inhaled through the respiratory tract and colonize the nasal passages. In cutaneous mucormycosis, the spores are inoculated directly into abraded skin. In patients with normal immune function, the spores are quickly ingested by neutrophils and alveolar macrophages.

The mechanisms for the increased susceptibility to mucormycosis of patients with impaired host defenses are not completely understood. However, defects in macrophage and neutrophil function are clearly important in controlling infection. Despite severe immunosuppression with advanced HIV disease, mucormycosis is rare, attesting to the importance of neutrophil function. In diabetics with ketoacidosis, the spores can germinate in the sinuses, and tissue invasion by hyphae occurs, producing the very serious disorder, rhinocerebral mucormycosis. Once tissue necrosis and invasion through blood vessels develops, the organism can penetrate cerebral tissue. This form of infection also occurs in patients who have prolonged periods of neutropenia and is associated with high mortality. Pulmonary mucormycosis can also develop in neutropenic patients and is characterized by fever, dyspnea, and hemoptysis. Cutaneous mucormycosis generally occurs following contamination of necrotic tissue in association with major trauma.

## Diagnosis

Rhinocerebral mucormycosis is recognized by the presence of a black eschar in the nasal passages of a patient with diabetic ketoacidosis or neutropenia. Facial pain and severe headache are frequent complaints in these patients. There can be progression to involvement of the orbit with protrusion of the eye that may mimic orbital cellulitis. Brain abscess is a complication of mucormycosis if the infection spreads posteriorly. Diagnosis requires a prompt biopsy demonstrating tissue invasion so that aggressive débridement and antifungal therapy can be administered. Pulmonary mucormycosis should be suspected in a neutropenic patient with progressive pulmonary infiltrates despite appropriate antimicrobial therapy. Cutaneous infection is manifested by cellulitis secondary to direct inoculation of the skin by the fungus or as a result of contaminated adhesive bandages.

In tissue, these fungi appear as broad, nonseptate hyphae that branch at right angles. This histologic appearance distinguishes mucormycosis from *Aspergillus*. Despite the tendency for invasion of blood vessels, the agents of mucormycosis are rarely cultured from blood or other tissue. Currently, investigators are developing antigen detection systems to facilitate the diagnosis of mucormycosis.

## Treatment

Therapy for mucormycosis requires a joint medical and surgical approach. In patients with diabetic ketoacidosis, initial management should include aggressive control of hyperglycemia. For immunocompromised patients, tapering of immunosuppressive medications should be attempted. Antifungal treatment with amphotericin B should be initiated as soon as the diagnosis of mucormycosis is confirmed. Since these fungi are less susceptible to amphotericin B, a higher dose is usually required. The currently available oral antifungal agents do not have activity against the agents of mucormycosis. Because response rates with amphotericin B alone are poor, surgical débridement of necrotic tissue is necessary. There is no known method to prevent this infection; however, in severely immunocompromised patients, the use of rooms with high-efficiency particulate air (HEPA) filters can reduce the risk of both mucormycosis and aspergillosis.

## SUMMARY

Fungi can produce a wide range of diseases in both healthy and immunocompromised individuals. In normal hosts, inhalation of the endemic organisms such as *Histoplasma capsulatum*, *Blastomyces dermatitidis*, or *Coccidioides immitis* can result in asymptomatic infection, pneumonitis, or dissemination, although the majority of cases are self-limited. In compromised hosts, these organisms are more commonly associated with dissemination as is infection with the opportunistic fungi such as *Candida*, *Aspergillus*, and *Cryptococcus neoformans*. Diagnosis of fungal infections requires a high index of suspicion in the appropriate clinical setting. Amphotericin B remains the treatment of choice for serious fungal infections; however, fluconazole and itraconazole have excellent activity against the endemic fungi. In the future, new formulations of amphotericin B with less toxicity will be available.

## CASE HISTORIES

### CASE HISTORY 1

A 32-year-old man with HIV-1 infection presented with severe bifrontal headache that had increased in intensity over the past 3 weeks. He had no other complaints, although his family had noted increased memory loss. His past medical history was significant for *Pneumocystis carinii* pneumonia, rectal herpes, and oral thrush. His last CD4+ count was 34/mm$^3$. Medications included zidovudine, trimethoprim-sulfamethoxazole, acyclovir, and rifabutin. On physical examination, his temperature was 38°C with a pulse of 108/min, a respiratory rate of 16/min, and a blood pressure of 134/86 mm Hg. He had mild thrush in his oropharynx and scattered cervical adenopathy. His neck was soft and supple without meningeal signs. A CT scan of his head revealed no mass lesions or hemorrhage. A lumbar puncture was performed. The opening pressure was mildly elevated. The fluid was clear, but there were 112 white cells/mm$^3$ with 74% lymphocytes. The CSF glucose was 48 mg/dL (serum glucose 104 mg/dL) and the protein was 125 mg/dL. The Gram's stain of the CSF showed no organisms and the acid-fast bacillus (AFB) smear was negative. A cryptococcal latex agglutination was positive at a titer of 1:1024. All bacterial cultures were negative, but the fungal culture of CSF grew *Cryptococcus neoformans* at 48 h.

After the result of the cryptococcal antigen test was known, amphotericin B 0.5 mg/kg/day was begun. Because of the known toxicities of this medication, he required frequent monitoring of his hemoglobin, white blood cell count, electrolytes, and renal function. After 2 weeks of therapy, his headache had resolved and his sense of well-being improved. Antifungal susceptibility testing revealed that his organism was susceptible *in vitro* to all antifungal agents tested. Due to his marked improvement, he was changed from amphotericin B to fluconazole to complete an 8-week course of induction therapy. A repeat lumbar puncture done at this time revealed improvement in his CSF cell counts and chemistries, his cryptococcal antigen had fallen to 1:16, and fungal cultures were negative. The patient was then placed on fluconazole 200 mg/day for life-long maintenance therapy.

### CASE 1 DISCUSSION

This is the typical presentation of cryptococcal meningitis in a patient with AIDS. In the United States, this infection is relatively common, occurring in 6–10% of HIV-infected individuals and in up to 30% in Africa. Of AIDS patients who are infected with *C. neoformans*, 90% develop meningitis. Amphotericin B remains the mainstay of therapy for patients with severe infection or altered mental status. For patients with mild disease, fluconazole can be considered. Factors associated with a poor prognosis include a cryptococcal antigen titer above 1:1024, a low CSF white cell count (<20 cells/mm$^3$), hyponatremia, and altered mental status. After induction therapy, HIV-infected patients require life-long maintenance therapy to prevent relapse. An unresolved issue is the role of antifungal prophylaxis in the primary prevention of cryptococcal meningitis in patients at high risk.

### CASE HISTORY 2

A 62-year-old man with hypertension and coronary artery disease recently retired and moved to Southern California. He visited his physician for a regular check-up but complained of a "flu-like" illness that had persisted for several months. He also noted joint aches, mild dyspnea, and a rash. His medications included nifedipine and enalapril. On physical examination, his temperature was 100.4°F with a pulse of 96/min, a respiratory rate of 20/min, and a blood pressure of 148/92 mm Hg. His skin revealed an erythematous rash that was slightly raised, but not papular. The remainder of the physical was normal. Because of the suspicion of coccidioidomycosis, his physician performed a coccidioidal skin test, which was positive and confirmed by serology. Complement-fixing IgM antibody was positive at 1:16. A chest x-ray demonstrated mild cardiomegaly without infiltrates. Blood, urine, and sputum cultures were negative. The patient was reassured that most cases of coccidioidomycosis in immunocompetent hosts are self-limited and that no therapy was indicated at this time. A follow-up evaluation 6 weeks later revealed that he had returned to his normal state of health.

### CASE 2 DISCUSSION

Coccidioidomycosis is a disease acquired by people who live in endemic areas, primarily the southwestern United States and Brazil. Recently, there has been a marked increase in coccidioidomycosis in people residing in endemic areas related to drought conditions, earthquakes, and dust storms that have aerosolized the spores. Most cases of primary infection occur via inhalation of the fungus and are self-limited. Antifungal treatment is generally reserved for patients with severe symptoms, progressive infection, dissemination, or meningitis. Although amphotericin B is the treatment of choice for severe infections, itraconazole is a reasonable alternative in patients with mild to moderate infection. There is no proven method to prevent infection, but avoidance of endemic areas and proper protection of laboratory personnel is critical.

## REFERENCES

**Books**

Holmberg, K., and Meyer, R., eds. *Diagnosis and Therapy of Systemic Fungal Infections.* New York: Raven Press, 1989.

Niederman, M. S., Sarosi, G. A., and Glassroth, J. G., eds. *Respiratory Infections: A Scientific Basis for Management.* Philadelphia: W. B. Saunders Co., 1994.

Patterson, R., Greenberger, P. A., and Roberts, M. L. *Allergic Bronchopulmonary Aspergillosis.* Providence, R.I.: OceanSide Publications, Inc., 1995.

Rippon, J. W. *Medical Mycology: The Pathogenic Fungi and the Pathogenic Actinomycetes.* 3rd ed. Philadelphia: W. B. Saunders Co., 1988.

**Articles**

Allende, M. C., Lee, J. W., Francis, P., et al. Dose-dependent antifungal activity and nephrotoxicity of amphotericin B colloidal dispersion in experimental pulmonary aspergillosis. *Antimicrob. Agents Chemother. 38*:518–522, 1994.

Brown, J. Mucormycosis. *Semin. Respir. Med. 9*:175–191, 1987.

Como, J. A., and Dismukes, W. E. Oral azole drugs as systemic antifungal therapy. *N. Engl. J. Med. 330*:263–272, 1994.

Denning, D. W., Follansbee, S. E., and Scolaro, M., et al. Pulmonary aspergillosis in patients with the acquired immunodeficiency syndrome. *N. Engl. J. Med. 324*:654–662, 1991.

Denning, D. W., Lee, J. Y., and Hostetler, J. S., et al. NIAID Mycoses Study Group multicenter trial of oral itraconazole therapy for invasive aspergillosis. *Am. J. Med. 97*:135–144, 1994.

Galgiani, J. N. Susceptibility testing of fungi: Current status of the standardized process. *Antimicrob. Agents Chemother. 37*:2517–2521, 1993.

Gerson, S. L., Talbot, G. H., and Lusk, E. Invasive pulmonary aspergillosis in adult acute leukemia. *J. Clin. Oncol. 3*:1109–1115, 1985.

Goodwin, R., Loyd, J., and DesPrez, R. Histoplasmosis in normal hosts. *Medicine 60*:231–266, 1981.

Klein, B. S., Vergeront, J. M., Weeks, R. J., et al. Isolation of *B. dermatitidis* in soil associated with a large outbreak of blastomycosis in Wisconsin. *N. Engl. J. Med. 314*: 529–540, 1986.

Rex, J. H., Bennett, J. E., Sugar, A. M., et al. A randomized trial comparing fluconazole with amphotericin B for the treatment of candidemia in patients without neutropenia. *N. Engl. J. Med. 331*:1325–1330, 1994.

Rinaldi, M. Invasive aspergillosis. *Rev. Infect. Dis. 5*:1061–1077, 1983.

Stansell, J. D. Pulmonary fungal infections in HIV-infected persons. *Semin. Resir. Infect. 8*:116–123, 1993.

Terrell, C. L., and Hughes, C. E. Antifungal agents used for deep-seated mycotic infections. *Mayo Clin. Proc. 67*: 69–91, 1992.

Thales, M., Tastakia, B., Shawker, T., et al. Hepatic candidiasis in cancer patients: The evolving picture of the syndrome. *Ann. Intern. Med. 108*:88–100, 1988.

Wey, S. B., Motomi, M., Pfaller, M. A., et al. Risk factors for hospital-acquired candidemia. *Arch. Intern. Med. 149*:2349–2353, 1989.

Wheat, J. Histoplasmosis and coccidioidomycosis in individuals with AIDS: A clinical review. *Infect. Dis. Clin. North Am. 8*:467–482, 1992.

Williams, D. M., Krick, J. A., and Remington, J. Pulmonary infection in the compromised host. *Am. Rev. Respir. Dis. 114*:359–394, 1976.

Zuger, A., Louie, E., and Holzman, R. S., et al. Cryptococcal disease in patients with acquired immunodeficiency syndrome. Diagnostic features and outcome of treatment. *Ann. Intern. Med. 104*:234–240, 1986.

# IV GENITOURINARY TRACT INFECTIONS

# 15

# URINARY TRACT INFECTIONS: CYSTITIS AND PYELONEPHRITIS

ANTHONY J. SCHAEFFER, M.D.

It is well established that the urine within the normal urinary tract is sterile, and consequently it appears likely that bacteria rarely colonize the mucosa lining the urinary tract. Recognition of the resistance of the normal urinary tract to infection is essential. Conversely, identification of bacteria in urine collected from the urinary tract is a probable indicator of bacterial colonization of the urinary tract mucosa and is highly predictive of subsequent infection, although the absence of associated pyuria occasionally leads observers to question this concept. Unresolved or recurrent bacteriuria must be assumed to reflect a predisposition resulting from a local or systemic abnormality.

Bacteriuria may result in a wide variety of clinical presentations. Asymptomatic bacteriuria probably reflects restriction of bacteria to the mucosal surface of the bladder or bladder urine. Asymptomatic bacteriuria is associated most frequently with a foreign body such as a urethral catheter and usually remits spontaneously once the foreign body is removed.

At the other end of the spectrum, bacteria may penetrate the deeper layers of the bladder and cause low-grade fever, frequent and urgent urination, and painful micturition, known as *dysuria*. These are the expected clinical manifestations of cystitis. The urine contains bacteria and leukocytes, a condition termed pyuria. In a very small proportion of patients, the bacteria in the bladder may gain access to the upper urinary tract, invade the mucosa of the renal pelvis, extend into the interstitial tissue of one or both kidneys, and cause acute pyelonephritis. Patients with acute pyelonephritis usually are very ill, with shaking chills, temperature spikes to approximately 40°C (104°–105°F), paralytic ileus of a degree simulating an acute surgical abdomen, and excruciating pain in one or both flanks.

Acute pyelonephritis often follows interference with normal urine flow secondary to mechanical obstruction caused by a renal or ureteral stone, tumor, congenital abnormality, or an enlarged prostate gland. Altered urine flow also may result from neurophysiologic dysfunction with impaired ureteral contractions and imperfect emptying of the bladder (e.g., diabetic neuropathy). If the flow of urine through a ureter becomes totally obstructed, a grave emergency can arise, since the obstruction must be relieved within at least 36 h if function of the affected kidney is to be preserved.

The histopathologic changes of acute pyelonephritis are relatively well defined. There is an accumulation of inflammatory cells consisting predominantly of segmented neutrophils that encroach upon and invade the renal tubules, giving rise to "white blood cell casts." The inflammatory cells also infiltrate the interstitial tissue of the renal medulla and extend into the cortex. The glomeruli usually are not involved and often stand out conspicuously against a background of interstitial fibrosis, tubular dilatation, and degeneration. In most instances, bacteria are demonstrable in the urine or in cultures of affected renal tissue.

In chronic pyelonephritis, the identifying histopathologic changes are far less distinct and are thus difficult to define. There is a striking paucity of inflammatory cells. Obstructed and dilated tubules are often filled with hyaline material resembling colloid. Obstruction and loss of collecting ducts and inevitable fibrosis eventually result in an irregularly scarred and lobulated kidney of ever-decreasing size, which for decades was considered to be prototypic of end-stage chronic renal infection. One of the enigmas of chronic pyelonephritis is the frequent lack of any direct evidence of infection. The urine may contain neither formed elements nor bacteria and may be considered abnormal only because of persistent traces of proteinuria. Furthermore, bacteria almost invariably cannot be demonstrated in grossly abnormal areas of affected kidneys. Indeed, the absence of direct evidence supporting a role for bacteria in active chronic pyelonephritis has led several laboratories to search for noninfectious mechanisms that would account for relentless progression of the disease. Results of these studies are of considerable interest and are briefly summarized in a later section of this chapter.

From a large number of studies involving experimental animals and patients, it is clear that all the foregoing histopathologic changes, once accepted as characteristic of chronic pyelonephritis, may occur in other diseases of the kidney that do not have an infectious origin. Ischemia secondary to progressive nephrosclerosis, persistent obstruction of the urine outflow tract due to an intrarenal or extrarenal lesion, and analgesic nephropathy all may result in peritubular mononuclear cell infiltration, dilation of tubules, fibrosis, and microscopically or grossly evident scarring unaccompanied at any time by evidence of bacterial infection. The fact that a multiplicity of pathogenic mechanisms can cause renal injury indistinguishable from that of chronic pyelonephritis explains why the incidence of chronic renal infection, based on autopsy surveys, has been exaggerated over the years. This new perspective also means that chronic pyelonephritis is probably less important than formerly believed as a determinant of elevated blood pressure and such complications of pregnancy as prematurity and increased morbidity and mortality of newborns.

## PREVALENCE, INCIDENCE, AND ECONOMIC IMPACT OF GENITOURINARY TRACT INFECTIONS

The prevalence of urinary tract infections appears to be influenced by many factors, including the age, sex, and personal habits of the patient. Asymptomatic bacteriuria is 10 times more common in male neonates than in females (incidences of 1.5% and 0.137%, respectively). Thereafter, the incidence of bacteriuria among children between the ages of 4 and 18 years is 1–2%. Noteworthy is the female-to-male ratio of 30:1, indicative of the predisposition of females to urinary tract infections. Recurrent urinary tract infections in girls usually become less frequent with onset of puberty, suggesting that hormonally induced alterations in the mucosal lining of the urogenital tract may be important. The prevalence of bacteriuria increases progressively among adult females and especially married women, presumably reflecting urethral trauma associated with sexual activity and pregnancy. It has been estimated that about 25% of women experience a urinary tract infection by their 30th year. In contrast, urinary tract infections are rare in young men. Structural or functional abnormalities in the urinary tract are much more common in men than in women with recurrent bacteriuria. The approximately 10% prevalence of infection in elderly women and men is frequently associated with anatomic or physiologic changes in the urinary tract that cause urinary stasis and calculi. The incidence of urinary tract infection is even higher among hospitalized men and women, particularly those with serious illnesses. Urinary tract infections account for 30–40% of all nosocomial (i.e., hospital-acquired) infections. The majority of these episodes are associated with urinary catheterization (see Chapter 25).

The potential sequelae of bacteremia due to gram-negative microorganisms are more frequently preceded by bacteriuria than by any other infection (see Chapter 32). It has been estimated that at least 25% of the 70,000–150,000 documented bacteremic episodes each year prove to be fatal. Other potential sequelae of urinary tract infections include pyelonephritis, chronic renal disease, and stones that are formed in alkaline urine caused by urea-splitting bacteria. The estimated economic impact of urinary tract infection is great. The cost of treatment for a single urinary tract infection ranges from $100 to $175 for an outpatient. Patients who suffer a postoperative urinary tract infection spend several additional days in the hospital, and the hospital costs increase by over $1000 compared with those of closely matched controls. Clearly, urinary tract infections pose a major health problem in terms of the pro-

portion of the population affected and the sequelae and cost of bacteriuric episodes. Fortunately, there is evidence that early detection and eradication of bacteriuria and prevention of recurrence reduce the incidence of subsequent life-threatening consequences of urinary tract infection.

## MICROBE–HOST RELATIONSHIPS

### Reservoir of Infection

Most urinary tract infections are caused by microorganisms that originate from the fecal flora of the lower bowel (see Chapter 2). Nearly 80% of infections occurring in nonhospitalized patients in the absence of obstruction are caused by *Escherichia coli*. Other gram-negative bacteria (e.g., *Klebsiella pneumoniae* and *Proteus* species) as well as gram-positive cocci (e.g., *Enterococcus faecalis* and *Staphylococcus saprophyticus*) are also potential uropathogens. There is no convincing evidence that the numerically superior anaerobic bacteria in the intestinal microflora play a significant etiologic role in urinary tract infections.

When identification of specific strains of bacteria is possible, the same strain can be found in most instances simultaneously in the patient's urinary and intestinal tracts. It is also well established that relatively few strains account for most urinary tract infections. The basic question of whether the common strains that cause urinary tract infections are uropathogenic or whether they are simply the prevalent *E. coli* in the bowel at the time of a bacteriuric episode remains controversial.

Nosocomial urinary tract infections are caused by a wider spectrum of microorganisms, including *Pseudomonas aeruginosa*. Hospital-acquired strains are usually resistant to multiple antimicrobial drugs and probably possess virulence factors that facilitate their entry into the urinary tract and make the nosocomial urinary tract infection more difficult to treat.

Epidemiologic studies indicate that surprisingly rapid shifts occur in the intestinal microbial flora following hospitalization. Within 1–2 days, specific strains of *E. coli* demonstrable in the intestinal flora at the time of admission to the hospital begin to be replaced by increasing numbers of "hospital strains." Similar changes have been observed in the urethral meatal flora of hospitalized patients with indwelling urethral catheters. The urethral meatus appears to be an important reservoir of infection, since the density of bacteria at the urethral meatus is significantly greater in hospitalized patients who acquire catheter-associated bacteriuria than in those who remain abacteriuric.

Pathogens from extraintestinal reservoirs may also cause urinary tract infections. These include parasites (see Chapter 18) such as *Echinococcus*, primarily in the kidney; *Schistosoma haematobium* and *S. mansoni*, primarily in the bladder; protozoa such as *Trichomonas*, primarily in the urethra; yeast, usually occurring in debilitated patients treated with antibiotics (see Chapter 25); and *Mycobacterium tuberculosis*. Subcellular forms of bacteria such as protoplasts may play a role in the persistence of urinary tract infections, and their presence and importance are currently the focus of investigation.

## Routes of Infection

Bacteria do not enter the urinary tract by filtration. Experiments in dogs, for example, have shown that during intravenous infusion of bacteria, the urine remains sterile. Recognized routes of entry allowing bacteria to gain access to the urinary tract include the following: (1) ascending, as in the presumed entrance of fecal bacteria into the bladder via the female urethra or into the kidney via the ureter; (2) hematogenous, as in staphylococcal infection of the renal cortex; and (3) direct extension, as in cystitis associated with an enterovesical fistula.

### Ascending Infection

Most urinary tract infections are caused by bacteria from the fecal reservoir that colonize the perineum, the vaginal introitus (the area inside the labia minora at the entrance of the vaginal canal) in the female, and the urethra prior to the occurrence of bacteriuria. Sexual activity, poor toilet habits, and fecal incontinence are thought to promote retrograde spread of bacteria and contribute to the higher prevalence of infection seen in married women, among infants and children who are not toilet trained, and in elderly individuals with poor sphincter control. Both the proximity of the urethral and anal orifices and the short urethral conduit in women are believed to contribute to the strikingly higher susceptibility of women to urinary tract infection throughout most of their lives.

What scientific evidence is there to support the ascending infection theory? Stamey and his associates performed frequent cultures of the vaginal vestibule and urethra in women with recurrent bacteriuria and observed that colonization of the vaginal introitus by specific serotypes of *Escherichia coli* occurred prior to development of bacteriuria with identical serotypes. Vaginal carriage of the same strain frequently persisted between episodes of bacteriuria. These data not only show the importance of persistence of the pathogenic strain on the vaginal mucosa in the pathogenesis of recurrent urinary tract infection, but also illustrate that recurrent infections caused by the same serotype may be separate events due to reentrance of bacteria into the urinary tract rather than "relapse" from a persistent renal bacterial focus. Thus, most recurrent urinary tract infections in women are probably due to persistence *outside* the urinary tract rather than relapse from a persistent focus *within* the kidney.

If vaginal colonization with uropathogenic bacteria plays a role in the pathogenesis of urinary tract infection, the vaginal mucosal flora in healthy women should differ significantly from that of patients with recurrent bacteriuria. Stamey and associates and Winberg and associates have shown that uropathogenic microorganisms rarely colonize the vaginal mucosa of women and girls. In contrast, between episodes of bacteriuria, the vaginal mucosa of women who have recurrent urinary tract infections frequently shows large numbers of these bacteria. Additional studies suggest that urethral colonization is in turn determined by the vaginal bacteria, presumably in part because the two mucosal surfaces are both derived embryologically from the urogenital sinus and are lined by squamous epithelial cells under the same hormonal control. Thus, susceptibility of the vaginal and urethral mucosa to colonization by urinary pathogens from the fecal flora clearly represents a major biologic alteration instrumental in the pathogenesis of urinary tract infections in females. There is considerably less evidence of retrograde spread of bacteria into the male urinary tract. Epidemiologic studies have demonstrated frequent colonization with *Proteus mirabilis* and other uropathogenic microorganisms of the anterior urethra in young uncircumcised boys with recurrent symptomatic bacteriuria. However, colonization of the adult male urethral mucosa with uropathogenic bacteria is infrequent in the absence of an anatomic abnormality such as a urethral stricture or anal intercourse and rarely has been implicated as the source of recurrent bacteriuria. Most episodes of recurrent bacteriuria in men appear to be associated with bacterial prostatitis or urinary stasis caused by benign or malignant prostate growth, which impedes the natural bladder-emptying mechanism.

Very little is known about the specific events by which bacteria migrate into the bladder, colonize the mucosa, and establish infection. Normal voiding mechanisms have been shown to eliminate over 99% of experimental organisms inoculated intravesically. However, urinary obstruction severe enough to cause residual urine clearly represents a major impairment to the bladder defense mechanism and frequently is associated with bacteriuria. Adherence of bacteria to the uroepithelial mucosa (as discussed later) also appears to be an important step in the development of urinary tract infection. Adherence appears to involve a specific interaction that is influenced by bacterial and epithelial cell-surface characteristics. Endogenous surface mucopolysaccharides of the bladder wall, which in animal models appear to reduce bacterial adherence to the vesicle mucosa, and hormonal and cell-mediated immune responses are probably also important urinary tract defense mechanisms. Once the bladder mucosa is infected, microorganisms begin to multiply in bladder urine. Urine can support limited bacterial growth above pH 5.5. At that pH, the stage is set for extension of the infection to the upper tract, that is, the ureter, renal pelvis, and kidney. Bacteriologic localization techniques involving ureteral catheters have shown that renal pelvic bacteriuria of either or both kidneys occurs in approximately 50% of men and women who have bladder bacteriuria and essentially normal intravenous urograms. Evidence of pyelonephritis, such as fever, chills, or flank pain, and destruction of renal tissue occurs rarely in these patients. In sharp contrast, upper tract bacteriuria in the presence of functional or anatomic obstruction of the urinary tract is frequently associated with symptoms of pyelonephritis, renal functional impairment, renal cortical scarring, and life-threatening urosepsis.

### Hematogenous Infection

Bacteria as well as fungi and mycobacteria may invade the kidneys, bladder, or prostate gland by hematogenous spread from a distant focus of infection. In fact, fungal and mycobacterial infections of the urinary tract usually occur by this mechanism. Similarly, renal cortical and perirenal abscesses due to staphylococci or group A streptococci are usually secondary to bacteremia associated with extensive infection of other organ sites.

### Direct Extension

Direct extension of bacteria from the enteric flora into the bladder, as in a colovesical fistula associated with diverticulitis of the colon, is an infrequent but important cause of recurrent bacteriuria. The infections are usually recurrent, caused by several different species of enteric bacteria, and accompanied by pneumaturia (air within the urinary tract).

## HOST SUSCEPTIBILITY AND BACTERIAL VIRULENCE FACTORS

Clearly, contamination by fecal bacteria cannot be the sole determinant of urinary tract infections. As Chapters 3 and 4 emphasize, both host and bacterial factors must be instrumental in the pathogenesis of urinary tract infection. With regard to the host, both systemic and local factors may affect susceptibility to urinary tract infection. Any systemic abnormality decreasing host resistance (e.g., malnutrition, diabetes mellitus, or impairment of the immune system) may contribute significantly to the development and persistence of infection. Various studies discussed later also indicate that systemic changes in the adhesive characteristics of epithelial cells are associated with female susceptibility to urinary tract infections. The local factors usually considered of prime importance are urinary stasis and the presence of a calculus, essentially a foreign body. Urinary stasis may result from obstruction, such as with benign prostatic hypertrophy, external pressure, such as from a tumor, neuromuscular dysfunction, or a congenital or acquired abnormality, such as vesicoureteral reflux. It is essential to recognize that the presence of any foreign body such as an indwelling catheter or calculus can act as a nidus for microorganisms and make eradication of infection extremely difficult, if not impossible. Trauma is an additional local factor that experimentally permits development of infection and that has probable clinical significance in urinary tract infections developing after instrumentation and in the common occurrence of so-called honeymoon cystitis.

Certain species of microorganisms have a far greater capacity than others to initiate urinary tract infection, irrespective of how they gain access to this organ system. For example, *E. coli* represents a clear minority of the intestinal microflora, yet it is the most frequent and important urinary pathogen in humans, presumably because of virulence factors that enhance its propensity to cause infection.

## Bacterial Adherence

Numerous studies have demonstrated that bacteria may selectively adhere to mucosal surfaces and that the extent to which they adhere can influence the degree of colonization (see discussion in Chapter 2). Adhesion allows the microorganisms to resist being washed away by the fluids and secretions that bathe mucosal surfaces. There is now evidence to suggest that specificity is involved in the adherence process and that adhesion is an important virulence factor for a number of pathogenic bacteria.

The ability of bacteria to adhere to specific epithelial cell surfaces is probably influenced by the characteristics both of cell types and of the secretions bathing them. Most studies of gram-negative bacteria have focused on hair-like surface proteins (pili). The first to be characterized were found in late stationary-phase cultures, commonly numbered between 100 and 400 per bacillus, and were over 7.0 nm in diameter and 1.5 $\mu$m long (type 1). They conferred on the organism the ability to adhere to a wide variety of cells, including guinea pig erythrocytes and squamous epithelial cells. Agglutination and adhesion by type 1 pili were inhibited by the monosaccharide D-mannose. These and other studies suggested that binding of some bacterial strains could occur via pili that act like lectins and presumably bind to mannose-containing receptors on the epithelial cell surface. Other types of pili, such as the P pilus of pyelonephritogenic *E. coli*, specifically agglutinate human erythrocytes, and such hemagglutination cannot be inhibited by D-mannose. The receptor sites frequently are sugar residues of glycolipids or glycoproteins in the cell membrane that may be genetically determined.

Nonspecific bacterial adhesion factors have also been identified, and they include (1) short-range attractive forces that act to overcome the repulsive forces between the negatively charged epithelial cells and bacteria, and (2) hydrophobicity. Studies have shown that adherence of nonfimbriated gonococci can be increased to the level of fimbriated organisms by chemical modification of the surface charges of the nonfimbriated bacteria. It

has been suggested that fimbriae increase adherence by simply counteracting repulsive electrostatic forces. In other experiments, Smyth and associates found that *E. coli* strains possessing the K88 antigen were hydrophobic because they adsorbed to hydrophobic gels in interaction chromatography, whereas K88-negative strains did not adsorb to the gels.

### Bacterial Adherence in Urinary Tract Infections

The role of bacterial adherence in urinary tract infections has been studied by *in vitro* assays in which the number of bacteria adhering to vaginal and uroepithelial cells is determined directly by light microscopy or indirectly by radiometric labeling techniques. Several groups of investigators observed that *Escherichia coli* strains isolated from urine adhere significantly better to uroepithelial and vaginal cells from women and children with recurrent urinary tract infections than to similar cells from healthy women who have never had an infection. This increased adherence in patients persisted despite temporary remission of infection, a finding that is consistent with the clinical observation that urinary tract infections in women usually recur despite spontaneous or pharmacologically induced remissions. Day-to-day variation was observed in all individuals studied, but the degree of variation was significantly greater in patients than in healthy controls. Similar results were obtained when buccal epithelial cells obtained from the same women were tested. Thus, susceptibility to recurrent urinary tract infection is associated with a widespread alteration in the surface characteristics of mucosal epithelial cells. Vaginal fluid is the medium in which bacterial adhesin bind to epithelial cell receptors.

The concept that vaginal fluid might modulate adherence of bacteria to epithelial cells is supported by the observation that type 1 piliated *E. coli* bound to vaginal fluid and that binding was greater to fluid from women demonstrating vaginal colonization with *E. coli* *in vivo* than from noncolonized women. Furthermore, vaginal fluid from colonized women generally enhanced adherence of *E. coli* to epithelial cells, whereas fluid from uncolonized women did not alter adherence.

Scandinavian investigators have suggested that bacterial adhesive capacity is a factor both for selecting *E. coli* from the fecal flora that are capable of causing urinary tract infections and for determining the level of infection within the urinary tract. For example, strains of *E. coli* that cause pyelonephritis adhered better *in vitro* to uroepithelial cells from healthy women than did either strains causing cystitis or asymptomatic bacteriuria or fecal isolates from healthy individuals. The ability of the pyelonephritogenic *E. coli* strains to adhere to uroepithelial cells correlated with their ability to agglutinate human erythrocytes in the presence of mannose and their inability to agglutinate guinea pig erythrocytes. Thus, it was suspected that the uroepithelial cells and human erythrocytes had a common structural receptor site in their membrane. Subsequent studies showed that at least one of these receptors is a disaccharide that is a part of the antigenic determinants of the human P blood group system. Ninety-one percent of *E. coli* strains isolated from children with acute pyelonephritis had surface pili that reacted specifically with the P blood group–specific receptor (P pili). P-specific recognition was found in only 19% of the strains causing cystitis, 14% of the strains associated with asymptomatic bacteriuria, and 7% of fecal *E. coli* isolates from healthy controls. These studies suggest that P pili are markers of bacterial virulence in early episodes of acute pyelonephritis in children, but whether they contribute to pathogenicity in the kidney by promoting tissue invasion or by mediating adherence to vaginal cells remains to be established. Studies comparing the density of renal pelvis mucosa receptor with that of urethral or vaginal receptor density have not been reported. No similar studies have been reported in adults.

In contrast, other studies have failed to show an association between *E. coli* adherence to vaginal cells from normal women and clinical pathogenicity. Fecal strains that never caused infection in women with recurrent urinary tract infections adhered as well as strains isolated from urine. Over 90% of the fecal and urinary isolates adhered. Unfortunately, fecal isolates from healthy women were not tested. Controlled studies of the fecal isolates from healthy women and patients with urinary tract infections are needed to determine whether there is a relationship between adherence and pathogenicity. Various studies have shown a strong association between adherence and pathogenicity for vaginal isolates. *E. coli* strains that had the same O serotype as those later isolated from bladder urine adhered avidly to vaginal epithelial cells, whereas strains not associated with urinary tract infection adhered poorly or not at all. The possibility that bacteria exposed to the vaginal environment may undergo modulation that alters their ability to adhere to and multiply on the vaginal mucosa and subsequently invade the urinary tract warrants further investigation.

These data must be interpreted with consideration of the potential differences between *in vitro* assays and *in vivo* infections. Over 80% of the epithelial cells used in these assays are nonviable and may not be representative of the vaginal or uroepithelial cell lining that bacteria encounter in the patient. Furthermore, substances associated with the surfaces of transitional epithelial cells *in vivo* and Tamm-Horsfall mucoprotein, also called uromucoid, which is formed by and excreted from the ascending loop of Henle into the urine, may enhance or diminish adherence *in vivo*. *In vitro* growth conditions and duration of storage of bacteria can appreciably affect the number and type of bacterial adhesins as well as their ability to attach to epithelial cells. To avoid artifacts induced by laboratory culture techniques, investigators have assessed adherence of fresh bacteria from urine of patients with acute cystitis. The fresh isolates adhered to uroepithelial cells and expressed type 1 and/or P pili.

The bacterial population was frequently heterogeneous, in that both piliated and nonpiliated cells were seen. The ability of bacteria to express or not express (phase vary) pili and other factors *in vivo* may enhance their virulence. For example, pili aid binding to epithelial cells, but also enhance phagocytosis. Therefore, pili would be beneficial in the initial phases of infection, and later their absence would be useful to protect against host defense mechanisms.

## Bacterial K Antigens

Strains of *Escherichia coli* elaborate envelope or capsular acidic polysaccharide antigens called *K antigens*. Specific K antigens are associated with *E. coli* strains implicated in infections of many different tissues, including those of the urinary tract, particularly pyelonephritis. In several experimental studies of urinary tract infection in mice, it is quite clear that *E. coli* strains elaborating specific K antigens have a striking propensity to cause pyelonephritis, in contrast to other strains that elaborate either no K antigens or K antigens of other serotypes. These observations collectively suggest that certain K antigens endow strains of *E. coli* with enhanced pathogenic potential; that is, either they are themselves virulence factors or they serve as reliable markers for the presence of other determinants intimately associated with virulence of the specific bacterial strains.

Studies from several laboratories indicate that it is not merely the presence of certain K antigens but the quantity of K antigen synthesized by a given strain of *E. coli* that determines the degree of virulence of that strain. Production of K antigens appears to correlate with relative resistance of such microbial strains to the bactericidal activity of normal serum mediated by immunoglobulins in concert with complement.

### Host Immune Response

Gram-negative microorganisms undergo dissolution when coated with specific antibody and exposed to serum complement. This antibody-complement–dependent bacteriolytic effect, observed with most normal sera, is the result of activation of the complement cascade, with C8 and C9 producing breaks in the integrity of the bacterial cell wall and membrane that lead to loss of internal contents, swift shifts in oncotic pressure, and bacterial lysis. From experimental studies in animals, deposits of bacterial antigen are known to persist in the kidney for long periods. Among infiltrating cells participating in the inflammatory response to infection are plasma cells that produce antibody specifically reactive with the bacterial antigen. An antibody response against the infecting organism occurs within the first week in patients with urinary tract infections. IgG and IgA are both synthesized by the bladder. IgM is synthesized only by kidney tissue.

Bacteria infecting the kidney are often coated by IgG as they pass down the ureter and into the bladder urine. Immunity induced by vaccination has been shown to protect against experimental hematogenous pyelonephritis in laboratory animals. The successful vaccines were boiled or formalin-killed whole bacteria and common pili. A protective effect in humans has not been demonstrated. Furthermore, the severity of infection has been shown to be unrelated to the rise in serum antibody during infection, and reinfections occur despite high serum antibody levels. Conspicuously lacking in most studies of urinary tract infection is attention to the role of cell-mediated immune responses. Delayed hypersensitivity reactions reaching peak intensity at 24 or 48 h can be demonstrated in bladder mucosa in the same manner in which one ordinarily performs a skin test. A transient, sparse T-cell infiltration occurs in the bladder, whereas in the kidney, T cells (mainly helper T cells) are persistent and abundant. Thus, it seems likely that cell-mediated immune responses play a role in host defense.

### Unique Susceptibility of Renal Medullary Tissues

*E. coli* and other gram-negative enteric microorganisms have an extraordinary propensity for infecting renal peritubular and interstitial tissues. There is a very high solute concentration in the medulla, with values of sodium reaching 425 mmol/L and those of urea reaching 850 mmol/L. Tubular fluid osmolality ranges from less than 50 to more than 1300 mOsm/L (i.e., from approximately one sixth to four times the osmolality of plasma). Leukocytes show decreased migration and phagocytic activity in fluids of such hypo- or hypertonicity, and the high solute concentrations as well as the hypertonicity of the medullary environment lead to partial inactivation of complement. Furthermore, the production of ammonia specifically inactivates C4, a critical component in the classic complement pathway. These factors may explain why the otherwise potent antibody-complement bacteriolytic system appears relatively ineffective in the milieu of the renal medulla. Survival of gram-negative microorganisms in the form of protoplasts or spheroplasts (devoid of their rigid cell walls) has been demonstrated to occur in bladder urine with an osmolality of at least 100 mOsm/L. Presumably such defective bacteria would readily survive in the even more hypertonic milieu of the renal medulla. It has been postulated that bacteria injured by antimicrobial agents or by the host antibody-complement bacteriolytic system might survive as cell-wall–injured or cell-wall–deficient bacteria and account for the persistence and remittency of infection. However, most studies attempting to demonstrate a capacity of bacterial protoplasts to invade and infect host tissues in animals have been unsuccessful. Furthermore, most protoplasts, even though devoid of most of their cell-wall material, still possess critical antigenic constituents, including K antigens capable of binding specific antibody. Thus, the host should be able to react with and dispose of bacteria irrespective of whether they are in their conventional or a defective form.

## Alternative Mechanisms of Renal Injury

Progression of pyelonephritis in the absence of bacteria in the urine or in biopsy specimens has led to the notion that mechanisms other than infection may be implicated in the production of renal damage. Experimental studies in mice and rats have revealed that microorganisms elaborating large amounts of urease, namely, strains of *Proteus mirabilis* and occasional *Klebsiella* species, may leave residual large deposits of this enzyme following their elimination from host tissues. The deposited enzyme may continue to create a high concentration of ammonia and a very high pH, approaching 8.0–8.5 or even greater, in extracellular fluids. Indeed, the presence of urine that contains bacteria and has a pH of 6.5–7.0 usually indicates infection due to *P. mirabilis* or another urea-splitting microorganism. An alkaline extracellular environment is well known to lead to cellular injury. Continued action of bacterial ureases may in this way lead to ongoing renal injury in the absence of any viable bacteria.

Mention has already been made of deposits of bacterial antigen within the kidney of animals with experimentally induced pyelonephritis. Using indirect immunofluorescence methods, some (but not all) groups of investigators have also demonstrated variable amounts of the so-called common antigen elaborated by most of the members of the family Enterobacteriaceae in human kidney biopsies or autopsy sections. Among the inflammatory cells in infected renal tissue are immunologically competent cells that actively elaborate antibodies specifically reactive with the bacterial antigenic constituents in question. In this manner, the stage could be set for renal cell injury caused by *in situ* antigen–antibody interactions (with or without complement) contributing to the injurious process.

Certain strains of *E. coli* have been found to elaborate antigenic constituents that cross-react with antigens of renal medullary cells of certain experimental animal species. Immune responses of the host to such bacterial antigens might well be expected to result in autoimmune renal damage. As yet, specific antibodies directed against kidney cells have not been found in the sera or renal tissue of animals with experimental pyelonephritis.

Pyelonephritis of rats induced by *Enterococ-* *cus faecalis* has reportedly been transferred to normal syngeneic Fisher rats by means of parabiosis. In this work, the prospective donors were infected with *E. faecalis* by a method previously established that regularly induces acute and chronic pyelonephritis in a high proportion of rats. The animals were subsequently treated with an antimicrobial regimen known to eradicate *E. faecalis* from renal tissues. The infected and treated rats were then placed in parabiotic union (cross-circulation) with normal Fisher recipients. Kidneys of the recipient parabionts were examined histologically at varying times during the 16-week period of parabiosis. Between 40% and 50% of the recipient Fisher rats developed histopathologic changes of pyelonephritis, including interstitial infiltration of mononuclear inflammatory cells, tubular and papillary distortion and degeneration, and fibrosis leading to significant scarring. Since antibodies reactive with normal rat kidney could be demonstrated in the sera of neither the donor rats nor the recipient parabionts, it was assumed that a cell-mediated immune mechanism was responsible for the pyelonephritis that was transferred.

## DIAGNOSIS OF URINARY TRACT INFECTION

Patients with urinary tract infections can be asymptomatic but generally have symptoms related to the site and severity of the infection. Symptoms may include the following, alone or in combination: (1) chills, fever, flank pain, and often nausea and vomiting (usually associated with acute pyelonephritis); and (2) dysuria, frequency or urgency of urination, suprapubic pain, and hematuria (usually associated with cystitis). Patients with chronic urinary tract infection may experience the symptoms associated with acute urinary tract infection chronically or periodically or, alternatively, may be virtually asymptomatic until renal failure develops. Most patients with asymptomatic bacteriuria can recall having had urinary tract symptoms in the past, and many develop acute symptomatic infection. There is general agreement that asymptomatic bacteriuria associated with pregnancy or due to urease-producing organisms capable of forming urinary calculi should be treated. In other instances, therapy is optional and, in the presence of a foreign body such as a urethral catheter, ineffective.

Physical findings such as flank mass and tenderness are characteristic of acute pyelonephritis, and prostatic or epididymal tenderness, swelling, and induration suggest acute prostatitis or epididymitis, respectively. However, the signs of urinary tract infection are usually ill defined.

Analysis and culture of the urine are essential to diagnosing urinary tract infection. Procurement of a urine sample that satisfactorily reflects the status of the bladder urine rather than urethral, vaginal, or skin contaminants is a challenging problem. Urine may be obtained by voiding, catheterization, or suprapubic aspiration. A voided urine sample should be obtained after satisfactory cleansing of the genitalia with a cotton swab and water. An antiseptic should not be utilized by women because it may contaminate the urine and produce a false-negative culture. Uncircumcised men should retract the foreskin, cleanse the glans with an antiseptic, and then remove the antiseptic with water before collection of the urine. No such preparation is necessary for circumcised men. In males, the first few milliliters of voided urine (first glass or urethral specimen) and a late midstream specimen (second glass or bladder specimen) should be obtained routinely. When prostatitis is suspected, secretions expressed by digital massage of the prostate and a subsequent few milliliters of voided urine should be collected. In women and children, the first specimen is frequently contaminated by bacteria from the vaginal or preputial mucosa. Therefore, only a late midstream urine specimen should be obtained. Catheterization of the urinary bladder produces more accurate specimens, but occasionally this technique yields contaminated urine, and it may induce bacteriuria but rarely bacteremia and septic shock. Urine obtained by direct suprapubic percutaneous needle aspiration reflects the bacteriologic status of the urine most accurately, since contamination from urethral organisms is eliminated. This method is suited particularly to infants and other individuals who cannot void voluntarily and carries minimal risk when performed by a physician who is skilled in this technique.

Bacteriuria and pyuria, as determined by microscopic examination, are characteristic of infection. Unfortunately, these findings are nonspecific. "Clean" voided urine specimens frequently are contaminated by periurethral bacteria and white blood cells. Conversely, about 50,000 bacteria per milliliter of urine (uncentrifuged) produce one microorganism per high-power field microscopically. Thus, failure to identify bacteria by light microscopy never excludes a urinary tract infection. A *quantitative urine culture* is the definitive laboratory test for establishing the presence of bacteria in the urine and for diagnosing urinary tract infections. Since urine frequently can support bacterial growth and because the bladder is a reservoir usually emptying at 3- to 4-h intervals, urine from patients with urinary tract infection generally shows more than 100,000 colonies per milliliter. Increased fluid intake with resultant diuresis and frequent emptying of the bladder can easily reduce the number of microorganisms per milliliter to fewer than 10,000 and sometimes to 1000. The presence of antimicrobial agents in the urine or infection by fastidious microorganisms also may lower the colony count. Rarely, in patients with unilateral renal infection, complete obstruction of the ureter on the same side prevents bacteria and white blood cells from entering the bladder. Occasionally, a localized infection such as perinephric or renal abscess may be present despite a sterile urine culture.

False-positive urine cultures are not uncommon, particularly when voided urine specimens are obtained from women with heavy bacterial colonization of the vaginal mucosa. If a urine specimen that contains even a few contaminating bacteria is allowed to stand at room temperature prior to culture, bacterial multiplication soon produces high bacterial counts. For this reason, urine should be plated out on appropriate culture media within 1 h of collection or stored in a refrigerator at 4°C for no longer than 24 h before plating.

The vast majority of urinary tract infections are produced by a single microbial species. In the absence of a foreign body such as a urethral catheter, growth of two or three types of bacteria usually represents improper collection or handling of the specimen. If the clinical situation permits, a repeat urine culture should be obtained to confirm the growth of the same microorganisms before definitive antimicrobial therapy is initiated.

## EVALUATION OF PATIENTS WITH BACTERIURIA

Appropriate evaluation of all patients with bacteriuria includes a complete history, physical examination, urinalysis, and urine culture. After the first infection in males and after the second or third infection in females, assessment of renal function by determination of serum creatinine and a search for congenital or acquired abnormalities by excretory urography or renal ultrasonography and cystoscopy are usually indicated. Excretory urography is not indicated in the vast majority of females with single or uncomplicated re-infections. Excretory urograms or sonograms are warranted, however, in high-risk patients with pyelonephritis, gross hematuria, obstruction, calculi, neurogenic bladder dysfunction, or renal damage associated with analgesic abuse or diabetes mellitus. Urethral calibration and measurement of postvoid residual urine should be performed on all women with recurrent infections. Cystoscopy should be used selectively in patients with hematuria or recurrent urinary tract infections at close intervals.

All the aforementioned radiographic studies are performed to find a surgically correctable lesion. Excretory urography is the most useful study for demonstrating potential foci of bacterial persistence such as a calculus or diverticulum, causes of urinary stasis such as a ureteropelvic junction obstruction or ureterocele, and evidence of chronic pyelonephritis or tuberculosis. Ultrasonography is less specific but safer than excretory urography because intravenous contrast is not required. Renal tomograms should be obtained when recurrent infections are caused by urea-splitting microorganisms because the associated alkalinization of the urine can rapidly lead to formation of calculi, which are relatively radiolucent and easily missed on routine plain film radiographs. In children, voiding cystourethrography is a useful procedure for identifying those patients who, because of abnormalities such as urethral valves, have vesicoureteral reflux or bladder outlet obstruction or both. Most ureteral reflux secondary to urinary tract infection responds to eradication of infection; however, severe reflux requires surgical reimplantation of the ureters.

## LOCALIZATION OF INFECTION SITE

Bacteriuria only confirms the presence of bacteria in bladder urine. The renal urine may be sterile. To determine the site of infection more accurately, investigators have devised various techniques and laboratory studies.

### Ureteral Catheterization

This procedure is the "gold standard" for evaluating other techniques that may indicate renal involvement and is the only way to localize a unilateral renal infection accurately. In this procedure a cystoscope is introduced into the bladder, the bladder is washed with sterile irrigating solution, catheters are passed to each midureter, and urine is collected from both kidneys for culture and urinalysis. Comparison of the washed bladder and kidney specimens permits accurate determination of the site of infection.

### Bladder Washout

In this procedure, a multilumen catheter is introduced into the bladder, and a baseline urine culture is obtained. The bladder is then filled for 30–45 min with a saline solution containing an aminoglycoside antibiotic, the solution is then washed out with saline, and serial urine cultures are obtained at 10-min intervals. In most cases of infection confined to the bladder, the postwashout cultures are sterile. If bacteria are detected, and especially if their numbers increase in the serial postwashout cultures, they are most likely emanating from the kidneys.

### Detection of Antibody-Coated Bacteria in Urine

Detection of bacteria coated with specific immunoglobulins by indirect immunofluorescence is a noninvasive technique for differentiating renal from bladder infections that has not gained popularity. In most bacteriuric specimens, bacteria either are all fluorescent (antibody-coated) and thus presumably associated with pyelonephritis or are all nonfluorescent (non–antibody-coated). However, a number of specimens from patients with pyelonephritis yield equivocal results, and excretion of antibody-coated bacteria occurs in a high proportion of patients with prostatitis or hemorrhagic cystitis.

Other techniques, such as renal biopsy, determination of maximum renal concentrating ability, and serologic titers, all fail as adequate criteria for detecting chronic pyelonephritis.

## MANAGEMENT OF URINARY TRACT INFECTIONS

### Classification

The following classification is based mainly on therapeutic and, to some extent, etiologic alternatives to management of the patient with urinary tract infection. This classification facilitates identification of high-risk and surgically curable patients and provides a rational framework for treating patients with recurrent urinary tract infection. All urinary tract infections are divided into the following three categories:

1. Isolated infections
2. Unresolved bacteriuria
3. Recurrent bacteriuria
   a. Bacterial persistence
   b. Reinfections

### Isolated Infections

Isolated infections represent either an initial event or a sporadic infection not preceded by infection in the previous year.

Approximately 80% of isolated infections are caused by *Escherichia coli*, are highly sensitive to many antimicrobial agents, and are eradicated by several days of empiric, inexpensive oral therapy. If the patient is hospitalized or has recently received oral antimicrobial agents, the bacteria may be more resistant and require specific therapy based on antimicrobial sensitivity patterns.

### Unresolved Bacteriuria

Unresolved bacteriuria indicates failure to sterilize the urine despite antimicrobial therapy. Unless bacteriuria is resolved, a urinary tract infection cannot be considered cured, and an infection cannot be classified as recurrent. The most common cause of unresolved bacteriuria during treatment is the presence of organisms that were initially resistant or that became resistant to the antimicrobial agent selected to treat the infection. Approximately 10% of isolated infections are unresolved for this reason. During therapy, rapid reinfection with a new, resistant microorganism rarely occurs. Adjustment of therapy, based on antimicrobial sensitivity testing, usually eradicates the infection. Another cause of unresolved bacteriuria is failure to achieve an adequate concentration of an appropriate antimicrobial agent in the urine of a patient with renal failure, analgesic nephritis, or an excessive mass of bacteria (such as with a giant staghorn calculus). These patients remain bacteriuric despite taking an antimicrobial agent to which the microorganism is sensitive.

### Recurrent Bacteriuria

Once bacteriuria has been resolved for several days and the antimicrobial drug stopped, the type of recurrent bacteriuria can be determined. Bacterial persistence *within* the urinary tract (e.g., in a renal calculus or in bacterial prostatitis) leads to recurrent infections with the same species. Surgery is usually required to eradicate the site of bacterial persistence and to cure the recurrent infections. Reinfections are caused by reintroduction of different bacteria from a reservoir *outside* the urinary tract. Most recurrent infections in females are reinfections and require antimicrobial prophylaxis rather than surgery. Vesicointestinal and vesicovaginal fistulae are uncommon causes of reinfection.

### Acute Symptomatic Infection

Initial evaluation should determine whether a patient has an uncomplicated infection that can be treated as an outpatient or whether the infection is complicated and hospitalization is necessary. Patients who have lower urinary tract infections, who are voiding adequately, and who are afebrile are judged to have uncomplicated infections and can be treated as outpatients. Patients with high fever and chills who are suspected of having bacteremia, as well as those with symptoms (e.g., colicky flank pain) or signs (e.g., palpable urinary bladder) of urinary tract obstruction have complicated infections and should be admitted to the hospital. Prompt evaluation by excretory urography or ultrasonography is frequently required, and drainage of obstruction (e.g., by passage of a urethral or ureteral catheter or ureterolithotomy) is mandatory. In addition to urinary tract obstruction, other major categories of increased risk of serious renal damage or poor response to therapy of urinary tract infection are (1) severe vesicoureteral reflux in children; (2) spinal cord injuries and other causes of neurogenic bladder, (3) pregnancy, (4) diabetes, (5) analgesic abuse, (6) congenital anomalies that become secondarily infected, (7) urea-splitting organisms that cause struvite "infection" renal stones, and (8) renal failure. Inappropriate response to antimicrobial therapy should alert the managing physician to the possibility that one or more of these conditions is associated with an episode of bacteriuria and should lead to further diagnostic studies.

Eradication of bacteria from the urine by antimicrobial agents depends on the concentration of active antimicrobial drug in the urine. Most antimicrobial agents excreted by the kidneys are concentrated in the urine at levels 10–100 times greater than their peak serum levels. When selecting an antimicrobial agent, first consider whether an agent is capable of achieving urinary levels that exceed the minimum inhibitory concentration for the infecting bacterial strain by a great margin. In urinary tract infections, it seems to make little difference whether the mode of action of the agent is bacteriostatic or bactericidal as long as the microorganism is sensitive to the agent chosen.

Both an increase in antimicrobial-resistant strains of Enterobacteriaceae and a proliferation of *Candida albicans* in the fecal flora that accompanies even short-term, oral administration of tetracycline, ampicillin, sulfonamides, (trimethoprim-sulfamethoxazole), and cephalosporins are well documented. A wide range of microorganisms that are resistant to antimicrobial agents is also encountered in hospitalized patients. Antimicrobial drugs such as nitrofurantoin and the fluoroquinolones, which are less likely to produce resistant microorganisms in the fecal flora, are particularly useful for empiric therapy in patients with recent antimicrobial therapy or with an increased susceptibility to recurrent urinary tract infections.

For most patients with an uncomplicated symptomatic infection, 3-day therapy with an inexpensive oral antimicrobial drug is effective. Several studies have advocated single-dose therapy for uncomplicated infections. Patients with evidence of systemic infection frequently require hospitalization for high-dose parenteral therapy. This is to ensure the attainment of therapeutic serum levels, should coexisting bacteremia be present. Therapy is generally begun with trimethoprim-sulfamethoxazole or a cephalosporin unless the patient acquired the infection while receiving antimicrobial agents or has some other underlying risk factor, in which case gentamicin or a third-generation cephalosporin drug is usually given. Outpatient therapy with a fluoroquinolone such as norfloxacin or ciprofloxacin may be used for less ill adult patients or when the results of bacterial antimicrobial sensitivity testing are available. Therapy is usually continued for 7–10 days. There is no convincing evidence that extension of therapy is necessary or that it improves the cure rate.

## Asymptomatic Bacteriuria

Although controversy exists about whether all patients with asymptomatic bacteriuria should be treated with antimicrobial drugs, there is agreement that children, young adults, and pregnant women should be so treated. Patients with asymptomatic bacteriuria associated with indwelling catheters should generally *not* be treated with antimicrobial drugs unless they become symptomatic or the catheter is to be removed within 24 h. Although the incidence of catheter-associated bacteriuria is reduced for the first 2 or 3 days of catheterization, the incidence of infection is the same thereafter, and the infecting microorganisms are usually highly resistant to antimicrobial drugs. Any patient with bacteriuria due to a urea-splitting organism such as *Proteus mirabilis* should be treated to prevent formation of a struvite "infection stone."

## Perinephric Abscess

Perinephric abscess formation is an uncommon but particularly serious problem. A mortality rate of over 50% has been reported; moreover, one third of the cases were undiagnosed before autopsy. The distinction between perinephric abscess and acute pyelonephritis is often difficult to make. Thorley, Jones, and Sanford, however, identified several distinctive features that aid differentiation between these two entities. Most patients with perinephric abscess, initially admitted with the diagnosis of acute pyelonephritis, were symptomatic and febrile for longer than 5 days. However, it should be noted that some patients with perinephric abscess have no urinary tract symptoms and are admitted to the hospital with a diagnosis of fever of unknown origin. A flank mass and an abdominal mass were noted in 27% and 35% of the patients, respectively.

The initiating event almost always is the rupture of an abscess within the renal parenchyma into the perinephric space. About two thirds of renal abscesses are believed to arise by direct extension from pyelonephritis and about one third by hematogenous spread. The etiologic bacteria reflect the pathogenesis. Perinephric abscesses associated with ascending infection are usually caused by Enterobacteriaceae; an abscess secondary to bacteremic spread is usually produced by *Staphylococcus aureus*. Occasionally, urine cultures are sterile. Any patient with presumed acute pyelonephritis who fails to improve as expected should be evaluated by ultrasound. On rare occasions, a computed tomography (CT) scan may be required for diagnosis. The treatment of perinephric abscess is surgical drainage and antibiotics. Antimicrobial therapy alone is of little value and frequently results in death.

## Recurrent Urinary Tract Infection

Recurrent urinary tract infections in men are usually associated with urinary stasis or bacterial prostatitis. Acute exacerbations of bacterial prostatitis are easy to recognize. Early symptoms include malaise, myalgia, and fever, often as high as 104°F (40°C). On rectal examination, the prostate is usually tense and exquisitely tender. Prostatic massage should be avoided to prevent bacteremia. Patients often respond dramatically to appropriate antimicrobial therapy, such as with an aminoglycoside or norfloxacin. Prostatic abscess is a rare complication that should be suspected if the prostate is fluctuant on rectal examination. Transurethral or perineal surgical drainage should be performed. A more common and more subtle sequela is chronic bacterial prostatitis. Between episodes of recurrent bacteriuria, the patients are asymptomatic, and the prostate is usually unremarkable by either rectal or cystoscopic examination. Comparison of quantitative cultures of urethral, bladder, and expressed prostatic fluid specimens is essential for documenting bacteria in the prostatic specimens that could not be accounted for by the urethral flora. Treatment is hampered by the inability of most antimicrobial drugs to diffuse from the plasma into prostatic fluid. Three-month therapy with trimethoprim-sulfamethoxazole or carbenicillin is effective in approximately 40% of patients. One-month therapy with a fluoroquinolone is effective in over 60% of patients. Those patients not cured may have prostatic calculi that act as a nidus for infection. Radical transurethral resection of the prostate and removal of prostatic calculi may be curative.

Recurrent urinary tract infections in women are due to reinfections in well over 95% of patients. Nevertheless, bacterial persistence associated with a structural or functional abnormality within the urinary tract should always be considered, particularly when the recurrent episodes are at close intervals, are caused by the same species of bacteria, or occur in young girls or elderly women. If bacterial persistence is suspected, evaluation by excretory urography, cystourography, and cystoscopy is indicated. Identification of a bacterial focus of infection is important because surgical removal and cure of recurrent bacteriuria can be accomplished in most cases.

Reinfection can be prevented by nightly low-dose antimicrobial prophylaxis with agents such as nitrofurantoin or trimethoprim-sulfamethoxazole, usually continued for 6 months. In some patients, the infection rate can be reduced by postcoital antimicrobial prophylaxis. Antimicrobial prophylaxis does not correct the basic underlying biologic abnormality; infections usually recur when the drug is discontinued.

Suppressive therapy should not be confused with prophylaxis. Suppressive therapy is given in the presence of bacterial persistence within the urinary tract, whereas preventive therapy is given after the urinary tract infection and focus of bacterial persistence have been eradicated. Suppressive therapy should be used when a focus of bacterial persistence such as a large calculus or bacterial prostatitis cannot be eradicated.

## CASE HISTORIES

### Case History 1

A 58-year-old man presented with a 2-day history of malaise, dysuria, urgency, and suprapubic pressure. He had his first urinary tract infection (UTI) 12 years earlier with urinary frequency, dysuria, nocturia, and fever. Acute prostatitis was diagnosed, and he responded to a few days of sulfonamide therapy. He was well for 7 years and had another UTI that responded to a short course of sulfonamide. A third UTI occurred 1 year prior to admission, initially responding to sulfonamide, but recurring within 3 weeks of stopping the medication. Several other antimicrobial agents failed to cure the infection permanently. With each episode, symptoms were severe and quite similar to those of the first UTI. Previous urologic evaluation included excretory urography and cystoscopy demonstrating bilateral ureteral reflux with dilatation and 100 mL of residual urine.

On examination, the patient was acutely ill. His temperature was 99°F (37.2°C). The abdomen was soft, without a mass, and the bladder was not palpable. The genitalia were unremarkable. The prostate was slightly enlarged with minimal diffuse induration. Urinalysis revealed 10 white blood cells per high-power field and numerous bacilli. Urine culture was obtained and oral ampicillin, 250 mg four times per day, was started. Urine culture subsequently showed greater than 100,000 *Escherichia coli* colonies per milliliter. The patient became asymptomatic within 24 h. Ampicillin was continued for 30 days. Cultures of the first and second voided urine specimens yielded no bacterial growth. Cultures of both expressed prostatic secretions and postmassage urine revealed 4000 and 40 colonies of *E. coli* per milliliter, respectively. Both urine and prostate fluid *E. coli* isolates were sensitive to ampicillin (< 1 $\mu$g/mL). Six months after discontinuation of therapy, another episode of dysuria, urgency, and frequency occurred. *E. coli* was again cultured in the midstream urine specimen. Sensitivities of the *E. coli* strain were ampicillin at 1 $\mu$g/mL and norfloxacin at less than 1 $\mu$g/mL. Norfloxacin was started at one 400-mg tablet twice daily for 30 days. He promptly became asymptomatic. Cultures of the urine and prostatic fluid showed no growth during therapy and for up to 6 months following therapy.

## CASE 1 DISCUSSION

Case 1 illustrates the value of segmented culture techniques in the adult male for localizing urinary infections to the prostate. Although the infecting strain of *E. coli* was sensitive to ampicillin, this drug was unable to eradicate *E. coli* from the prostate gland. The quinolone norfloxacin, however, appears to possess favorable diffusion characteristics that achieved a cure of recurrent prostatitis in this patient for up to 6 months. The presence of residual urine and bilateral ureteral reflux, however, place this patient at high risk for subsequent episodes of urinary tract infection.

## CASE HISTORY 2

A 34-year-old woman was admitted with a history of recurrent left pyelonephritis characterized by fever, chills, nausea, and vomiting. She had her first UTI 12 years earlier, with one or two infections per year over the next 10 years. The patient had her first episode of pyelonephritis 1 year prior to admission. Intravenous excretory urography at that time demonstrated bilateral nephrocalcinosis. Metabolic evaluation for causes of stone disease was negative. Six months prior to admission, she had an *Escherichia coli* UTI treated with empiric antimicrobial therapy for 10 days. Follow-up cultures were not obtained. She remained asymptomatic until 3 days prior to admission, when she developed left flank pain, fever, chills, nausea, and vomiting. Examination showed an acutely ill woman with blood pressure 120/75 mm Hg; pulse 105/min; respirations 20/min; and temperature 104°F (40°C). The rest of the examination was normal except for left costovertebral angle tenderness on palpation. Laboratory studies showed a white blood count of 15,000/mm$^3$ with a predominance of segmented neutrophils. Hemoglobin and hematocrit were normal. Urinalysis demonstrated pH of 7.0 and 30–40 leukocytes per high-power field in the centrifuged sediment. Midstream urine specimen was sent for culture.

Gentamicin, 60 mg every 8 h by intravenous infusion, was begun. Admission urine culture results reported on the second hospital day revealed *Proteus mirabilis* (100,000 colonies per milliliter), sensitive to gentamicin. The patient became afebrile, and subsequent cultures showed no growth. Repeat intravenous urogram demonstrated a 1 × 2 cm left renal pelvic calculus. Plain film tomograms showed another small calculus in the left renal pelvis. The patient underwent left extracorporeal shock wave lithotripsy. Stone analysis showed 82% struvite and 18% carbonate-apatite. The patient was treated with prophylactic antimicrobial therapy for 6 months postoperatively. Twenty-four-hour urine collections revealed idiopathic hypercalciuria, and diuretic therapy was started. Two episodes of *E. coli* lower UTI have occurred in the 3 years since discontinuation of prophylactic antibiotics. Repeat intravenous urograms demonstrated extensive bilateral nephrocalcinosis without evidence of struvite infection stones.

## CASE 2 DISCUSSION

This case illustrates how subtle an early struvite infection stone can be. Clearly, the easiest way to make the diagnosis is to recognize that repeated cultures that show *P. mirabilis* must be associated with an infection stone. This case also illustrates the value of plain film tomography in demonstrating the relatively radiolucent struvite stone. Despite recurrent urinary tract infections and evidence of increasing nephrocalcinosis, careful follow-up therapy has prevented recurrent formation of infection stones.

## REFERENCES

**Book**

Stamey, T. A. *Urinary Infections.* Baltimore: Williams & Wilkins Co., 1980.

**Review Articles**

Smith, H. Microbial surfaces in relation to pathogenicity. *Bacteriol. Rev. 41*:475–500, 1977.
Svanborg-Eden, C., and deMan, P. Bacterial virulence in urinary tract infection. *Infect. Dis. Clin. North. Am. 1*: 731–750, 1987.

**Articles**

Abrutyn, E., Mossey, J, Berlin, J. A., et al. Does asymptomatic bacteriuria predict mortality and does antimicrobial treatment reduce mortality in elderly ambulatory women? *Ann. Intern. Med. 120*:827–33, 1994.
Acar, J. F., and Francousal, S. The clinical problems of bacterial resistance to the new quinolones. *J. Antimicrob. Chemother. 26*(Suppl. B):207–213, 1990.
Carroll, K. C., Hale, D. C., vonBoerum, D. H., et al. Lab-

oratory evaluation of urinary tract infections in an ambulatory clinic. *Am. J. Clin. Pathol. 101*:100–103, 1994.

Hooton, T. M., and Stamm, W. E. Management of acute uncomplicated urinary tract infections in adults. *Med. Clin. North Am. 75*:339–375, 1991.

Johnson, J. R., Lyons, M. F., Pearce, W., et al. Therapy for women hospitalized with acute pyelonephritis: A randomized trial of ampicillin versus trimethoprim-sulfamethoxazole for 14 days. *J. Infect. Dis. 163*:325, 1991.

Johnson, J. R., and Stamm, W. E. Diagnosis and treatment of acute urinary tract infections. *Infect. Dis. Clin. North Am. 1* (4):773–791, 1987.

Komaroff, A. L. Urinalysis and urine culture in women with dysuria. *Ann. Intern. Med. 104*:212–218, 1986.

Leibovico, L., Greenshtain, S., Cohen, O., et al. Toward improved empiric management of moderate to severe urinary tract infections. *Arch. Intern. Med. 152*:2481–2486, 1992.

Mattsby-Baltzer, I., Hanson, L. A., Kaijser, B., et al. Experimental *Escherichia coli* ascending pyelonephritis in rats: Changes in bacterial properties and the immune response to surface antigens. *Infect. Immunol. 35*:634–646, 1982.

Norrby, S. R. Short-term treatment of uncomplicated lower urinary tract infections in women. *Rev. Infect. Dis. 12*:458–467, 1990.

Raz, R., and Stamm, W. E. A controlled trial in intravaginal estriol in postmenopausal women with recurrent urinary tract infection. *N. Engl. J. Med. 329*:753–756, 1993.

Ronald, A. R., Nicolle, L. E., and Harding, G. K. Standards of therapy for urinary tract infections in adults. *Infection 20*(Suppl. 3):S164-S170, 1992.

Schaeffer, J. K., Jones, J. M., and Dunn, J. K. Association of in vitro *E. coli* adherence to vaginal and buccal epithelial cells with susceptibility of women to recurrent urinary tract infections, *N. Engl. J. Med. 304*:1062–1066, 1981.

Sheinfeld, J., Schaeffer, A. J., Cordon-Cardo, C., et al. Association of the Lewis blood-group phenotype with recurrent urinary tract infections in women. *N. Engl. J. Med. 320*:773, 1989.

Stamm, W. E. Catheter-associated urinary tract infections: Epidemiology, pathogenesis, and prevention. *Am. J. Med. 91*(Suppl 3B):3B-65S–3B-71S, 1991.

Stamm, W. E., Wagner, K. F., Amsel, R, et al. Causes of the acute urethral syndrome in women. *N. Engl. J. Med. 303*:409–415, 1980.

Svanborg-Eden, C., Freter, R., Hagberg, L., et al. Inhibition of experimental ascending urinary tract infection by an epithelial cell-surface receptor analogue. *Nature 298*:560–562, 1982.

Vaisanen-Rhen, V., Elo, J., Vaisanen, E., et al. P-fimbriated clones among uropathogenic *Escherichia coli* strains. *Infect. Immunol. 43*:149–155, 1984.

Venegas, M. F., Navas, E. L., Gaffney, R. A., et al. Binding of type 1 piliated *Escherichia coli* to vaginal mucous from women. *Infect. Immunol. 63*(2):416, 1995.

Winberg, J., Bollgren, I., Kallenius, G., et al. Clinical pyelonephritis and focal renal scarring. A selected review of pathogenesis, prevention and prognosis. *Pediatr. Clin. North Am. 29*:801–814, 1982.

# 16

# SEXUALLY TRANSMITTED DISEASES

FRANK J. PALELLA, Jr., M.D. and ROBERT L. MURPHY, M.D.

During the past few decades, the clinical specialty of sexually transmitted diseases has evolved from a narrow field of inquiry including the "classic venereal diseases" of gonnorrhea, syphilis, chancroid, lymphogranuloma venereum, and granuloma inguinale to a much broader group of illnesses. This definition of sexually transmitted diseases encompasses virtually all pathogens that may be transmitted through human-to-human contact during intimate sexual activity, including those illnesses produced by bacteria, fungi, ectoparasites, protozoans, and viruses.

Historical references (even dating to antiquity) testify to the presence and clinical recognition of diseases that were sexually transmitted. However, the emergence of the study and treatment of these illnesses as a distinct medical specialty has been hastened by multiple social forces acting in response to the diverse and prevalent comorbid conditions and sequelae of the various sexually acquired infections. Millions of individuals are diagnosed while experiencing the acute symptoms associated with a sexually transmitted disease (STD), while many others develop later complications such as infertility, pelvic inflammatory disease, ectopic pregnancy, cancer, acquired immunodeficiency syndrome (AIDS), congenital infections, or death.

Patients with STDs may differ from other patients with communicable diseases in several important ways. First, many of them are asymptomatic, often for very long periods of time (as with syphilis or human immunodeficiency virus [HIV]). Such individuals may be undiagnosed but continue to transmit the infecting agent. In addition, multiple infections may occur simultaneously, and issues surrounding reluctance by patients to disclose intimate information about their sexual practices comprise a delicate challenge to the health care provider to appear objective, compassionate, and nonjudgmental. Dealing effectively with such issues is vital to allow for appropriate history-taking, evaluation, and treatment.

The emergence of HIV and AIDS has augmented the importance of the above factors and created new concerns (see Chapter 23). The potential consequences of sexual behavior are now more dire than ever, causing us to scrutinize sexual activity with the knowledge that it could have lethal consequences. Likewise, HIV impacts adversely on the natural history of other STDs (most notably syphilis and the herpesviruses), making them more difficult to diagnose and to treat. These realities resonate in ways that compel clinicians, educators, and public health authorities to reevaluate priorities and plans of action.

Notable trends in STDs in the past decade include the following:

1. Increasing incidence of genital ulcer disease. Herpes simplex continues to be the leading cause of genital ulcers in the United States. Increasing rates of syphilis and chancroid were noted in the mid-1980s and had an apparent association with the use of intravenous (IV) drugs and coexistent HIV-1 infection. Since 1990 the reported rates of both of these infections has declined in the United States but remain disproportionately high among African-Americans.

2. Continuing increase in the prevalence of antibiotic resistance among gonococcal isolates. Both plasmid and chromosomally mediated resistance have been noted.

3. *Chlamydia trachomatis* continues to be the the most common STD in the United States. Recent advances in diagnostic strategies (e.g., antigen and culture assays) have made this infection somewhat easier to confirm, yet it remains an underrecognized pathogen.

4. The clinical recognition of human papillomavirus and its pathogenic role in cervical carcinoma as well as genital squamous cell carcinoma has become clear.

5. The demographics of HIV in the United States are evolving to resemble more closely transmission patterns of the rest of the world (i.e., increasing heterosexual transmission). However, recrudescence of unsafe sexual practices among very young gay men has her-

alded what may become a "second wave" of HIV infection in this group.

6. Women and infants disproportionately suffer the long-term consequences of STDs. Increasing sexual activity among adolescent females in particular has led to greater likelihood of STD acquisition with adverse reproductive sequelae in this group.

## ULCERATIVE GENITAL DISEASES

### Syphilis

Syphilis is a human infectious disease caused by the spirochete *Treponema pallidum* (Fig. 16–1). It has been described as a distinct clinical entity since the early 1500s. Syphilis has been one of the most well-studied diseases of modern medicine, in large part because of its protean clinical manifestations, its prolonged and variable course, and its transmissibility. The successful early treatment of syphilis, achieved in the antibiotic era, has made later manifestations comparatively rare. Although nonvenereal transmission may occur, most cases of syphilis are spread by sexual contact. *T. pallidum* is indistinguishable by morphologic or laboratory methods from the treponemes that cause yaws (*T. pallidum* subsp. *pertenue*) and pinta (*T. carateum*). Other members of the genus *Treponema* are widely distributed in the environment and are not known to cause disease in humans. *T. pallidum* cannot be grown *in vitro*, a fact that has always severely limited the study of this organism and associated clinical syndromes. The organism can be cultivated in rabbit testes, and rabbits

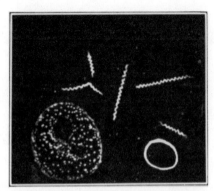

**FIGURE 16–1.** *Treponema pallidum.* Diagrammatic sketch of the appearance of this spirochete under darkfield illumination, drawn to scale in comparison with a red corpuscle and a leukocyte. (From Joklik, W. K., and Smith, D. T., eds. *Zinsser Microbiology.* 15th ed. New York: Appleton-Century-Crofts, Publishing Division of Prentice-Hall, Inc., 1972. With permission.)

can develop secondary but not tertiary lesions. All information concerning tertiary syphilis is derived from human data.

### Epidemiology

Approximately one third of those who have sexual intercourse with an infected person become infected. The incubation period ranges from 3 days to 3 months, averaging 3 weeks, and is probably related to the inoculum size. The natural history of untreated syphilis was studied in two large clinical trials, the Oslo study of 1890–1910 and the Tuskegee study of 1932–1972; more recently the latter has been criticized as racist and unethical. In that study, 412 black men with a history of untreated but inactive syphilis at the time of enrollment were followed until 1972. During that time they were not offered potentially curative therapy with penicillin and in fact actually were discouraged from such therapy. One of the original goals of the study was to examine whether syphilis had a course in blacks different from that in whites. This objective was achieved, and the additional information only confirmed the findings of the Oslo study.

Following World War II, the incidence of syphilis in the United States had generally declined until the late 1970s. After a brief period of increasing rates, the incidence again began to decline after 1982, primarily because urban homosexuals and bisexuals, fearing AIDS, adopted significantly less risky sexual practices. This contrasts to progressively increasing rates of primary and secondary syphilis among urban heterosexuals throughout the latter half of the 1980s (Fig. 16–2). Much of the increase was associated with the use of illicit drugs (especially crack cocaine) and the exchange of sexual services for drugs, particularly among ethnic/racial minorities. Concomitant increased rates of congenital syphilis were also observed. Although rates of primary and secondary syphilis have decreased among all ethnic/racial groups since 1990, there continues to be a wide discrepancy among African-Americans, Hispanics, and non-Hispanic whites. 86% of all reported cases of primary and secondary syphilis in 1993 occurred among African-Americans, with a greater than 60-fold higher rate than in non-Hispanic whites. Similar differences were seen in the rates of congenital syphilis.

### Clinical Manifestations

Syphilis has three classic stages of illness.

**Primary Syphilis.** *Primary syphilis* is the term applied to the disease during the first 2–4 weeks following infection and is best characterized by a firm, usually nontender, cutaneous ulcer with a well-defined margin and indurated base at the site of inoculation of the spirochete. The classic ulcer is referred to as

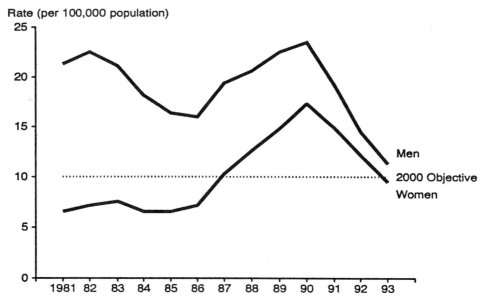

**FIGURE 16–2.** Primary and secondary syphilis—rates by gender, 1981–93 and the year 2000 objective. (From Centers for Disease Control. *Sexually Transmitted Disease Surveillance 1993*, December 1994. With permission.)

a *chancre.* Nontender regional lymphadenopathy is common and may be unilateral or bilateral. Because atypical ulcers have become more common, any ulcerative genital, oral, or anal lesion in sexually active patients should be suspected to be primary syphilis and evaluated appropriately. Untreated chancres persist 10–14 days before healing spontaneously without leaving a scar.

**Secondary Syphilis.**    The *secondary stage of syphilis* results from wide dissemination of the spirochete and is characterized by a variety of mucocutaneous eruptions. This stage occurs most typically 3–6 weeks following inoculation and may develop while the chancre is still present, though its characteristic clinical signs may be noted up to a year following initial infection.

The most common manifestation of this phase is the skin rash, occurring in 75–100% of patients (Fig. 16–3). The rash is characterized as erythematous and papular and may spread to involve the entire body including the palms and soles. Rashes may be atypical and resemble folliculitis, annular lesions, or viral warts (condylomata lata). If lesions are moist, vesicular, or ulcerated, spirochetes can be demonstrated by darkfield microscopy. Other manifestations of secondary syphilis include sore throat, fevers, hepatitis, diffuse lymphadenopathy, mucosal ulcerations, malaise, patchy alopecia, and thinning of the lateral one third of the eye brows.

LATENT SYPHILIS. *Latent syphilis* is defined as that occurring in those patients with a positive serologic test for syphilis but without signs or

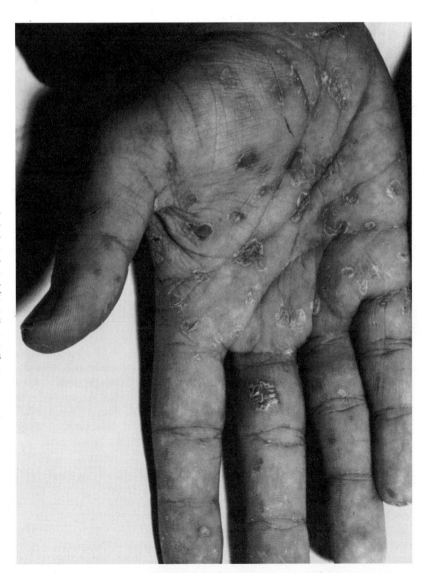

**FIGURE 16–3.** Secondary syphilis. For the past 6 weeks this 22-year-old student has had a scaling papular eruption of the palms and soles, an annular scaling plaque of the scrotum, and a mucous patch on the hard palate. Darkfield examination of the palmar lesions was negative. VDRL serologic test for syphilis was reactive. (From Shelley, W. B. *Consultations in Dermatology II.* Philadelphia. W. B. Saunders Co., 1974. Photo by Edward F. Gilfort.)

symptoms of the disease. Latent syphilis is further defined as *early latent* if infection is thought to have been present for less than 1 year, and *late latent* if present for more than 1 year. *Early latency* is considered potentially infectious, with approximately 25% of patients eventually developing signs of secondary syphilis, usually within the first year. Mothers giving birth during this time may deliver infants with congenital syphilis. *Late latent* syphilis is characterized by the development of immunity to relapse and acquired resistance to reinfection and a corresponding decrease in the likelihood of congenital syphilis. Because of the difficulty in differentiating late latent from asymptomatic neurosyphilis, examination of the cerebrospinal fluid (CFS) is essential to ensure that adequate therapy is prescribed.

**Tertiary Syphilis.** *Tertiary syphilis* is usually not apparent clinically until many years after the spontaneous clearing of the secondary stage. The typical lesions of tertiary syphilis are called *gummas*. They are granulomatous, often ulcerative lesions that may affect skin, soft tissue, or bones anywhere and, if left untreated, can permanently destroy the affected tissue. Some of the most dramatic examples occur in the cardiovascular, central nervous, or musculoskeletal systems.

The delayed onset of tertiary syphilis and its histology raise the possibility that tertiary lesions may be a manifestation of autoimmune disease.

CARDIOVASCULAR SYPHILIS. Cardiovascular manifestations occur in up to 80% of untreated patients, although clinically apparent disease is seen in only 10% after a latent period of 10–30 or more years. The three major clinical cardiac conditions attributable to syphilis include thoracic aortic aneurysm, aortic valve incompetence, and coronary ostial stenosis.

*Aortic Aneurysm.* This is the most common clinically apparent cardiac manifestation of tertiary syphilis. More than 60% of syphilitic aneurysms involve the ascending arch and 25% the transverse arch. Dissection does not occur. In general, patients are asymptomatic until the aneurysm has encroached on surrounding structures or has ruptured. Large numbers of spirochetes are demonstrable in the affected region at autopsy. Often, the earliest finding is an abnormal chest radiograph demonstrating a mediastinal mass with a typical but nonspecific eggshell calcification out-

lining the aneurysm. Surgical intervention may be required.

*Aortic Valve Incompetence.* Aortic regurgitation occurs in 30% of patients with tertiary syphilis and appears to be the result of aortic root dilation with stretching of the aortic valve, resulting in aortic valve incompetence. Patients are typically over 50 years of age and do not have other valvular conditions such as aortic stenosis. Aortic insufficiency is managed similarly to valvular disorders of other causes.

*Coronary Ostial Stenosis.* The proximal portions of the coronary arteries may also be involved by an obliterative endarteritis. Symptoms are the same as for other causes of ischemic coronary artery disease. Typically, only proximal involvement is seen. Surgical management may be more difficult when the aorta is also involved because cross-clamping of severely calcified sections may be riskier and grafting of the vascular graft into the aorta more difficult.

NEUROSYPHILIS. Clinically apparent central nervous system syphilis (CNS) occurs in 3–7% of untreated patients. It has become clear, however, that subclinical CNS involvement is quite common even in the earlier stages of the disease. Spirochetes have been recovered from 15–40% of CSF specimens in early syphilis. Abnormal CSF findings are noted in 13% of patients with untreated primary and in 25–50% with untreated secondary syphilis. Neurosyphilis is a chronic central nervous system infection capable of producing vascular and parenchymal lesions. The most common forms of neurosyphilis are asymptomatic and tabes dorsalis; paresis and vascular neurosyphilis are less common (Table 16–1).

*Asymptomatic Neurosyphilis.* Asymptomatic neurosyphilis is characterized by the absence of neurologic symptoms and the presence of CSF abnormalities. It can be categorized into early (<5 years) or late (>5 years). Asymptomatic neurosyphilis peaks at 12–18 months after initial infection and decreases with time. Progression to clinical neurosyphilis has been observed in 23–87% of untreated patients.

Serologic tests for syphilis are almost always positive in asymptomatic neurosyphilis. The CSF is characterized by modest (<100 cells/mm$^3$) lymphocytosis, normal or slightly elevated protein, and positive nontreponemal test.

*Meningeal and Cerebrovascular Syphilis.* Meningeal syphilis is quite rare and may mimic aseptic meningitis. The incubation pe-

## TABLE 16–1. SELECTED CLINICAL MANIFESTATIONS OF NEUROSYPHILIS*

Meningovascular
  Hemiparesis
  Hemiplegia
  Aphasia
  Seizures
Parenchymatous
General paresis
  Personality changes, cognitive dysfunction,
    alterations in affect and sensorium
  Hyperreflexia
  Pupillary dysfunction (Argyll Robertson)
  Speech dysfunction (difficulty in phonation,
    slurring)
  Tremors caused by optic atrophy (face, extremities)
Tabes dorsalis
  Ataxia
  Bowel/bladder disturbances
  "Lightning" pains
  Impotence
  Romberg's sign
  Cranial nerve (II–VII) dysfunction
  Peripheral neuropathy

*Modified from Mandell, G. L., Bennett, J. E., and Dolin, R., *Principles and Practice of Infectious Diseases*. New York: Churchill Livingstone, 1995. With permission.

riod is usually less than 1 year and patients are generally younger. Headache, fever, and stiff neck with lymphocytic pleocytosis are typical. Cranial nerve abnormalities or even hydrocephalus are not uncommon. The CSF nontreponemal tests are usually positive. Treatment with penicillin results in a prompt clinical response.

Cerebrovascular syphilis may involve the meninges or result in infarction secondary to syphilitic endarteritis. Most cases occur in the younger adult population, 5–12 years after the initial infection. Common clinical manifestations include hemiparesis or hemiplegia, psychologic or behavioral changes, aphasia, and seizures. The diagnosis should be suspected in a young adult with a stroke syndrome without obvious risk factors, with a positive syphilis serologic test and abnormal CSF exam.

*Paresis* refers to meningoencephalitis related to direct invasion of the cerebrum by *T. pallidum*. This occurs progressively over many years, and the clinical presentation may be insidious or acute. Chronic, progressive combined psychiatric and neurologic deterioration is typical. The most common focal neurologic findings are pupillary abnormalities such as the Argyll Robertson pupil, slurred speech, expressionless face, tremors, and deep-tendon reflex dysfunction. Serum nontreponemal serology is usually positive. In the instances where it may be negative, there is often a history of treated syphilis. CSF abnormalities are found in nearly all instances. The CSF nontreponemal tests are very specific for neurosyphilis but are only 30–70% sensitive. In contrast, the CSF fluorescent treponemal antibody (FTA) test may be more sensitive, but false-positive reactions occur in 0.5–4.5% of cases, possibly because of "contamination" of CSF with peripheral blood.

*Tabes Dorsalis.* Tabes dorsalis had accounted for about one third of all cases of neurosyphilis in the prepenicillin era but now is quite rare in the United States. It usually occurs after a latency period of at least 20–25 years. This diagnosis should be suspected in a patient with "lightning pains" in the lower extremities, ataxia, absent deep-tendon reflexes, paresthesias or hyperesthesias, Argyll Robertson pupil, a positive Romberg's sign, and bladder dysfunction. CSF abnormalities are common, but blood and CSF serologies may revert to normal in treated and inactive cases with continuing symptoms.

CONGENITAL SYPHILIS. Congenital syphilis was described in early medical writings as the "the French disease." The risks of developing congenital syphilis were well described in the Oslo study, which documented that 26% of babies born to infected mothers were disease-free or recovered spontaneously, 25% remained seropositive but well, and 49% were symptomatic. Typical symptoms include hepatomegaly, splenomegaly, anemia, jaundice, rash, petechiae, "snuffles," abnormal long bone radiographs, lymphadenopathy, and pseudoparalysis.

The diagnosis of congenital syphilis can be categorized as definite, compatible, or unlikely. A definite diagnosis requires confirmation of *T. pallidum* by darkfield examination, immunofluorescence, or histologic examination. A compatible diagnosis can be made by serologic testing, although sensitivity and specificity issues exist because of passive transplacental transfer of maternal antibody to the baby. Serial observation of the child's clinical condition, serologic and CSF status, and bone findings are often the most effective ways to identify congenital syphilis.

The mother of a baby with congenital syphilis is likely to have a history of other STDs. A leading risk factor, however, is lack of prenatal care, which is associated with being single, young, poor, from a rural area, and with a lack of formal education. Congenital syphilis cases in U.S. children less than 1 year of age dropped below 200 in 1980 but had risen to over 600 by 1989. Since 1990, the rate of congenital syphilis has declined annually in the United States. Between 1992 and 1993 the overall rate dropped from 94.7 to 79.0 cases per 100,000 live births, yet increases were seen in nine states.

## Syphilis and Human Immunodeficiency Virus Infection

When co-infection with syphilis and HIV exists, several issues make the management more complex.

First, it is clear from several large African and North American studies that the presence of genital ulcers caused by syphilis (or by any STD) enhances the likelihood of transmission or acquisition of HIV and other STDs. Intravenous drug use, prostitute contact, history of other genital ulcer disease, and lack of circumcision are all independent risk factors for the acquisition of HIV. The mechanism for the relation between HIV infection and prior genital ulcer disease is unknown. Disruption of epithelial or mucosal surfaces may provide a more efficient portal of entry, and the base of syphilitic ulcerations likely contains large numbers of activated lymphocytes and macrophages, the potential target for HIV. The Centers for Disease Control (CDC) has recommended HIV testing in all patients with newly diagnosed syphilis.

The clinical course of syphilis appears accelerated in HIV–co-infected persons, and the manifestations of syphilis may be atypical. Earlier and more frequent neurologic involvement is strongly suggested. Earlier forms of CNS involvement—that is, acute syphilitic meningitis or meningovascular syphilis (as opposed to tabes dorsalis)—seem to predominate. Because of these concerns, CSF needs to be evaluated in any HIV-infected person with serologic or clinical evidence of syphilis.

The CDC recommends that penicillin regimens be used for the treatment of all stages of syphilis in the HIV-infected patient, especially among those with neurosyphilis, syphilis in pregnancy, or congenital syphilis, as no proven therapeutic alternatives exist. There are reports of higher syphilis treatment failure rates in HIV-infected patients treated with benzathine penicillin. Although *T. pallidum* is highly sensitive to penicillin, the CSF levels achieved after intramuscular benzathine penicillin do not reach spirocheticidal levels. In general, because of concerns about neuro-

logic relapse and/or persistence of treponemes in the CSF, many experts advise that all HIV-infected persons with serologic evidence of syphilis and CSF abnormalities should be treated with high-dose intravenous penicillin for 10–14 days. The CDC has recommended serologic follow-up at 1–2 weeks after completion of treatment and at months 1, 2, 3, 6, 9, and 12.

### Treatment

The treatment of syphilis varies according to the stage of disease and allergic history of the patient. Table 16–2 outlines the current CDC recommendations.

### Diagnosis

**Microscopy.** Since *T. pallidum* is very difficult to culture *in vitro*, the diagnosis of syphilis in the primary stage is based on demonstrating motile treponemes from the chancre. Treponemes can usually be found in a chancre of any stage, but they are very sensitive to penicillin and cannot be found within 4 h after the drug is given. Demonstration of treponemes by darkfield examination is important in the initial stage of the disease, because diagnostic serologic changes usually do not begin to appear until 14–21 days after contact. Darkfield examinations are easily done. The surface of the chancre is cleaned with a saline-moistened swab to clear away exudate and bacterial contamination. Another swab is then applied to the chancre to cause an outpouring of serous fluid containing treponemes. Serous fluid is then removed from the surface of the chancre by a small pipette or cover slip and placed on a microscope slide, protected by the coverslip, and examined with darkfield illumination within 10–15 min. *T. pallidum* exhibits rapid and purposeful corkscrew-like motion across the microscopic field. Treponemes are susceptible to a decrease in temperature and soon stop moving; their characteristic shape is not apparent when they are motionless. Motile treponemes can also be found in smaller numbers in both skin lesions and enlarged lymph nodes of patients with secondary syphilis. Both primary and secondary lesions are contagious. Nonpathogenic treponemes are commonly isolated from the oral cavity and resemble *T. pallidum* morphologically.

**Serology.** Unfortunately, the cutaneous manifestations of primary and secondary syphilis may be inconsistent, and the first symptom of the disease may be appearance of

## TABLE 16–2.  SYPHILIS—TREATMENT GUIDELINES*

**EARLY SYPHILIS**
Primary and Secondary Syphilis and Early Latent Syphilis of Less Than 1 Year's Duration
*Recommended Regimen*

**Benzathine penicillin G,** 2.4 million units IM, in one dose.

*Alternative Regimen for Penicillin-Allergic Patients (Nonpregnant)*
  **Doxycycline,** 100 mg orally two times a day for 2 weeks; **or**
  **Tetracycline,** 500 mg orally four times a day for 2 weeks.
  **Doxycycline** and **tetracycline** are equivalent therapies. There is less clinical experience with doxycycline, but compliance is better. In penicillin-allergic patients who cannot tolerate doxycycline or tetracycline, three options exist:

1. If follow-up or compliance cannot be ensured, the patient should have skin testing for penicillin allergy and be desensitized if necessary.
2. If compliance and follow-up are ensured, **erythromycin,** 500 mg orally four times a day for 2 weeks, can be used but is less effective than other regimens.
3. Patients who are allergic to penicillin may also be allergic to cephalosporins; therefore, caution must be used in treating a penicilin-allergic patient with a cephalosporin.

Data evaluating the effectiveness of **ceftriaxone** are inadequate to establish optimal dose and duration of therapy. Because 8–10 days of blood treponemocidal activity is needed, single-dose ceftriaxone therapy is not adequate for syphilis.
*Follow-Up*
  Because failures can occur with any regimen, patients should be reexamined clinically and serologically at 3 and 6 months. If nontreponemal antibody titers have not declined fourfold by 3 months in primary or secondary syphilis, or by 6 months in early latent syphilis, or if signs or symptoms persist and reinfection has been ruled out, patients should have a CSF examination and be retreated appropriately. HIV-infected patients should have more frequent follow-up, including serologic testing at 1, 2, 3, 6, 9, and 12 months. Any patient with a fourfold increase in titer at any time should have a CSF examination and be treated with the neurosyphilis regimen unless reinfection can be established.
*Lumbar Puncture in Early Syphilis*
  CSF abnormalities are common in adults with early syphilis, but very few patients develop neurosyphilis when the treatment regimens described above are used. Therefore, lumbar puncture is not recommended routinely in early syphilis. Since CSF abnormalities are common in HIV-infected individuals with primary or secondary syphilis and are of unclear prognostic significance, many recommend CSF evaluation before therapy in all HIV patients with syphilis.
*HIV Testing*
  All patients diagnosed with syphilis should be tested for HIV, and in areas of high prevalence of HIV infection repeated HIV testing should be 3 months later.

**LATE LATENT SYPHILIS OF MORE THAN 1 YEAR'S DURATION, GUMMATOUS SYPHILIS, AND CARDIOVASCULAR SYPHILIS**
CSF examination is indicated clearly in the following specific situations:

1. Neurologic signs or symptoms.
2. Treatment failure.
3. Serum nontreponemal antibody titer ≥1:32.
4. Other evidence of active syphilis (aortitis, gumma, iritis).
5. Nonpenicillin therapy planned.
6. Positive HIV antibody test.

If CSF examination reveals findings consistent with neurosyphilis, patients should be treated for neurosyphilis (see below). Some experts also treat cardiovascular syphilis with a neurosyphilis regimen.
*Recommended Regimen*

**Benzathine penicillin G,** 7.2 million units total, administered as three doses of 2.4 million units IM.

*Alternative Regimen for Penicillin-Allergic Patients (Nonpregnant)*
  **Doxycycline,** 100 mg orally twice a day for 4 weeks; **or**
  **Tetracycline,** 500 mg orally four times a day for 4 weeks.
Alternative drugs should be used only in penicillin-allergic patients after CSF examination has excluded neurosyphilis.
*Follow-Up*
  Quantitative nontreponemal serologic tests should be repeated at 6 and 12 months. If titers increase fourfold, if an initially high titer (≥1:32) fails to decrease, or if the patient has signs or symptoms attributable to syphilis, the patient should be evaluated for neurosyphilis and retreated appropriately (see below).
**NEUROSYPHILIS**
  Clinical evidence of neurologic involvement during any stage of syphilis warrants CSF examination.

*Table continued on following page*

**TABLE 16–2.   SYPHILIS—TREATMENT GUIDELINES*** *Continued*

*Recommended Regimen*

**Aqueous crystalline penicillin G,** 2–4 million units every 4 h IV for 10–14 days.

*Alternative Regimen (if Outpatient Compliance Can Be Ensured)*
**Procaine penicillin,** 2.4 million U IM daily; **and**
**Probenecid,** 500 mg orally four times a day for 10–14 days.
Many recommend **benzathine penicillin G,** 2.4 million units IM weekly for three doses after completion of these neurosyphilis treatment regimens. Patients who cannot tolerate penicillin should be skin tested and desensitized, if necessary.

*Follow-Up*
If pleocytosis was present initially, CSF examination should be repeated every 6 months until the cell count is normal. If it has not decreased at 6 months, or is not normal by 2 years, retreatment should be strongly considered.

SYPHILIS IN PREGNANCY
*Screening*
Pregnant women should be screened early in pregnancy, and those seropositive considered infected unless treatment history and sequential serologic titers show an appropriate response. In populations with suboptimal prenatal care, patients should be screened, and if necessary, treated immediately. In areas of high syphilis prevalence, or in patients at high risk, screening should be repeated in the third trimester and again at delivery. Seropositive women must be assumed to be infected unless appropriate treatment is clearly documented and follow-up titers demonstrate adequate decline. Delivery of a stillborn infant after 20 weeks' gestation should prompt testing of its mother.

*Treatment*
Patients should be treated with the penicillin regimen appropriate for the woman's stage of syphilis. Tetracycline and doxycycline are contraindicated in pregnancy, and erythromycin should not be used because of its failure to cure fetal infection. Pregnant women with histories of penicillin allergy should first be carefully questioned and, if necessary, skin tested and then either treated with penicillin or desensitized.

*Follow-Up*
Monthly serologic follow-up is mandatory so that retreatment can be given if needed.

CONGENITAL SYPHILIS
An infant should be evaluated if born to a confirmed seropositive woman who:

Has untreated or poorly documented treatment of syphilis; **or**
Was treated for syphilis <1 month before delivery; **or**
Was treated for syphilis during pregnancy with a nonpenicillin regimen; **or**
Does not exhibit the expected decrease in nontreponemal antibody titer after appropriate treatment for syphilis; **or**
Was treated but had insufficient serologic follow-up during pregnancy to assess disease activity.

**An infant should not be released from the hospital until the serologic status of its mother is known.**
The clinical and laboratory evaluation of infants born to women described above should include:

1. A thorough physical examination.
2. Nontreponemal antibody titer.
3. CSF analysis for cells, protein, and VDRL.
4. Long-bone x-rays.
5. Other tests as clinically indicated.
6. Specific antitreponemal IgM antibody in infants without evidence of congenital syphilis by the above criteria.

Infants should be treated if they have

1. Any clinical evidence of active disease; **or**
2. A reactive CSF-VDRL **or** an abnormal CSF examination regardless of CSF serology; **or**
3. Quantitative nontreponemal titer at least fourfold greater than that of the mother; **or**
4. Positive antitreponemal-ABS-IgM.

Even if their evaluation is negative, infants should be treated if their mothers have untreated syphilis or evidence of relapse or reinfection after treatment. Incompletely evaluated infants should be assumed to be infected and should be treated.

*Treatment*
Treatment should consist of 100,000–150,000 units/kg of **aqueous crystalline penicillin G** daily (50,000 units/kg IV every 8–12 h) **or** 50,000 units/kg of IM **procaine penicillin** once daily for 10–14 days.
Infants who do not meet the criteria listed for treatment are at **low** risk for congenital syphilis. If their mothers had been treated with **erythromycin** during pregnancy, or treated <1 month before delivery, or did not have an adequate serologic response to treatment, **benzathine penicillin G,** 50,000 units/kg IM, should be given as a one-time dose.

*Follow-Up*
Seropositive untreated infants should be followed closely through 12 months of age. In the absence of infection, nontreponemal titers should be decreasing by 3 months and should have disappeared by 6 months of age. If they are stable or increasing, the child should be reevaluated and fully treated. Additionally, in the absence of infection, treponemal antibodies may be present up to 1 year. If they persist beyond 1 year, the infant should undergo reevaluation and be treated for congenital syphilis.

*Table continued on opposite page*

## TABLE 16–2.  SYPHILIS—TREATMENT GUIDELINES *Continued*

Treated infants should also be observed to ensure decreasing nontreponemal antibody titers, with disappearance by 6 months. Treponemal tests may remain positive despite effective therapy. Infants with CSF pleocytosis should be reexamined every 6 months or until the cell count is normal, with retreatment if the cell count is still abnormal after 2 years. If the CSF-VDRL at 6 months is persistently reactive, the infant should be retreated.

*Therapy of Older Infants and Children*
Children discovered to have syphilis after the newborn period should have a CSF examination to rule out congenital syphilis. Any child thought to have congenital syphilis or with neurologic involvement should be treated with 200,000–300,000 units/kg/day of **aqueous crystalline penicillin G** (50,000 units/kg every 4–6 h) for 10–14 days. Older children with definite acquired syphilis and a normal neurologic examination may be treated with **benzathine penicillin G,** 50,000 units/kg IM, up to the adult dose of 2.4 million units. Follow-up should be performed as described previously.

### SYPHILIS IN HIV-INFECTED PATIENTS
*Diagnosis*
All sexually active patients with syphilis should undergo counseling and testing for HIV. Neurosyphilis should be considered in the differential diagnosis of neurologic disease in HIV-infected persons. When clinical findings suggest that syphilis is present but serologic tests are negative or confusing, alternative tests (biopsy of lesions, darkfield examination, and DFA staining of lesion material) should be used. In cases of congenital syphilis, the mother should be tested for HIV; if her test is positive, the infant should be referred for follow-up.

*Treatment and Follow-Up*
Penicillin should be used whenever possible for all stages of syphilis in HIV-infected patients. Patients may need to be desensitized before treatment with penicillin.
No alteration in therapy for early syphilis is recommended for HIV–co-infected patients. However, some advise CSF examination and/or treatment with a regimen appropriate for neurosyphilis for all patients co-infected with syphilis and HIV. Close clinical and quantitative nontreponemal serologic (VDRL, RPR) follow-up is necessary for 12 months after treatment. Patients with early syphilis whose titers fail to decrease fourfold within 6 months should undergo CSF examinaion and be retreated.

*Modified from Centers for Disease Control. Sexually transmitted diseases treatment guidelines. *MMWR 42*(RR-14): 1993. With permission.

the tertiary form. Since the lesions of tertiary syphilis may be irreversible, it is very important to diagnose and treat primary and secondary syphilis. This can be done with a high level of accuracy by using a variety of serologic tests for syphilis (STS).

In the discussion of serologic tests for syphilis, sensitivity and specificity of assays are important. *Sensitivity* is the ability of the test to be reactive in cases of syphilis in all stages. Highly sensitive tests are useful for preliminary screening. *Specificity* refers to the ability of a test to be negative in cases that are not syphilis. The ideal approach to the serologic diagnosis of syphilis is to use a highly sensitive test for screening purposes followed by a highly specific test to discriminate between syphilis and nonsyphilitic conditions.

Serologic tests for syphilis are divided into two broad categories: (1) nontreponemal (cardiolipin) antibody tests, the so-called Wassermann antibody; and (2) treponemal antibody tests. In general, nontreponemal tests are useful as screening tests, and the treponemal antibody tests establish a specific diagnosis of syphilis.

WASSERMANN TEST. In 1906, 1 year after the treponeme causing syphilis was identified, August Paul von Wassermann employed an aqueous extract of liver from an infant who died of congenital syphilis as an antigen for a complement fixation test. The liver contained large numbers of motile treponemes that Wassermann theorized would serve as antigen to combine with antibody in the serum of infected persons. Although the liver extract showed reactivity with sera of patients with syphilis, years later it was recognized that the observed reactivity was not with treponemes but with intracellular, nontreponemal hepatocyte components, probably a component of mitochondrial membranes, now termed *cardiolipin.* Antibody to cardiolipin is known as *Wassermann antibody,* or reaginic antibody (not to be confused with IgE reaginic antibody).

*VDRL Test.* In 1922, R. L. Kahn developed the first precipitin cardiolipin test for syphilis. In 1941, lecithin and cholesterol were combined with cardiolipin, improving both the sensitivity and specificity of the test, and leading to a slide microflocculation test developed by the Venereal Disease Research Laboratory of the U.S. Public Health Service (hence, the VDRL test). The VDRL test is simple, inexpensive, and easy to perform on large numbers of sera in a short time. Thus it has been a mainstay for screening sera for syphilis for over five decades.

Wassermann antibody is quantitated by making twofold dilutions of the serum until the reaction disappears, and results are reported as the reciprocal of the highest dilution of serum that precipitated with antigen. It is necessary to inactivate complement and other inhibitors by preheating the serum to be tested to 58°C for 30 min, limiting the use of VDRL in the field. More recently, the cardiolipin–lecithin–cholesterol complex has been stabilized with the addition of ethylenediamine tetraacetic acid (EDTA) and choline chloride to inactivate the inhibiting substances in unheated sera, permitting screening of large numbers of sera with minimal laboratory facilities. Several commercial variants of this test are available (e.g., the Plasmacrit and rapid plasma reagin [RPR] card test). The RPR test has equal and possibly better sensitivity and specificity than the VDRL test.

Tests for Wassermann antibody are used to screen large numbers of individuals for active syphilis (e.g., tests for marriage license applications or prenatal blood tests). Positive tests are considered to be diagnostic for syphilis when there is a high or increasing titer or when careful history-taking and physical diagnosis reveal symptoms or lesions consistent with primary or secondary syphilis. Wassermann tests are also useful in the investigation of patient contacts to find unrecognized active syphilis. In addition, Wassermann antibody tests may be of prognostic aid in following the response to therapy, since the VDRL titer falls over a 6- to 8-month period following adequate therapy.

*Nonsyphilitic Wassermann Antibodies.* Because the Wassermann antigen is found in the mitochondrial membranes and related antigenic material is present in mycoplasma, other bacteria, and some yeasts, antibodies to the Wassermann antigen appear in other diseases, such as infectious mononucleosis, hepatitis, leprosy, and in patients with autoimmune disorders. These reactions are termed *biologic false-positive* (BFP) serologic tests for syphilis.

TREPONEMAL ANTIBODY TESTS. These are based on the use of whole treponemes or treponemal extracts as antigen. The treponeme used is either the virulent *T. pallidum*, grown only in rabbit testes, or a nonvirulent treponeme that can be cultivated in a special medium.

*TPI Test.* The first successful treponemal antibody test was developed in 1949, the *T. pallidum* immobilization (TPI) test. The antibody responsible for treponemal immobilization differs from Wassermann antibody because it persists in high titer for many years. The TPI test is both sensitive and quite specific, but it is difficult to perform and requires closely supervised animal colonies and highly trained personnel. The exacting conditions necessary to carry out the TPI test have limited it to only a few research laboratories.

*The FTA and FTA-ABS Tests.* In 1957, the Venereal Disease Research Laboratory developed an antitreponemal antibody test based on indirect immunofluorescence to replace the more cumbersome TPI test. A suspension of virulent *T. pallidum* from infected rabbit testes is placed on a glass microscope slide, overlaid with patient serum, and then exposed to anti–human gamma globulin tagged with fluorescein and viewed under ultraviolet light. Human antitreponemal antibody bound to the spirochete will fluoresce, outlining the treponeme. This is the fluorescent treponemal antibody. Because small amounts of antibody to endogenous treponemes normally-present in humans can give a false-positive FTA test, sera are first absorbed with extracts of nonpathogenic treponemes; this is the FTA absorption test (FTA-ABS). The FTA-ABS can be performed in most clinical laboratories, and results are often available within a day. Although this test is not difficult, it is too complex to serve as a screening test.

*Microhemagglutination Tests.* Within recent years, three microhemagglutination (MHA) tests have been developed to test for treponemal antibodies. These tests are based on the principle of indirect hemagglutination using antigens of *T. pallidum* adsorbed onto erythrocytes and include the hemagglutination treponemal test for syphilis (HATTS), the *T. pallidum* hemagglutination assay (TPHA), and the MHA assay for antibodies to *T. pallidum* (MHA-TP). These three tests show similar reactivity at each stage of syphilis, with comparable sensitivities. Ease of performance, cost, and lack of need for expensive equipment are major factors in the popularity of the MHA tests compared with the FTA-ABS.

REACTIVITY OF SEROLOGIC TESTS. Table 16–3 lists the results of various serologic tests using sera from patients with well-documented primary or secondary syphilis. The FTA-ABS test is reactive in significantly more patients with primary syphilis than other serologic tests, and detects more than 90% of cases of darkfield-positive primary syphilis. If the FTA-ABS test is negative in a patient

## TABLE 16–3. REACTIVITY OF NONTREPONEMAL AND TREPONEMAL TESTS FOR SYPHILIS*

| TEST | STAGE | | |
| --- | --- | --- | --- |
| | **1** | **2** | **LATE** |
| Nontreponemal serology | | | |
|   VDRL | 70[†] | 99[†] | 1[‡] |
|   RPR | 80 | 99 | 0 |
| Treponemal serology | | | |
|   FTA-ABS | 85 | 100 | 98 |
|   TPHA, MHA-TP | 65 | 100 | 95 |
|   TPI | 50 | 97 | 95 |

*Modified from Mandell, G. L., Bennett J. E., and Dolin, R. *Principles and Practice of Infectious Diseases.* New York: Churchill Livingstone, 1995. With permission.

[†]The percentage of patients having positive serology with treated or untreated primary or secondary syphilis.

[‡]Treated late syphilis.

thought to have primary syphilis, it should be repeated 7–10 days later. The FTA-ABS test is clearly the most reactive in all stages of syphilis.

All tests give acceptable results with secondary syphilis. After specific therapy for primary syphilis is instituted, a positive Wassermann test becomes negative within 6–8 months. If therapy is delayed until the onset of secondary syphilis, 90–95% of adequately treated patients are seronegative within 12 months. This characteristic is very useful in monitoring the patient's response to therapy. If therapy is not begun until at least 2 years after the onset of disease, treatment does not affect the Wassermann test, although about half of active syph-

ilis cases become Wassermann antibody–negative over 15–25 years.

These findings are in sharp contrast to treponemal antibody tests. Of these, the TPI and FTA-ABS tests remain positive in a much higher percentage of cases (depending upon the stage at which therapy was started). Other than their lower sensitivity in primary syphilis, the MHA tests compare favorably with the FTA-ABS. The MHA fails to detect antibodies in a few individuals with late syphilis, so it is prudent to perform serum FTA-ABS tests in suspected late syphilis if the MHA test is negative.

Both the FTA and MHA tests have been applied to the detection of antibody against *T. pallidum* in CSF, since treponemal tests are more specific than nontreponemal tests. Both tests are oversensitive, in that many persons without symptoms or other CSF findings have positive tests. There is no satisfactory explanation for these false-positive tests. Currently, the best approach in diagnosing CNS syphilis is to perform the VDRL test on CSF. This test is rarely positive in the absence of neurosyphilis, but it may lack sensitivity.

Recently, it has been recognized that sera from up to 10% of patients with systemic lupus erythematosus (SLE) may give an atypical, beaded fluorescence with the FTA-ABS (Fig. 16–4).

### Chancroid

Chancroid is an acute, ulcerative disease caused by the gram-negative, facultative an-

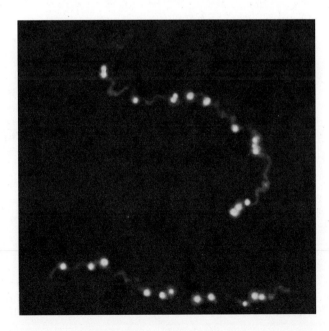

**FIGURE 16–4.** Atypical "beaded" spirochete fluorescence in FTA-ABS test with serum from patients with lupus erythematosus. (From Kraus, S. J., Haserick, J. R., and Lantz, M. A. Atypical FTA-ABS test fluorescence in lupus erythematosus patients. *JAMA 211*:2140, 1970. Copyright © 1970, American Medical Association.)

aerobic bacillus *Haemophilus ducreyi*. Chancroid is transmitted from person to person (usually during intercourse) and is more common in lower socioeconomic groups and uncircumcised men. Men are up to 10 times more likely to develop clinical disease than women. In contrast to syphilis, there are no latent or tertiary stages of disease. *H. ducreyi* can be cultured from approximately 50% of lesions.

### Epidemiology

In the United States, the annual incidence of chancroid was less than 1000 cases in the early 1980s. By 1990, 5000 cases were reported, but its incidence has declined since. It is endemic in many areas of the United States yet may also occur in discreet outbreaks. Chancroid is a major public health problem in many third world countries. Like other ulcerative genital diseases, it is a well-established cofactor in the transmission of HIV. Co-infection with *T. pallidum* or herpes simplex may occur in up to 10% of patients with chancroid.

### Clinical Manifestations

The incubation period for chancroid is usually between 4 and 7 days. There is no prodromal period, and clinical infection begins with a tender genital papule surrounded by erythema that evolves into a pustular eroded ulceration, or chancre. The ulcer is well demarcated, has ragged undermined edges, and is without induration. Up to five discreet, tender concomitant ulcerations are typical. There is little inflammation of the surrounding skin. Painful inguinal lymphadenitis is seen in up to 50% of cases and is usually unilateral. Buboes can progress and may suppurate. *H. ducreyi* does not disseminate further and is not known to be an opportunistic pathogen in HIV-infected individuals. Untreated infections may persist for several months.

### Diagnosis

The diagnosis of chancroid is made by isolating *H. ducreyi* from a genital ulcer or bubo. *H. ducreyi* is a small, nonmotile, non–spore-forming organism that requires hemin for growth. Gram's stain reveals typical streptobacillary chaining. The selective culture media required for definitive diagnosis is not commercially available. Rapid diagnostic techniques such as enzyme immunoassays and polymerase chain reaction (PCR) are being de-

veloped. A presumptive diagnosis can be made if the Gram's stain shows the characteristic features. A clinical diagnosis is based on a compatible history, a painful genital ulcer, and exclusion of other genital ulcer diseases, such as syphilis, herpes, lymphogranuloma venereum, and donovanosis.

### Treatment

Treatment regimens include intramuscular ceftriaxone, oral erythromycin, or azithromycin in a single oral dose. Ceftriaxone may be suboptimal treatment in HIV-infected individuals. None of the current treatment regimens has been evaluated systematically in women.

## Granuloma Inguinale

### Clinical Manifestations and Epidemiology

Granuloma inguinale (donovanosis) is a chronic, progressively destructive genital ulcer disease caused by *Calymmatobacterium granulomatis*, a gram-negative bacterium. The primary lesion begins as an indurated nodule that slowly evolves into a granulomatous heaped ulcer that may coalesce with adjacent ulcerative lesions. The pathognomonic histologic feature of granuloma inguinale is the large infected mononuclear cell that contains intracytoplasmic cysts within which deeply staining Donovan bodies are visible. Hematogenous dissemination to bony structures and viscera may occur.

Granuloma inguinale is rare in developed countries but is highly endemic in certain parts of the developing world. The role of sexual transmission remains unclear, and the disease is only mildly contagious. Usually lesions cannot be found in the sexual partners of known cases.

The incubation period may be as long as 80 days. Lesions are usually sharply defined, painless, and bleed readily on contact. Secondary infection may occur, although surrounding cellulitis is rare. Inguinal involvement is usually due to primary infection rather than to lymphangitic spread and may seem "bubo-like" in appearance (pseudobuboes.)

### Diagnosis and Treatment

The diagnosis is usually made clinically and can be confirmed by preparing a crush preparation from the lesion and observing clusters of blue- or black-staining organisms, referred to as Donovan bodies. No multinucleated giant cells and few lymphocytes are usually seen. The differential diagnosis of suspected granuloma inguinale includes carcinoma, chancroid, condylomata lata of secondary syphilis, and amebiasis. Concurrent infections with other STDs such as gonorrhea or syphilis are not uncommon.

First-line treatment in developed countries is tetracycline. Chloramphenicol is most appropriate for resistant cases, and erythromycin is adequate in pregnancy. Medication should be continued until complete healing is achieved.

### Genital Herpes

Genital herpes infection is caused primarily by herpes simplex virus type 2 (HSV-2), which is distinct from HSV-1, the agent generally responsible for herpes labialis. Newer serologic assays avoid the cross-reactivity between HSV-1 and HSV-2 observed with older methods of testing. Seroepidemiologic surveys with the newer assays reveal a wide disparity between antibody prevalence and history of clinical infection, indicating that subclinical infection is common.

#### Epidemiology

Herpes simplex viruses are worldwide in distribution. The ability of these viruses to establish life-long latent infections with intermittent reactivation and viral shedding ensures their survival.

The prevalence of genital herpes has increased over the past three decades, with parallel increase of neonatal infection. Antibody to HSV-1 is present in about 50% of the U. S. population, but prevalence may be as high as 80% in lower socioeconomic groups. Antibody to HSV-2 is usually not detected before puberty but rises to 50% in men and women attending STD clinics, nearly double that observed in the general population. Higher rates are reported in females, female prostitutes, homosexual men, and persons in lower socioeconomic groups.

#### Clinical Manifestations

Infection takes place after close personal contact when virus in infected secretions or at an infected mucocutaneous surface comes into direct contact with a mucous membrane or nonintact skin surface of a susceptible individual. There is no evidence that fomite or aerosol transmission takes place. Clinically apparent initial infection is characterized by focal necrosis and inflammation with ballooning degeneration of cells. Concomitantly, HSV-2 ascends peripheral sensory nerves and enters the nerve root ganglia where latency is established (in both symptomatic and asymptomatic infections). A large minority of initial infections are asymptomatic. The latent infection more likely leads to asymptomatic viral shedding than to overt disease. Thus, the number of persons shedding HSV asymptomatically at any time greatly outnumbers those with active disease. Reinfection with new strains occurs but is thought to be rare. Recrudescence may or may not be symptomatic and remains incompletely understood. It is known that stimuli that activate viral replication in the ganglion are diverse and include hormonal or immunologic alterations.

#### Symptoms and Signs

The symptoms and signs of genital herpes vary greatly. Initial episodes of genital herpes can be classified as primary or nonprimary. Primary herpes is more likely to be associated with systemic symptoms, severe local involvement of longer duration, and more prolonged viral shedding. Patients with first episodes of genital herpes but who have clinical or serologic evidence of prior HSV-1 infection have a much milder clinical course (nonprimary first episode). HSV-1 was reported to cause 5–15% of all first-episode genital herpetic infections. There is no clinical difference in the presentation of primary genital HSV-1 or HSV-2 infection.

Primary infection occurs after an incubation period of 5–14 days and is manifest by pain, itching, dysuria, vaginal discharge, and tender inguinal adenopathy. The lesions usually start as erythematous papules or vesicles that spread rapidly to the surrounding area. Frequently, the vesicles coalesce and become pustular. Eventually, the lesions break, leaving tender, shallow ulcers that heal spontaneously without scarring. The mean duration of viral shedding is 12 days and time to reepithelialization of the affected skin is 16–20 days. Healing may take longer in women. Ninety percent of women with primary HSV-2 infection have concomitant HSV cervicitis, explaining why symptoms may persist longer and more complications are seen in women. In recurrent attacks, the rate of cervical involvement drops to 12–29%. Rarely, even pelvic inflammatory disease occurs. Dysuria, urethritis, and a urethral discharge related to primary genital herpes is most common in women but may be present in up to one third of men, in whom it is often accompanied by disproportionately severe dysuria. In women such involvement may be clinically consistent with the acute urethral syndrome. Extragenital lesions (e.g., thigh, buttock, or groin) with primary genital outbreaks are noted during the second week of disease and are thought to occur via autoinoculation. The clinical course of primary genital herpes infection is illustrated in Figure 16–5.

Pharyngitis may be present in patients with primary genital herpes and is usually accompanied by fever, headache, mucosal ulcerations, and cervical lymphadenopathy. Aseptic meningitis is seen in more than one third of women and in approximately 10% of men with primary genital HSV-2 infection. There are usually no residual effects. Encephalitis is much more likely to be caused by HSV-1 than HSV-2.

Episodes of recurrent genital herpes range from 8–12 days in duration or less. About 50% of patients experience a prodromal phase characterized by a tingling, burning, or shooting pain in the region of the outbreak 1–48 h prior to eruption of the vesicular lesions. Symptoms and signs tend to be localized to the genital region. In a given individual lesions tend to arise at the same site with each recurrence. Shorter duration of disease and of viral shedding, fewer constitutional symptoms, and rarer complications are characteristic. Possible reasons for this include the presence of neutralizing antibody to HSV and cellular immune responses that inactivate extracellular virus.

Asymptomatic viral shedding is one of the least understood aspects of HSV infection. The source of viral shedding in women is the cervix and/or vulva and occurs in 4% during the first year following a primary infection but drops to 0.5–2.0% in the following years. In men, the anatomic site is less well understood but is most likely due to unrecognizable or atypical genital lesions.

Another poorly understood aspect of HSV infection is the genital recurrence rate, which varies greatly. Following primary HSV-2 infection, 90% have a recurrence within 12 months, with a median of five recurrences in the 2 years following primary infection. Rates are lower following HSV-1 genital infection, and they are higher in those with high titers of complement-independent neutralizing antibody.

Recently, a syndrome of anorectal pain, discharge, constipation, and tenesmus was noted in a group of sexually active homosexual males. These symptoms and findings are characteristic of HSV proctitis. Serologic evidence indicates that 85% of men with herpes proctitis are experiencing a primary HSV-2 infection. Other symptoms of herpes proctitis include sacral paresthesias, difficulty in urinating, as well as signs of perianal skin and mucous membrane ulceration extending into the distal rectum. Rarer complications of genital HSV infection include transverse myelitis and autonomic nervous system abnormalities.

### Diagnosis

The diagnosis of herpesvirus infection can be established by recovery of the virus in cell culture. The virus grows in a wide range of diploid fibroblasts, including human embryonic tonsil, MCR-5, and WI-38. Growth is prompt, with early HSV cytopathic effect appearing in some cells by 24 h, in more than half by 48 h, and in almost all by 96 h.

Giemsa-stained smears from the base of ulcerated skin or mucous membrane lesions show multinucleated giant cells, many with intranuclear inclusion bodies, in about 50% of patients who ultimately have positive cultures. The use of fluorescein-tagged herpesvirus antibodies (immunofluorescence [IF] test) on smears from ulcerated lesions detects about 70% of patients who have positive cultures.

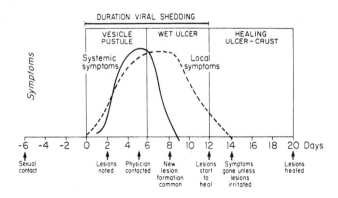

**FIGURE 16–5.** The clinical course of infection by primary genital herpes simplex virus. (From Corey, L., Adams, H. G., Brown, Z. A., et al. Genital herpes simplex virus infections: Clinical manifestations, course, and complications. *Ann. Intern. Med. 98*:958, 1983. With permission.)

Immunoperoxidase (IP) staining has a sensitivity and specificity similar to that of the immunofluorescence technique and uses light microscopy. Another rapid antibody-based diagnostic method is the enzyme-linked immunosorbent assay (ELISA), which may be as sensitive as virus isolation for detection of HSV-2 antigen. These immunologic techniques (IF, IP, and ELISA) distinguish between HSV-1 and HSV-2 and produce the same results as the more time-consuming restriction endonuclease analysis.

Despite seroprevalence rates of between 30 and 70% in women attending prenatal clinics, clinical evidence of HSV is much less frequent. Although neonatal herpes is not a reportable disease, the estimated frequency of infection in the United States is approximately 1 in 7500 births, or about 700 cases annually. Recent studies indicate that most clinical manifestations of recurrent genital herpes are similar in pregnant and nonpregnant women. Visceral dissemination of herpes during primary infection in pregnant women has been reported, but fortunately appears to be rare. Pregnancy morbidity has been observed principally in primary cases.

The major identifiable source of HSV infection of the newborn is through contact with an infected birth canal, especially the cervix. Approximately 70% of babies with neonatal HSV are born to mothers who were asymptomatic at delivery. The relative risk of neonatal HSV is much higher when the mother is experiencing primary infection. The risk of transmission by a mother with recurrent herpes ranges from 0 to 8%. In a remarkably large percentage of patients with neonatal herpes, the source is unknown.

Managing pregnant women with history of genital herpes remains problematic. Women should undergo a thorough examination of the vulvar area and cervix early in labor. A viral culture of the cervix and vulvar area should be taken. If no obvious lesions are present, the baby should be delivered vaginally. If any suspicious abnormality is present, a cesarian section should be performed as long as membranes have not been ruptured greater than 4–6 h (in which case considerable fetal exposure to maternal secretions has probably already taken place). Only 1–6% of infants exposed to HSV-infected maternal secretions develop neonatal herpes. Infants born to mothers with suspected active herpes should be cultured, placed in isolation, and observed closely for signs of herpes infection.

The benefit of early empiric antiviral therapy with acyclovir has not yet been determined.

### Herpes and Human Immunodeficiency Virus Infection

HIV infection often alters the course of HSV disease. Recurrences are reported to be more frequent, more severe, and more difficult to treat as the HIV-related disease progresses. The genital, rectal, or oral HSV lesions may become quite large, painful, and chronic. Patients with HSV ulcerations in which activated lymphocytes are present may be at the same increased risk of acquiring HIV as patients with chancres. Many HIV-infected patients with active HSV may benefit from chronic suppressive therapy with acyclovir. *In vitro* data demonstrate the ability of gene products of HSV to transactivate regulatory genes of HIV, thereby increasing the latter's replication. The clinical significance of this is unclear.

### Treatment

Acyclovir, valacyclovir, famciclovir, foscarnet, and topical fluoridines are the only antiviral agents with a positive therapeutic effect in genital herpes. Acyclovir is selectively phosphorylated by cells infected with HSV. Virus-specific thymidine kinase converts acyclovir to acyclovir monophosphate, which is then phosphorylated to acyclovir triphosphate, the active drug that inhibits HSV DNA polymerase. Mutants of HSV that lack thymidine kinase are resistant to acyclovir but are often susceptible to the parenteral agent foscarnet.

Topical acyclovir initiated after the appearance of skin lesions significantly shortens viral shedding but has little effect upon the time to crusting and healing, pain, or upon the subsequent number of new skin lesions. This contrasts to intravenous acyclovir (every 8 h for 5 days) in the treatment of first-episode genital herpes, which results in decreased viral shedding from genital lesions, pharynx, cervix, and urethra, and in urine. In addition, the duration of local and systemic symptoms is shortened, and complications such as extragenital lesions and urinary retention are avoided. However, its use as a parenteral agent remains impractical.

Oral acyclovir is the mainstay of primary therapy, is nearly as effective as the intravenous preparation, and is much more convenient. Treatment of recurrent herpes with short courses of acyclovir may benefit some patients. Long-term suppressive therapy for

### TABLE 16–4.    GENITAL HERPES SIMPLEX VIRUS INFECTIONS—TREATMENT GUIDELINES*

**FIRST CLINICAL EPISODE OF GENITAL HERPES**
Acyclovir, 200 mg orally five times per day for 7–10 days or until clinical resolution occurs.

**FIRST CLINICAL EPISODE OF HERPES PROCTITIS**
Acyclovir, 400 mg orally five times per day for 10 days or until clinical resolution occurs.

**FOR PATIENTS WITH SEVERE DISEASE OR COMPLICATIONS NECESSITATING HOSPITALIZATION**
Acyclovir, 5 mg/kg body weight IV every 8 h for 5–7 days or until clinical resolution occurs.

**RECURRENT EPISODES**
Most episodes of recurrent herpes in immunocompetent hosts are not benefitted by acyclovir. In severe recurrent disease, some who start therapy at the begining of the prodrome or within 2 days after onset of lesions may experience limited benefit.
Acyclovir, 200 mg orally five times a day for 5 days; **or**
Acyclovir, 400 mg orally 3 times daily for 5 days; **or**
Acyclovir, 800 mg orally twice a day for 5 days.

**DAILY SUPPRESSIVE THERAPY**
Daily treatment reliably reduces the frequency of recurrences by at least 75% in patients with frequent (more than six per year) recurrences but does not entirely eliminate viral shedding or the potential for transmission. Daily therapy for up to 5 years is safe and effective. Acyclovir-resistant HSV has been isolated after long-term suppressive therapy but not associated with treatment failure among immunocompetent patients. After 1 year of suppression, acyclovir should be discontinued to assess the recurrence rate.
Acyclovir, 400 mg orally 2 times a day; **or**
Acyclovir, 200 mg orally three to five times a day.

**GENITAL HERPES AMONG HIV-INFECTED PATIENTS**
Higher than standard doses of oral acyclovir are needed among those HIV infected. Regimens such as 400 mg orally three to five times daily (as used in other immunocompromised patients) are effective. Immune status, not HIV infection alone, predicts disease severity and response to therapy. The indications for suppressive therapy among immunocompromised patients, and the dose required, are controversial. Clinical benefits must be weighed against the potential for selecting acyclovir-resistant HSV strains. For severe disease caused by proven or suspected acyclovir-resistant strains, treatment with IV foscarnet 40 mg/kg every 8 h may be the best treatment.

*Adapted from Centers for Disease Control. Sexually transmitted disease treatment guidelines. *MMWR 42*(RR-14): 1993. With permission.

up to 1 year in patients with frequent recurrences can significantly reduce the number of outbreaks and may diminish the incidence of neurologic complications. The drug appears to be well tolerated (Table 16–4). Valacyclovir, an oral "pro-drug" rapidly metabolized to acyclovir, appears to have efficacy similar to oral acyclovir. Famciclovir, a similar agent, is now approved for treatment of varicella zoster virus infections and for HSV infections.

## GENITAL MUCOSAL DISEASES

### Gonorrhea

Gonorrhea is one of the oldest known infectious diseases with primary involvement of the genitourinary tract. The pharynx, rectum, eye, joints, and other organs may be involved as well. Hippocrates may have been the first to write on the subject, in the fourth and fifth centuries B.C. He referred to gonorrhea as "strangury" and associated it with "the pleasures of Venus" even though it was not clear until relatively recently that urethral discharge in men was linked to illness among women. The term *clap*, which is still commonly used, first appeared in print in 1378 A.D. and most probably referred to the *Les Clappier* district of Paris, where prostitutes commonly worked. Prior to Neisser's description of *Neisseria gonorrhoeae* in 1879, it was thought that gonorrhea and syphilis were different manifestations of the same disease.

### Clinical Manifestations

*Neisseria gonorrhoeae* is a small, gram-negative diplococcus whose only natural host is humans. Gonococci survive for only a very brief time outside the human body, and there are no documented cases of transmission except through intimate physical contact. *N. gonorrhoeae* initially infects the mucosal surfaces of the genitourinary tract, primarily the urethra in males and the cervical endothelium in females. The rectum, pharynx, and conjunctivae can also be infected primarily. Ascending genital infection, salpingitis in females and epididymitis in males, and bacteremic dissemination, are relatively common and account for most of the serious morbidity.

More than 70 different types of *N. gonorrhoeae* can be differentiated by auxotyping (ascertaining nutritional requirements), serotyping, or by antimicrobial sensitivities. The most useful and widely available method is serotyping with monoclonal antibodies specific for various epitopes expressed on the outer membrane protein I, important for epidemiologic purposes.

For infection to occur, gonococci must adhere effectively to mucosal surfaces and survive the usual mechanical forces present in the genitourinary system (Fig. 16–6). Adherence is mediated by pili interacting with host proteins on the mucosal surface. Gonococci are also capable of mucosal invasion and entering the bloodstream. Repeated infections in the same person by one strain indicates that gonococci evade local immune mechanisms or change surface antigens frequently. The considerable tissue damage following gonococcal salpingitis suggests that gonococci may produce a tissue toxin or evoke an immune response that results in damage to host tissues.

### Epidemiology

Approximately 1 million new infections with *N. gonorrhoeae* occur in the United States each year. The incidence of gonorrhea varies considerably with age, sex, and race. Factors increasing risk include lower socioeconomic status, urban residence, unmarried marital status, and a past history of gonorrhea. Over 80% of reported cases occur in patients 15–29 years of age. The highest reported incidence is among sexually active adolescent females, who have nearly twice the rate of sexually active women aged 20–24. The rate of gonococcal infection in sexually active African-American females is dramatically higher than in other groups (81% of all cases in 1993). In the 1980s, prostitution and illicit drug use appeared as new risk factors for gonorrhea, and male homosexuality and bisexuality declined as risk factors because of the changing sexual practices in this group. During the period 1975–1993, gonorrhea rates decreased 65% in the United States, most dramatically from 1990–1993. A national gonorrhea control program and the behavioral changes induced by the HIV epidemic probably account for much of the observed decline.

The efficiency of transmission depends on the site of inoculation and the number of exposures. The best data are for men exposed to infected women: the transmission rate after one such unprotected exposure during intercourse is 20% and rises to 60–80% following four exposures. The rate among women exceeds 50% following one exposure to an infected man. Rates of infection following other types of sexual contact are less well defined. Barrier contraception with condoms, diaphragms, and spermicides clearly are partially protective.

Acute gonorrhea in men is associated with anterior urethritis 1–8 days (mean 3–4 days) following exposure. Typical symptoms are dysuria and discharge, often purulent and profuse. Up to 10% never develop symptoms, partly related to the infecting strain type. Since most infections among men produce readily apparent symptoms, treatment is usually sought early enough to prevent serious sequelae. Untreated gonorrhea spontaneously resolves over a period of weeks. Complications of urethritis include epididymitis, acute or chronic prostatitis, and infections of Cowper's and Tyson's glands.

Acute gonorrhea in women involves infection of the endocervical canal. Colonization of the urethra is common but rarely without concomitant endocervical involvement. Skene's and Bartholin's glands may also be infected. When present, symptoms include increased vaginal discharge, dysuria, abnormal uterine bleeding, and menorrhagia. The cervix may have obvious purulent discharge, erythema, or areas of easily induced bleeding. Coexisting infection with other STDs is common. Extension to the rectum occurs frequently (20–50%) in women with genital gonorrhea, but in contrast to homosexual men is usually asymptomatic. Acute salpingitis, or pelvic inflammatory disease (PID), is the most severe complication of gonorrhea, occurring in up to 40% of infected women. This high rate reflects that many infections among women do not produce early symptoms and are undetected and untreated until serious complications have arisen. Salpingitis is the most important complication of gonorrhea because of the potential severity of the acute disease and secondary complications of infertility and ectopic pregnancy. Clinical findings of acute salpingitis include any combination of abdominal pain, dyspareunia, abnormal menses, adnexal or cervical tenderness, abnormal cervical discharge, and fever.

Pharyngeal infection occurs in up to 20%

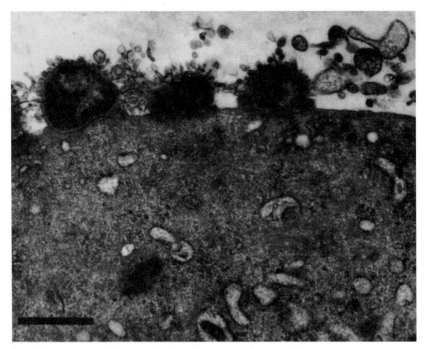

**Figure 16–6.** Electron micrograph showing gonococci closely attached to the surface of a urethral epithelial cell. The membrane of the host cell appears pushed up around the gonococcus to form cushion-like structures. The bar represents 500 nm × 46,000. (From Ward, M. E., and Watt, P. J. Adherence of *Neisseria gonorrhoeae* to urethral mucosal cells: An electron-microscopic study of human gonorrhea. *J. Infect. Dis. 126*:601, 1972. The University of Chicago Press, © 1972 by the *Journal of Infectious Diseases.*)

of heterosexual women and up to 25% of homosexually active men. Fellatio appears to be a more efficient mode of transmission than cunnilingus. It is unclear whether there is an increased risk of dissemination among those with pharyngeal involvement.

Acute hematogenous dissemination of gonorrhea occurs in 1–3% of untreated patients, with arthritis, tenosynovitis, and dermatitis the most common findings. Disseminated infection occurs more commonly in women than in men, in pregnancy, and in those with terminal complement component deficiency.

### Diagnosis

**Culture.** The diagnosis of gonorrhea depends on culture of the microorganism. Gonococcal isolation is aided by a selective culture medium that suppresses the growth of other microorganisms that might mask the appearance of *N. gonorrhoeae*, Thayer-Martin (TM) medium. It is composed of "chocolate" agar with vitamins and cofactors and the antibiotics vancomycin, colistin, and nystatin (VCN). The terms TM and VCN refer to the same culture medium for isolation of both *N. gonorrhoeae* and *N. meningitidis.*

A modification of the VCN medium containing trimethoprim in a small prescription bottle and capped under an atmosphere of 10% carbon dioxide (Transgrow) can be used for transport to laboratories. *N. gonorrhoeae* is very sensitive to cold temperatures and can be killed if inoculated onto medium just removed from a refrigerator.

**Enzyme-Linked Immunosorbent Assay.** Recently, an ELISA test for specific gonococcal antigens has resulted in a rapid (3–4 h) and sensitive method for identifying patients with gonorrhea, with 70–80% sensitivity in men and women. The ELISA test is significantly more sensitive than the cervical Gram's stain (78 vs. 48%). Neither prolonged transport nor refrigeration up to 30 days affects ELISA results. Thus, immunologic antigen detection for gonorrhea has certain advantages over cultures.

**Serology.** For many years there has been a need for a serologic test to detect infection with *N. gonorrhoeae*. In part because of the wide variety of potential antigens, including pili, polysaccharide capsules, and membrane and somatic proteins, and considerable variation in strain specificity, the single best gonococcal antigen for serologic testing has not been determined. In contrast, culture of the infected site has an approximately 80% sensitivity and almost 100% specificity for both symptomatic and asymptomatic infections. Although culture is considerably more expensive than most serologic procedures, its sensitivity and specificity ultimately make it a more economical screening procedure.

### Treatment

Sulfanilamide was the first antimicrobial used for treatment of gonorrhea in the mid-1930s. This was replaced by penicillin in 1946, as many gonococcal strains had become resistant. By the early 1970s, "low-level" chromosomally mediated penicillin resistance was observed in many parts of the world, particularly in Southeast Asia. Effective therapy with penicillin was maintained by increasing the dose and/or by administering probenecid to block renal tubular secretion of penicillin. In 1976, the first two cases of infection with penicillinase-producing *Neisseria gonorrhoeae* (PPNG) were detected, and by 1980 PPNG had be-

come endemic in many areas of the United States. In 1983, "high-level" chromosomally mediated penicillin- and tetracycline-resistant strains were identified in North Carolina. By 1989, penicillin was no longer effective in many parts of the United States, and the CDC recommended intramuscular ceftriaxone therapy. In 1993, 30.4% of gonococcal isolates reported in the United States were resistant to penicillin, tetracycline, or both.

Spectinomycin, an aminoglycoside used exclusively for treatment of gonorrhea, is very effective in uncomplicated infections with PPNG, and spectinomycin resistance remains rare in the United States. One disadvantage of spectinomycin is its failure to eradicate gonococcal pharyngitis.

In 1989, the third-generation cephalosporin ceftriaxone became the treatment of choice because it eradicates gonorrhea from all potentially infected sites and single intramuscular injection is highly effective (Table 16–5).

A number of oral agents, including the third-generation cephalosporin cefixime and

### TABLE 16–5.   GONOCOCCAL INFECTIONS—TREATMENT GUIDELINES*

Because of the great number of antimicrobial therapies safe and effective against *N. gonorrhoeae*, these guidelines are not comprehensive. Factors considered when selecting a treatment regimen include the anatomic site of involvement, resistance patterns, the likelihood of concurrent infection with *C. trachomatis*, and side effects and costs of various regimens.

**TREATMENT OF ADULTS**
*Uncomplicated Urethral, Endocervical, or Rectal Infections*
Single-dose efficacy is a major consideration, as is coexisting chlamydial infection. Persons with gonorrhea should also be treated for presumptive chlamydial infections simultaneously.
  **Ceftriaxone,** 125 mg or 250 mg IM once; **or**
  **Cefixime,** 400 mg orally in a single dose; **or**
  **Ciprofloxacin,** 500 mg orally in a single dose; **or**
  **Ofloxacin,** 400 mg orally in a single dose;
                              **PLUS**
A regimen effective against *C. trachomatis* such as doxycycline 100 mg orally two times a day for 7 days.
  Oral cefixime does not achieve a bactericidal level as high nor as sustained as with ceftriaxone. Quinolones are contraindicated for use during pregnancy and among nursing women, as well as in persons <17 years of age.

**ALTERNATIVE REGIMENS**
For patients who cannot take a tetracycline (e.g., pregnant women) for chlamydia, **erythromycin** may be substituted (**erythromycin** base or stearate at 500 mg orally four times a day for 7 days **or erythromycin ethylsuccinate,** 800 mg orally four times a day for 7 days).
  Among nonpregnant patients, **azithromycin** in a single 1 g dose is equivalent to 1 week of doxycycline for uncomplicated chlamydial urethritis or cervicitis.

**SPECIAL CONSIDERATIONS**
All patients with gonorrhea should be tested for syphilis and should be offered HIV counseling and testing. Most patients with incubating syphilis will be cured by regimens containing beta-lactams (e.g., ceftriaxone) or tetracyclines, but not by spectinomycin or the quinolones (ciprofloxacin, norfloxacin).
*Treatment of Sex Partners*
Persons exposed to gonorrhea within the preceding 30 days should be examined, cultured, and treated presumptively. If the index patient was asymptomatic, any of his/her sexual contacts over the preceding 60 days should be evaluated and treated.

*Adapted from Centers for Disease Control. Sexually transmitted disease treatment guidelines. *MMWR 42*(RR-14): 1993. With permission.

the quinolones ciprofloxacin and ofloxacin, are effective in single-dose regimens for gonococcal infections. These therapies are widely used, largely to avoid the parenteral route. In 1993 the CDC adopted these three agents as first-line alternatives to ceftriaxone for acute uncomplicated gonococcal infections. Either of the quinolones is an effective oral regimen in the beta-lactam–intolerant patient. Spectinomycin has become little used now.

## Chlamydia

Infections caused by *Chlamydia trachomatis* are the most prevalent STDs in developed nations. The reported rates of chlamydia infections in the United States increased dramatically from 1984 to 1992 (now estimated at 4 million infections annually), reflecting increased screening and recognition of asymptomatic infection, and improved reporting. Reported rates in women greatly outnumber those in men.

*Chlamydia trachomatis* is an obligate intracellular parasite that cannot be cultured on artificial media. Chlamydiae are distinct from all other microorganisms and have been placed in their own order, Chlamydiales, and family, Chlamydiaceae. Chlamydiae are responsible for several recognized forms of disease in humans: trachoma, pneumonitis, sexually transmitted lymphogranuloma venereum, and genital mucosal disease (Table 16–6).

### Epidemiology

The prevalence of *C. trachomatis* ranges from 3–5% in asymptomatic men and women in general medical settings to greater than 20% in STD clinics. During pregnancy, 5–7% of women are reported to be culture-positive for chlamydia. Neonates may acquire infection after passing through an infected birth canal. Teenage females have the highest seroprevalence rates and may have physiologically increased susceptibility to infection related to

cervical ectopy and lack of immunity. Use of oral contraceptives is also associated with increased likelihood of chlamydial infection. Increased sexual activity at younger ages over the past two decades has created a large pool of young women at risk.

### Clinical Manifestations

The two principal modes of transmission of *C. trachomatis* are sexual and congenital. In western society, the vast majority is sexually transmitted. Clinical features of infection closely parallel those seen with gonorrhea. Chlamydial infection has a longer incubation period (7–21 days), less frank purulence from inflamed sites, and is more likely to be asymptomatic than gonorrhea. Although both infections can become systemic, the manifestations associated with systemic chlamydial infection are more likely to result from antigen–antibody complex formation rather than from hematogenous spread as in gonorrhea.

In men, urethritis is the most common clinical condition associated with chlamydia. Although symptoms are generally milder than with gonorrhea, there is enough overlap to prevent clinical determination of the responsible agent. Chlamydia is the most common cause of nongonococcal urethritis, and 60–75% of female partners of culture-positive men are infected.

Epididymitis may result from ascending chlamydial infection, and chlamydia is the most common etiology in sexually active men under 35 years of age. Coliforms are the usual cause in men over 35. Chlamydial epididymitis presents as unilateral scrotal pain, swelling, and tenderness of the epididymis. Therapy with tetracycline, macrolides, or fluoroquinolones is usually rapidly effective. It is unlikely that chlamydia causes other forms of local infection, such as prostatitis.

The D, K, and LGV strains of chlamydia can

### TABLE 16–6. CHLAMYDIAL SPECIES AND THEIR ASSOCIATED HUMAN DISEASES*

| SPECIES | BIOVAR | MODE OF SPREAD | HUMAN DISEASE |
|---------|--------|----------------|---------------|
| *C. psittaci* | Many | Aerosol (sexual in animals) | Pneumonia, endocarditis, abortions |
| *C. trachomatis* | LGV (L-1, L-2, L-3) | Sexual | Lymphogranuloma venereum (LGV) |
| | (A, B, Ba, C) | Fomites, flies | Trachoma |
| | (B, Ba, D–K) | Sexual, hand to eye | Oculogenital disease; infant pneumonia |
| *C. pneumoniae* | TWAR | ?Aerosol | Bronchitis, pneumonia, ?coronary artery disease |

*Modified from Mandell, G. E., Bennett, J. E., and Dolin, R. *Principles and Practice of Infectious Diseases.* New York: Churchill Livingstone, 1995. With permission.

produce proctitis that may be asymptomatic or appear as a purulent form indistinguishable from that caused by gonorrhea. In one large STD center up to 15% of homosexual men with proctitis had chlamydia. Treatment with tetracycline is quite effective.

The most severe consequence of chlamydial infection is Reiter's syndrome (urethritis, conjunctivitis, and arthritis), a form of reactive tenosynovitis. Like postenteric arthritis syndrome, HLA-B27–positive patients are at greatest risk. Reiter's syndrome is unlikely to occur if appropriate therapy is initiated promptly.

Asymptomatic infections account for about 70% of infections in women. Such infections can persist for up to 15 months, during which time transmission to others and/or the development of serious upper tract disease leading to infertility can occur.

The most common symptomatic manifestation in women is cervicitis with a mucopurulent discharge. The presence of more than 30 polymorphonuclear leukocytes per high-power field strongly suggests chlamydial or gonococcal cervicitis. Infection with chlamydia may persist for many months or resolve spontaneously.

Local extension or infection of the female urethra, Bartholin's glands, or endometrium is common and responds to usual treatment regimens. Up to 40% of women infected with chlamydia or gonorrhea develop PID. Among these women, salpingitis and subsequent tubal scarring or tuboovarian abscess result in involuntary infertility in 20%, ectopic pregnancy in 9%, and chronic pain in 18%. Another serious consequence of chlamydial infection is perihepatitis, or Fitz-Hugh–Curtis syndrome, also seen in gonococcal infections.

### Diagnosis

The diagnosis of chlamydial infection can be made by inoculation of infected secretions onto McCoy or Hela cell-tissue culture, which is relatively expensive and may require as long as 5–10 days. Rapid, nonculture methods include direct immunofluorescence staining of smears with monoclonal antibodies, use of DNA probes, and detection of chlamydial antigen by ELISA. Presumptive clinical diagnosis is relatively easy if pyuria (>4 polymorphonuclear leukocytes [PMNs] per high-power field) is present in men, or more than 30 PMNs are seen on endocervical Gram's stain. Strategies that combine screening of first-void urine by the leukocyte esterase test followed

by specific testing using electroimmunoassay (EIA) with direct fluorescent antibody (DFA) confirmation among sexually active males are effective and cost-conscious. PCR-based diagnostic techniques are highly sensitive and specific in diagnosing chlamydial cervicitis and urethritis.

The CDC recommends chlamydial screening for (1) all women with mucopurulent cervicitis; (2) all sexually active women less than 20 years of age; (3) women 20–24 years old who fail to use barrier contraception or who have a new sexual partner in the 3 months prior to evaluation; and (4) women older than 24 years old who do not use barrier contraception and have a new partner within 3 months prior to the evaluation.

### Treatment

Tetracycline or doxycycline for 1 week has been standard therapy. No tetracycline resistance has been documented. Other effective agents include the macrolides and the quinolones. Azithromycin, an extended-spectrum macrolide, is as effective as doxycycline for uncomplicated chlamydial urethritis and cervicitis. It is administered in a single 1-g oral dosage, enabling directly observed therapy. The CDC treatment guidelines have adopted azithromycin as a first-line treatment, equivalent to doxycycline. Effective second-line treatment options include ofloxacin or erythromycin for 1 week.

## Mycoplasmas

Mycoplasmas are small gram-negative organisms that are not seen on routine Gram's-stained clinical specimens. They can be grown in special media, but clinicians do not have 251ready access to this culture media. Three of the 12 human mycoplasmal species cause clinical disease in the genitourinary tract of sexually active patients, *M. hominis, M. genitalium,* and *Ureaplasma urealyticum.*

### Epidemiology

*U. urealyticum* appears to cause 20–40% of the gonorrhea-negative, chlamydia-negative urethritis in men. Recovery of *U. urealyticum* from the male urethra does not necessarily implicate ureaplasmas as the cause of urethritis because these organisms may colonize the genital tract without causing illness. Colonization occurs as a consequence of sexual activity and increases proportionally with the number of sexual partners. Ureaplasmas may also cause acute prostatitis. The possible role of *M. genitalium* as a cause of urethritis is unclear, and the role of the mycoplasmas in epididymitis, prostatitis, and Reiter's syndrome is unknown. Data suggest that *M. hominis*, *M. genitalium*, and *U. urealyticum* may cause PID. The data concerning local abscess formation, vaginitis, and cervicitis are not convincing.

### Treatment

The recommended treatment for *M. genitalium* or *U. urealyticum* infection is doxycycline, with erythromycin being the alternate agent. However, 10% of ureaplasmas are resistant to tetracycline and about 40% of the tetracycline-resistant strains are also resistant to erythromycin. Alternative therapy in this situation includes the quinolones, particularly ofloxacin, spectinomycin, and probably azithromycin.

## EPIDERMAL DISEASES

### Human Papillomavirus

Anogenital warts are caused by specific types of human papillomaviruses (HPVs), small naked viruses with icosahedral symmetry and double-stranded circular DNA. Warts are benign, self-limited tumors of the epithelium. Although both are caused by different strains of HPV, there is no clinical or virologic association between genital warts and the common skin wart. Exophytic genital and anal infection is caused primarily by HPV types 6 and 11. Other viral types that may be present in the genital or anal region (types 16, 18, 31, 33, and 35) have a strong association with genital dysplasia and carcinoma. Types 16 and 18 in particular are incontrovertibly linked with the development of cervical and vulvar carcinoma 5–30 years after infection.

### Epidemiology and Clinical Manifestations

Anogenital warts are the most common viral STD. They are three times more common than genital herpes and are exceeded in incidence only by gonorrhea and chlamydial infection. HPV is transmitted during direct sexual contact, and the incubation period is 2–6 months. Infection may occur anywhere there has been direct physical contact, including the anus and oral cavity. Behaviors associated with increased risk for genital warts include sex with a person with symptomatic or asymptomatic infection, smoking, and the long-term use of oral contraceptives.

Genital warts in men can occur anywhere on the external genitalia, urethra, rectum, or bladder, particularly areas likely to be traumatized during intercourse. Most commonly, genital warts are exophytic and referred to as condylomata acuminata. Warts are usually multiple and vary in size from 1–5 mm in diameter, though they can be larger. They may be flat and inconspicuous, making diagnosis and treatment difficult.

In women, condylomata usually appear first on the vulva and in 20% of cases then rapidly spread to the perineum and perianal area. Subclinical infection of the cervix is common but is difficult to recognize without colposcopy. Studies with colposcopy, using cytologic, histologic, and other assays to detect HPV DNA or antigen demonstrate that HPV can be found in over 70% of precancerous cervical lesions and in over 90% of overtly malignant lesions.

### Diagnosis

Diagnosis of anogenital warts can be difficult. The cutaneous manifestations of HPV are diverse. Condylomas may appear flat, exophytic, verrucous (rough), or smooth. Lack of skin changes discernible to the naked eye does not rule out the prescence of HPV. Warts must be distinguished from normal anatomic variants, tumors, and other infectious agents. Lesions resemble condylomata lata, a manifestation of secondary syphilis. Diagnosis is usually made on clinical, cytologic, or histologic grounds. The potential for the use of specific DNA probes appears promising.

### Treatment

Treatment objectives are resolution of signs and symptoms in that no therapy has been demonstrated to eradicate HPV. Normal-appearing tissue adjacent to visible lesions can be subclinically infected and serve as a viral reservoir likely to give rise to clinical recurrence.

Treatment may be topical, surgical, or intralesional. Topical modalities include cryotherapy with liquid nitrogen or chemical ablation with agents like podophyllin, trichloroacetic acid (TCA), or 5-fluorouracil. More complex cases involving greater warty burden may require surgery, electrocautery, or $CO_2$ laser treatment. Intralesional interferon requires frequent injections, making this potentially less well tolerated and impractical. Systemic interferon may prove beneficial, especially as an adjunct to treatment of refractory or recurrent warts.

## Molluscum Contagiosum

### Epidemiology and Clinical Manifestations

Molluscum contagiosum is a benign papular lesion of the skin caused by the molluscum contagiosum virus, a member of the poxvirus family. Molluscum contagiosum is spread by sexual or nonsexual routes. The incubation period ranges from 1 week to 6 months. The lesions are very characteristic: 3–5 mm in diameter, smooth, firm, dome-shaped, and grayish white in color with an umbilicated center.

### Diagnosis and Treatment

Diagnosis is usually made clinically. Biopsy reveals characteristic large round intracytoplasmic molluscum bodies. Treatment is generally readily accomplished by excisional curettage. An alternative is cryotherapy with liquid nitrogen. Podophyllin or TCA are probably less effective. In severely immunosuppressed patients, such as those with AIDS, therapy may not be as effective. Often, new lesions appear more quickly than existing lesions and can be removed safely.

## Ectoparasitic Diseases

### Lice

*Phthirus pubis*, the crab louse, is transmitted from one person to another primarily during intimate contact but also, less frequently, after sharing bedding. It is more difficult to transmit than the other species of lice that infect man, *Pediculus humanus corporis*, the body louse, and *Pediculus humanus capitis*, the head louse. Lice need human blood to survive.

Clinical manifestations of infection with the crab louse are not likely to be apparent until at least 5 days after the initial bite. When allergic sensitization has taken place, itching occurs, leading to scratching and signs of inflammation. Superinfection may occur. The diagnosis is made by careful visual inspection and identification of adult lice and their eggs (nits), which are firmly attached to the pubic hair.

The treatment for lice is permethrin 1% or lindane 1%. These pediculocides need to remain in contact with the eggs for at least 1 hour to be effective. Ridding the patient's clothing and linens of nits and adult lice is also an important part of the treatment program. Household contacts and sexual partners should also be evaluated.

### Scabies

*Sarcoptes scabiei* is the mite responsible for scabies. Mites actually move quite rapidly and are quick to burrow into the horny layer of the skin and to begin laying eggs. Scabies may be transmitted by close personal contact, although prolonged (e.g., overnight) contact is most likely to result in transmission. Household outbreaks are common, making this one of the few STDs with frequent nonsexual household-wide outbreaks. Scabies may also be transmitted by animals, particularly dogs. Animal mites are very similar to human mites but differ biologically: their incubation period is shorter, typical burrows are absent, and household contacts need not be treated, since the condition is not transmissible between humans.

The hallmark of scabies is pruritus, usually worse at night or after a hot shower or bath. The lesions associated with scabies may appear papular or eczematous. The hands are often the first place of involvement, particularly the finger webs. Skin folds are a common site of infection. Lesions on the penis may appear nodular or mimic a chancre or superficial fungal infection. The pathognomonic burrow is a short, wavy, dirty-appearing line. Scabies often coexists with other STDs, especially syphilis and gonorrhea. Especially when penile lesions lead to the diagnosis of scabies, it is important to undertake evaluation for these other STDs.

Diagnosis is often made clinically but can be confirmed by examination of a skin scraping or by prying a mite from its burrow with a needle. Treatment is relatively easy, with lindane being the most common preparation used in the United States.

## ENTERITIS/DIARRHEAL SYNDROMES

Infections with pathogens that commonly cause enteritis or diarrhea are increasingly recognized to occur following sexual exposure, particularly when a history of oroanal or anogenital contact is present. Although primary enteric infection with many sexually transmitted agents is possible (e.g., HSV, HPV, gonorrhea, chlamydia, and syphilis), enteritis is generally associated with *Shigella* species, *Salmonella* species, and *Campylobacter* species.

The protozoans *Entamoeba histolytica* and *Giardia lamblia* are also known to cause diarrhea and be sexually transmitted.

## VAGINAL DISEASES

### Vulvovaginal Candidiasis

Vulvovaginal candidiasis or candida vaginitis is most likely not an STD of women. However, 20% of women with this infection have a male partner who exhibits penile colonization with *Candida* but who may or may not be symptomatic. *Candida* species are found in up to 55% of asymptomatic women of childbearing age. Generally those with symptomatic vaginitis have a predisposing factor such as pregnancy, recent antibiotic use, diabetes, immunosuppression, or oral contraceptive use. It is unclear whether HIV-infected women are more likely to develop symptomatic candida vaginitis. Women in warmer climates and those who wear tight-fitting, ill-ventilated clothing are also at higher risk for this infection.

Diagnosis is made by examination of vaginal secretions by wet saline or 10% potassium hydroxide preparation or by culture. This is important not only to identify yeast but also to ensure the absence of motile trichomonads, clue cells, or many white blood cells, any of which would suggest other etiologies or mixed infection.

Treatment is uncomplicated, with a variety of locally administered antifungal agents such as miconazole and clotrimazole or systemic therapy with oral imidazoles such as fluconazole.

### Trichomoniasis

Trichomoniasis is a common STD caused by the flagellated protozoan, *Trichomonas vaginalis*. The clinical syndrome in women ranges from asymptomatic carriage to frank vaginitis. Men are usually asymptomatic but may develop urethritis.

The prevalence of trichomoniasis in women attending STD clinics ranges from 7–32%. Its presence is associated with nonuse of barrier or oral contraceptives. The organism is identified in up to 40% of male partners and 85% of female partners of infected index cases. Fewer than 5% of urethritis in men is attributable to trichomonas. Hence, asymptomatic infections among men likely comprise an important reservoir. Approximately 5% of girls born to infected mothers may become infected, manifested as vaginitis. The high prevalence of trichomonads noted among individuals with gonorrhea warrants routine screening for other STDs among individuals in whom trichomonas is isolated.

Clinically, women present with a malodorous, frothy vaginal discharge and may have diffuse vaginal erythema. A wet preparation of vaginal fluid reveals the typical motile trichomonads and an excessive number of polymorphonuclear leukocytes. Treatment of the patient and sexual partners with one 2-g dose of metronidazole is effective.

### Bacterial Vaginosis

Bacterial vaginosis is the most common vaginal disease in women of childbearing age. Formerly referred to as nonspecific vaginitis, *Gardnerella* vaginitis, and *Haemophilus* vaginitis, this condition was viewed as an inconsequential disease by many primary care providers. More recent evidence, however, suggests an association between bacterial vaginosis and prematurity, chorioamnionitis, and PID.

Bacterial vaginosis is present in up to one third of women visiting STD clinics and in approximately 5% of those being seen for general medical reasons. Although originally thought to be caused by the anaerobe *Gardnerella vaginalis*, bacterial vaginosis is now understood to be due to the interaction of *G. vaginalis* with other anaerobic bacteria and genital mycoplasmas that have replaced *Lactobacillus*, the normal vaginal flora. Male partners may or may not be colonized with *G. vaginalis*.

Vaginal discharge exhibiting an amine-like (fishy) odor when treated with potassium hydroxide and having a pH greater than 4.7 is common, as are the presence of "clue cells" on a wet preparation. Clue cells are epithelial cells whose margins are obscured by adherent bacteria. Treatment recommendations are for 1 week of metronidazole. Routine treatment of male partners is not beneficial nor recommended.

## CASE HISTORY

### CASE HISTORY 1

A 15-year-old African-American female from Chicago was referred to the City of Chicago Social Hygiene Center (STD clinic) by a disease intervention specialist who had phoned her. The reason for referral was that a recent sexual partner had been diagnosed with trichomonas urethritis and had listed her as a sexual partner.

The patient had no significant prior medical or STD history. She denied intravenous drug use. No sexual partners were known to be bisexual, drug users, or hemophiliac. She had been sexually active for 3 years with fewer than five partners, including a new partner (index case) during the prior 3 months. She had never undergone a pelvic examination. She had no known allergies.

The patient denied vaginal discharge, dyspareunia, dysuria, abdominal pain, rash, or pruritus. Menstrual periods were regular; she had not missed a cycle. She did not use any form of contraception.

Physical examination revealed a thin teenaged female in no acute distress who appeared healthy. She was afebrile. The oral cavity, lymph nodes, skin, and abdomen were normal. The external genitalia were normal. The vagina was remarkable for the presence of a frothy, grayish white, malodorous discharge. The vaginal mucosa appeared beefy red. The cervix was erythematous and bleeding was easily induced. There was cervical motion tenderness and an endocervical whitish yellow discharge. Palpation of the adnexa was remarkable for left-sided tenderness, but no mass was appreciated. Rectovaginal exam also revealed some tenderness with abdominal palpation, but no discharge or intrarectal lesions were noted.

Laboratory evaluation was remarkable for the following: the wet preparation demonstrated trichomonas and ''clue cells'' but no yeast or hyphal elements; the Gram's stain of endocervical secretions had greater than 50 PMNs per high-power field, but no predominant microorganisms and specifically no gram-negative intra- or extracellular diplococci; an RPR and urine pregnancy test were negative. An HIV antibody test was advised, but the patient declined.

Gonorrhea cultures of throat, cervix, and rectum were obtained. An ELISA test for chlamydia was obtained from an endocervical specimen. A herpesvirus culture was taken from cervical secretions.

The patient was treated empirically with cefixime (400 mg) and 1 g of azithromycin, both orally (under direct observation in clinic). She was also given a supply of metronidazole (500 mg twice daily for 7 days), and was instructed to return to the clinic within 48 h and to refer her sexual partners from the prior 3 months for evaluation and therapy.

After 48 h, she returned to the clinic for evaluation. She still had no signs or symptoms. Examination revealed less cervical motion and adnexal tenderness but was otherwise unchanged. The gonorrhea cultures from the cervix and rectum were positive for *Neisseria gonorrhoeae*. The chlamydia and herpes assays were negative. A follow-up visit in 1 week was remarkable only for the presence of greater than 50 cells per high-power field

without other laboratory or clinical abnormalities. A repeat gonorrhea culture was negative.

## CASE 1 DISCUSSION

This case highlights many of the features seen in a variety of STD patients. The patient was initially referred for therapy by public health authorities as part of their routine contact tracing of a male with an atypical form of urethritis due to trichomonas. Although the patient admitted to no signs or symptoms of disease, her examination was quite abnormal. She was ultimately diagnosed with three separate infections: trichomonas vaginitis, bacterial vaginosis, and gonococcal cervicitis with salpingitis and rectal colonization. Infections such as these are common, particularly in patients with multiple sexual partners, who do not use barrier contraceptive methods, who become sexually active at a very early age, and who are from lower socioeconomic groups. Asymptomatic and multiple infections are likely, especially in this high-risk patient. Bacterial vaginosis, the most common infection in women attending STD clinics, may predispose patients to salpingitis. Fortunately in this case, the infection was easily treated as an outpatient. Many patients with salpingitis require hospitalization and even surgery if a tuboovarian abscess forms. She is still at risk for potential infertility and ectopic pregnancy even though she received adequate therapy before becoming symptomatic. With continued unprotected sexual activity and recurrent episodes of salpingitis the risks of tubal scarring, which can lead to ectopic pregnancy or permanent infertility, increase dramatically.

## REFERENCES

### Books

Holmes, K. K., and Mardh, P. A., Sparling, P. F., et al. *Sexually Transmitted Diseases.* New York: McGraw-Hill, 1990.
Jones, J. H. *Badblood.* New York: Free Press, 1981.
Merritt, H. H., et al. *Neurosyphilis.* New York: Oxford University Press, 1946.

### Review Articles

Centers for Disease Control, Division of STD/HIV Prevention. *Sexually Transmitted Disease Surveillance 1993*, December 1994.
Centers for Disease Control, Sexually Transmitted Diseases Treatment Guideline, September 1993. *MMWR* 42(RR-14): 1993.
Chapel, T. A. The signs and symptoms of secondary syphilis. *Sex. Transm. Dis.* 7:161, 1980.
Corey, L. Genital herpes. In: Holmes, K. K., Mardh, P. A., Sparling, P. F., et al., eds. *Sexually Transmitted Diseases.* New York: McGraw-Hill, 1990:391.
Healy, B. P. Cardiovascular syphilis. In: Holmes, K. K., Mardh, P. A., Sparling, P. F., et al., eds. *Sexually Transmitted Diseases.* New York: McGraw-Hill, 1990.
Hook, E. W., and Handsfield, H. H. Gonococcal infections in the adult. In: Holmes, K. K., Mardh, P. A.,

Sparling, P. F., et al., eds. *Sexually Transmitted Diseases.* New York: McGraw-Hill, 1990:150.

Merritt, H. H. Early clinical and laboratory manifestations of syphilis of the central nervous system. *N. Engl. J. Med. 223*:446, 1940.

Moran, J. S., and Levine, W. C. Drugs of choice for the treatment of uncomplicated gonococcal infections. *Clin. Infect. Dis. 20*(Suppl. 1):S47–65, 1995.

Musher, P. M. Biology of *Treponema pallidum.* In: Holmes, K. K., Mardh, P. A., Sparling, P. F., et al., eds. *Sexually Transmitted Diseases.* New York: McGraw-Hill, 1990:205.

Rolfs, R. T., Treatment of syphilis, 1993. *Clin. Infect. Dis. 20*(Suppl. 1):S23–38, 1995.

Schulte, J. M., and Schmid, G. P. Recommendations for treatment of chancroid. *Clin. Infect. Dis. 20*(Suppl. 1): S39–46, 1995.

Sparling, P. F. Biology of *Neisseria gonorrhoeae.* In: Holmes, K. K., Mardh, P. A., Sparling, P. F., et al., eds. *Sexually Transmitted Diseases.* New York: McGraw-Hill, 1990:131.

Stamm, W. E., and Holmes, K. K. *Chlamydia trachomatis* infection of the adult. In: Holmes, K. K., Mardh, P. A., Sparling, P. F., et al., eds. *Sexually Transmitted Diseases.* New York: McGraw-Hill, 1990:184.

Stone, K. M. Human papillomavirus and genital warts: Update on epidemiology and treatment. *Clin. Infect. Dis. 20*(Suppl. 1):S91–97, 1995.

Swartz, M. N. Neurosyphilis. In: Holmes, K. K., Mardh, P. A., Sparling, P. F., et al., eds. *Sexually Transmitted Diseases.* New York: McGraw-Hill, 1990:150.

Weber, J. T., and Johnson, R. E., New treatments for *Chlamydia trachomatis* genital infection. *Clin. Infect. Dis. 20*(Suppl. 1):S66–71, 1995.

**Original Articles**

Daling, J., et al. Sexual practices, sexually transmitted diseases, and the incidence of anal cancer. *N. Engl. J. Med. 317*:973, 1987.

Dowdle, W. R., et al. Association of antigenic type of herpesvirus hominis with site of viral recovery. *J. Immunol. 99*:974, 1967.

Greenblatt, R. M., Lukehart, S. A., Plummer, F. A., et al. Genital ulceration as a risk factor for human immunodeficiency virus infection. *AIDS 2*:47, 1988.

Guinan, M. E., et al. Genital herpes simplex virus infection. *Epidemiol. Rev. 7*:127, 1988.

Jaschek, G., et al. Direct detection of *Chlamydia trachomatis* in urine specimens from symptomatic and asymptomatic men by using a rapid polymerase chain reaction assay. *J. Clin. Microbiol. 31*(5):1209–1212, 1993.

Madiedo, G., et al. False positive VDRL and FTA in cerebrospinal fluid. *JAMA 244*:688, 1980.

Ohye, R., et al. Decreased susceptibilty of *Neisseria gonorrhoeae* to fluoroquinolones—Ohio and Hawaii, 1992–94. *MMWR 43*:18, 1994.

Olansky, S., et al. Untreated syphilis in the male Negro. X: Twenty years of clinical observation of untreated syphilitic and presumably nonsyphilitic groups. *J. Chronic Dis. 4*:177, 1956.

Rockwell, D. H., et al. The Tuskegee study of untreated syphilis. *Arch. Intern. Med. 114*:792, 1964.

Sellors, J. W., et al. Comparison of cervical, urethral, and urine specimens for the detection of *Chlamydia trachomatis* in women. *J. Infect. Dis. 164*:205–208, 1991.

Shafer, M. A., et al. Evaluation of urine-based screening strategies to detect *Chlamydia trachomatis* among sexually active asymptomatic young males. *JAMA 270*:2065–2070, 1993.

Stamm, W. E., Handsfield, H. H., Rompalo, A. M., et al. The association between genital ulcer disease and acquisition of HIV infection in homosexual men. *JAMA 260*:1429, 1988.

Taylor-Robinson, D., et al. Human intra-urethral inoculation of ureaplasmas. *Q. J. Med. 46*:309, 1977.

# V GASTROINTESTINAL TRACT INFECTIONS

# 17

# INFECTIOUS DIARRHEA

STUART JOHNSON, M.D. and STANFORD T. SHULMAN, M.D.

Infectious diarrhea is a leading cause of morbidity and mortality worldwide, particularly for young children living in developing or underdeveloped countries. Diarrheal diseases in these areas reflect socioeconomic factors such as lack of clean drinking water, inefficient disposal of sewage, and malnutrition. Significant improvement in these basic public health measures may need to be preceded by some form of economic and political stability such as that achieved in more developed countries. In 1900, the annual death rate from diarrheal disease in New York City was 5603 per 100,000 infants. In 1980, in the United States it was 3.5 per 100,000 infants, a decrease of more than 1000-fold. However, economic progress and modernization in this country has, paradoxically, exposed large segments of the population to increased risk of diarrhea and enteric disease. Large-scale food production and preparation with subsequent widespread product distribution has facilitated major outbreaks of salmonellosis, enterohemorrhagic *Escherichia coli* infection, and other enteric infections. Breakdowns in technique or equipment in metropolitan water treatment facilities in this country and abroad have also led to massive outbreaks of cryptosporidiosis and cholera. Therefore, most people in both developed and underdeveloped countries are at significant risk for enteric disease. This chapter describes the major bacterial and viral agents associated with enteric infection and compares the pathogenesis of the diseases they produce.

## BACTERIAL DIARRHEA

As a background for this discussion, it should be kept in mind that the gastrointestinal tract facilitates huge fluxes of water. Approximately 9 L of fluid (primarily from the salivary, gastric, biliary, and pancreatic secretions) enters the adult upper intestinal tract each day and, yet, fecal water content is typically less than 200 mL/day. The majority of this fluid is absorbed in the small intestine. The absorptive and secretory functions of the intestine are also separated spatially; secretion occurs primarily through the crypt cells, whereas absorption occurs through cells in the villus tips. The flow of water across the intestinal mucosa follows osmotic gradients that are produced by ionic gradients. Therefore, water content of the stool is intimately dependent on intestinal electrolyte transport. It follows that large-volume, watery stools can be a consequence of either anatomic disruption of villus tips as is seen in viral enteritis, or they can be a consequence of increased luminal chloride secretion as is seen in cholera. The site of both these infections is in the small intestine, where the major fluxes of fluid occur.

Bacteria cause disease in the intestinal tract by several mechanisms: toxin production, including "pure" enterotoxins with resultant fluid secretion but without epithelial disruption and various types of tissue destructive cytotoxins; adherence and effacement of the intestinal brush border; decreased intestinal motility; and epithelial invasion with elicitation of host inflammatory responses. Several virulence factors are often employed by an individual pathogen, but regardless of specific virulence determinants, all enteric pathogens must overcome important nonspecific host defenses (e.g., gastric acidity, proteases, mucin, and intestinal motility) and colonize the host first. One exception to this dogma involves ingestion of preformed toxins, exemplified by botulism and staphylococcal and clostridial food poisoning.

Despite the diverse pathogenic mechanisms employed by individual species, infectious enteritides can be classified as one or both of two basic syndromes: inflammatory diarrhea and noninflammatory or secretory diarrhea. Pathogens that produce secretory diarrhea syndromes colonize the small intestine and typically elaborate an enterotoxin, leading to luminal fluid accumulation manifested clinically by large-volume, watery stools. The prototypical secretory pathogen is *Vibrio cholerae*. The other syndrome, inflammatory diarrhea, is typified by the dysentery produced by *Shigella* species. Dysentery refers to the passage of frequent, small-volume stools accompanied by blood and mucus, abdominal cramping, and tenesmus. These symptoms are associated with bacterial invasion of the intestinal wall, usually the distal colon, with epithelial necrosis, focal mucosal ulceration, and an acute inflammatory response as manifested by red blood cells and large numbers of neutrophils in the stool.

An additional enteric disease syndrome involves penetration of intact mucosa with bacterial multiplication in the lymphatic, reticuloendothelial system. This syndrome is referred to as enteric fever and is exemplified by infection with *Salmonella typhi*. Systemic symptoms such as fever and headache are prominent in this syndrome, and diarrhea is often not present. If present, diarrhea often occurs well after the onset of systemic symptoms. A brief summary of the characteristic distinguishing features of the most common causes of bacterial enteric disease is given in Table 17–1.

Screening fecal specimens for leukocytes and occult blood has been proposed as a rapid, simple test to differentiate inflammatory and noninflammatory diarrheas and to reduce the number of specimens submitted for culture. If inflammatory cells are present, identification of the type (e.g., neutrophils or mononuclear cells) may also be helpful in determining the kind of diarrhea syndrome involved. Typically, dysentery due to shigellosis results in stool smears showing 80–90% neutrophils, reflecting the acute inflammatory reaction following mucosal penetration. Typhoid fever is associated with a large number of mononuclear inflammatory cells on smear. Cholera and infection with enterotoxigenic *E. coli* or viral agents are characterized by the absence of fecal inflammatory cells. However, the sensitivity and specificity of these tests for detecting inflammatory diarrhea is low, particularly for inflammatory pathogens other than *Shigella* species. When interpreted in the context of clinical findings, examination of mucus from a fresh stool specimen stained with methylene blue can be helpful in the evaluation of community-acquired diarrheas, but has no role in the evaluation of nosocomial diarrhea.

In addition to the more common bacterial etiologies of acute infectious diarrhea listed in Table 17–1, several "new" pathogens have been recognized. *Aeromonas hydrophila* has been recovered from children with acute diarrhea and adults with more chronic symp-

## TABLE 17–1.    CHARACTERISTICS OF ENTEROPATHOGENIC BACTERIAL INFECTIONS

| Organism | Enteric Syndrome* | Site of Infection | Bloody Stools† | Fecal WBCs† | Risk of Person–Person Transmission‡ | Pathogenic Mechanism | Extraintestinal Manifestations |
|---|---|---|---|---|---|---|---|
| *Escherichia coli* (EC) | | | | | | | |
| Enteropathogenic EC | Secretory | Small bowel | 0 | 0 | Low | Epithelial effacement | Rare |
| Enteroadherent EC | Secretory | Small bowel | 0 | 0 | Low | ? | Rare |
| Enterotoxigenic EC | Secretory | Small bowel | 0 | 0 | Low | Enterotoxin production | Rare |
| Enteroinvasive EC | Inflammatory | Colon | + | ++ | Low | Invasion | Rare |
| Enterohemorrhagic EC | Inflammatory | Colon | ++ | 0 | High | Epithelial effacement? | Hemolytic-uremic syndrome, thrombocytopenic purpura |
| *Salmonella typhi* | Enteric fever | Small bowel (ileum) | 0 | ± | Low | Replication within macrophages | Bacteremia, hepatitis, splenomegaly |
| *Salmonella typhimurium* | Inflammatory | Small bowel & colon | ± | ± | Mod§ | Invasion | Abscess, osteomyelitis |
| *Shigella dysenteriae* type 1 | Inflammatory | Colon | ++ | ++ | High | Invasion | Hemolytic-uremic syndrome, protein-energy malnutrition |
| *Shigella sonnei/flexneri* | Inflammatory | Colon | 0 | + | High | Invasion | Rare |
| *Vibrio cholerae* | Secretory | Small bowel | 0 | 0 | Low | Enterotoxin production | Rare |
| *Yersinia enterocolitica* | Inflammatory Enteric fever? | Small bowel (ileum) & colon? | + | ± | Low | Invasion? Resistance to phagocytosis | Mesenteric adenitis, bacteremia, abscess, reactive arthritis, erythema nodosum |
| *Campylobacter jejuni* | Inflammatory | Small bowel & colon | ± | + | Low | Invasion? | Occasional bacteremia, reactive arthritis, Guillain-Barré syndrome |
| *Clostridium difficile* | Secretory & inflammatory | Colon | 0 | ± | High§ | Enterotoxin (cytotoxin?) production | Rare |

*See text for definitions.

†++, very common; +, frequently present; ±, variably present; 0, uncommon or rare.

‡Risk of direct person-to-person contact usually relates to the infectious inoculum required to cause disease (e.g., $10^2$ for *Shigella*, $10^8$ for *Vibrio cholerae*).

§High risk of transmission for *Clostridium difficile* (and for nontyphoidal salmonellae to a lesser extent) applies to contacts who have had prior or current antimicrobial treatment as often occurs in the hospital setting.

toms and a history of drinking untreated water. *Plesiomonas shigelloides* has been associated with self-limited inflammatory diarrhea syndromes in association with raw shellfish consumption or foreign travel. More recently, enterotoxin-producing strains of *Bacteroides fragilis* have been associated with noninflammatory diarrhea in Apache children in Arizona.

In contrast to these aforementioned causes of community-acquired diarrheas, *Clostridium difficile* is a major and the only important recognized cause of nosocomial, or hospital-acquired, diarrhea. This pathogen, which produces features of both secretory and inflammatory diarrheas, is discussed in more detail in Chapter 27. Early on it was speculated that this organism was part of the normal human bacterial flora, present in the intestine in low numbers, and that it proliferated following antimicrobial therapy. Antimicrobial therapy functions to ablate the colonization resistance afforded by other enteric flora. It is now clear that *C. difficile* infections are primarily acquired, similar to other enteric infections, but this pathogen is unique with respect to its strong association with antimicrobial therapy and reservoirs of infection.

In addition to acute infectious diarrhea, persistent diarrhea, often defined as more than 14 days in duration, is a major cause of morbidity and mortality in underdeveloped regions. In many studies comparing etiologies, the same pathogens have been found in children with acute (self-limited) and persistent diarrheal illnesses, and it appears that these children are susceptible to reinfections with new pathogens. Other studies have noted certain pathogens, such as enteroaggregative *E. coli*, in association with persistent diarrhea. Although most bacterial pathogens that cause acute self-limited diarrhea occasionally cause prolonged episodes, *C. difficile* is one of the few agents that frequently cause chronic symptoms when not recognized and treated appropriately.

## Infection with *Escherichia coli*

Recognition of *Escherichia coli* as a human pathogen was complicated by the fact that this organism is also the most common facultative anaerobic bacterium of normal human colonic flora. Early serotyping studies, however, revealed an association of certain *E. coli* strains with infantile diarrhea. These strains, originally designated O111:B4 and O55:B5, were associated with a number of outbreaks of lethal diarrhea in infants in England, Mexico, and Scotland in the 1940s. In the years following these outbreaks, additional serotypes also isolated from babies with severe diarrhea were described. Serotyping involves three distinct *E. coli* antigens: lipopolysaccharide, the O or heat-stable somatic antigen; heat-labile capsular "K" antigen; and the heat-labile flagellar "H" antigen. The pathogenic mechanism by which most of these serologically identified "enteropathogenic" strains cause diarrhea was not enterotoxin production or mucosal invasion, but rather was the consequence of specific types of epithelial adhesion. It was subsequently shown that other strains of *E. coli* cause diarrhea by producing various enterotoxins and cytotoxins, by direct epithelial cell invasion, as well as by epithelial adhesion. In light of the marked diversity of enteric pathogens in general, it is remarkable that this one species, *E. coli*, demonstrates nearly the entire variety of mechanisms by which enteric pathogens cause diarrhea. Diarrheagenic *E. coli* are now classified as enteropathogenic, enteroadherent (or enteroaggregative), enterotoxigenic, enteroinvasive, and enterohemorrhagic.

## *Enteropathogenic* Escherichia coli

Enteropathogenic *E. coli* (EPEC) now refers to diarrheagenic *E. coli* of specific serotypes that do not produce classic virulence factors. The pathogenic mechanism for many of these strains involves a particular type of epithelial adherence. These strains adhere to and efface the brush border of small intestinal epithelium. *In vitro* they adhere to Hep-2 cells in a focal manner; other pathogenic strains adhere to Hep-2 cells in a diffuse pattern.

The most common disease association of EPEC is the syndrome of epidemic infantile diarrhea. Classically, this disease is seen in hospital nurseries where infants develop the sudden onset of severe, watery diarrhea leading to dehydration and shock; a high mortality rate accompanies the disease. During 1960 and 1961 in Chicago, more than 1300 cases of gastroenteritis with 77 deaths occurred in infants and young children. The highest attack rate was in newborn infants, who also had the highest death rate (16%). The basis of the unique susceptibility of infants to EPEC is not clear but the risk is lower in breast-fed infants, and susceptibility may involve, at least in part, the lack of specific immunity. Hospital nursery outbreaks are now uncommon in developed countries but still occur in the developing world. EPEC is also responsible for sporadic cases of acute diarrhea.

### Enteroadherent Escherichia coli

In contrast to EPEC, enteroadherent *E. coli* (EAEC) are classified by their virulence factors rather than by serotype. This distinction from EPEC is somewhat confusing, as the pathogenesis of disease due to both EAEC and EPEC primarily involve adherence. In contrast to EPEC, most EAEC strains *in vitro* exhibit aggregative adherence patterns on Hep-2 cells. EAEC has been implicated in traveler's diarrhea and sporadic cases of diarrhea in children. Recently, aggregative EAEC has been associated with persistent diarrheal disease in children.

### Enterotoxigenic Escherichia coli

Enterotoxigenic *E. coli* (ETEC) produce one or both of two protein toxins, one heat-labile (LT), which activates adenylate cyclase and is inactivated by heat, and the other heat-stable (ST), which activates guanylate cyclase. The biochemical and physiologic characteristics of these two toxins are given in Table 17–2. ETEC also produce structural pili, which are necessary for the attachment of the organism to intestinal epithelial cells. In distinction from most other *E. coli*, these pili are mannose resistant. Although some ETEC strains may produce adherence factors other than pili, adherence of the organism is a critical step in the pathogenesis of diarrhea, allowing for colonization and subsequent toxin elaboration. At least five antigenically distinct pili or colonization factors (CFA I–V) are produced by ETEC. Both LT and ST, as well as the CFAs, are encoded by transferable plasmids.

LT is a large (MW=86,000) subunit toxin that is immunologically similar to cholera toxin and has the same subunit structure of five B units and one A unit. Similar to cholera toxin, the B subunit of LT binds to the $GM_1$ ganglioside initiating the chain of events that leads to adenylate cyclase activation and chloride secretion. ST is a much smaller molecule than LT (MW~2000) composed of a single peptide that is less antigenic than LT. There are two variants of ST (STaI and STaII) that are important in human disease and a variant (STb) that is important in porcine disease. The mechanism of action of ST also involves enterocyte receptors but with subsequent activation of guanylate cyclase.

Individual *E. coli* strains may produce one or both of the enterotoxins, depending on their plasmids. Organisms carrying both types of plasmids usually are associated with more severe diarrhea for a longer period than are those carrying plasmids only for ST. There is some association between serotype and enterotoxin type. *E. coli* strains associated with enterotoxin formation and watery diarrhea are only rarely found in infections of the urinary tract, wounds, meningitis, or other nonenteric sites.

Assays for the detection of ETEC are available as research tools and are based on the phenotypic or genotypic demonstration of the enterotoxins. These assays include the isolated rabbit ileal loop model, a suckling mouse assay, cell culture assay, immunologic assays that demonstrate LT in the stool or culture fluid specimens, and the identification of enterotoxin-producing genes using oligonucleotide probes. Culture of *E. coli* for unique biochemical or colonial characteristics is of little value.

ETEC is the most common bacterial etiology of acute bacterial diarrhea worldwide, both in regard to traveler's diarrhea and the acute diarrhea of residents of those areas in which traveler's diarrhea is acquired. Children under 2 years of age are most commonly affected in these areas, but ETEC may also

**TABLE 17–2.  COMPARISON OF HEAT-LABILE (LT) AND HEAT-STABLE (ST) TOXINS OF *ESCHERICHIA COLI***

| | | | ASSAY MODEL | | | |
|---|---|---|---|---|---|---|
| | **HEAT RESISTANCE (100°C)** | **IMMUNOLOGICALLY RELATED TO *VIBRIO CHOLERAE*** | *Y1 Hamster/Adrenal Tumor Cell Culture* | *Chinese Hamster Ovary Cell Culture* | *Rabbit Ileal Loop* | *Suckling Mouse* |
| *E. coli* Labile toxin | − | + | + | + | + | − |
| *E. coli* Stable toxin | + | − | − | − | + | + |

produce cholera-like diarrhea in the adult residents of these regions. The most common mode of spread of ETEC is through contaminated food. Between 1975 and 1994, 13 U.S. outbreaks of ETEC gastroenteritis were reported to the Centers for Disease Control (CDC), of which 9 were food-borne. Humans are the only known source of ETEC and asymptomatic carriage may be the most important reservoir of this infection.

Certain of the serologically defined "enteropathogenic" E. coli strains also produce enterotoxins. Because the genes for enterotoxin and pili are located on plasmids, these virulence determinants can be transferred to other E. coli strains and other gram-negative bacteria. A nursery outbreak of epidemic infantile diarrhea has been described in which enterotoxigenic E. coli, Klebsiella, and Citrobacter of different serotypes were isolated. It appears that certain E. coli serotypes are particularly well adapted to accept and maintain these plasmids.

### Enteroinvasive Escherichia coli

A number of well-studied outbreaks of dysentery caused by E. coli have been described, particularly in adults, and usually associated with contaminated food. These outbreaks are similar to those caused by Shigella, and the symptoms include severe abdominal cramping with bloody diarrhea. In these outbreaks, the isolated E. coli strains have the ability to penetrate and replicate within epithelial cells to cause focal epithelial necrosis, characteristics not possessed by enterotoxin-producing strains. The histologic differences between disease produced by ETEC and enteroinvasive E. coli are apparent in Figure 17–1. As in Shigella, a large plasmid (140 MD [megadalton]) encodes for invasiveness.

### Enterohemorrhagic Escherichia coli

Enterohemorrhagic E. coli (EHEC) strains produce one or more shiga-like, or verotoxins, that are bacteriophage encoded. Shiga-like toxin 1 is nearly identical to the shiga toxin produced by Shigella dysenteriae type 1. The pathogenesis of EHEC disease is unknown but may involve direct effects of the toxins on epithelial and endothelial cells or may be mediated by the host inflammatory response. EHEC strains are associated with a few specific serotypes.

In 1982, two outbreaks of acute hemorrhagic enteritis occurred in Oregon and Michigan in association with hamburger patties served by a fast-food chain. At least 47 people were affected by an unusual syndrome characterized by severe crampy abdominal pains, grossly bloody copious diarrhea without fecal leukocytes, and little or no fever. No previously recognized pathogens were recovered from stool specimens. However, a rare E. coli serotype, O157:H7, was isolated from 9 of 20 cases (but not from controls) and from an implicated meat patty. Since that original outbreak, E. coli O157:H7 has been associated with multiple food-borne outbreaks and sporadic cases of bloody diarrhea. Although other foods have been implicated, consumption of undercooked ground beef is the most frequently documented vehicle. The major reservoir appears to be healthy cattle whose meat becomes contaminated with intestinal contents during slaughter and processing. One outbreak in 1993 was associated with more than 500 laboratory-confirmed cases and four deaths involving people in four states who consumed hamburgers at one restaurant chain.

Although bloody diarrhea with severe abdominal cramping is the most common clinical manifestation, the spectrum of illness includes asymptomatic infection, nonbloody diarrhea, the hemolytic-uremic syndrome (HUS), thrombotic thrombocytopenic purpura (TTP), and death. Patients at the extremes of age are at increased risk for symptomatic illness and the more severe manifestations such as HUS and TTP. E. coli O157:H7 was isolated from 46% of children with HUS in Minnesota, and the incidence of HUS increased from 1979 to 1988. Attendance at day-care centers was one risk factor in that study; evidence of secondary transmission in family contacts of infected patients suggests that a low inoculum size may be sufficient to cause disease with E. coli O157:H7.

E. coli O157:H7 isolates can be identified presumptively by lack of sorbitol fermentation on MacConkey-sorbitol agar culture plates sent for serotyping at reference laboratories. Antimicrobials have not yet been shown to be effective in treatment of E. coli O157:H7 infections, and some agents such as trimethoprim-sulfamethoxazole increase toxin production, at least in vitro.

### Salmonellosis

Salmonellae display marked antigenic diversity as evidenced by the identification of more than 2000 serotypes. Molecular analysis, however, indicates there is only one Salmonella

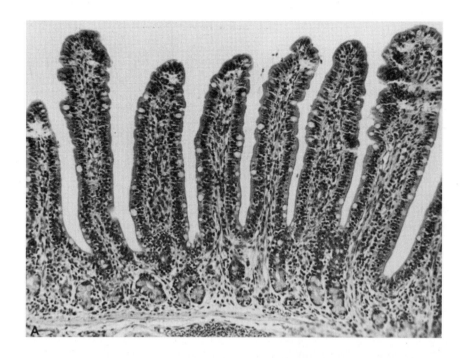

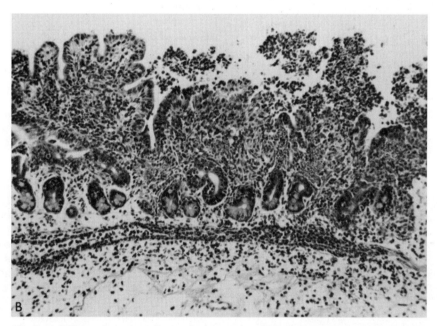

**FIGURE 17-1.** *A,* Effects of enterotoxin-producing strains of *Escherichia coli* on rabbit ileum (× 170). Section of ligated small bowel loop 7 h after inoculation with enterotoxin-producing organisms shows normal morphology. *B,* Effect of epithelium-penetrating strains of *E. coli* on rabbit ileum. Section of ligated loop 7 h after inoculation with penetrating organisms shows marked mucosal disarray, with necrosis, ulceration, and intense acute inflammatory reaction. (From DuPont, H. L., Formal, S. B., Hornick, R. B., et al. Pathogenesis of *Escherichia coli* diarrhea. *N. Engl. J. Med. 285*:1, 1971. Reprinted by permission from the *New England Journal of Medicine.*)

species with multiple strains or variants based on differences in somatic cell-wall lipopolysaccharide (O) and flagellar protein (H) antigens. The Kauffman-White classification recognizes nine serogroups (A through I) defined by O antigens and serotypes within the groups defined by H antigens. A clinically useful categorization groups *Salmonella* according to host preference: those whose natural host is humans (*S. typhi* and *S. paratyphi*), those adapted primarily to animals (*S. choleraesuis*), and those capable of inducing disease in animals and man (>2000 serotypes). A recent new isolate in Chicago has been named *Salmonella mjordan* after a prominent Chicagoan. Despite the great diversity in this last group, 10 serotypes generally account for about 70% of clinical isolates (Table 17–3). The similarity of serotypes between human and animal isolates illustrates the pattern of spread between humans and their food supply.

The widespread dissemination of *Salmonella* in this country reflects, in part, a vicious circle in the food-processing industry, particularly in egg and poultry production. Poultry growers use high-protein additives as food supplements. These additives are obtained from slaughterhouse by-products and mixed with feed grains. Many of the by-products are derived from animals with a high incidence of infection with salmonellae. Once ingested, the salmonellae proliferate within the bird's gastrointestinal tract. Varying numbers of salmonellae remain in the region of the cloaca, contaminating the surface of eggs and remaining in the bird after evisceration and

dressing. For example, the incidence of salmonella contaminating 50-lb cans of pooled, frozen eggs has been found on occasion to be greater than 50%. Transovarian contamination of eggs has also been postulated as the mechanism for the frequent large outbreaks of *S. enteritidis* in the northeast United States.

The frequency of salmonellae in our food supply suggests that although more than 40,000 isolates of salmonella were recorded from humans in recent years, the actual incidence of salmonellosis is considerably greater. The possibility that most of the population in the United States has had mild clinical or subclinical infection, and therefore has been actively immunized by salmonella early in life, is suggested by Figure 17–2, in which the rate of isolation of salmonellae from humans is plotted against age. The large number of isolates from children under 10 years of age and the uniformly low incidence after age 10 may indicate a high proportion of immune persons, particularly in view of the potentially widespread exposure. As seen in Figure 17–3, the reported number of cases of salmonella infection in the United States has risen steadily since 1960.

### Clinical Syndromes

In humans, salmonella infection occurs in one of three forms: (1) most commonly, acute gastroenteritis; (2) enteric fever, such as typhoid or paratyphoid fever; and (3) extraintestinal focal infections, such as osteomyelitis, abscess, empyema, and local infection at the site of peripheral vascular prostheses. Several virulence factors for *Salmonella* have been studied, but the features that determine the particular disease manifestation is unknown. A moderately large inoculum ($10^6$–$10^9$) is necessary to infect normal volunteers, making person-to-person transmission somewhat difficult. However, in patients with compromised host defenses the critical inoculum size may be lower. Conditions that lower gastric acidity, decrease gastrointestinal motility, and alter intestinal flora (e.g., antimicrobials) predispose patients to infection. Person-to-person transmission or cross-infection by nontyphoidal salmonellae occurs in hospitals; antimicrobial treatment is a significant associated risk in this setting. The ability to survive within macrophages following phagocytosis is an important feature of salmonellae, and conditions associated with macrophage dysfunction may further predispose patients. Several diseases in which functional "blockage" of macrophages

**TABLE 17–3.   TEN MOST COMMON *SALMONELLA* SEROTYPES FROM HUMANS, U.S. 1992***

| RANK | SEROTYPE | No. | PERCENTAGE |
|---|---|---|---|
| 1 | S. typhimurium | 7894 | 23 |
| 2 | S. enteritidis | 6547 | 19 |
| 3 | S. heidelberg | 2519 | 7 |
| 4 | S. hadar | 1526 | 4 |
| 5 | S. newport | 1478 | 4 |
| 6 | S. agona | 748 | 2 |
| 7 | S. thompson | 689 | 2 |
| 8 | S. javiana | 646 | 2 |
| 9 | S. oranienburg | 595 | 2 |
| 10 | S. montevideo | 558 | 2 |
| 2000 | S. mjordan | 1 | 0 |
|  | Total | 23,201 | 67 |
|  | Total (all serotypes) | 34,520 |  |

*From Centers for Disease Control, Annual Summary 1992, Salmonella Surveillance, 1993. With permission

occurs show an increased incidence and severity of salmonellosis. These diseases include sickle cell anemia, malaria, bartonellosis, louse-borne relapsing fever, and disseminated histoplasmosis. The specific role of enterotoxins, outer membrane lipopolysaccharide, and the Vi antigen are unknown. The capsular polysaccharide Vi antigen seen in most *S. typhi* strains correlates with virulence experimentally and may function by inhibition of complement-mediated phagocytosis, similar to the role of capsular polysaccharides in *Streptococcus pneumoniae* and *Haemophilus influenzae* infections.

**Gastroenteritis.** Acute gastroenteritis varies from very mild to severe infection and may occasionally be associated with bacteremia or bacteriuria. In mild or moderate cases, prudent withholding of antibiotics does not slow the clinical recovery and results in more rapid clearing of the microorganism from the stool. The decision to withhold antibiotics depends on the severity of the illness in the individual patient and the presence of underlying disease, such as cancer, immunologic defects including acquired immunodeficiency syndrome (AIDS), and sickle cell disease, which could impair host defense mechanisms. Recent experience in several studies with quinolones confirms older observations that antimicrobial treatment of *Salmonella* gastroenteritis often prolongs fecal excretion.

Signs and symptoms of salmonella gastroenteritis vary widely but usually include nausea, abdominal cramps, and diarrhea, which sometimes becomes bloody. The microorganisms may invade focal areas of the small and large intestine, where they are ingested by neutrophils and macrophages in the lamina propria (Fig. 17–4). Sigmoidoscopic and biopsy studies of humans with salmonellosis may show active colitis, with focal ulceration and submucosal microabscesses.

**Enteric Fever.** In contrast to nontyphoidal salmonellae, *Salmonella typhi* causes gastrointestinal symptoms only late in the course of the disease, usually after prolonged fever. *S. typhi* is an example of a facultative intracellular parasite that survives well within macrophages, and enteric fever is primarily a systemic infection involving the reticuloendothelial system. *S. paratyphi* A, *S. schott-*

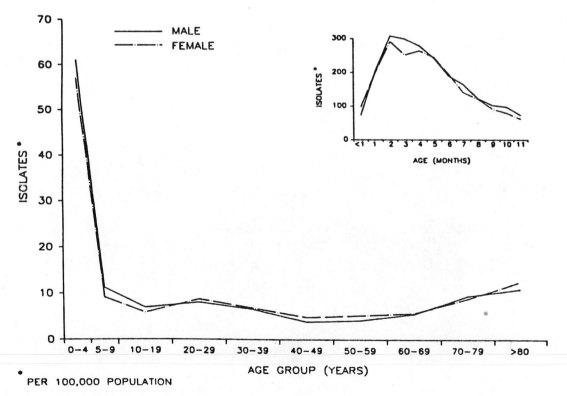

**FIGURE 17–2.** Rate of reported isolates of *Salmonella*, by age in the United States in 1980. (From Centers for Disease Control. *Salmonella Surveillance, Annual Summary 1980*, U.S. Department of Health and Human Services, Public Health Service, December 1982, p. 3. With permission.)

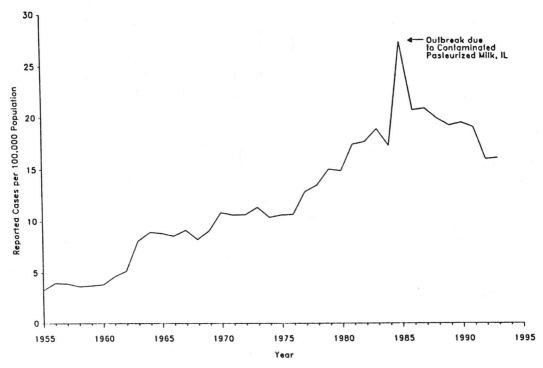

**FIGURE 17–3.** Salmonellosis (excluding typhoid fever): data for 1955–1993 (by year) for the United States. (From *Morbidity and Mortality Weekly Report.* Summary of notifiable disease, United States 1993. October 21, 1994, p. 50. With permission.)

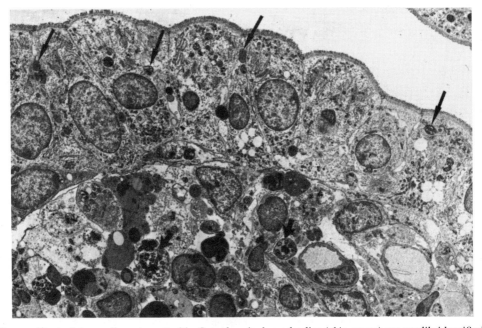

**FIGURE 17–4.** Salmonella gastroenteritis. Cytoplasmic dense bodies (*thin arrows*) are readily identified. Bacteria are absent from epithelium. In contrast, many phagocytosed bacteria (*thick arrows*) are present in neutrophils and macrophages in the lamina propria (× 2500). (From Takeuchi, A., and Sprinz, H. Electron-microscope studies of experimental *Salmonella* infection in the preconditioned guinea pig. *Am. J. Pathol. 51*:137, 1967. With permission.)

*muelleri,* and *S. hirschfeldii* may also cause a clinical syndrome of enteric fever similar to that of *S. typhi.*

Once the defense mechanisms of the upper gastrointestinal tract are overcome, *S. typhi* penetrate the distal small intestine at the site of Peyer's patches, localized lymphoid structures which hypertrophy during the course of infection. Complications of this lymphoid hyperplasia include necrosis and ulceration that may lead to hemorrhage or intestinal perforation, which usually manifests during the second week of illness. After infection of the Peyer's patches, the organisms migrate (likely in phagocytized cells) to regional lymph nodes, which in turn hypertrophy. Subsequently, they reach the systemic circulation and localize in reticuloendothelial organs such as the liver and spleen.

Clinically, enteric fever is insidious in onset, with stepwise increase in temperature over the first several days, then becoming sustained. Although not a specific sign of enteric fever, the pulse is typically slow, out of relation to the temperature elevation. The natural course of untreated typhoid fever demonstrates sustained fever for 3–4 weeks with gradual resolution. Systemic symptoms, such as headache, predominate over gastrointestinal symptoms, and constipation is often present rather than diarrhea. A faint maculopapular, salmon-colored rash, refered to as rose spots, may be recognized on the trunk of light-skinned patients early in the illness. *S. typhi* may be cultured from the stool early and late during the course of infection and from the blood, liver, and bone marrow. Serologic diagnosis has traditionally involved the Widal test (febrile agglutinins), which measures agglutinating antibodies against O and H antigens, but is neither sensitive nor specific.

*S. typhi* is spread by contaminated food or polluted water supplies in underdeveloped countries and primarily by contaminated food in the United States. As humans are the only known hosts, outbreaks of typhoid fever can usually be traced to an infected individual ("Typhoid Mary") who is invariably asymptomatic but fecally shedding. The nidus of chronic carriage is within the biliary tree, and asymptomatic carriers often have abnormalities of the biliary system, such as stones. Chronic carriers can be identified serologically, as they typically have high titers of antibody to the Vi antigen.

The incidence of typhoid fever in the United States has been falling since 1900, although it has plateaued since the late 1960s. Approximately 500 cases occur annually in the United States, but it is estimated that 33 million cases with 500,000 deaths occur annually worldwide.

Antimicrobial therapy for typhoid fever has traditionally been with chloramphenicol because of its predictable response, relative safety, and low cost. Ampicillin, trimethoprim-sulfamethoxazole, cefoperazone, ceftriaxone, cefotaxime, and ciprofloxicin have also been effective. *In vitro* susceptibility does not always correlate with clinical response, and clinical trials are important to establish efficacy and duration of therapy needed. Despite good *in vitro* susceptibility, the aminoglycosides are not clinically useful, presumably because of their inactivity in the acid pH environment within the phagolysosomes where the salmonellae reside. In addition, antibiotic resistance has been increasing worldwide. An outbreak of multi–drug-resistant *S. typhi* occurred in 1990 in India in which 81% of strains were resistant to ampicillin, streptomycin, tetracyline, and chloramphenicol and 40% of strains were resistant to trimethoprim-sulfamethoxazole. To date, resistance to quinolones has not been a problem, and they remain the drug of choice for multi–drug-resistant strains, at least in adults. Furazolidone may also be an acceptable alternative agent.

Although improved hygiene and sanitation are important public health priorities in regards to prevention of typhoid fever, vaccination has shown moderate success and may become a more important intervention in the future (see Chapter 40).

**Extraintestinal Infection.** Extraintestinal infections with salmonellae are frequently associated with other chronic disease or with a defect in host defenses. Neonates and young infants more frequently develop sepsis and extraintestinal foci of infections with salmonella (e.g., meningitis). Therefore, antibiotic therapy is indicated for gastroenteritis in this age group. Patients with sickle cell disease are more susceptible to infection (particularly osteomyelitis) with salmonella, and patients with metastatic cancer are more prone to develop extraintestinal infections than the normal population. The increased incidence of salmonella disease in cancer and in sickle cell patients may be in part related to localization of microorganisms in foci of poor perfusion.

A variety of nontyphoidal salmonellae have been found to produce infections of peripheral vascular grafts. Grafts of abdominal aortic and femoral arterial bypasses frequently yield salmonella if individuals with these prostheses develop any form of salmonella infection. This may reflect periodic bacteremia following subclinical or mild intestinal infections. Intravascular salmonellae tend to localize at sites of atheromatous ulceration and to set up foci of proliferation and infection. Two serotypes, *S. choleraesuis* and *S. typhimurium*, are most commonly involved. The presence of foreign bodies in the vascular system, as elsewhere, predisposes to colonization by smaller numbers of microorganisms than otherwise are needed to initiate infection.

## Shigellosis

The four species of *Shigella*, *S. dysenteriae* (10 subtypes), *S. boydii*, *S. flexneri* (eight subtypes), and *S. sonnei* (one type), all cause invasive, inflammatory bowel disease of varying severity. For reasons that are not apparent, the incidence of various species has varied in different parts of the world over cycles of several years. For many years, *S. flexneri* was the most common species isolated in the United States, but for the past 15 years, *S. sonnei* has been dominant. Several years ago, the appearance of the very virulent *S. dysenteriae* type 1 (Shiga's bacillus) from an endemic focus in Central America produced several outbreaks of severe disease in the southwestern United States.

In contrast to *Salmonella*, all *Shigella* species are restricted to humans as both a natural reservoir and as the major mode of dissemination. Shigellosis is transmitted by the fecal–oral route, primarily by hand-to-mouth contact, but also by food handlers and insect vectors (e.g., flies) in areas of food preparation. Where outdoor latrines are prevalent, the incidence of the disease is sometimes directly related to the large number of flies attracted to the latrines. The availability of water for frequent washing of hands is of importance in controlling outbreaks. As few as 10 bacilli are said to be capable of causing shigellosis, in contrast to the $10^6$ organisms necessary to induce salmonella enteric fever. Because of inadequate sanitary precautions, both shigellosis and hepatitis A are endemic in institutions for the care of mentally retarded children. Reflecting both the mode of fecal–oral transmission and perhaps some element of local immunization, the highest isolation rates for shigella are in children younger than 5 years old. Fatality rates are highest in young malnourished children. The incidence of bacillary dysentery in older age

groups is similar to that for salmonellosis. In contrast to salmonellosis, the reported incidence of shigella has been stable in the United States, after an earlier decline (Fig. 17–5).

Infections with *Shigella* involve direct tissue invasion, but in contrast to *Salmonella* they are usually limited to the epithelial cells lining and possibly the submucosa of the colon. Severe cases of shigella dysentery may be associated with focal mucosal destruction and deep ulceration, but the infection does not extend beyond the intestinal tract. Shigellae are rarely found in blood cultures. The limited exposure of shigellae to deep structures in the body may account for the minimal amounts of circulating antibody found in convalescent patients.

Epithelial cell invasion by *Shigella* involves multiple virulence determinants that are chromosomal and plasmid-encoded. Large virulence-associated plasmids (~140 MD) are present in all virulent *Shigella*. Once the organism attaches to the epithelial membrane, it is internalized by membrane-bound vesicles accompanied by actin polymerization, similar to the process involved in phagocytosis. The organism is then able to lyse the vesicle, multiply in the cytoplasm, and migrate to the cell periphery leaving a "trail" of F-actin deposition. Shigella is then able to invade adjacent cells, extending the destructive epithelial lesion. Several genes involved in this process have been characterized, including the *ipa* (invasion plasmid antigen) genes, *inv* (invasion) genes, and *virG* (involved in phagocytic vesicle release and cell-to-cell spread).

Shiga toxin is a potent cytotoxin produced in *S. dysenteriae* type 1 and some other *Shigella* strains, but its role in the pathogenesis is not clear. The toxin is a subunit protein (MW=74,000) composed of one A subunit and five B subunits with binding specificity for a specific microvillus membrane glycolipid receptor. The A subunit enzymatically cleaves the 28S ribosomal RNA of the 60S ribosomal subunit in eukaryotic cells with resultant inhibition of protein synthesis. The glycolipid receptor for the B subunits are located on the villus cells and not the crypt cells, thereby impairing sodium absorption without affecting chloride secretion and leading to net luminal fluid accumulation. This mechanism could explain the watery diarrhea syndromes seen in shigellosis, particularly early in the course of illness, but small bowel involvement has not been proven in shigellosis. Shiga toxin may

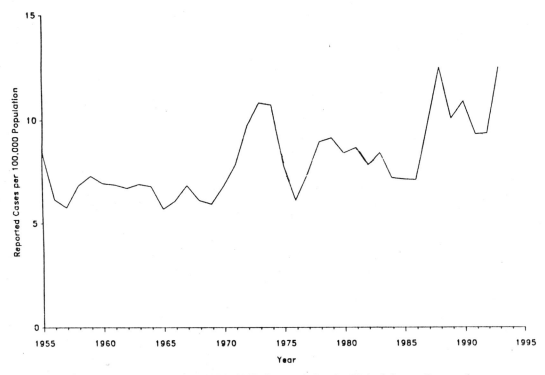

**FIGURE 17–5.** Shigellosis: data for 1955–1988 (by year) for the United States. Reported cases per 100,000 population. Data are from the National Shigella Surveillance System. (From *Morbidity and Mortality Weekly Report,* Summary of notifiable disease, United States 1993. October 21, 1994, p. 51. With permission.)

also be involved in HUS complicating *S. dysenteriae* type 1 infection by its effect on endothelial cells with resultant microangiopathic hemolysis.

Clinically, shigellosis is manifested by fever with subsequent watery diarrhea. Progression to bloody diarrhea and dysentery syndromes is primarily dependent on the *Shigella* species involved. Ulcerative lesions are most prominent in the distal colon and rectum, explaining the symptoms of pain and tenesmus. Occasionally, rectal prolapse occurs in young children. Hyponatremia and toxin-mediated encephalopathy and seizures often accompany shigellosis. More severe complications such as toxic megacolon, intestinal obstruction, and HUS are usually associated with infection by *S. dysenteriae* type 1. An important sequela of shigellosis is protein-losing enteropathy with loss of serum proteins. Shigellosis has a profound impact on protein-energy malnutrition in underdeveloped countries. Dysentery, not watery diarrhea, correlates best with growth impairment in Bangladeshi infants.

Diagnosis of *Shigella* enteritis is based on culture of the organism and clinical findings.

Examination of fecal mucus for leukocytes is also helpful to distinguish shigellosis from amebiasis, the major differential of adult dysentery in the tropics. Fecal leukocytes are present in shigellosis and are typically absent in amebiasis, probably secondary to leukocyte toxic affects of the trophozoite.

Whereas treatment of *Salmonella* gastroenteritis is generally not recommended, treatment of shigellosis shortens the duration of symptoms and is always indicated for treatment of *Shigella*-associated dysentery. Ampicillin and trimethoprim-sulfamethoxazole (TMP/SMZ) have been used traditionally for treatment of shigellosis because of their efficacy and safety in children. Increasing resistance to these agents, including recent reports of rates of 80% resistance to TMP/SMZ in India and Thailand, has led to search for alternate agents. Nalidixic acid has been used with apparent safety in children, but resistance to this agent develops rapidly. Currently, all *Shigella* strains are susceptible to the newer flouroquinolones, but their use in children has been cautioned because of the risk of arthropathy. A recent, large study of ciprofloxacin found that a single 1-g dose was effective for adult infections due to *Shigella* species other than *S. dysenteriae* type 1. Six of 25 patients who received one or two doses failed therapy, whereas none of 15 patients with *S. dysenteriae* type 1 infections who received 500 mg twice daily for 5 days failed. Ciprofloxacin in combination with loperamide has been used safely for dysentery not due to *S. dysenteriae* type 1. Ceftriaxone is an effective alternate therapy as is amidinocillin pivoxil.

## Cholera

*Vibrio cholerae* are gram-negative, curved, rod-shaped, motile bacteria with a single polar flagellum. The species consists of more than 70 serogroups based on differences of the O antigen. With one newly recognized exception, only strains in serogroup O1 have been capable of causing epidemic cholera. *V. cholera* O1 strains are further differentiated into two biotypes: "El Tor" associated with the 7th cholera pandemic, and "classic" which was predominant previously. There are also two serotypes within serogroup O1: *Inaba* and *Ogawa*.

Cholera is a disease only of humans. People and water contaminated by human feces are the major reservoirs of infection. Cholera is an ancient disease, having been known for thousands of years; epidemics consistent with cholera were described in early Sanskrit writings. The disease has been endemic in Asia for centuries and is most prevalent along the great rivers of the Indian subcontinent. Since the 19th century, seven pandemics of cholera have appeared, each claiming large numbers of lives. In England in 1849, John Snow, a perceptive physician, became convinced that the disease was being spread by the drinking water in London. To stop the use of drinking water from one well in an area of high infection, Snow removed the handle of the communal water-pump on Broad Street and succeeded in reducing the number of new cases, thereby helping to establish the importance of water-borne transmission of cholera. The "Broad Street pump" incident stands as one of the earliest examples of interventional epidemiology.

The reappearance of cholera in Indonesia in 1960 and its subsequent spread to Asia, Africa, Oceania, and the Middle East over the next 30 years heralded the 7th cholera pandemic. During the massive population shifts resulting from the Pakistani–Indian War in 1971, thousands of deaths from cholera occurred. Scattered epidemics involving the El Tor strain occurred in Europe but did not persist there. In 1970 the pandemic reached Africa, affecting 29 countries in less than 2 years involving more than 150,000 cases and 20,000 deaths.

A single case of cholera occurred along the Texas Gulf Coast in August 1973, in a shrimp fisherman who had not traveled out of the United States and had no known contact with foreign travelers. In August and September of 1978, 11 cases of cholera occurred in residents living along the Louisiana coast. Most cases were associated with the ingestion of steamed crabs and were due to a unique strain of *V. cholerae* biotype El Tor. The organism could be recovered from crabs boiled or steamed for 8 min but not from those cooked for 10 min. This small outbreak emphasizes the role of food-borne transmission of cholera in the United States and by undercooked shellfish in particular. Since 1973, 65 cases associated with this endemic focus have been reported, but no epidemics have occurred likely due, in part, to the availability of clean water and well-maintained sanitation systems in the United States.

In January 1991, cholera appeared simultaneously in several cities along the Peruvian coast, marking the spread of the 7th pandemic to the Americas and the first time in this century that epidemic cholera was seen in South America. At the peak of the epidemic, 20,000 cases were reported per week in Peru, half of whom were hospitalized. Serosurveys showed that 30–50% of the coastal population was infected. One year later more than 500,000 cases and more than 4500 deaths were reported in 19 South American countries. A case-control study in Trujillo, Peru, implicated drinking unboiled water and water from household storage containers as risk factors. The aging municipal water system characterized by clandestine taps into the water lines, low pressure, frequent cut-offs, and lack of chlorination played a major role in cholera transmission. In 1991, 17 U.S. cases related to this epidemic occurred in persons who had traveled to South America or eaten crabs brought back from Equador.

In late 1992, massive outbreaks of cholera started appearing in India and Bangladesh along the Bay of Bengal that marked a major shift in the epidemiology of cholera. The first reports of what will likely be referred to as the 8th cholera pandemic can be traced to Madras, India, in October 1992. Similar to the recent outbreak in South America, but distinctly different from endemic cholera in this region, most of the cases occurred in adults. Cholera has been endemic for many years in the Indian subcontinent and most adults have acquired immunity to *V. cholerae* O1. *V. cholerae* strains from these outbreaks did not agglutinate with O1 antisera and are now assigned to O139 serogroup and referred to as Bengal. Despite the lack of reactivity to O1 antisera, molecular genetic typing indicate that these strains are closely related to the pandemic O1 El Tor strain and unrelated to sporadic non-O1 strains. This new epidemic challenges previous notions about epidemic determinants of *V. cholerae* and immunity to this pathogen.

## Pathophysiology and Clinical Disease

In contrast to the pathogenesis of salmonellosis and shigellosis, *V. cholerae* does *not* penetrate the epithelial surface of the gastrointestinal tract nor does it incite any significant inflammatory response. Similar to salmonellosis, a relatively large inoculum of *V. cholerae* is necessary to overcome the natural defenses of the upper gastrointestinal tract. Following ingestion of a significant inoculum, *V. cholerae* colonizes the small intestine and then secretes a potent enterotoxin, sometimes referred to as choleragen, which results in a massive outpouring of isotonic fluid from the mucosal surface of the small intestine. Grossly, the bowel may be slightly edematous, but histologically it appears normal (Fig. 17–6). Although occasional inflammatory cells can be seen, there is no significant cellular response, either within the mucosa or in the intestinal lumen.

Although most of the pathophysiology of cholera can be attributed to the effects of cholera toxin, colonization of the small intestine by *V. cholerae* is a crucial event both in terms of toxin elaboration and in regards to the host immune response. The genetic basis for cholera toxin production and adherence of the organism, which is mediated by the toxin-coregulated pili (Tcp), emphasize the importance of both virulence determinants. The expression of cholera toxin and TcpA (major subunit component of Tcp) are under

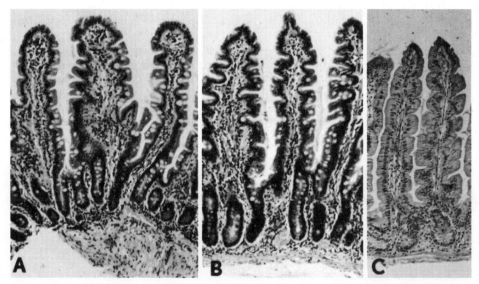

**FIGURE 17–6.** Three jejunal biopsies. All hematoxylin and eosin (× 200). *A*, Small bowel biopsy from a 32-year-old Pakistani male with acute cholera of 38-h duration. Patient had received intravenous fluids for 24 h. The epithelium is intact and the goblet cells, especially toward the tips of the villi, have discharged their mucus. A moderate inflammatory infiltrate composed of lymphocytes, monocytes, and plasma cells is present in the lamina propria. The subepithelial capillaries are hyperemic. *B*, Small bowel biopsy of a 28-year-old asymptomatic Pakistani male who served as a control. Biopsies *A* and *B* are almost identical. A similar degree of inflammatory infiltration is present in the lamina propria of both of these biopsies. (Pakistani biopsies courtesy of the Department of Experimental Pathology, Walter Reed Army Institute of Research.) *C*, Small bowel biopsy from a 30-year-old asymptomatic North American male. Very few inflammatory cells are present in the lamina propria of this biopsy. The villi are shorter in length, indicating that the biopsy was taken more distally than the biopsies in *A* and *B*. (From Barua, D., and Burrows, W., eds. *Cholera.* Philadelphia, W. B. Saunders Co., 1974. With permission.)

the control of the same transcriptional activator, ToxR.

The mode of action of cholera toxin has been worked out in considerable detail. Cholera toxin is an oligomeric protein toxin with a molecular weight of 84,000 D and is made up of one A (27,000 D) and five B subunits (11,000 D). In addition, the A subunit is composed of two fragments, $A_1$ and $A_2$, held together by a disulfide bond (Fig. 17–7). Since the toxin is produced extracellularly and intraluminally, it first must bind to the mucosal cell surface. The B subunits arranged in a doughnut-like structure bind to $GM_1$ ganglioside, a receptor on the epithelial cell membrane. The A subunit, located in the center of the doughnut, passes through the cell membrane where the disulfide bond is hydrolyzed and $A_1$ is separated from $A_2$. The $A_1$ subunit possesses adenosine diphosphate (ADP)–ribosyl transferase activity and stimulates the transfer of ADP-ribose from nicotinamide-adenone dinucleotide (NAD) to a guanosine triphosphate (GTP)–binding protein (Gs-alpha) that controls adenylate cyclase activity. Gs-alpha, when freed from its beta-gamma subunit, migrates to the basolateral membrane where it exerts positive control on adenylate cyclase. ADP ribosylation of Gs-alpha prevents its inactivation by GTPase (a negative control) resulting in a sustained increase of adenylate cyclase activity. This permanent activation of adenylate cyclase results in increased intracellular cyclic adenosine monophosphate (cAMP), which then opens chloride channels in the luminal membrane. The end result is secretion of isotonic fluid from the intestinal epithelial cell into the lumen of the small intestine. In addition to its effect on cAMP production, cholera toxin may also mediate some of its secretory activity through platelet-activating factor and prostaglandins.

Although cholera is notorious for producing severe, dehydrating diarrhea, 75% of cholera infections are subclinical, and most of the symptomatic cases are mild. Clinically, the patient first notices a slight fullness in the abdomen and loss of appetite. The hands and feet become cold, and the patient may vomit. Shortly thereafter the patient begins to have large numbers of liquid stools, first brown and then almost clear, which contain small amounts of mucus and are classically described as "rice water" stools. Vomiting and leg cramps are common and are the result of acidosis and hypokalemia, respectively. If fluids are not restored by aggressive oral or intravenous therapy, death from severe dehydration and hypovolemic shock can occur within hours or a few days (Fig. 7–8). In severe cases, a stool volume of up to 24 L/day may occur. In the acute disease, 50% or more of patients die unless proper fluid therapy is given.

Despite the profound secretory effects of cholera toxin on the intestine, absorptive mechanisms remain intact and can be utilized therapeutically. Bound cholera toxin does not block or prevent reabsorption of sodium and water by the small intestine or the colon. However, the secretion of water and ions from the mucosal cells of the small intestine exceeds the capacity of the colon to absorb the

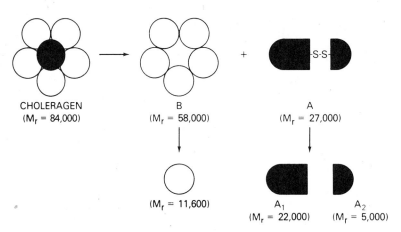

**FIGURE 17–7.** Subunit structure of choleragen. (From Fishman, P. H. Mechanism of action of cholera toxin: Events on the cell surface. In: Field, M., Fordtran, J. S., and Schultz, S. G., eds. *Secretory Diarrhea. Clinical Physiology Series, American Physiological Society.* Baltimore: Williams & Wilkins, 1981:86. With permission.)

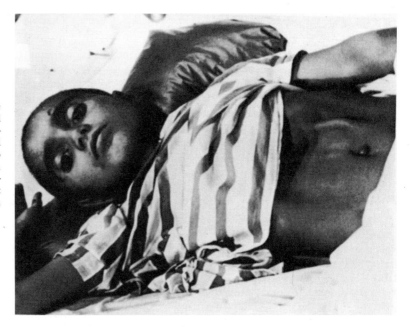

FIGURE 17–8. A child with severe cholera. Note markedly diminished turgor of abdominal skin, which remains elevated after being released by the examiner's hand. Note also apathetic expression and sunken eyes. (From Barua, D., and Burrows, W., eds. *Cholera*. Philadelphia: W. B. Saunders Co., 1974. With permission.)

loss. In mild to moderate cases, fluid balance can be achieved and water reabsorption facilitated by the use of oral rehydration solutions. The recognition that intestinal sodium absorption is coupled to glucose or nutrient transport represented a major advance in the understanding and treatment of dehydrating diarrheal illnesses. Oral rehydration solutions utilize this principle by including glucose in an electrolyte supplementation package that, when added to 1 L of clean water and ingested, promotes water and electrolyte absorption (Fig. 17–9). The concentrations of glucose and electrolytes are critical to optimize absorption and avoid hyperosmolarity. Inclusion of rice powder or other glucose polymers and amino acids in place of glucose has also proved effective. These solutions have been very successful in maintaining hydration in patients in parts of the world where intravenous fluids are not available. Widespread use of oral rehydration solutions, promoted by the World Health Organization, has very substantially reduced mortality from gastrointestinal infections, particularly in young children.

Cholera is a self-limited disease, provided that the patient does not die from dehydra-

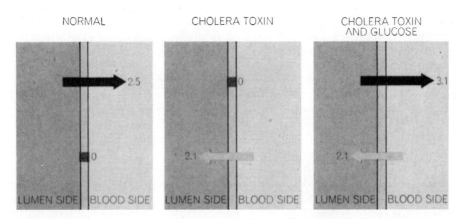

FIGURE 17–9. Net ion flow across intestinal tissue is given in microequivalents per square centimeter per hour. The normal flow of sodium ion (*top*) and chloride ion (*bottom*) is reversed (*center*) if cholera toxin is added to fluid. Adding glucose on lumen side helps restore balance (*right*). (From Hirschhorn, N., and Greenough, W. B., III. *Cholera. Sci. Am. 225*:15, 1971. Copyright © 1971 by Scientific American, Inc. All rights reserved.)

tion or shock before recovery. Although *V. cholerae* is susceptible to tetracycline and other agents, the permanent activation of intracellular adenylate cyclase by cholera toxin results in little or no evidence of clinical effect from an antibiotic for at least the first 24–36 h. Between 24 and 48 h are needed for new epithelial cells to extend from the mucosal crypts in the small intestine to the tips of the villi, replacing those cells that have bound cholera toxin and thus are secreting large amounts of water and electrolytes.

### Immunity and Vaccine Development

Natural infection with *V. cholerae* is a highly immunizing process. Recurrent infections are rare, and long-lasting immunity appears to develop. Humans produce both circulating antibodies and local secretory IgA antibodies directed against cholera toxin and other vibrio antigens. The systemic or circulating antibody response to natural infection, however, is of low magnitude in comparison with the high level of toxin-neutralizing IgG produced in response to parenteral vaccination with cholera toxin.

Early experience with parenteral vaccines using a variety of approaches, including killed whole-cell, toxoid, and lipopolysaccharide preparations, provided little protection against natural infection, despite high levels of circulating antibodies. These vaccine failures emphasized the relative importance of secretory antibodies over systemic antibodies in protection from cholera and provided further evidence that the mucosal and systemic immune systems are largely separate entities, responding to different routes of antigen exposure.

In addition to the method of vaccine delivery, recent trends in cholera epidemiology may point to the importance of specific vibrio antigens to which protective immunity is directed. The importance of immunity to vibrio antigens and virulence determinants other than cholera toxin is inferred by the recent appearance of *V. cholerae* O139 on the Indian subcontinent. Large numbers of cases occurred in the adult population despite widespread immunity in that population to *V. cholerae* O1. Both serogroups of *V. cholerae* produce virtually the same toxin but differ in the somatic antigens expressed.

In recognition that effective immunity could be stimulated best by imitating the route of exposure in natural infection, most modern vaccine trials have involved oral preparations. The two main approaches have included the combination of the nontoxic B subunit of cholera toxin and whole killed *V. cholerae* cells (BS-WC) and live, attenuated *V. cholerae* organisms. The BS-WC vaccine demonstrated efficacy in a large, randomized field trial in Bangladesh, showing 85% protection in all age groups for 6 months. However, protection fell to approximately 50% by $1^{1}/_{2}$ years, and there was reduced efficacy against El Tor strains. For unclear reasons, the vaccine shows reduced efficacy for persons with blood group O. Live, attenuated vaccines have the theoretical advantage of more closely mimicking natural infection with a replicating organism and potentially presenting a different set of antigens that are produced *in vitro*. Early candidate attenuated vaccines demonstrated efficacy but also elicited significant side effects (diarrhea, loose stools, abdominal cramps, vomiting, and fever). Although some strains show less reactogenicity, they may be less able to colonize the recipients. Currently, a large field trial is underway in Indonesia with the CVD103-HgR live, cholera vaccine in which the *ctx*A genes have been deleted from a *V. cholerae* strain of the classic biotype.

### Infection with Non-O1 *Vibrio cholerae* and Other Vibrios

Non-O1 *V. cholerae* (also referred to as non-agglutinating vibrios or noncholera vibrios) differs in the laboratory from *V. cholerae* O1 by its failure to agglutinate in O1 antiserum. Despite the production of a cholera-like toxin by some strains, non-O1 *V. cholerae* does not produce epidemic cholera. The organism is not uncommon in the brackish water of bays and estuaries and has been isolated from both domestic animals and humans. Some human patients with infection give a history of foreign travel, whereas others report having recently ingested raw oysters. Symptoms include diarrhea, abdominal cramps, fever and, in about one third of patients, bloody diarrhea. Other *Vibrio* species associated with gastroenteritis include *V. parahaemolyticus*, *V. hollisae*, *V. mimicus*, *V. fluvialis*, and *V. furnissii*.

*V. alginolyticus*, *V. damsela*, *V. metschnikovii*, *V. mimicus*, and *V. vulnificus* have been associated with infections of the external ear canal or with soft tissue wounds contaminated by either sea or brackish water. Although in the past most such isolates have been found in halophilic environments such as seawater, several patients in New Mexico and Oklahoma have developed wound infections following contamination with brackish water. Therefore, such infections are not limited to coastal communities. Species of *Vibrio* should be suspected in any serious wound or ear infection contaminated with brackish or sea water.

*V. parahaemolyticus* is commonly recovered from marine environments and is a frequent cause of food-borne outbreaks. For many years it has been the most common cause of food poisoning in Japan, usually transmitted by sashimi (raw fish). Although sporadic cases are not common in the United States, within the last two decades *V. parahaemolyticus* has caused several outbreaks of food poisoning along the Atlantic or Gulf Coasts involving steamed crabs. Other shellfish have also been found to contain the microorganism, and its survival in frozen shrimp has been described. Typical symptoms include watery diarrhea, abdominal cramps, nausea, and vomiting, and a dysentery syndrome has been reported in other countries. Strains that are hemolytic on Wagatsuma's agar (Kanagawa's phenomenon) are pathogenic for humans.

*V. vulnificus* is a particularly virulent member of this genus that can cause a primary septicemia syndrome in patients with underlying liver disease (particularly alcoholic cirrhosis and hemochromatosis) or other chronic illness. Although this syndrome can originate from a wound, the usual source is the gastrointestinal tract, and a common risk factor is the consumption of raw oysters. A distinctive clinical finding seen in about 70% of cases is the presence of bullous skin lesions. The disease is usually fulminant with a high mortality.

## Infection with *Yersinia enterocolitica*

*Yersinia enterocolitica* is a gram-negative bacillus capable of producing a wide spectrum of disease ranging from enterocolitis to bacteremia and death. The disease has been reported more frequently in Scandinavia and other European countries than in the United States. Symptoms include fever, diarrhea, and severe abdominal pain. Occasionally, infection with *Y. enterocolitica* has been recognized only after surgery for suspected appendicitis or on culture of mesenteric lymph nodes. The organism has been found in wild and domestic animals and has been isolated from water, raw milk, and food. Recovery of *Yersinia enterocolitica* by culture is greatly improved by "cold enrichment"; for example, incubation of a rectal swab at 4°C for 2–3 weeks before inoculation to culture media. Unfortunately, this procedure, although providing valuable retrospective information, delays the prompt identification of this organism. Incubation of streaked plates at 4°C also enhances recovery within 3–7 days.

*Y. enterocolitica* causes diffuse enterocolitis with focal mucosal ulcers and diffuse mesenteric lymphadenitis. The organism is invasive, and this process is chromosomally mediated. Although a heat-stable toxin similar to the ST of *E. coli* is elaborated by most clinical isolates, this enterotoxin does not correlate with virulence. Clinical isolates also carry plasmids (40–48 MD in size) that are related to the virulence plasmids of *Y. pestis* and *Y. pseudotuberculosis*. Outer membrane proteins encoded by these plasmids are important virulence factors for *Y. enterocolitica* and are associated with resistance to complement-mediated phagocytosis and serum bactericidal activity. *Y. enterocolitica* is able to utilize siderophores produced by other bacteria or administered therapeutically. Iron overload states and desferoxamine therapy predispose patients to systemic infections with *Y. enterocolitica*.

Clinically, patients can present with enterocolitis (most often in children), a pseudoappendicitis syndrome or terminal ileitis, focal extraintestinal infections, or bacteremia. Of particular interest are the postinfectious sequelae of erythema nodosum (seen in 20–25% of cases), reactive arthritis (strongly associated with HLA-B27), and occasionally Reiter's syndrome. Reactive arthritis has also been reported in association with several other enteric pathogens including *Salmonella*, *Shigella*, *Campylobacter*, and *Clostridium difficile*.

The following description of one large outbreak demonstrates the wide range of disease manifestations in response to one epidemic strain of *Y. enterocolitica*. Between June 11 and July 29, 1982, a large interstate outbreak of enteritis occurred in association with milk consumption. One hundred seventy-two culture-positive *Y. enterocolitica* infections were identified in and around Little Rock, Arkansas; Memphis, Tennessee; and Greenwood, Mississippi. One hundred forty-eight patients (86%) had diarrhea and/or abdominal pain, usually accompanied by fever; 24 patients had extraintestinal infections of the throat, blood, urinary tract, central nervous system, and wounds. Forty-one percent of cases occurred among children younger than 5 years of age. Most patients required hospitalization, and 17 underwent appendectomies. Separate case-control studies in each city showed that drinking milk pasteurized by a plant in Memphis was associated with illness, and contamination of a single lot was suspected. A telephone survey indicated that the number of people affected was much higher than the 172 cases reported.

Most *Y. enterocolitica* infections are self-limited, and antimicrobial treatment of enterocolitis and the pseudoappendicitis syndrome has not been proven effective. However, systemic and extraintestinal infections as well as infections in immunocompromised hosts clearly should be treated with antimicrobials. Most strains are susceptible to the tetracyclines, aminoglycosides, trimethoprim-sulfamethoxazole, third-generation cephalosporins, and quinolones. Penicillin and first-generation cephalosporins are not effective.

### Infection with *Campylobacter* Species

*Campylobacter jejuni* is the most frequent bacterial cause of enteritis in developed countries, and isolation rates in the United States show a distinct peak in the summer months (Fig. 17–10). In the Unites States, two peaks in age-specific rates are seen (<1 and 15–29 years), whereas in developing countries children under the age of 2 are affected disproportionately. Campylobacter are small, curved gram-negative rods with polar flagellae. They are highly motile and exhibit a corkscrew-like motion, which may represent a virulence fac-

tor for the organism. Isolation of the organism usually requires incubation at 42°C in a microaerobic atmosphere. A selective medium containing vancomycin, polymyxin B, trimethoprim, amphotericin B, and cephalothin facilitates the recovery of this fastidious pathogen.

*C. jejuni* is widely dispersed in the environment, and animal sources are the main reservoir for human infection. *C. jejuni* has been isolated from the feces of 30–100% of chickens, turkeys, water fowl, and wild birds. Handling and consuming poultry are the most important risk factors for campylobacter enteritis in the United States. *C. jejuni* has also been isolated from healthy swine, cattle, sheep, and horses, and they are likely the source for environmental contamination. Household dogs and cats, especially young ones, are commonly infected and occasionally implicated in direct transmission to humans. In contrast to contaminated foods, which are implicated in most sporadic cases, contaminated water (surface water or unchlorinated water supplies) and raw milk tend to cause outbreaks.

Although many virulence mechanisms for *C. jejuni* have been proposed, including enterotoxin, flagellae, and lipopolysaccharides, the important pathogenic features have not been delineated. Because campylobacter enteritis demonstrates an inflammatory diarrhea syndrome and bacteremia occasionally results, mucosal invasion may be involved. The stool contains many segmented neutrophils and

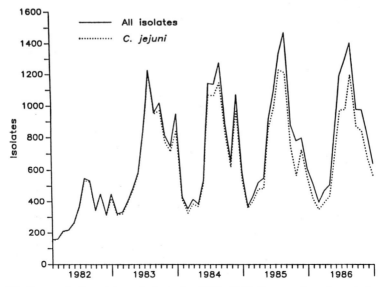

**FIGURE 17–10.** Reported *Campylobacter* isolates for 1982–1986 (by month and year) for the United States. (From Centers for Disease Control. *MMWR 37*, (SS-2):1987. With permission.)

frequently red blood cells. Both the small intestine and colon appear to be involved, with fatal cases showing hemorrhagic necrosis of the small intestine and numerous hyperplastic mesenteric lymph nodes.

Signs and symptoms of infection with *C. jejuni* overlap with other inflammatory enteritides such as salmonellosis and shigellosis. Typically symptoms include fever and malaise followed by diarrhea, often with severe, cramping abdominal pain. The stools can be watery or grossly bloody. Bacteremia and extraintestinal infections occasionally occur, particularly in immunocompromised hosts. Noninfectious sequelae include reactive arthritis, hepatitis, and nephritis. *Campylobacter* infection may also predispose to the Guillain-Barré syndrome. The clinical picture of campylobacter enteritis is quite different in underdeveloped countries, where symptomatic infections tend to be milder with less features of inflammatory diarrhea. These differences may be due to intense exposure in early life, with the development of specific immunity. Supporting this theory is that campylobacter-specific serum IgA levels increase linearly with age in Bangladeshi and Thai children as the incidence of infection decreases.

Similar to infection with *Salmonella* or *Shigella*, enteric infection with *C. jejuni* is frequently self-limiting, and antibiotic infection should be reserved for those with moderate to severe symptoms and for immunocompromised hosts. Erythromycin is still the drug of choice for most infections, but the organism is usually susceptible to other macrolides, tetracyclines, aminoglycosides, and chloramphenicol. Cephalosporins and penicillins are not effective and rapidly increasing resistance to ciprofloxacin has limited the utility of quinolones.

Other *Campylobacter* species, including *C. coli*, *C. cinaedi*, and *C. fennelliae*, also cause a milder form of enteritis. *C. fetus* is an uncommon cause of self-limiting enteritis but causes a systemic illness in immunocompromised hosts. High-molecular-weight surface-array proteins in this species inhibit complement-mediated killing and phagocytosis and are the mechanism by which *C. fetus* bacteremia occurs.

## VIRAL GASTROENTERITIS

Acute viral gastroenteritis is one of the most frequent causes of illness in our society, second only to the common cold. This probably accounts for most of the nonspecific episodes of vomiting and diarrhea seen in the United States as well as in other parts of the world, particularly the tropics. It is estimated that, worldwide, rotavirus infects nearly every child in the first few years of life.

Two clinically distinct forms of viral gastroenteritis have been noted. One form, exemplified by Norwalk virus, is associated with epidemic outbreaks of gastroenteritis and affects both children and adults. Outbreaks commonly occur in schoolchildren, members of families, or groups involved in a gathering at which a common meal is consumed. There is no seasonality associated with this form of viral enteritis. Patients have a rapid onset of gastroenteritis that lasts for 1–2 days. They usually develop diarrhea, vomiting, headache, fever, and muscle aches.

The second form of viral gastroenteritis, exemplified by rotavirus, is most often sporadic in nature but typically occurs in the winter months in North America. Sporadic viral enteritis occurs most frequently in children between 6 and 24 months of age. Symptoms include severe diarrhea lasting from 4–8 days, which may also be associated with vomiting and fever. Infants often suffer severe dehydration and may require hospitalization. Marked diarrhea can also occur in adults but is less common.

In addition to classification by epidemiologic patterns, enteric viruses can also be grouped morphologically. Rotaviruses and enteric adenoviruses are larger virions (70–80 nm in diameter) and have been cultivated *in vitro*. In contrast, Norwalk virus, Norwalk-like viruses, calicivirus, and astrovirus are smaller (27–40 nm in diameter) with round, less-distinct features and most have not been cultured *in vitro*.

### Norwalk Virus

The first identification of this virus came from studies conducted on specimens obtained during an outbreak of "winter vomiting disease" in Norwalk, Ohio, in October 1968. The Norwalk agent was recovered during an outbreak of illness at an elementary school where about half of the students became ill. Attempts to identify known bacterial or viral agents or filterable enterotoxins were unsuccessful. Three serial passages with stool filtrates from sick patients were made through human volunteers, with a resulting attack rate of 67%. The disease was characterized by an incubation period of 16–48 h, with symptoms lasting from 24–48 h, including low-grade fever and combinations of diarrhea, vomiting, abdominal cramps, malaise, and headache. Manifestations of the disease varied from one volunteer to another; vomiting was seen in some, and diarrhea in others (Fig. 17–11). Immunity to the agent, as shown by subsequent challenge of previously infected volunteers, showed two forms, one of short and the other of long duration.

Despite the inability to culture Norwalk virus, the virus has been partially characterized (including cloning of the entire genome) by purification of the agent from stool specimens. Norwalk virus is a single-stranded RNA virus that appears related to the caliciviruses. The virus is spread by the fecal–oral route; however, air-borne transmission has been suggested by the short incubation period and rapid secondary transmission seen in outbreaks. Multiple contaminated vehicles have been implicated in outbreaks, including poorly cooked shellfish from contaminated coastal waters, prepared foods (e.g., salads and cake frosting), and drinking and swimming water sources.

The pathology of Norwalk enteritis is located in the proximal small intestine. Histopathologic changes of the mucosal architecture at the duodenal-jejunal junction were studied by biopsy in a group of volunteers given the Norwalk agent. The mucosal villi became shortened, the crypts hypertrophied, and the interstitial tissue of the villi became more cellular, containing both mononuclear cells and segmented neutrophils. Abnormal changes persisted for several days but cleared by 6–8 weeks after the acute illness (Fig. 17–12). Transient functional abnormalities of the small intestine include abnormal D-xylose absorption, intestinal lactase deficiency, and malabsorption of fat. Gastric emptying was also delayed.

### Other Small, Round Enteric Viruses

Several small, round, structured viruses that appear morphologically similar to Norwalk virus have also been associated with the epidemic form of viral gastroenteritis. These Norwalk-like viruses have been named after the location of their respective outbreak (e.g., Snow Mountain, Montgomery County). These agents share some immunologic cross-reactiv-

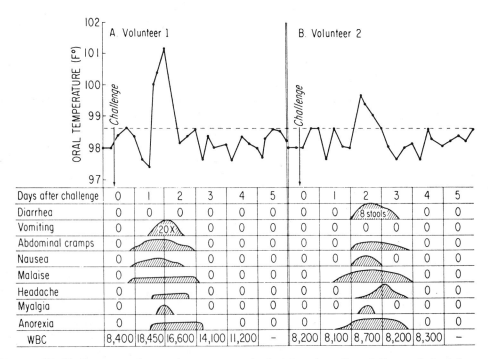

| Days after challenge | 0 | 1 | 2 | 3 | 4 | 5 | 0 | 1 | 2 | 3 | 4 | 5 |
|---|---|---|---|---|---|---|---|---|---|---|---|---|
| Diarrhea | 0 | 0 | 0 | 0 | 0 | 0 | 0 | 0 | 8 stools | | 0 | 0 |
| Vomiting | 0 | 20X | 0 | 0 | 0 | 0 | 0 | 0 | 0 | 0 | 0 | 0 |
| Abdominal cramps | 0 | | | 0 | 0 | 0 | 0 | 0 | | | 0 | 0 |
| Nausea | 0 | | | 0 | 0 | 0 | 0 | 0 | | 0 | 0 | 0 |
| Malaise | 0 | | | 0 | 0 | 0 | 0 | | | | 0 | 0 |
| Headache | 0 | | | 0 | 0 | 0 | 0 | 0 | | | 0 | 0 |
| Myalgia | 0 | | | 0 | 0 | 0 | 0 | 0 | | 0 | 0 | 0 |
| Anorexia | 0 | | | | 0 | 0 | 0 | | | | 0 | 0 |
| WBC | 8,400 | 18,450 | 16,600 | 14,100 | 11,200 | – | 8,200 | 8,100 | 8,700 | 8,200 | 8,300 | – |

**FIGURE 17–11.** Response of two volunteers to oral administration of stool filtrate derived from a volunteer who received original Norwalk rectal-swab specimen. The height of the *shaded curve* is roughly proportional to the severity of the sign or symptom. (From Dolin, R., Blacklow, N. R., DuPont, H., et al. Transmission of acute infectious nonbacterial gastroenteritis to volunteers by oral administration of stool filtrates. *J. Infect. Dis. 123*:307, 1971. With permission.)

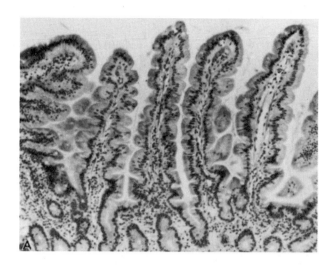

**FIGURE 17–12.** Biopsies of the small intestine before and after oral ingestion of Norwalk agent. Before ingestion (*A*), villi are tall, and the cellularity of the lamina propria is normal. Two days after ingestion (*B*), the villi are shortened, the crypts are hypertrophied and contain increased numbers of mitoses, and the cellularity of the lamina propria is increased. Six days after ingestion (*C*), shortened villi, hypertrophied crypts, and increased mitoses persist. (Hematoxylin and eosin stain, × 100.) (From Schreiber, D. S., Blacklow, N. L., and Trier, J. S. The mucosal lesion of the proximal small intestine in acute infectious nonbacterial gastroenteritis. *N. Engl. J. Med. 288*:1318, 1973. Reprinted by permission from the *New England Journal of Medicine.*)

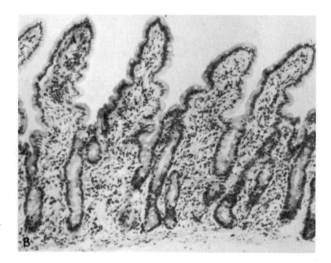

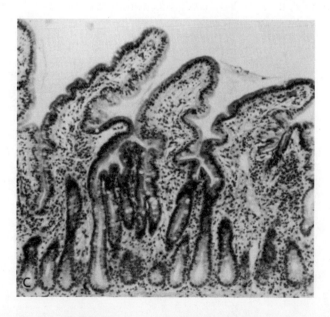

ity, but only the Snow Mountain virus has been characterized to any significant extent. Like Norwalk virus, Snow Mountain virus is a single-stranded RNA virus.

As mentioned above, caliciviruses appear to be related to Norwalk virus. However, the usual enteritis syndrome involves sporadic diarrhea in young children, and the clinical picture is similar to mild rotavirus diarrhea. In contrast to the other small, round enteroviruses, astrovirus has been cultured *in vitro*. This single-stranded RNA virus also produces a sporadic watery diarrhea syndrome in young children. A large, controlled study in Thailand indicates that astrovirus gastroenteritis is common in children, second in frequency to rotavirus.

## Rotavirus

Rotavirus is the most common cause of severe diarrhea in children, both in underdeveloped and developed countries. Since the identification of this wheel-shaped virus by electron microscopy in 1973, the virus has been characterized in detail. The name of the rotavirus group is derived from the Latin word *rota*, meaning wheel, because the circular outer capsid resembles the rim of a wheel connected to short spokes that radiate from a wide hub (Fig. 17–13). Rotaviruses are double-stranded RNA viruses belonging to the Reoviridae family. The genome consists of 11 segments, each coding for a separate protein. Four of these proteins are structural proteins and two (VP4 and VP7) are located on the surface of the outer viral capsid. VP4 is a spike-shaped hemagglutinin that is cleaved into two fragments by trypsin and is involved in cell entry. VP7 is a glycoprotein that determines the viral serotype. Rotaviruses are divided into three major antigenic groupings, A (most common), B (associated with epidemics in China), and C. There are four common serotypes within group A.

Epidemiologic studies of rotavirus infections have shown that gastroenteritis caused by this group of agents shows a distinct predilection for infants between 6 and 24 months of age. Infection is common in patients hospitalized for acute gastroenteritis, with up to 50% of infants and young children positive for rotavirus in stool. Infection follows a characteristic seasonal pattern, with most infants hospitalized between November and April. This seasonal pattern also follows a regional sequence starting in Mexico and the southwestern United States in early winter and end-ing in the northeastern United States and Canada in the spring. Often nearly 80% of infants hospitalized with acute gastroenteritis during December and January shed the virus. Concurrent studies on the parents of clinically ill children show up to 40% to be infected, although most infections in adults are subclinical.

Clinically, rotaviral gastroenteritis is a watery, dehydrating diarrheal syndrome. In addition to diarrhea, vomiting can be a serious problem contributing to dehydration. The disease is usually not fatal unless there has been severe dehydration or (in developing countries) is associated with preexisting malnutrition. Diarrhea begins somewhat later than vomiting and may reflect infection of the intestine at different levels. Mucosal abnormalities are similar to those seen in patients with Norwalk virus infections. Treatment is symptomatic, with fluid replacement being the most important factor. In general there are numerous virus particles in the stools of patients with rotavirus infections and the diagnosis can be made by immunoelectron microscopy, counterimmunoelectrophoresis, radioimmunoassay, or by enzyme-linked immunosorbent assay (ELISA). A commercially available ELISA test has been most useful for the rapid and apparently specific identification of viral antigen in the stool.

Most children have acquired antibody to rotaviruses by the time they are 2 years of age. In studies of children who develop reinfection, repeated illness is usually due to infection with a different serotype. Infection with one serotype does not appear to provide cross-protection from illness due to the other. As a consequence of its segmented genome, reassortment of rotaviral genes can occur naturally in the setting of mixed infections, resulting in new strains. Vaccine development has mimicked this strategy by substituting one of the 11 genes in an animal strain of rotavirus with VP7 gene from a human rotaviral strain, the so-called jennerian approach. Two reassortant vaccines, one containing the VP7 gene from rotavirus serotype 1 and a tetravalent vaccine with four reassortant strains representing all four common serotypes, are under study. The vaccine efficacy was modest overall (40% vs. 57%, monovalent vs. tetravalent vaccine) but showed better efficacy against severe disease (73% and 82%) and reduced medical visits (67% and 78% reduction). Only the tetravalent vaccine was efficacious against non–serotype 1 infections

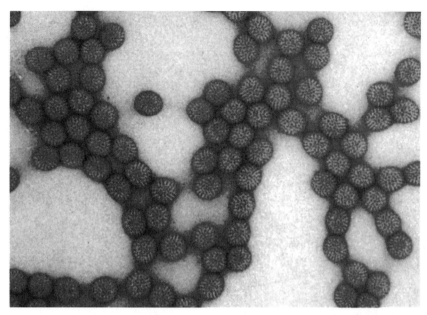

**FIGURE 17–13.** Purified rotavirus stained with 2% phosphotungstic acid ( × 124,875). (From Gomez-Barreto, J., et al. Acute enteritis associated with reovirus-like agents. *JAMA 235*:1857, 1976. Copyright © 1976, American Medical Association.)

during the second year, reflecting either the lack of heterotypic immunity or a difference in duration of effect by the two vaccines.

### Enteric Adenovirus

A subgroup of fastidious adenoviruses, group F serotypes 40 and 41, have specific tissue culture growth characteristics and are associated with acute gastroenteritis. These double-stranded DNA viruses do not grow in the conventional cell lines used for other adenoviruses. Adenovirus diarrhea tends to be mild and self-limited, but can be very severe on occasion. Symptoms include low-grade fever, watery stools, emesis, and occasionally respiratory symptoms. Infants are particularly susceptible to these agents.

## TRAVELER'S DIARRHEA

Traveler's diarrhea is the most frequent infectious and medical problem encountered by persons visiting Latin America, Asia, or Africa. The chances of developing traveler's diarrhea depend on the traveler's country of origin, his or her destination, and what he or she does, particularly regarding dietary precautions. The clinical illness is highly variable, reflecting the diverse causative agents. Typically, patients experience watery diarrhea, cramps and nausea; vomiting, bloody diarrhea, and fever

are less common. Diarrhea lasts a mean of 3 days. A study of a large group of American students on a 3-week visit to Mexico revealed that 30% developed diarrhea during the trip. Cultures of both sick and asymptomatic students yielded enterotoxin-producing strains of *Escherichia coli* in 72% of the sick and 15% of the nonsick students. Most enteropathogens are found in a certain proportion of symptomatic and nonsymptomatic patients who are exposed to the agent. The ratio of symptomatic to nonsymptomatic is lower for permanent residents of the endemic regions, likely reflecting acquired immunity.

In a study involving gastroenterologists traveling to a Latin American country for an International Congress, approximately 50% of the physicians and their family members developed traveler's diarrhea. An etiologic agent was identified in almost two thirds of those with diarrhea; the agents identified included enterotoxicogenic *E. coli*, salmonellae, shigellae, invasive *E. coli*, *Vibrio parahaemolyticus*, *Giardia lamblia*, and rotaviruses. Consumption of salads containing raw vegetables was significantly associated with enterotoxicogenic *E. coli* infection. Overall, about 80% of cases of traveler's diarrhea are caused by bacterial pathogens, explaining the efficacy of antimicrobial therapy for the prevention and treatment of this complication of foreign travel.

Although prophylaxis of traveler's diarrhea

is possible, the history of developing antimicrobial resistance in enteropathogens and infectious agents in general emphasizes that with few exceptions this approach should not be advocated. Doxycycline was the first agent used for prophylaxis but was efficacious only in relation to the rate of local enteropathogen susceptibility to doxycycline. TMP/SMZ was initially very effective, but because of widespread resistance, particularly in *E. coli* and *Shigella,* TMP/SMZ is only reliably effective at the present time in inland Mexico during the summer. Although quinolones are now effective therapies for traveler's diarrhea worldwide, resistance in *Campylobacter* has been increasing rapidly. Other reasons not to recommend prophylaxis include the risk of antimicrobial side effects (e.g., photosensitivity, allergic skin reactions, bone marrow hypoplasia, antibiotic-associated diarrhea, and candida vaginitis) and the potential for selection of antibiotic-resistant pathogens requiring alternate therapeutic agents. More important preventative measures include counseling regarding dietary precautions, which are often summarized by the maxim "boil it, cook it, peel it, or forget it." Contaminated food is the main vehicle for transmission of traveler's diarrhea, but water has also been implicated, particularly for viral pathogens. Bismuth subsalicylate (Pepto-Bismol) is an alternative to antimicrobial prophylaxis but needs to be given four times daily and the traveler needs to follow dietary precautions carefully to maximize the benefit.

Early treatment after symptoms develop is a reasonable alternative to prophylaxis with antimicrobial drugs. Antimicrobial treatment of traveler's diarrhea reduces the duration of symptoms from a range of 50–93 h without treatment to 16–30 h. Quinolone antimicrobials are the drugs of choice for nonpregnant adults, except for diarrhea that develops in inland Mexico during the summer. All of the available fluoroquinolones, norfloxacin, ciprofloxacin, ofloxacin, and fleroxacin appear to be equally efficacious. Three-day regimens have been effective and the inclusion of loperamide (Imodium) to the regimen offers some additional improvement early on. However, the use of agents such as paregoric, tincture of opium, diphenoxylate-atropine (Lomotil), or loperamide (Imodium) to reduce intestinal motility may block an important natural defense mechanism of the body and are cautioned against if fever or dysentery is present. Ciprofloxacin and loperamide have

been used successfully without complications in one study of dysentery. However, only 1 of the 88 cases in that study involved *Shigella dysenteriae* type 1, the more virulent species of *Shigella,* and anecdotal evidence has implicated other antimotility agents in complications of invasive enteric infections, such as toxic megacolon. Recently, single-dose quinolone regimens have been shown to be effective for nondysenteric episodes when started early. Other antimicrobial agents that show promise for the treatment of traveler's diarrhea include bicozamycin and aztreonam, agents which are poorly absorbed from the intestine.

## CASE HISTORY

### CASE HISTORY 1

A 26-year-old Hmong male presented with diarrhea and fever of several weeks' duration. This man, who was part of a hill-tribe group from Northern Laos, had immigrated to the United States 4 months previously and had no known chronic illnesses. He described the gradual onset of watery-loose, nonbloody stools without nausea, vomiting, or abdominal pain, although he did complain of "bloating." He noted a decreased appetite with a 10-lb weight loss in addition to generalized weakness and lightheadedness over this same time period. Although he had not taken his temperature at home, he had seen a physician the previous week who noted fever and prescribed diphenoxylate-atropine (Lomotil) and acetaminophen. He was married, with five children, none of whom were ill. He was not currently employed.

On physical examination the patient appeared thin, flushed, and in mild distress. He was febrile (104.5°F) without tachycardia (pulse, 84/min) or hypotension (blood pressure, 102/60) and his respiratory rate was 20/min. His abdomen was soft, nontender, and the bowel sounds were hypoactive. Brown-yellow liquid, guaiac-negative stool was noted on rectal examination. No hepatosplenomegaly was present and the rest of the examination was noncontributory.

The white blood cell count was 4100/mm³ with 66% neutrophils, 24% lymphocytes, and 10% monocytes. The hemoglobin was 12.8 g/dL and the platelet count was 118,000/mm³. The aspartate transaminase (AST) was 305 IU/L (eight times the upper limit of normal) and the alkaline phosphatase and bilirubin levels were within normal limits. The plain film of the abdomen was notable for mild generalized gaseous distention of the small intestine. Thick and thin blood smears for malaria were negative.

The patient was admitted to the medicine ward and intravenous fluids were administered. After blood and stool cultures were obtained, ceftazidime and gentamicin were administered intravenously. A tuberculin skin test was negative. Despite antibiotic administration, he remained febrile (103°–105°F) over the next 5 days. Blood cultures from admission grew *Salmonella typhi*.

## CASE 1 DISCUSSION

This patient with typhoid fever illustrates several important points regarding this enteric disease syndrome and the evaluation of fever in a recent immigrant. Enteric fever is an insidious disease with a gradual, stepwise increase in temperature over the first week, after which it becomes sustained. Although not specific for this syndrome, the pulse–temperature dissociation noted here (inappropriately low pulse for the degree of fever) is classic for enteric fever. Systemic symptoms such as fever and headache usually overshadow gastrointestinal symptoms and often diarrhea is not present or develops sometime after the onset of illness. The symptoms of abdominal bloating and the finding of distended loops of small bowel in this patient is consistent with enteric fever; often a "doughy" abdomen with palpable loops of air- and fluid-filled bowel is described. Other tip-offs to the diagnosis in this patient include the relative leukopenia and elevated AST, indicating hepatic parenchymal inflammation.

Two points regarding this patient's apparent lack of response to antimicrobial therapy are worth mentioning. Although gentamicin displays excellent *in vitro* activity against *S. typhi*, this agent is not effective clinically, presumably because typhoid fever is an intracellular infection and the aminoglycosides are not effective in the low-pH environment of the phagolysomes in which *S. typhi* reside. On the other hand, third-generation cephalosporins such as ceftriaxone (and likely, ceftazidime) are effective therapeutic agents. The resolution of signs and symptoms in enteric fever is gradual, similar to the onset of symptoms, and it is not unusual to remain febrile several days after the initiation of effective therapy.

How does this patient's illness relate to his recent immigration from a tropical, third world country? Most tropical diseases have relatively short incubation periods and most parasites do not survive long outside of the endemic area, where the particular environment or the intermediate hosts are not present. Therefore, the list of tropical diseases in the differential of this presentation, 4 months after leaving Southeast Asia, is relatively short. Important diagnoses to consider would be vivax malaria and tuberculosis, both of which were considered in this case. Other diseases endemic to Southeast Asia that could occur many months to years later include: paragonimiasis, strongyloidiasis, *Opisthorchis* infection, amebic liver abscess, melioidosis, or complications of hepatitis B infection. In contrast to the United States, the HIV epidemic

in Thailand and surrounding countries has spread beyond the usual high-risk groups and affects large segments of the whole population. Finally, the incubation period for typhoid fever is usually 7–14 days. Therefore, he acquired his infection in the United States, and an asymptomatic carrier, possibly a food preparer, was suspected as the source.

## REFERENCES

**Books**

Blaser, M. J., Smith, P. D., Greenberg, H. B., and Guerrant, R. L., eds., *Infections of the Gastrointestinal Tract*. New York: Raven Press, 1995.

Tzipori, S. *Infectious Diarrhea in the Young*. Amsterdam: Elsevier, 1985.

**Review Articles**

Blacklow, N. R., and Greenberg, H. G. Viral gastroenteritis. *N. Engl. J. Med.* 325:252, 1991.

Chalker, R. B., and Blaser, M. J. A review of human salmonellosis. *Rev. Infect. Dis.* 10:111, 1988.

Claeson, M., and Merson, M. Global progress in the control of diarrheal diseases. *Pediatr. Infect. Dis. J.* 9:345, 1990.

Cover, T. L., and Aber, R. C. *Yersinia enterocolitica*. *N. Engl. J. Med.* 321:16, 1989.

DuPont, H. L., and Ericsson, C. D. Prevention and treatment of traveler's diarrhea. *N. Engl. J. Med.* 328:1821, 1993.

Field, M., Rao, M. C., and Chang, E. B. Intestinal electrolyte transport and diarrheal disease. *N. Engl. J. Med.* 321:800, 1989.

Geurrant, R. L. Lessons from diarrheal diseases: Demography to molecular pharmacology. *J. Infect. Dis.* 169:1206, 1994.

Hedberg, C. W., MacDonald, K. L., and Osterholm, M. T. Changing epidemiology of food-borne disease: A Minnesota perspective. *Clin. Infect. Dis.* 18:671, 1994.

Keusch, G. T., and Bennish, M. L. Shigellosis: Recent progress, persisting problems and research issues. *Pediatr. Infect. Dis. J.* 8: 713, 1989.

Levine, M. M. *Escherichia coli* that cause diarrhea: Enterotoxigenic, enteropathogenic, enteroinvasive, enterohemorrhagic, and enteroadherent. *J. Infect. Dis.* 155: 377, 1987.

Mekalanos, J. J., and Sadoff, J. C. Cholera vaccines: Fighting an ancient scourge. *Science* 265:1387, 1994.

Robins-Browne, R. M. Traditional enteropathogenic *E. coli* of infantile diarrhea. *Rev. Infect. Dis.* 9:28, 1987.

Ryan, C. A., Hargrett-Bean, N. T., and Blake, P. A. *Salmonella typhi* infections in the United States, 1975–84: Increasing role of foreign travel. *Rev. Infect. Dis.* 11:1, 1989.

**Original Articles**

Bennish, M. L., Harris, J. R., Wojtyniak, B. J., et al. Death in shigellosis: Incidence and risk factors in hospitalized patients. *J. Infect. Dis.* 161:500, 1990.

Bennish, M. L., Salam, M. A., Khan, W. A., and Khan, A. M. Treatment of shigellosis: Comparison of one- or two-dose ciprofloxacin with standard 5-day therapy. A randomized, blinded trial. *Ann. Intern. Med. 117:*727, 1992.

Berche, P., Poyart, C., Abachin, E., et al. The novel epidemic strain O139 is closely related to the pandemic strain O1 of *Vibrio cholerae. J. Infect. Dis. 170:*701, 1994.

Bernstein, D. I., Glass, R. I., Rodgers, G., Davidson, B. L., and Sack, D. A. Evaluation of rhesus rotavirus monovalent and tetravalent reassortant vaccines in US children. *JAMA 273:*1191, 1995.

Blaser, M. J., Black, R. E., Duncan, D. J., and Amer, J. *Campylocacter jenuni*–specific serum antibodies are elevated in healthy Bangladeshi children. *J. Clin. Microbiol. 21:*164, 1985.

Centers for Disease Control. Multistate outbreak of *Escherichia coli* O157:H7 infections from hamburgers. *MMWR 42:*258, 1993.

Clemens, J. D., Sack, D. A., Harris, J. R., et al. Field trial of oral cholera vaccines in Bangladesh: Results from three-year follow-up. *Lancet 335:*270, 1990.

Cholera Working Group. Large epidemic of cholera-like disease in Bangladesh caused by *Vibro cholerae* O139 synonym Bengal. *Lancet 342:*387, 1993.

DuPont, H. L., Reves, R. R., Galindo, E., et al. Treatment of traveler's diarrhea with trimethoprim-sulfamethoxazole and with trimethoprim alone. *N. Engl. J. Med. 307:*841, 1982.

Griffin, P. M., Ostroff, S. M., Tauxe, R. V., et al. Illnesses associated with *Escherichia coli* O157:H7 infections. *Ann. Intern. Med. 109:*705, 1988.

Hermann, J. E., Taylor, D. N., Echeverria, P., and Blacklow, N. R. Astroviruses as a cause of gastroenteritis in children. *N. Engl. J. Med. 324:*1757, 1991.

Ho, M. S., Glass, R. I., Pinsky, P. F., et al. Rotavirus as a cause of diarrheal morbidity and mortality in the United States. *J. Infect. Dis. 158:*1112, 1988.

Johnston, J. M., Martin, D. L., Perdue, J., et al. Cholera on a Gulf Coast oil rig. *N. Engl. J. Med. 309:*523, 1983.

Kapikian, A. A., Kim, H. W., Wyatt, R. G., et al. Human reovirus-like agent as the major pathogen associated with "winter" gastroenteritis in hospitalized infants and young children. *N. Engl. J. Med. 294:*965, 1976.

LeBaron, C. W., Lew, J., Glass, R. I., et al. Annual rotavirus epidemic patterns in North America. *JAMA 264:* 983, 1990.

Lee, L. A., Gerber, A. R., Lonsway, D. R., et al. *Yersinia enterocolitica* O:3 infections in infants and children associated with the household preparation of chitterlings. *N. Engl. J. Med. 322:*984, 1990.

Levine, M. M., Taylor, D. N., and Ferreccio, C. Typhoid vaccines come of age. *Pediatr. Infect. Dis. J. 8:*374, 1989.

Martin, D. L., MacDonald, K. L., White, K. E., Soler, J. T., and Osterholm, M. T. The epidemiology and clinical aspects of the hemolytic uremic syndrome in Minnesota. *N. Engl. J. Med. 323:*1161, 1990.

Merson, M. H., Morris, G. K., Sack, D. A., et al. Traveler's diarrhea in Mexico: A prospective study of physicians and family members attending a congress. *N. Engl. J. Med. 294:*1299, 1976.

Murphy, G. S., Bodhidatta, L., Echeverria, P., et al. Ciprofloxacin and loperamide in the treatment of bacillary dysentery. *Ann. Intern. Med. 118:*582, 1993.

Ormand, J. E., and Talley, N. J. *Helicobacter pylori:* Controversies and an approach to management. *Mayo Clin. Proc. 65:*414, 1990.

Palmer, D. L., Koster, F. T., Islam, A. F. M. R., et al. Comparison of sucrose and glucose in the oral electrolyte therapy of cholera and other severe diarrheas. *N. Engl. J. Med. 297:*1107, 1977.

Petruccelli, B. P., Murphy, G. S., Sanchez, J. L., et al. Treatment of traveler's diarrhea with ciprofloxacin and loperamide. *J. Infect. Dis. 165:*557, 1992.

Salam, I., Katelaris, P., Leigh-Smith, S., and Farthing, M. J. G. Randomised trial of single-dose ciprofloxacin for travellers' diarrhoea. *Lancet 344:*1537, 1994.

Sansonetti, P. J., Ryter, J. A., Clerc, P., Mauvelli, A. T., and Mourier, J. Multiplication of *Shigella flexneri* within HeLa cells: lysis of the phagocytic vacuole and plasmid-mediated contact hemolysis. *Infect. Immun. 51:*461, 1986.

St. Louis, M. E., Morse, D. L., Potter, M. E., DeMelfi, T. M., and Guzewich, J. J. The emergence of grade A eggs as a major source of *Salmonella enteritidis* infections. New implications for the control of salmonellosis. *JAMA 259:*2103, 1988.

Swerdlow, D. L., Mintz, E. D., Rodriguez, M., et al. Waterborne transmission of epidemic cholera in Trujillo, Peru: Lessons for a continent at risk. *Lancet 340:*28, 1992.

Wanke, C. A., Schorling, J. B., Barrett, L. J., Desouza, M. A., and Guerrant, R. L. Potential role of adherence traits of *Escherichia coli* in persistent diarrhea in an urban Brazilian slum. *Pediatr. Infect. Dis. J. 10:*746, 1991.

# 18

# COMMON INTESTINAL PARASITIC INFECTIONS

BORIS REISBERG, M.D.

Parasitic infection of the human gastrointestinal tract is common, especially in those parts of the world where poor sanitation and an unprotected water supply exist. Although parasitic infection of the intestinal tract is rarely fatal, these infections contribute greatly to the global problem of diarrheal illness, malnutrition, and human suffering. Worse perhaps is the fact that infants and children bear the brunt of the morbidity and mortality associated with these infections. It is impossible to discuss all of the human intestinal parasitic infections in this chapter; therefore, the reader is referred to the references for texts devoted to parasitic infections. This chapter covers common intestinal infections found in the United States.

The first part of this chapter deals with those parasites that are mainly responsible for diarrheal illness, namely *Entamoeba histolytica, Giardia lamblia, Isospara belli, Cryptosporidium,* and *Microsporidia*. The second half of this chapter discusses common nematode infections.

## *ENTAMOEBA HISTOLYTICA* INFECTION

Infection with the protozoan *Entamoeba histolytica* occurs throughout the civilized world but is most commonly seen in countries with a warm climate where people live in poverty and sanitation is poor. In these tropical and semitropical areas of the world, there are an estimated 400 million infections and 30,000 deaths annually. On a global scale, death due to amebiasis is exceeded only by the parasitic infections malaria and schistosomiasis. Estimates of the incidence of *E. histolytica* infection in the United States have varied between 3 and 10%. With increasing international travel, amebiasis may occur in visitors to the United States from highly endemic areas, as well as in United States citizens who have traveled abroad.

### Life Cycle of *Entamoeba histolytica*

*Entamoeba histolytica*, *E. hartmanni*, *E. coli*, *E. polecki*, and *E. gingivalis* are all capable of colonizing the mouth and intestinal tract of humans, but only *E. histolytica* is capable of producing disease. Man is the definitive host of *E. histolytica* and the only reservoir of infection.

*Entamoeba histolytica* exists in two distinct forms: as a cyst and as a motile, actively feeding trophozoite. Cysts are produced when the local conditions become unfavorable for trophozoite viability, which occurs when the stool is dehydrated in its passage from the colon to the rectum. In transforming into a cyst, the ameba discharges ingested food and rounds up to form a precyst, containing a single nucleus. As the cyst matures, it forms a tough outer membrane and the nucleus divides. Immature cysts contain two nuclei; mature cysts, which measure 10–18 μm in diameter, have

four nuclei. Cysts of *E. histolytica* are usually found in asymptomatic individuals whose stools are well formed. Infected individuals may excrete as many as 45 million cysts per day. The disease is spread by ingestion of food or water contaminated with *E. histolytica* cysts.

Once swallowed, the cysts, which are resistant to gastric juice, enter the small bowel. It is here that excystation occurs, liberating four trophozoites, which pass into the large intestine, their natural habitat. *Entamoeba histolytica* trophozoites are 12–50 μm in size and have a glassy green tinge when observed with a microscope. The nucleus is round, and on the inner surface of the thin nuclear membrane are minute deposits of chromatin (see Figs. 18–1 and 18–2). In the center of the nucleus is a prominent karyosome (nucleolus). The structure of the nucleus is the most important morphologic feature in distinguishing *E. histolytica* from other intestinal amebae, with the exception of *E. hartmanni*, which has a similar appearing nucleus. Differentiation between these two amebae is made by size. Both the trophozoites and cysts of *E. hartmanni* are smaller than those of *E. histolytica*. The upper limit of the size of *E. hartmanni* cysts is 10 μm, and of the trophozoites, 12 μm.

*E. histolytica* trophozoites viewed in wet mount move rapidly and in one direction. This typical ameboid movement is accomplished utilizing pseudopodia. Multiplication is by binary division, as long as local conditions remain favorable. *Entamoeba histolytica*

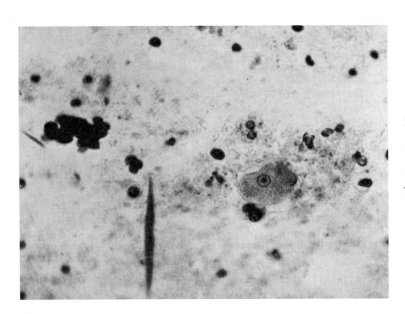

**FIGURE 18–1.** Trophozoite of *Entamoeba histolytica* stained with iron hematoxylin. Note Charcot-Leyden crystals and clumped red blood cells. (From Hunter, G. W., Shwartzwelder, J. C., and Clyde, D. F. *Tropical Medicine*. 4th ed. Philadelphia: W. B. Saunders Co., 1966. With permission.)

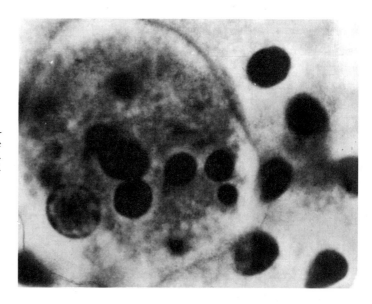

**FIGURE 18–2.** *Entamoeba histolytica* trophozoite. Note ingested red cells (trichrome stain). (From Markell, E. K., and Voge, M. *Medical Parasitology.* 7th ed. Philadelphia: W. B. Saunders Co., 1992. With permission.)

grow in and multiply best under anaerobic conditions. When they have invaded the bowel wall, the trophozoites reach sizes near the upper end of their size spectrum and are frequently observed to have ingested red blood cells. As metabolic conditions become unfavorable, precysts are formed, and the cycle begins again.

### Pathogenesis of Infection

The initial step in the pathogenesis of amebiasis is the adhesion of *E. histolytica* trophozoites to the epithelium of the colon. Mechanically, this seems to be accomplished by formation of filopodia—long filamentous elements that extend outward from the amebic cell surface. Inhibition of this process by conditions known to prevent microfilament formation causes a marked reduction in amebic adherence. Adherence of *E. histolytica* is also dependent on a specific carbohydrate-binding protein (lectin) on the amebic cell surface. The lectin of *E. histolytica* seems to bind preferentially to those polysaccharides and glycoconjugates that contain *N*-acetylgalactosamine. Attachment of *E. histolytica* to intestinal epithelial cells is also dependent on temperature, the amount of time elapsed since incubation, and pH. Experimentally, the optimal temperature has been found to be 35°–37°C; maximal adherence to a fixed epithelial cell monolayer is reached after 15 min of incubation and at a pH of 5.7–6.0.

Viable *E. histolytica* trophozoites are cytolethal to numerous tissue culture cell lines, and attachment is quickly followed by destruction of the intestinal epithelial monolayer. Although *E. histolytica* produces numerous proteases, hyaluronidase, and other hydrolytic enzymes, cell-free cytotoxicity has not been demonstrated *in vitro*. Contact between the target cell and the intact trophozoite is required for cytolytic effect. At the same time that cellular destruction is occurring, phagocytosis of viable or killed target cells also occurs. *E. histolytica* trophozoites are capable of destroying leukocytes on contact. Examination of tissue specimens obtained from patients reveals the presence of leukocytes only at the periphery of established lesions.

For many years, it has been recognized that different strains of *E. histolytica* vary in pathogenicity. Amebae isolated from asymptomatic intestinal carriers do not produce lesions on intrahepatic inoculation of hamsters, whereas those strains isolated from symptomatic patients do. Sargeaunt and Williams demonstrated that amebae isolated from patients with invasive disease had a different mobility pattern of their isoenzymes (zymodemes) on starch gel electrophoresis than did amebae isolated from asymptomatic carriers. This is a consistent difference confirmed by other investigators. Recently, genomic DNA differences between pathogenic and nonpathogenic strains of *E. histolytica* have been reported. These genomic differences are perhaps reflective of differences in constituent isoenzymes and explain why in the United States invasive amebiasis is a rare disease even though 5% of the population is infected.

## Acute Intestinal Amebiasis

Disease is initiated by ingestion of food or water contaminated with fecal matter containing cysts of *E. histolytica*. Cysts are able to survive in moist soil for at least 1 week at temperatures of 28°–34°C, and even longer in colder temperatures. Cysts may also live for several days to weeks in water and are not killed by the concentration of chlorine usually present in municipal water. In many areas of the world, water used for drinking and washing may be contaminated by surface runoff into shallow wells, streams, or even by the discharge of untreated sewage into lakes and rivers. In the United States, several large epidemics of amebiasis have occurred in the past from the cross-contamination of fresh-water pipes by waste water. Cysts are killed by boiling water, desiccation, direct sunlight, heat, or by 200 ppm of iodine.

Contamination of food and water with direct person-to-person spread is usually related to a totally asymptomatic cyst passer. In the majority of infected persons, *E. histolytica* lives as an asymptomatic commensal organism in the lumen in the large bowel. Invasion of the colonic epithelium with the production of symptomatic disease occurs in less than 10% of infected individuals.

In patients who develop symptomatic disease, the onset of infection is usually gradual, with the patient complaining of abdominal pain and discomfort associated with frequent bowel movements. Rectal pain and urgency to defecate are also common. The stool is often noted to be loose and watery and to contain varying amounts of blood and mucus. Patients may have anywhere from a few bowel movements per day to several movements per hour. The combination of bloody diarrhea, abdominal pain, and urgency is the classic presentation of amebic dysentery.

Fever and other constitutional symptoms are frequently absent, facts that are sometimes helpful in differentiating bacillary dysentery produced by *Shigella* from amebiasis. In approximately a third of patients with amebiasis, the onset of illness is acute, with profuse diarrhea containing blood and mucus, accompanied by high fever and signs of toxicity. These patients present in a manner identical to those with bacillary dysentery, and differentiation on clinical grounds alone is impossible. The abdominal pain is frequently most intense in the lower abdomen, and most commonly in the right lower quadrant. Abdominal tenderness is a frequent finding on physical examination. The combination of right lower quadrant pain and lower abdominal tenderness may be confused with acute appendicitis.

The characteristic colonic lesions produced by trophozoites of *E. histolytica* are discrete ulcers separated from each other by normal-appearing intestinal mucosa. The ulcers vary in size from 2–3 mm to 1–2 cm. As trophozoites penetrate the submucosa, they spread out laterally, creating an ulcer shaped like an "inverted flask," the edges of which are thickened and shaggy and overhang the ulcer crater. The base of the ulcer is coated with a necrotic exudate (see Figs. 18–3 and 18–4). Invasion of the bowel wall by trophozoites produces little in the way of an acute inflam-

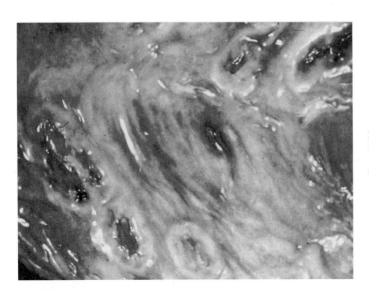

**FIGURE 18–3.** Amebic ulcers of the large intestine. Note raised margins of ulcers. (Courtesy of the Louisiana State University School of Medicine, New Orleans.)

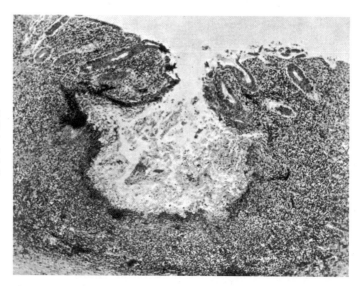

FIGURE 18–4. Section of colon showing flask-shaped chronic amebic ulcer involving the mucosa and submucosa. The neutrophilic infiltration of the border of the lesion suggests secondary bacterial invasion. (From Medical Museum Collection, Armed Forces Institute of Pathology. With Permission.)

matory reaction. Rarely, the ulcers may extend through the muscular layers of the intestine into the serosa. This is usually followed by frank intestinal perforation and amebic peritonitis.

A second local complication of amebic dysentery is massive lower intestinal hemorrhage, which occurs when the base of an ulcer crater erodes into an arteriole. Lower gastrointestinal hemorrhage usually responds to supportive care and specific antiamebic chemotherapy. Surgical exploration is not indicated. The majority of amebic ulcers are present in the cecum and rectosigmoid areas of the colon, but they may be found throughout the colon and even in the terminal ileum. Sigmoidoscopy is frequently helpful for diagnostic purposes. The presence of discrete ulcers with normal intervening mucosa makes ulcerative colitis and bacillary dysentery unlikely possibilities.

Although dysentery is the classic presentation of acute amebiasis, some patients may experience only mild diarrhea and abdominal pain, with no evidence of ulcerative lesions on sigmoidoscopy. Stools may be watery or soft but are free of blood and mucus. In these mild cases, the diagnosis is often overlooked because examination of the stool for amebic trophozoites and cysts is not requested by the physician.

### Chronic Intestinal Amebiasis

Many patients with acute amebiasis, if left untreated, improve spontaneously, only to have a relapse within a short time. Such patients, especially if they reside in regions of low endemicity, such as the United States, may see several physicians before the possibility of amebiasis is considered. Physicians often neglect the possibility of amebiasis because in the United States intrinsic inflammatory bowel conditions, such as ulcerative colitis and regional enteritis, are fairly common, and the signs and symptoms associated with these diseases may be indistinguishable from those of chronic amebiasis.

The patient with chronic amebiasis usually has frequent episodes of blood-tinged diarrhea, weight loss, and abdominal pain. These symptoms may be present for several months. Repeated examination of the stool may be negative for trophozoites, especially when they are sought following antibiotic therapy or barium contrast studies of the bowel. Barium roentgenograms of the colon in patients with chronic amebiasis may mimic those seen in patients with ulcerative colitis and regional enteritis, including the presence of skip lesions, thumbprinting, and loss of haustral markings. Rarely, toxic megacolon may develop in patients with acute or chronic amebiasis. This complication previously had been thought to occur almost exclusively in patients with ulcerative colitis. On sigmoidoscopy, characteristic ulcers may be seen. Biopsies and smears made of the ulcerative lesions may be positive for trophozoites at a time when stools have been negative on repeat examinations. Patients with chronic amebiasis almost always have a positive serologic test for amebiasis.

Other intestinal complications of amebiasis include intestinal stricture formation and amebomas. Strictures are usually asymptomatic but occasionally produce abdominal pain or difficulty with defecation. When present, they most frequently occur in the rectum, anus, and sigmoid colon. Strictures usually resolve following therapy with a tissue amebicide. Amebomas are tumors consisting of granulation tissue that arise from the colon; they are most commonly found in the cecum but may occur anywhere in the colon and rectum. Symptoms, if present, may include abdominal pain, alternating diarrhea and constipation, weight loss, and rarely, a mass that can be palpated on abdominal examination. On barium enema examination, an ameboma may appear as a polypoid lesion, a napkin ring deformity, or an area of bowel-wall infiltration, all of which may easily be mistaken for carcinoma of the colon, especially if the patient has no prior history of dysentery. Amebomas, like strictures, resolve with specific chemotherapy.

### Extraintestinal Amebiasis

The most common extraintestinal site of *E. histolytica* infection is the liver, to which the trophozoites gain access via the portal circulation. Once infection is established in the liver, abscesses form. Almost all of the other extraintestinal sites of amebic infection follow the establishment of a liver abscess. Diagnosis of extraintestinal amebiasis is notoriously difficult, for most patients do not give a history of concomitant diarrhea or dysentery and may recall no gastrointestinal illness in the recent past. Stools are frequently negative on repeated examinations for trophozoites and cysts.

#### *Liver Abscess*

For reasons unknown, most patients who develop amebic liver abscess are male. The abscess is usually solitary and located in the right lobe of the liver. Pain and fever are the most common presenting symptoms. The pain is usually localized to the right upper quadrant, but may be present in the epigastrium or appear pleuritic in character over the right lower chest. Almost all patients are febrile. Occasionally, fever is the only presenting complaint, and the initial impression is that of fever of unknown origin.

On physical examination, the most frequent finding is tenderness in the right upper quadrant of the abdomen. The liver is usually palpable in those patients with a subacute or chronic presentation but is palpable in only one third or fewer of those patients with an acute illness.

Routine laboratory studies are not helpful. The white blood count is usually elevated but may be normal. There is no eosinophilia. Serum liver enzyme tests are nonspecific; the most consistent abnormality is an elevated serum alkaline phosphatase. High serum transaminase levels (ALT, AST) correlate with more aggressive disease with multiple liver abscesses. Hyperbilirubinemia and jaundice are uncommon. Trophozoites or cysts are found in the stools of only 10% of patients. Most helpful in determining the extent and localization of amebic abscess has been the use of ultrasonography and computed tomography (CT) of the liver and abdomen. Most patients are found to have a solitary abscess in the right lobe of the liver, but young patients with an abrupt onset of infection frequently are found to have multiple liver abscesses.

A definitive diagnosis may be made by performing needle aspiration of the abscess cavity and finding brown to brownish red, necrotic, non–foul-smelling material (the so-called anchovy paste) that is negative for bacterial growth. Trophozoites should be looked for in the aspirated material, especially in the final portions of the aspirate, although they are not commonly demonstrated. Fortunately, almost all patients with amebic liver abscess as well as other extraintestinal forms of amebiasis have a positive serologic test for amebiasis (see later discussion under Diagnosis).

Treatment consists of antiamebic chemotherapy, with or without needle aspiration of the abscess cavity. The major indications for therapeutic aspiration are the presence of an abscess cavity greater than 10 cm in diameter, an expanding abscess with rupture appearing imminent, or an abscess that has responded poorly to medical therapy. Small cavities respond well to medical therapy and do not need to be aspirated routinely.

#### *Other Extraintestinal Sites of Infection*

Less frequent complications of liver abscess are lung abscess and pericarditis. Lung abscess and empyema are almost always found in the right lower lobe and result from extension of an amebic liver abscess through the diaphragm. Amebic pericarditis is a rare complication of amebic liver abscess. Spread of infection to the pericardial sac is usually from an abscess in the left lobe of the liver, although pericarditis may be produced by contiguous spread from an adjacent lung abscess. Very rarely trophozoites reach the brain via the bloodstream to produce a brain abscess. Cutaneous amebiasis, usually of the perianal area, develops in a few individuals following prolonged contact of the perianal skin with *E. histolytica* trophozoites.

The vast majority of patients with invasive amebic infection develop circulating antibody within 1 week of infection. Specifically, antibody activity resides predominantly in the IgG fraction. Unfortunately, IgG plays little, if any, role in the intraluminal defense against invasive amebic disease. Population studies of individuals living in highly endemic areas also fail to provide evidence of protective immunity with advancing age. In fact, quite the contrary is found, with morbidity and mortality from *E. histolytica* infection increasing up to the age of 40–70 years.

### Diagnosis

A definitive diagnosis of amebiasis is dependent on the demonstration of trophozoites or cysts in the stool or trophozoites in aspirated pus or tissue specimens. All patients suspected of amebiasis should have at least three stool specimens examined for trophozoites and cysts. The stool should be collected directly in a paper cup to prevent lysis of the trophozoites by water. Examination for motile trophozoites should be done within 1 h of obtaining the specimen. Specimens of stool that cannot be examined within 1 h should be kept in the refrigerator. If routine stool examinations are negative and the diagnosis of amebiasis is still strongly suspected, a stool specimen should be obtained by saline purge if the patient can tolerate this procedure.

The initial examination of the stool should be a wet-mount preparation. A small sample of stool is placed on a microscope slide and emulsified with saline. A coverslip is added, and the slide is scanned under low power. The microscope should be equipped with an ocular micrometer so that the smaller trophozoites of *E. hartmanni* can be differentiated from *E. histolytica*, since, except for size, these organisms are morphologically identical. A second wet mount using a dilute iodine solution should also be used. Specimens that are negative on direct examination should be reexamined after concentration by the formol ether technique.

Identification of *E. histolytica* trophozoites requires an experienced technician. Trophozoites are usually only found in loose, watery, or dysenteric stools. White blood cells and macrophages with ingested red blood cells may be confused with trophozoites. *Entamoeba histolytica* trophozoites must also be differentiated from nonpathogenic amebae that may colonize the colon. Whenever possible, it is recommended that all parasitology laboratories preserve a portion of the stool with both 5% formalin and polyvinyl alcohol. Polyvinyl alcohol preserves the trophozoites, and the specimen preserved with 5% formalin can be examined for cysts. The preserved material can also be stained with either an iron hematoxylin or a Gomori-Wheatley trichrome stain, procedures which greatly aid in the differentiation of *E. histolytica* trophozoites from other protozoal trophozoites and white blood cells.

In patients with invasive intestinal amebiasis, the diagnosis may be strongly suspected by the finding of characteristic ulcers separated by normal-appearing intestinal mucosa during sigmoidoscopy. Scraping of the exudate overlying the ulcer and material aspirated through the sigmoidoscope should also be submitted for parasitologic examination. At the time of sigmoidoscopy, a biopsy may also be obtained from an area of ulceration and serial sections of the biopsied tissue stained with periodic acid–Schiff (PAS) stain. Occasionally, the biopsy is positive when multiple stool examinations fail to demonstrate trophozoites.

If three stool specimens are examined, trophozoites will be demonstrable in 70–95% of patients with intestinal amebiasis. Unfortunately, many medications and roentgenographic contrast media interfere with the ability to find trophozoites and cysts in the stool. Among the substances that interfere with the diagnosis of amebiasis are antimicrobial, antiprotozoal, and antihelmintic drugs; bismuth; barium; kaolin; magnesium hydroxide; soap; and hypertonic salt enemas. These agents may cause the temporary disappearance of trophozoites and cysts from the stool for several weeks.

In recent years, serologic testing has played an important role in the diagnosis of amebiasis. The serologic diagnosis of amebiasis has been especially useful in cases of amebic liver abscess and other extraintestinal foci of infection in which the absence of trophozoites and cysts in the stool is quite common.

Of the several serologic tests currently available for diagnosis of amebiasis, indirect hemagglutination (IHA) seems to be the most sensitive. Of patients with amebic liver abscess, 90–100% have a titer of 1:128 or greater by IHA. Most patients (80–90%) with invasive intestinal amebiasis also have an elevated IHA titer. Antibody titers measured by IHA usually revert to normal within 12 months of diagnosis and therapy. Complement fixation and gel diffusion titers usually return to the normal range within 6 months. Some individuals, however, continue to have elevated titers for several years without evidence of continued infection. Thus, a single serologic test is only suggestive of the diagnosis. Recently, newer diagnostic tests based on the detection of the galactose-specific adhesion by a monoclonal antibody technique and the detection of *E. histolytica* antigen in feces and serum show promise, and may even replace stool examination and culture.

## Treatment

Drugs used for the treatment of amebiasis can be divided into two major groups. The first encompasses those agents effective against the cyst form of the parasite, which are classified as intraluminal agents. The second group consists of those agents that are effective against the trophozoite, which are classified as tissue amebicides. Of all the effective agents in use, only metronidazole (Flagyl) is effective against both cysts and trophozoites and is therefore listed as both an intraluminal agent and an amebicide. Outlined below is a therapeutic plan found clinically useful.

### Intestinal Noninvasive Disease

Because of the potential for asymptomatic cyst passers to infect others, the consensus is that these individuals should be treated. The two major drugs effective against *E. histolytica* cysts are diloxanide furoate (Furamide), which is given orally in doses of 500 mg three times a day for 10 days. Diiodohydroxyquin (Di-Quinol) in adult doses of 650 mg three times a day for 20 days is also an effective intraluminal agent and is usually preceded by a 10-day course of oral tetracycline, 250 mg four times a day. Of the two drugs, diloxanide furoate is better tolerated but more difficult to obtain. Diiodohydroxyquin has the potential to produce optic neuritis. Side effects of both drugs are mostly limited to gastrointestinal upset and hypersensitivity reactions.

### Intestinal Invasive Disease

In recent years, metronidazole has been found to be a very effective agent in the therapy of amebiasis. It is effective against trophozoites present in tissue and relatively effective against cysts in the stool. Since the failure rate in treating asymptomatic cyst passers is between 12 and 19%, most clinicians combine metronidazole with either diiodohydroxyquin or diloxanide furoate, the dosages for which have already been outlined. Metronidazole is given orally in an adult dose of 750 mg three times a day for 5–10 days.

### Extraintestinal Amebiasis: Liver Abscess

Although there have been some treatment failures, metronidazole administered as outlined above is the drug of choice. Some patients with extraintestinal amebiasis may be so ill that they are unable to take or cannot tolerate oral medication. For these patients, the same dose of metronidazole can be administered intravenously. If after 72 h the patient is still febrile and the response to metronidazole is perceived by the physician to be less than satisfactory, chloroquine phosphate and emetine hydrochloride should be added to the treatment regimen. Chloroquine phosphate is given at an adult dose of 1 g orally each day for the first 2 days, then 0.5 g daily for 2 weeks; emetine hydrochloride is given as well at an adult dose of 65 mg per day intramuscularly for 2 weeks. Treatment of the liver abscess is usually followed by an agent active against intraluminal cysts.

Eradication of amebiasis can ultimately be accomplished only by governmental initiatives aimed at the elimination of poverty, poor sanitation, and the unsatisfactory living conditions of a vast portion of the world's population; unfortunately, these goals are unlikely to be achieved in the near future.

## INFECTION WITH *GIARDIA LAMBLIA*

*Giardia lamblia* is a flagellated protozoan that inhabits the upper portion of the human small intestine. Both trophozoite and cyst stages of the parasite are found in humans. Trophozoites are usually found in duodenal aspirates and biopsy specimens of the duodenum and jejunum and are infrequently seen in stools. The trophozoite of *G. lamblia* has a characteristic pear shape and measures 10–18 $\mu$m in length and 5–15 $\mu$m in width. There are two anterior nuclei and two slender median rods (axostyles). Four pairs of flagella are attached to the ventral side, and

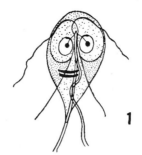 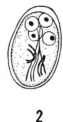 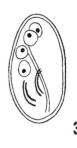

**1**        **2**        **3**

FIGURE 18–5. *1, Giardia lamblia* trophozoite; *2 and 3, G. lamblia* cysts. (From Markell, E. K., and Voge, M. *Medical Parasitology.* 4th ed. Philadelphia: W. B. Saunders Co., 1976. With permission).

attachment to the intestinal epithelium is mediated by a mannose-binding lectin as well as a large ventral sucking disc (see Fig. 18–5). Trophozoites are acid-intolerant and live optimally in the alkaline environment usually present in the upper small intestine.

Cysts of *G. lamblia* are thick walled and oval in shape. Initially, the cyst contains two nuclei that divide, forming four nuclei as the cyst passes down the intestinal tract and matures (Fig. 18–5). The cysts are the infective form of the parasite. Following ingestion, the cysts undergo excystation in the duodenum, forming two daughter trophozoites, completing the cycle.

### Epidemiology

*Giardia lamblia* has a worldwide distribution; it has been reported in almost 100 different countries. There are, however, certain geographic areas where the incidence of infection is fairly high. In the United States, giardiasis is more common in residents of and travelers to the Rocky Mountain states than in the rest of the country. Giardiasis is the most commonly reported parasitic disease in the United States.

*Giardia lamblia* is the pathogen most frequently responsible for water-related outbreaks of diarrheal illness in the United States. Cysts are capable of remaining viable in cold or tepid water for 1–3 months and are able to survive in the concentrations of chlorine usually present in municipal water. Most community-acquired infections have occurred where surface water (streams, rivers, lakes) is the principal water source, and chlorination the principal method for disinfection. There is highly suggestive evidence that these surface waters may be contaminated by fecal material from infected beavers and perhaps other wild animals. Smaller outbreaks have been reported in campers and backpackers in the Rocky Mountains who drank from mountain streams or ponds. To eliminate the

transmission of giardial infection from municipal water, filtration and coagulation–flocculation should be performed in addition to chlorination.

Infection may also occur by fecal–oral transmission. It does not take ingestion of many cysts to cause infection. When human volunteers were fed known numbers of giardial cysts in gelatin capsules, ingestion of 100 or more cysts produced infection in all volunteers, and as few as 10–25 cysts produced disease in 8 of 22 (36%) volunteers. Fecal–oral transmission occurs most commonly in sexually active male homosexuals but also occurs in children confined in institutions. Indirect modes of transmission include contamination of food by asymptomatic cyst passers.

### Pathogenesis of Infection

The low pH of gastric secretions is probably somewhat protective against infection with *G. lamblia*, and it has been observed that individuals with achlorhydria and hypochlorhydria are at increased risk of developing infection. Genetic factors may also play a role in susceptibility to infection, since giardiasis is seen more frequently in persons with type A blood and less frequently in persons with type O blood.

The mechanism by which *G. lamblia* produces diarrhea is not fully understood. From biopsy studies of the duodenum and jejunum, trophozoites of *G. lamblia* are most frequently found attached to the microvillus layer of the epithelium. In patients with severe disease, partial or subtotal villous atrophy is seen. Accompanying this change in villous architecture is a variable inflammatory infiltrate in the lamina propria consisting of both lymphocytes and neutrophils. It is not known whether this inflammatory response is protective, pathogenic, or perhaps both. Rarely, trophozoites are found within the mucosa and lamina propria of the upper small intestine. Direct invasion of the mucosa is felt to be only coincidental and not responsible for the symptoms of infection.

There is good evidence for epithelial cell dysfunction of the upper small intestine. Quite commonly, the microvilli of the upper small intestine are found to be temporarily deficient in disaccharidase activity. Also, fat and vitamin $B_{12}$ malabsorption are commonly observed, indicating that the absorptive dysfunction extends into the ileum. So far, no toxin has been found to explain the epithelial cell dysfunction, nor are there enough trophozoites present to mechanically block the enormous absorptive capacity of the small intestine. In many symptomatic patients with giardiasis, the biopsy of the upper small intestine is normal. This may be due in part to the patchy nature of the mucosal abnormalities, which can easily be missed when only a single biopsy is performed.

### Host Response to Infection

Specific antibody to both cyst and trophozoite antigens can be found in the majority of patients recovering from *Giardia lamblia* infection. Even patients who are asymptomatic cyst passers have detectable circulating antibody. It has also been observed that residents of endemic areas are less commonly infected than are visitors. In the human intestine, it is quite possible that secretory antigiardial IgA may interfere with adherence of this parasite to the gut epithelium and thus prevent the establishment of a new infection. There seems to be a definitely increased incidence of giardiasis in patients with common variable immunodeficiency. Not only is there an increased incidence of disease in such patients, but the illness is usually prolonged and more severe than in normal hosts.

Cellular immunity also appears to play a role in host defense against giardial infection. In the experimental mouse model, lymphocytes from an immune animal protect nonimmune mice from *G. muris* infection (a rodent strain of giardia). Athymic nude mice when infected with *G. muris* experience prolonged and severe infection suggesting that the host response to giardial infection involves cellular, as well as humoral, immunity. Patients with acquired immunodeficiency syndrome (AIDS), when infected with giardia, experience a severe and prolonged diarrheal illness.

### Acute Symptomatic Infection

Following an incubation period of 1–3 weeks, an acute diarrheal illness lasting 5–7 days is the most common presentation of giardiasis. The acute illness is quite variable in severity. Some patients have an abrupt, explosive onset with frequent watery, foul-smelling stools, whereas others have only a few loose bowel movements. Most commonly, the patient also has abdominal cramps and complains of nausea, anorexia, and increased flatulence. Less often, fever, vomiting, and abdominal distention may be present. Blood or mucus is rarely present in the stool. In 86% of experimentally infected volunteers, cysts can no longer be found in the stool after 6 weeks. In some patients the acute illness may be prolonged, lasting 1–2 months. An even smaller percentage of infected individuals develop a subacute or chronic illness.

### Chronic Giardiasis

In patients who have chronic giardiasis, diarrhea is often intermittent and less severe than in the acute illness. Stools are frequently foul smelling, and foul-smelling gas may be passed from the rectum. Substernal burning, nausea, and anorexia may occur. Because of these symptoms, peptic ulcer disease, hiatal hernia, and gallbladder disease may be suspected.

Signs and symptoms of intestinal malabsorption are commonly present in patients with chronic giardiasis. As a result of chronic malabsorption, weight loss is frequently reported by the patient. These symptoms, in association with persistent or intermittent diarrhea, often lead first to a diagnosis of pancreatic insufficiency, celiac disease, regional enteritis, ulcerative colitis, or intestinal malignancy. In some patients frank steatorrhea develops, as evidenced by the passage of bulky, greasy, foul-smelling stools. In patients with steatorrhea, the absorption of vitamin A and folate are also frequently impaired. In some patients, absorption of vitamin $B_{12}$ is abnormally low, implying that the absorption defect extends into the ileum. In addition to fat malabsorption, defects in the absorption of carbohydrates are found in up to 50% of patients with giardiasis, as indicated by decreased absorption of D-xylose. Intestinal biopsy also shows reduced activity of the disaccharidases, lactase, maltase, and sucrase, which may persist for some time even after completion of medical therapy.

Very rarely, there is extraintestinal extension of infection into the biliary tract. In patients so affected, the signs and symptoms of infection are identical to those seen in patients with classic, acute, or chronic cholangitis or cholecystitis.

## Asymptomatic Carriers

Most people who become infected with *G. lamblia* do not recall experiencing a diarrheal illness. These individuals are usually discovered only when epidemiologic investigations are carried out. It has been found that in some regions of the United States, 5–10% of the population excrete cysts in their stools. The duration of asymptomatic carriage of *G. lamblia* is unknown.

## Diagnosis

The diagnosis of giardiasis is most commonly made by finding cysts in the stool. Since the cysts passed in some patients may be intermittent or low in number and thus difficult to find, a stool specimen should be examined every other day for a total of three or four occasions. Stools should be examined directly and after concentration with formol ether or zinc sulfate and stained with Lugol's solution or iron hematoxylin. In the acute phase of the disease, when diarrhea is severe and transit time is short, trophozoites may also be found in the stool. In a small number of patients, cysts cannot be found in the stool, but a diagnosis can usually be made by duodenal intubation and aspiration, since trophozoites are frequently present in the fluid and mucus that is obtained. To increase the yield even further, biopsy of the duodenal and jejunal mucosa may be performed. A less invasive procedure is the "string test," in which the patient swallows a weighted capsule attached to a nylon line (Enterotest: available from Hedeco Co., Mountain View, California) long enough to pass into the upper small intestine. The capsule and line are removed after several hours, and the mucus adherent to the distal line is scraped onto a glass slide along with a few drops of saline and examined for trophozoites.

Recently, the detection of surface specific giardial antigen in the stool by enzyme-linked immunosorbent assay (ELISA) and fluorescein-tagged monoclonal antibody has been described. These techniques are able to detect very small numbers of organisms that are present in the stool or are seen only on duodenal aspiration and biopsy. In addition, these techniques require less skilled technician time and are more suitable to mass screening and epidemiologic studies than is routine stool examination.

## Treatment

Although not approved by the U.S. Food and Drug Administration (FDA), metronidazole (Flagyl) has proven over the past several years to be a well-tolerated and effective agent in the treatment of giardiasis. Cure rates with metronidozole are in the range of 85–90%. The usual adult dose is 250 mg three times a day for 7 days. Because of possible mutagenic potential in laboratory animals (not shown in humans), children are often treated with furazolidone (Furoxone). This agent is not quite effective in the elimination of infection as metronidozole but is available as a pleasant-tasting liquid suspension, which improves pediatric patient compliance.

Quinacrine (Atabrine) is also an effective agent in the treatment of giardiasis but is very difficult to obtain and may be available only from the Centers for Disease Control (CDC).

## INFECTION WITH *ISOSPORA BELLI*

*Isospora belli* is a coccidian protozoa that is capable of producing a diarrheal illness in both immunocompetent and immunocompromised hosts. Infection is initiated by swallowing food or water contaminated with sporocysts of *I. belli*. A higher incidence of *I. belli* infection has been observed in homosexual men, also suggesting that transmission of this parasitic infection may occur sexually. Excystation occurs in the upper small intestine with the release of four sporozoites from each sporocyst. Asexual development (schizogony) occurs within the cystoplasm of the epithelial cell with the development of trophozoites, schizonts, and finally, merozoites.

The merozoites are then released by the disintegrating schizont to invade other epithelial cells, and this cycle is repeated. At least 1 week later the sexual cycle (gametogony) begins with the production of micro- and macrogametocytes. Following fertilization of the macrogametocytes by the microgametocytes, the zygote, or oocyst, is formed. The oocyst, when shed into the bowel lumen, initially contains a single sporoblast. Following fecal passage of the oocyst, the sporoblast divides in two and secretes a cyst wall around itself (sporocyst). Within each sporoblast, four sporozoites develop. Ingestion of the sporocyst containing the sporozoites initiates the infection in the duodenum and upper jejunum.

## Acute and Chronic Intestinal Infection

The most common symptom complex of *Isospora belli* infection is a self-limited diarrheal illness that lasts from 1–3 weeks. Watery diarrhea is frequently associated with cramping abdominal pain, fever, and weight loss. Some patients develop a chronic diarrheal illness frequently associated with malabsorption. *Isospora belli* infection in patients with AIDS is a much more serious illness that follows a protracted course of diarrhea, debility, weight loss, and wasting.

On pathologic examination of the small bowel, villus shortening; hypertrophic crypts; and infiltration of the lamina propria with lymphocytes, plasma cells, and lymphocytes are frequently observed. Whether these mucosal changes alone are enough to account for the diarrheal illness is as yet unknown.

### Diagnosis

Oocysts may be few in number or shed only intermittently in the stool. The cysts have an ovoid shape and measure 20–33 $\mu$m in length by 10–19 $\mu$m in width. Stools are best examined following a concentration technique. Identification of the cysts is also easier when the stool concentrate is stained with a modified Kinyoun stain. With this stain the oocysts of *Isospora belli* stain bright red on a green background. If repeated stool examinations are negative, sometimes the only way to confirm the diagnosis of *I. belli* infection is by intestinal biopsy.

### Treatment

Most infections with *Isospora belli* can be successfully treated with trimethoprim-sulfamethoxazole (Bactrim, Septra). In adults the usual dose is one double-strength tablet every 6 h by mouth for 10 days followed by one double-strength tablet every 12 h for an additional 3 weeks. An alternative regimen for the treatment of *I. belli* infection is pyrimethamine plus sulfadoxine (Fansidar) given orally. Patients with AIDS may require chronic suppression of this infection with weekly administration of trimethoprim-sulfamethoxazole.

## INFECTION WITH *CRYPTOSPORIDIUM*

*Cryptosporidium*, like *Isospora belli*, is a coccidian protozoan capable of infecting the human intestinal tract, producing a diarrheal illness.

Prior to 1976, infection with *Cryptosporidium* was felt to be confined to young farm animals (pigs, lambs, calves). In 1976, the first human case of cryptosporidiosis was described, and until 1982 there were only a handful of reported human cases. In the past 6–8 years, several large outbreaks of cryptosporidiosis have been described affecting thousands of normal individuals following contamination of municipal water treatment plants. The oocyst is resistant to chlorination, and filtration of these very small parasites is the primary mechanism of exclusion of contaminated surface waters from the drinking supply. With the development of the AIDS epidemic, numerous cases of cryptosporidiosis have been described. This protozoan is now recognized as a major enteric pathogen of patients with AIDS, producing a severe, protracted diarrheal illness.

With the increased awareness of this protozoan as a cause of diarrheal illness and increased skill in routine identification of this parasite by parasitology laboratories, cryptosporidial infections have also been identified with increased frequency in normal hosts. The overall frequency of cryptosporidial infection in the United States has been estimated at 2.6%. A higher incidence of infection was found when children attending selected day-care centers were sampled. Both human-to-human and animal-to-human transmission can occur. Nosocomial transmission between hospital staff and patients has been described, as well as an increased incidence of infection among household contacts of an infected patient. Individuals who work with animals, such as farm workers and veterinarians, also are at increased risk to develop infection.

### Life Cycle

Infection is initiated by ingestion of small (2–5 $\mu$m) spherical oocysts. Excystation occurs in the upper intestinal tract with the liberation of four sporozoites. The entire asexual (schizogony) development of the parasite, with the production of trophozoites, schizonts, and merozoites, as well as the sexual cycle (gametogony), with the production of gametes, all occurs in a single host. This monoxenous life cycle lends itself to perpetuation of infection. The merozoites liberated from the schizonts within the intestinal tract are able to infect more enterocytes. Oocysts are excreted in the stool and are capable of infecting other humans or susceptible animals.

The life forms of *Cryptosporidium* are confined to the microvillus border of the intestinal epithelial cell. The parasite is enclosed in a vacuole, the membrane of which appears to be of host origin. Thus, the parasite is intracellular but extracytoplasmic. In patients with AIDS, cryptosporidia are found throughout the entire intestine and occasionally invade the gallbladder and biliary tree. Rarely, the respiratory epithelium may become infected with this parasite.

### Acute and Chronic Intestinal Infection

In the normal host after an incubation period of 7–8 days, a self-limited watery diarrheal illness without blood or mucus ensues. Patients may also experience abdominal cramps and low-grade fever. The diarrheal illness usually resolves after 1 or 2 weeks, but excretion of oocysts may persist for 2–4 weeks after symptoms abate. In young children, a self-limited diarrhea illness lasting 3–5 days is common. In immunocompromised hosts, particularly in patients with AIDS, *Cryptosporidium* infection is severe and protracted. The diarrheal illness is often watery and voluminous, with fluid losses of up to 20 L/day described. This is often associated with malabsorption, significant weight loss, electrolyte imbalance, marked suffering, and poor quality of life for the patient. It has been estimated that 11–21% of patients with AIDS and diarrhea are infected with *Cryptosporidium*. The mechanism causing the diarrhea is unknown, although jejunal biopsies often show partial villus atrophy with or without crypt hyperplasia.

### Diagnosis

Oocysts can be easily demonstrated (after stool concentration) by a modified acid-fast stain, such as a cold Kinyoun stain. In the normal host, fewer oocysts are excreted during the diarrheal illness and several concentrated stools may need to be examined to establish a diagnosis. Recently, monoclonal and polyclonal fluorescent antibody and ELISA tests have been developed to aid in the rapid diagnosis of this parasitic infection.

### Treatment

Currently there is no established effective therapy for cryptosporidiosis. Although the macrolide antibiotic spiramycin initially was felt to be efficacious, subsequent studies have failed to confirm that benefit. Several small studies treating patients with the oral amino-glycoside antibiotic paromomycin seem promising but need to be confirmed by larger prospective controlled trials.

## INFECTION WITH *MICROSPORIDIA*

*Microsporidia* are obligate intracellular spore-forming parasites belonging to the order Microsporidia of the phylum Microsporia. Similar in size to cryptosporidia, microsporidia have recently been found to be a fairly common cause of chronic diarrhea in patients with AIDS.

### Epidemiology

By electron microscopy the spores of microsporidia species are found to have distinctive polar tubes coiled around electron lucent inclusions and an endospore layer just outside the plasma membrane. Of the several genera of microsporidia capable of producing infection in man, *Enterocytozoon bieneusi* is the most frequently found.

Microsporidia are capable of producing infection in a wide variety of mammals, fish, birds, and even insects. Animal-to-man transmission probably occurs, but most people become infected by coming in contact with bodily fluids, especially stool and to a much lesser extent respiratory secretions and urine.

### Intestinal Infection

In patients with AIDS and low CD4 counts (i.e., <100/mm$^3$) infection with microsporidia often results in chronic watery diarrhea with weight loss and debility. In one study of chronic diarrhea in patients with AIDS, 22% of the patients had microsporidia present on stool examination. These parasites can also be diagnosed by light and electron microscopic studies of small intestine biopsies. Infection in patients with AIDS is not limited to the small intestine. Infection of the gallbladder, biliary ducts, liver, kidney, peritoneum, trachea, bronchi, and conjunctiva has been described.

### Diagnosis

Diagnosis can be accomplished by examination and staining stool specimens or biopsy material with May-Grünwald-Giemsa.

### Treatment

Clinical trials of various therapeutic agents are in progress. At times, intestinal disease responds to metronidozole. Albendazole therapy may also be of benefit.

# COMMON INTESTINAL NEMATODE INFECTIONS

Of the more than half million different species of roundworms, many of which infect animals and plants, only about 12 species are parasitic for humans. On a global scale, infection with nematodes (roundworms) is more common than infection with any other group of pathogens. *Enterobius* and *Ascaris* each account for a billion infections worldwide. Not far behind are infections with *Trichuris* and hookworm, which each cause a half billion infections annually. In the United States, it has been estimated that 54 million people, mostly children, are infected with nematodes. The intestinal nematodes are unsegmented roundworms with a cylindric shape that is tapered at both ends. They are large parasites, all of which can be seen by the naked eye without magnification. The sexes of the roundworms are separate, with the male usually smaller than the female. Each roundworm has a complete digestive tract with an oral opening at one end and a distal anal opening.

## *Trichuris trichiura* Infection

Trichuriasis, infection with *Trichuris trichiura* (or whipworm), is a common infection in the United States, especially in the southeastern portion of the country. It has been estimated that in the United States there are 2.2 million individuals infected with trichuris. Worldwide, the incidence of infection is even greater in tropical and subtropical areas of the world where there is overcrowding and poor sanitation.

## Life Cycle

The life cycle of *Trichuris trichiura* is simple, and no intermediate host is required. Infection is initiated by the ingestion of the embryonated eggs present in soil that has been contaminated by human feces. The eggs are hardy and may remain viable in moist soil for years. In the small intestine the male and female larvae emerge and pass to the large intestine and cecum. Adult male and female worms develop in the large intestine. The adult worms have a characteristic appearance with a thin whiplike anterior portion and a stout hind portion, "the whip handle." The adults measure 30–50 mm in length. The slender anterior portion of the worm penetrates the mucosa of the large intestine, anchoring the parasite while the posterior portion of the body protrudes into the bowel lumen facilitating copulation and oviposition. After the adult worms mature, the female is capable of laying 1000 eggs per day. The unsegmented eggs, passed into the feces, require about 2 weeks to embryonate in warm moist soil. Adult worms may live as long as a year in the intestinal tract.

### *Clinical Manifestations of Trichuriasis*

Like all nematode infections, symptomatology is directly proportional to the extent of the infection (worm burden) and to the age and general health of the host. Most infections with trichuris are light to moderate. In these individuals symptoms of infection are uncommon. With heavy infections in children, complaints of abdominal pain, bloody or mucoid diarrhea, and weight loss may be experienced. Rarely, appendicitis secondary to appendiceal obstruction and prolapse of the rectum may occur.

### *Diagnosis*

Diagnosis of *Trichuris trichiura* infection is made by finding the characteristic ovoid-shaped eggs with clear mucus plugs at each pole. Infections can be quantitated by counting the number of eggs found in a direct fecal smear. In light infections fewer than 10 eggs are present. In heavy infections 50 or more eggs are present in the fecal smear.

### *Treatment*

Trichuris infections can be effectively treated with mebendazole 100 mg twice a day for 3 days. Mebendazole (Vermox) is poorly absorbed from the intestinal tract and has insignificant side effects.

## *Enterobius vermicularis* Infection

Enterobiasis, infection with the pinworm *Enterobius vermicularis*, is the most common helminthic infection in the United States. An estimated 42 million individuals, mostly children, are infected with pinworms. Infections tend to spread within the family setting, especially if several children live in the same household or sleep in the same bed. Transmission of enterobius infection is by the fecal–oral route. This may be direct, from the unwashed hands of one child to the mouth of another, or indirect, by fecal contamination of sheets, linen, and night clothes.

### *Life Cycle*

The life cycle of *Enterobius vermicularis* is very similar to that of *Trichuris trichiura* because it is direct, requiring no intermediate host.

Infection is initiated by swallowing the embryonated egg, which passes into the small intestine, releasing the enclosed larvae. The larvae migrate down the intestinal tract to the cecum and colon where the adult worms develop in about a month. The adult male is very small, measuring 2–5 mm in length, but the adult female is much larger, 8–13 mm long with a sharply pointed posterior end (pin). The fertilized females migrate at night to the perianal and perineal skin and deposit their eggs in this location. Each female pinworm is capable of laying 11,000 ovoid eggs, which are surrounded by a thick wall and flattened on one side. The embryonated eggs, which develop within 6 h, are picked up by the child's hands or contaminate the bed clothes or linen and can initiate a new infection.

### Clinical Manifestations of Enterobiasis

Most pinworm infections are asymptomatic. When symptoms are reported, the most frequent complaints are perianal itching and restless sleep produced by the deposited eggs. Rarely, in young girls vaginitis or even salpingitis has been reported. Another rare complication of pinworm infection is appendicitis.

### Diagnosis

Since eggs are rarely deposited into the stool, the most common method of confirming enterobius infection is the recovery of the characteristic eggs from the perianal skin. The most commonly employed method is the "Scotch-tape" swab. A piece of transparent adhesive tape backed by a tongue blade is pressed around the perianal skin early in the morning. The transparent tape is then transferred to a glass slide and examined under the microscope. A single Scotch-tape swab picks up eggs from at least 50% of those infected, and three swabs on consecutive days pick up eggs from 90%. In families with multiple children, all family members should be examined in this manner.

### Treatment

Enterobius infection is effectively treated with a single 100-mg oral dose of mebendazole and repeated again in 1 week. Alternatively, pyrantel pamoate can be utilized as a single dose of 11 mg/kg and repeated again at 2 weeks. Frequently, physicians treat all chil-

dren in the family if one child is discovered to have pinworms. Bed clothes and linen can be decontaminated by ordinary washing in hot water.

### *Ascaris lumbricoides* Infection

Infection with *Ascaris lumbricoides* is the most common helmintic infection in the world, with over a billion humans infected. Infection is most common in tropical or subtropical areas of the world, where poor sanitation and overcrowding exist, but is not uncommon in temperate regions. In the United States, an estimated 4 million people are infected with ascaris, mostly in the southeastern and Gulf states. Children bear the major brunt of this parasitic infection, with symptoms related to migration of the parasite through the lungs and to intestinal disease. Ascaris is the largest of the intestinal roundworms, with the female worm measuring 20–35 cm in length and the mature male 15–30 cm. The average life span for the adult worms is about 6 months.

### Life Cycle

Infection is initiated by ingestion of embryonated eggs present in the soil. The larvae emerge in the small intestine and penetrate the bowel wall and into the portal circulation. They are carried via the bloodstream to the lungs, where they increase in size and molt twice. The larvae next break into the bronchial tree and travel up into the trachea and then into the esophagus. The swallowed larvae reach the small intestine, where they develop into mature adults. From ingestion of the embryonated egg to the development of a gravid female takes about 8–12 weeks. Each female is capable of laying 200,000 eggs per day. Fertilized eggs require 2–3 weeks to develop in the soil before they are mature and are infective.

### Clinical Manifestations of Ascariasis

In heavy infections, pulmonary infiltrates associated with peripheral eosinophilia may develop when the larvae migrate through the lungs. This self-limited pneumonia is associated with cough, dyspnea, fever, and scattered pulmonary infiltrates on chest x-ray. On repeated exposure to ascaris, allergic reactions may be responsible for bronchospasm (asthma) and cutaneous urticaria.

The symptoms of small-intestine infection are directly dependent on worm burden, with light infections being asymptomatic. In heavy infections with worm loads of several hundred to a thousand worms, abdominal pain, diarrhea, anorexia, and malnutrition may be experienced. Malnutrition is due to impaired absorption of carbohydrates and fat in the small intestine. In heavy infections, symptoms may be secondary to a mass of tangled worms that can produce intestinal obstruction. Ascaris worms may also migrate into the common bile duct or pancreatic duct to produce obstructive cholecystitis and pancreatitis, or into the appendix with resulting appendicitis.

### Diagnosis

Finding the characteristic ovoid eggs covered with an albuminoid shell in the feces is the most common method of confirming ascaris infection. On occasion adult worms may crawl out the nose, be vomited, or pass into the stool. In families with several children, all family members should have their stool examined for the presence of eggs.

### Treatment

Mebendazole, 100 mg twice a day by mouth for 3 days, or pyrantel pamoate (Antiminth) as a single dose (11 mg/kg up to a maximum of 1 g) are both equally effective agents in treating ascariasis.

## Infection with *Necator americanus* and *Ancylostoma duodenale*

Infection with the hookworms *Necator americanus* and *Ancylostoma duodenale* dates to prehistoric times. These parasites are common in the tropical and subtropical areas of the world where there is overcrowding and poor sanitation. *Ancylostoma duodenale* (Old World hookworm) has been mostly found in southern Europe, the north coast of Africa, northern India, and China, and is not discussed at length in this section.

*Necator americanus* (New World hookworm) is present in the United States, mostly in the southeastern portion of the country, but is more frequently found in Central and South America, the Caribbean, Africa, and Asia. Together, hookworm infection affects half a billion people throughout the world.

Hookworms derive their name from the teeth (*Ancylostoma*) or cutting plates (*Necator*) in the anterior buccal capsule, which allow the hookworm to attach to the intestinal mucosa and account for the significant blood loss experienced by heavily infected individuals.

### Life Cycle

The life cycle of *Necator americanus* has been described as the skin-penetrating type. Infection is acquired by walking barefooted or in sandals in soil containing the filariform hookworm larva. The skin is penetrated by the larva, often producing a papular eruption and severe pruritus of the skin ("ground itch"). The filariform larva then enters the venous circulation and is carried to the pulmonary capillary bed. In the lungs *N. americanus* does not evoke an intense reaction as occurs in infection with ascaris or strongyloides (see description later in this chapter). The larva then breaks into the bronchial tree, migrates up into the trachea and then into the esophagus and is swallowed. In the small intestine the filariform larvae molt (third molt) and develop a temporary bacial capsule for attachment to the mucosa. Here the larvae grow and develop into adult male and female worms. After about a period of 5 weeks from initiation of infection, the female hookworms begin to oviposit. The hookworm eggs deposited with the feces into warm moist soil first develop into the rhabditiform larvae, which are free-living and feed on bacteria and organic debris. By about a week the rhabdoid larvae develop into the nonfeeding filariform larvae capable of invading a new human host.

The life cycle of *Ancylostoma duodenale* is almost identical to that of *N. americanus* with the exception that infection can also be initiated by swallowing the filariform larva and that a developmental stage in the lungs is not required.

### Clinical Manifestations of Hookworm Infection

As with most intestinal parasitic infections, symptoms are largely dependent on worm burden. In the United States most infections with *Necator americanus* are light and infections are usually asymptomatic. In heavy infections the major symptoms are secondary to anemia and hypoalbuminemia. Blood loss occurs because of ingestion of blood by the parasite, but is much more related to loss into the bowel lumen from the bleeding laceration created by the attachment of the cutting plates or teeth of the hookworm. It has been estimated that 0.03 mL of blood is lost per day for each adult *N. americanus* worm and 0.15 mL for each *A. duodenale* adult. In heavy infections, over 1000 adult worms may be present in the small intestine. The resulting anemia and hypoalbuminemia may be compounded in those individuals consuming diets poor in protein and iron. Occasionally, a transient pulmonary infiltrate develops during the stage of pulmonary migration, associated with eosinophilia.

Humans may also develop a cutaneous eruption if they come in contact with the dog and cat hookworm larvae, *Ancylostoma braziliense* or *A. caninum.* These larvae penetrate the skin and migrate through the subcutaneous tissue, forming serpiginous tunnels associated with intense itching. Infection with these hookworms and this cutaneous eruption has been termed *cutaneous larva migrans.* The larva cannot complete the life cycle as human hookworms do and essentially remain trapped in the skin until they die, which may take several weeks.

### Diagnosis

The diagnosis of hookworm infection rests on the demonstration of the characteristic eggs in the stool. The number of eggs can be quantitated, and egg counts greater than 2000/g of stool in children is considered clinically significant.

### Treatment

Hookworms are very effectively treated with oral mebendazole, 100 mg twice a day for 3 days.

### Strongyloides stercoralis Infection

Infection with *Strongyloides stercoralis* is most common in warm climates, but it is also present in temperate areas of the world. Strongyloides infection somewhat parallels hookworm infection. Infection in the United States has been reported mostly from the southeastern portion of the country. In addition to children being the most common target for infection, *S. stercoralis* may produce severe infection (hyperinfection) in the compromised host.

### Life Cycle

The life cycle of *Strongyloides stercoralis* is very similar to that of the hookworm in that infection is usually initiated when the infective filariform larvae penetrate the skin and make their way to the lung via the bloodstream. From the lungs the larvae migrate up the tracheobronchial tree and into the esophagus, and then into the upper small intestine. In the duodenum and upper jejunum the larvae mature into the adult worms, the female measuring about 2.5 mm in length. The

gravid female lays her eggs, which usually hatch in the mucosal epithelium, producing rhabdoid larvae. The rhabdoid larvae are passed into the feces and in areas of poor sanitation are deposited in the soil. The rhabdoid larvae of strongyloides may exist in the soil as a free-living form or develop into nonfeeding, infective filariform larvae.

For reasons that are poorly understood, in some individuals, usually those who are immunologically compromised, the progression from rhabdoid to filariform larvae may occur in the lower intestine. The infectious filariform larvae thus produced are able to enter the host's circulation in the large intestine and rectum or through the perianal or perineal skin. This autoinfection (hyperinfection) leads to both persistence of infection and large numbers of worms infecting the host.

### Clinical Manifestations of Strongyloidiasis

At the site of skin penetration, a local pruritic inflammatory reaction may develop, but this occurs less frequently and is less symptomatic than with hookworm infection. When larvae penetrate the perianal skin, they may produce a serpiginous trail associated with urticaria. This creeping eruption has been termed *larva currens.* During the larval migration through the lung, patchy infiltrates associated with peripheral blood eosinophilia may develop—Löffler's pneumonia.

With heavy intestinal infection, complaints of abdominal pain, weight loss, and diarrhea are common. The abdominal pain may be epigastric and burning in nature, similar to the pain produced by peptic ulcer disease.

Patients who are immunocompromised because of an underlying hematologic malignancy, corticosteroid therapy, malnutrition, or AIDS are prone to develop hyperinfection. In these individuals infective filariform larvae develop from the rhabdoid larvae as the latter pass down the gastrointestinal tract. The filariform larvae penetrate the vascular system in the colon and rectum or through the perianal or perineal skin. Not infrequently after entering the host's circulation, these larvae follow an aberrant course and settle in various organs, producing local inflammatory disease. The lung is commonly involved in this process, but any organ may be affected. There may also be local ulcerations of the bowel, with the development of bacterial sepsis.

## Diagnosis

The diagnosis of strongyloides infection rests on the demonstration of larvae in the stool, in bronchial secretions, or in duodenal fluid. Multiple stools should first be examined after concentration; if persistently negative, a duodenal aspirate obtained by intubation or material obtained by a "string test" (see diagnosis of giardiasis above) should be examined for the presence of larvae.

## Treatment

Strongyloides infection can be effectively treated with thiabendazole (Mintezol), 25 mg/kg twice a day by mouth for 2 days. In patients with hyperinfection, treatment with thiabendazole should be extended for at least 2–3 weeks.

## CASE HISTORY

### CASE HISTORY 1

A 4-year-old child living in South Carolina complained to his mother of abdominal cramps for several days. There was no associated fever or diarrhea. When the symptoms persisted the child was seen in the pediatric clinic where the physical examination was completely normal except for some mild discomfort on palpation of the abdomen. Examination of the urine was normal, as was the white blood cell count, but the differential count revealed 18% eosinophils. This prompted an examination of a stool specimen, which revealed characteristic eggs of *Ascaris lumbricoides*. Treatment twice each day for 3 days with mebendazole resulted in cure.

### CASE 1 DISCUSSION

Infection with helminthic worms in the United States produces mild disease, often with nonspecific intestinal symptoms. As in this case the findings of eosinophils prompted an examination of the stool for evidence of parasites. Occasionally, ascaris organisms crawl out of the rectum, nose, mouth or up the biliary tract. In third world countries, most children suffer from malnutrition, and ascariasis is associated with increased morbidity.

## REFERENCES

### Books

Bogitsh, B. J., and Cheng, T. C., eds. *Human Parasitology.* Philadelphia: Saunders College Publishing, 1990.

Cook, G. C. *Parasitic Disease in Clinical Practice.* New York: Springer-Verlag, 1990.

Leech, J. H., Sande, M. A., and Root, R. K., eds. *Parasitic Infections.* New York: Churchill Livingstone, 1988.

### Original Articles

Adams, E. B., and MacLeod, I. N. Invasive amebiasis. I. Amebic dysentery and its complications. *Medicine 56:* 315–323, 1977.

Adams, E. B., and MacLeod, I. N. Invasive amebiasis. II. Amebic liver abscess and its complications. *Medicine 56:*325–334, 1977.

DeHovitz, J. A. Management of *Isospora belli* infections in AIDS patients. *Infect. Med. 10:*437–440, 1988.

Fichenbaum, C. J., Ritchie, D. J., and Powderly, W.G. Use of paromomycin for treatment of cryptosporidiosis in patients with AIDS. *Clin. Infect. Dis. 16:*298–300, 1993.

Hague R., Kress, K., Wood, S., Terry, F. H. G., et al. Diagnosis of pathogenic *Entamoeba histolytica* infection using a stool ELISA based on monoclonal antibiodies to the galactose-specific adhesion. *J. Infect. Dis. 167:*247–249, 1993.

Hayes, E. B., Matte, T. D., O'Brien, T. R., McKinley, T. W., et al. Large community outbreak of cryptosporidiosis due to contamination of filtered public water supply. *N. Engl. J. Med. 320:*1372–1376, 1989.

Heyworth, M. F. Immunology of *Giardia* and *Cryptosporidium* infections. *J. Infect. Dis. 166:*465–472, 1992.

Ravdin, J. I. Pathogenesis of disease caused by *Entamoeba histolytica:* Studies of adherence, secreted toxins, and contact-dependent cytolysis. *Rev. Infect. Dis. 8:*247–260, 1986.

Soave, R., and Johnson, W. D., Jr. *Cryptosporidium* and *Isospora belli* infections. *J. Infect. Dis. 157:*225–229, 1988.

Strachen, W. D., Spice, W. M., Chiodini, P. L., Moody, A. H., and Ackers, J. P. Immunological differentiation of pathogenic and nonpathogenic isolates of *Entamoeba histolytica.* Lancet 1:561–562, 1988.

Tannich, E., Horstmann, R. D., Knoblock, J., and Arnold, H. H. Genomic DNA differences between pathogenic and nonpathogenic *Entamoeba histolytica. Proc. Natl. Acad. Sci. USA 86:*5118–5122, 1989.

Weber, R., Bryan, R. T., Owen, R. L., Wilcox, C. M. et al. Improved light-microscopical detection of Microsporidia spores in stool and duodenal aspirates. *N. Engl. J. Med. 326:*161–166, 1992.

# 19

# VIRAL HEPATITIS

STANFORD T. SHULMAN, M.D.

*Viral hepatitis* is the term applied to those viral infections in which the liver is the dominant target organ. The many other viral illnesses that may affect the liver but in which hepatic involvement does not usually dominate the clinical picture are not discussed here. That jaundice could occur in an epidemic form was known to the Greeks and Romans of 2500 years ago. During the 18th century, at least nine well-defined epidemics of jaundice were described in Central Europe, some including remarkably astute clinical observations. Subsequently, the infectious nature of hepatitis was clearly established by studies that strongly suggested fecal–oral transmission in some circumstances and transmission by blood or serum in other situations. An example of the latter was the early World War II outbreak of 50,000 cases of hepatitis among American soldiers who had received injections of yellow fever vaccine that contained human serum. The fecal–oral form of hepatitis became known as *infectious hepatitis,* and the latter variety was termed *serum hepatitis.*

In the past 25 years, there has been truly remarkable progress in identifying and characterizing the specific etiologic agents of viral hepatitis. We now recognize *hepatitis A virus* (HAV) as the etiology of infectious hepatitis;

*hepatitis B virus* (HBV) as the etiology of serum hepatitis; the *delta hepatitis agent* as a novel defective viral pathogen; *hepatitis C virus* (HCV) as another usually parenterally transmitted agent that often causes chronic liver disease; and *hepatitis E virus* (HEV), another agent transmitted by the fecal–oral route. The latter two agents account for a large portion of the viral hepatitis not associated with either HAV or HBV, often referred to as *non-A, non-B hepatitis.* This form of hepatitis includes infection by HCV and HEV and probably several additional agents.

All of the hepatitis viruses except HBV have a single-stranded RNA genome. Diagnostic tests to measure specific well-characterized serologic markers now enable accurate identification of infection with HAV, HBV, the delta virus, and HCV. A highly effective HBV vaccine is available, and HAV vaccines have been licensed for use in many countries. Because similarity of the clinical manifestations of the several forms of viral hepatitis frequently makes differentiation on clinical grounds alone somewhat difficult, an accurate history of potential sources of infection together with serologic testing are required for accurate diagnosis of the specific type of viral hepatitis. Table 19–1 summarizes informa-

281

**TABLE 19–1.   CHARACTERISTICS OF VIRAL HEPATITIS**

|   | **HEPATITIS A** | **HEPATITIS B** | **DELTA VIRUS** | **HEPATITIS C** | **HEPATITIS E** |
|---|---|---|---|---|---|
| Causative agent | 27-nm RNA virus | 42-nm DNA virus with surface and core components | 36-nm RNA defective virus with HBsAg coat | Small 10-kb ss–RNA virus | 27–34-nm RNA virus |
| Transmission | Fecal—oral | Parenteral | Parenteral | Parenteral; sporadic also (fecal—oral?) | Fecal—oral; contaminated water supply |
| Incubation | 15–50 days | 45–180 days | 28–180 days | About 60–150 days | 14–63 days |
| Period of infectivity | Late incubation to early clinical phase | When HBsAg positive | When anti-HDV seropositive | Unknown | Unknown |
| Fulminant hepatitis | Rare | Uncommon | Common | Uncommon | Common in third trimester; otherwise uncommon |
| Chronic hepatitis or carrier state | No | Common (5–10%) | Common | Common | No |
| Prophylaxis | Hygiene; ISG | Hygiene; HBIG; HBV vaccine | Hygiene; HBIG; HBV vaccine | Screening blood; hygiene | Hygiene; safe water supply |

tion about the five hepatitis virus–related illnesses.

## HEPATITIS A: INFECTIOUS HEPATITIS

### Virology

HAV was initially identified by electron-microscopic study of feces from patients with acute infectious hepatitis in 1973. By 1979, the virus had been propagated in primate cell cultures, and by 1983 more than 99% of the viral genome had been cloned. HAV is classified as a picornavirus (genus *Enterovirus*) and morphologically is a nonenveloped spherical particle 27 nm in diameter with icosahedral symmetry; its genome is single-stranded RNA (Fig. 19–1*A* and *B*). Marmosets, chimpanzees, and owl monkeys have been experimentally infected, and viral particles can be visualized subsequently in the hepatocyte cytoplasm. HAV is one of the hardiest viruses: it is stable at 60°C for 1 h, withstands exposure to 10% ether at 4°C for 20 h, and can be stored at −20°C for at least 1¹/₂ years. It is destroyed by boiling for 15 min or by autoclaving, and HAV can be inactivated but retain its antigenicity by boiling for 5 min, by exposure to ultraviolet light, or by exposure to 1:4000 formalin at 37°C for 3 days.

The single-stranded RNA genome of HAV is 7478 nucleotides long with a poly(A) tail, and a viral protein is covalently linked to the 5′ terminus. The genome encodes a single protein that cleaves into three structural and nonstructural protein precursors that are further cleaved into three structural proteins. Only a single serotype of HAV is known even though there are four human genotypes, and the serologically recognized epitope of HAV is expressed on VP1 and probably on VP3. Vaccine development has focused on inactivated HAV that appears to induce lasting immunity, and the U.S. Food and Drug Administration (FDA) licensed this vaccine in early 1995.

### Serology and Immunity

The serologic response to HAV infection is characterized by a brief IgM–anti-HAV response, with subsequent prolonged synthesis of IgG–anti-HAV. The first available serologic test measured total serum anti-HAV, and thus reflected either recent or remote infection without distinguishing between them. The current assay is specific for IgM–anti-HAV and is very useful in clinical diagnosis of acute hepatitis A, because, unlike most other viral infections, IgM–anti-HAV is almost always detectable in serum at the time of clinical presentation of hepatitis A and persists for several months. In contrast, IgG–anti-HAV is present in convalescence and persists for an extended time, often for life (Fig. 19–2). Detectable se-

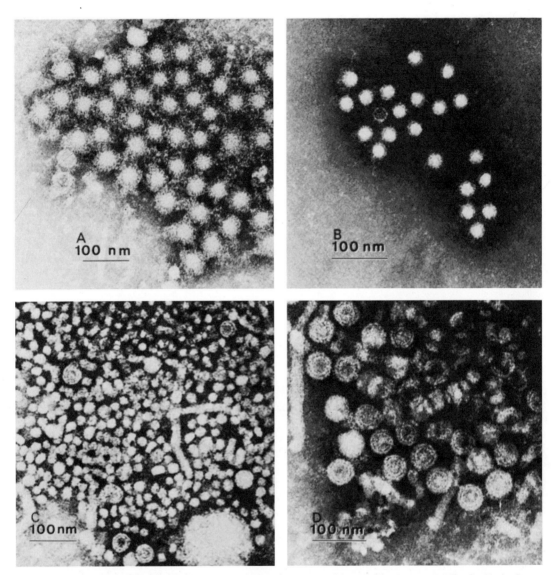

**FIGURE 19–1.** *A,* Hepatitis A viruses from human stool, aggregated by human antibody (4+). *B,* Hepatitis A viruses from chimpanzee stool, aggregated by human antibody (2+). *C,* Tubular and small diameter spherical forms of hepatitis B surface antigen and the larger entire hepatitis B virus (Dane particle) aggregated by chimpanzee antibody. *D,* Aggregate of hepatitis B viruses concentrated by differential centrifugation. (From WHO Collaborating Centre for Reference and Research on Viral Hepatitis, Centers for Disease Control, Bureau of Epidemiology, Hepatitis Laboratories Division, Phoenix, Arizona. Photograph courtesy of Dr. Clifford Gravelle.)

rum IgG–anti-HAV confers immunity to reinfection with HAV.

### Pathogenesis and Infectivity

HAV replicates *in vitro* in human hepatoma cells and diploid fibroblasts without producing cytopathic changes; this also appears to be the case in hepatocytes *in vivo.* After oral inoculation, viral replication occurs in the enteric mucosa accompanied by a brief viremic period during which virus is excreted into stool and spread to liver. In acute human and experimental infections, HAV is found in the hepatocyte cytoplasm and disappears coincident with recovery from hepatic injury. HAV appears to enter hepatocytes after binding to a viral receptor on the cell membrane. Subsequently, uncoating occurs, viral RNA polymerase and viral protease are produced, viral RNA and proteins are synthesized, and new viral particles are assembled and leave the hepatocyte without producing cell lysis. The pre-

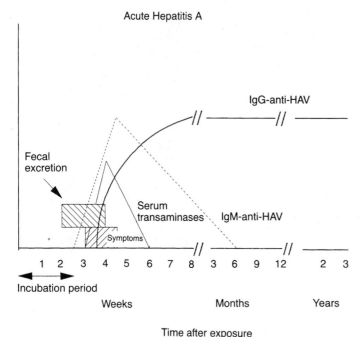

**FIGURE 19–2.** The course of acute hepatitis A. After a relatively brief incubation period, virus is excreted in feces, elevated serum transaminase levels develop, and symptoms may occur. IgM–anti-HAV is present in serum when symptomatic patients seek medical attention, and levels then wane. Serum IgG–anti-HAV is detectable relatively early and persists for decades, serving to protect against recurrent infection.

cise mechanisms of hepatocyte damage are unclear, although lymphocytic infiltration occurs and cytokines are released, suggesting that liver injury may be immunopathologically mediated. HAV-specific CD8+ T lymphocytes isolated from liver in acute hepatitis A are specifically cytotoxic for HAV-infected cells. Hepatocyte injury is reflected by elevated serum levels of alanine aminotransferase (ALT or serum glutamic-pyruvic transaminase [SGPT]) and other hepatic enzymes and is apparent 15–50 days after infection. This becomes maximal within 3–7 days and, except for the relatively few patients who develop fulminant hepatitis A, patients typically recover completely. Fulminant hepatitis A has an approximately 50% mortality rate. Chronic infection with HAV does not develop.

Stool excretion of HAV occurs late in the incubation period and prior to onset of the clinical illness and, although somewhat variable, typically diminishes rapidly with the onset of clinical illness. It is most likely that fecal HAV is derived from virus released by hepatocytes into the biliary tree. Viral excretion is quite uncommon once serum transaminase levels have peaked. Therefore, patients are most infectious late in the incubation period, that is, before it is apparent that they are sick. This clearly complicates control of spread of HAV.

## Clinical Disease

HAV infection in susceptible (anti-HAV–negative) individuals very frequently results in asymptomatic, subclinical infection. This is particularly true in children. Symptomatic infection occurs at all ages but is much more likely to occur in adults. The most common symptoms include the abrupt onset of nausea, vomiting, fever, and vague abdominal discomfort, developing 15–50 days (median is 30 days) after exposure. Smokers may lose their desire for tobacco. Headache and myalgias may occur, and some patients have shaking chills, high fever, and prostration, resembling acute bacteremia. On the other hand, symptomatic children frequently are only mildly ill, with nonspecific symptoms; the diagnosis of infectious hepatitis is made only if serum liver enzymes are measured. During the early preicteric phase of acute hepatitis A, few physical findings are apparent. Hepatomegaly with mild tenderness or right upper quadrant fullness may be noted. Laboratory studies show evidence of increasing hepatic dysfunction, with rising serum transaminase and other hepatic enzyme levels. Leukopenia is common, and atypical lymphocytes may be seen. IgM–anti-HAV is detectable, and total serum IgM levels are elevated (Fig. 19–2).

In many HAV-infected individuals, particularly children, symptoms subside after 3–7 days and recovery quickly ensues, with serum enzyme levels returning to normal. In others, however, particularly adults, an icteric phase often occurs. The frequent absence of icterus in children contributes to their serving as efficient unsuspected transmitters of infection. Icterus is associated with increased serum bilirubin and enzyme levels, especially ALT (or SGPT) and aspartate aminotransferase (AST, or serum glutamic-oxaloacetic transaminase [SGOT]). Frequently, patients manifest improved appetite and decreased nausea and vomiting even as their icterus is worsening. Recovery ensues, and clinical and biochemical findings resolve within a few weeks. The exception to this pattern is the relatively infrequent patient with hepatitis A who develops fulminant hepatitis A, which has a very high fatality rate and which may require liver transplantation. Only a small fraction of all acute fulminant hepatitis is related to HAV, and a fatality rate of 0.14% for hospitalized patients with HAV has been reported. Unlike other forms of viral hepatitis, chronic hepatitis does not follow acute hepatitis A, even though occasional patients manifest elevated serum enzymes or intrahepatic cholestasis and icterus for several months, always with resolution. There is no known chronic carrier state, unlike hepatitis B and hepatitis C.

## Epidemiology

HAV is present worldwide and is quite contagious. The dominant mode of transmission is the fecal–oral route, either through direct person-to-person spread or by ingestion of contaminated food or water. Thus, the epidemiology of hepatitis A is similar to that of other enteric infections, including poliomyelitis. As in the past with polio, seroepidemiologic studies in the United States show that prior HAV infection is more common in those of lower socioeconomic status. Although common source outbreaks are described, most cases are acquired through sporadic or endemic transmission, particularly from individuals in the preicteric phase of acute hepatitis A, when fecal excretion is maximal. In developing areas of the world where sanitation may be inadequate, transmission is widespread, with most infections occurring in the early years of life as subclinical or anicteric illnesses. Thus, long-lived immunity is acquired in childhood, and adults are protected. As sanitation improves, the risk of childhood infection decreases, and susceptibility more frequently extends to adulthood, when infection is likely to be more severe. Paradoxically, as sanitation improves, HAV can emerge as an increasing problem in developing nations.

In developed areas, such as the United States, hepatitis A is particularly endemic in day-care centers and institutions for the retarded, where fecal contamination is more common. Food-borne transmissions in these circumstances usually result from breaches in the usual sanitary safeguards. From 1983 to 1989, a 58% increase in the incidence of hepatitis A was recorded by the Centers for Disease Control (CDC) in the United States. An estimated 143,000 cases occur in the United States. annually at a cost of over $200 million. Specific identified risk factors associated with hepatitis A in the United States include contact with another person known to be infected with hepatitis, male homosexuality, foreign travel, and contact with a child attending a day-care center. Many community hepatitis A outbreaks can be traced to preschool day-care centers, particularly those large centers with long hours and a high proportion of children who are not toilet-trained. Transmission is common among these young children, who experience clinically inapparent infections but who efficiently transmit infection to older siblings, parents, and day-care center staff, who are much more likely to develop symptomatic, icteric hepatitis A. This form of transmission can account for a very substantial proportion of hepatitis A in a community, and intervention in day-care centers in which HAV transmission appears likely may reduce overall community rates of infection substantially.

Sexual transmission of HAV is common among homosexual men, and viral hepatitis that occurs in such patients who have been immunized against hepatitis B virus is most often due to HAV. HAV is similar to other enteric pathogens that can be transmitted sexually. Parenteral HAV transmission is uncommon but can occur because of the brief viremic phase early in the incubation period. Thus, posttransfusion hepatitis A has occurred, but only rarely. Nosocomial (hospital-acquired) HAV infections can occur if diarrhea or incontinence is accompanied by poor hygienic practices (i.e., insufficient handwashing).

## Prevention

### Sanitation

Careful disposal of excreta and avoidance of contamination of the water supply greatly reduce the risk of fecal–oral transmission of infectious agents like HAV. Handwashing is highly effective in preventing person-to-person spread. HAV transmission is particularly difficult to prevent completely because of both the high incidence of subclinical cases (particularly in children) and the maximal viral excretion prior to onset of symptoms in those who become symptomatic.

### Passive Immunization

Pooled human immune serum globulin (ISG) has been known since 1945 to provide protection against infectious hepatitis (hepatitis A), but its effectiveness depends on dosage and time of administration. When ISG is given in proper dosage (0.02 mL/kg) to household contacts within 2 weeks of exposure, up to 87% effective prevention of symptomatic hepatitis A is documented. ISG may prevent infection completely (particularly if given very soon after exposure) or may ameliorate symptoms, resulting in subclinical infection as well as in resultant long-term active immunity (''passive-active'' immunity). ISG is recommended for all household contacts of individuals with hepatitis A and should be administered as soon as possible after exposure, since its prophylactic value decreases with time. ISG is generally *not* recommended for school exposures to HAV, but it is valuable in limiting epidemics in institutions for the retarded and in day-care centers, as well as in preventing hepatitis A in travelers to foreign countries with high risk for endemic HAV infection.

### Active Immunization

Serum IgG antibody correlates with immunity to hepatitis A. An effective vaccine against hepatitis A has been the goal of recent research. The possibilities under study have included an inactivated vaccine such as formalin-inactivated HAV, an attenuated live vaccine that lacks virulence but retains immunogenicity, and recombinant vaccines consisting of a viral surface polypeptide that possesses a critical neutralization epitope. Inactivated vaccine has been tested most extensively and demonstrated to be safe, immunogenic, and protective, and has recently been licensed in the United States after being licensed in 36 other countries.

## HEPATITIS B: SERUM HEPATITIS

### Virology

The etiologic agent of hepatitis B is the hepatitis B virus (HBV), which was discovered serendipitously in 1965 during studies of genetic polymorphism, was associated with hepatitis in 1967, and led to the Nobel Prize in Medicine for Dr. Baruch Blumberg in 1976. The World Health Organization recently estimated that a *billion* individuals alive have been infected with HBV, that approximately 300 million people worldwide are chronically infected, and that 1–2 million deaths each year are attributed to HBV. HBV was considered the ninth leading cause of death worldwide. Hepatitis B virus is the single most important cause of persistent viremia in humans, and there are more than 1 million HBV-infected people in the United States. Some 200,000–300,000 new HBV infections occur in the United States each year, with about 6000 deaths per year attributed to HBV and its complications.

This agent is responsible for almost 80% of cases of primary hepatocellular carcinoma (hepatoma); it is second only to tobacco as a known human carcinogen. By electron microscopy there are three distinct kinds of particles in the serum of patients with HBV infection (Fig. 19–1 *C* and *D*). The intact virion, known as the Dane particle, is a 42-nm-diameter sphere with an outer shell 7-nm thick comprised of hepatitis B surface antigen (HBsAg) and an inner core 28 nm in diameter possessing the hepatitis B core antigen (HBcAg), hepatitis B e antigen (HBeAg), DNA polymerase, and a small (3200 bases), circular, mostly double-stranded DNA genome. HBV is the smallest known DNA virus. Smaller 22-nm spherical particles and tubular particles with a 22-nm cross-sectional diameter represent HBsAg produced in great excess. HBV proved to be the prototype for a group of viral agents now termed the *hepadnaviruses* that include several animal viruses, such as the woodchuck hepatitis virus, duck hepatitis B virus, and ground-squirrel hepatitis virus, and agents that infect Taiwanese snakes, Himalayan marmots, and European herons; they all have similar structures and hepatotropism and are characterized by the unique presence of DNA polymerase and double-stranded DNA. HBV and several of the animal viruses are clearly oncogenic, leading to primary hepatic carcinoma (hepatoma), and all hepadnaviruses can produce either acute or chronic infections of the liver. HBV is resistant to many conditions that inactivate most viruses and bacteria, surviving storage at 60°C for 4 h, at room temperature for 6 months, or $-10°$ to $-20°C$ for $4^{1}/_{2}$ years. It is inactivated by being kept at 60°C for 10 h or by boiling. HBV is phenol resistant but is inactivated by chlorine (10,000 ppm for 10 min) or formalin and by heat or steam sterilization.

## HBV Markers

The presence or absence of the various HBV antigens and the corresponding antibodies in patient serum specimens at different stages of HBV infection provides information regarding the stage of the infection, the presence of immunity, and the degree of infectivity.

### Surface Antigen: HBsAg

This antigen was known previously as Australian antigen and hepatitis-associated antigen (HAA), but it is now termed the HBsAg, since it forms the outer coat of the intact HBV virus (Dane particle). HBsAg occurs in three forms: HBsAg; pre-S2, which is made up of HBsAg plus 55 additional amino acids encoded by the pre-S2 region of the envelope gene and which is important for hepatocyte attachment; and pre-S1, containing the sequence of pre-S2 and 119 additional amino acids encoded by the pre-S1 region of the envelope gene and also containing a liver-attachment site. The pre-S2 encoded sequence also carries a receptor for polymerized human albumin that may be important in viral entry, and serum expression of pre-S1 antigen correlates with active HBV replication. The small spherical and the tubular particles seen by electron microscopy of serum represent HBsAg produced in great excess during HBV replication. Excessive envelope protein production is also characteristic of other hepadnaviruses. HBsAg expresses a single common group-specific antigen (a), as well as either of two subtype antigens (d or y) and one of two allelic groups (r or w), resulting in four possible antigenic subtypes: adr, adw, ayr, and ayw. The subtype of the infecting strain of HBV does not appear to be a determinant of the severity or outcome of infection but is useful in epidemiologic studies. HBsAg is measured in blood and other body fluids by radioimmunoassay (RIA) or enzyme-linked immunosorbent assay (ELISA); current assays detect 5–10 ng protein/per milliliter, or $10^{10}$ particles per milliliter. HBsAg is widely distributed in body fluids including blood, saliva, semen, and breast milk, but not feces, and its presence generally correlates with infectivity. HBsAg typically appears in serum late in the incubation period and persists through most or all of the clinical stages of acute hepatitis B (Fig. 19–3). Its disappearance almost always signals termination of hepatitis B infection and is shortly thereafter followed by detectable serum anti-HBsAg (Fig. 19–3). HBsAg in the liver is localized to the cytoplasm and to the nuclear membrane, cisternae, and endoplasmic reticulum. Individuals who fail to clear HBsAg from serum have chronic HBV infection, either associated with chronic liver disease or as a chronic HBsAg carrier without liver disease (Fig. 19–4). Chronic HBV infection is considered present generally if HBsAg-positivity persists longer than 6 months.

### Core Antigen: HBcAg

This distinct protein of 21 kD with kinase activity is important for viral packaging and is associated with the core of the Dane particle in serum or in hepatocytes and with disrupted Dane particles. HBcAg is denser than HBsAg, having a buoyant density of 1.32 g/cc³ in CeCl₂, compared with 1.20 g/cc³ for HBsAg. In hepatocytes, exclusively nuclear localization of HBcAg is generally associated with viremia but rarely with active liver disease, whereas cytoplasmic HBcAg correlates with viremia and active liver disease. Unlike HBsAg, HBcAg is *not* found in serum. Anti-HBc, on the other hand, is readily demonstrable in serum by RIA and other techniques shortly after HBsAg is detectable (see below) and represents the earliest humoral immune response to HBV antigens (Fig. 19–3).

### e Antigen: HBeAg

The core gene of HBV, which includes a pre-core region, encodes the core antigen (HBcAg) and a cleavage product, HBeAg. When pre-core is transcribed, HBcAg moves to the endoplasmic reticulum where it is cleaved and HBeAg is secreted and circulates in a soluble form in some HBsAg-positive sera. Although there are two distinct HBeAg specificities, the biologic function of HBeAg remains obscure. While it is not essential for viral replication, HBeAg is a good marker of active HBV replication. The pre-core mutant strains of HBV lack HBeAg and have been associated with fulminant hepatitis.

The clinical importance of HBeAg relates to the fact that it serves as a marker for in-

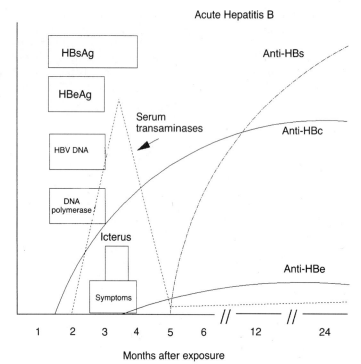

**FIGURE 19–3.** Time course of acute hepatitis B (HBV) infection. After an incubation period of several months, serum becomes positive for HBsAg, HBeAg, and markers of viral replication—HBV DNA and DNA polymerase. Shortly thereafter, serum transaminase levels rise, reflecting hepatocellular damage and then symptoms (often including icterus) develop. The earliest antibody response is anti-HBc, often preceding clinical manifestations. With successful resolution of infection, serologic markers of active infection and viral replication disappear, and serum transaminases return to normal. Anti-HBc persists, whereas HBsAg and HBeAg are replaced by anti-HBs and anti-HBe, respectively. The appearance of anti-HBs generally confirms recovery from HBV infection and provides long-lived immunity against subsequent infection.

creased risk of significant chronic liver disease and for increased infectivity. As a marker reflecting active HBV replication, HBeAg correlates with DNA polymerase activity. Loss of HBeAg-positivity and appearance of anti-HBe in serum generally indicates lower infectivity and decreased severity of HBV-associated liver disease, but the absence of HBeAg does not equate with lack of infectivity.

### DNA Polymerase and HBV DNA

Active HBV replication is reflected by the presence of serum DNA polymerase and HBV DNA (Fig. 19–3). The sustained disappearance of these markers of replication, whether spontaneous or as a consequence of therapeutic regimens (e.g., interferon-alpha [IFN-alpha] is evidence of terminated HBV infection. Loss of viral replication is soon followed by evidence of sustained remission of chronic hepatitis B.

### Antibodies against HBV Antigens

The earliest evidence of a humoral response to HBV is the presence of serum *anti-HBc* late in the incubation period, generally coinciding with the appearance of HBsAg (Fig. 19–3). Anti-HBc declines to low values with convalescence and can persist at low levels for many years. IgM–anti-HBc occurs early

except in young infants and strongly suggests acute HBV infection. *Anti-HBs* is first detectable later in convalescence, often considerably after HBsAg has disappeared, and generally signifies termination of infection (Fig. 19–3). Anti-HBs lasts many years and protects against reinfection. Anti-HBc may be the only marker of HBV infection in the interval between the decline of HBsAg and the appearance of anti-HBs; this interval is termed the "core window." Anti-HBe usually appears shortly after HBeAg disappears in the early convalescent period. In individuals who develop chronic HBV infection, HBeAg usually persists and anti-HBe does not appear (Fig. 19–4).

### Pathogenesis

The pathogenesis of hepatitis B infection is very complex. HBV is not hepatotoxic, as demonstrated by the fact that most chronic carriers of HBV, whose sera contain very high concentrations of viral particles, lack evidence of liver disease. Rather, it appears that the host response to HBV characterized by cytotoxic T cells and natural killer cells leads to hepatocyte necrosis, resulting in either *acute hepatitis* that subsides after a period of weeks to several months, or *chronic hepatitis* that may

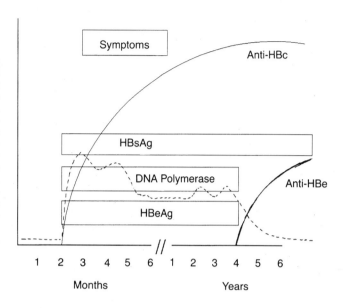

Chronic Hepatitis B Infection

**FIGURE 19–4.** One of the patterns of chronic hepatitis B infection. After an incubation period of about 2 months, serum transaminase levels (*dashed line*) abruptly rise coincident with the appearance of several serologic markers (HBsAg, HBeAg, anti-HBc, HBV DNA and DNA polymerase) before the onset of symptoms. Serum transaminase levels fluctuate and eventually normalize, although serum HBsAg persists as a marker of chronic hepatitis B virus infection. DNA polymerase and HBeAg are no longer detectable in serum after 4 years, the latter replaced by anti-HBe. Anti-HBs never develops, since surface antigenemia never clears. Most such patients remain infected for many decades, and some develop chronic active hepatitis B, cirrhosis, and even hepatocellular carcinoma.

persist for many years. Apparently, HBV replication in the liver eventually ceases in some chronically infected individuals, even though viral DNA may remain integrated into the hepatocyte DNA and cells may continue to express HBsAg.

Late in the long (45- to 180-day) incubation period of HBV, at or shortly before the onset of hepatic inflammation and necrosis, some individuals develop hypersensitivity-like symptoms (arthralgia, skin rash, vasculitis) that are the result of circulating antigen–antibody complexes. A particularly severe form of HBV immune complex disease is adult periarteritis nodosa. In this disease a sizable fraction of patients have evidence of HBsAg and immunoglobulin deposits within vessel walls.

Hepatocyte necrosis is probably a consequence of T-cell cytotoxicity directed against HBV or the hepatocyte membrane antigens expressed on the hepatocyte surface. The pre-S2 portion of HBsAg has been suggested to be the target of T cells infiltrating the liver in chronic hepatitis B. Individuals with some degree of impairment of T-cell function (such as those with Down syndrome, uremia, malignancy, human immunodeficiency virus [HIV] infection, neonates, etc.) are more likely to have a relatively mild degree of necrosis, incomplete elimination of HBV, and persistent

smoldering chronic HBV infection. This situation is in contrast to individuals with normal T-cell function, who tend to have a more severe acute illness that results in termination of the infection, clearance of HBsAg from liver and serum, and development of anti-HBs. This host–virus relationship is further complicated by the fact that HBV DNA can be found integrated into the genome of primary hepatocellular carcinoma (hepatoma) cells in HBsAg-positive individuals and into the genome of other nontumor host cells. This DNA integration is not associated with viral replication and suggests that, at least in some circumstances, integration inhibits replication and promotes malignant transformation. Individuals deficient in B-cell immunity are capable of developing acute or chronic hepatitis.

Chronic HBV infection in individuals also infected with HIV is associated with less severe histologic changes and lower serum transaminase levels. However, this milder hepatic involvement is associated with evidence of greater viral replication, including higher serum levels of HBeAg, HBV DNA, and HBV DNA polymerase and increased HBcAg and HBeAg expression on hepatocyte nuclei. These findings support the immune-mediated pathogenesis of hepatitis B and suggest that HBV in HIV-infected individuals will be more resistant to antiviral therapy; the latter has been confirmed in treatment trials. Concurrent HIV infection is associated with decreased survival of HBV-infected patients, but HBV infection does not adversely affect survival in HIV-positive patients.

## Clinical Disease

The clinical picture of *acute hepatitis B* is similar in some respects to that of acute hepatitis A but tends to be a more serious illness, has a more insidious onset, has a propensity to linger or to become chronic, and typically affects somewhat older individuals. The incubation period between infection and onset of symptoms varies between 45 and 180 days, with HBsAg becoming detectable in serum several weeks before the clinical onset. Some patients develop hypersensitivity symptoms as noted above, whereas others manifest anorexia, fatigue, chills, and fever prior to the onset of jaundice. Coincident with the onset of symptoms, serum transaminases increase to reflect hepatocyte necrosis, and anti-HBc becomes detectable—initially of the IgM class and later of the IgG. Prior to the increase in serum transaminases, markers associated with the Dane particle (DNA polymerase, HBV DNA, HBeAg) are detectable in serum.

The icteric phase of acute hepatitis B lasts 2–6 weeks, generally peaking in severity by 14 days and resolving over a variable period. As jaundice worsens, fever, malaise, and weakness improve. Hepatomegaly frequently is present in the icteric phase, often with splenomegaly, and persists for some time after icterus clears. In children the illness is shorter and recovery is generally faster. In approximately 90% of acutely infected individuals, Dane particle markers in the serum clear shortly after the serum transaminases peak and anti-HBe may become detectable, serum HBsAg disappears as transaminases reach near-normal values, and shortly thereafter, anti-HBs becomes detectable, signaling the successful termination of infection and establishment of long-term immunity against reinfection.

Hepatitis B infection is very different from hepatitis A in that a significant minority of HBV-infected individuals do not terminate their infection but become chronically infected, frequently for life. In these patients, HBsAg persists in serum, as do anti-HBc, HBeAg or anti-HBe, and Dane particle markers, such as DNA polymerase and HBV DNA. Chronic hepatitis B may take the histologic form of *chronic persistent hepatitis B*, which is associated with mild portal triaditis and mildly elevated serum transaminases. This form resolves within 1 year without development of cirrhosis. The more serious form of chronic hepatitis B is *chronic active (or aggressive) hepatitis B*, which is associated usually with more elevated transaminase levels and histologic evidence of T-cell inflammation that spills out of the portal triad, across the limiting plate, and into the lobules. This form has a tendency to produce bridging fibrosis and cirrhosis, leading in turn to portal obstruction and its complications. Patients with cirrhotic chronic hepatitis B are at dramatically increased risk for development of hepatoma. Treatment with IFN-alpha for chronic hepatitis B infection has been successful in about one third of patients, with those with low HBV DNA levels and high transaminases and relatively short duration of infection showing the highest response rates.

Fulminant acute hepatitis B is relatively rare but is more common than other viral causes of fulminant acute liver failure, particularly in adults. These patients develop massive necrosis of virtually all hepatocytes, and 80% mortality is common. Fulminant hepatitis A is associated with a lower mortality rate, while fulminant non-A, non-B hepatitis has a higher mortality rate. Many such patients have been salvaged by hepatic transplantation in recent years, although HBV infection of the transplanted liver is common.

The *chronic HBsAg carrier*, in striking contrast, is classically an asymptomatic individual with minimal or no liver disease, who may or may not have had a symptomatic illness at the time of acquisition of HBV. Serum of such patients is chronically positive for HBsAg, anti-HBc, HBeAg or (more often) anti-HBe, HBV DNA, and DNA polymerase. Chronic HBsAg carrier rates as high as 20% or more are seen in some Asian populations. In the United States and Western Europe, chronic carrier rates are less than 1%.

## Epidemiology

In a recent serologic survey representative of the entire U.S. urban (noninstitutionalized) population 6 months to 74 years of age, serologic markers of HBV were found in 4.8% (3.2% of whites, 13.7% of blacks). No gender differences were noted but serologic markers increased in frequency with age. Overall, 0.3% were HBsAg-positive (0.19% in whites, 0.85% in blacks), indicating active infection.

HBV epidemiology resembles that of the HIV in many aspects. Transmission of HBV occurs primarily by parenteral, sexual, or vertical (maternal–infant) routes, and the fecal–oral route is relatively unimportant. This transmission pattern reflects the fact that HBV is present in virtually all body fluids of an infected individual, including blood, semen, saliva, and urine. Transmission generally requires either direct inoculation (transfusion of a blood product, injection with a contaminated needle, accidental needle-stick injury) or intimate personal contact (between sexual partners, or mother and neonate). Groups at particularly high risk for HBV infection include intravenous (IV) drug abusers who share needles, male homosexuals, the sexually promiscuous, health care workers, transfused patients, and hemophiliacs. In addition, certain geographic areas are known to be associated with relatively high rates of chronic HBsAg carriage and HBV-related liver disease with their concomitant risk of infectivity, including Southeast Asia (particularly China and Taiwan), sub-Saharan Africa, Oceania, and the Mediterranean region. In these regions, the role of vertical transmission from mother to neonate, resulting in long-term or even life-long HBV infection, is thought to be crucial in maintaining high rates of HBsAg-positivity. This is particularly true in Southeast Asia. In the United States, the incidence of chronic HBsAg-positivity is approximately 0.3% but is higher in selected subgroups with specific ethnic or behavioral risk factors (see above). HBV can contaminate all blood components except for preparations of gamma globulin, but the screening of blood products for HBsAg in order to exclude positive material has very substantially, but not completely, eliminated the problem of posttransfusion hepatitis B infection. Recent epidemiologic surveys suggest that homosexual activity has become a somewhat less important risk factor and that IV drug abuse and heterosexual activity have become relatively more important risk factors for acute hepatitis B infection. Even with extensive inquiry, however, the source of acute hepatitis B infection remains unknown in about 30% of instances.

Vertical transmission of HBV is an extremely important public health problem worldwide and contributes very substantially to the high rates of chronic HBV infection in many areas and to the resulting prevalence of chronic liver disease and hepatoma. For example, Beasley demonstrated that hepatoma was 223 times more common in middle-aged HBsAg-positive men in Taiwan than in HBsAg-negative controls, with hepatoma and cirrhosis accounting for 54% of deaths in HBsAg carriers but only 1.5% in noncarriers. Vertical transmission is possible from any HBsAg-positive mother to her offspring but is particularly efficient when the mother is HBeAg-positive or when she experiences acute hepatitis B in the third trimester of pregnancy or in the early postpartum period. IgM–anti-HBc rarely develops after perinatal transmission of HBV and cannot be used for diagnosis in this situation. Prompt administration of anti-HBs (HBIG) and HBV vaccine to neonates born to HBsAg-positive women is highly effective in preventing vertical transmission.

Hepatitis B is an occupational risk for medical personnel as well as a potential nosocomial risk. Staff and patients in dialysis, oncology, and transplantation units are at higher risk because exposure to blood products is common and HBV-infected patients are more likely to be asymptomatic chronic carriers.

## Prevention

Highly significant advances have occurred regarding prevention of HBV infection, including the development both of vaccines composed of purified HBsAg and of an immune globulin containing high-titer anti-HBs (HBIG).

### *General Measures*

Even though HBV is much less commonly transmitted by the fecal–oral route than is HAV, the general hygienic measures noted above for hepatitis A are a necessary part of prophylaxis against HBV. In addition, used needles and other blood-contaminated materials must be discarded properly, and needle-recapping should be avoided. Barrier protection against splashes with blood-contaminated secretions by dentists, surgeons, and others is effective. Routine screening of blood donors to exclude HBV-infected individuals from the donor pool and utilizing volunteer blood donors rather than paid donors have been highly effective in reducing the incidence of posttransfusion hepatitis B. The risk of transmission of HBV by heterosexual and homosexual activity can be substantially reduced by the use of condoms. Recommendations for prevention of HBV after percutaneous expo-

**TABLE 19–2.   HEPATITIS B PROPHYLAXIS AFTER PERCUTANEOUS EXPOSURE TO BLOOD**

| | SOURCE STATUS | | |
|---|---|---|---|
| EXPOSED PERSON | *HBsAg-Positive* | *HBsAg-Negative* | *Unknown* |
| Unvaccinated | HBIG × 1 plus HBVax | HBVax | HBVax |
| Vaccinated | | | |
|   Known responder | Test exposed person for anti-HBs<br>If ≥10 mIU, no treatment<br>If <10 mIU, HBVax booster | None | None |
|   Known nonresponder | HBIG × 2 or HBIG × 1 plus 1 dose HBVax | None | If known high-risk source, may treat as if source were HBsAg-positive |
|   Unknown response | Test exposed person for anti-HBs<br>If ≥ 10 mIU, no treatment<br>If <10 mIU, HBIG × 1 plus HBVax booster | None | Test exposed person for anti-HBs<br>If ≥10 mIU, no treatment<br>If <10 mIU, HBVax booster |

HBIG, hepatitis B immune globulin (0.06 mL/kg IM); HBVax, hepatitis B vaccine (for adults 10 μg Recombivax HB or 20 μg Energix-B).

sure to blood containing (or possibly containing) HBsAg are shown in Table 19–2.

### Passive Immunization

Serum globulin preparations enriched in HBIG are used in certain circumstances to provide prompt passive immunity to HBV infection. These circumstances include (1) following an inadvertent needle-stick from a HBsAg-positive patient or accidental transfusion of HBsAg-positive blood products; (2) after an eye-splash or contamination of an open skin wound with HBsAg-positive material; (3) following accidental ingestion of HBsAg-positive material, (e.g., a pipetting accident); (4) for sexual partners of patients with acute hepatitis B within 14 days of contact; (5) household contacts under 1 year of age of patients with acute hepatitis B; and (6) infants born to HBsAg-positive mothers. In certain of these circumstances, active immunization with HBV vaccine is also indicated (see below). Ideally, it is best to document that the "donor" is HBsAg-positive (and therefore infected) and that the "recipient" is anti–HBs-negative (and therefore susceptible) before administering HBIG, which is expensive. This is not always possible or practical, however. In families of an acute hepatitis B patient, it is generally not indicated to give HBIG to children older than 1 year of age, since the risk of spread other than sexually is low; children younger than 1 year are given

HBIG and HBV vaccine because their risk of developing chronic HBV infection is greater.

### Active Immunization

A safe and highly effective HBV vaccine consisting of HBsAg purified from chronic carrier donor plasma became available in 1983, and this has been replaced by more recent HBsAg vaccines that contain recombinant HBsAg synthesized by yeast (*Saccharomyces cerevisiae*) transfected with the gene for HBsAg subtype adw. A regimen of three doses (at 0, 1, and 6 months) generally elicits protective anti-HBs. Intramuscular injection is important, and sites with considerable adipose tissue (e.g., gluteus) should be avoided to achieve optimal immune responses. The need for reimmunization has not been established. HBV vaccine is indicated for high-risk individuals, including health professionals (especially those at highest risk, such as dentists and their assistants, surgeons, dialysis staff), susceptible dialysis patients, hemophiliacs, certain residents and staff of chronic-care institutions, IV drug abusers, sexual and household contacts of a chronically HBsAg-positive individual, Alaskan Eskimos, Pacific Islanders, and other susceptible populations, and homosexual males. HBV vaccine should be combined with HBIG in the following circumstances: (1) after accidental needle-stick or splash exposures with HBsAg-positive or high-risk material, (2) for prevention of vertical transmission to neonates, and (3) for sexual contacts and for infant contacts younger than 1 year of patients with acute hepatitis B. About half of HBV infections among children born in the United States to Southeast Asian refugees are not attributable to perinatal transmission, indicating that child-to-child transmission may occur commonly. It has been suggested that HBV vaccine should be given to all infants and young children of Southeast Asian ethnicity in the United States, regardless of whether there is HBV infection in family members.

Administration of HBV vaccine to individuals who are already immune is not harmful but represents an unnecessary expense. Approximately 90% of vaccine recipients develop anti-HBs, and about 10% appear to be unresponsive. Recombinant vaccine leads to early and high production of antibody to pre-S2 determinants of HBsAg and perhaps to earlier immunity than serum-derived vaccine. Although a primary antibody response is not detectable in about 70% of recipients, secondary and tertiary responses are very common after the second and third vaccine doses. Several dozen countries, including China, Korea, Taiwan, and the United States have initiated programs for universal newborn vaccination, and other high-risk ethnic groups are receiving widespread vaccine, including Aborigines in Australia, Maoris in New Zealand, and Eskimos in North America.

## HEPATITIS DELTA VIRUS

The hepatitis delta virus (HDV) is a unique defective spherical 36-nm virus composed of a core containing a circular, single-stranded, negative-polarity RNA genome of about 1750 bases; the delta antigen, a phosphoprotein that interacts with virion RNA and is possibly involved in viral replication; and a lipoprotein envelope made up of HBsAg. HDV appears to replicate through an RNA that is complementary to the viral genome. There is a strong analogy between HDV and certain pathogenic RNA agents of plants, including the viroids, virusoids, and satellite RNAs. Delta was first discovered as a novel antigen in hepatocyte nuclei of certain patients chronically infected with HBV, and viral replication appears to take place in hepatocyte nuclei. Replication of HDV is completely dependent upon the presence of HBV (or, experimentally, another hepadnavirus) as a "helper virus" and curiously

is associated with suppression of HBV replication.

Thus, HDV causes infection *only* in individuals with coexistent active infection with HBV. Italian researchers have found evidence of HDV infection in some patients with inapparent HBV infection that is manifested only by IgM–anti-HBc, particularly in drug abusers. The presence of HDV infection is reflected by delta antigen and HDV RNA in liver and by serum anti-delta antibody. In acute HDV infection IgM–anti-delta is demonstrable in serum. Newer techniques that demonstrate serum HDV antigen (HDAg) and HDV RNA appear to correlate with active replication. Transmission of HDV is by the identical routes that HBV is transmitted. Vertical transmission has been described from HBeAg-positive HDV-infected mothers but appears uncommon. The delta antigen comprises two major proteins of 24–27 kD and 27–29 kD, the functions of which are unknown.

HDV is important clinically in two circumstances. As a *co-infecting agent* with HBV in a previously non–HBV-infected individual, HDV is associated with more severe acute hepatitis as reflected, for example, by a higher rate of fulminant hepatitis and a higher fatality rate, as well as with a substantially increased risk for development and severity of chronic hepatitis B liver disease. As a co-infecting agent, the incubation period of HDV is the same as that of HBV. On the other hand, well-established HBV infection promotes efficient replication of HDV. Therefore, as a *superinfecting agent* in an already HBV-infected individual, HDV infection may produce an acute exacerbation of previously stable chronic hepatitis, increase the tendency for development of significant chronic active hepatitis B and cirrhosis, or accelerate the course of chronic liver disease. In this situation, the incubation period is about 4–8 weeks. The relationship of HDV to hepatoma is less clear. In both chronic active hepatitis B and chronic active delta hepatitis, T cells predominate in the liver inflammatory infiltrate, with helper T cells particularly in the portal tracts and suppressor/cytotoxic T cells particularly in the areas of piecemeal necrosis.

HDV is found worldwide but is uncommon in some HBV-infected populations, including male homosexuals and Southeast Asians. In the United States and Western Europe it is common only in IV drug abusers and their sexual partners and less in hemophiliacs and homosexuals. Very high HDV rates are reported among HBV-infected individuals in the Amazon River Valley, the Middle East, Oceania, and Southern Europe. It has been estimated that there are about 70,000 HDV-infected individuals in the United States and that this has a large inpact on morbidity and mortality because chronic HDV infection is severe. Screening of blood donors for HBsAg is highly effective in the prevention of transfusion-related HDV. Studies evaluating the efficacy of IFN-alpha in treatment of chronic HDV have demonstrated biochemical and histologic improvement in about half of recipients but frequent relapses after termination of therapy.

## NON-A, NON-B HEPATITIS

The term *non-A, non-B hepatitis* (NANB) has been used to connote viral hepatitis that is not due to infection with HAV, HBV, Epstein-Barr virus, or cytomegalovirus. Experimental transmissibility to primates, epidemic occurrence, and an unequivocal relationship to transfusions provided support for the existence of additional viral agents, ultimately leading to the identification of hepatitis C virus (HCV) and hepatitis E virus (HEV).

That at least two distinct modes of transmission exist for NANB suggested the presence of at least two distinct viral agents, one transmitted parenterally, causing both posttransfusion hepatitis and sporadic cases in developed countries, and a water-borne form with fecal–oral transmission producing epidemics in developing countries.

### Hepatitis C

Within the past decade, a small positive-stranded RNA virus in the Flaviviridae family with a genome of about 10,000 nucleotides was implicated as the cause of about 85% of transfusion-transmitted NANB. This agent has been termed hepatitis C virus.

CDC surveillance studies have found that only 5–10% of HCV cases are related to blood transfusions, that 40% are associated with IV drug abuse, 5% to health care occupational exposure, and 10% to heterosexual activity with multiple partners or household or sexual contact with an individual with hepatitis. In about 40% there is no identifiable source of infection. Perinatal transmission occurs occasionally. HCV infection is characterized by a long incubation period (60–150 days), frequent subclinical or anicteric illnesses (25% become icteric), development of a chronic carrier state, and about 50% risk for development of chronic liver disease, including chronic active hepatitis and/or cirrhosis. This illness resembles hepatitis B in many respects but is generally milder with lower serum transaminase and bilirubin levels. However, when HCV manifests a fulminant course, up to 90% mortality has been reported.

Seroconversion to HCV may not occur for as long as 6 months after infection and 4 months after onset of clinical hepatitis. Seroepidemiologic studies indicate that HCV is a major cause of blood-borne NANB hepatitis throughout the world as well as a common cause of sporadic or community-acquired NANB hepatitis among patients with no identified parenteral exposure. About 50% of the latter group are positive for HCV antibody within 6 weeks of illness onset and 90% by 6 months. It appears that HCV-infected patients without history of transfusion are just as likely as posttransfusion HCV patients to develop significant chronic liver disease. HCV RNA can be detected in serum within 1–2 weeks of infection and persists throughout the course of infection. At least five distinct HCV genotypes exist.

IFN-alpha treatment of chronic hepatitis C has been shown to be effective in transiently suppressing the activity of hepatitis and in improving hepatic histologic features, but lasting responses following discontinuation of therapy are uncommon. Clinical trials combining IFN-alpha with antiviral agents are in progress.

### Prevention

Efforts to prevent posttransfusion hepatitis C have focused upon exclusion of paid blood donors and screening donors for anti-HCV, which has dropped the risk of posttransfusion hepatitis to about 3 per 10,000 units transfused. Immune serum globulin in the United States does not contain antibiotics to HCV and therefore is unlikely to prevent HCV infection. Organ, semen, and tissue donors should also be screened for anti-HCV.

Vaccine development will be hampered significantly by the fact that HCV infection does not appear to confer protective immunity against homologous or heterologous strains of HCV. Certain HCV genotypes such as HCV type 1b (II) appear to be associated with particularly severe liver disease.

## Hepatitis E

A distinctive form of NANB hepatitis is characterized by fecal–oral transmission, and a short incubation period (usually 2–9 weeks, mean of 6 weeks), occurring either endemically over a period of months or in explosive water-borne epidemics related to fecal contamination of the water supply. This was first documented in a water-borne outbreak involving 29,000 icteric people in New Delhi, India. This is now known as hepatitis E and appears to account for over 50% of sporadic acute hepatitis in developing countries.

Hepatitis E characteristically occurs shortly after the onset of the rainy season in developing countries when the water supply can be contaminated by fecal material. Clinical attack rates are highest among young adults. The fatality rate in epidemic water-borne hepatitis E, which is reported primarily from India, Africa, Mexico, and Southeast Asia, is particularly high (about 20%) in pregnant women in the third trimester and is related to fulminant hepatitis; in other individuals the disease has a fatality rate of 1–2%. Endemic HEV infection has not been reported in the United States or Western Europe. Chronic liver disease has not been demonstrated following enterically transmitted hepatitis E. Spherical, nonenveloped viral particles 32–34 nm in diameter are seen in feces of patients with hepatitis E, and they react with convalescent sera from many geographic areas, as assessed by immune electron microscopy. Reactivity with patient sera from many geographic areas indicates that HEV is responsible for enteric NANB hepatitis worldwide.

The genome of HEV is a single-stranded polyadenylated RNA of 7600 bases with three open reading frames. Hepatitis E virus has not officially been classified but resembles caliciviruses. The virus has been serially transmitted in cynomolgus monkeys and other primates, virus-like particles have been demonstrated in bile and feces, and an associated antigen has been identified in hepatocyte cytoplasm. HEV appears to replicate in liver cells.

It is unclear how long infected patients remain infective, but chronic hepatitis has not been demonstrated. There is no commercially available serologic test. Research studies have demonstrated that serum IgM–anti-HEV is present from 2 weeks before to 6 weeks after the acute illness and that IgG–anti-HEV peaks 2–4 weeks after onset of illness and persists, conferring immunity. Passive administration of immune globulin prepared in the United States is not effective against hepatitis E.

## CASE HISTORY

### CASE HISTORY 1

A 19-year-old man with a life-long history of mild factor VIII deficiency presented with a 5-day history of jaundice, malaise, anorexia, and low-grade fever. He had recently visited rural areas of India, returning 4 weeks prior to examination. Examination demonstrated low-grade fever of 101°F (38.5°C), mild scleral icterus, a tender liver palpable 4 cm below the right costal margin, and evidence of previous intraarticular hemorrhages. The remainder of the examination was normal. Laboratory tests showed serum alanine aminotransferase and aspartate aminotransferase each about 1000 units/L (normal for each <40), total bilirubin of 9.3 mg/dL, with direct bilirubin of 4.0 mg/dL. Serologic studies were anti–HIV-negative, IgG–HAV-positive, IgM–HAV-negative, anti–HCV-negative, HABsAg–negative, anti–HBs-positive, anti–HBc-positive, and anti–HBe-negative. What kind of hepatitis does he have?

### CASE 1 DISCUSSION

This patient falls into the category of the multitransfused subject who is at risk for HIV, hepatitis B, and hepatitis C. Many develop chronic hepatitis B infection that is most often manifested serologically as HBsAg-positive, anti–HBs-negative, and anti–HBc-positive. In contrast, this patient's HBV serologic studies indicated resolved HBV infection. Similarly, his hepatitis A serologic studies indicate past HAV infection with resolution. He has no serologic evidence of HCV infection, although seroconversion may be delayed for up to 6 months after infection. This patient's clinical illness is highly suggestive of enterically transmitted acute hepatitis E infection acquired in India, although parenterally or nonparenterally transmitted hepatitis C infection is not ruled out by the information provided.

## REFERENCES

**Books**

Gerin, J. L., Purcell, R. H., and Rizzetto, M., eds. The *Hepatitis Delta Virus.* New York: Wiley-Liss, 1991.

Gust, I. D., and Feinstone, S. M., eds. *Hepatitis A.* Boca Raton, FL: CRC Press, 1989.

Hadziyannis, S. J., Taylor, J. M., Bonino, F., eds. *Hepatitis Delta Virus.* New York: Wiley-Liss, 1993.

Hollinger, F. B., Lemon, S. M., Margolis, H. S., eds. *Viral hepatitis and liver disease.* Baltimore: Williams & Wilkins, 1991.

Zuckerman, A., ed. *Viral Hepatitis and Liver Disease.* New York: Alan R. Liss, 1988.


## Review

Hollinger, F. B. ed. An overview of the clinical development of hepatitis A vaccine. *J. Infect. Dis. 171*(Suppl. 1):S1–S77, 1995.


## Articles

Alter, H. J., Purcell, R. H., Shih, J. W., et al. Detection of antibody to hepatitis C virus in prospectively followed transfusion recipients with acute and chronic non-A, non-B hepatitis. *N. Engl. J. Med. 321*:1494–1500, 1989.

American Academy of Pediatrics. *Report of the Committee on Infectious Diseases.* 23rd ed. 1994:221–241.

Beasley, R. P., Hwang, L-Y., Lin, C. C., et al. Hepatocellular carcinoma and hepatitis B virus: A prospective study of 22,707 men in Taiwan. *Lancet*:1129–1133, 1981.

Beasley, R. P., Hwang, L-Y., Lee, G. C., et al. Prevention of perinatally transmitted hepatitis B virus infections with hepatitis B immune globulin and hepatitis B vaccine. *Lancet*:1100–1102, 1983.

Beasley, R. P., Hwang, L-Y., Stevens, C. E., et al. Efficacy of hepatitis B immune globulin for prevention of perinatal transmission of the hepatitis B virus carrier state. *Hepatology 3*:135–141, 1983.

Beasley, R. P. Hepatitis B virus, the major etiology of hepatocellular carcinoma. *Cancer 10*:1942–1956, 1988.

Bergmann, K. F., Cote, P. J., Moriarity, A., et al. Hepatitis delta antigen. *J. Immunol. 143*:3714–3721, 1989.

Bryan, J. P., Tsarev, S. A., Iqbal, M., et al. Epidemic hepatitis E in Pakistan: Patterns of serologic response and evidence that antibody to hepatitis E virus protects against disease. *J. Infect. Dis. 170*:517–521, 1994.

Chauhan, A., Dilawar, J.B., Kaur, V., et al. Hepatitis E virus transmission to a volunteer. *Lancet 341*:149–150, 1993.

DiBisceglie, A. M., and Negro, F. Diagnosis of hepatitis delta virus infection. *Hepatology 10*:1014–1016, 1989.

Farci, P., Alter, H. J., Govindarajan, S., et al. Lack of protective immunity against reinfection with hepatitis C virus. *Science 258*:135–140, 1992.

Farci, P., Mandas, A., Coiana, A., et al. Treatment of chronic hepatitis D with interferon alfa-2a. *N. Eng. J. Med. 330*:88–94, 1994.

Hadler, S. C., Francis, D. P., Maynard, J. E., et al. Long-term immunogenicity and efficacy of hepatitis B vaccine in homosexual men. *N. Engl. J. Med. 315*:209–214, 1986.

Innis, B. L., Snitbhan, R., Kunasol, P., et al Protection against hepatitis A by an inactivated vaccine. *JAMA 271*:1328–1334, 1994.

Lau, J. Y. N. and Wright T. L. Molecular virology and pathogenesis of hepatitis B. *Lancet 342*:1335–1340, 1993.

Lettau, L. A. The A, B, C, D, and E of viral hepatitis: Spelling out the risks of healthcare workers. *Infect. Control. Hosp. Epidemiol. 13*:77–81, 1992.

Maynard, J. E., Kane, M. A., and Hadler, S. C. Global control of hepatitis B through vaccination. *Rev. Infect. Dis. 11*:S574–578, 1989.

Miller, R. H. Proteolytic self-cleavage of hepatitis B virus core protein may generate serum e antigen. *Science 236*:722–725, 1987.

Nousbaum, J-B., Pol, S., Nalpa, S. B., et al. Hepatitis C virus type 1b (II) infection in France and Italy. *Ann. Int. Med. 122*:161–168, 1995.

Perrillo, R. P. The management of chronic hepatitis B. *Am. J. Med. 96*:(Suppl. 1A):34S–40S, 1994.

Reyes, G. R., Purdy, M. A., Kim, J. P., et al. Isolation of a cDNA from the virus responsible for enterically transmitted non-A, non-B hepatitis. *Science 247*:1335–1339, 1990.

Vallbracht, A., Maier, K., Stierhof, Y-D., et al. Liver-derived cytotoxic T cells in hepatitis A virus infection. *J. Infect. Dis. 160*:209–217, 1989.

# VI  CENTRAL NERVOUS SYSTEM INFECTIONS

## 20

# INTRODUCTION TO INFECTIONS OF THE CENTRAL NERVOUS SYSTEM

RAM YOGEV, M.D. and MOSHE ARDITI, M.D.

The central nervous system (CNS) is unlike other organs in its closed confinement within rigid borders, its sequestration from the rest of the body by various barriers, and its relatively immunocompromised status. The brain is surrounded by the leptomeninges and bathed in the cerebrospinal fluid (CSF) which, in the case of infection, provides both a culture medium for the infecting organisms and a rapid means of disseminating the infection throughout the CNS.

The CNS is susceptible to a large number of infectious agents, and many viruses, bacteria, parasites, and fungi are implicated as the cause of CNS infections. CNS infections can be broadly divided into (1) *meningitis,* infection of the leptomeninges and the CSF; and (2) *encephalitis,* infection of the brain parenchyma. However, although these two conditions can be distinguished in many cases on clinical grounds, they frequently coexist and are referred to as *meningoencephalitis.* Three of the reasons for this phenomenon are:

1. During bacterial meningitis, the inflammatory mediators and toxins produced in the subarachnoid space diffuse into the brain parenchyma and cause an inflammatory response of the brain tissue.

2. In encephalitis, the inflammatory reaction reaches the CSF and produces symptoms of meningeal irritation in addition to those related to encephalitis.

3. Some etiologic agents may attack both the meninges and the brain.

Infections of the CNS, especially those that are bacterial, are often life-threatening situations that represent medical emergencies. There are very few other infections that demand such urgent medical attention and skill in differential diagnosis and antibiotic selection to effect a favorable outcome.

## CLASSIFICATION AND PATHOGENESIS

### Acute Bacterial Infections

Acute bacterial infections of the CNS can be divided into focal infection of the brain parenchyma (abscess) or diffuse inflammatory processes mainly involving the leptomeninges (meningitis) (Table 20–1). Brain abscesses usually develop from contiguous or adjacent anatomic tissues. Acute mastoiditis and sinusitis are examples of infections which, if not promptly treated, may serve as the source for direct bacterial invasion of the brain, causing focal cerebritis and later an abscess. Traumatic head injury or wound infections following neurosurgical or orthopedic procedures involving the calvarium or the spine may also lead to the formation of a brain abscess.

"Metastatic" infections (e.g., bacteria from other areas of the body seeding to the brain via the bloodstream) may lead to a brain ab-

**TABLE 20–1.    CLASSIFICATION OF INFECTIONS OF THE CENTRAL NERVOUS SYSTEM**

| TYPE OF INFECTION | EXAMPLE | PATHOGENESIS | MOST FREQUENT CAUSATIVE MICROORGANISMS |
|---|---|---|---|
| Acute bacterial ("suppurative"*) | Abscesses: brain, epidural, subdural | Hematogenous (lung, intestinal tract) or Direct invasion (trauma, ENT, sinuses, neuroorthopedic surgery) | Peptostreptococci *Bacteroides* sp. Staphylococci Group A or D streptococci |
| | Meningitis: neonates and young infants† | Hematogenous | *Escherichia coli* Group B streptococci *Listeria monocytogenes* |
| | Infants and young children‡ | Hematogenous (nasopharynx) or Direct invasion—rarely | *Streptococcus pneumoniae* *Neisseria meningitidis* (*Haemophilus influenzae* rare) |
| | Adults children‡ | Hematogenous (nasopharynx) or Direct invasion—rarely | *Streptococcus pneumoniae* *Neisseria meningitidis* (*Haemophilus influenzae* rare) |
| | All ages | Direct invasion (head trauma, congenital, neuromalformations, neurodiagnostic procedures, neuroorthopedic surgery) | Staphylococci Group A streptococci *Streptococcus pneumoniae* *Pseduomonas aeruginosa* *Escherichia coli* Other Enterobacteriaceae |
| Granulomatous meningitis | Tuberculous Cryptococcal | Hematogenous (lung) Hematogenous (lung) | *Mycobacterium tuberculosis* *Cryptococcus neoformans* |
| Acute viral ("aseptic") | Meningitis | Hematogenous (intestinal tract, oropharynx) | Enteroviruses Mumps virus Arboviruses Adenoviruses |
| | Encephalitis | Hematogenous (intestinal tract, arthropod vector feeding, respiratory tract) | Herpesvirus Enteroviruses Mumps virus Arboviruses Epstein-Barr virus |

*Refers to predominance of neutrophils in the CSF.
†Less than 2–3 months of age.
‡2–3 months to 5 years of age.

scess. Usually these bacteria originate from the mouth flora, and microaerophilic bacteria (such as *Haemophilus aphrophilus*) or anaerobic bacteria (such as *Peptostreptococcus*) are the most common etiologic agents. Congenital cyanotic heart disease is a common predisposing risk factor for brain abscess. Although bacteremia with *Streptococcus pneumoniae* is common, especially in children (and in certain cases leads to meningitis), this bacterium very rarely causes brain abscesses. This observation suggests that specific receptors (yet unidentified) exist in the target tissue that allow the bacteria to adhere, multiply, and cause infection. These receptors apparently play a major role in the pathogenesis of infection by determining what type of bacteria produces infection in the brain or in the meninges.

Acute bacterial meningitis most commonly occurs in the very young and the very old. In the preantibiotic era, fatality rates from bacterial meningitis ranged from 70 to 100%. Some progress was achieved when antiserum treatment was used. However, the most dramatic decrease in mortality occurred with the introduction of penicillin, whereupon mortality was reduced to 6% in infants and children and to 25–30% in neonates and the elderly. These mortality rates are still too high, and bacterial meningitis remains a life-threatening illness in all age groups. The mortality and morbidity of bacterial meningitis have not changed significantly in the five decades since the introduction of penicillin. Even the use of recently developed and more potent antibiotics has not substantially improved the outcome. This unexpected fact, despite seemingly more effective antimicrobial therapy as judged by more rapid sterilization of the CSF, may result from the harmful interaction between host inflammatory cells and bacterial components released into the CSF by multiplying bacteria or by antibiotic-induced bacterial lysis. This interaction, which continues despite bacteriologic cure, is believed to be the reason for the high percentage of neurologic sequelae currently observed in patients who recover from meningitis. As many as 25–40% of those who survive the infection may develop long-term sequelae. The major sequelae of meningitis consist of cognitive defects, hearing loss, motor lesions (including seizures, spasticity, and paresis), cranial nerve lesions, and behavioral disturbances. Sensorineural hearing loss, which occurs in 5–10% of cases, is the most serious neurologic sequela because in the very young it is likely to

impair speech acquisition and learning. It has been estimated that approximately 40% of all hearing defects acquired postnatally are due to bacterial meningitis. Recent routine immunization of infants with *H. influenzae* type b conjugate vaccine has resulted in the near disappearance of invasive diseases (including meningitis) due to this agent, which was the most common cause of bacterial meningitis.

A wide variety of microorganisms can cause acute bacterial infection of the meninges (Table 20–2). In adults and children *Streptococcus pneumoniae* and *Neisseria meningitidis* are the most common causes of bacterial meningitis. In recent years the number of infections due to gram-negative bacilli has increased significantly. This trend is not surprising, since gram-negative bacillary meningitis is usually hospital acquired and remains a major problem. In elderly patients (older than 60 years of age), *S. pneumoniae* is the most common cause of meningitis followed by gram-negative bacilli. Susceptibility to bacterial meningitis is affected not only by age (i.e., most cases occur in the very young or the very old) and genetics but also by acquired or congenital deficiencies in host defense mechanisms. Individuals with IgG or complement deficiencies, patients who have undergone splenectomy, or those with congenital or functional asplenia have an increased incidence of septicemia and meningitis caused by *S. pneumoniae* and *H. influenzae* type b. Patients with sickle cell anemia and other hemoglobinopathies are also at increased risk for developing meningitis (usually with *S. pneumoniae*) because of poor splenic function and a defect in the alternative complement pathway. Meningococcal infections occur with increased frequency in individuals who have a deficiency of the terminal components of the complement system (i.e., C5–C9).

Certain environmental situations can increase the probability of acquiring meningitis. A higher incidence of *N. meningitidis* meningitis has been reported in crowded households, day-care centers, and college and military dormitories. Because the bacteria are transmitted from person to person through the air, the proximity of susceptible individuals in these situations facilitates the spread of infection and the occurrence of secondary cases.

Recurrent bacterial meningitis often suggests the presence of a communication between the subarachnoid space and the paranasal sinuses, nasopharynx, or middle ear.

**TABLE 20–2.    ETIOLOGIC AGENTS OF BACTERIAL MENINGITIS BY AGE GROUP\***

| ORGANISM | 0–2 MONTHS | 2 MONTHS–4 YEARS | 5–29 YEARS | >30 Years |
|---|---|---|---|---|
| *Streptococcus pneumoniae* | 3% | 40% | 20% | 40% |
| *Neisseria meningitidis* | — | 30% | 42% | 10% |
| *Haemophilus influenzae* | 4% | 25% | 8% | 4% |
| Group B streptococcus | 50% | — | 1% | 4% |
| *Listeria monocytogenes* | 10% | — | 2% | 5% |
| Other† | 33% | 5% | 27% | 37% |

\*Modified from Wenger, J. D., Hightower, A. W., Facklam, R. R., et al. *J. Infect. Dis. 162*:1316–1323, 1990. With permission.
†Includes *S. aureus, E. coli,* streptococci, klebsiella, etc.

This communication results from fractures or congenital fistulae that transverse through the paranasal sinuses, cribriform plate of the ethmoid bone, or petrous bone. Some individuals have experienced more than 10 episodes of meningitis as a result of such lesions, which can be difficult to identify precisely. The most common bacterium recovered in such instances is *S. pneumoniae.* Therefore, any individual with a history of head trauma who develops meningitis should be promptly examined for excessively watery nasal or otic discharge, which is the result of intermittent or continuous drainage of CSF into the nasal cavities or into the ear through the fracture line. These conditions are called CSF rhinorrhea or CSF otorrhea.

Communication of the subarachnoid space with the skin is usually associated with congenital midline defects of the skull or spine, such as cranial or lumbosacral dermal sinus, dermoid cyst, and myelomeningocele. The meningitis resulting from these lesions is often caused by gram-negative bacilli or staphylococci.

### Acute Viral Meningitis and Encephalitis

Acute viral infections of the CNS are usually designated as aseptic meningitis, myelitis, or encephalitis (the last being characterized by altered cerebral function). However, a single satisfactory localization on the basis of clinical findings alone is often difficult. Thus, compound terms such as meningoencephalitis or encephalomyelitis are used to describe the spectrum of the disease. The term *aseptic* was used initially to describe an illness characterized by an acute onset, fever, CSF pleocytosis, with sterile bacterial cultures. With the use of viral isolation methods and new culture techniques to define other microorganisms, it has become clear that *aseptic* is not synonymous with *viral,* and that additional multiple etiologic agents can produce such syndromes (see Chapter 22).

Many viral pathogens cause CNS infections in humans. Some of the most common viruses are listed in Table 20–1. With the exception of *Herpes simplex* encephalitis, the specific viruses causing CNS syndromes are frequently difficult, and sometimes impossible, to identify. Until recently, this lack of specific identification was moot because no useful antiviral therapy was available. With the development of antiviral therapy, increased attention has been focused on the pathogenesis and prompt and specific diagnosis of the various viral infections of the CNS (especially *Herpes simplex* encephalitis) so that appropriate therapy can be initiated promptly.

Viral CNS infections are common. Although all ages are involved, more than 90% of the patients are under 30 years of age. The viral etiology varies with the season of the year, the age of the patient, and the geographic location. In the United States, about 70% of cases are due to enteroviruses. Most cases occur in children and in the late summer and early fall. Arboviral meningoencephalitis occurs mostly during the summer months because virus transmission occurs by an arthropod such as a mosquito or a tick active during this time of the year. Mumps virus infections are more frequent in the late winter and early spring. Herpesvirus and human immunodeficiency virus (HIV) infections occur sporadically during the year. In immunocompromised patients other viruses such as adenovirus and cytomegalovirus may cause meningoencephalitis. Poliovirus and lymphocytic choriomeningitis virus, which are important causes of meningoencephalitis worldwide, cause remarkably few cases in the United States.

Viruses gain access to the CNS by one of two routes, hematogenous or neuronal. Most viruses that cause CNS infection do so hematogenously. Following multiplication at the site of entry or in regional lymph nodes that drain the entry site, the virus enters the bloodstream and reaches the CNS. For example, in arthropod-borne viral disease, the virus is transmitted by an insect bite to the skin, where the virus undergoes local replication. Transient viremia occurs with seeding of the virus to the reticuloendothelial system, particularly the liver, spleen, and lymph nodes. Following multiplication in these organs, a secondary viremia occurs leading to further seeding of the virus to other sites, including the CNS. Alternatively, viruses reach the CNS by peripheral intraneuronal routes as occurs with herpes simplex virus. Studies in animals and in humans have suggested that the olfactory tract may be a common route to the brain in cases of *Herpes simplex* encephalitis. Another example of intraneuronal transmission of virus to the CNS is rabies. In this case, the limbic system is involved. Once the rabies virus has reached the CNS, subsequent replication can remain within the neurons or result in cell-to-cell or extracellular transmission.

The precise mechanisms by which viruses reach the CSF and produce neurologic damage are still under investigation. The pathologic findings in acute viral encephalitis are striking. Inflammation of cortical capillary vessels occurs primarily in the gray matter or at the junction of the gray and the white matters, and lymphocytic infiltration is seen in the perivascular areas. As the disease progresses, astrocytosis and gliosis become prominent histopathologic findings.

Viral meningitis is usually an acute, self-limiting illness which, in many instances, mimics other treatable life-threatening CNS infections. Therefore, it is important to recognize the similarities among viral meningitis, partially treated bacterial meningitis, tuberculous meningitis, and fungal meningitis.

As indicated above, the term *encephalitis* is used when there is clinical or pathologic evidence of cerebral involvement. Approximately 20,000 cases of encephalitis occur in the United States each year, with *Herpes simplex* encephalitis accounting for approximately 10% of these cases. The arthropod-borne viruses (arboviruses), such as St. Louis encephalitis, eastern or western equine encephalitis, and La Crosse virus, cause sporadic and epidemic CNS infections in the United States. Japanese B encephalitis is the most common epidemic CNS infection outside of North America. In China alone, for example, more than 10,000 cases occur annually.

In general, viral encephalitis can be divided into four pathogenic categories: (1) acute primary viral encephalitis, (2) postinfectious encephalomyelitis, (3) slow viral infections of the CNS, and (4) chronic degenerative diseases of the CNS of presumed viral origin.

The acute primary form occurs when the virus directly invades and replicates within the CNS, causing encephalitis.

Postinfectious encephalomyelitis is thought to be an autoimmune phenomenon initiated by a viral pathogen. There is a latent phase between the acute viral illness and the onset of neurologic symptoms. Histopathologic studies demonstrate perivascular inflammation and demyelination, but the virus cannot be recovered from the CNS. Postinfectious encephalomyelitis is most commonly associated with varicella and influenza in the United States. The exact mechanisms that determine why only certain patients develop postinfectious encephalomyelitis are as yet unknown.

Neurodiagnostic techniques, including electroencephalography (EEG), computed tomography (CT), and magnetic resonance imaging (MRI), may be of diagnostic help in cases of suspected encephalitis. Brain scan and EEG are especially of value in patients with herpes encephalitis. In these patients, characteristic periodic high-voltage spike activity, particularly emanating from the temporal regions, and a background of slow-wave complexes are highly suggestive of *Herpes simplex* infection of the brain. Brain biopsy or CSF polymerase chain reaction (PCR) for HSV are the most sensitive and specific means of diagnosis for differentiating between *Herpes simplex* encephalitis and other diseases that mimic it.

### Granulomatous Meningitis

In granulomatous meningitis the term *granulomatous* refers to the histopathologic characteristic of this infection—formation of granulomata. The granuloma is a collection of lymphocytes and histiocytes derived from mononuclear cells, epithelioid cells, and multinucleated giant cells. Granulomatous meningitis is characterized by a subacute and progressive clinical course and may be remittent, with definite remissions and relapses.

*Mycobacterium tuberculosis* and *Cryptococcus neoformans* are the most common causes of granulomatous meningitis. Both organisms usually infect the CNS in the course of hematogenous dissemination of infection originating in the lungs. Meningitis may be the initial clinical manifestation of tuberculosis or cryptococcal disease when dissemination of the organisms to the CNS is intense. In such cases chest roentgenograms may show little or no evidence of underlying infection.

Recently, strains of *M. tuberculosis* have developed resistance to many drugs, which has caused increased treatment failure rates. Drug-resistant tuberculosis is especially common in HIV-infected patients, the homeless, drug users, and previously treated patients who had a cavitary lesion.

Tuberculous meningitis in adults frequently results from reactivation of an old tuberculous CNS focus that had developed many years earlier and then spread to the subarachnoid space. Tuberculous meningitis is typically associated with active, progressive systemic disease. Tuberculosis of the CNS may also present as a tuberculoma of the brain, which is a well-circumscribed intraparenchymal mass that may slowly enlarge (up to several centimeters in diameter) and may significantly increase intracranial pressure because of its mass. Biopsy of such a lesion usually shows a central core of caseous necrosis surrounded by a typical tuberculous granulomatous reaction. Organisms can often be seen with acid-fast stains, and calcification frequently occurs in inactive lesions. Although seen less frequently in the United States and Europe, tuberculomas still constitute up to 25% of intracranial masses in India and South America. In about 25% of the cases, multiple lesions are found. In children, tuberculomas are usually found in the posterior fossa, whereas in adults they are predominantly supratentorial. History of exposure to a patient with tuberculosis may give an important clue to this treatable disease.

In contrast, exposure history for cryptococcus is of little value, since this fungus is a widespread saprophyte. Evidence of underlying cellular immune dysfunction is more important because it predisposes the patient to this infection. The development of subacute or chronic meningitis in patients with Hodgkin's disease or lymphosarcoma, in those receiving high-dose daily corticosteroids, or in those at risk for acquired immunodeficiency syndrome (AIDS) should raise the possibility of cryptococcal meningitis. Initial manifestations of cryptococcal meningitis may be unexplained fevers and chronic headaches.

Chronic meningitis in the immunosuppressed patient with impaired cellular immunity requires special consideration because of the distinctive differential diagnosis. *Listeria monocytogenes; Mycobacterium avium-intracellulare; Toxoplasma gondii;* and *Nocardia, Histoplasma,* and *Coccidioides* species are some of the other etiologic agents of chronic meningitis in such patients that should be considered in the differential diagnosis. The list of opportunistic agents associated with chronic meningitis in individuals with AIDS is even longer, including papovavirus, cytomegalovirus, *Treponema pallidum, Candida* species, and the human immunodeficiency virus itself.

## CLINICAL ASPECTS

### Manifestations of Meningitis

Fever, headache, vomiting, impairment of consciousness, and stiff neck and back are common manifestations of meningeal irritation in adults, irrespective of its etiology. The headache is usually generalized and persistent. Unfortunately, it is a manifestation that children younger than 2 years of age cannot communicate; they are usually irritable, which is not as specific an indicator of a CNS process. Nuchal rigidity (the most pathognomonic sign of meningitis in adults) is resistance to flexion of the neck caused by cervical and upper thoracic paraspinal muscle spasm as a result of meningeal inflammation. True nuchal rigidity, which usually indicates meningeal inflammation, should be distinguished from meningismus (e.g., painful or difficult flexion or rotation of the head), which is caused by posterior cervical or shoulder girdle muscle spasm related to acute pharyngitis/tonsillitis, especially peritonsillar abscess, or acute posterior or anterior cervical lymphadenitis. Torticollis and other processes in the neck can cause symptoms that simulate nuchal rigidity.

Meningitis presents as two symptom patterns in infants and young children. The first is insidious and develops progressively over several days; it may be preceded by a nonspecific febrile illness or an upper respiratory–like infection. In this setting, it is usually difficult, if not impossible, to time the exact onset of meningitis, especially if another infection, such as otitis media, is diagnosed and oral antibiotics given. The second pattern is acute and fulminant, with the manifestations of sepsis and meningitis developing rapidly over a few hours. This rapidly progressive form may be associated with severe brain edema that can provoke herniation of the cerebellar tonsils, resulting in death.

In children, the presenting symptoms are often nonspecific. Fever, listlessness, sleepiness, irritability, and vomiting are commonly found, and there is a higher incidence of seizures. In neonates as well as in very old patients, the signs and symptoms of meningitis may be even more subtle, consisting of only fever, confusion, and poor feeding; unstable or low temperature is not rare. Stiff neck or fullness of the anterior fontanelle are relatively late signs of meningitis in infants and may not be present in all cases. It is important to consider the possibility of meningitis in any patient with fever and unexplained alteration in mentation or level of alertness and consciousness. Whereas judgment based upon clinical findings is certainly important, the adage "If you think about doing a spinal tap to verify the diagnosis, do it" still holds. The potential diagnostic value of a lumbar puncture when indicated far outweighs the very small risk of harm from the procedure.

Several features that may be found during the physical examination warrant specific mention. Petechiae, especially in association with fever, should always raise the possibility of bacteremia and meningitis. Although petechiae classically are associated with meningococcal infection, they can occur with *H. influenzae, S. pneumoniae,* and many viral infections. It is important to note that pediatric patients with meningitis may also have an extrameningeal focus of infection, such as buccal or periorbital cellulitis, otitis media, or pneumonia. Therefore, if such a focus is found, the patient's status (e.g., age, immune compe-

tence, severity of symptoms in relation to the identified focus, and symptoms unexplained by the known focus) should be carefully assessed before a decision is made not to do studies for determining the presence of meningitis. Focal neurologic signs, such as hemiparesis, quadriparesis, or cranial nerve palsy, occur in about 15% of patients with meningitis and reflect the possible presence of cortical venous or arterial thrombosis secondary to edema and inflammation. Papilledema is uncommon early in the course of acute meningitis and, when present, should prompt an evaluation for venous sinus thrombosis, subdural collection of fluid, or brain abscess.

## Differential Diagnosis of CNS Infections

Because the signs and symptoms of CNS infection are very diverse and are not pathognomonic, many other diseases should be considered in the differential diagnosis (Table 20–3). Even distinguishing among the various infectious processes that may occur in the CNS, such as viral meningitis, fungal meningitis, tuberculous meningitis, brain abscess, early bacterial meningitis, subdural empyema, and others, may be difficult. In some instances, the initial laboratory findings are nonspecific and serial cerebrospinal fluid evaluation is necessary to identify the etiologic agent or the response to therapy. Clues to the specific diagnosis may come from careful history of potential exposure (e.g., tuberculosis, or specific viral, bacterial, or fungal exposure), lack of haemophilus immunization in young children, meticulous physical examination (e.g., lesions outside the CNS with potential to spread, systemic manifestations of noninfectious diseases), careful ex-

## TABLE 20–3.　A PARTIAL LIST OF DIFFERENTIAL DIAGNOSES OF CNS INFECTIONS

| NONINFECTIOUS | INFECTIOUS |
|---|---|
| Brain tumors | Viral meningoencephalitis |
| Leukemia | Bacterial meningitis |
| Lymphoma | Tuberculosis |
| Subarachnoid hemorrhage | Brain abscess |
| Subdural hematoma | Parameningeal infections |
| Systemic lupus erythematosus | Lyme disease |
| Malignant hypertension | Syphilis |
| Multiple sclerosis | Brucellosis |
| Sarcoidosis | Toxoplasmosis |
| Mollaret's (recurrent) meningitis | Cysticercosis |
| Behçet's disease | Cryptococcosis |
| Ruptured dermoid cyst | Fungal meningitis |
| Ruptured spinal ependymoma | Rickettsial infections |

amination of cerebrospinal fluid, immunologic studies, and roentgenographic studies.

Brain tumors and brain abscesses are frequently indistinguishable by their clinical presentation alone. Increased intracranial pressure may be the only presenting neurologic
sign, and lumbar puncture may not be helpful
in differentiating between these two entities
because the CSF may be entirely normal, except for the fact that its pressure is increased.
Epidural or subdural spinal abscesses usually
present with spinal cord compression, symptomatology that can simulate noninfectious
diseases such as Guillain-Barré syndrome, spinal cord tumor, meningioma, and herniated
disc. Emergency myelography is often essential to differentiate spinal cord compression
from other processes. The urgency of myelography cannot be overemphasized because,
when abscess formation occurs within the spinal canal, the spinal cord must be decom-
pressed promptly by appropriate neurosurgical means if return of normal neurologic
function is to be expected.

Neoplastic metastases involving the meninges may produce the same clinical manifestations as granulomatous meningitis. The CSF
abnormalities may also be identical to those
that are typically seen in tuberculous or cryptococcal meningitis. Only special studies such
as careful examination of the cells in the CSF,
special staining procedures (e.g., acid-fast or
India ink), and biopsy may be helpful in the
diagnosis.

## CEREBROSPINAL FLUID
## ABNORMALITIES

Analysis of CSF (usually obtained by lumbar
puncture) is essential for the evaluation of a
patient with CNS infection. There are very
few conditions that contraindicate the prompt
performance of a lumbar puncture. These
conditions include (1) the presence of obvious signs of increased intracranial pressure
(e.g., papilledema, sixth nerve palsy, altered
pupillary responses, increased blood pressure
with bradycardia), (2) significantly unstable
cardiopulmonary status (e.g., with severe sepsis) that might be aggravated by the procedure, and (3) infection in the area that the
needle must traverse to obtain CSF. If signs of
increased intracranial pressure are present,
removal of even small amounts of CSF (3–4
mL) may result in downward displacement of
the brain into the foramen magnum, com-

pressing the cerebellar peduncles against
the lower medulla and leading to brainstem
compression. Sudden removal of CSF under
increased pressure may also cause shifting of
the brain with transtentorial herniation of
some portion of the cerebral hemispheres
into the posterior fossa. Foraminal or
transtentorial herniation of the brain is an
extreme emergency situation that requires
immediate neurosurgical decompression to
save the patient. For the above reasons, if increased intracranial pressure is suspected,
noninvasive neurodiagnostic procedures
such as a CT scan or MRI should be performed before lumbar puncture is
performed.

The typical CSF abnormalities associated
with types of CNS infections are shown in
Table 20–4. When the CSF is obtained, it
should be examined immediately. The total
number of white blood cells should be
counted in a counting chamber and, following centrifugation, a differential cell count
should be performed on a Wright-stained
smear of the sediment. Normally, the CSF has
fewer than 5–10 mononuclear leukocytes/
mm$^3$ and no polymorphonuclear neutrophils
(PMNs). Therefore, the presence of a single
PMN is abnormal and suggests the possibility
of CNS infection. In addition, if the number
of mononuclear cells is higher than 10, a CNS
process (including infection) should be suspected. Although the differential count is
more likely to disclose a predominance of
PMNs in bacterial meningitis and a predominance of mononuclear cells in viral, tuberculous, or fungal meningitis, there is an overlap
between these groups. Up to one third of
cases with tuberculous or viral meningitis
demonstrate a predominance of PMNs, and
as many as 10% of cases of early or partially
treated bacterial meningitis have a predominance of lymphocytes. The CSF protein concentration (normally <40 mg/dL) and the
CSF glucose concentration (normally >40
mg/dL) and its ratio to the simultaneous
blood glucose concentration (normally >0.4)
may help in the diagnosis.

The CSF abnormalities associated with tuberculous, fungal, and viral meningitis overlap even more, and it may be impossible to
separate one from the other (see Table 20–
4). The CSF findings in tuberculous meningitis usually consist of a lymphocytic pleocytosis (25–500 cells/mm$^3$), increased protein
concentration, and depressed glucose level.
CSF acid-fast smears are positive in 10–22%

**TABLE 20—4.  CEREBROSPINAL FLUID ABNORMALITIES OFTEN ASSOCIATED WITH CNS INFECTIONS**

| | LEUKOCYTES | | CEREBROSPINAL FLUID FINDINGS | | |
| CONDITION | No. Per mm³ | Predominant Cell | Glucose | Protein | Stained Smear | Result of Culture |
|---|---|---|---|---|---|---|
| Bacterial meningitis ("purulent") | 0–60,000 | Segmented neutrophils | Very low (<5–20 mg/dL) | Elevated | Usually positive* | Usually positive* |
| Partially treated meningitis | 0–2500 | Neutrophils and mononuclear cells | Normal to slightly reduced | Elevated | Often negative | Often negative |
| Tuberculous meningitis | 25–500 | Mononuclear cells | Low (<10–30 mg/dL) | Elevated | Usually negative | Usually negative |
| Fungal meningitis | 0–1000 | Mononuclear cells | Low | Elevated | Often positive | Usually positive |
| Viral meningitis ("aseptic") | 0–1000 | Mononuclear cells (neutrophils in early phase) | Normal (65–70 mg/dL) | Slightly elevated | Negative | Negative |
| Brain abscess | 10–200 | Lymphocytes or neutrophils | Normal | Elevated | Usually negative | Usually negative |
| Syphilis | 30–500 | Lymphocytes | Normal | Elevated | Usually negative | Usually negative |
| Sarcoidosis | 50–200 | Mononuclear cells | Normal | Elevated | Negative | Negative |

*A major exception is bacterial meningitis caused by *Neisseria meningitidis*, in which the Gram's stain of cerebrospinal fluid sediment often fails to reveal microorganisms, and cultures may be negative for growth.

of the cases, and CSF cultures are positive in 38–88% of the cases.

Antituberculous therapy should be initiated promptly if the clinical setting suggests infection with *M. tuberculosis*, since delay in treatment may preclude full recovery. Typical CSF findings in cryptococcal meningitis include a mild lymphocytic pleocytosis (0–400 cells/$mm^3$) and a depressed glucose level in 55% of cases. It is important to note that in AIDS patients, currently the most common patients with this infection, the CSF often shows little evidence of an inflammatory reaction. India ink staining of CSF is positive in over half of the cases, demonstrating the cryptococcal cells with their large capsules. The yield is highest in patients with acute infection. More than 85% of patients have cryptococcal polysaccharide antigen in the CSF. Although the initial CSF culture is positive in only three quarters of the patients, additional CSF cultures increase the yield and are indicated.

Because it is not justified to exclude bacterial meningitis and to defer antimicrobial therapy solely on the basis of the CSF parameters, the sediment of centrifuged CSF should be Gram's stained and examined thoroughly. A positive Gram's stain provides helpful information, but a negative stain does not rule out bacterial meningitis. The probability of visualizing bacteria on a Gram's stain is dependent upon the number of organisms present. The percentage of positive Gram's-stained smears is less than 25% when there are fewer than $10^3$ organisms/mL. The percentage is higher (up to 40–50%) when there are $10^4$–$10^5$ organisms/mL. When more than $10^5$ organisms/mL are present, 97% of Gram's stains are positive. Staining of the CSF with acridine orange and examination with fluorescence microscopy may increase the sensitivity of the method, and bacteria not observed by the usual Gram's stain may be found. Pretreatment with oral antibiotics may only slightly modify the results of Gram's stains and cultures with some bacteria (e.g., *H. influenzae*), but with others (e.g., *S. pneumoniae* and *N. meningitidis*) the changes are significant. Rapid tests (within 1 h) are available to detect bacterial antigens associated with *H. influenzae* type b, *S. pneumoniae*, *N. meningitidis*, and group B streptococcus in both CSF and urine. The most sensitive test is the latex agglutination test. Various latex agglutination tests typically demonstrate sensitivity of 90–100% as compared with 65–75% for counterimmunoelectrophoresis (CIE). These

tests are especially helpful for patients in whom pretreatment has rendered the interpretation of bacterial cultures difficult (partially treated meningitis). However, failure to detect antigen in the CSF using these tests does not rule out bacterial meningitis. Again, the sensitivity of the test is in direct correlation to the number of bacteria in the CSF; if they are below $10^2$–$10^3$/mL, the test result is usually negative.

Detection of endotoxin in the CSF or measurement of CSF C-reactive protein, lactate acid concentration, and lactate dehydrogenase (LDH) activity have been reported to be helpful in differentiating bacterial from viral meningitis. The accuracy and usefulness of these tests are uncertain because they have not been extensively used and thus need further evaluation.

In addition to CSF cultures, blood cultures should be obtained for every patient with suspected bacterial meningitis. These cultures are positive in 80% of children with *H. influenzae* meningitis, in 50% with *S. pneumoniae* meningitis, and in a third of patients with *N. meningitidis* meningitis.

From the above discussion of the CSF findings in CNS infections, it should be obvious that, despite the availability of many sensitive tests for detecting various etiologic agents, the differential diagnosis relies heavily on the physician's ability to consider these tests in the context of the clinical setting of the individual patient. Only then can reasonable decisions concerning antimicrobial therapy be made.

## THEORETICAL AND PRACTICAL CONSIDERATIONS OF ANTIBIOTIC THERAPY

### General Approach to Antimicrobial Therapy

Prompt treatment of bacterial meningitis with an appropriate antibiotic is essential to minimize the occurrence of additional nervous system damage. The development of serious neurologic complications such as seizures, hemiplegia, hearing impairment, and cognitive dysfunction is correlated with the type of bacteria causing the meningitis, with its concentration in the CSF, and with very low CSF glucose concentrations (<20 mg/dL). The initial antimicrobial regimen chosen for treatment should be sufficiently broad to affect all likely pathogens that commonly cause meningitis in the patient's age group. Remember that the Gram's stain can be misinterpreted and that rapid antigen tests do not provide information regarding antimicrobial susceptibility. Therefore, the preferred initial antimicrobial regimen varies with the expected pathogens, their susceptibilities, and the age of the patient.

## Entry of Beta-Lactam Antibiotics into the CSF

A number of new beta-lactam antibiotics have been evaluated recently for the treatment of meningitis, and several have been shown to be very effective in eradicating bacteria. Multiple factors influence the penetration of beta-lactam antibiotics into the CSF. The blood-brain barrier and the blood-CSF barrier restrict penetration of most antimicrobial drugs into the brain and CSF, respectively. Concentration of antibiotics in these two CNS areas in normal volunteers and in experimental animals are approximately 1/200–1/500 those achieved in the serum. Penetration of antibiotics into the CSF is by passive diffusion, and inflammation of the pia-arachnoid during infection enhances the permeability of the barrier, with subsequent increase in CSF antibiotic concentrations. The blood-brain barrier acts like a lipid layer. As a result, highly lipophilic substances (e.g., drugs such as chloramphenicol, rifampin, isoniazid) enter readily into the CSF, whereas certain cephalosporins and aminoglycosides do not.

Most antibiotics that diffuse into the CSF are removed from the subarachnoid space by "bulk-flow" mechanisms across the arachnoid villi. In addition, penicillins, cephalosporins, and aminoglycosides are transported out of the CSF to the intravascular region by an energy-requiring exit pump in the choroid plexus. This active exit pump of the choroid plexus rapidly moves antimicrobial agents back into the systemic circulation, making it even more difficult to achieve and maintain high concentrations of antibiotics in the CSF or brain tissues.

Two other considerations are relevant to the penetration of antibiotics into the CSF following the disruption of the blood-brain barrier.

1. The penetration of antibiotics declines as meningeal inflammation subsides during the course of treatment of meningitis. For example, on the first day of therapy for bacterial meningitis, ampicillin levels in CSF are about 40% of serum levels, but after 7 days of treatment the CSF level is less than 20% of the serum level; therefore, the dosage of the antimicrobial agents must not be reduced during therapy.

2. Experimental meningitis studies in animals show that antiinflammatory agents, such as corticosteroids, decrease meningeal inflammation and thus may reduce permeability of the blood-brain barrier.

## Need for Bactericidal Activity in CSF

The blood-brain barrier and the blood-CSF barrier restrict delivery of antibodies and complement to the nervous system. Thus, host immune responses outside the CNS have a very limited effect on the invading pathogen after it enters the CNS. Some evidence exists that active production of IgM and IgG by antibody-secreting B lymphocytes that have entered the CNS as part of the inflammatory response may be important in combating invading bacteria. However, phagocytosis of encapsulated meningeal pathogens is inefficient in CSF *in vivo*, resulting in unhindered bacterial proliferation and ultimately in high bacterial concentrations within the CSF. These observations suggest that antibiotics are of paramount importance in treatment of bacterial CNS infections. Unfortunately, an antibiotic not only must reach the affected area of the CNS but also must achieve concentrations that exceed the minimum bactericidal concentration (MBC) of the antibiotic for the invading bacteria (as determined *in vitro*).

The need for high bactericidal activity in the CSF to effect a desirable outcome has been demonstrated in experimental models of meningitis. CSF concentrations of beta-lactam or an aminoglycoside agent that are at least 10 times higher than the MBC of the infecting pathogen were necessary to achieve optimal bacterial eradication.

An innovative approach to assist in the choice of an effective antibiotic is to combine *in vitro* data (e.g., the MBC) with *in vivo* data (e.g., CSF antibiotic levels) to produce an index that reflects the degree to which the achievable CSF antibiotic levels exceed the MBC of the bacteria. This ratio, called the inhibitory quotient, should exceed 10 if the desired bactericidal effect is to be achieved. For example, an *H. influenzae* isolated from a patient with meningitis was found to be killed *in vitro* (MBC) by drug A at a concentration of 0.5 $\mu$g/mL and by drug B at 0.05 $\mu$g/mL concentration. From data in the literature, it is known that drug A produces CSF levels of 4

$\mu$g/mL and drug B only 2 $\mu$g/mL. From the equation inhibitory quotient = CSF drug level ÷ MBC, the inhibitory quotient for drug A is 8 (4 ÷ 0.5), and for drug B it is 40 (2 ÷ 0.05). Although drug A achieves absolute CSF levels higher than drug B, drug B is predicted to be more efficient in eradicating the bacteria (e.g., inhibitory quotient >10) and should be the preferred drug.

### Antimicrobial Drug Resistance

In the last 5 years, *S. pneumoniae*, which had been highly sensitive to penicillin, has gradually become more resistant. The bacteria have undergone mutations in the penicillin-binding proteins (PBPs), resulting in increased resistance to penicillin, and, to a lesser extent, to cephalosporins. Ten to 30% of *S. pneumoniae* strains isolated from patients in the United States (most commonly serotypes 6B, 14, 19F, and 23) are relatively resistant to penicillin (MIC 0.1–1.0 $\mu$g/mL), and about 1–3% are highly resistant to penicillin (MIC ≥2.0 $\mu$g/mL). In addition to increased resistance to penicillin, the rate of resistance to other antibiotics such as trimethoprim-sulfamethoxazole (TMP/SMZ), erythromycin, tetracycline, and clindamycin is also increasing in the penicillin-resistant strains. Since resistance to penicillin is caused by altered PBPs, it is not surprising that treatment failures with the newer cephalosporins (i.e., cefotaxime and ceftriaxone) have been reported. Currently, all *S. pneumoniae* strains in the United States are sensitive to vancomycin, and thus it should be added to the therapy of suspected *S. pneumoniae* meningitis until the sensitivity of the bacteria is known.

Some other bacteria that cause meningitis have changed their susceptibility to antibiotics. For example, a substantial proportion of strains of *H. influenzae* type b have become resistant to ampicillin and, to a lesser extent, to chloramphenicol. Most of the resistant strains contain a plasmid that mediates production of a beta-lactamase that hydrolyzes penicillins and some cephalosporins. Thus, the initial therapy for *H. influenzae* meningitis should be ceftriaxone or cefotaxime, which are highly active against *H. influenzae*, including organisms that produce beta-lactamase or that are multiresistant.

### Need for Adjunctive Antiinflammatory Therapy

A major goal of antimicrobial therapy has been to achieve sterilization of the CSF as rapidly as possible. However, there have been concerns that rapid lysis, particularly of gram-negative bacteria, may result in a massive release of endotoxin that could be harmful to the host. Studies in animals and humans have shown that products of bacterial lysis, such as cell fragments and lipopolysaccharides (e.g., endotoxin) induced by cell-wall–active antibiotics, can cause a transient increase of locally produced cytokines. These proinflammatory agents may amplify and augment tissue injury. In fact, although the newer antibiotics are much more efficient in sterilization of the CNS compared with older agents, there has been little improvement over earlier treatment trials. In animal experiments, use of the corticosteroid dexamethasone (given prior to or concomitant with the first dose of antibiotic) was found to be effective in preventing the antibiotic-induced burst of cytokines in the CSF, and thus augmentation of the inflammatory response was aborted. The addition of dexamethasone to antimicrobial therapy for patients with *H. influenzae* meningitis was shown to be beneficial in reducing neurologic complications. However, its addition to the treatment regimen of patients with other pathogens causing meningitis (i.e., *S. pneumoniae*, group B streptococcus, *Escherichia coli*) is controversial, and further confirmatory studies are needed.

### Duration of Therapy

Regimens used for the therapy of bacterial meningitis are largely empiric and are based upon antibiotic pharmacokinetic data and clinical experience. The duration of antibiotic therapy for meningitis continues to be somewhat controversial: the patient needs to be treated long enough to effect permanent cure but not any longer. For example, in neonates, the suggested duration of therapy for *Escherichia coli* meningitis is the longer time of (1) 14 days after the documentation of sterile CSF, or (2) 21 days total. In older infants, children, and adults, shorter courses of therapy are used. The clinical and bacteriologic responses of patients with meningococcal meningitis and *H. influenzae* type b meningitis suggest that a 7- to 10-day course of therapy is sufficient in the majority of cases.

## VACCINE IMMUNOPROPHYLAXIS OF MENINGITIS

Capsular polysaccharides appear to be the major antigenic determinants of many of the major bacterial pathogens that play an important role in causing meningitis. Vaccines employing some of these bacterial polysaccharides have proved to be highly immunogenic and protective, especially in adults. Currently, vaccines for protection against *H. influenzae* type b and selected strains of *S. pneumoniae* and *N. meningitidis* are available.

In the last decade, several *H. influenzae* type B polysaccharide–protein conjugate vaccines have been developed. In such conjugates, the polysaccharide is converted from being a T-cell–independent antigen to a T-cell–dependent antigen. This conversion not only increases the B-cell response to the polysaccharide moiety but also induces memory T cells, which enhance amnestic responses to the antigen. Conjugate vaccines of *H. influenzae* type b (such as PRP conjugated to diphtheria or tetanus toxoid or PRP conjugated to an outer membrane protein of *N. meningitidis*) are highly immunogenic even in children as young as 2 months of age. Since approximately 60% of all *H. influenzae* type b meningitis in the United States had occurred in children younger than 15 months of age, these vaccines have reduced the incidence of *H. influenzae* disease dramatically since routine immunization was instituted several years ago. The enormous success of the *H. influenzae* type B conjugate vaccine in preventing disease suggests that other vaccines against pneumococcus, meningococcus, and group B streptococcus should be developed using the same concept (i.e., polysaccharide–protein conjugation).

The available meningococcal vaccines are monovalent serogroup A or C, bivalent A/C, and quadrivalent A/C/Y/W-135. The monovalent A or C vaccines are recommended for use in epidemics caused by these two serotypes. The immunogenicity of these vaccines differs in various age groups. For example, monovalent serogroup A polysaccharide vaccine is highly immunogenic in children 3 months of age and older and is effective in preventing meningitis. In contrast, the serogroup C polysaccharide vaccine is immunogenic only in adults and children 2 years of age or older. The use of this vaccine in army recruits decreased the incidence of meningococcal meningitis by 90%. An outer membrane vesicle vaccine against group B meningococcus failed to protect 40% of those inoculated. Therefore, no highly effective vaccine against serogroup B is available.

Pneumococcal vaccine was first licensed in the United States in 1978 and was composed of 14 common capsular serotypes. It has now been reformulated to include 23 common serotypes. Despite this broader spectrum of serotypes, pneumococcal vaccine still does not prevent all pneumococcal infections, because many pneumococcal serotypes are not included and because insufficient responses to serotypes included in the vaccine occur, especially in very young and very old patients. The pneumococcal vaccine is recommended for individuals older than 2 years of age who are at increased risk of developing disseminated infection with *S. pneumoniae*. This targeted population includes those patients with functional asplenia (e.g., sickle cell disease) or traumatic asplenia, nephrotic syndrome, HIV infection, and other individuals with increased risk for serious pneumococcal infections. More immunogenic pneumococcal vaccines are currently being investigated in children younger than 2 years of age. A heptavalent polysaccharide–protein (i.e., toxoid, outer-membrane protein) conjugate vaccine has been shown to elicit a good antibody response in infants as young as 2 months of age, but further studies are needed to evaluate its effectiveness in reducing morbidity and mortality.

## REFERENCES

### Books

Schoenfeld, H., and Helwig, H. *Bacterial Meningitis.* Basel: Karger, 1992.

Yogev, R. *Meningitis.* In: Jenson, H. B., and Baltimore, R. S., eds. *Pediatric Infectious Diseases: Principles and Practice.* New York: Appleton & Lange, 1995:781–807.

### Review Articles

Connolly, K. J., and Hammer, S. M. The acute aseptic meningitis syndrome. *Infect. Dis. Clin. North Am.* 4: 599–622, 1990.

Greenlee, J. E. Anatomic considerations in central nervous system infections. In: Mandell, G. L., Douglas, R. G., and Bennett, J. E., eds. *Principles and Practice of Infectious Diseases.* 3rd ed. New York: Churchill Livingstone, 1990:732–741.

Gutman, L. T. Extrapulmonary tuberculosis. *Semin. in Pediatr. Infect. Dis.* 4:250–260, 1993.

Quagliarello, V. J., and Scheld, W. M. New perspectives on bacterial meningitis. *Clin. Infect. Dis.* 17:603–610, 1993.

Toltzis, P. Viral encephalitis. *Adv. Pediatr. Infect. Dis.* 6: 111–136, 1991.

Whitley, R. J., and Arvin, A. M. Herpes simplex virus infections. In: Remington, J. S., and Klein, J. O., eds. *Infectious Diseases of the Fetus and Newborn Infant.* Philadelphia: W. B. Saunders Co., 1995:354–376.

# 21

# COMMON ETIOLOGIC AGENTS OF BACTERIAL MENINGITIS

## MOSHE ARDITI, M.D. and RAM YOGEV, M.D.

During the last decade, advances in the understanding of the pathophysiology of bacterial meningitis and development of appropriate vaccines have provided opportunities to improve the outcome of this disease. Although bacterial meningitis can be caused by virtually any organism, *Streptococcus pneumoniae, Haemophilus influenzae* type b (Hib), and *Neisseria meningitidis* are by far the most common pathogens isolated. Until recently, *H. influenzae* type b was the most common cause of bacterial meningitis in children. However, the introduction of conjugate Hib vaccines had a dramatic impact on reducing the incidence of invasive Hib. Various predisposing host factors, such as age, race, immunodeficiency, and specific environmental situations, are discussed in Chapter 20. In this chapter we discuss the common bacteria causing meningitis, their virulence factors, the interactions between the host and the infecting organism, and the emergence of antibiotic resistance.

## STREPTOCOCCUS PNEUMONIAE

### Bacteriology

*Streptococcus pneumoniae* (the pneumococci) are encapsulated, gram-positive cocci that ap-

pear in pairs (diplococci). On occasion, organisms that have been exposed to antibiotics may appear gram-negative and be morphologically distorted. Capsules are critical for pathogenic effect; however, they cannot be seen in usual Gram's stain preparations. *S. pneumoniae* is a fastidious organism that requires a complex medium for isolation. The characteristics of the pneumococci are described in Chapter 11. The most important virulence factor of *S. pneumoniae* is the surface capsule, which is composed of a high-molecular-weight polysaccharide complex. The polysaccharide capsule is antigenic, and at present 84 pneumococcal serotypes have been identified. While certain serotypes are more prevalent in adults, others are more prevalent in children. Serotypes of interest, 14, 6, 18, 19, 23, 4, 9, 7, 1, and 3 cause most childhood pneumococcal infections. Of importance is that serotypes 6, 14, 19, and 23 are most frequently associated with resistance to penicillin.

### Epidemiology

Pneumococci are the most common cause of acute otitis media and sinusitis and are a frequent cause of pneumonia and meningitis in children. They are also now the most common cause of bacteremia in infants 1–24 months of age. The most recently reported prospective, multistate surveillance study of bacterial meningitis in the United States, conducted in 1986, showed that Hib was the most common etiologic agent overall (45%), followed by *S. pneumoniae* (18%) and *Neisseria meningitidis* (14%). However, since the recent introduction and widespread use of polysaccharide-protein conjugate Hib vaccines, Hib meningitis has dramatically decreased, making *Streptococcus pneumoniae* the leading cause of bacterial meningitis in children.

Pneumococci are ubiquitous; many persons carry these organisms in the upper respiratory tract without symptoms. Transmission is from person to person, presumably by respiratory droplet contact. Patients with increased risk for developing severe pneumococcal disease because of impaired immunologic response to *S. pneumoniae* include those with congenital or acquired immunodeficiency, Hodgkin's disease, nephrotic syndrome, sickle cell anemia, splenectomy, and organ transplantation. Pneumococcal infections are most prevalent when respiratory diseases are most common, usually during the winter months. Of the 84 known serotypes defined by the capsular polysaccharide, only 10 are commonly associated with meningitis. *S. pneumoniae* causes meningitis in all age groups, with a higher incidence in the very young and old. In patients older than 15 years of age it is the most common etiologic agent (30–50%). There are approximately 5000 cases of pneumococcal meningitis in adults each year in the United States. The disease is most commonly seen in elderly males, particularly African-Americans and Native Americans. The native Alaskan population has an extremely high incidence of pneumococcal meningitis.

Mortality from pneumococcal disease is highest in patients who have bacteremia or meningitis. Meningitis due to *S. pneumoniae* is associated with a higher case-fatality rate (19%) than is seen with *N. meningitidis* (13%) or *H. influenzae* (3%). The case-fatality rate for *S. pneumoniae* meningitis varies between age groups; it is 10–12% in children less than 5 years old, whereas in adults over age 60 years it is more than 30%.

## Pathogenesis and Pathophysiology

The polysaccharide capsule that is a component of each of the major meningeal pathogens (i.e., *S. pneumoniae*, *N. meningitidis*, and *H. influenzae*) inhibits phagocytosis by neutrophils, and also interferes with opsonizing activity of the alternate complement pathway. Anticapsular antibodies produce type-specific immunity to infection. When antibody binds to the capsule, C3b generated by the classic complement pathway attaches and the opsonized organisms are phagocytosed and killed.

The usual sequence of events in the development of bacterial meningitis caused by the three common bacterial agents starts with initial mucosal colonization, followed by bloodstream invasion, penetration of the blood-brain barrier (BBB), and multiplication of the bacteria within the cerebrospinal fluid (CSF) (Fig. 21–1). While the most frequent way for the bacteria to reach the meninges is through bacteremia, some bacteria can also reach the meninges by spread from contiguous infections such as mastoiditis or sinusitis, or by direct invasion through communication between the upper respiratory tract and the meninges. This communication may be congenital (e.g., an otic communication or a sinus tract) or the result of a skull fracture, especially if the fracture involves the paranasal sinuses. If the communication persists, recurrent episodes of meningitis may result. The incidence of acute bacterial meningitis after head injury ranges from 0.2–18%. If there is a continuous CSF leak, meningitis occurs in 3–50% of patients. *S. pneumoniae* accounts for more than half of these cases. A CSF leak is likely to be a more frequent predisposing factor for pneumococcal meningitis in adults. In children, acute otitis media is a common predisposing factor for pneumococcal meningitis. In this instance, the meningitis follows bacteremia rather than direct invasion through the mastoid.

Once infection is introduced into the CSF, bacteria multiply rapidly because of inadequate local defenses. The bacteria release toxins such as neuraminidase that contribute to its ability to invade the meninges by splitting membrane glycoprotein and glycolipids. Teichoic acid polymers of the pneumococcal cell wall are important in eliciting the inflammatory response in the CFS. It is the intense host inflammatory response provoked by the bacterial cell-wall components that account for many of the adverse effects observed in meningitis. The ability of certain bacteria to invade the CSF is due to several virulence factors that allow the bacteria to escape specific host defense mechanisms. Mucosal colonization is facilitated by IgA proteases that cleave

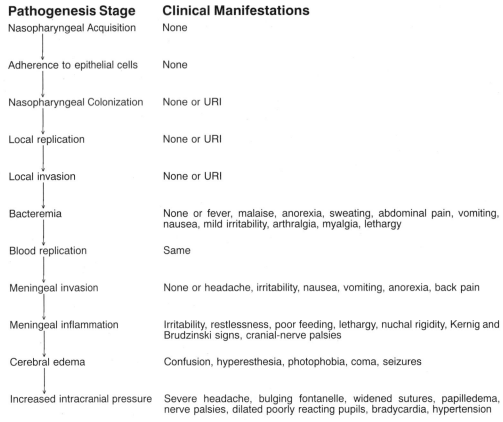

**Pathogenesis Stage**

Nasopharyngeal Acquisition

Adherence to epithelial cells

Nasopharyngeal Colonization

Local replication

Local invasion

Bacteremia

Blood replication

Meningeal invasion

Meningeal inflammation

Cerebral edema

Increased intracranial pressure

**Clinical Manifestations**

None

None

None or URI

None or URI

None or URI

None or fever, malaise, anorexia, sweating, abdominal pain, vomiting, nausea, mild irritability, arthralgia, myalgia, lethargy

Same

None or headache, irritability, nausea, vomiting, anorexia, back pain

Irritability, restlessness, poor feeding, lethargy, nuchal rigidity, Kernig and Brudzinski signs, cranial-nerve palsies

Confusion, hyperesthesia, photophobia, coma, seizures

Severe headache, bulging fontanelle, widened sutures, papilledema, nerve palsies, dilated poorly reacting pupils, bradycardia, hypertension

FIGURE 21–1. Sequential steps in the pathogenesis and clinical manifestations of bacterial meningitis.

the principal defensive immunoglobulin of the mucosal surfaces, the mucosal secretory IgA. The exact mechanism by which the bacteria move from the surface of the nasopharyngeal epithelial cells into the blood is unknown. One explanation may be an inflammatory response to a "trivial" viral infection. It was shown, in animal models, that with the increase in inflammatory cells in the nasopharynx following influenza virus infection other host protective mechanisms were adversely affected. This includes reduced bacterial killing due to a defect in phagosome-lysosome fusion, reduced macrophage function, and decreased neutrophil chemotaxis. Once bacteria invade the bloodstream, their survival is attributed to the polysaccharide capsule, which helps the bacteria evade the serum complement activity. The rate of bacterial growth in the blood is controlled by host defenses. In young children and nonimmune adults, serum bactericidal activity against *S. pneumoniae* (and other meningeal pathogens such a *H. influenzae*) is diminished because of the lack of specific antibodies against the bacteria polysaccharides or membrane proteins. In addition, animal experiments have shown that the reticuloendothelial system and the alternative complement pathway are very important components in the host defenses against *S. pneumoniae*. If these components are nonfunctional (e.g., because of splenectomy, sickle cell anemia, or C3 deficiency), both the incidence and the magnitude of bacteremia increase. If the primary bacteremia is of low magnitude ($10–10^3$ organisms/mL of blood), it is clinically represented only as low-grade fever with relative paucity of symptoms. This type of low-grade bacteremia is relatively common in children with otitis media or pneumonia. However, if the magnitude of bacteremia reaches greater than $10^3–10^4$ organisms/mL of blood, spread of infection to serous surfaces such as joints frequently occurs. If bacteremia continues unabated, then invasion of the CSF can occur. However, the precise mechanisms of bacterial invasion of the BBB, (i.e., activation of specific receptors by specific bacterial proteins that may exist on the brain microvessel endothelial cells, and/or specific topographic locations in the BBB) remain unknown. After bacteria invade the CSF by breaching the BBB, the lack of effective local humoral immunity in this closed space containing CSF allows for unrestricted bacterial replication. Early in the course of meningitis, changes take place in meningeal and cerebral capillaries. These microvessels, which constitute the BBB by virtue of their tight intercellular endothelial junctions, undergo morphologic changes such as opening of tight junctions, and become permeable to proteins. In experimental meningitis models, the bacterial titer in the CSF correlates with the subsequent increase in permeability in the BBB. The major physiologic consequence of altered vascular permeability is cerebral edema (vasogenic). Brain edema may also have cytotoxic (induced by inflammatory mediators in the CSF) and interstitial (impaired CSF absorption secondary to arachnoid villus dysfunction from blockage by leukocytes and fibrin) components.

Investigations in animal models of pneumococcal meningitis have shown that bacterial cell wall or its components (i.e., teichoic acid and peptidoglycan in *S. pneumoniae* and lipopolysaccharide [LPS] of *H. influenzae* and *N. meningitidis*) induce meningeal inflammation (Fig. 21–2). The inflammatory response is begun by local production and secretion of cytokines with the CSF, in particular interleukin-1 (IL-1), IL-6, and tumor necrosis factor (TNF). The action of these cytokines in the CSF results in activation of cerebral microvessel endothelial cells and induction of a complex cascade of adhesion molecules (glycoproteins) on the surface of the endothelium and of leukocytes. Subsequently, the interaction between activated leukocytes and endothelial cells leads to adherence and transmigration of leukocytes through the BBB endothelial cells into the CSF. Both experimental and human studies revealed that the rapid bactericidal activity of currently used antibiotics (especially beta-lactam agents) causes lysis of bacteria with release of proinflammatory cell fragments (e.g., *S. pneumoniae* cell-wall fragments and LPS fragments from gram-negative bacteria) into the CSF. Because of the closed subarachnoid space where the CSF circulates, this mechanism causes a brisk but transient increase in local cytokine production, which is associated with enhanced CSF inflammation and BBB disruption. This observation may explain why many patients treated for bacterial meningitis worsen clinically before they improve.

During meningitis, the subarachnoid space, which normally absorbs CSF, contains purulent material that may interfere with the normal flow of CSF, resulting in obstructive hydrocephalus. Since the subarachnoid space is transversed by vascular structures that bring blood to and from the brain, these vessels are

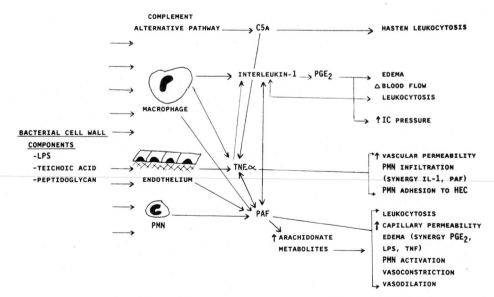

**FIGURE 21–2.** Hypothetical scheme for the generation in bacterial meningitis. HEC, human endothelial cell; $PGE_2$, prostaglandin $E_2$; IC, intracranial; PMN, polymorphonuclear cells; LPS, lipopolysaccharide; TNF, tumor necrosis factor; PAF, platelet activating factor.

frequently involved in the inflammatory process and areas of focal vasculitis can develop. Cortical venous thrombosis causes areas of hemorrhagic cortical infarction, and arteritis of major vessels leads to foci of ischemic cerebral infarction. In addition, venous obstruction resulting from purulent material in the veins can contribute to cerebral swelling. A vicious cycle then develops in which cerebral edema contributes to further venous obstruction and stasis, and phlebitis further accelerates cerebral swelling. Focal cerebral ischemia may lead to permanent neurologic impairment. The reduction in cerebral blood flow is also associated with regional hypoxemia and lactate production related to a shift to anaerobic glycolysis.

Local production of vasoactive mediators (oxygen radicals and nitrogen intermediates) is associated with the loss of cerebrovascular autoregulation. The resulting reduction in cerebral blood flow can impair oxygen and glucose delivery to the brain and result in neurologic sequelae.

Increased intracranial pressure (ICP) is a common acute phenomenon in bacterial meningitis. Increased ICP manifests itself as headache in adults, but the fontanelle bulges in about 60% of cases in infants with an open anterior fontanelle. Papilledema, a common finding of increased ICP in adults, is rarely found in children, but when present in an infant, other complications of meningitis, such as venous sinus thrombosis, brain abscess, or subdural empyema, should be ruled out. Several mechanisms may contribute to increased ICP: (1) the increased fluid leakage through the BBB affected by the cytokines; (2) abnormal patterns of cerebral blood flow due to loss of autoregulation; (3) hypoventilation (which occurs in some patients with meningitis) causing hypercarbia, which increases cerebral blood flow through its effect on cerebral vascular tone; (4) abnormal collection of subdural fluid or development of hydrocephalus; and (5) interstitial cerebral edema as a result of metabolic abnormalities in brain cells. Severely increased ICP can cause transtentorial herniation of the brain. This complication is relatively frequent in adult patients with meningitis, but is found in less than 5% of pediatric patients. When transtentorial herniation occurs, the patient's respiratory and hemodynamic patterns worsen, pupillary reaction to light becomes sluggish, and the patient responds only to noxious stimuli. The presence of these features defines patients with serious morbidity and higher mortality rate. It has been suggested that diagnostic lumbar puncture in patients whose cardiorespiratory system is unstable or who suffer from advanced symptoms of increased ICP can cause a sudden decrease in CSF pressure. In addition, the neck flexion required for performing a lumbar puncture may decrease cerebral venous return and increase cerebral blood flow. These effects may shift brain substance through the tentorium or the foramen magnum, causing herniation.

## Clinical Features of Meningitis

The clinical manifestations of *S. pneumoniae* meningitis are indistinguishable from those of meningitis due to other bacteria (see Chapter 20). A definitive diagnosis is made by examining the CFS. Gram's stain shows the typical gram-positive diplococci in 70–90% of untreated meningitis, and the latex agglutination test is positive for *S. pneumoniae* in approximately 79% of cases. However, it is important to note that, in contrast to *H. influenzae* in which previous treatment with antibiotics rarely affects the Gram's stain and culture results, such therapy may cause the Gram's stain to be negative and organisms difficult to culture in pneumococcal meningitis. In addition, certain strains of *S. pneumoniae* (types 6, 15, 29, and 35) have some immunologic cross-reactivity with *H. influenzae* type b, which may produce a positive result for *H. influenzae* type b instead of pneumococcus by latex agglutination. Other possible misinterpretations of Gram's-stained smears include mistaking pneumococci for *H. influenzae* because of bipolar gram-positive staining of the organism due to inadequate decolorizing, or mistaking *Listeria* for pneumococci. The acridine orange stain may be slightly more sensitive than Gram's stain for detecting bacteria in CSF specimens.

With the effective antimicrobial therapy currently available, most patients with *S. pneumoniae* meningitis survive, but they frequently have complications. All studies of bacterial meningitis support the conclusion that *S. pneumoniae* meningitis has the highest case-fatality rate for community-acquired meningitis. Mortality has been reported to be as high as 30–40%, although studies using active surveillance generally report mortality of 20% or lower. Almost 50% of patients who survive the infection have some hearing loss. Visual problems, paralysis, and mental or neurodevelopmental impairments occur.

## Emergence of Penicillin Resistance

Until recently, penicillin G was the drug of choice for the treatment of most pneumococcal infections. However, S. pneumoniae strains with resistance to penicillin G have been identified from many regions of the United States and elsewhere with increasing frequency in recent years. The most common penicillin-resistant pneumococcal strains are types 6, 9, 14, 19, and 23. Penicillin resistance is due to mutations and alterations in penicillin-binding proteins of the organism, resulting in a cell wall with lower affinity for penicillin. As summarized in Table 21–1, strains that are inhibited *in vitro* (i.e., minimal inhibitory concentration [MIC]) by less than $0.1 \mu g/mL$ of penicillin are considered susceptible, strains with an MIC of $0.1–1 \mu g/mL$ are defined as having intermediate or relative resistance, and strains with an MIC greater than $1 \mu g/mL$ are resistant. In recent years the frequency of penicillin-resistant isolates has ranged from almost 0 to 33% in various regions of the country. The highest frequencies of penicillin-resistant pneumococcal isolates were reported from Houston, Dallas, and San Diego. Even more concerning are the recent reports of emergence of resistance to the extended-spectrum cephalosporins (such as ceftriaxone and cefotaxime) with clinical failure in the treatment of pneumococcal meningitis. As a result, the National Committee for Clinical Laboratory Standards (NCCLS) recently amended the definition of resistance to ceftriaxone, cefotaxime, and other cephalosporins. Strains with an MIC of $0.25 \mu g/mL$ or more for these agents are defined as susceptible, those with an MIC of $0.5–1 \mu g/mL$ are regarded as moderately susceptible, and organisms with a MIC of $2.0 \mu g/mL$ or more are defined as resistant. At present, these definitions apply only to meningeal isolates of S. pneumoniae. Unfortunately, penicillin-resistant pneumococci, particularly highly resistant strains, are often also resistant to non–beta-lactam antibiotics such as erythromycin, tetracycline, and trimethoprim-sulfamethoxazole.

From the previous discussion it is obvious that penicillin and ampicillin are likely to be ineffective for treatment of meningitis caused by penicillin-resistant pneumococci. Resistance to the extended-spectrum cephalosporins (ceftriaxone and cefotaxime), which are widely used to treat meningitis, have been associated recently with treatment failures in children with pneumococcal meningitis. Such treatment failures suggest that the initial empiric treatment of these infections of meningitis may need to be altered after considering local patterns of resistance. The increasing resistance of S. pneumoniae to commonly used antimicrobial agents is a cause for great concern, and there is a strong likelihood that the already high morbidity and mortality associated with S. pneumoniae meningitis will increase if multi–drug-resistant infection becomes more widespread.

## Immunity and Vaccine

A 23-valent pneumococcal vaccine is composed of purified capsular polysaccharide antigens of 23 pneumococcal serotypes, and is available for the prevention of invasive pneumococcal infection. This vaccine includes the most common serotypes of S. pneumoniae that cause infections in humans. In addition, the vaccine also includes those strains most commonly associated with antimicrobial resistance. Unfortunately, the vaccine is ineffective in children younger than 2 years of age. Although greater use of pneumococcal polysaccharide vaccine may reduce the incidence of resistant pneumococcal disease in adults and older children, newer pneumococcal conjugate vaccines should have a much more substantial impact on the problem of pneumococcal resistance in all age groups. Linking a polysaccharide covalently to a protein carrier allows the polysaccharide to be processed as a T-cell–dependent antigen, greatly increasing its immunogenicity in young children and enabling booster (memory) responses in all age groups. A polysaccharide–protein conjugate vaccine against *Haemophilus influenzae* type b has dramatically reduced infections with this bacteria in immunized children. This remarkable experience has encouraged a major effort to prevent pneumococcal disease using similar technology. Several pneumococcal conjugate vaccines are being tested currently for efficacy in children younger than 2 years of age.

## TABLE 21–1.  *STREPTOCOCCUS PNEUMONIAE*, PENICILLIN SUSCEPTIBILITY

|  | MIC FOR PENICILLIN |
|---|---|
| Susceptible | $<0.1 \mu g/mL$ |
| Relatively resistant | $0.1–1.0 \mu g/mL$ |
| Resistant | $>1 \mu g/mL$ |

## NEISSERIA MENINGITIDIS

Epidemic cerebrospinal meningitis was first described in 1805, and since then meningococcal meningitis has continued to be a cause of endemic and epidemic disease worldwide, with a propensity for afflicting young children and military recruits. *Neisseria meningitidis* also may produce fulminating sepsis and death within a very short time. The rapid onset of the disease, its often fulminant course, and its high mortality evoke anxiety among both laymen and physicians.

### Morphology

*Neisseria meningitidis* is a nonmotile, non–spore-forming, gram-negative coccus that typically appears in pairs with the opposing sides flattened or indented, giving them the appearance of ''kidney bean'' diplococci. Other gram-negative cocci include bacteria from the genera *Moraxella* and *Veillonella*. On suitable solid media, *N. meningitidis* isolates from blood or cerebrospinal fluid form transparent or semilucent, nonpigmented, nonhemolytic colonies approximately 1–5 mm in diameter. In contrast, organisms isolated from the nasopharynx of healthy individuals often grow as opaque colonies. Colonies are convex and, if large amounts of polysaccharide are present, appear mucoid rather than smooth.

### Growth

Many *Neisseria* strains are considered fastidious and require the use of appropriate media and conditions. The *Neisseria* are aerobic and prefer a humid environment at a temperature of 37°C for optimal growth; isolation and growth are enhanced by a concentration of 5–10% $CO_2$. Some *Neisseria* species such as *N. meningitidis* and *N. gonorrhoeae* require a specially treated medium to improve their growth. Heavy metals, fatty acids, and other heat-labile components are some of the growth inhibitors that should be eliminated. Therefore, most clinical laboratories prepare chocolate agar plates by heating sheep blood in molten agar at 80°–90°C for the isolation and propagation of the sensitive *Neisseria* strains. Another medium (devised by Mueller and Hinton) is particularly good as a basic culture medium for cultivating *N. meningitidis*. The genus *Neisseria* includes six important species: *N. gonorrhoeae, N. meningitidis, N. flavescens, N. subflava, N. mucosa,* and *N. sicca*. They are distinguished by a series of biochemical tests. *N. meningitidis* ferments glucose and

### TABLE 21–2. SUGAR FERMENTATION BY *NEISSERIA* SPECIES

| SPECIES | SUGAR | | |
| --- | --- | --- | --- |
| | Glucose | Maltose | Sucrose |
| *Neisseria gonorrhoeae* | + | − | − |
| *N. meningitidis* | + | + | − |
| *N. sicca* | + | + | + |
| *N. flavescens* | − | − | − |
| *N. mucosa* | + | + | + |
| *N. subflava* | + | + | ± |

maltose, whereas *N. gonorrhoeae* ferments only glucose (Table 21–2). *N. meningitidis* also produces catalase and indophenol oxidase. To perform the oxidase test, colonies are flooded with a solution of dimethyl- or tetramethyl-paraphenylenediamine, and if they turn pink or dark blue (depending on which reagent is employed), the test is positive. A positive oxidase test is often cited as useful for identifying *N. meningitidis;* however, nonpathogenic *Neisseria* also may give a positive test result. Thus, the identification of *N. meningitidis* from nasopharyngeal cultures should not rely on the results of the catalase test alone.

### Antigenic Structure

The cell wall of *N. meningitidis* is typical of gram-negative bacteria; it contains a peptidoglycan backbone and LPS (endotoxin) complexed with protein in the outer membrane (Fig. 21–3). The organism produces a polysaccharide capsule which is the basis of the serogroup typing system. There are 16 different polysaccharide groups, the most important 9 of which are listed in Table 21–3. Capsules of *N. meningitidis* strains can be identified by the quelling reaction in the presence of appropriate serogroup antibody. Almost all isolates from invasive disease can be grouped based on the capsular polysaccharide, with the most important groups being A, B, C, W-135, and Y. Group A strains historically have been responsible for worldwide epidemic outbreaks involving large numbers of individuals and occurring cyclically. Therefore, group A *N. meningitidis* has traditionally been considered to be the epidemic type. In contrast, groups B and C *N. meningitidis* tended to cause sporadic cases or limited outbreaks of meningococcal disease. Thus, group B and C strains were considered to be the endemic serotypes. However, a progressive shift in the relative importance of these serotypes and other serotypes has occurred since the early

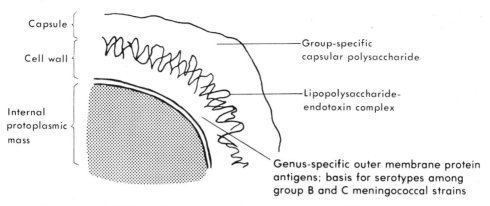

**FIGURE 21–3.** Major antigenic and virulence determinants of *Neisseria meningitidis.*

1960s. Group B strains increasingly have been the cause of the majority of community-acquired cases of meningococcal disease, and new groups have been reported more often. Since 1980, group W-135 has been the second most frequent strain causing invasive disease. In addition, the spectrum of *N. meningitidis* infections has changed. The W-135 strains appear to have a propensity for causing bacteremia, whereas serogroup Y frequently induces pulmonary infections.

In addition to the group-specific polysaccharide antigens, subgrouping is possible within groups B and C meningococci based on differences in outer membrane proteins (OMP). Group B can be subgrouped to at least 12 different serotypes on this basis. Interestingly, serotype 2 is the most frequently isolated (>50% of serogroup B) and is also an antigenic determinant in group C strains. The importance of the subgrouping based on OMP pattern relates to epidemiologic studies and vaccine development. Another principal outer membrane antigen is the lipooligosac-

charide (LOS), which is analogous to LPS, of enteric gram-negative bacilli. The LOS is serologically diverse, with at least 12 different serotypes. Again, this diversity of LOS can be used as an epidemiologic tool to show that various isolates are related or nonrelated.

## Pathogenesis and Immunity

The meningococcus is an exclusively human parasite. It can exist as an apparently harmless member of the normal flora of the nasopharynx or it can produce acute disease. Carrier rates of *N. meningitidis* in the upper respiratory tract are usually 5–15% in healthy adults and children. Higher colonization rates can be found in closed populations such as in military recruit camps or boarding schools. A close relationship has been noted between the carrier rate in a population and the onset and decline of an epidemic. It has been suggested that when the carrier rate exceeds 20% in a community, the danger of an epidemic (due to the predominant serotype) increases. Recent studies have indicated that pili, which have been demonstrated on the surface of many meningococci, provide a means for meningococci to attach selectively to nonciliated human pharyngeal mucosal cells. Although the organisms appear to attach selectively to the nonciliated columnar epithelium, they also cause damage to the ciliated cells, possibly by direct action of meningococcal LOS. *N. meningitidis* preferentially colonizes the nasopharyngeal region of the upper respiratory tract, rather than the oropharynx. Although the nasopharynx provides a significantly more humid environment with a higher $CO_2$ content than the oropharynx, a more likely explanation for this preferential colonization seems to be the presence of a higher density

### TABLE 21–3.  CAPSULAR POLYSACCHARIDES OF *NEISSERIA MENINGITIDIS* GROUPS*

| Group | Capsular Polysaccharide |
|-------|-------------------------|
| A | O-Acetylated 2-acetamido-deoxy-D-mannose-6-phosphate |
| B | Alpha-2,8,N-Acetylneuraminic acid |
| C | Alpha-2,9,O-Acetylneuraminic acid |
| L | N-Acetylglucosamine phosphate |
| W-135 | Alternating sequence of D-galactose and N-acetylneuraminic acid |
| X | D-Glucose-4-phosphate |
| Y | O-Acetylated alternating sequence of D-glucose and N-acetylneuraminic acid |

*Partial list.

of specific receptors for *N. meningitidis* pili on nasopharyngeal epithelial cells. The preference of *N. meningitidis* to attach to the nasopharynx has a practical diagnostic application; cultures of the nasopharynx are the best way to determine if a person is a carrier of *N. meningitidis*. Carriers can be divided into three groups: chronic (constantly colonized for up to 2 years), intermittent, and transient. Coincidental viral infection may affect acquisition of meningococcal nasopharyngeal carriage. Household contacts of a patient with *N. meningitidis* infection who have a recent history or symptoms of upper respiratory infection have significantly higher carriage rates compared with household members without such symptoms. Many studies suggest that the vast majority of people exposed to a pathogenic strain of *N. meningitidis* become carriers rather than develop active infection.

It is possible that viral infection may initiate invasive meningococcal disease. This was suggested because both diseases have peak incidence in the winter, and patients with invasive meningococcal disease statistically more often are found to have serologic evidence of viral infection (such as influenza). Once the attached bacteria start to invade, the organisms penetrate the epithelial cells and enter the subepithelial spaces and adjacent lymphoid tissue, subsequently reaching the systemic circulation. A possible mechanism for the survival of *N. meningitidis* is induction of secretory IgA production. Group C polysaccharide induces secretory IgA antibody, which blocks the bacteriolytic effect of IgG or IgM antibodies plus complement. Such a mechanism enables the bacteria to reside in the nasopharynx or to initiate penetration without being eradicated. In addition, many meningococcal strains produce IgA1 protease, which degrades mucosal IgA and facilitates access of the bacteria to the vascular system. Although the circumstances that determine whether an individual remains a carrier or progresses to invasive disease are not known, the capsular polysaccharide of *N. meningitidis* is an important virulence factor that helps the bacteria to invade the blood and survive by inhibiting complement activation, thus making the bacteria more resistant to opsonization and phagocytosis.

Protective antibodies are usually acquired as a result of carriage, subclinical, or overt infection. However, natural immunization may not require infection or colonization with each serogroup or even with *N. meningitidis*.

Antibodies may be produced in response to cross-reacting antigens of other *Neisseria* species and even of other nonrelated bacteria that carry cross-reactive antigens. Susceptibility or resistance to clinical meningococcal disease is determined by the absence or presence of serum bactericidal, that is, bacteriolytic activity. This killing effect is mediated by specific IgG or IgM antibodies in concert with the terminal components (C5–C9) of the complement system. These circulating bactericidal antibodies appear to prevent multiplication and dissemination to other tissues (particularly the central nervous system) of *N. meningitidis* that have invaded the bloodstream. The importance of the complement system in protection against *N. meningitidis* is evident from the striking association of recurrent meningococcemia in patients with congenital deficiency of a terminal complement components. Circulating group-specific opsonic and bactericidal antibody are present in the serum of many adults. This explains why the peak incidence of serious *N. meningitidis* infections (like that of *H. influenzae* infections) is between 6 months and 2 years of age, which corresponds to the time between loss of transplacental antibodies and the appearance of naturally acquired antibodies. Infections later in life appear in populations in which many people carry a virulent strain and are in close contact with susceptible individuals who lack specific antibodies.

Group C and group A capsular polysaccharides induce specific antibodies of either IgG or IgM class. These antibodies have a bactericidal effect in two ways. First, IgG and perhaps IgM act as opsonic antibody to augment phagocytosis and subsequent killing by polymorphonuclear neutrophils. Second, following binding of IgG or IgM antibodies to *N. meningitidis* capsular antigen, activation of the complement cascade via the classic pathway causes a point injury of the bacterial cell wall and membrane.

Group B capsular polysaccharide is relatively nonimmunogenic. Data suggest that humans are immunologically unresponsive, or "tolerant," to group B meningococcal polysaccharide because of its extraordinary similarity to host autologous tissue constituents (e.g., neuraminic acid residues of mammalian cell membranes and polysialosyl glycoproteins of nervous tissue). Even after full recovery from group B *N. meningitidis* infection, only low titers of IgM antibodies can be found. These antibodies have low binding affinity and only modest bacteriolytic activity against the offending bacteria.

Currently, a tetravalent vaccine is available that contains the groups A, C, Y, and W-135 polysaccharides. This vaccine is less immunogenic in infants and young children. There is no vaccine against group B. New vaccines, OMPs or LPSs from various meningococcal serotypes, are under intense investigation. Conjugates of LPS and OMP are also being investigated with promising results.

A significant portion of the meningococcal cell wall consists of lipopolysaccharide or endotoxin complex (see Fig. 21–3). During the growth phase of *N. meningitidis* or with its death, endotoxin is released into the extracellular environment. Group C meningococci, more than other serotypes, release capsular polysaccharide and endotoxin into the extracellular environment during growth. Therefore, detection and quantitation of capsular polysaccharide or endotoxin in blood or cerebrospinal fluid can be useful in assessing the severity of infection in an individual patient. Such information can be of considerable diagnostic and prognostic importance. Multiple *in vitro* and *in vivo* studies show that endotoxin is directly responsible for the fulminant course of *N. meningitidis* sepsis and its high mortality rate. Endotoxin derived from *N. meningitidis* has been used extensively in studies of tissue injury caused by gramnegative bacillary endotoxins. Many of the pathophysiologic and immunohistopathologic changes observed in patients who develop meningococcal sepsis and shock are elicited by endotoxin, which in turn induces host inflammatory mediators. These events include: (1) activation of the clotting system with extensive deposits of fibrin in glomerular arterioles and small vessels of other tissues; (2) hemorrhage of the adrenal glands (Waterhouse-Friderichsen syndrome) and hemorrhagic necrosis of other organs; and (3) altered peripheral vascular resistance, circulatory failure, and death.

## Epidemiology

Infection due to *N. meningitidis* remains an important worldwide health problem. It has been estimated that almost 300,000 cases of meningococcal disease occur in the world every year and that more than 30,000 are fatal. Relatively more cases are reported in children and adolescents (up to age 19) during an epidemic than during nonepidemic circumstances. Therefore, careful surveillance of age distribution patterns may be valuable in recognizing an epidemic early. Currently, serogroups B and C are the most common agents causing meningococcol disease in the United States. The remainder are primarily serogroup Y and serogroup W-135. Meningococcal infections occur primarily as isolated cases, sporadic small epidemics, or closedpopulation outbreaks (such as military recruits). However, group A strains have the potential to cause widespread epidemics, which have appeared in 8- to 12-year cycles. Between the peaks of the cycle, group A meningococci almost disappear and cause only 1–2% of reported cases. It has been more than 40 years since an epidemic due to group A *N. meningitidis* occurred in the United States, but serious epidemics with this serogroup have occurred in Brazil and South Africa in recent years.

The fatality rate varies depending upon the prevalence of disease, the nature of the infection, and socioeconomic conditions. In industrialized countries during endemic periods, the fatality rate can be as low as 7% for meningitis and exceed 19% for meningococcemia without meningeal involvement. However, during epidemics, mortality from meningitis is 2–10% and death rates from meningococcemia can be as high as 70%, particularly in developing countries.

Asymptomatic colonization of the upper respiratory tract is frequent and provides the focus from which the organism is spread. Transmission is from person to person through droplets of respiratory tract secretions. As discussed above, colonization of the upper respiratory tract of a new host is an immunizing process, and circulating bactericidal and hemagglutinating antibodies are generally detectable within 7–10 days. From a variety of studies it is clear that only a brief period of colonization by *N. meningitidis* is needed before invasive disease occurs. The incubation period is 1–10 days, most commonly less than 4 days. Disease occurs most often in children younger than 5 years of age; the peak attack rate occurs in the 3- to 5-month age group.

## Clinical Aspects of Meningococcal Disease

The clinical manifestations of *N. meningitidis* infection range from transient bacteremia to fulminant sepsis with death within hours. A few patients may present with an upper respiratory illness or viral-like exanthem and recover without specific antimicrobial therapy;

only later are blood cultures reported positive for *N. meningitidis*. The most frequent disease due to *N. meningitidis* is meningococcemia, which may follow a fulminant course with rapid progression to septic shock (Waterhouse-Friderichsen syndrome) or a much slower course producing meningitis. Some patients present with features of both sepsis and meningitis. In most series, the peak incidence of invasive disease occurs in the late winter and early spring. The disease has been reported in all age groups, but the majority of cases occur in infants younger than 2 years of age.

The patient with sepsis usually presents with skin rash, malaise, weakness, headache, and hypotension on admission or shortly thereafter. The patient with meningitis presents with fever, headache, meningeal signs, and mental status varying from fully alert to comatose. Variations of these manifestations can occur, and patients can progress from one syndrome to the other during the course of the disease. Because of the wide range of clinical expression of *N. meningitidis* infection, a high index of suspicion and a careful search for clues of disease are required for early diagnosis. Erroneous diagnosis and inappropriate therapy can have fatal consequences.

Meningococcal sepsis is commonly accompanied by cutaneous lesions of a petechial or purpuric nature (Fig. 21–4). The rash initially may be urticarial, maculopapular, or petechial. Occasionally, if the patient is not completely undressed when examined, these important lesions can be missed. Purpura, which is separate and distinct, is a feature of fulminating disease and does not arise from the petechiae seen in milder cases. The petechial rash is manifested as discrete lesions 1–2 mm in diameter on the extremities and trunk. The wrist and forearm are frequently involved as well as the lower leg and ankles. The petechiae may spare the palmar and plantar surfaces. They are commonly seen in clusters under areas where pressure has been applied to the skin by the elastic in underwear or stockings. These petechial lesions can coalesce to form larger lesions that appear ecchymotic. The petechiae correlate with the degree of thrombocytopenia present, and they are important as a clinical indicator of the severity of disease and of development of disseminated intravascular coagulation (DIC). It is important to follow the progression of petechial lesions, both to monitor the effectiveness of therapy and to assess whether additional therapies become necessary. A simple way of accomplishing this is to circle areas of petechiae and to document the number of petechial lesions and time of the count on a flow sheet. Counts within each circle should be performed periodically until the patient's condition stabilizes.

Several other diseases may produce skin lesions resembling the petechiae of *N. meningitidis* septicemia. These diseases include Rocky Mountain spotted fever, rubella, rubeola, sec-

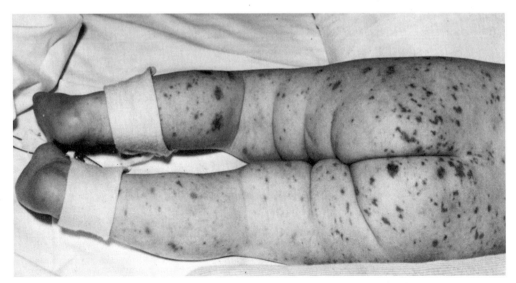

**FIGURE 21–4.** Representative cutaneous eruption of acute meningococcemia in a young child with meningococcal meningitis. (From Bell, W. E., and McCormick, W. F. *Neurologic Infections in Children.* 2nd ed. Philadelphia: W. B. Saunders Co., 1981. With permission.)

ondary syphilis, bacterial endocarditis, and cutaneous eruptions associated with drug allergies. Moreover, in infants and children, *Haemophilus influenzae* type b or, very rarely, pneumococcal sepsis can also present with similar clinical manifestations of petechial or purpuric skin lesions, DIC, and shock. Therefore, the therapeutic approach to pediatric patients with this syndrome must include antimicrobial therapy effective against *N. meningitidis*, *H. influenzae*, and *S. pneumoniae*. To facilitate identification of the etiologic agent, a urine sample should be tested by the latex agglutination technique for specific bacterial antigens (see Fig. 21–5). In addition, a representative skin lesion can be incised under sterile conditions, and two or three drops of tissue fluid expressed for Gram's stain and culture. The presence of polymorphonuclear neutrophils with gram-negative cocci or diplococci within or outside of these phagocytic cells is highly suggestive (even pathognomonic) of *N. meningitidis* infection. Although rarely performed, culture of the fluid from the incised lesion is best done by placing one or two drops directly onto chocolate agar at the bedside. Isolation of *N. meningitidis* from skin lesion or blood provides a definitive diagnosis of meningococcemia.

The shock state that frequently develops in patients with meningococcemic sepsis dominates the clinical picture and is an ominous prognostic sign. These patients are poorly responsive, showing both peripheral vasoconstriction and cyanotic, poorly perfused extremities. There is evidence of acidosis, hypoxia, and DIC. Clinical evidence of DIC includes increased numbers of petechiae within circumscribed areas, gastric or gingival bleeding, or oozing at the sites of venipuncture or intravenous infusions. Myocardial failure as evidenced by congestive heart failure and pulmonary edema may occur, and histologic evidence of myocarditis is present in more than 50% of patients who die of meningococcal disease.

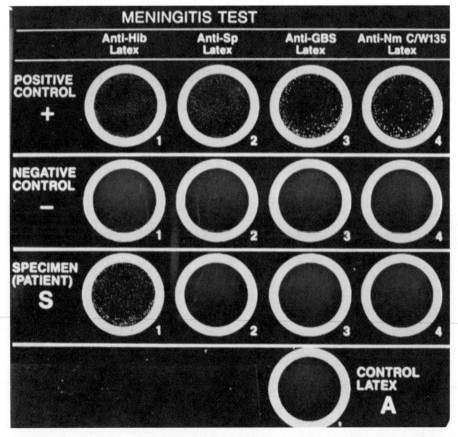

**FIGURE 21–5.** Results of latex agglutination test of CSF from a child with *Haemophilus influenzae* type b meningitis. Note the positive agglutination in the left-hand well in the third (patient specimen) row.

The clinical manifestations of meningococcal meningitis are indistinguishable from those of acute meningitis caused by *H. influenzae* type b or *S. pneumoniae*. These manifestations are discussed in Chapter 20.

Meningococcal pneumonia has been reported in as many as 10–20% of patients with meningococcemia or meningitis. However, primary meningococcal pneumonia, once considered a rare disease, is now recognized as one of the more common forms of meningococcal disease in military recruits, and it has been reported to cause 4.5% of all bacterial pneumonias in a general hospital population. Pulmonary infection is probably disseminated via air-borne droplets. Thus, respiratory isolation of patients with pneumonia is indicated. Most primary meningococcal pneumonia is caused by serogroup Y, whereas groups B and C are mostly involved in pneumonia associated with meningitis or septicemia. Usually, the onset of primary *N. meningitidis* pneumonia is gradual and the clinical symptoms do not differ from those of other pneumonias. The chest x-ray examination generally shows lung consolidation with patchy alveolar infiltrates. Establishing the diagnosis is difficult. Because nasopharyngeal carriage of meningococci is common, isolation of the bacteria from the sputum does not establish the diagnosis. Pleural effusion culture and blood culture yielding *N. meningitidis* are accepted confirmatory diagnostic tests.

Chronic meningococcemia is defined as persistent meningococcal bacteremia associated with low-grade fever, chills, rash, arthralgia, and headache but without clinical evidence of sepsis. The reported mean duration of illness is 6–8 weeks. Symptoms tend to be intermittent; the rash often appears in association with fever and then disappears. Bacteremia and arthralgias also tend to be intermittent. The pathophysiology of chronic meningococcemia is not well understood, but a defect in host immunity that allows the bacteria to survive, rather than a change in bacterial virulence, seems to be a reasonable explanation. Interestingly, the skin changes suggest a hypersensitive reaction secondary to antigen–antibody complexes.

### Other Diseases and Complications

Infections of the genitourinary tract with *N. meningitidis* have been reported. These infections include proctitis, urethritis, vaginitis, and cervicitis. That some infected patients have pharyngeal colonization with the same strain suggests that sexual habits may be related to the genitourinary infections.

Approximately 50 cases of primary meningococcal conjunctivitis have been reported, most in children. Meningitis, corneal ulceration, and corneal opacity are the most frequent complications.

Serous membranes are sometimes involved in *N. meningitidis* disease, leading to pleuritis, pericarditis, peritonitis, or arthritis. Aspiration of the affected area often reveals predominance of mononuclear cells, and Gram's stain and culture are negative. These findings suggest an immune-complex–mediated hypersensitivity phenomenon that usually occurs when the patient with invasive meningococcal disease is otherwise improving.

## HAEMOPHILUS INFLUENZAE

### Morphology

*Haemophilus influenzae* is a small, nonmotile, non–spore-forming, gram-negative, pleomorphic bacterium (rod). Many other bacteria also have a gram-negative pleomorphic appearance on Gram's stain. A partial list of these bacteria is given in Table 21–4.

### Growth

*Haemophilus influenzae* belongs to the genus Haemophilus (from the Greek: *haima* = blood, *philein* = to love). Members of this genus require enriched media for growth, and most must have available either one or both of two growth factors, referred to as X and V. X factor has been identified as hemin (or related protoporphyrins), and V factor is found to be replaceable by nicotinamide adenine dinucleotide ($NAD^+$) or nicotinamide adenine dinucleotide phosphate (NADP). Table 21–5 lists the members of this genus, their requirements for X and V factors, their capacity to lose red blood cells, and their increased $CO_2$ requirement. A biotyping system

### TABLE 21–4. PARTIAL LIST OF GRAM-NEGATIVE COCCOBACILLI

*Actinobacillus actinomycetemcomitans*
*Bordetella pertussis*
*Brucella melitensis*
*Cardiobacterium hominis*
*Eikenella corrodens*
*Francisella tularensis* (also called *Pasteurella tularensis*)
*Haemophilus* species
*Campylobacter fetus*
*Streptobacillus moniliformis*

**TABLE 21–5. DIFFERENTIAL GROWTH CHARACTERISTICS OF THE *HAEMOPHILUS* GROUP**

| SPECIES | GROWTH FACTORS | | HEMOLYSIS |
|---|---|---|---|
| | X | V | |
| *Haemophilus influenzae* | + | + | − |
| *H. parainfluenzae* | − | + | − |
| *H. aegyptius* | + | + | − |
| *H. ducreyi* | + | − | + |
| *H. suis* | + | + | − |
| *H. Haemolyticus* | + | + | + |
| *H. parahaemolyticus* | − | + | + |
| *H. aphrophilus* | + | − | − |

**TABLE 21–6. THE CARBOHYDRATE COMPONENTS OF *HAEMOPHILUS INFLUENZAE* CAPSULES**

| SEROTYPE | CARBOHYDRATE |
|---|---|
| a | Glucose |
| b | Ribose, ribitol |
| c | Galactose |
| d | Hexose |
| e | Hexosamine |
| f | Galactosamine |

is also very helpful in epidemiologic studies. For example, Brazilian purpuric fever (BPF), a life-threatening infection that presents as an acute febrile illness in children 3 months to 10 years of age with abdominal pain or vomiting and hemorrhagic skin lesions, was recognized during 1984 in the state of São Paulo, Brazil. Epidemiologic investigations could not identify a pathogen, but a history of conjunctivitis in the 30 days preceding the fever was identified as a common denominator in all 10 children who died of BPF. When conjunctival cultures from children with acute febrile illnesses became positive for *H. influenzae* biotype III (*aegyptius*) this agent was identified as the cause of BPF. Further investigation confirmed that this "new" disease arose probably from a single clone of *H. influenzae* biogroup *aegyptius* with unique invasive potential. Other epidemiologic studies found that most cases of *H. influenzae* meningitis are caused by biotype I, which is rarely isolated from the respiratory system of well children.

### Antigenic Structure

*H. influenzae* strains can be encapsulated or nonencapsulated. The major antigenic capsular component of encapsulated strains is a polysaccharide. Six distinct antigenic types have been identified and are labeled a–f (Table 21–6). Serologic tests such as precipitation, agglutination, or quelling (capsular swelling) can be used to differentiate the various serotypes. The most common test used clinically is latex agglutination (Fig. 21–5). Virulence appears to be related to the specific antigenic component. For example, *H. influenzae* type b, by far the most frequent cause of serious infection in humans (e.g., meningitis, arthritis) as compared to other antigenic types, which are more commonly found in the nasopharynx of children and cause otitis media and sinusitis.

Protection against *H. influenzae* type b develops slowly during infancy and is mediated by anticapsular antibody (see below). In most cases the formation of these natural antibodies is due to cross-reacting polysaccharides from other bacteria. For example, type b cross-reacts with *S. pneumoniae* types 6, 15, 29, and 35 as well as with antigens found in *Staphylococcus aureus*, *Bacillus subtilis*, and some strains of *Escherichia coli*. The antigen in *E. coli* that cross-reacts with the *H. influenzae* polyribose phosphate capsule is a surface-stable, acidic capsular polysaccharide that is part of the *E. coli* K antigen.

### Epidemiology

Before the availability of effective vaccines, *Haemophilus influenzae* type b was the most common cause of bacterial meningitis and invasive infections in infants and children in the United States. It was estimated that 12,000 cases of meningitis per year were caused by this bacteria with an additional 10,000 cases of other invasive diseases, such as epiglottitis, septic arthritis, and pneumonia. Widespread vaccination of infants with the Hib conjugate vaccine has dramatically reduced the incidence of Hib disease in the United States.

*H. influenzae* is a normal inhabitant of the upper respiratory tract of humans. Sixty to 90% of children of various ages carry unencapsulated *H. influenzae* in the nose or throat, but only 5% of them are colonized with type b. Even lower percentages are now reported since the introduction of conjugate vaccination. As with meningitis caused by *N. meningitidis*, *H. influenzae* type b meningitis is primarily a disease of pharyngeal carriers. The mode of transmission is presumably person to person, by direct contact, or through inhalation of droplets of respiratory tract secretions containing the organisms.

As with other respiratory pathogens, family size and living conditions may also affect risk. Secondary cases of meningitis are more common in household contacts of primary meningitis cases than in the general population. The incidence of Hib disease has been higher in certain groups, including Native Alaskans and some Native Americans, infants and young children who attend day-care centers, African-Americans, Hispanics, and patients with immunodeficiencies. The disease was most common in children 3 months to 3 years of age, with peak incidence for meningitis between 6 and 12 months of age, and for epiglottitis in children older than 2 years. Most cases of *H. influenzae* septic arthritis, cellulitis, and pneumonia also occurred in infants younger than 2 years old. The reasons for this age difference are not clear.

## Pathogenesis

The sequential steps in the pathogenesis and pathophysiology of *H. influenzae* meningitis are similar to those described for pneumococcal or meningococcal meningitis (Fig. 21–1). The exact mechanism by which *H. influenzae* moves from the surface of the nasopharyngeal epithelial cells into the blood is unknown. Probable mechanisms are similar to those utilized by *S. pneumoniae*. For example, studies in infant rats showed that preinoculation of the nose with virus increased nasal colonization with *H. influenzae* and led to a higher rate of bacteremia.

In patients with nontypable (nonencapsulated) *H. influenzae,* the bacteria may spread locally to the sinuses, middle ear, bronchi, or lung, probably following a viral infection or when other underlying conditions that modify the host defense mechanisms exist. Although *H. influenzae* is one of the most common causes of suppurative otitis media in children (about 20% of all cases), most *H. influenzae* strains isolated from this condition are nontypable, with *H. influenzae* type b responsible for only 5–10% of otitis media caused by *H. influenzae.*

Bloodstream invasion by encapsulated *H. influenzae* type b is associated with more serious diseases. The bacteria multiply in the blood rapidly, reaching levels of $10^3$–$10^5$ organisms/mL of blood within 12–48 h. The rate of bacterial growth is controlled by the host defenses, as previously discussed for *S. pneumoniae.* If the magnitude of bacteremia reaches $10^3$–$10^4$ organisms/mL of blood, spread of infection to serous surfaces (e.g.,

meninges, pericardium, joints) or other tissues (e.g., skin and bone) frequently occurs.

## Meningitis

One of the most frequent manifestations of bacteremic spread of *H. influenzae* is meningitis. The factors that lead to meningeal localization of *H. influenzae* are not completely clear. One possibility is that the polysaccharide capsule of *H. influenzae* type b possesses unique neurotropism. This is suggested by the observation that only certain capsular types of *S. pneumoniae, N. meningitidis, H. influenzae,* and *E. coli* cause meningitis. These observations also suggest the presence of specialized receptors on endothelial cells lining the blood vessels supplying the brain.

The specific pathophysiologic changes leading to cerebral dysfunction and damage during bacterial meningitis are probably induced both by bacterial products and by the host inflammatory response, as described previously for pneumococcal meningitis, and are generally well underway by the time a clinical diagnosis of meningitis can be made. *H. influenzae* LPS is probably the first molecule to be recognized by the host. This recognition triggers an intense inflammatory reaction, which includes the induction and release of several inflammatory mediators (i.e., cytokines) (Fig. 21–2). Some investigators suggest that limiting the number of white blood cells (WBCs) in the CSF during meningitis may be beneficial to the patient with respect to neurologic sequelae. Thus, therapeutic strategies to down-modulate the host inflammatory response may play a major role in future attempts to improve the outcome of bacterial meningitis.

No specific clinical signs and symptoms differentiate *H. influenzae* meningitis from that caused by other organisms. Usually, the symptoms of meningitis develop relatively slowly (2–3 days). However, in some cases, a fulminant course with less than 24 h from the onset of symptoms to death is observed. The CSF findings (WBC and differential, protein, glucose, and lactate) in patients with *H. influenzae* meningitis are similar to those seen with other bacterial meningitis (see Chapter 20). Gram's stain is positive in more than 80% of cases, and the latex agglutination test is positive in more than 90% of cases. About 50% of patients with *H. influenzae* meningitis do well in all respects. An additional one fourth to one third of the surviving patients have a significant disability, the most common being hearing loss, followed by language disorders and mental retardation. The mortality rate is less than 5%.

### Other Systemic Infections

Other systemic diseases caused by *H. influenzae* type b include pneumonia, epiglottitis, septic arthritis, and cellulitis. Rarely, *H. influenzae* type b causes osteomyelitis, abscess, endocarditis, peritonitis, pericarditis, or neonatal sepsis. About one quarter to one third of documented bacterial pneumonia in children was caused by *H. influenzae* type b. The age distribution was similar to that of meningitis, with most cases occurring in infants younger than 2 years of age. In older children and adults, *H. influenzae* type b is rarely the cause of pneumonia, except in patients with chronic obstructive pulmonary disease. The best diagnostic test is blood culture, which is positive for *H. influenzae* in almost 80% of the cases. Gram's stain of the pleural fluid may be helpful in diagnosis but is prone to possible misinterpretation. Detection of capsular polysaccharide (PRP) in urine or pleural fluid by the latex agglutination test is rapid and reliable and, thus, should always be performed. Usually the outcome is excellent, with a negligible mortality rate.

A less common but even more serious disease caused by *H. influenzae* type b is epiglottitis. Epiglottitis is a rapidly progressive cellulitis of the epiglottis. The typical patient is a child between 2 and 5 years old who develops a sore throat with the abrupt onset of fever and toxicity. The disease progresses rapidly over the first 12–24 h and includes respiratory distress, dysphagia, and drooling. To keep the airway open the patient insists on sitting and breathes with an open mouth. In most cases bacteremia is documented, although it is unclear if infection of the epiglottis occurs directly from the colonized nasopharynx or follows bacteremia. The diagnosis is based on the clinical presentation. Direct observation of the epiglottis should be avoided because it may trigger acute airway obstruction. Lateral neck x-ray emphasizing the soft tissue is very useful in confirming the diagnosis. Early nasotracheal intubation for 2–3 days is probably the most important treatment. Antibiotics should be added but they are secondary to respiratory support. Rarely, other manifestations of *H. influenzae* infection present concomitantly with epiglottitis, including pneumonia, cervical adenitis, and very rarely, meningitis.

Although *Staphylococcus aureus* is a very common cause of septic arthritis in children, in infants younger than 2 years of age *H. influenzae* is common. There are no clinical or laboratory features that can distinguish between the two pathogens except Gram's stain and culture of joint fluid or the latex agglutination test of urine and joint fluid. The larger joints are usually involved, and if the hip joint is involved, emergency surgical drainage is required to save the intracapsular blood supply to the head of the femur.

Cellulitis (an acute infection of the skin) is usually caused by *S. aureus* and group A streptococcus. In infants 6 months to 3 years of age, cellulitis of the face, head, or neck may be due to *H. influenzae*. An acute cellulitis of the cheeks with violet discoloration is highly suggestive of *H. influenzae* infection, but *S. pneumoniae* can also present in this way. Because a high percentage of patients with *H. influenzae* cellulitis are also bacteremic, initial antibiotic therapy should be given intravenously to prevent spread of bacteria to other organs (especially the meninges).

### Immunity

Immunity to infection with *H. influenzae* is related directly both to age and to the amount of serum bactericidal antibodies directed against capsular PRP. The increased immunity to *H. influenzae* infections that occurs with age is accompanied by an increase in antibody to PRP capsular polysaccharide. It has been assumed that the development of antibody with increasing age is due to subclinical exposure to *H. influenzae* residing in the nasopharynx or to cross-reacting polysaccharides of other bacteria.

The fact that the most serious infections caused by *H. influenzae* occur in infants and young children should particularly recommend these individuals for vaccination with PRP. Coupling of PRP to OMP from *N. meningitidis* (PRP-OMP) or to nontoxic diphtheria toxoid (PRP-CRM) or to tetanus toxoid (PRP-T) results in immune responses to PRP in infants when given at 2, 4, and 6 months of age. For example, PRP-OMP proved to be protective in Navajo infants in whom 22 episodes of *H. influenzae* type b meningitis occurred in 2500 infants who received placebo but in only 1 of 2500 infants who received the vaccine. Evidence from another population with high rates of Hib vaccine coverage in Finland suggests that elimination of Hib disease is possible with universal infant Hib conjugate vaccine immunization, in part because of the ability of Hib vaccination to decrease Hib nasopharyngeal colonization rates. Because Hib conjugates are very effective in preventing HIB infections, all children should be immunized with an Hib conjugate vaccine beginning at 2 months of age.

## REFERENCES

**Book**

Yogev, R. Meningitis, In: Jenson, H. B. and Baltimore, R. S., eds. *The Practice of Pediatric Infectious Diseases.* New York: Appleton & Lange, Inc. 1995:781–807.

**Articles**

Arditi, M., and Yogev, R. Convalescent therapy for selected children with acute bacterial meningitis. *Semin. Pediatr. Infect. Dis.* 1:404–410, 1990.

Ashwal, S., Perkins, R. M., Thomason, J. R., et al. Bacterial meningitis in children: Current concepts of neurologic management. *Adv. Pediatr. 40:* 185–215, 1993.

Beutler, B., and Cerami, A. Cachectin: More than a tumor necrosis factor. *N. Engl. J. Med. 316:*379–385, 1987.

Friedland, I. R., and McCracken, G. H., Jr. Management of infections caused by antibiotic-resistant *Streptococcus pneumoniae. N. Engl. J. Med. 331:*377–381, 1994.

Haven, P. L., Garland, J. S., Brook, M. M., et al. Trends in mortality in children hospitalized with meningococcal infection, 1975 to 1987. *Pediatr. Infect. Dis. J. 8:*8–11, 1989.

Klein, J. O., Feigen, R. D., and McCracken, G. H., Jr. Report of the task force on diagnosis and management of meningitis. *Pediatrics 78*(Suppl.):959–982, 1986.

Lambert, H. P. Meningitis. *J. Neurol. Neurosurg. Psychiatry 57:*405–415, 1994.

Lebel, M. H., Freij, B. J., Syrogiannopoulos, G. A., et al. Dexamethasone therapy for bacterial meningitis. Results of two double-blind, placebo-controlled trials. *N. Engl. J. Med. 319:*964–971, 1988.

Quagliarello, V. J., and Scheld, W. M. New perspectives on bacterial meningitis. *Clin. Infect. Dis. 17:*603–610, 1993.

Sande, M. A., Tauber, M. G., Scheld, W. M., et al. Report of a second workshop: Pathophysiology of bacterial meningitis. *Pediatr. Infect. Dis. J. 8:*901–933, 1989.

Scheld, W. M., and Wispelwez, B. Meningitis. *Infect. Dis. Clin. North Am. 4*(4):555–584, 1990.

Smith, A. L. Neurologic sequelae of meningitis. *N. Engl. J. Med. 319:*1012–1014, 1988.

# 22

# VIRAL INFECTIONS OF THE CENTRAL NERVOUS SYSTEM

MICHELE TILL, M.D.

*Viral meningitis* is generally a benign illness of limited duration characterized by signs and symptoms of fever, headache, photophobia, and meningeal irritation. The term *aseptic meningitis* is often used to indicate viral meningitis but includes a variety of nonviral clinical syndromes indistinguishable from viral meningitis. These conditions, which cause pleocytosis in the cerebrospinal fluid (CSF) with no detectable bacteria on Gram's stain or routine culture, include partially treated bacterial meningitis; suppurative parameningeal infections; infective endocarditis; mycoplasmal, treponemal, rickettsial, and parasitic infections; meningeal metastases; intracranial tumors; vasculitides; sarcoidosis; and Mollaret's, Behçet's, and Vogt-Koyanagi-Harada recurrent meningitides. Therefore, the term *aseptic meningitis* is not synonymous with viral meningitis but encompasses other entities as well.

*Viral encephalitis,* unlike viral meningitis, is generally a very serious disease with significant morbidity and mortality. The characteristic features of viral encephalitis are the prominent clinical findings of cerebral dysfunction, reflecting infection and inflammation of the cerebral parenchyma. Signs and symptoms include confusion, stupor, coma, and seizures, in addition to fever, headache, and meningeal irritation. The term *meningoencephalitis* is used to connote a syndrome, usually viral in etiology, that combines encephalitic features with clinical and/or laboratory evidence of meningeal involvement.

Subacute sclerosing panencephalitis (SSPE), progressive multifocal leukoencephalopathy (PML), and the transmissible spongiform encephalopathies comprise a group of clinical syndromes characterized by a prolonged incubation period followed by progressive deterioration of neurologic function. The diverse clinical signs and symptoms that occur with these diseases of the central nervous system (CNS) reflect the regional foci of myelin destruction and neuronal loss. SSPE and PML each have a defined viral etiology, whereas transmissible spongiform encephalopathies, such as Creutzfeldt-Jakob disease (CJD), are caused by prions, small proteinaceous infectious particles. These clinical entities are considered separately from viral meningitis and encephalitis.

## VIRAL MENINGITIS AND ENCEPHALITIS

### Etiology

Table 22–1 lists pathogenic viruses associated with meningitis and meningoencephalitis in the United States. The most common of these agents are the enteroviruses, mumps, herpes simplex virus (HSV), Epstein-Barr virus (EBV), and the arthropod-borne agents. These viruses differ in their primary tropism and modes of transmission. The enteroviruses are usually acquired by fecal–oral transmission and generally remain localized to the gastrointestinal tract. Respiratory viruses are usually acquired by respiratory, hand-to-nose, or hand-to-eye transmission. These viruses generally remain confined to the respiratory tract (see Chapters 8 and 12). The arthropod-borne viruses, or arboviruses, are transmitted by a bite from an infected blood-feeding insect. Following viremia in the inoculated host, other blood-feeding insects can become infected and subsequently perpetuate the infectious cycle. Viruses can also be transmitted congenitally; by inoculation, including by animal bites and intravenous drug use; and by sexual contact.

### Enteroviruses

Enteroviruses are small, nonenveloped RNA viruses that belong to the Picornaviridae family. The enteroviruses are divided on the basis of antigenic relationships into polioviruses, coxsackievirus groups A and B, and echoviruses. The echovirus serotypes 4, 6, 9, 11, 16, and 30 and the coxsackievirus serotypes A7, A9, B2, B3, B4, and B5 are most frequently implicated in sporadic and community outbreaks of viral meningitis. Enteroviral infections occur primarily in late summer and early fall.

### Respiratory Viruses

**Adenoviruses.** The viruses that belong to the Adenoviridae family have a double-stranded, linear DNA genome in an icosahedral virion. Subgroup A, hemagglutination group IV (serotype 12, among others) and subgroup B, hemagglutination group I (serotypes 3 and 7, among others) have been most closely associated with sporadic meningoencephalitis. Serotypes 1, 6, 7, and 12 have been associated with

### TABLE 22–1.   VIRAL CAUSES OF MENINGITIS AND MENINGOENCEPHALITIS

**Togaviridae**
Alphaviruses
  Eastern equine encephalitis virus
  Western equine encephalitis virus
  Venezuelan equine encephalitis virus
Rubivirus
  Rubella
**Flaviviridae**
St. Louis encephalitis virus
Powassan virus
**Bunyaviridae**
California encephalitis viruses
  La Crosse virus
  Jamestown Canyon virus
  Other bunyaviruses
**Paramyxoviridae**
Paramyxoviruses
  Mumps virus
  Parainfluenza virus
Morbillivirus
  Measles virus
**Orthomyxoviridae**
Influenza A
Influenza B
**Arenaviridae**
Lymphocytic choriomeningitis virus
**Picornaviridae**
Enteroviruses
  Polioviruses
  Coxsackievirus A
  Coxsackievirus B
  Echoviruses
**Reoviridae**
Orbivirus
  Colorado tick fever virus
**Rhabdoviridae**
Rabies virus
Vesiculoviruses
**Retroviridae**
Lentiviruses
  Human immunodeficiency virus type 1
  Human immunodeficiency virus type 2
Oncornaviruses
  Human T-lymphotropic virus type 1
  Human T-lymphotropic virus type 2
**Herpesviridae**
Herpes simplex virus type 1
Herpes simplex virus type 2
Varicella-zoster virus
Epstein-Barr virus
Cytomegalovirus
Human Herpesvirus-6
Herpes B virus
**Adenoviridae**
Adenoviruses

meningoencephalitis complicating respiratory epidemics. Adenovirus serotypes 7, 12, and 32 can cause chronic meningoencephalitis in patients with hypogammaglobulinemia.

**Paramyxoviruses.** The Paramyxoviridae family includes the paramyxovirus (mumps, parainfluenza), the morbillivirus (measles), and the pneumovirus genera. These viruses have a linear RNA genome encapsidated in a cylindric nucleocapsid that is surrounded by an envelope. These viruses vary greatly in size. The viral envelope, which is partially derived from the cytoplasmic membrane of the host, contains both neuraminidase and hemagglutinin activity (paramyxoviruses) or hemagglutinin activity alone (measles). After the enteroviruses, mumps is the second most common cause of viral meningitis, although the institution of a mumps vaccine program has dramatically decreased the incidence in the United States. Measles commonly infects the central nervous system. Most infections are asymptomatic; however, 0.1–0.2% of patients develop clinical signs and symptoms ranging from mild to severe. A large number of patients who recover from measles encephalitis have neurologic sequelae. SSPE is now a rare, chronic, fatal, and progressive encephalitis associated with natural measles infection early in life (see below).

**Orthomyxoviruses.** The Orthomyxoviridae family includes influenza virus type A and influenza virus type B. These viruses have a segmented single-stranded RNA genome encapsidated in a nucleoprotein capsid that is surrounded by a lipid bilayer containing neuraminidase and hemagglutinin glycoproteins. The orthomyxoviruses have been associated with some cases of encephalitis and with Reye syndrome, which is a postinfectious noninflammatory encephalopathy and hepatic disorder.

**Togaviruses.** Rubella has been classified in the Togaviridae family on the basis of its RNA genome (see below). Unlike the alphaviruses, which are transmitted by vectors, rubella is spread by respiratory droplets and has been placed in its own genus, *Rubivirus*. Acute encephalitis complicating acquired rubella is rare, 1 in 5000 cases, but the mortality rate is high (20–50%).

### Arboviruses

Arboviruses were originally named for their *ar*thropod-*bo*rne mode of transmission. The arthropod vector, including mosquitos, ticks, and flies, becomes infected by ingesting the blood of a vertebrate host during the viremic phase of infection. The infected arthropod then transmits the disease by biting a new susceptible host. Arbovirus infections occur most often in the summer and fall months.

Viruses transmitted by arthropod vectors are chiefly members of the Togaviridae, Flaviviridae, Reoviridae, and Bunyaviridae families. These viruses, with the exception of members of the Reoviridae family, have a single-stranded RNA genome in an enveloped nucleocapsid. Reoviruses are nonenveloped particles that have a double-stranded RNA genome in an icosahedral capsule.

The Togaviridae family contains the alphavirus genus that is transmitted by arthropod vectors. The alphaviruses include the eastern, western, and Venezuelan equine encephalitis species. Encephalitis caused by the eastern equine encephalitis virus generally has a more severe course and a higher fatality rate than encephalitis caused by the other viruses. The mortality rate in the United States averages higher than 30%. Neurologic sequelae including mental retardation, behavioral changes, and seizure disorders are common following encephalitis caused by alphaviruses. Vertebrate reservoirs include horses and birds.

The Flaviviridae family includes St. Louis encephalitis virus, Powassan virus, yellow fever, and Dengue. Yellow fever primarily involves the liver, kidney, and heart. Dengue is associated with backache and arthralgia and is termed breakbone fever. Repeated infections with Dengue result in a devastating hemorrhagic fever and shock. Encephalopathy is a rare occurrence in patients with Dengue infection. Japanese B encephalitis virus is a major mosquito-transmitted cause of encephalitis in the Far East. St. Louis encephalitis virus has been associated with major epidemics of viral meningitis and encephalitis. In general, neurologic sequelae from St. Louis encephalitis are rare. St. Louis encephalitis has a predominantly avian reservoir, whereas the reservoir for Powassan virus is small mammals, particularly groundhogs.

The Reoviridae family contains the orbivirus genus. Colorado tick fever is the only known human disease caused by an orbivirus in the United States. Generally, Colorado tick fever is a self-limited disease. However, CNS infection in children may produce serious neurologic sequelae.

The Bunyaviridae family contains the California encephalitis viruses, including the La Crosse, Jamestown Canyon, and several other unnamed bunyaviruses. After St. Louis encephalitis, these agents, particularly the La Crosse virus, are the major cause of mosquito-borne encephalitis in the United States. Encephalitis primarily occurs in children. Seizures are a common clinical manifestation, occurring in almost 60% of affected children. Overall, bunyavirus infections are relatively mild, although fatalities have occurred. Fewer than 20% of patients experience sequelae, which include behavioral disturbances, headaches, cognitive deficits, and occasionally seizures.

The arthropod-borne viruses of the Rhabdoviridae family include the vesiculoviruses. Vesicular stomatitis virus (VSV) commonly infects domesticated animals and is occasionally transmitted to humans as an incidental host. Infection with VSV in humans generally produces a self-limited flu-like syndrome or may be asymptomatic. Although neurologic involvement is rare, two cases of severe encephalitis have been reported, both occurring in children.

### Sexually Transmitted Viruses

**Retroviruses.** The Retroviridae family includes the Oncovirinae, Spumavirinae, and Lentivirinae subfamilies. The retrovirus virion consists of a lipid-containing envelope surrounding an icosahedral capsid that contains two copies of a single-stranded RNA genome. The Oncovirinae (human T-lymphotropic virus types I [HTLV-I] and II [HTLV-II]) and Lentivirinae (human immunodeficiency virus types 1 [HIV-1] and 2 [HIV-2]) infect the CNS and are transmitted by sexual contact, transfusion, perinatal exposure, and use of contaminated needles (see Chapter 23).

**Herpesviruses.** The Herpesviridae family includes the herpesvirus and cytomegalovirus genera. Herpesviruses known to cause infections of the central nervous system include herpes simplex virus types 1 (HSV-1) and 2 (HSV-2), varicella-zoster virus (VZV), Epstein-Barr virus (EBV), human herpesvirus-6 (HHV-6), human cytomegalovirus (CMV), and herpes B virus. Viruses in the Herpesviridae family have a double-stranded DNA genome encapsidated in an icosahedral capsid and surrounded by a lipid-containing envelope. A characteristic of viruses in this family is their ability to establish a latent state in the host cell they infect. Herpesviruses are transmitted sexually or by exposure to infected body fluids. Herpes B virus is a simian virus transmitted to humans via bite from an infected monkey. It can cause a severe hemorrhagic encephalitis in humans. HHV-6 usually causes a benign febrile disease in children (roseola) but has been associated with febrile seizures in young children and rare cases of meningitis and encephalitis in children and adults. Of all the herpesvirus CNS infections, those caused by herpes simplex viruses are most common, specifically HSV-1 encephalitis and HSV-2 meningitis.

### Viruses with Other Modes of Transmission

The Rhabdoviridae family contains rabies and the rabies-related viruses. The surface glycoprotein is capable of inducing virus-neutralizing antibody. Immunization with this glycoprotein has been shown to be protective in animals against a subsequent rabies virus challenge. Antinucleocapsid antibodies are useful for detecting the intracytoplasmic eosinophilic inclusions, or Negri bodies, which are characteristic of rabies infection in tissues. Transmission occurs mainly by animal bite with salivary inoculation into the wound.

The Arenaviridae family contains the lymphocytic choriomeningitis (LCM) virus. The arenavirus genome consists of two single-stranded RNA molecules joined in a circle. The genome is encapsidated in a circular nucleocapsid surrounded by a lipid envelope. LCM virus primarily infects mice and hamsters, with humans being an incidental host. Transmission modes appear to include aerosols, direct rodent contact, and rodent bites.

## Epidemiology

The etiology of the viral meningitides and encephalitides differs with the geographic location, season, and age of the patient. Encephalitides transmitted by mosquitos, ticks, flies, and other insect vectors are limited to the location and time of year that these insects are feeding, particularly the late summer and autumn months. Mumps infections peak in the late winter and early spring but occur year-round. Enterovirus spread is facilitated by close family and school contacts. Enteroviral meningitis, as well as the other viral meningitides, is usually a disease of the young, rarely occurring in adults older than 40.

Worldwide, rabies virus is primarily transmitted by domestic animal bites (approximately 80%), with wild animal bites, particularly those of bats, skunks, raccoons, and foxes, accounting for the remainder of the cases. Small rodents, reptiles, and birds have not been found to be reservoirs of this virus in nature. Transmission has also occurred via mucous membrane or conjunctival contact with high concentrations of aerosolized rabies, usually occurring in bat caves or in medical laboratories. A few cases have been transmitted by infected corneal transplants. The rabies vaccine program for domestic pets has significantly decreased the incidence in the United States.

LCM and poliovirus are very infrequent causes of meningitis in the United States but are significant etiologic agents in other geographic locations. LCM virus infection is more prevalent in the winter months and is spread among persons living in rodent-infested regions. Mice, laboratory animals, and some household pets, such as hamsters, excrete the virus in their stool and urine. Since immunization against poliovirus has eradicated naturally occurring disease in the Western hemisphere, poliovirus infection in the United States occurs almost exclusively in recipients of live polio vaccine or their contacts. Poliovirus encephalitis occurs rarely, primarily in infants.

Geographic location and travel history facilitate the diagnosis of encephalitis transmitted by an arthropod-borne vector. For example, St. Louis and California encephalitides are most common in the midwestern United States, whereas eastern equine encephalitis is found primarily in the regions bordering the Atlantic and Gulf coasts. Colorado tick fever is confined to the western United States.

Viral meningitis caused by HSV-2 and HIV occurs sporadically throughout the year without seasonality.

### Pathogenesis (Fig. 22–1)

Clinical manifestations of CNS infection can be produced by either direct infection of the neural parenchyma or infection of contiguous tissues. In addition, some manifestations reflect the effect of host immune responses upon infected neural elements. Neurotropic viruses most commonly enter the central nervous system by hematogenous spread from an extraneural site of viral replication. The primary site of replication is usually the respiratory tract for measles, mumps, and influenza viruses; the gastrointestinal tract for enteroviruses; and the subcutaneous tissues for the arboviruses. Thus, inhalation of respiratory droplets, fecal–oral contamination, and direct inoculation of the host either by an animal bite or an insect bite are the major routes of infection. Transplacental infections can occur with rubella or cytomegalovirus and involve the fetal central nervous system and other tissues as well. Sexual transmission occurs with HIV and HSV.

During the course of many viral infections, initial virus replication at an extraneural site is followed by hematogenous dissemination. Viral particles are then cleared by the reticuloendothelial system. This mechanism of viral clearance may be detrimental to the host if a population of these reticuloendothelial cells is susceptible to viral infection. In this situation, virus may replicate in these cells and further disseminate. Viruses in the Orthomyxoviridae and Paramyxoviridae families escape clearance by the reticuloendothelial system by adsorption to red blood cells. The paramyxoviruses and morbilliviruses propagate within leukocytes, where they remain in an immunologically privileged site.

Viruses enter the central nervous system by one of several mechanisms. Most commonly, viruses cross the cerebral capillary endothelial cells of the blood-brain barrier. Some viruses can directly infect the endothelial cells of the cerebral microvasculature and subsequently contiguous neural tissue. Infected leukocytes can also transport viruses into the central nervous system. The epithelium of the choroid plexus may represent another portal of entry.

Alternatively, viruses can enter the central nervous system by retrograde migration within sensory or motor axons. Rabies and poliovirus infections can reach the central nervous system by this route. Herpes simplex virus and varicella-zoster virus invade sensory axons from the skin or mucous membranes at the time of the primary infection and ascend to ganglia. During typical exacerbations, the infection is reactivated at the primary site after antegrade transport from the ganglia to the periphery. Reactivated virus also reaches the central nervous system by retrograde transport. Retrograde transport of HSV from the trigeminal ganglia to the brain appears to account for the preferential localization of infection with this virus to the temporal lobes.

The olfactory pathway received early attention as a possibly important route of spread of viruses to the central nervous system. Fibers of the olfactory nerve extend through the nasal submucosa and epithelial cells and thus make direct contact with the environment. Togaviruses and herpesviruses have been shown to infect the olfactory and frontal lobes of experimental animals after inoculation into the nasal mucosa. However, spread of infectious organisms via the olfactory route has been found to be of clinical significance only in the entry of free-living amoebas, such as *Naegleria*.

Following entry of virus into the central nervous system, selected cells may become infected. Infection of specific cells (neuronal or

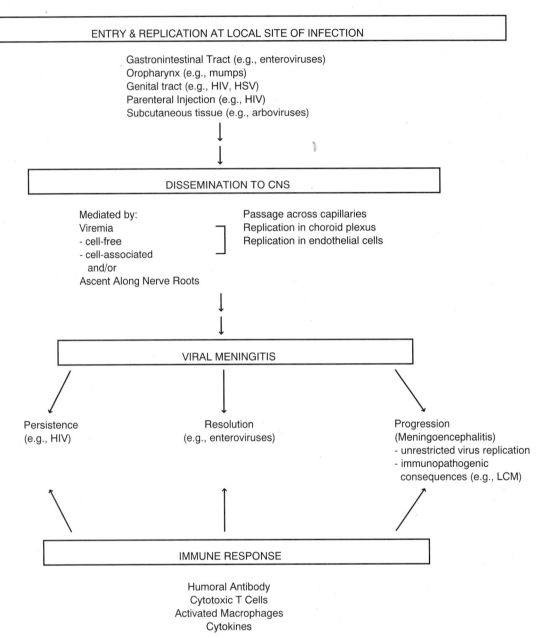

**FIGURE 22–1.** Pathogenesis of viral meningitis. (Adapted from Hammer, S. M., and Connolly, K. J. Viral aseptic meningitis in the United States: Clinical features, viral etiologies and differential diagnosis. *Curr. Clin. Top. Infect. Dis. 12*(1):1, 1992. With permission.

oligodendrial) is contingent upon the presence of suitable cell-surface receptors for virus attachment and the ability of the virus to replicate within the infected cell. The virus may then disseminate by spread to contiguous cells, either through extracellular gaps, or along the extensive network of neural axons and dendrocytes.

The immune response of the central nervous system to viral infection is not fully understood. Inflammation is mediated predominately by lymphocytes sensitized by the infecting agent and primarily distributed perivascularly. The sensitized lymphocytes are activated by locally released cytokines. Some polymorphonuclear cells are evident in the inflammatory infiltrate. As the inflammatory response develops, the blood-brain barrier is altered to allow immunoglobulins and other serum proteins to enter the CSF. B lymphocytes, which also enter the CSF, differentiate into plasma cells, which synthesize immunoglobulins locally. Locally synthesized immunoglobulins have been found for mumps, measles, varicella-zoster, and HIV when they infect the central nervous system.

In general, T-lymphocyte–mediated responses are more important than B-lymphocyte responses for viral clearance. Failure to clear the infecting virus often occurs in patients with depressed cell-mediated immunity, and they may develop a chronic, active encephalitis, such as HIV and CMV encephalitis in patients with acquired immunodeficiency syndrome (AIDS).

## Neuropathology

Viral meningitis is an inflammatory process involving the leptomeninges. Since this is usually a benign, self-limiting illness, its pathologic correlates are not as well characterized as those of viral encephalitis. The usual histologic appearance of viral meningitis when it is associated with fatal encephalitis consists of an inflammatory infiltrate that is generally confined to the leptomeninges. The inflammatory infiltrate consists primarily of mononuclear cells with some neutrophils.

Encephalitis is a diffuse inflammatory process involving the brain parenchyma and usually, although not invariably, the leptomeninges as well. Hematogenous dissemination of a virus to the brain results in a predominantly perivascular inflammatory reaction within the brain parenchyma. The inflammatory reaction is primarily composed of mononuclear cells, although a few polymorphonuclear cells may be present. Polymorphonuclear cells may also predominate early in the course of infection. Neurons may show changes ranging from minimal swelling and hyalinization to complete destruction. Neuronal engulfment and phagocytosis by macrophages may be observed. In severe cases, destruction of nerve and supporting cells may be so complete that cystic areas of necrosis and hemorrhage may develop in the brain, a condition termed *porencephaly.* Cerebral edema may occur as a direct consequence of infection or as a result of inappropriate antidiuretic hormone (ADH) secretion.

The viruses associated with encephalitis generally do not produce characteristic pathologic changes that enable precise histologic diagnosis. HSV, poliovirus, and rabies are commonly localized to certain parenchymal regions. HSV, CMV, adenovirus, rabies virus,

and some forms of measles virus infections have characteristic intranuclear inclusion bodies that can be diagnostic. Brains of patients with the AIDS-related dementia complex (ADC) or HIV encephalopathy demonstrate glial nodules, focal necrosis, perivascular inflammation, multinucleated giant cells, and demyelination. Meningeal involvement may also occur. This pathology is felt in part to be mediated by the secretion of neurotoxic substances by HIV-1–infected macrophages. CMV encephalitis produces ependymal and periventricular necrosis with intranuclear or intracytoplasmic inclusions.

Rabies and LCM virus produce disease without pathologic evidence of an acute cytolytic effect on cells of the central nervous system. In the case of LCM virus, relatively few cells are infected, and they usually do not lyse or die as a result of infection. Rather, they survive in an antigenically altered state that reflects virus-induced changes in the outer cell membrane. Because these cells have been modified by viral antigen(s) present within or on their surfaces, they are recognized as "non-self" by the immune system of the infected host. A vigorous immune-mediated attack may ensue against virus-infected host cells, including those within the central nervous system. This immune response may induce injury or death of virus-infected host cells, which in turn may result in tissue injury and inflammation extending to nearby noninfected cells. Therefore, the host immune response in fact contributes to tissue injury and disease. The virus–host reaction to LCM virus serves as an example of viral central nervous system disease that is immunopathologically mediated.

Postinfectious encephalomyelitis as a complication of respiratory or exanthematous viral infections and postvaccinal encephalomyelitis may occur without direct infection of the central nervous system. The pathogenesis of Guillain-Barré syndrome and postinfectious myelitis or encephalomyelitis appears to involve the immune response induced by sensitization of the patient to peripheral or central myelin, respectively. Demyelination results from this response. A similar demyelinating syndrome was seen with the early rabies vaccines originally formulated from virus cultivated in neural tissue. These vaccines could sensitize the recipient to neural antigens and lead to tissue damage. An animal model of immune-mediated demyelination, termed *experimental autoimmune encephalitis,* has clarified a number of issues related to these disorders. Perivascular infiltration by mononuclear cells and perivenous demyelination are the characteristic pathologic changes of postinfectious and postvaccinal encephalomyelitis. The fibrinoid necrosis, hemorrhage, and perivenous demyelination seen in acute hemorrhagic leukoencephalitis probably represent a more severe form of postinfectious encephalomyelitis.

Reye's syndrome is characterized by acute noninflammatory cerebral edema and fatty liver and usually follows a respiratory, cutaneous, or enteric viral infection in children. The pathogenesis of Reye's syndrome is not known, but it appears to be a postinfectious encephalopathy rather than an encephalitis. Influenza A and B and varicella virus infections are most commonly associated with Reye's syndrome. This syndrome is also associated with salicylate ingestion during the viral infection. In recent years, the incidence of Reye's syndrome has declined sharply, paralleling the sharp decline in administration of aspirin to children.

### Clinical Manifestations (Table 22–2)

Viral meningitis is usually a benign disease of limited duration lasting 1–2 weeks. Common prodromal symptoms of viral meningitis include fever, malaise, anorexia, myalgia, and sore throat. After a period of 3–14 days, signs of meningeal irritation including headache and stiff neck become apparent. Other symptoms of meningitis may include fever, severe frontal or retroorbital headache, photophobia, lethargy, nausea, and vomiting. Infants may only manifest fever and irritability. Mucocutaneous manifestations of infection include a nonpruritic, maculopapular rash associated with enterovirus infections, herpangina associated with group A coxsackievirus infection, and vesicular eruptions associated with HSV-2 infection.

The characteristic clinical presentation of viral encephalitis is evidence of cerebral dysfunction, which can distinguish it from meningitis. The signs and symptoms of encephalitis include altered state of consciousness, abnormal behavior, seizures, and deterioration in cognitive function accompanied by prominent memory deficit. Signs of temporal lobe dysfunction, including bizarre behavior and visual or auditory hallucinations, are commonly associated with herpes simplex encephalitis. In addition, signs and symptoms of meningeal irritation as well as fever, headache, malaise, nausea, vomiting, and anorexia are also frequently present in acute encephalitis. A much more insidious onset is characteristic of the chronic encephalitis of Creutzfeldt-Jakob disease, AIDS-related dementia, and PML. Depending on the region of the brain affected, neuronal involvement may result in focal or generalized seizures. Coma or respiratory failure can occur if there is brainstem involvement or profound cerebral edema.

Physical findings may include frank neurologic defects such as pathologic reflexes, cranial nerve deficits, seizures, tremors, altered consciousness, and obvious meningeal signs with nuchal rigidity. Papilledema and third- and sixth-nerve cranial palsies can result from increased intracranial pressure. Involvement of the hypothalamic region can contribute to disturbances of temperature, water, and electrolyte regulation.

### Laboratory Findings

Laboratory studies of the peripheral blood are of limited value in diagnosing viral meningitis or encephalitis. The peripheral white blood cell count is normal or somewhat elevated. Other routine hematologic and chemical tests are usually normal. The serum amylase may be elevated if mumps virus is the cause of meningitis. Serum transaminases may be elevated in illnesses due to CMV, EBV, LCM, adenovirus, and some arboviruses.

Examination of the CSF obtained by lumbar puncture is the single most useful procedure for the diagnosis of viral meningitis. The CSF opening pressure is usually elevated, and there is a lymphocytic pleocytosis in the range of 50–500 cells/mm³. There may be atypical lymphocytes present. As a general rule, cell counts exceeding 250 cells/mm³ give the CSF a slightly hazy appearance to the naked eye. CSF counts seldom exceed 1000 cells/mm³ in patients with viral central nervous system infection. Exceptions occur, particularly with LCM, mumps, eastern equine encephalitis, and California encephalitis, in which CSF counts can exceed 1000 cells/mm³. Usually, the differential cell count reveals a predominance of mononuclear cells. However, early in the course of infection (within the first 24 h), the CSF may have a predominance of segmented neutrophils. Repeat examination of the CSF shows that lymphocytes have become the dominant inflammatory cell. Red blood cells may be found in CSF of patients with HSV encephalitis, California encephalitis, and Colorado tick fever. Other CSF abnormalities may include a moderately elevated protein,

**TABLE 22–2.   CLINICAL FEATURES OF THE MORE COMMON VIRAL CAUSES OF MENINGITIS***

| AGENT | SEASON | AGE | EXPOSURE HISTORY | CLINICAL SYNDROME | CSF PROFILE | DIAGNOSTIC TESTS |
|---|---|---|---|---|---|---|
| Enteroviruses | Summer, early fall | Children, young adult | Known outbreak of enteroviral disease | May have exanthem, conjunctivitis, pleurodynia, myo- or pericarditis, herpangina, hand-foot-and-mouth disease | May see polymorphonuclear pleocytosis with early shift to mononuclear cells | Culture of CSF, blood, stool, throat |
| HSV-2 | No seasonal pattern | Young adult | Sexually active, new partner | Genital herpes, urinary retention, radioculopathy | | HSV-2 may be isolated in the CSF in patients with primary HSV, rarely with recurrences; culture of genital lesions; seroconversion, CSF PCR |
| HIV-1 | No seasonal pattern | Any age, peak may be in young adults | Sexual history, intravenous drug use, transfusion, specific exposure (needle-stick, etc.) | May have associated mononucleosis-like illness | | Serum ELISA may be negative; need for follow-up testing. Special techniques: plasma, PBML,[†] and CSF cultures, serum HIV antigen, PCR, antibody in CSF |
| Mumps | Late winter to spring | Classically peaks in 5- to 9-year-olds. In vaccine era adolescents now a more significant proportion | Known outbreak in the community | Parotitis in 50% of cases; orchitis, pancreatitis may be present | May cause hypoglycorrhachia in 1/4; leukocyte counts may be >1000/mm$^3$ | CSF culture, serology |
| LCM virus | Late fall to early winter | Young adults | Contact with pet hamsters, mice, or their excreta | May have alopecia, arthritis, orchitis, parotitis | May cause hypoglycorrhachia in 1/4 | CSF; blood culture, urine culture later; serology |

*From Hammer, S. M., and Connolly, K. J. Viral aseptic meningitis in the United States: Clinical features, viral etiologies and differential diagnosis. *Curr. Clin. Top. Infect. Dis. 12*(1):1, 1992. With permission.
[†]PBML, peripheral blood mononuclear leucocytes.

usually 65–150 mg/dL. Normal CSF glucose concentration is common. However, in about 10% of patients with mumps meningitis and occasionally in other viral meningitides such as LCM and rarely with HSV-2 infection, a low glucose concentration may be seen. Histochemical staining and microscopic examination of the centrifuged CSF sediment reveals neither bacteria nor fungi. However, bacterial cultures of the blood and CSF should be obtained. Virus can occasionally be isolated from the CSF early in the course of infection with enteroviruses and with HIV, but CSF viral cultures overall are of low yield. Throat washings, blood, urine, and stool have higher yield on viral culture, and acute and convalescent sera should be tested for antibody titers to the suspected virus or the agent isolated from culture. Computed tomography (CT) and magnetic resonance imaging (MRI) studies are useful for ruling out other clinical situations that can mimic viral meningitis, including parameningeal, brain, subdural, and epidural abscesses; neoplasia; and viral encephalitis.

## Diagnosis

It is important to emphasize that the frequency with which a specific virus can be identified as responsible for meningitis depends on the thoroughness with which virologic studies have been pursued and the time after onset of illness when CSF or other specimens for culture are collected. The success rates for isolating an enterovirus from the CSF of patients of various ages vary inversely with age. Although some series report as high as 75% recovery for a virologic agent using standard virologic techniques, most consider the usual recovery rate to be 25–33% of those infected. Even these percentage figures are rather high, since they reflect the results of virologic studies initiated in carefully selected patient populations. For example, results of viral studies by the Centers for Disease Control (CDC) on CSF specimens from a more general population group indicate that, overall, the specific etiology of aseptic meningitis is established in only 20% of cases.

In general, it is important to obtain both acute and convalescent serum specimens to assess antibody titer changes. Both serum specimens should be obtained so that a diagnostic fourfold or greater increase in titer can be documented. The timing of specimen acquisition is critical. The first serum specimen should be obtained as soon as the suspicion of viral meningitis arises, and the convales-

cent serum specimen should then be obtained 2–3 weeks later. Inability to recover a specific virus in viral meningitis results in part from the rapid elimination of virus from the central nervous system. Finally, throat washings and especially stool specimens should also be obtained for virus isolation in the acute stage, irrespective of whether there have been symptoms or signs implicating the gastrointestinal tract as the organ system primarily infected. Since enteroviruses are the leading cause of viral meningitis, and stool specimens contain relatively large amounts of enterovirus for at least several days after the onset of clinical signs of disease, there is a reasonable probability of recovering the etiologic agent from the stool.

If an enterovirus is isolated by viral culture, serum can then be tested for antibody against the specific enterovirus; a fourfold rise in antibody titer provides a reasonably certain diagnosis of enteroviral meningitis. Without an enteroviral isolate from throat washings or stool specimens, attempts at serologic tests are not practical because of the large number of possible serotypes. Because enterovirus may be shed from stool for several weeks, virus isolation from the stool cannot absolutely verify an enterovirus as the etiology of meningitis, since a prior asymptomatic infection may have occurred. Polymerase chain reaction (PCR) assays of CSF have shown promise as a diagnostic tool for enteroviral meningitis.

Mumps virus and arboviruses are the agents most frequently recovered from confirmed cases of viral encephalitis. When epidemics of viral encephalitis occur, arboviruses are the agents most frequently recovered. During nonepidemic periods, sporadic cases of viral encephalitis are often caused by HSV-1. Unfortunately, figures for prevalence of specific viruses are imprecise because a specific viral agent is identified in only 30% or less of the 1000–2000 annual reported cases of encephalitis in the United States.

HSV antigen is not detected in CSF reliably enough to be very useful. Detection of viral DNA or RNA by molecular hybridization techniques or by PCR holds great promise for the early diagnosis of several forms of viral encephalitis, especially HSV.

The electroencephalogram (EEG) may be useful for localizing cerebral lesions. Characteristic periodic epileptiform foci that localize to the temporal lobe are found in some patients with herpes simplex encephalitis.

Definitive diagnosis of herpes encephalitis

depends on prompt brain biopsy (usually of the frontal lobe) and demonstration of the virus or viral antigens within biopsied brain tissue. The most reliable method of demonstrating HSV is to isolate the etiologic agent in suitable tissue culture lines. Alternatively, one may detect HSV antigen by immunofluorescence, using highly specific antibody probes. Detection of antigen is more rapid but is not as sensitive or specific as virus isolation. Opinions vary widely regarding the advisability of brain biopsy in patients suspected of having herpetic encephalitis. However, with improved CT-guided stereotactic biopsy techniques, the complication rate is low, and a biopsy may be performed if the diagnosis is in question.

### Differential Diagnosis

Since meningitis and encephalitis may be life-threatening diseases, it is often desirable to establish the specific etiologic agent producing the infection. It is particularly important to differentiate between bacterial and viral meningitis, but this sometimes is difficult. The CSF findings can be extremely helpful. In general, bacterial meningitis is associated with high numbers of neutrophils in the CSF ($>1000$ cells/mm$^3$), hypoglycorrhachia (low CSF glucose), and elevated protein. The Gram's stain of CSF in bacterial meningitis due to *Streptococcus pneumoniae* and *Neisseria meningitidis* can be diagnostic. However, if the patient has received antimicrobial therapy, the Gram's stain can be negative. Identification of bacterial antigens with counterimmunoelectrophoresis (CIE) can sometimes be helpful; however, latex agglutination using beads coated with specific antibody is more rapid and sensitive than CIE. CSF lactic acid concentrations greater than 35 mg/dL suggest bacterial infection. The overlap of CSF findings in viral central nervous system infections and those due to bacteria, mycobacterium, or fungi can be confusing, and the initial evaluation may not distinguish the differing infections. In such cases, it is necessary to initiate empirical antimicrobial therapy and sometimes to evaluate a second CSF specimen before reaching a final diagnosis.

Nonviral causes of aseptic meningitis also need to be considered in the differential diagnosis (Tables 22–3 and 22–4). Leptospirosis, an uncommon disease, may manifest clinically as an aseptic meningitis syndrome. Usually, the initial symptoms of fever, chills, meningismus, and nausea and vomiting are followed by signs of renal and hepatic injury.

The diagnosis can be substantiated by a history of exposure to water that also has been in contact with rodents, and established by serologic tests documenting a fourfold rise in agglutinin titers.

An aseptic meningitis-like syndrome can be associated with infective endocarditis. Meningeal inflammation occurs either because of emboli or as a result of immune-complex–mediated vasculitis in the vicinity of the leptomeninges. Clinical findings resembling aseptic meningitis may divert attention from subtle cardiac abnormalities, allowing the underlying endocardial infection to be overlooked. In all instances of so-called aseptic meningitis in adults, blood cultures are advisable.

Neoplasms and dermoid or epidermoid cysts adjacent to the subarachnoid space can present clinically as aseptic meningitis. Certain drugs, such as trimethoprim-sulfamethox-

### TABLE 22–3. NONVIRAL INFECTIOUS CAUSES OF ASEPTIC MENINGITIS*

**More prominent as causes of aseptic meningitis:**
  *Borrelia burgdorferi* (Lyme disease)
  *Leptospira* sp.
  *Mycobacterium tuberculosis*
  *Cryptococcus neoformans*
  *Treponema pallidum* (syphilis)
**Less commonly present as aseptic meningitis:**
  *Mycoplasma pneumoniae*, rarely *M. Hominis* and
    *Ureaplasma urealyticum*
  *Rickettsia* sp., *Coxiella burnetii*, *Ehrlichia* sp.
  *Chlamydia psittaci* and *trachomatis* (LGV)
  *Listeria monocytogenes*, *Brucella* sp., *Norcardia* sp.,
    *Actinomyces*, cat-scratch bacillus (*Bartonella*)
  *Coccidioides immitis*, *Histoplasma capsulatum*
**Rarely other fungal pathogens such as:**
  *Aspergillus* sp., *Blastomyces dermatitidis*, *Candida*
    sp., *Cladosporium* sp., *Paracoccidioides*
    *brasiliensis*, *Sporothrix schenkii*, *Zygomycetes*
**Parasitic agents that more commonly present in the CNS as chronic infection, encephalitis, or focal lesions but which may rarely present initially as aseptic meningitis:**
  *Angiostrongylus cantonensis*, *Toxoplasma gondii*, *Taenia solium*, *Echinococcus granulosus*, *Strongyloides stercoralis*, *Schistosoma* sp., *Gnathostoma* sp.,
  *Multiceps multiceps*, *Acanthamoeba*, *Naegleria floweri*, *Entamoeba histolytica*, *Trypanosoma* sp., *Paragonimus* sp.
**Infectious syndromes:**
  Parameningeal infections
  Endocarditis/bacteremia
  Partially treated bacterial meningitis
  Postinfectious syndromes following viral infection
    (more typically encephalitis)
  Bacterial toxins: toxic shock syndrome; streptococcal
    pharyngitis, scarlet fever, pertusis, diptheria

*Adapted from Hammer, S. M., and Connolly, K. J. Viral aseptic meningitis in the United States: Clinical features, viral etiologies and differential diagnosis. *Curr. Clin. Top. Infect. Dis.* 12(1):1, 1992. With permission.

**TABLE 22–4. NONINFECTIOUS ETIOLOGIES OF ASEPTIC MENINGITIS\***

**Adverse reactions to medications:**
  *Antibiotics*—trimethoprim-sulfamethoxazole, trimethoprim, sulfamethoxazole, penicillin, isoniazid
  *Nonsteroidal antiinflammatory agents*—ibuprofen, tolmetin, sulindac, naproxen
  *Foreign proteins*—OKT3, intravenous human immune globulin
  *Miscellaneous*—azathioprine, high-dose cytosine arabinoside, phenazopyridine, carbamazepine
**In association with serum sickness**
**Associated with medical procedures:**
  Neurosurgery, intrathecal injections, spinal anesthesia, chymopapain injection
**Systemic Illnesses:**
  Systemic lupus erythematosus, sarcoidosis, Behçet's disease, Sjögren's syndrome, rheumatoid arthritis, polymyositis, familial Mediterranean fever, Wegener's and lymphomatoid granulomatosis, polyarteritis nodosa, granulomatous angiitis and other cerebral vasculitides, Kawasaki disease, Vogt-Koyanagi-Harada syndrome
**Heavy metal poisoning:**
  Arsenic, lead, mercury
**Intracranial tumors and cysts, lymphomatous or carcinomatous meningitis**

\*Adapted from Hammer, S. M., and Connolly, K. J. Viral aseptic meningitis in the United States: Clinical features, viral etiologies and differential diagnosis. *Curr. Clin. Top. Infect. Dis.* 12(1):1, 1992. With permission.

azole, azathioprine, and nonsteroidal antiinflammatory agents have been associated with a clinical syndrome resembling aseptic meningitis. Recurrent meningitides (including Mollaret's and Behçet's) and meningitis associated with systemic lupus erythematosus, vasculitides (including Kawasaki disease), sarcoidosis, tumor necrosis, and Lyme borreliosis have laboratory findings consistent with an aseptic meningitis syndrome.

Encephalitis must be differentiated from CNS tumors, intracranial abscesses, and hemorrhage. The availability of imaging techniques has greatly aided the ability to distinguish these forms of intracranial disease.

### Course and Treatment

Treatment of viral meningitis is symptomatic except when caused by a herpesvirus, which can be treated with acyclovir or ganciclovir. When appropriate supportive care is administered, the prognosis is excellent, with full clinical recovery and low mortality the rule. Complications such as weakness of a specific motor group may occur, but they are usually mild and self-limited. Since antibody is known to restrict or inhibit cell-to-cell spread of echoviruses, intravenous administration of large amounts of high-titer antibody has been used to treat chronic echovirus meningoencephalitis in children with hypogammaglobulinemia. The results have been disappointing because of the inability of antibody to penetrate the blood-brain barrier and gain access to the central nervous system compartment in significant amounts. The benefit of periodic intraventricular infusions of echovirus antibody–containing immunoglobulin was reported for a boy with sex-linked hypogammaglobulinemia who had persistent, progressive type 5 echovirus encephalitis. These data provide support for the suggestion that intraventricular antibody infusions might be of benefit in other viral encephalitides such as rabies.

Supportive treatment is indicated for comatose patients with encephalitis, since recovery can occur after a prolonged period of unconsciousness. Supportive measures include monitoring and correction of electrolyte imbalances, control of seizure activity, and thermal regulation. Corticosteroids and/or mannitol may be useful to reduce cerebral edema and increased intracranial pressure.

It is important to have a high index of suspicion for HSV encephalitis, since treatment with acyclovir significantly decreases mortality when initiated early. Acyclovir has also been used to treat serious CNS infections caused by HHV-6, herpes B virus, and VZV. For rabies, preexposure or postexposure prophylaxis (rabies vaccine, hyperimmune serum) prior to the onset of signs and symptoms has been shown effective. It is possible that antiretroviral agents such as zidovudine (AZT) may benefit HIV-1–infected patients who have neurologic involvement. Two antiviral agents with activity against CMV are now available (ganciclovir and foscarnet) and have been used to treat CMV encephalitis with variable results. Foscarnet can be used to treat infections with acyclovir-resistant HSV and VZV and ganciclovir-resistant CMV. Foscarnet also has some activity against HIV-1 *in vitro*, but its clinical efficacy in CNS infections has not been studied.

## SLOW VIRUS INFECTIONS

### Etiology

#### Measles-like virus

SSPE is caused by a measles-like virus that has been isolated from cultures of brain cells from SSPE patients. The SSPE paramyxovirus differs from measles virus by mutations in genomic RNA that cause defects in the formation of structural and envelope proteins. Although SSPE is a chronic infection of the CNS, viral progeny are usually not produced. Patients with SSPE have very high serum and CSF levels of antibodies to measles.

### Papovaviruses

The JC polyomavirus is a member of the Papovaviridae family, which includes the papillomaviruses and polyomaviruses. These viruses have a double-stranded DNA genome encapsidated in a nonenveloped icosahedral particle. The majority of viruses isolated from pathologic specimens from patients with PML have been strains of the JC virus.

## Epidemiology

SSPE is a very rare disease, with fewer than 40 new cases reported annually in the United States. The majority of cases occur in the first and second decades of life. The decreasing incidence has been associated with the increasing use of measles vaccination and the resulting decreased prevalence of wild measles. One epidemiologic study indicated that the majority of SSPE patients had a history of measles much earlier in life (mean age of 15 months) than a matched control group (mean age of 48 months).

PML is a rare disease of immunocompromised hosts. It has been reported in patients with collagen vascular diseases, acquired immunodeficiency syndrome (AIDS), Hodgkin's lymphoma, and in renal transplant recipients. PML has a worldwide distribution, with the age of first clinical manifestation between the fifth and seventh decades of life in non-AIDS patients and between the third and fourth decades for adult AIDS patients.

## Pathogenesis

The pathogenesis of SSPE is not known. The host immune response and the variant measles virus play important roles in the causation of this disease.

The pathogenesis of PML is associated clearly with the underlying immunoincompetence of the host. Antibodies to the JC virus are common in the general population. The development of PML may be related to activation of latent virus in the brain parenchyma.

## Neuropathology

SSPE is characterized by a diffuse infiltrate of lymphocytes and plasma cells with neuronal destruction in the white and gray matter of the brain and brainstem. Gliosis and myelin degeneration are seen in more chronic cases. Cowdry type A intranuclear inclusion bodies composed of paramyxovirus-like nucleocapsids are seen in neurons, oligodendrocytes, and astrocytes. Therefore, SSPE is a fatal, progressive subacute encephalitis that causes nonselective loss of cells in the brain parenchyma.

PML is characterized by discrete foci of demyelination, which become confluent and form large plaques. Within the plaques, oligodendrocytes show characteristic nuclear enlargement with basophilic inclusions, and giant astrocytes develop that are morphologically similar to the predominant cell type seen in glioblastoma. Viral particles and antigens can be detected in the lesions by electron microscopy and immunofluorescence, respectively.

## Clinical Manifestations

SSPE generally has two stages of neurologic decline. The first is characterized by the insidious deterioration of intellectual performance and the onset of behavioral abnormalities. Following a period of several weeks to months, the patient has the sudden onset of severe intellectual deterioration, seizures, myoclonus, and visual disturbances which rapidly progress to multifocal myoclonus, depression of consciousness, and development of a decorticate state.

Patients with PML deteriorate rapidly; death occurs usually within 6 months after the presenting neurologic symptoms. Signs and symptoms are diverse, reflecting the random distribution of lesions in the central nervous system. Personality changes, paresis, and cortical blindness progress to quadriparesis, dementia, and coma. A small subset of patients experience fluctuations in their clinical course that can continue for 2–3 years.

## Laboratory Findings

Patients with SSPE have elevated IgG concentrations and very high levels of measles antibody in both serum and CSF. Antibody levels are substantially higher in SSPE patients than in patients who have had measles or have been vaccinated. Patients have characteristic EEG and CT abnormalities.

Patients with PML usually have normal CSF. The EEG shows diffuse nonspecific slowing. Cranial CT can detect the large demyelinated foci, although MRI is more sensitive for detecting PML lesions. Clinical symptoms are often more severe than suggested by the extent of involvement on radiologic studies. Definite diagnosis requires identification of the characteristic pathology on brain biopsy. Since antibodies for JC are prevalent in the general population, serologic studies are not useful.

### Course and Treatment

There is no current treatment for SSPE, although a few patients have had remissions with the use of interferon. SSPE can be prevented by immunization to prevent measles. There is no known method of preventing PML. Trials of cytosine arabinoside by intravenous and intrathecal routes are ongoing for treatment of PML in AIDS patients. Some clinical improvement has also been reported with the use of AZT and with interferon.

## PRION DISEASES (TRANSMISSIBLE SPONGIFORM ENCEPHALOPATHIES)

### Etiology

While originally thought to be viral in origin, considerable research has led to the identification of prions as the cause of several neurodegenerative diseases in humans and animals referred to as transmissible spongiform encephalopathies (Table 22–5).

A prion is a small proteinaceous infectious particle that resists inactivation by procedures that modify nucleic acids. The prion was first discovered in scrapie, a neurodegenerative disorder of sheep. The scrapie prion ($PrP^{sc}$) has been shown to transmit disease to a variety of species. When the gene for this protein was cloned, it was found to encode for a normal cellular protein ($PrP^{c}$). Studies in transgenic mice have shown that the presence of $PrP^{c}$ is necessary for $PrP^{sc}$ to cause disease. Because it is difficult to understand how an infectious agent can replicate without the presence of nucleic acid, the prion theory was met with much skepticism. Recent research, however, suggests that the introduction of $PrP^{sc}$ may induce conformational changes in native $PrP^{c}$, converting it to $PrP^{sc}$. Prion diseases are unique in that they are both infectious and genetic. Specific mutations in the human $PrP^{c}$ gene have been linked to Creutzfeldt-Jakob disease and Gerstmann-Sträussler-Scheinker syndrome (GSS), with certain mutations associated with specific phenotypic disease characteristics. This is particularly evident in GSS, a rare inherited neurodegenerative disorder with variable clinical presentations. Kuru is a unique prion disease in that transmission is believed to have occurred solely from the consumption of brain tissue from humans who died of kuru.

### Epidemiology

Kuru is confined to the Fore people of eastern New Guinea. Transmission was associated with ritualistic cannibalism of dead relatives, which was practiced as a rite of mourning. Consumption of brain tissues was limited to children and adult women, thus accounting for the unusual age and sex distribution of the disease. The incidence of kuru has declined greatly since the cessation of ritualistic cannibalism by 1960. Therefore, the patients most recently diagnosed with kuru demonstrate very long incubation periods.

Currently, CJD has three recognized forms: infectious, sporadic, and inherited. There is a worldwide distribution, with an estimated prevalence of 1 case per million persons. The majority of cases occur in the fifth to seventh decades of life. Most cases are sporadic, while 10–15% of cases are familial with autosomal dominance and variable penetrance. Epidemiologic studies have failed to confirm the ingestion of scrapie-infected meat as a cause of CJD in humans. Iatrogenic transmission has occurred by corneal transplantation, contaminated CNS electrode implantation, dura mater grafts, and cadaveric pituitary hormone injections.

Bovine spongiform encephalopathy (BSE) emerged in cattle in Great Britain in 1987, presumably related to a change in processing methods of sheep remains used in cattle feed. The new method did not inactivate scrapie prions, which were then ingested by cattle. Whether BSE can be transmitted to humans is still uncertain. Measures have been undertaken to prevent animals and humans from being exposed to BSE; however, due to the prolonged incubation period of transmissible spongiform encephalopathies, the risk of

### TABLE 22–5.   PRION DISEASES

Human diseases
    Kuru
    Creutzfeldt-Jakob disease (CJD)
    Gerstmann-Sträussler-Scheinker syndrome (GSS)
    Fatal familial insomnia
Animal diseases
    Scrapie (sheep and goats)
    Transmissible mink encephalopathy
    Chronic wasting disease (mule deer, elk)
    Bovine spongiform encephalopathy

transmission to humans cannot be excluded for many years. Recently, 10 cases of CJD with unique neuropathologic features were diagnosed in Great Britain, raising fears that they could be related to beef consumption. Additional research is needed to assess this issue.

## Pathogenesis

While it is now accepted that the prion PrP[sc] is the transmissible agent that causes human spongiform encephalopathies, the mechanism remains unclear. However, the prion protein is an integral neuronal membrane sialoglycoprotein that accumulates during the course of the disease and may be responsible for the neuropathologic findings.

## Neuropathology

Spongiform encephalopathy is characterized by diffuse neuronal loss, proliferation of astrocytes, and vacuolization of astroglial and neuronal processes. This last finding corresponds to the spongy histopathologic state. Demyelination and inflammation are conspicuously absent. Amyloid plaques are often present, particularly in GSS and kuru. These plaques stain with antisera to PrP[27-30], the insoluble core of PrP[sc].

## Clinical Manifestations

Creutzfeldt-Jakob disease is characterized by rapidly progressive dementia with fatal outcome. The duration varies from 3 weeks to several years, but most patients die within 6 months. The most common presentation begins with malaise, altered personality, and sleep disturbances followed by progressive dementia, ataxia, myoclonus, and cortical blindness. In the rare amyotrophic form, patients also exhibit lower motor neuron signs and neurogenic muscle atrophy.

Gerstmann-Sträussler-Scheinker disease produces cerebellar ataxia, pyramidal signs, and dementia, although patients may have diverse clinical manifestations. The average duration of disease is 5 years, considerably longer than in CJD.

The clinical presentation of kuru was remarkable for its uniformity. Patients first developed headache and joint pain, with the onset of difficulty walking 6–12 weeks later. Death occurred in all patients within 2 years of the onset of symptoms. Dementia occurred at a later disease stage than with CJD.

## Laboratory Findings

In CJD the CSF is usually normal. Serial CT or MRI scans may show progressive cerebral atrophy but are more useful to exclude other disease processes. Characteristic patterns are found on EEG in two thirds of patients, which can aid in diagnosis. Diagnosis is usually confirmed by staining brain tissue with antiprion antibody.

## Treatment

There is no treatment for CJD or GSS. Since CJD is transmissible from human to human, precautions are necessary for handling potentially infectious material and caring for patients. CJD patients must not be permitted to donate organs or blood. Accidental exposure to infected material should be treated by washing with sodium hydroxide for 5–10 min, followed by copious washing with water. Surgical instruments and electrodes should be autoclave sterilized and exposed surfaces cleaned with 1% hypochlorite solution.

## CASE HISTORIES

### CASE HISTORY 1

A 36-year-old white male with a 10-year history of intravenous drug abuse was hospitalized with a 3-day history of malaise, myalgia, anorexia, and nausea. On the day of admission he had developed a severe headache and photophobia. He had been previously well except for a history of acute hepatitis B several years earlier. He was taking no medications and had last used intravenous cocaine 2 weeks prior to admission. There was no history of recent travel.

The patient was alert and responded appropriately to questions. Temperature was 39°C, pulse was 118/min, and respirations were 20/min. Physical examination was significant for mild nuchal rigidity and pain with neck flexion and a fine maculopapular exanthem distributed over the trunk. There were no other physical or neurologic abnormalities.

Laboratory studies included a peripheral leukocyte count of 4800 cells/mm³, with 68% segmented neutrophils, 25% lymphocytes, 5% monocytes, and 2% atypical lymphocytes. Heterophile antibody and Venereal Disease Research Laboratories (VDRL) were negative. Lumbar puncture revealed an opening pressure of 120 mm of $H_2O$ (normal <180 mm of $H_2O$) and clear, colorless fluid. Microscopic examination revealed 188 leukocytes/mm³, of which 86% were mononuclear cells. Protein was 60 mg/dL (normal <45 mg/dL), and the glucose was normal. Gram's stain and India ink analysis failed to demonstrate any microorganisms. Blood cultures and cerebrospinal fluid cultures were negative. An enzyme-linked immunosorbent assay (ELISA) for HIV-1 antibody was negative. However, serum was positive for HIV-1 p24 core antigen.

The patient's fever slowly disappeared over a 5-day period. His symptoms also resolved, and he was discharged and followed as an outpatient. Six weeks later, a repeat serum ELISA was positive for antibodies to HIV-1.

## CASE 1 DISCUSSION

No specific antimicrobial therapy was given to this patient, since his clinical presentation and laboratory findings were consistent with an acute viral syndrome. In addition, the patient's history of intravenous drug abuse placed an HIV-1–related acute retroviral syndrome in the differential diagnosis. Symptoms of this syndrome include fever, night sweats, meningismus, myalgias, anorexia, nausea, vomiting, diarrhea, and a nonexudative pharyngitis. Signs include a maculopapular or urticarial exanthem in 25–50% of patients, generally localized to the trunk.

The acute retroviral syndrome usually occurs 1–6 weeks after exposure to the virus. The incidence is unknown, since symptoms can be mild and resemble a minor flu-like illness. Although this syndrome occurs prior to antibody production, p24 core antigen of HIV can often be detected in the serum or CSF. Occasionally, the virus can be cultured from CSF. HIV-1 antibody is generally detectable 6–12 weeks later, by which time antigenemia has usually cleared.

The differential diagnosis of an acute retroviral syndrome includes influenza, infectious mononucleosis, measles, mumps, cytomegalovirus infection, secondary syphilis, and rarely, acute viral hepatitis.

## CASE HISTORY 2

A 21-year-old college student was hospitalized in January after a few days of malaise, headache, and low-grade fever. The patient was brought to the hospital after friends found him behaving strangely and having difficulty speaking. On examination in the emergency room, the patient was confused, oriented to person only, and complaining of a severe headache. His speech was moderately impaired. His temperature was 40°C. The remainder of the physical and neurologic examinations were unremarkable. There were no nuchal signs.

Routine laboratory studies and cranial CT were normal. Lumbar puncture revealed an opening pressure of 280 mm $H_2O$ and slightly cloudy fluid. There were 300 white cells/mm$^3$ and 53 red cells/mm$^3$. Ninety-eight percent of the white cells were lymphocytes. The glucose was 65 mg/dL (serum glucose was 88 mg/dL) and protein was 95 mg/dL. No organisms were visible on Gram's stain or by India ink. CSF for HSV PCR study was sent. An EEG showed a spike and slow wave pattern localized to the left temporal lobe.

The patient was treated with intravenous acyclovir at 10 mg/kg every 8 h. After 2 days, the patient was less confused, but still had spiking fevers and difficulty speaking. After the fifth day of therapy, fever had disappeared. Although his speech improved, he complained of difficulty with his memory. The patient completed a 14-day course of intravenous acyclovir and was discharged in good condition. Some memory problems persisted.

## CASE 2 DISCUSSION

This patient's clinical course is typical of herpes simplex type 1 encephalitis. His illness was heralded by malaise, headache, and low-grade fevers, which progressed to spiking fevers with behavioral changes. The virologic diagnosis is presumptive because a brain biopsy was not performed. However, the clinical and laboratory findings, EEG results, and apparent good clinical response to acyclovir are consistent with HSV-1 infection of the central nervous system. HSV PCR was reported positive. MRI would have been more sensitive than CT for demonstrating an early abnormality, and it can also be used to localize a lesion if a biopsy is performed.

This patient responded to antiviral therapy. Early treatment with acyclovir, which is well tolerated with few side effects, has significantly reduced mortality in herpes encephalitis. However, residual neurologic deficits are still common. Therefore, patients with a clinical presentation consistent with viral encephalitis are often treated empirically with acyclovir. Several HSV isolates have been found to be resistant to acyclovir, particularly in individuals receiving long-term acyclovir. This emerging resistance may complicate treatment in the future. Foscarnet has been used with success to treat some acyclovir-resistant HSV infections.

Although testing CSF for HSV by PCR is very useful for diagnosis of herpes encephalitus, the most definitive study is a brain biopsy. This differentiation is particularly important when dealing with the immunocompromised host, such as AIDS patients who may be co-infected with other pathogens.

## REFERENCES

### Books

Johnson, R. T., ed. Pathogenesis of CNS infections. In: *Viral Infections of the Nervous System.* New York: Raven Press, 1982.
Mandell, G., Bennett J., and Dolin, R., eds. Viral diseases. In: *Principles and Practice of Infectious Diseases.* New York: Churchill Livingstone, 1995.

### Review Articles

Bale, J. F., Jr. Viral encephalitis. *Med. Clin. North Am.* 77(1):25, 1993.
Berger, J. R., Kaszovitz, B., Post, M. J., et al. Progressive multifocal leukoencephalopathy associated with hu-

man immunodeficiency virus infection. A review of the literature with a report of sixteen cases. *Ann. Intern. Med. 107:*78, 1987.

Brew, B. J. HIV-1 related neurological disease. *J. AIDS 6*(Suppl. 1):S10, 1993.

Drew, W. L. Cytomegalovirus infection in patients with AIDS. *Clin. Infect. Dis. 14:*608, 1992.

Dupont, J. R., and Earle, K. M. Human rabies encephalitis: A study of forty-nine fatal cases with a review of the literature. *Neurology 15:*1023, 1965.

Esmonde, T. F. G., and Will, R.G. Transmissible spongiform encephalopathies and human neurodegenerative disease. *Br. J. Hosp. Med. 49*(6):400, 1993.

Hammer, S. M., and Connolly, K. J. Viral aseptic meningitis in the United States: Clinical features, viral etiologies and differential diagnosis. *Curr. Clin. Top. Infect. Dis. 12*(1):1, 1992.

Hollander, H., and Stringari, S. Human immunodeficiency virus-associated meningitis. *Am. J. Med. 83:*813, 1987.

Kelsey, D. S. Adenovirus meningoencephalitis. *Pediatrics 61:*291, 1978.

Lantos, P. L. From slow virus to prion: A review of transmissible spongiform encephalopathies. *Histopathology 20:*1, 1992.

McKinney, R. E., Katz, S. L., and Wilfert, C. M. Chronic enteroviral meningoencephalitis in agammaglobulinemic patients. *Rev. Infect. Dis. 9:*334, 1987.

Pachner, A. R. Neurologic manifestations of Lyme disease, the new "great imitator." *Rev. Infect. Dis. 11*(Suppl. 6):S1482, 1989.

Prusiner, S. B. Genetic and infectious prion diseases. *Arch. Neurol. 50:*1129, 1993.

Rennels, M. B. Arthropod-borne virus infections of the central nervous system. *Neurol. Clin. 2:*241, 1984.

Rubeiz, H., and Roos, R. P. Viral meningitis and encephalitis. *Semin. Neurol. 12*(3):165, 1992.

Shimizu, T., Ehrlich, G., Inaba, G., et al. Behçet's disease (Behçet's syndrome). *Semin. Arthritis Rheum. 8:*223, 1979.

Sperber, S. J., and Schleupner, C. J. Leptospirosis: A forgotten cause of aseptic meningitis and multisystem febrile illness. *South. Med. J. 82:*1285, 1989.

Tenser, R. B. Herpes simplex and herpes zoster nervous system involvement. *Neurol. Clin. 2:*215, 1984.

## Articles

Chonmaitree, T., Menegus, M. A., and Powell, K. R. The clinical relevance of CSF viral culture. *JAMA 247:*1843, 1982.

Cizman, M., Mozetic, M., Radescek-Rakar, R., et al. Aseptic meningitis after vaccination against measles and mumps. *Pediatr. Infect. Dis. J. 8:*302, 1989.

Cohen F. E., Pan, K. M., Huang Z., et al. Structural clues to prion replication. *Science 264:*530, 1995.

Dagan, R., Jenista, J. A., and Menegus, M. A. Association of clinical presentation, laboratory findings, and virus serotypes with the presence of meningitis in hospitalized infants with enterovirus infection. *J. Pediatr. 113:*975, 1988.

Dwyer, J. M., and Erlendsson, K. Intraventricular gamma-globulin for the management of enterovirus encephalitis. *Pediatr. Infect. Dis. J. 7:*S30, 1988.

Hall, C. B., Long, C. E., Schnabel, K. C., et al. Human herpesvirus-6 infection in children. *N. Engl. J. Med. 331*(7):432, 1994.

Hemachudha, T., Griffin, D. E., Giffels, J. J., et al. Myelin basic protein as an encephalitogen in encephalomyelitis and polyneuritis following rabies vaccination. *N. Engl. J. Med. 316:*369, 1987.

Johnson, R. T. Slow infections of the central nervous system caused by conventional viruses. *Ann. N. Y. Acad. Sci. 724:*6, 1994.

Johnson, R. T. The pathogenesis of acute viral encephalitis and post-infectious encephalomyelitis. *J. Infect. Dis. 155:*359, 1987.

Johnson, R. T., Griffin, D. E., Giffels, J. J., et al. Measles encephalomyelitis—clinical and immunologic studies. *N. Engl. J. Med. 310:*137, 1984.

Kessler, H. A., Blaauw, B., Spear, J., et al. Diagnosis of human immunodeficiency virus infection in seronegative homosexuals presenting with an acute viral syndrome. *JAMA 258:*1196, 1987.

Lipton, S. A., and Gendelman, H. E. Dementia associated with the acquired immunodeficiency syndrome. *N. Engl. J. Med. 332*(14):934, 1995.

Mehta, P. D., Thormar, H., Kulczycki, J., et al. Immune response in subacute sclerosing panencephalitis. *Ann. N. Y. Acad. Sci. 724:*378,1994.

Rowley, A. H., Whitley, R. J., Lakeman, F. D., et al. Rapid detection of herpes-simplex-virus DNA in cerebrospinal fluid of patients with herpes simplex encephalitis. *Lancet 335:*440, 1990.

Soong, S-J., Watson, N. E., Caddell, G. R., et al. Use of brain biopsy for diagnostic evaluation of patients with suspected herpes simplex encephalitis: A statistical model and its clinical implications. *J. Infect. Dis. 163:*17, 1991.

# VII INFECTION IN THE IMMUNOCOMPROMISED HOST

# 23

## HUMAN IMMUNODEFICIENCY VIRUS INFECTION AND AIDS

JOHN P. PHAIR, M.D. and ELLEN GOULD CHADWICK, M.D.

In 1981, several investigators reported the occurrence of opportunistic infections due to intracellular microbial pathogens and a rare cancer, Kaposi's sarcoma (KS), in epidemiologically restricted populations. This illness, first noted in mid-1979 and characterized by profound immune defects, was later termed acquired immunodeficiency syndrome (AIDS). Initially, cases were reported in homosexually active males and injection drug users (IDU). Individuals who received blood transfusions or blood component therapy, children born to mothers who were IDUs, and sexual contacts of bisexual males and IDUs subsequently were identified as having similar defects and

clinical manifestations. Many persons with AIDS have a prodromal illness of varying duration characterized by fever, generalized lymphadenopathy, malaise, weight loss, oral thrush, and diarrhea. Investigation of symptomatic and asymptomatic individuals in the high-risk groups documented that an altered immunoregulatory state precedes the development of AIDS. The diagnosis of AIDS was based upon the clinical findings of an opportunistic infection, KS, or non-Hodgkin's lymphoma (usually of the B-cell type, if localized to the central nervous system [CNS]), or severe wasting—conditions suggestive of a defect in cell-mediated immunity. Since January

1993, an absolute T-helper cell count less than 200/mm$^3$, tuberculosis, cervical cancer, and recurrent pneumonia have been added to the surveillance definitions of AIDS.

The most common presentation of AIDS has been pneumonia due to *Pneumocystis carinii* (PCP), which has accounted for 55% of cases. KS alone, and both KS and PCP are common in homosexual men. Other presenting illnesses include central nervous system toxoplasmosis, mycobacteriosis (especially infections due to *Mycobacterium avium* complex [MAC]), and disseminated fungal or progressive herpes virus infection. Finally, a small group of patients present with encephalopathy or wasting.

This chapter reviews the etiology, epidemiology, immunopathogenesis, diagnosis, natural history, and treatment of patients with infection due to the human immunodeficiency virus (HIV) and AIDS. Specific issues relevant to maternal–fetal transmission, manifestations, and management of HIV infection in children are also addressed.

## ETIOLOGY

The cause of the immune dysfunction that leads to AIDS is infection with a retrovirus, HIV-1 or HIV-2. These agents are related to a number of primate retroviruses that cause a similar syndrome in specific species of Old World monkeys. HIV-1 was the first to be recognized and was isolated in three laboratories in 1983–1984. Initially, it was called the lymphadenopathy-associated virus, human T-cell lymphotropic virus type III (HTLV-III), or AIDS-related virus (ARV). Genetic analysis indicated that HIV-1 and HIV-2 are closely related to the lentivirus group of retroviruses and by consensus the name human immunodeficiency virus (HIV) was assigned to these new human viruses. HIV-1 is epidemic in central and east Africa, Europe, North America, Oceania, and Asia. HIV-2 is found primarily in west Africa and is the cause of imported cases of AIDS in western Europe and in North America.

HIV are RNA viruses. The genetic material is contained within a protein core of 24,000 D termed p24. Closely associated with the RNA genome are three viral enzymes—reverse transcriptase, which transcribes DNA from RNA after the virus core enters the cytoplasm of a human cell; an integrase; and protease. Surrounding the core is a multilay-

ered outer envelope composed of an inner protein coat of 17,000 D termed p17. This protein lines a lipid layer into which is inserted a glycosylated protein of 41,000 D (gp41). Attached to gp41 is a larger glycosylated protein, gp120, of 120,000 D. The gp120 protein contains a sequence of amino acids that recognize and adhere to surface CD4 surface molecules of a number of kinds of human cells, most prominently the helper T (CD4+) lymphocytes. A subset of monocytes/macrophages and B lymphocytes also bears small numbers of CD4 molecules. There is evidence suggesting that endothelial cells, rectal mucosal cells, and possibly lymphocyte progenitor cells can be infected even though CD4 molecules have not been identified on the surface of these cells.

Once the virus attaches to the CD4+ surface molecule, its core is internalized, the RNA uncoated and, through the action of reverse transcriptase, viral DNA is transcribed. The DNA is circularized and integrated through the action of the viral integrase into the DNA of the infected cell. This proviral DNA can remain in a latent state in the cell for months to years, but most often cells are productively infected. The proviral DNA transcribes viral mRNA, which encodes the specific viral components. Specifically, there is a region that transcribes the precursor protein (p55) of the internal structural proteins (gag), the viral enzymes (pol), and the outer envelope components (env). The virion is assembled in the cytoplasm of the infected cell and buds from the cell surface. Coincident with budding, p55 is proteolytically cleaved into the core, p24, p6, and p17 by the viral protease.

## EPIDEMIOLOGY

AIDS was first recognized in homosexual men and IDUs in New York, San Francisco, and Los Angeles in 1979–1980. Since the initial recognition of the syndrome, persons with AIDS have been diagnosed in all 50 states and all inhabited continents. In the United States the proportion of AIDS cases occurring in homosexual or bisexual men during the 1980s and 1990s has slowly decreased, whereas the number of cases among IDUs, their sexual contacts, and children born to infected women has increased. A small number of cases continue to be reported among recipients of contaminated blood and blood component therapy. For the most part such individuals were infected with HIV before donors of blood were screened for high-risk behavior, symptoms related to HIV and antibody to the virus (before March 1985).

The majority of persons with AIDS are male and between the ages of 20 and 44, and AIDS represents the most common cause of death in men of this age group. Infection in older adults generally has been associated with receipt of HIV-infected blood. Since the latter half of the 1980s and 1990s an increasing number of women have been diagnosed with AIDS as a result of drug use or sexual contact with men who are bisexual or drug users. Heterosexual transmission is the most common cause of HIV-1 infection in women in the United States. All racial groups are represented among cases reported to the Centers for Disease Control (CDC) as part of the national surveillance program.

It is estimated that approximately 1 million residents of the United States are infected. The coincident epidemic of injection drug use and crack cocaine use in this country has resulted in an increasing number of economically disadvantaged people from the inner cities being infected and developing AIDS. Thus, African-Americans and Hispanics, especially women and children, are disproportionately represented among those persons with AIDS.

## IMMUNOLOGY AND IMMUNOPATHOGENESIS

The primary targets of HIV are the CD4-bearing lymphocytes (helper T cells), macrophages/monocytes, and B cells. The CD4+ lymphocytes play a central role in the regulation of the immune system, releasing a number of cytokines necessary for normal function of this response. HIV infection results in depletion and dysfunction of the CD4+ lymphocytes. The infection of the mononuclear phagocytes does not apparently produce cell death, but the depletion of CD4+ lymphocytes results in decreased serum concentrations of lymphokines, such as interleukin-2 (IL-2) and interferon-gamma, with consequent macrophage/monocyte dysfunction. Infection of B lymphocytes induces autonomous production of immunoglobulins and hypergammaglobulinemia. Paradoxically, however, the loss of CD4+ lymphocytes and B-cell infection induce a state in which the infected

individual responds poorly to new antigens with specific antibody production.

The depletion of CD4+ lymphocytes is associated with the overwhelming retroviral infection. Replication of the virus results in cell death. Infection with HIV *in vitro* induces cell fusion and giant cell formation, but this is not a consistent or prevalent finding upon histologic examination of tissues from infected individuals. Antibody-mediated cell cytotoxicity or lymphocytotoxic antibody possibly mediate destruction of some HIV-infected lymphocytes, and both forms of antibody have been associated with decreasing CD4+ cell numbers as infection advances.

The result of the immunologic perturbation is a defect in both cell- and antibody-mediated responses. In adults, the first defect predominates, and infection with intracellular pathogens such as fungi, protozoa, mycobacteria, and herpesvirus is characteristic of advanced HIV infection. The failure to produce specific antibody clinically is most significant in children and is associated with bacteremic infections due to encapsulated pyogenic organisms, such as *Streptococcus pneumoniae* and *Haemophilus influenzae*.

## DIAGNOSIS OF HIV INFECTION

Following the isolation of HIV-1, an immunoassay was developed to detect serum antibodies to the virus. The later formulations of the enzyme-linked immunoassay (EIA), originally developed to screen blood donors, are highly sensitive, able to detect more than 99% of infected individuals. The assays are also highly specific, giving a false-positive rate of less 1%. However, the estimated infection rate in such low-risk populations in the United States is 0.2% or less. Widespread testing in low-risk populations results in 5–10 persons falsely identified as infected for every truly infected individual. Therefore, a confirmatory assay is required before a definitive diagnosis of HIV-1 infection can be established. The most commonly used confirmatory test is the Western blot assay (Fig. 23–1). The EIA primarily detects antibody to the core protein, p24, and to the glycosylated envelope protein, gp41. The EIA is relatively inexpensive and is semiautomated. In contrast, the Western blot can detect antibody to all viral proteins but is more expensive and labor-intensive, relying upon a subjective interpretation by a technician. By consensus, the Western blot is not

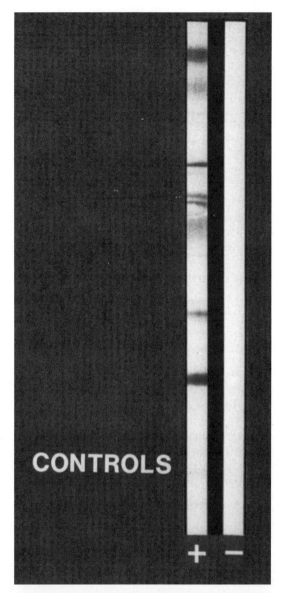

**FIGURE 23–1.** Positive and negative Western blot result. In the positive specimen on the left, serum has reacted with HIV proteins that have been separated by electrophoresis and transferred to a nitrocellulose paper strip. From the top, the bands represent antibody to gp160, gp120, p66, p55, p51, gp41, p24, and p17. The right lane shows that this normal (negative) serum does not react with any HIV antigen.

is as widely used as the Western blot, and neither offers an improvement in terms of convenience or expense.

A major limitation of the assays for HIV antibody is the variable length of time during which antibody cannot be detected in serum following infection. This period is analogous to the "window" seen in persons recently infected with hepatitis B virus. There have been documented instances of individuals in the window period donating blood that resulted in HIV-1 infection in recipients. It is presumed that sexual contact with a person in the window period also could result in transmission of HIV-1.

Other techniques are able to detect infection before antibody can be measured. Following infection and during the window period, the core protein, p24, circulates in blood for a period of several weeks and can be detected with an enzyme-linked assay using antibody for p24. Once antibody to the virus is produced by the infected patient, p24 is usually cleared from the blood. Studies of this assay's potential usefulness in blood donors and retrospective testing of stored serum obtained from high-risk individuals who later developed antibody indicate that this technique has limited utility as a means of detecting infected individuals who are antibody-negative. Virus also has been isolated by culture of peripheral blood lymphocytes from seronegative individuals at high risk of infection. In addition, the polymerase chain reaction (PCR) enzymatically can be used to amplify proviral DNA from lymphocytes or RNA from plasma of antibody-negative individuals before seroconversion.

## NATURAL HISTORY OF HIV-1 INFECTION

Following infection with HIV-1 there is a period of intense viral replication in the lymphoreticular tissues followed by viremia. With onset of the immune response, virus is cleared from the plasma but remains sequestered in the lymphoreticular system. As with many viral infections, at the onset of infection the proportion and number of CD8+ lymphocytes increase and the proportion and number of CD4+ lymphocytes decrease. Approximately 50% of individuals experience a self-limited mononucleosis-like syndrome manifested by fever, malaise, sore throat, and generalized lymphadenopathy. A few individ-

interpreted as positive unless there is evidence of antibody to products of at least two of the three major gene regions, gag, pol, or env. Blots that have no bands are negative, whereas those with bands but not enough to be diagnostic are termed indeterminate. Alternative confirmatory tests include a radioimmune precipitation assay (RIPA) and an immunofluorescent assay. At present neither

uals develop aseptic meningitis. A large number of HIV-1–infected individuals, however, are asymptomatic immediately after infection and remain asymptomatic for a prolonged period. A subset of asymptomatic individuals develop generalized lymphadenopathy.

During this period of clinical latency, there is an equilibrium between viral replication and host cell death; it is estimated that $10^9$ virions are produced every 24 h, and CD4+ lymphocytes are destroyed. The destruction of these cells is a consequence of direct viral replication or possibly of immune-mediated cytotoxic responses.

With time, the majority of infected individuals demonstrate a progressive decrease in numbers of CD4+ lymphocytes, but in some the numbers of these cells plateau at relatively normal values. Other infected persons demonstrate a rapid fall in CD4+ cell counts. The rapidity and degree of the decrease serves as an accurate prognostic indicator for the development of the opportunistic diseases that define AIDS. The normal helper T cells approximate $1000 \pm 300/mm^3$ in adults and represents 40–45% of T cells in the peripheral circulation. As infection progresses and CD4+ cell counts approach $200/mm^3$, symptoms such as unexplained fever, malaise, weight loss, diarrhea, oropharyngeal thrush, or hairy leukoplakia are noted in approximately one third of patients. At or below counts of $200/mm^3$ helper T cells, there is an increasing risk of developing *Pneumocystis carinii* pneumonia, or other AIDS-defining conditions.

In association with the fall in CD4+ cells, serum concentrations of beta$_2$-microglobulin and neopterin increase. Both are nonspecific markers of immune activation of lymphocytes and monocytes/macrophages. In addition, approximately 20–25% of HIV-infected persons with CD4+ cell counts between $200/mm^3$ and $400/mm^3$ demonstrate p24 antigen in serum in association with a decline in antibody to this core protein. Knowledge of the level of these markers adds prognostic information, because increases in p24 concentrations are associated with an increased risk of developing AIDS.

Although it is not known whether all HIV-infected adults will progress to AIDS, it has been estimated that 50% of those who do develop AIDS do so within 10 years and that up to 15% may be AIDS-free at 20 years. In adults, it is very uncommon to establish a diagnosis of AIDS within the first 12 months following seroconversion, and 90% of infected adults are AIDS-free 4 years after the appearance of specific antibody. Once an individual's CD4+ count approaches $200/mm^3$, the occurrence of fever and thrush adds significantly and independently to the risk of developing AIDS.

## TREATMENT OF HIV INFECTION

A rational approach to therapy should be based upon the goal of reducing the rate of viral replication. Early intervention could interact synergistically with immune surveillance, prolong the period of immune stability, and prevent clinical progression. Later intervention has a beneficial, although transitory, effect to lower viral burden but results in the selection of resistant viral mutants. If therapy in patients with advanced infection results in a mutant that is less capable of rapid replication, then clinical latency may be prolonged.

The substituted nucleosides, such as zidovudine (ZVD, AZT), zalcitabine (ddC), didanosine (ddI), stavudine (d4T), and lamivudine (3TC), inhibit the viral enzyme reverse transcriptase (RT) and terminal chain transcription. These agents interfere with transcription of proviral DNA from viral RNA that occurs after cellular internalization of the viral core. Although ZVD has been shown to have a virologic benefit when given to HIV-1 infected persons, clinical trials have documented that a combination of nucleoside RT inhibitors reduce viral burden more effectively than ZVD monotherapy. In addition, the combinations of ZVD plus ddI, and ZVD plus ddC, as well as ddI monotherapy decrease progression to AIDS or death more effectively than ZVD monotherapy.

Three protease inhibitors that block cleavage of the polyprotein that is the precursor of HIV-1 structural proteins and viral enzymes have been approved for clinical use. These agents, saquinavir, indinavir, and ritonavir, reduce viral burden dramatically as indicated by decreases in plasma levels of HIV-RNA. The combination of RT inhibitors and the protease inhibitors give promise of providing the most effective therapy for HIV-1 infection yet available.

Non-nucleoside RT inhibitors are also under study and should be available for use in the near future. These agents lower viral burden but select resistant virions within 4–8 weeks of initiation of therapy and will be used in combination with RT inhibitors and/or protease inhibitors.

The question of whether or not combination anti-retroviral therapy should be initiated during early HIV-1 infection or withheld until CD4+ lymphocyte counts drop to $500/mm^3$ remains unanswered but is the subject of intense study. Clearly, all infected persons with fewer than $500/mm^3$ CD4+ lymphocytes should have some combination of RT inhibitors with or without a protease inhibitor initiated.

All of the available antiretroviral agents are associated with adverse effects. ZVD and 3TC can suppress the bone marrow; ddI, ddC and d4T produce neuropathy; and ddI has been associated with pancreatitis. Indinavir therapy can lead to development of renal stones and asymptomatic hyperbilirubinemia, and ritonavir produces gastrointestinal side effects. Finally, all three protease inhibitors have an affinity for hepatic cytochrome P450 isoenzymes to varying degrees. This requires avoidance of administration, or alteration in dosage, of other drugs metabolized by these isoenzymes to reduce the possibility of potentially dangerous drug-drug interactions.

## MANAGEMENT OF OPPORTUNISTIC INFECTIONS

The most common AIDS-defining complication of HIV-1 infection during the first 10 years of the epidemic has been pneumonia due to *Pneumocystis carinii,* accounting for up to 55% of AIDS diagnoses. It is estimated that approximately 70% of patients with AIDS ultimately develop this form of pneumonia during their HIV-1 infection. Widespread use of prophylaxis has reduced the frequency of PCP, which represents a reactivation of infection originally established in early childhood. Eighty percent of children have serum antibody to *P. carinii* by age 6. Failure of the immune system allows replication of *Pneumocystis carinii* and development of pneumonia. Prophylaxis in the form of single monthly administration of pentamidine by aerosol or oral administration of trimethoprim-sulfamethoxazole (TMP/SMZ) or dapsone has proved effective. Inhaled pentamidine produces mild to moderate respiratory symptoms and is not as effective as the oral prophylactic regimens. The systemic agents, however, are associated with frequent allergic reactions. Prophylaxis

should be initiated in adults when the CD4+ cell count falls to $200/mm^3$.

Diagnosis of PCP requires a high degree of suspicion, for the pneumonitis can present as fever of unknown origin with or without respiratory symptoms or as a life-threatening pulmonary infection. Induction of sputum can be used to demonstrate the cysts of pneumocystis, but up to 50% of cases require bronchoscopy with lavage to demonstrate the agent. The chest x-ray can be normal but more commonly demonstrates bilateral interstitial pneumonia. Therapy is generally initiated with intravenous TMP/SMZ. The high rate of adverse reactions (approximately two thirds of patients develop rash, fever, or neutropenia) requires that intravenous pentamidine, trimetrexate, or the combination of clindamycin and primaquine frequently be substituted in order to complete the required 3 weeks of therapy. Adjunctive use of corticosteroids is associated with improved survival from an episode of acute PCP if begun within the first 2–3 days of antibiotic therapy. With early diagnosis and aggressive management, survival from an initial episode of PCP should approach 90%. Recurrent PCP has a higher mortality. All patients surviving PCP should receive prophylaxis to reduce the frequency of recurrences.

Cryptococcal meningitis and cerebral toxoplasmosis are treated with amphotericin B and sulfadiazine-pyrimethamine, respectively. These infections of the central nervous system should be suspected when an HIV-infected individual presents with headache or focal neurologic findings. Cerebral imaging techniques are utilized to detect masses due to toxoplasma or B-cell lymphoma. In the absence of such findings, a lumbar puncture should be performed to determine if cryptococcal antigen is present in the cerebrospinal fluid (CSF). This immunoassay is more sensitive than the India ink test to demonstrate the fungus in CSF. Culture for cryptococci and mycobacteria, as well as the usual cell counts and assays for protein and sugar, are also necessary. If the diagnosis of cryptococcal meningitis is established and initial treatment is successful, life-long maintenance fluconazole is required to prevent relapse.

Antibiotic therapy for presumptive cerebral toxoplasmosis should be administered for 2 weeks to individuals with multiple mass lesions identified by computed tomography (CT) or magnetic resonance imaging (MRI). After completion of the initial therapy, the CT or MRI should be repeated. If the lesions have diminished in size, a full course of treatment should be completed and followed by maintenance therapy to prevent relapse. If the lesions are unchanged after 7–10 days or if there is a solitary lesion, a brain biopsy is necessary to rule out cerebral lymphoma. The use of TMP/SMZ as prophylaxis for PCP also lowers the prevalence of toxoplasma infections in persons with advanced HIV infection. The combination of dapsone and pyrimethamine also is an effective form of prophylaxis for both toxoplasma cerebritis and PCP.

Infections due to herpes simplex or herpes zoster generally can be managed successfully with acyclovir. Acyclovir-resistant herpes simplex and herpes zoster increasingly have been isolated from HIV-infected patients. Such infections require treatment with foscarnet. Ganciclovir and foscarnet are now available for therapy of cytomegalovirus (CMV) infection. Although successful in slowing the progression of sight-threatening retinitis, discontinuation of an antiviral agent is associated with relapse. Unfortunately, ganciclovir therapy is not as effective in treatment of CMV pneumonitis and induces neutropenia when given with zidovudine. Although disseminated fungal infections such as histoplasmosis and blastomycosis can be treated successfully with amphotericin B and the triazole itraconazole, sufficient experience has accumulated to determine that maintenance therapy is required to prevent relapses. Disseminated mycobacterial infection due to tubercle bacilli can be managed with the usual antituberculous agents unless the organism is multi–drug-resistant. The most common mycobacterial infection in persons with AIDS is due to the MAC, organisms resistant to isoniazid and rifampin. Combination therapy with the macrolides, clarithromycin, or azythromycin plus ethambutol is associated with clinical improvement.

Opportunistic infections that cannot be cured because of the lack of effective agents include cryptosporidiosis, a protozoal infection of the gastrointestinal tract, and progressive multifocal leukoencephalopathy due to JC papovavirus.

## LATE MANIFESTATIONS OF HIV INFECTION AND AIDS

A problem unrelated to opportunistic infections is dementia directly resulting from HIV infection of the CNS. Studies indicate that neurologic manifestations are uncommon among HIV-infected individuals before the diagnosis of AIDS. However, up to 40% of persons with AIDS develop CNS disease, and a significant proportion is due to HIV encephalopathy. Ninety percent of autopsied cases show evidence of HIV effects upon the CNS, and CSF pleocytosis is common even in asymptomatic HIV-infected individuals. The neurons are not infected, although virus can be demonstrated in mononuclear phagocytes, microglia, and multinucleated giant cells of CNS. The pathogenesis of dementia has not been elucidated completely. The dementia presents with memory and motor defects, and in untreated patients progresses to coma and death in weeks or months. There are reports of responses to zidovudine therapy.

A second condition increasing in frequency is severe wasting. In Africa this is especially common and has been termed "slim disease." The pathogenesis of this manifestation of HIV infection is unknown but may be related to malabsorption due to viral effects upon the mucosal epithelial cells of the small intestine and/or alteration in metabolism resulting from this retroviral infection.

Other less common manifestations of HIV-1 infection include a poorly understood cardiomyopathy and renal disease. These conditions are more fully described in the later section, Pediatric HIV-1 Infection.

### Dermal Manifestations

A wide variety of skin diseases occur in HIV-infected persons. Some conditions are more common in HIV-1–infected persons such as KS, and others occur with greater severity such as psoriasis and seborrheic dermatitis. *Staphylococcus aureus* is the most common skin pathogen and is manifest as folliculitis, impetigo, ecthyma, cellulitis, or abscess formation. Bacillary angiomatosis due to infection with *Bartonella quintana* or *henselae* can be confused with KS. Infection with these organisms is also seen in bone, lymph nodes, and internal organs. Molluscum contagiosum represents an extremely common and persistent problem for HIV-1–infected individuals, requiring repeated cryotherapy or electrosurgery for control. The herpetic complications of HIV-1 infection have been discussed previously.

## NEOPLASTIC AND HEMATOLOGIC MANIFESTATIONS OF HIV INFECTION

Until the outbreak of AIDS, KS of endothelial cell origin was seen rarely in North America and Europe, occurring infrequently in men over the age of 60. The lesions are found on the lower extremities, and the disease is indolent in nature. In central Africa, in contrast, KS is most commonly seen in young men, is widely disseminated, and involves the viscera, including the bronchi and gastrointestinal tract. KS represents the second most common tumor of males in this region of Africa. The virulence of KS in persons with AIDS resembles that of the African type. In the decade before the recognition of AIDS, KS was increasingly reported in patients with renal allografts, emphasizing the role of an altered immune response in the pathogenesis of this tumor. Although KS is used to establish the diagnosis of AIDS, there is recent evidence to indicate that it is due to infection with a second sexually transmitted agent, possibly a member of the herpes virus family, and can occur in the absence of HIV-1 infection in homosexual or bisexual men.

B-cell lymphomas have become increasingly prevalent as a presenting, AIDS-defining condition as effective prophylaxis for opportunistic infections is implemented. Similar neoplastic complications have been recorded in transplant patients. Epstein-Barr virus co-infection accounts for a subset of B-cell lymphomas of the CNS that occur as a result of the profound immunosuppression induced by HIV.

Thrombocytopenia mediated by immunologic mechanisms is also common in advanced HIV disease. Autoantibodies directed at either platelet antigens or immune complexes adhering to the platelet surface have been demonstrated in thrombocytopenic HIV-infected persons. Some patients with thrombocytopenia respond to antiretroviral therapy with increases in platelet counts.

## PEDIATRIC HIV-1 INFECTION

### Transmission

One of the major features differentiating HIV infection in children from that in adults is the mode of transmission. Among children younger than 13 years of age who have AIDS, more than 90% have been perinatally infected during gestation or delivery from an HIV-seropositive mother.

Perinatal HIV transmission occurs by three routes: (1) transplacental infection *in utero,* (2) exposure to blood and cervical secretions during delivery, and (3) postpartum ingestion of breast milk containing the virus. *In utero* HIV infection has been demonstrated by isolating the virus from aborted 13- to 20-week fetuses. The virus has been isolated from cord blood, and the placenta has been shown to contain cell-surface CD4 that serves as receptor for HIV. Therefore, HIV may directly infect the placenta, facilitating transplacental spread of the virus. The ability to recover HIV from cervical secretions supports the possibility of intrapartum transmission, similar to the mechanism seen in infection by hepatitis B virus. Although both free and cell-associated virus have been detected in breast milk from HIV-infected mothers, the least common route of vertical transmission is breast feeding. A metaanalysis of several prospective studies found that the additional risk of transmission through breast feeding by women with established HIV infection is 14%. In contrast, in women who breast-feed after acquiring HIV postnatally, the risk was 29%. This suggests that the maternal viremia during primary infection places the infant at an increased risk of infection. It is recommended that HIV-infected mothers in the United States refrain from breast-feeding; however, in developing countries, where it is the cornerstone of infant nutrition and prophylaxis against diarrheal disease, the advantages of breast-feeding appear to outweigh the risk.

The rate of HIV transmission from infected mother to infant has been studied in numerous centers throughout the world and approximates 25%. Risk factors influencing the rate of vertical transmission are incompletely defined. Several prospective studies have identified maternal features that appear to promote transmission, including p24 antigenemia, depressed CD4 counts ($<700/mm^3$), increased CD8 counts ($>1800/mm^3$), placental membrane inflammation, and delivery before 34 weeks' gestation. Although several studies showed increased transmission rates with advanced maternal disease stage or AIDS, many transmitting mothers in each series were asymptomatic.

Important recent data suggest that interruption of perinatal transmission is possible. A multicenter, placebo-controlled trial utilizing ZDV therapy in pregnant women as early as 14 weeks' gestation through delivery and in their newborns for the first 6 weeks of life demonstrated reduction of the rate of vertical transmission from 25.5% in the placebo recipients to 8.3% in ZDV recipients. Toxicity from ZDV in both the mothers and infants was minimal. Studies utilizing HIV-antibody concentrate (HIVIG) to reduce perinatal transmission further are in progress. In addition, several reports evaluating the route of delivery demonstrated a slightly decreased transmission rate among women delivered by cesarean section, although the difference was marginal statistically.

Transfusions of infected blood and/or blood products have accounted for 9% of pediatric AIDS cases diagnosed through 1994. The period of highest risk of exposure to HIV was between 1978 and 1985, prior to the availability of HIV antibody–screened blood products. Surveys among hemophiliacs followed between 1985 and 1989 found that 70% with severe factor VIII deficiency and 50% with severe factor IX deficiency were HIV-seropositive. However, since 1984 with heat-treatment of factor VIII concentrate, and since 1985 with HIV antibody screening, HIV transmission has been virtually eliminated from this population.

Although HIV rarely can be isolated from saliva, it is present in very low titer (<1 infectious particle/mL) and has not been implicated as a vehicle for transmission. Studies of household contacts of HIV-infected adults, children, toddlers, and infants have found that HIV has not been transmitted through nonsexual contact. Rare instances of household transmission have been documented when there was contact with blood.

In the pediatric population, sexual contact is an infrequent route of HIV transmission, but some cases resulting from sexual abuse have been reported. In contrast, sexual contact is a major route of transmission in the adolescent population, responsible for more than one third of cases.

## DIAGNOSIS

Demonstration of IgG antibody to HIV by a repeatedly reactive EIA and confirmatory test (e.g., Western blot or immunofluorescence assay) establishes the diagnosis of HIV infection in any child at least 18 months of age. In younger infants, diagnosis is more difficult because maternal HIV antibody passively crosses the placenta during gestation, and serum tests for IgG antibody to HIV do not differentiate between maternal and infant antibody. Virtually all infants born to HIV-infected mothers have a positive HIV antibody test at birth, but most infants who are not infected will lose maternal antibody between 6

and 12 months of age. Because a small proportion of uninfected infants continue to test HIV antibody–positive for up to 18 months, IgG antibody tests cannot be used to make a definitive diagnosis of HIV infection in infants under this age. In contrast, the presence of IgA or IgM anti-HIV in the infant's circulation can indicate HIV infection, as these immunoglobulin classes do not cross the placenta. However, because detectable serum IgA anti-HIV is not generally present until 3–6 months of age, this test is less useful in young infants (sensitivity 50–60% at 3 months and 60–100% at 6 months). IgM anti-HIV assays have been both insensitive and nonspecific and need further improvement before being useful clinically.

Tests that identify viral presence, such as HIV culture and HIV DNA or RNA PCR, are considerably more valuable in young infants. These tests are highly specific (>98%) and have sensitivity of 40–50% in the first month of life, 80–100% by 2–3 months, and 90–100% by 6 months. Demonstration of p24 antigen in the infant's blood, also very specific, is limited by the test's low sensitivity; p24 antigen is often bound by the high levels of maternally derived antibody to produce immune complexes that are undetectable by the standard p24 antigen assays. A modification of the test in which immune complexes are dissociated and then p24 is sought has improved the sensitivity of the test to 85% by 3 months and greater than 90% by 6 months of age.

## Clinical Manifestations

Early reports describing the natural history of perinatally acquired HIV infection were primarily retrospective series of children who had an early onset of symptoms and were therefore biased towards more rapidly progressive disease. More recent longitudinal studies have demonstrated a bimodal distribution of disease expression, with 20–30% of HIV-infected children developing significant immune deficiency and AIDS-defining illnesses before the age of 1 year and two thirds having a more slowly progressive course with at least 5-year survival.

The CDC has developed a pediatric HIV classification system to stratify the clinical stage of disease and degree of immunologic impairment (Table 23–1). Among the clinical categories, "mildly symptomatic" (A) includes children with nonspecific findings such as lymphadenopathy, parotitis, hepatosplenomegaly and recurrent/persistent sinusitis or otitis media. "Moderately symptomatic" (B)

## TABLE 23–1. PEDIATRIC HUMAN IMMUNODEFICIENCY VIRUS (HIV) CLASSIFICATION*

| IMMUNOLOGIC CATEGORIES | CLINICAL CATEGORIES | | | |
|---|---|---|---|---|
| | N: NO SIGNS/ SYMPTOMS | A: MILD SIGNS/ SYMPTOMS | B: MODERATE SIGNS/ SYMPTOMS[†] | C. SEVERE SIGNS/ SYMPTOMS[†] |
| 1. No evidence of suppression | N1 | A1 | B1 | C1 |
| 2. Evidence of moderate suppression | N2 | A2 | B2 | C2 |
| 3. Severe suppression | N3 | A3 | B3 | C3 |

*Children whose HIV infection status is not confirmed are classified by using the above grid with a letter E (for perinatally exposed) placed before the appropriate classification code (e.g., EN2).
[†]Both category C and lymphoid interstitial pneumonitis in category B are reportable to state and local health departments as acquired immunodeficiency syndrome.

includes children with a variety of organ-specific dysfunctions and/or infections, and "severely symptomatic" (C) includes children with illnesses fitting the 1987 CDC definition of AIDS. Children whose HIV infection is not yet confirmed are classified using the same clinical categories with a letter E (vertically exposed) placed in front of the classification (e.g., E/N2).

The immune category classification is based on the absolute CD4 count or the percentage of CD4 cells (CD4 percent) (Table 23–2). Age adjustment of the absolute CD4 count is necessary because normal counts, which are relatively high in infants, decline steadily until 6 years of age, when they reach adult norms.

The spectrum of clinical manifestations of HIV infection is quite variable in infants and children, with the majority having a normal physical examination at birth. Presenting symptoms may be subtle, such as failure to thrive, lymphadenopathy and hepatosplenomegaly, diarrhea, interstitial pneumonitis, and oral thrush, and may be notable only for their persistence. Recurrent bacterial infections, chronic parotid swelling, lymphocytic interstitial pneumonitis (LIP), and the early onset of progressive neurologic deterioration are characteristic of children with AIDS but are less common in adults.

### Infections

One of the more common problems associated with HIV infection in children is recurrent bacterial infections, such as pneumonia, sepsis, and meningitis. Encapsulated organisms, such as *Streptococcus pneumoniae* and *Haemophilus influenzae*, are most commonly observed—a pattern similar to that seen in primary antibody deficiency syndromes. A laboratory hallmark of pediatric HIV infection is polyclonal hypergammaglobulinemia; however, paradoxically, many symptomatic HIV-infected children fail to mount primary or secondary antibody responses to antigens they have not previously encountered. Recurrent hematogenous infections occur in approximately 20% of children with AIDS, whereas these infections are considerably more rare in adults.

Opportunistic infections (OIs) begin to occur as the CD4 count declines. In adults, OIs usually represent reactivation of a latent infection acquired early in life. In contrast, young children generally experience primary infection and, lacking prior immunity, have a more fulminant course of disease. This principle is best illustrated by PCP, the most common OI in the pediatric population. The peak incidence of PCP occurs between the ages of 3 and 6 months, with a median survival of 1

## TABLE 23–2. IMMUNOLOGIC CATEGORIES BASED ON AGE-SPECIFIC CD4+ T-LYMPHOCYTE COUNTS AND PERCENT OF TOTAL LYMPHOCYTES

| IMMUNOLOGIC CATEGORY | <12 MONTHS* | | 1–5 YEARS* | | 6–12 YEARS* | |
|---|---|---|---|---|---|---|
| | $\mu L$ | (%) | $\mu L$ | (%) | $\mu L$ | (%) |
| 1. No evidence of suppression | ≥1500 | (≥25) | ≥1000 | (≥25) | ≥500 | (≥25) |
| 2. Evidence of moderate suppression | 750–1499 | (15–24) | 500–999 | (15–24) | 200–499 | (15–24) |
| 3. Severe suppression | <750 | (<15) | <500 | (<15) | <200 | (<15) |

*Age of child.

month. The classic clinical presentation of PCP includes acute onset of fever, tachypnea, dyspnea, and marked hypoxemia. Chest x-ray findings include interstitial infiltrates or diffuse alveolar disease; however, nodular lesions, lobar infiltrates, or effusions may occasionally be seen. Diagnosis is made by demonstration of *P. carinii* in bronchoalveolar lavage fluid; rarely, an open lung biopsy is necessary.

Atypical mycobacterial infection, particularly with MAC, has been diagnosed with increasing frequency as HIV-infected children live longer, with the incidence estimated to be 24% in children with fewer than 100 CD4 cells/$mm^3$. Disseminated MAC infection is characterized by fever, malaise, night sweats, and weight loss; diarrhea, anemia, and granulocytopenia are often present. Diagnosis is made by isolation of MAC from blood, bone marrow, or tissue. While the contribution of MAC infection to mortality is not well established, it is a major contributor to morbidity.

Oral candidiasis is the most common fungal infection seen in HIV-infected children. It progresses to involve the esophagus in approximately 20% of children, causing anorexia, dysphagia, vomiting, and fever. Intestinal cryptosporidiosis is another OI that occurs commonly. Although a self-limited infection in healthy hosts, it causes severe chronic diarrhea and malnutrition in HIV-infected children. Infection persists indefinitely, especially in children with significantly depressed CD4 counts, as there is no effective therapy for this agent. Medications that have been used empirically, such as spiramycin or paromomycin, have been only partially effective.

Viral infections, especially herpes viruses, pose significant problems for HIV-infected children. Herpes simplex virus (HSV) causes recurrent gingivostomatitis, which may be complicated by local and distant cutaneous dissemination. Primary varicella-zoster virus (VZV) infection (chickenpox) may be severe, prolonged, and complicated by bacterial superinfection or visceral dissemination, including life-threatening pneumonitis. Recurrent, atypical, or chronic episodes of herpes zoster are often debilitating and require prolonged therapy with acyclovir; in rare instances, VZV has developed resistance to acyclovir in this setting, requiring the use of foscarnet. CMV infection occurs after severe CD4 depletion (usually <50/$mm^3$) and may involve any organ. Epstein-Barr virus (EBV) seropositivity is common and has been postulated to be etiologically related to LIP, parotitis, non-Hodg-

kin's lymphoma, and soft tissue tumors such as leiomyoma and leiomyosarcoma. Measles may occur despite previous immunization; it can present without a typical rash and is generally fatal when it disseminates to the lung or brain.

### Central Nervous System

The prevalence of CNS involvement in vertically infected children is estimated to be 20–50%, and it may be the initial manifestation of the disease. The most common presentation is progressive encephalopathy with loss or plateau of developmental milestones, cognitive deterioration, and impaired brain growth. With progression, apathy, spasticity, and weakness may occur, as well as loss of language and motor skills. The encephalopathy may progress intermittently with periods of deterioration followed by transiently stable plateaus. Associated abnormalities identified by neuroimaging techniques include cerebral atrophy, basal ganglia calcifications and, less frequently, leukomalacia.

### Respiratory Tract

Recurrent upper respiratory tract infections such as otitis media and sinusitis are common. Although the etiologic agents are usually the same as those in normal children, unusual pathogens (e.g., *P. aeruginosa* and anaerobes) may be present in chronic infections and result in complications such as mastoiditis.

LIP is the most common chronic lower respiratory tract abnormality, occurring in one fourth to one third of children with AIDS. LIP is a chronic interstitial process with nodular lymphoid hyperplasia in the bronchial and bronchiolar epithelium that often leads to progressive alveolar-capillary block over months to years. Its characteristic persistent diffuse reticulonodular pattern allows a presumptive diagnosis to be made radiologically before the onset of symptoms in most instances. Clinically, there is insidious onset of tachypnea, cough, and mild to moderate hypoxemia with normal auscultatory findings or minimal rales. Progressive disease is accompanied by digital clubbing and symptomatic hypoxemia that often responds to oral corticosteroid therapy. The etiology of LIP is not well established, although several studies suggest that it is associated with a primary EBV infection in the setting of HIV infection. EBV capsid antibody titers typically are elevated, and EBV

DNA has been found in lung tissue of children with LIP.

Infectious complications of the lung are common, and bacterial pneumonias occur frequently. *S. pneumoniae* is the most common pathogen, but gram-negative bacteria may also be a problem. PCP is the most common opportunistic infection, but other pathogens include CMV, aspergillus, cryptococcus, and histoplasma. Common respiratory viruses, including respiratory syncytial virus, parainfluenza, influenza, and adenovirus, may occur simultaneously and have a protracted course. Pulmonary and extrapulmonary tuberculosis have been reported with increasing frequency in HIV-infected children, but are considerably more common in HIV-infected adults.

### Cardiovascular System

The incidence of cardiac disease in HIV infection has not been well established, but approximately 20% of HIV-infected children have some cardiac involvement. The pathogenesis of cardiomyopathy may be multifactorial including pulmonary insufficiency, anemia, nutritional deficiencies (e.g., selenium), specific viral infections such as CMV, immunologic disturbances, and drug toxicities. Left ventricular dysfunction appears to be the most common cardiac manifestation, followed by congestive heart failure, dilated cardiomyopathy, arrhythmias, and rarely, pericardial effusion and coronary arteriopathy. Electrocardiography and echocardiography may be helpful in assessing cardiac function before the onset of clinical symptoms.

### Gastrointestinal and Hepatobiliary Tract

The gastrointestinal (GI) tract is commonly involved in HIV infection. AIDS enteropathy, a syndrome of malabsorption with partial villous atrophy not associated with a specific pathogen, has been postulated to be a result of direct HIV infection of the gut. In addition, a variety of pathogens characteristically cause GI disease including bacteria (salmonella, nontuberculous mycobacteria, campylobacter), protozoa (cryptosporidia, microsporidia, isospora, giardia), viruses (CMV, rotavirus), and fungi (candida). Infections may be localized or disseminated and may affect any part of the GI tract. The most common GI symptoms are chronic or recurrent diarrhea with malabsorption, abdominal pain, dysphagia, and failure to thrive (FTT). The "wasting syndrome," a loss of more than 10% of body weight, is not as common as FTT in pediatric patients.

Chronic liver inflammation manifested by fluctuating serum levels of transaminases with or without cholestasis is relatively common, often without identification of an etiologic agent. In some patients, chronic hepatitis caused by CMV, hepatitis B or C, or nontuberculous mycobacteria may lead to portal hypertension and liver failure. Antiretroviral drugs such as ZDV and ddI may also cause reversible elevation of transaminases.

Pancreatitis with elevated serum pancreatic enzyme levels may be the result of drug therapy (e.g., pentamidine or ddI) or, rarely, opportunistic infection.

### Renal Disease

AIDS nephropathy is an unusual presenting symptom of HIV infection, more commonly occurring in older symptomatic children. A wide range of histologic abnormalities has been reported: focal glomerulosclerosis, mesangial hyperplasia, segmental necrotizing glomerulonephritis, and minimal change disease. Nephrotic syndrome is the most common manifestation of renal disease with edema, hypoalbuminemia, proteinuria, and azotemia with normal blood pressure. Children with focal glomerulosclerosis generally progress to renal failure within 6 months to 1 year, but those with other histologic abnormalities may be stable for prolonged periods of time.

### Skin

Many cutaneous manifestations seen in HIV-infected children are inflammatory or infectious disorders that are also common in healthy children. These disorders tend to be more widespread and respond less consistently to conventional therapy than in the well child. Seborrheic dermatitis, eczema, recurrent or chronic episodes of HSV, herpes zoster, molluscum contagiosum, anogenital warts, and candidal infection are common and may be difficult to control. Allergic drug eruptions are also common, in particular related to sulfonamides, and generally respond to withdrawal of the drug.

### Neoplastic and Hematologic Manifestations

In contrast to adults, malignancies have been reported infrequently in HIV-infected children, representing only 2% of AIDS-defining illnesses. It is likely, however, that the incidence of malignancies will increase as more children are infected and their life expectancy is prolonged. Non-Hodgkin's lymphoma and primary CNS lymphoma are the most commonly reported malignancies in children. Recently, there have been several reports of multiple soft tissue tumors such as leiomyoma, leiomyosarcoma, and rhabdosarcoma in HIV-infected children. Kaposi's sarcoma is exceedingly uncommon in the pediatric population.

Hematologic abnormalities are common and are caused by multiple factors including bone marrow suppression by HIV and by other infections, malnutrition, and adverse reactions to drugs. Thrombocytopenia, anemia, leukopenia, and/or granulocytopenia occur frequently, even in otherwise asymptomatic HIV-infected children. Autoimmune thrombocytopenia may be the presenting manifestation of HIV and is usually responsive to antiretroviral drugs or intravenous immunoglobulin (IVIG) with or without corticosteroids. Anemia may be drug-induced (ZDV, dapsone, or antibiotics), or the result of iron or vitamin $B_{12}$ deficiency or chronic infection. Neutropenia may also be drug-induced or due to chronic infection, and absolute lymphopenia occurs less frequently in the pediatric population than in HIV-infected adults.

## PROGNOSIS

In children with perinatal infection, survival from the onset of clinical disease depends on multiple factors. Factors associated with a poor prognosis include onset of symptoms before the first birthday, opportunistic infections (especially infantile PCP), and progressive encephalopathy. Laboratory findings suggesting disease progression are absolute CD4 lymphopenia, hypogammaglobulinemia, and progressively elevated p24 antigen levels in the blood.

### Specific Therapy

Although there has been great progress in our understanding of the pathogenesis of HIV and its disease manifestations, the currently available treatments against HIV are quite limited. All experts agree that antiretroviral therapy should be offered to HIV-infected children with evidence of significant immunodeficiency or HIV-associated symptoms. The major parameter reflecting significant immunodeficiency is a depressed CD4 lymphocyte count. Because normal CD4 counts

in young children are higher than in adults, the following thresholds for initiation of antiretroviral therapy are recommended:

1. For infants <1 year of age: <1750 CD4 cells/mm$^3$.
2. For infants 1–2 years of age: <1000 CD4 cells/mm$^3$.
3. For children 2–6 years of age: <750 CD4 cells/mm$^3$.
4. For children >6 years of age: <500 CD4 cells/mm$^3$.

Regardless of the CD4 count, any symptom that fulfills the CDC criteria for AIDS (i.e., encephalopathy, opportunistic infections, severe failure to thrive or wasting syndrome, recurrent severe bacterial infections, and HIV-associated malignancy) is considered an indication for specific therapy. Thrombocytopenia (<75,000/$\mu$L) and hypogammaglobulinemia (IgG <250 mg/dL) are also indications to begin antiretroviral therapy. There is some controversy about whether to initiate antiretroviral therapy in HIV-infected children who present with LIP, parotitis, persistent thrush, recurrent or persistent diarrhea, cardiomegaly, nephrotic syndrome, neutropenia (<750/$\mu$L), or severe anemia (Hgb <7g/dL). In these cases, most experts agree that, if the potential benefit from antiretroviral therapy seems to be greater than its potential side effects, therapy should be offered.

ZDV is the antiretroviral with the greatest clinical experience in pediatrics, and historically has been used as first-line therapy. However, preliminary results of a multicenter treatment protocol performed by the AIDS Clinical Trial Group have caused clinicians to rethink this approach. This study compared ZDV monotherapy, ddI monotherapy, and the combination of ZDV plus ddI in children with symptomatic HIV infection; those children receiving ZDV monotherapy experienced more rapid disease progression and drug toxicity than those in the other two treatment arms. There was no survival difference for subjects receiving the three treatment regimens. While there is no consensus regarding the antiretroviral drug of choice at this writing, most clinicians prescribe ddI or ddI plus ZDV for children with symptomatic HIV infection. It is important to recognize that this study did not evaluate prevention of vertical transmission or treatment of asymptomatic infants and children, where ZDV may still play a major role. Another drug that may be used in combination with ZDV is ddC, although there is considerably less pediatric experience with this agent.

New agents being investigated in HIV-infected children include nonnucleoside reverse transcriptase inhibitors and protease inhibitors.

## Supportive and General Treatment

Children who are HIV infected should be followed closely by a multidisciplinary team of specialists. Frequent checkups promote early recognition of neurologic deterioration or failure to thrive. Aggressive nutritional support is very important, with calorie-enriched formulas, supplemental nasogastric feedings and, in some cases, intravenous hyperalimentation. Diphtheria, pertussis, and tetanus immunizations should proceed normally, and the inactivated polio vaccine should be substituted for the live attenuated (oral) polio vaccine (see Chapter 40). Because of the severe morbidity and mortality associated with measles in these children, it has been recommended that most HIV-infected children receive the measles-mumps-rubella vaccine, regardless of their degree of immune deficiency, even though it is a live virus vaccine. *Haemophilus influenzae* type b vaccine should be given on a routine schedule, and pneumococcal vaccine at 2 years in an effort to prevent some of the invasive infections common in pediatric AIDS. It is important to recognize, however, that the antibody response to many of these immunizations may be impaired.

## Prophylaxis against Specific Infections

Prevention of PCP is one of the most important goals of HIV management. Because the peak age at which PCP has occurred in the pediatric population (3–6 months) is often before a definitive diagnosis of HIV infection has been established, guidelines for initiation of PCP prophylaxis were issued in 1991. These recommendations were based on age-related changes in normal CD4 lymphocyte values in the first years of life and on studies that correlated CD4 counts in infants with development of PCP. Unfortunately, PCP cases continue to occur sporadically in infants younger than 1 year of age with CD4 counts above the threshold for prophylaxis. Therefore, revised guidelines indicate that all infants between 6 weeks and 1 year of age either (1) born to HIV-infected mothers or (2) proved to be HIV infected should receive prophylaxis regardless of the CD4 count or percentage (Table 23–3). When the infant is older than 1 year of age the previously established guidelines should be utilized. The best prophylactic regimen is $150/750$ mg/m$^2$/day

### TABLE 23–3. RECOMMENDATIONS FOR PCP PROPHYLAXIS AND MONITORING OF CD4+ CELL NUMBERS FOR HIV-EXPOSED INFANTS AND HIV-INFECTED CHILDREN

| AGE | PCP PROPHYLAXIS | CD+ MONITORING |
|---|---|---|
| Birth to 4–6 weeks | No prophylaxis | 1, 3, 6, 9, 12 months of age |
| 4–6 weeks to 4 months | Prophylaxis for all | 1, 3, 6, 9, 12 months of age |
| 4–12 months | Prophylaxis for all | 1, 3, 6, 9, 12 months of age |
|   HIV-infected or indeterminate | | |
|   HIV infection reasonably excluded* | No prophylaxis | None |
| 1–5 years, HIV-infected | Prophylaxis if CD4+ count <500 or CD4+ percent <15%[†‡] | Every 3–4 months[§] |
| 6–12 years, HIV-infected | Prophylaxis if CD4+ count <500 or CD4+ percent <15%[‡] | Every 3–4 months |

*≥2 negative HIV diagnostic tests (culture or PCR), both of which are performed at ≥1 month of age and one of which is performed at ≥4 months of age, or ≥2 negative HIV IgG antibody tests performed at >6 months of age in a child who has no clinical evidence for HIV disease.

[†]Children 1–2 years of age who were on PCP prophylaxis and had a CD4+ count >750 or percent >15% in the first year of life should continue on prophylaxis.

[‡]Prophylaxis should be considered on a case-by-case basis for children who may otherwise be at risk for PCP, such as children with rapidly declining CD4+ counts or percents with category C conditions (16).

[§]More frequent monitoring (e.g., monthly) is recommended for children whose CD4+ counts or percents are approaching the threshold of prophylaxis.

of TMP/SMZ divided into two daily doses 3 days a week. For severe adverse reactions to TMP/SMZ, alternative therapies include dapsone, aerosolized or intravenous pentamidine, or possibly atovaquone (which is currently being tested in children).

Intravenous gammaglobulin was used empirically for prophylaxis against recurrent bacterial infections during the late 1980s, and a subsequent placebo-controlled trial found that it was beneficial in children whose CD4 count was above $200/mm^3$. However, a recent study found that in HIV-infected children taking ZDV who also received TMP/SMZ for PCP prophylaxis, monthly IVIG provided no additional benefit in preventing serious bacterial infections.

## Social Issues

The social complexities of treating a child with AIDS are frequently formidable. Many infected children have parents who live in poverty, are ill or dying, or have a history of drug abuse. The variety of medical specialties necessary to care for a medically complex child may be overwhelming to the parent, and the financial burdens may be staggering. Finally, many families feel isolated. For these reasons, the role of the social worker in coordinating the care of a child with AIDS may be equally important to that of the medical providers.

The issues that relate to infected adolescents are different. Although only several hundred teenagers in the United States between the ages of 13 and 19 years have been recorded as having AIDS, the 10-year median incubation period in adults suggests that 15% of adult HIV infections were acquired during adolescence. The risk-taking attitudes of teenagers and the growing number of teen runaways (many of whom engage in prostitution to support themselves) signal this as a target population for whom education on AIDS prevention is critical.

## CASE HISTORIES

### Case History 1

A 35-year-old homosexual man is seen for advice regarding possible exposure to HIV. He is asymptomatic, but has a history of repeated sexual contacts with individuals who are infected. Serologic studies reveal a positive EIA for antibody to HIV that is confirmed by Western blot. T-cell phenotyping demonstrates that CD4 (helper T) cells account for 22% of his peripheral blood lympho-

cytes; the absolute CD4 count is $360/mm^3$. The proportion of CD8 (T-cytotoxic) cells is 33% with an absolute count of $540/mm^3$. A repeat study 1 month later reveals similar T-cell proportions and numbers. Although offered therapy with zidovudine (ZVD or AZT) he refuses because he is asymptomatic and worried about adverse effects. Repeat evaluation in 3 months reveals a decrease in the CD4 cell number to $300/mm^3$. Physical examination now reveals thrush. He again refuses AZT therapy. Prophylaxis to prevent PCP is discussed, and he agrees to take TMP/SMZ daily. In addition, a course of ketoconazole is begun to treat oropharyngeal candidiasis. Three months later he is asymptomatic, but the CD4 count is $270/mm^3$. With the evidence that the CD4 number is continuing to fall, he agrees to begin AZT at 500 mg/day. Two weeks later he reports mild nausea but otherwise no difficulties with the therapy, and his hemoglobin has remained stable. One month later, however, he reports development of a rash over his back and chest that is associated with itching and fever. He is diagnosed as hypersensitive to TMP/SMZ, and monthly aerosolized pentamidine is substituted for the oral antibiotic. With AZT therapy, the CD4 cell count has risen to $400/mm^3$, and with clearance of the drug rash he feels well. He is monitored by obtaining an interval history, physical examination, CD4 counts, and complete blood counts every 3 months for the next 15 months. At that point his CD4 count drops to $200/mm^3$. Serologic studies reveal the presence of p24 HIV antigen. The decision is made to discontinue AZT and begin therapy with ddI. The patient is warned about the possible development of peripheral neuropathy and pancreatitis with this inhibitor of viral reverse transcriptase. He tolerates the drug, p24 antigenemia clears, and the CD4 count rises to $280/mm^3$.

### Case 1 Discussion

This case illustrates the prolonged course and need for close monitoring of HIV-infected patients. The psychologic problems of acceptance of potentially toxic therapy is an issue the physician must consider. In addition to anti-HIV therapy, treatment of intercurrent infections and institution of prophylaxis is indicated at specific times in the natural history of the infection. Generally, PCP prophylaxis is indicated in adult patients with fewer than $200/mm^3$ CD4 cells; however, the risk of PCP is great in individuals who have CD4 counts between 200 and $350/mm^3$ and who also have minor infections, such as thrush. Many physicians, therefore, begin PCP prophylaxis before the CD4 cell count reaches $200/mm^3$. AZT is effective in stabilizing the immunodepletion induced by HIV for 12–24 months. Resistance through mutation of the viral reverse transcriptase is associated with declining efficacy of the drug, as manifested by a decrease in CD4 cell number and development of antigenemia. Fortunately, the newer substituted nucleosides, such as ddC and ddI, continue to be effective inhibitors of reverse transcriptase and can be substituted for AZT. With time it is likely that this patient will develop a serious complication of HIV-induced immunosuppression, such as disseminated fungal infection, lymphoma, HIV-wasting syndrome, or encephalopathy, despite antiretroviral therapy.

## CASE HISTORY 2

A 15-month-old boy is referred for evaluation of recurrent infections. He was the 7-lb, 8-oz full-term product of an uncomplicated pregnancy and delivery, born to a 23-year-old single woman who had no known risk factors for HIV infection. In the first year of life, the baby experienced four episodes of diarrhea, recurrent otitis media, and one episode of bronchiolitis. He grew parallel to the fifth percentile curve, although his weight and height were never greater than the fifth percentile. At 14 months of age, he developed a fever of 104°F without localizing signs, and a blood culture revealed *S. pneumoniae*. He recovered uneventfully with intravenous penicillin and was referred for evaluation.

On initial examination the child was small for his age, but appeared healthy. Remarkable physical findings included dull tympanic membranes, mild bilateral parotid enlargement, and diffuse lymphadenopathy measuring 0.5–1 cm in the anterior and posterior cervical chains and in the axillary and inguinal regions. Pulmonary and cardiac examinations were normal, and the liver and spleen were enlarged (5 cm and 3 cm below the costal margins, respectively). The diaper area revealed an erythematous rash typical of candida infection. Neurologic examination revealed decreased tone and inability to stand unsupported.

Laboratory examination revealed a WBC of $8600/mm^3$ with a normal differential, hemoglobin of 9.5 g/dL, and positive HIV antibody by EIA and Western blot. Serum immunoglobulins revealed IgG of 1696 mg/dL (normal is 345–1213 mg/dL), and the total CD4 count was $1044/mm^3$. Chest x-ray revealed a diffuse bilateral reticulonodular pattern involving all lobes of the lung, but a pulse oximetry test demonstrated normal blood oxygen saturation.

ddI therapy was initiated, and the child was followed monthly. Three months later, he developed another bacteremic illness with *S. pneumoniae* and was again treated uneventfully with antibiotics. A screening chest x-ray at 20 months of age revealed an increase in the reticulonodular infiltrates, which was not associated with pulmonary symptoms.

When the parents of the child were tested for HIV antibody, the mother was found to be positive by EIA and Western blot; the father was negative. The mother then recalled that a previous sexual partner may have used recreational drugs and, therefore, may have been HIV infected.

## CASE 2 DISCUSSION

This case illustrates a variety of features of pediatric HIV infection. Many HIV-positive women, especially those who are asymptomatic, may not recognize that they have been exposed to HIV through sexual contact and, therefore, do not report having risk factors. It is not uncommon for the child to be the first family member recognized to be HIV-positive. Developmental delay and recurrent diarrhea accompanied by poor growth in the first year of life are common presentations of perinatally acquired HIV infection. One of the hallmarks of pediatric HIV infection is recurrent serious bacterial infections. Although antiretroviral therapy appears to lessen the frequency of some opportunistic infections, it does not modify the frequency of bacterial infections. Helper T-cell counts in normal children tend to be higher than those in adults and may be correspondingly higher in HIV-infected children than in HIV-infected adults. Although a helper T-cell count of $1044/mm^3$ is not normal for a child this age, it is not so low that he is at particularly high risk for an opportunistic infection. Children with LIP are more likely to have generalized enlargement of the salivary glands and lymph nodes and may remain asymptomatic for prolonged periods despite marked chest x-ray abnormalities. It is highly likely that this child will eventually develop poor oxygenation and respiratory distress as a result of progressive LIP, but this usually can be successfully reversed with administration of systemic corticosteroids, such as prednisone.

## REFERENCES

### Books

Leoung, G., and Mills, J., eds. *Opportunistic Infections in Patients with Acquired Immunodeficiency Syndrome.* New York and Basel: Marcel Dekker, Inc., 1989.

Levy, J. A., ed. *AIDS Pathogenesis and Treatment.* New York and Basel: Marcel Dekker, Inc., 1989.

Yogev, R., and Connor, E., eds. *Management of HIV Infection in Infants and Children.* St. Louis: Mosby Year Book, Inc., 1992.

Pizzo, P. A., and Wilfert, C. M., eds. *Pediatric AIDS.* 2nd ed. Baltimore, MD: Williams & Wilkins, 1994.

Sande, M. A., and Volberding, P. A., eds. *The Medical Management of AIDS.* 4th ed. Philadelphia: W. B. Saunders Co., 1995.

### Review Articles

Detels, R. Epidemiologic contribution to the HIV and AIDS literature. *Curr. Op. Infect. Dis.* 8:51–53, 1995.

Haviler, D., and Richman, D. D. Antiretroviral therapy. *Curr. Op. Infect. Dis.* 8:66–73, 1995.

McArthur, J. Neurologic disease associated with HIV-1 infection. *Curr. Op. Infect. Dis.*, 8:74–84, 1995.

Coffin J. M. HIV population dynamics in vitro: Implication for genetic variation, pathogenesis and therapy. *Science* 267:483, 1995.

Chadwick, E. G., and Yogev, R. Pediatric AIDS. *Pediat. Clin. North Am. 42*:969–992, 1995.

## Original Articles

Blanche, S., Tardieu, M., Duliege, A. M., et al. Longitudinal study of 94 symptomatic infants with perinatally acquired human immunodeficiency virus infection. *Am. J. Dis. Child. 144*:1210–1214, 1990.

Bozzette, S. A., Finkelstein, D. M., Spector, S. A., et al. A randomized trial of three antipneumocystis agents in patients with advanced human immunodeficiency virus infection. *N. Engl. J. Med. 322*:693–699, 1995.

Centers for Disease Control and Prevention. Zidovudine for the prevention of HIV transmission from mother to infant. *MMWR 43*:285–288, 1994.

Centers for Disease Control and Prevention. 1994 Revised classification system for human immunodeficiency virus infection in children less than 13 years of age. *MMWR 43*:RR-12:1–10, 1994.

Chadwick, E. G., Connor, E. J., Hanson, C. G., et al. Tumors of smooth-muscle origin in HIV-infected children. *JAMA 263*:3182–3184, 1990.

Concorde Coordinating Committee. MRC/ANRS randomized double-blind controlled trial of immediate and defined zidovudine in symptom-free HIV infection. *Lancet 343*:871–881, 1994.

Duliege, A. M., Messiah, A., Blanche, S., et al. Natural history of HIV type 1 infection in children: Prognostic value of laboratory tests on the bimodal progression of the disease. *Pediatr. Infec. Dis. J. 11*:630–635, 1992.

Dunn, D. T., Newel, M. L., Ades, A. E., et al. Risk of human immunodeficiency virus type 1 transmission through breast-feeding. *Lancet 340*:585–588, 1992.

Epstein, L. G., Sharer, L. R., Oleske, J. M., et al. Neurological manifestations of human immunodeficiency virus infection in children. *Pediatrics 78*:678–687, 1986.

European Collaborative Study. Risk factors for mother-to-child transmission of HIV-1. *Lancet 339*:1007–1012, 1992.

Gabiano, C., Tovo, P. A., deMartino M., et al. Mother-to-child transmission of human immunodeficiency virus type 1: Risk of infection and correlates of transmission. *Pediatrics 90*:369–374, 1992.

Hoover, D. R., et al. Clinical manifestations of AIDS in the era of *Pneumocystis* prophylaxis. *N. Eng. J. Med. 329*:1922–1926, 1993.

Lewis, L. L., Butler, K. M., Husson, R. N., et al. Defining the population of human immunodeficiency virus-infected children at risk for *Mycobacterium avium-intracellular* infection. *J. Pediatr. 121*:677–683, 1992.

Lindegren, M. L., Hanson, C., Miller, K., et al. Epidemiology of human immunodeficiency virus infection in adolescents, United States. *Pediatr. Infect. Dis. J. 13*:525–535, 1994.

Masur, H., Ognibene, P., Yarchoan, R., et al. CD4 counts as predictors of opportunistic pneumonia in human immunodeficiency virus (HIV-1) infection. *Ann. Intern. Med. 111*:223–231, 1989.

Nightingale, S. D., et al. Two controlled trials of rifabutin prophylaxis against mycobacterium avium complex infection in AIDS. *N. Engl. J. Med. 329*:828–833, 1993.

Pantaleo, G., et al. HIV infection is active and progressive in lymphoid tissue during the clinically latent stage of disease. *Nature 362*:355–359, 1993.

Persaud, D., Chandwani, S., Rigaud, M., et al. Delayed recognition of human immunodeficiency virus infection in preadolescent children. *Pediatrics 90*:688–691, 1992.

Phair, J., Munoz, A., Detels, R., et al. The risk of PCP among men infected with HIV-1. *N. Engl. J. Med. 322*: 161–165, 1990.

Phair, J., and Wolinsky, S. Diagnosis of infection with the human immunodeficiency virus. *Clin. Infect. Dis. 15*: 13–17, 1992.

Pizzo, P. Pediatric AIDS: Problems within problems. *J. Infect. Dis. 161*:316–325, 1990.

Powderly, W. G., et al. A randomized trial comparing fluconazole with clotrimazole troches for the prevention of fungal infections in patients with advanced human immunodeficiency virus infection. *N. Engl. J. Med. 322*: 700–705, 1995.

Quinn, T. C., Kline, R. L., Halsey, N., et al. Early diagnosis of perinatal HIV infection by detection of viral-specific IgA antibodies. *JAMA 266*:3439–3442, 1991.

Saint Louis, M. E., Kamenga, M., Brown, C., et al. Risk for perinatal HIV-1 transmission according to maternal immunologic, virologic, and placental factors. *JAMA 269*:2853–2859, 1993.

Salsseta, K., et al. Human immunodeficiency virus type 1 mRNA expression in peripheral blood cells predicts disease progression independently of the members of CD4+ lymphocytes. *Proc. Natl. Acad. Sci. USA 91*:1104–1108, 1994.

Schoenbaum, E., Hartel, D., Selwyn, P., et al. Risk factors for human immunodeficiency virus infection in intravenous drug users. *N. Engl. J. Med. 321*:874–879, 1989.

Selwyn, P., Feingold, A., Hartel, D., et al. Increased risk of bacterial pneumonia in HIV-1 infected intravenous drug users without AIDS. *AIDS 2*:267–272, 1988.

Selwyn, P., Hartel, D., Lewis, N., et al. A prospective study of the risk of tuberculosis among intravenous drug users with human immunodeficiency virus infection. *N. Engl. J. Med. 320*:545–550, 1989.

Simonds, R. J., Lindegren, M. L., Thomas, P., Hanson, D., et al. Prophylaxis against *Pneumocystis carinii* pneumonia among children with perinatally acquired human immunodeficiency virus infection in the United States. *N. Engl. J. Med. 332*(12):786–790, 1995.

Spruance, S. L., et al. Didanosine compared with combination of zidovudine in HIV-infected patients with signs of clinical deterioration while receiving zidovudine. A randomized double-blind clinical trial. *Ann. Intern. Med. 120*:360–368, 1994.

Thomas, P. A., Weedon, J., Krasinski, K., et al. Maternal predictors of perinatal HIV transmission. *Pediatr. Infect. Dis. J. 13*:489–495, 1994.

Tovo, P. A., De Martino, M., Gabiano, C., et al. Prognostic factors and survival in children with perinatal HIV-1 infection. *Lancet 339*:1249–1253, 1992.

Working Group on Antiretroviral Therapy. National Pediatric HIV Resource Center: Antiretroviral therapy and medical management of the human immunodeficiency virus-infected child. *Pediatr. Infect. Dis. J. 12*: 513–522, 1993.

# 24

# DIAGNOSIS AND MANAGEMENT OF INFECTION IN THE IMMUNOCOMPROMISED HOST

GARY A. NOSKIN, M.D., JOHN P. PHAIR, M.D., and
ROBERT L. MURPHY, M.D.

In health, an individual is protected from disease due to invasive microorganisms both by barriers to invasion and by nonspecific and specific mechanisms of host defense. Compromise of any of these systems can result in increased susceptibility to infection and/or a more severe and difficult to treat infectious disease.

With increasing medical technology and prolonged survival of individuals with immune deficiencies, infections in compromised hosts can be anticipated to increase. In the future, immunocompromised patients with infections will account for a substantial percentage of all admissions to acute-care hospitals. Immunocompromised hosts are often indiscriminately grouped together; however, their underlying conditions may be inherited, acquired, or the result of treatment (iatrogenic).

Accurate evaluation of the status of a patient's immune system provides important information both prognostically and therapeutically.

The "compromised host" is generally defined as a person who has one or more defects in the usual defense mechanisms against infection. These defects may range from mild and subclinical to severe and life threatening. Patients with impaired host defenses are at increased risk for *opportunistic infections*. These are infections caused by organisms that are generally considered nonpathogenic in immunocompetent individuals (e.g., *Pneumocystis carinii, Aspergillus fumigatus*) or whose clinical course is accentuated in patients with impaired host defenses (e.g., disseminated varicella in a child with leukemia or recurrent *Salmonella* bacteremia in a patient with acquired immunodeficiency syndrome [AIDS]).

This chapter provides a basis for the laboratory assessment of immunocompetence, various syndromes of immunodeficiencies, and describes infections in the compromised host.

## BARRIERS TO INFECTION

Barriers to infection include an intact integument, respiratory and gastrointestinal tract mucosa, and gastric acidity. Breaks in the skin, due to either trauma, unrelieved pressure leading to decubitus ulcers, or iatrogenic intervention such as surgery or placement of intravascular lines, are commonly associated with local or systemic infection. As discussed in Chapter 7, the upper airway protects the lower respiratory tract from infectious agents and the development of pneumonia or bronchitis. Viral respiratory tract infection, alcoholism, and endotracheal intubation to assist ventilation alter or bypass these local defenses, leading to an increased occurrence of lower respiratory tract infections. The acidity of the stomach also serves as a barrier to infectious microbes. Raising the gastric pH results in a dramatic lowering of the number of *Salmonella typhi* required to infect volunteers with this organism. Inhibition of gastric acidity also has been associated with an increased prevalence of hospital-acquired (nosocomial) pneumonia in patients in intensive care units. The intact mucous membrane of the gastrointestinal tract serves to protect the host against disease due to bacteria normally resident in the compartment. Trauma, including surgery, and cytotoxic therapy are associated with breaks in this important barrier and severe infectious disease problems.

## LABORATORY ASSESSMENT

In concert with antibody and complement, leukocytes are the cells that play a critical role in protection against and control of infection. Defective function or deficient numbers of segmented neutrophils, lymphocytes, phagocytic mononuclear cells, or complement components have been associated with infection. The laboratory assessment of host defenses begins with the determination of the total peripheral white blood cell (WBC) count and differential. Granulocytopenia is probably the most common host defect that predisposes patients to infection. Quantitative immuno-

globulin levels and isohemagglutinin levels are assays of the amount and function of the immunoglobulin-producing B cells. Specific antibody responses to common vaccines are secondary measures of immune responses and can be helpful in some circumstances. In children, responses to vaccines can often be used to assess primary antibody responses. The simplest and most available screening tests of cell-mediated (T-cell) function are skin tests using common antigens such as mumps, *Candida*, or *Trichophyton*. A positive response indicates that T cells and macrophages are functioning properly. Assessment of the number and subtype of T lymphocytes is routinely performed using flow cytometry and serves as a method of monitoring immune function in patients with human immunodeficiency type 1 (HIV-1) infection.

In patients with recurrent infections, the studies listed in Table 24–1 should be performed. If there are abnormal white cell counts or differential, altered immunoglobulin levels, or negative skin-test reactions (*anergy*), additional evaluation is required. In infants, a chest radiograph is useful in determining whether the thymus is present. If the result of the initial assessment is normal, a

## TABLE 24–1.   ROUTINE ASSESSMENT OF HOST DEFENSES

| | NORMAL VALUES (ADULTS)* |
|---|---|
| **COMPLETE BLOOD COUNT (CBC)** | |
| Leukocytes | 5000–10,000 |
| Neutrophils | 2000–6000 |
| Lymphocytes | 1000–3500 |
| Helper T cells (CD4 lymphocytes) | 700–1300 |
| Suppressor T cells (CD8 lymphocytes) | 350–700 |
| **HUMORAL ASSAYS** | |
| Immunoglobulins (mg/dL) | |
| IgG | 600–1750 |
| IgM | 50–210 |
| IgA | 110–400 |
| Complement components | |
| C3 | 70–176 mg/dL |
| C4 | 20–50 mg/dL |
| $CH_{50}$ | 25–50 units |
| **DELAYED SKIN TESTS (CELL-MEDIATED IMMUNITY)†: COMMONLY AVAILABLE ANTIGENS** | |
| Purified protein derivative (PPD) | |
| Candida | |
| Trichophyton | |
| Mumps | |
| Histoplasmin | |
| Coccidioidin | |

*Number per mm³.
†One tenth (0.1) mL should be injected *intradermally*. Reactions should be read at 48 h. Diameters of the area of induration should be measured.

well-defined defect in host defenses is unlikely. Additional testing generally requires the sophistication of a reference laboratory or major university medical center.

## Segmented Neutrophils

To protect against infection, neutrophils must be produced in appropriate numbers and travel to the site of infection. The peripheral blood contains the majority of neutrophils available for delivery to tissue. Approximately one half of these cells are in the so-called marginal pool and are not enumerated by peripheral white cell counts. The cells in the marginal pool readily adhere to and migrate between the endothelial cells of postcapillary venules, thus entering the extravascular space. Entry of neutrophils and mononuclear cells into the skin occurs approximately 2 h following acute injury, peaks by 12 h, and by 24 h the predominant cells are mononuclear. Movement of neutrophils in tissue is dependent upon both the contractile elements in the cytoplasm of these cells and the cell's ability to respond to chemotactic stimuli. Such stimuli are generated by specific bacteria, direct bacterial activation of complement via the alternative pathway, or activation of the classic pathway by antigen–antibody reactions.

After reaching the microorganisms in the extravascular space, neutrophils must engulf and kill the invaders. Phagocytosis of encapsulated bacteria requires coating of the organism with specific opsonic antibody and/or complement. The observation that certain complement defects are associated with the failure of phagocytosis of *Staphylococcus aureus* but normal uptake of *Escherichia coli* emphasizes the complex relationship among opsinins, phagocytes, and bacteria. The measurement of functional activity of the classic complement pathway can be determined by assaying total hemolytic complement activity by the $CH_{50}$ end-point method. This test is useful in the evaluation of patients with suspected congenital deficiencies or patients with infections such as recurrent disseminated gonococcemia or meningococcemia, who often lack functional terminal complement components (C5–C9).

The prototypic example of the inability of neutrophils to kill ingested bacteria is seen in chronic granulomatous disease (CGD). Neutrophils harvested from a child with this disease cannot kill catalase-positive organisms such as *Staphylococcus aureus* (Fig. 24–1). In other diseases, the difference in microbial killing between cells obtained from healthy volunteers and neutrophils from patients varies, as is the case for the wide range of values produced by neutrophils obtained from individuals with diabetes (Fig. 24–2).

Neutrophils kill bacteria by both oxidative bactericidal mechanisms and by releasing cationic proteins from cytoplasmic granules into the phagolysosome that contain bacteria. A number of tests have been developed that assess the burst of oxidative metabolic activity that occurs with phagocytosis. A widely available assay measures either the quantitative or qualitative reduction of the dye nitroblue tetrazolium (NBT). This reduction is an indirect measure of hexose monophosphate shunt activity, which is responsible for the oxidative burst. NBT reduction by neutrophils is dependent on the production of superoxide; consequently, a negative test indicates a congenital defect in neutrophil function such as CGD.

Finally, it should be reemphasized that the single most important assay relevant to the neutrophil and infection is the absolute neutrophil count. The risk of developing infection is inversely proportional to the neutrophil count. Although the risk of infection is significant for patients with neutrophil counts below $1000/mm^3$, the risk is particularly high in those with neutrophil counts below $100/mm^3$. Neutropenia secondary to disease or to cytotoxic chemotherapy is the most common cause of infection related to defects in host resistance. Recently, the widespread use of granulocyte colony-stimulating factors (G-CSFs) has significantly shortened the period of neutropenia in patients undergoing chemotherapy or bone marrow transplantation. As a result of the use of these cytokines, length of hospital stay as well as number of infectious complications have decreased. If the etiology of a deficient number of neutrophils is not readily discernible, a bone marrow aspiration and biopsy should be performed.

## Lymphocytes

The lymphocyte has been established as the major cellular element responsible for the immune response. There are two major components of cellular immunity: antibody-producing B lymphocytes and the thymic-dependent lymphocytes (T cells). These subpopulations of human lymphocytes were recognized initially by the presence of surface immunoglobulins (B cells) or receptors for sheep erythrocytes (T cells). The most convenient method

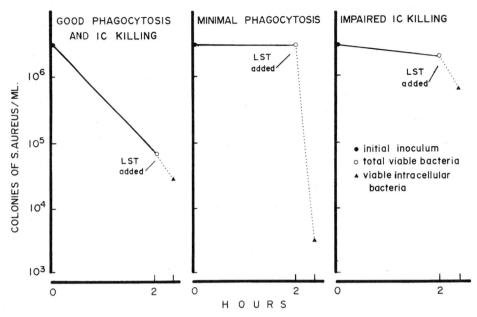

**FIGURE 24-1.** Examples of phagocytosis and intracellular (IC) killing of *Staphylococcus aureus* by polymorphonuclear neutrophils. LST = lysostatin, a staphylocidal chemical. Patients with chronic granulomatous disease manifest impaired IC killing, as shown in the right panel.

currently available for identifying the subsets of lymphocytes is to direct monoclonal antibodies at specific cell-surface antigens and use flow cytometry to count them. B lymphocytes, T lymphocytes (OKT3, CD3), and T-cell subsets (helper [OKT4, CD4], suppressor [OKT8, CD8] cells, and others) can be enumerated by this method. These techniques are now used routinely in most medical centers throughout the United States. The most common use for these assays is to assess immune status in HIV-1–infected individuals and to monitor response to therapy (see Chapter 23). The normal ratio of one cell type to another is altered in many disease states, both trivial and serious. HIV-1 infection, for example, is associated with a depletion of helper T (CD4 cells) lymphocytes. While the normal adult number of CD4 cells in peripheral blood ranges from 750–1250/mm³, individuals with HIV-1 infection have a gradual decline in number of these lymphocytes. Once the CD4 cell count falls below 200/mm³, these patients are at increased risk for *Pneumocystis carinii* pneumonia and other opportunistic infections.

Immunoglobulins (Ig), the secretory products of B lymphocytes, exist in several classes and subclasses in serum and bodily secretions. IgG and IgM mediate immune reactions against microorganisms by such means as comple-

ment fixation, often necessary for opsonization. Toxins are neutralized by IgG as well. Specific secretory IgA produced as a result of infection or local immunization prevents adherence of virus and bacteria to mucosal surfaces, the initial step required for colonization and, presumably, for tissue invasion. The function of IgD is unknown, but this immunoglobulin may act as a surface receptor on B lymphocytes that triggers antibody production. IgE mediates immediate hypersensitivity reactions by activating release of vasoactive substances from mast cells following interaction of allergens with antigen-specific cell-bound IgE.

The functional capacity of B lymphocytes is assessed by determining immunoglobulin concentrations in serum. This should be determined in patients suspected of having a deficiency. The function of T lymphocytes can be evaluated using intradermal antigens to determine skin test reactivity. This is commonly performed with mumps, *Candida*, and *Trichophyton* or by use of a multitest applicator of eight different antigens. Variation in observer measurements of the degree of induration elicited by intradermal injection of antigen, failure to inject the antigen properly, and failure to use appropriate commercially available antigens can obscure the assessment of response. Positive reactions indicate an intact

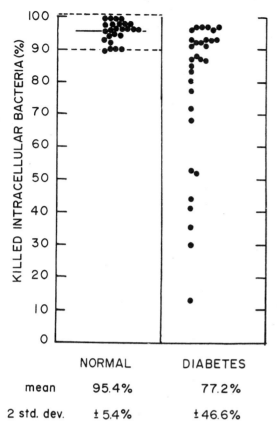

**FIGURE 24–2.** Killing of *Staphylococcus aureus* by polymorphonuclear neutrophils obtained from diabetic patients and normal volunteers, demonstrating impairment in microbicidal mechanisms in diabetes.

system; a negative reaction to several antigens (*anergy*) is less easily interpreted.

## Monocytes/Macrophages

The mononuclear phagocytes are cells derived from bone marrow that exist in two distinct populations: the circulating monocyte and the tissue histiocyte, or macrophage. The tissue macrophages make up the reticuloendothelial system found in the liver, spleen, and pulmonary alveoli. The macrophages play a central role in the immune and inflammatory response. In their initial contact with foreign microorganisms, macrophages ingest, process, and present antigens to lymphocytes in order to stimulate a primary immune response and the production of cytokines, which modulate the immune and inflammatory response. In addition, monocytes produce specific components of the complement system. Laboratory evaluation of the function of this component of host defense is less well

developed than the assessment of the cells previously discussed.

Mononuclear cells from peripheral blood can be separated from lymphocytes by density gradient centrifugation or by their adherence to plastic surfaces. Nonadherent lymphocytes are removed by washing. The phagocytic and bactericidal capacity of these cells can be assessed after establishment of monolayers in culture. Studies have demonstrated that monocytic phagocytosis and killing of microorganisms is slower than by neutrophils. The function of the reticuloendothelial system, an indirect measurement of macrophage capacity, can be determined by uptake of radiolabeled particles and scanning of liver and spleen, or by determining clearance rates of particles from blood. Currently, a major difficulty in assessing the contribution of mononuclear cells to host defense is the lack of a readily available simple test of function.

### Summary

While most defects in host defense are readily identifiable, available methods of measuring host immunity are not sufficiently refined, however, to delineate subtle defects in resistance. The complete blood count determines if a patient is neutropenic, the reaction to skin test antigens indicates an intact T-lymphocyte–macrophage system, and measurement of immunoglobulin concentrations assesses B-cell function. A major contribution to patient well-being is ruling out serious disease by obtaining a thorough history, a complete physical examination, and the results of the readily available tests outlined in Table 24–1. The remainder of this chapter addresses the infectious complications of impaired host defenses.

## SYNDROMES OF HOST IMMUNOCOMPETENCE

The observation of Major Ogden Burton in 1952 that hypogammaglobulinemia was associated with repeated infection by encapsulated organisms represented the first recognition of a defined failure of immunocompetence. Later studies of children with a variety of deficiencies provided further insight into the relationship of immunity to specific infections, led to the recognition of the T-cell and B-cell systems, and to the interaction of the immune response with the inflammatory response. The evaluation of immunocompetence begins with a thorough history. Thus, the absence of recurrent childhood infection is important evidence against a congenital defect in antibody synthesis, cell-mediated immunity, or another aspect of the immune system. In contrast, the history of a splenectomy or sickle cell disease should alert the physician to the possibility of overwhelming infection due to encapsulated bacteria such as *Streptococcus pneumoniae, Neisseria meningitidis,* or *Haemophilus influenzae.* Postsplenectomy sepsis due to these organisms is associated with disseminated intravascular coagulation (DIC) and death in as many as 50% of patients. This susceptibility is most apparent within the first 2 years following splenectomy and emphasizes the importance of administering pneumococcal vaccine to patients prior to elective splenectomy. Other important pieces of historical information include a history of malignancy, high-risk sexual activity, organ transplantation, immunosuppressive medications, or injection drug use, any of which should alert the physician to a possible defect in host immunocompetence. In addition, isolation of an unusual pathogen such as *Aspergillus, Cryptococcus, Toxoplasma gondii, Mycobacterium avium-intracellulare,* or *Pneumocystis carinii* should prompt systematic investigation of host defense mechanisms.

The physical examination in a patient suspected of having impaired host defenses should be complete with particular attention to the lymph nodes, liver, and spleen. The routine laboratory assessment of the immune response is discussed earlier in this chapter.

A difficult and common clinical problem is recurrent minor infections, such as upper respiratory tract infections, bronchitis, or staphylococcal skin infections in either an adult or a child. In the great majority of these patients, a careful evaluation of immune function fails to reveal an etiology. Alternatively, one of the nonimmunologic disorders associated with recurrent infections such as Kartagener's syndrome, in which an anatomic abnormality in the structure of the dynein arms of the respiratory epithelial cilia exists, may be present.

It should be noted that many organisms that rarely cause disease in an individual with a normal immune or inflammatory response can produce severe, or even life-threatening, infection in the compromised host. Thus, *P. carinii* is known to infect 80% of children within the first several years of life and may account for some pneumonitis in the infant. In the overwhelming majority of infants and young children, the infection is self-limited or

## TABLE 24–2.　COMMON DISORDERS ASSOCIATED WITH SECONDARY HOST DEFENSE ABNORMALITIES

Neutropenia
　Leukemia
　Rheumatoid arthritis and Felty's syndrome
　Cytotoxic therapy
Neutrophil dysfunction
　Solid tumors
　Hodgkin's disease
　Cirrhosis
　Diabetes mellitus
　Uremia
　Systemic lupus erythematosus
　Corticosteroid therapy
　Alcoholism
Hypogammaglobulinemia/defective opsonins
　Chronic lymphocytic leukemia
　Paraproteinemias
　Multiple myeloma
　Sickle cell disease
　Thermal injury
Depressed cell-mediated immunity
　Leukemia
　Non-Hodgkin's lymphoma
　Solid tumors
　Sarcoidosis
　Aging
　Major surgery
　Protein-calorie malnutrition
　Systemic lupus erythematosus
　AIDS
　Idiopathic CD4 lymphopenia
　Acute viral infections
　Bone marrow or solid organ transplantation

asymptomatic. The organism, however, is not eradicated by the immune system and persists indefinitely. If the immune status of the individual is impaired at a later date, either by infection with HIV-1 or by immunosuppressive therapy, the organism can replicate and produce a severe form of pneumonia. A similar phenomenon occurs with reactivation of tuberculosis in elderly individuals in association with loss of their previously fully effective cell-mediated immunity. Table 24–2 lists common defects and the diseases associated with specific deficiencies, and Table 24–3 details the infections associated with defective function of specific cells. Although these tables provide a useful framework, it must be understood that there is often overlap and that patients frequently manifest multiple defects.

## Defenses in Neutrophil Number and Function

### Neutropenia

The most prevalent defect in host defense is a deficiency in the number of neutrophils

## TABLE 24–3.  INFECTIONS ASSOCIATED WITH SPECIFIC DEFECTS

| DEFECT | TYPICAL INFECTION |
|---|---|
| Polymorphonuclear neutrophils | Staphylococcus aureus |
| | Streptococcus pyogenes |
| | Enterococci |
| | Enteric gram-negative bacilli |
| | P. aeruginosa |
| | Candida species |
| | Aspergillus |
| | Trichosporon |
| | Fusarium |
| | Mucoraceae |
| B-cell (hypogammaglobulinemia) | Streptococcus pneumoniae |
| | Haemophilus influenzae |
| | Neisseria meningitidis |
| T-cell and macrophage deficiencies | Listeria monocytogenes |
| | Salmonella species |
| | Mycobacterium species |
| | Legionella |
| | Rhodococcus equi |
| | Rochalimea species |
| | Disseminated fungal infections |
| | Coccidioidomycosis |
| | Cryptococcosis |
| | Blastomycosis |
| | Histoplasmosis |
| | Pneumocystis carinii |
| | Toxoplasma gondii |
| | Strongyloides stercoralis |
| | Cryptosporidium |
| | Isospora belli |
| | Leishmania species |
| | Herpes simplex virus |
| | Varicella-zoster virus |
| | Cytomegalovirus |
| | Adenovirus |
| | Parvovirus B19 |
| | Epstein-Barr virus |
| Complement deficiency, splenectomy | Staphylococci |
| | Neisseria species |
| | S. pneumoniae |
| | H. influenzae |
| | Babesia species |
| | Plasmodium species |

totoxic chemotherapy or bone marrow transplantation has been shortened significantly. On the other hand, the depth of neutropenia has increased (ANC commonly <100/mm$^3$), and patients who previously were not considered candidates for aggressive chemotherapy are now offered this option.

Fever in neutropenic patients must be considered related to infection even if other potential causes of temperature elevation, such as atelectasis or blood transfusions, are present. More than half of temperature elevations in neutropenic adults are due to infection, despite identifying the etiologic organisms in less than half. This percentage is even lower in children. Bacterial or fungal infections in the neutropenic host may progress rapidly and result in death within hours. Therefore, prompt evaluation, including appropriate cultures, should be completed rapidly and empiric broad-spectrum antibiotics initiated without waiting for culture results. Approximately 20% of febrile neutropenic adults (and a lower percentage of children) prove to be bacteremic or fungemic. Another fifth of the patients have bacteriologically documented nonbacteremic infection, such as pneumonia, urinary tract, or soft tissue infection. A further 20% have clinical signs and symptoms consistent with infection, but cultures are negative. When a positive culture is obtained, the empiric antibiotics that had

## TABLE 24–4.  COMMON PATHOGENS IN NEUTROPENIC PATIENTS

Gram-negative bacilli
  Escherichia coli
  Klebsiella sp.
  Pseudomonas aeruginosa
  Enterobacter cloacae
  Serratia sp.
  Proteus sp.
  Salmonella sp.
Gram-positive cocci and bacilli
  Staphylococcus aureus
  S. epidermidis (and other coagulase-negative staphylococci)
  Streptococcus pneumoniae
  S. pyogenes
  Enterococcus faecalis
  E. faecium
Anaerobes
  Bacteroides sp.
  Clostridium sp.
  Fusobacterium sp.
Fungi
  Candida sp.
  Aspergillus sp.

(neutropenia) due to diseases such as leukemia, congenital or cyclic neutropenia, or cytotoxic therapy. Infections that occur in patients with neutropenia include those due to aerobic gram-negative bacilli, staphylococci, and certain fungi, especially Candida and Aspergillus (Table 24–4). It is uncommon for patients to develop clinically significant infections until the absolute neutrophil count (ANC) falls below 1000/mm$^3$, and the great majority of individuals do not become infected until the ANC decreases to less than 500/mm$^3$. With the recent availabilty of G-CSFs, the period of neutropenia for most patients undergoing cy-

been started should be altered based on *in vitro* susceptibility.

Diagnosing infection in the neutropenic patient can be a challenge even to experienced clinicians. These patients generally do not produce purulent sputum, develop pulmonary infiltrates, demonstrate pyuria or purulent drainage from infected catheter sites, or show many of the classic findings of the inflammatory response. Therefore, although withholding antimicrobial therapy while awaiting culture results is often reasonable in the immunocompetent host, it may be lethal in the neutropenic host.

In patients with chemotherapy-induced neutropenia, bacteremia often develops from an occult site, usually as a consequence of cytotoxic chemotherapy-induced mucositis that allows bacteria to invade the mucosal layers of the oral cavity and the intestinal tract. Therefore, enteric gram-negative bacilli and *Pseudomonas aeruginosa* are important pathogens in these patients. Staphylococci and streptococci can also cause bacteremia, generally in association with skin or catheter infections. Emerging pathogens in neutropenic patients are coagulase-negative staphylococci (e.g., *S. epidermidis*), enterococci, and diphtheroids. Although difficult to detect, anaerobic infections can also develop in neutropenic patients. The most common sites for anaerobic pathogens are the mouth (gingivitis) and rectum (perirectal abscess). An infection unique to patients with neutropenia or AIDS is *typhlitis*, an inflammation of the cecum due to enteric gram-negative bacilli and anaerobes.

Fungal infections now account for significant morbidity and mortality in patients with malignancies. Fungal colonization occurs within several days following the initiation of broad-spectrum antibiotics. Candidal infections may be superficial, that is, localized to the oral mucosa or skin, or systemic. Catheter-related fungal infections generally require removal of the central venous access device to avoid dissemination. However, in neutropenic patients, fungemia may be present for several days before microbiologic confirmation. Therefore, the clinician must have a high index of suspicion and initiate antifungal therapy empirically in patients who remain febrile despite 3–5 days of broad-spectrum antibiotics. Patients with documented fungemia should have a careful funduscopic examination to look for candidal endophthalmitis. Another manifestation of disseminated fungemia is erythematous, raised skin lesions. Although rashes are common in neutropenic patients, any suspicious lesion should be biopsied. In neutropenic patients with fungemia, the mortality rate may approach 80%; consequently, antifungal prophylaxis has gained in popularity.

The lungs represent another important site of infection in patients with neutropenia. The most common organisms are those seen in association with nosocomial pneumonia; however, as the duration of neutropenia increases, *Aspergillus* species increase in likelihood. Fungal pneumonia due to *Aspergillus* or *Mucor* portends a very poor prognosis unless there is recovery of neutrophils. Angioinvasive infection and pulmonary infarction can occur with both of these fungi. These fungi can also colonize the nasopharynx and result in rhinocerebral infection. Mucormycosis should be suspected in a patient with sinusitis or orbital cellulitis that fails to respond to appropriate antibacterial therapy. A careful examination of the nares may reveal a necrotic eschar, which can be cultured for fungi.

The antimicrobial treatment of febrile neutropenic patients is constantly in evolution. Therapy is based on the predominant organisms and antibiotic susceptibility profiles within each institution. In general, the administration of a synergistic combination of bactericidal antibiotics is preferred for patients who appear toxic or are hemodynamically unstable. The most widely used therapy combines a broad-spectrum penicillin, such as piperacillin, azlocillin, or mezlocillin, with an aminoglycoside. Equally good results are seen with the combination of an extended-spectrum cephalosporin with an aminoglycoside. The availability of third-generation cephalosporins and imipenem has led to the use of monotherapy with these agents. Despite initial reluctance to use only one agent for empiric therapy, several well-controlled clinical trials have documented that monotherapy is reasonable in this patient population. The major concern with monotherapy is the selection of antibiotic-resistant organisms. Ceftazidime, the most commonly used drug for monotherapy, is associated with the development of enterococcal infections, and imipenem predisposes patients to bacterial and fungal superinfection. Vancomycin should not be used for initial therapy unless there is evidence of a catheter infection or documented staphylococcal infection. In patients who remain febrile despite broad-spectrum antibiotics, amphotericin B should be added to the regimen empirically. Early empiric use of antifungal therapy is appropriate because fungal infections may be difficult to diagnose in these patients and prompt initiation of therapy improves outcome. Amphotericin B remains the antifungal agent of choice for immunocompromised patients. In order to provide coverage against *Aspergillus* species the usual dose in 1.0 mg/kg/day. Liposomal preparations of amphotericin B are currently under investigation, and preliminary data reveal that they have similar efficacy but less toxicity than conventional amphotericin B. Fluconazole, a triazole antifungal agent, has been shown to be effective for the prevention of candidal infections in patients with leukemia or undergoing bone marrow transplantation. While effective in preventing infections due to *C. albicans*, fluconazole can select for more resistant organisms such as *C. krusei*.

The use of hematologic growth factors or cytokines has revolutionized the treatment of patients with neutropenia. These agents are glucoproteins that send messages to cells of the immune system and hematopoietic precursors. The most commonly used agents are granulocyte-macrophage colony-stimulating factor (GM-CSF) and G-CSF. GM-CSF exerts its major activity on neutrophils in which it increases phagocytic activity, superoxide production, bactericidal activity, and antibody-dependent cell cytotoxicity. GM-CSF also increases antifungal activity of monocytes/macrophages and facilitates the oxidative burst. In clinical trials, use of this cytokine has resulted in decreased duration of hospitalization and antibiotic usage in patients undergoing bone marrow transplantation. G-CSF has effects on neutrophils similar to those of GM-CSF but has no effect on mononuclear cells. In patients with chemotherapy-induced neutropenia, G-CSF has been shown to accelerate neutrophil recovery and improve their function. In a study of patients with small cell carcinoma of the lung, patients treated with G-CSF had a decreased period of neutropenia, fewer days of fever, and fewer documented infections than untreated controls.

Other cytokines with potential usefulness in the treatment of patients with neutropenia include monocyte colony-stimulating factor (M-CSF); interferon-gamma (IFN-gamma); and interleukin-1 (IL-1), IL-3, and IL-6. M-CSF causes marked increases in the number and antimicrobial properties of monocytes. In animal models, this cytokine proved effective in the prevention of disseminated candidiasis and invasive aspergillosis. Currently, it is being investigated as adjuvant therapy in patients with systemic fungal infections. IFN-gamma enhances neutrophil phagocytosis as well as bactericidal and fungicidal activity. In animal models of infection, this cytokine did not stimulate hematopoiesis and its future role in neutropenic patients is uncertain. It is very effective in CGD (see below). IL-1 and IL-3 result in increased numbers of neutrophils and facilitate their migration; IL-3 also increases the number of eosinophils and monocytes. IL-6 has no direct effect on neutrophils; however, this cytokine has potent antimycobacterial properties. In addition to antimicrobial therapy, the future treatment of febrile neutropenic patients may include various combinations of cytokines that stimulate the hematopoietic and immune systems in a complementary fashion.

## Chronic Granulomatous Disease

The classic congenital defect in neutrophil function is CGD, a genetic failure of intracellular killing of phagocytosed catalase-positive bacteria. In these individuals, the normal microbicidal oxidants are not synthesized because of defects in NADPH oxidase, rendering patients susceptible to severe, recurrent chronic infection that leads to formation of granulomata in all tissues, especially the lungs, liver, and spleen. When catalase-negative organisms are phagocytosed, microbial $H_2O_2$ production contibutes to bacterial killing, but catalase-positive organisms destroy $H_2O_2$ and escape killing.

Four genetic forms of NADPH oxidase deficiency exist, the most common being x-linked, while the other three are autosomal recessive. When CGD is suspected clinically, an NBT dye reduction slide test and a quantitative measurement of the oxidative burst by activated neutrophils should be performed. These tests should be performed on the affected child and mother, as knowledge of the genetic subtype is important for family counseling.

The clinical manifestations of CGD can be variable in severity, and some patients with a milder variant may not be identified until adulthood. This congenital defect should be suspected in patients with unexplained pneumonia due to catalase-positive organisms such as *S. aureus*, *Serratia marcescens*, *Burkholderia* (*Pseudomonas*) *cepacia*, *Nocardia*, or *Aspergillus*. Recurrent skin or soft tissue infections due to staphylococci or *Serratia* should also increase the index of suspicion.

An important aspect of care for these children is the prevention of infection. Although their activities and social interactions should not be restricted, prompt disinfection of any wound is important. The use of daily prophylactic trimethoprim-sulfamethoxazole has been shown to reduce the risk of bacterial infections significantly. A major advance recently has been evidence that administration of IFN-gamma thrice weekly substantially decreases infections in these patients. This is currently the standard therapy for patients with CGD.

### Chediak-Higashi Syndrome

Chediak-Higashi syndrome (CHS) is one of the most severe of all congenital immune defects. This syndrome is transmitted in an autosomal recessive fashion and results in profound abnormalities in the formation of intracellular granules. This defect affects all granule-containing cells including neutrophils, platelets, melanocytes, renal tubular cells, thyroid follicle cells, and mast cells. As a result of dysfunctional granules, these patients have multiple abnormalities in neutrophil and natural killer lymphocyte function. Patients with CHS experience recurrent bacterial infections, usually involving the skin and respiratory tract. Viral, fungal, and parasitic infections are also common. Since the precise abnormality in this syndrome is not known, no specific therapy exists. Bone marrow transplantation has been successful in a small number of patients, but follow-up is limited.

## DEFICIENCIES IN THE COMPLEMENT SYSTEM

For neutrophils to be effective, serum opsonins (activated complement or antibody) must be available and functional. Absence of the third component of complement is associated with the same bacterial spectrum of infections noted in neutropenic patients. Other congenital defects in the complement cascade have been described. A terminal complement component deficiency involving one of the components from C5–C9 leads to a defect in the attack complex and is associated with recurrent meningococcal and disseminated gonococcal infections. These organisms are sensitive to the bactericidal (lytic) activity of fresh serum, which is mediated by these complement components.

Other than C1 inhibitor and properidin deficiencies, all primary complement deficiencies are inherited in an autosomal recessive manner. Patients with these disorders are at increased susceptibility to infection, rheumatic disorders, or angioedema. Patients with C3 deficiency are at a greater risk for infections caused by bacteria that require C3b-dependent opsonization, such as *Haemophilus influenzae* type b and *Streptococcus pneumoniae*. On the other hand, patients with one of the terminal complement deficiencies have normal resistance to pneumococci and *H. influenzae* type b because C3b is intact, but are at increased risk for infections due to *Neisseria* species. Terminal complement deficiencies are relatively common, as evidenced by studies suggesting that 15% of patients with a systemic meningococcal infection have genetic impairment of these components.

C1q deficiency is associated with a lupus-like syndrome and increased susceptibility to bacterial meningitis and sepsis. Patients with C4 deficiency frequently develop a lupus-like syndrome with only a mildly increased risk of infection. C2 deficiency is the most common genetic defect of the complement system, occurring in approximately 1 in 10,000 individuals. The clinical manifestations of this defect are varied and range from asymptomatic to severe infections due to encapsulated organisms.

While the above-mentioned defects are congenital, there are several acquired abnormalities in complement that predispose patients to infection. Newborn infants usually have mild defects in serum opsonizing and chemotactic activities and complement levels that are between 50 and 80% of adult levels. The impairment in complement is even greater for preterm infants. Patients with nephrotic syndrome are susceptible to infections due to encapsulated bacteria and *E. coli* in part because of loss of complement. Sickle cell disease is another condition that predisposes patients to infection. These individuals are at high risk of infection with *S. pneumoniae* because of two defects—functional asplenia and decreased serum opsonizing activity. Finally, patients with severe burns often develop overwhelming sepsis due to abnormalities in the alternative complement pathway leading to decreased serum opsonic and chemotactic activity.

## DEFICIENCIES IN NUMBER AND FUNCTION OF B LYMPHOCYTES

Lymphocytes derived from bone marrow (B cells) are the antibody-producing precursors of plasma cells. Absent B-cell progenitors, defects in B-cell maturation, B-cell dysfunction, or lack of helper T-cell activity all can lead to agammaglobulinemia, hypogammaglobulinemia, inability to produce specific antibody class or subclass (dysgammaglobulinemia), or failure to respond to specific antigens. Thus, there are a variety of clinical syndromes associated with B-cell defects to review.

## X-Linked Agammaglobulinemia (Bruton's Disease)

X-linked agammaglobulinemia was the first immunodeficiency disorder described and is characterized by absent B-cell precursors or the failure of B cells to mature. No B cells, therefore, can be found in the peripheral blood or lymphoid tissue. There is virtual absence of the immunoglobulins IgG, IgA, and IgM in serum and body secretions. The defect has been mapped to the long arm of the X chromosome at Xq22, and mutations of the cytoplasmic tyrosine kinase gene. Both are now known to be responsible for X-linked agammaglobulinemia. This enzyme is important in B-cell signaling.

Affected infants are usually asymptomatic until maternal antibodies disappear around 6 months of age. At that time, hypogammaglobulinemia results in recurrent infections of the middle ear, respiratory tract, and gastrointestinal tract. These infections can be complicated by bacteremia or central nervous system (CNS) involvement. The presence of lower respiratory tract disease at the time of diagnosis is a poor prognostic sign. Vaccination with inactivated antigen is of no help in these patients because of their inability to mount an antibody response, and live virus immunization is absolutely contraindicated because of risk of active infection.

As this defect is X-linked, boys are affected and their mothers (who are healthy) are carriers. Therefore, suspicion of the diagnosis is based on a family history of recurrent infections in boys on the maternal side. IgG levels are very low, less than 100 mg/dL and frequently undetectable. This deficiency can be confirmed by the absence of antibody production following routine vaccination. If the diagnosis remains uncertain, a lymph node biopsy can be performed that demonstrates a complete absence of plasma cells and germinal centers. Treatment involves regular replacement with intravenous gammaglobulin infusions every 2–3 weeks, to keep the serum IgG level above 200 mg/dL.

## Common Variable Immunodeficiency

Common variable immunodeficiency (CVI) occurs in both children and adults but is more frequently diagnosed in adults. Although this disorder most commonly occurs in adulthood, it is often referred to as *acquired hypogammaglobulinemia*, but familial clusters suggest a genetic predisposition. Some patients have only intrinsic B-cell defects, but most also have T-cell activation abnormalities and deficient secretion of IFN-gamma and IL-2, IL-4, and IL-5. Many are also deficient in a 34-kD B-cell differentiation factor. It is thought that the lack of essential cytokines contributes to the defective B cells. These patients have variable patterns of low but not absent serum levels of IgG, IgA, and usually IgM.

The clinical manifestations of CVI are different than X-linked agammaglobulinemia. CVI affects both sexes equally, and infections are less frequent and less severe than in patients with X-linked agammaglobulinemia. IgG levels are usually below 250 mg/dL but not as low as in patients with X-linked agammaglobulinemia. Interestingly, patients with CVI are at a significantly higher risk for cancer than the general population. A recent study found that the increased risk of lymphoma is 438-fold.

The treatment of CVI is similar to that of other forms of acquired hypogammaglobulinemia, that is, aggressive antibiotic treatment of bacterial infections and supplemental intravenous immunoglobulin (IVIG). Because of the association of CVI with autoimmune diseases and malignancies, patients should be screened for these on a regular basis. Experimental administration of IL-2 has been associated with clinical benefit in a small number of patients, but it is unclear if IL-2 exerts its effect on T cells or B cells in CVI.

## Hypogammaglobulinemia

A delay in the onset of production of IgG in infants has been termed *transient hypogammaglobulinemia of infancy*. IgM and IgA are present in normal concentrations in serum, and usually there is recovery within the first several years of life. Prior to recovery, otitis media and upper respiratory tract infections are common; severe infections such as pneumonia, bacteremia, and meningitis are uncommon.

In addition to these forms of agammaglobulinemia and hypogammaglobulinemia, children have been described with selective IgG2 subclass deficiency. Such children fail to respond to immunization with polysaccharide vaccines. They have recurrent middle ear infections, sinusitis, and pneumonia caused by organisms with polysaccharide capsules. Another group of children have been described who have normal IgG subclass concentrations but manifest recurrent infections, such as those seen with IgG2 subclass deficiency. These children fail to respond to *H. influenzae* type b vaccines but usually respond to pneumococcal vaccine and to protein antigens, such as diphtheria and tetanus toxoids. IgG subclass deficiency is present in a sizable minority of patients with food allergy, asthma, diabetes mellitus, Henoch-Schönlein purpura, Friedreich's ataxia, and autoimmune diseases. Patients with malignancies, HIV-1 infection, and protein wasting states (e.g., severe burns, nephrotic syndrome) also may have deficiencies in IgG or its subclasses, related to excessive losses.

Relatives of persons with IgA deficiency and of patients with common variable immunodeficiency often have IgG subclass deficiencies. These patients may be asymptomatic, but some have frequent sinopulmonary infections, recurrent herpes simplex infections, osteomyelitis, and urinary tract infections. In addition, primary T-cell deficiencies can be associated with hypogammaglobulinemia.

A number of other disorders are associated with deficiencies of immunoglobulin and/or specific antibody responses. Some clearly benefit from replacement IgG therapy, while in others the relevance of the immunoglobulin deficiencies to infection is not well established. As an example, group B streptococcal sepsis and meningitis of the newborn is associated with low maternal levels of anti–group B streptococcal type-specific opsonic antibodies. Although preliminary studies indicated that IVIG therapy may be effective in preventing neonatal sepsis due to this organism, larger trials have not confirmed this observation.

It is not clear what lower limits of IgG subclass levels are compatible with freedom from infection. Although IgG2 deficiency is definitely associated with poor responses to bacterial polysaccharide, no correlation of deficiencies of other IgG subclasses is well defined. Frequent viral upper respiratory infections may be associated with IgG3 deficiency, but this is not firmly established.

Following trauma or major surgery, changes in the immune status, including depressed serum immunoglobulin levels, depressed serum subclass concentrations, low serum levels of complement components, and altered T-cell phenotypes, have been noted. The direct relevance of these changes to infection in these patients has not been defined. Many hematologic malignancies of adults including multiple myeloma, the paraproteinemias, and chronic lymphocytic leukemia are complicated by hypogammaglobulinemia. Infections with encapsulated organisms frequently occur in these patients; however, the neutropenia associated with the chemotherapy these patients receive also predisposes them to these infections.

It has been recognized for years that replacement therapy with immunoglobulin preparations such as IVIG benefit some hypogammaglobulinemic patients. The widespread availability of preparations that can be administered safely intravenously has led to renewed interest in exploring the benefits of this therapy in a wide variety of immunodeficiencies.

## DEFICIENCIES IN NUMBER AND FUNCTION OF T LYMPHOCYTES

The contribution of thymic-dependent lymphocytes (T cells) to host defense is complex. Cooperation between T and B cells is required for maturation of antibody production by B lymphocytes; for example, isotype switching of secretion from IgM to IgG. IgA and IgE production also requires interaction between helper T cells and B lymphocytes. The expansion of the B-cell response involves well-characterized soluble factors produced by T lymphocytes (interferons and interleukins, primarily IL-2) and by macrophages. In addition to processing antigen for induction of an immune response, the macrophage produces IL-1, an endogenous pyrogen, which stimulates B cells directly, up-regulating T-cell "helper" function, and serves to augment delivery of phagocytic cells to sites of inflammation. Suppressor T cells, alone or in combination with monocytes, dampen antibody production and T-helper activity, thus serving as modulators of humoral and cellular immune responses.

Other cytokines produced by T and B cells under specific conditions act to amplify the host response by interacting with macrophages and neutrophils (see Chapter 3). Interferons are antiviral factors released following exposure to virus-specific antigen, or nonspecifically after exposure of lymphocytes to mitogens. IFN-alpha also enhances IgG2 and IgG3 production, inhibits IgE production, and stimulates activity of natural killer (NK) cells. IFN-beta also enhances NK function. IFN-gamma has activities similar to other interferons but also facilitates macrophage activation.

An example of the importance of the role of interferons in viral infections is found with disseminated herpes zoster infection occurring in patients with malignancy or HIV-1 infection. In such patients there is impaired production of local interferon at the time of dissemination. Early systemic administration of interferon to patients with disseminated cutaneous zoster is successful in limiting further spread of infection, suggesting that interferon therapy corrects a host deficiency. Clinical trials also have demonstrated the potential efficacy of interferon treatment of cytomegalovirus, chronic hepatitis B, chronic hepatitis C, human papilloma virus infections, and chronic granulomatous disease. Recombinant DNA technology now enables large-scale production of interferons, and clinical investigations examining the utility of these agents for these and other infectious diseases is currently underway.

Defects in cell-mediated immunity are due to multiple causes. Congenital thymic aplasia (*DiGeorge's syndrome*) represents an embryologic failure of development of the thymus and parathyroid glands from the third and fourth pharyngeal clefts. The clinical manifestations of this syndrome are quite variable and many patients have little or no permanent abnormality in immunologic activity. Some, however, are severely deficient in T-cell function. DiGeorge patients frequently have malformations of the cardiac outflow tract, abnormal facies, and hypoparathyroidism. The inheritance of this syndrome is unknown, although partial monosomy of 22q11 is found in some patients.

The prototypic T- and B-lymphocyte disorder, *severe combined immunodeficiency* (SCID), is due to failure of hematopoietic stem cells to differentiate normally. SCID is actually a group of rare disorders that are X-linked or inherited as an autosomal recessive deficit. In the X-linked form, T cells and NK cells are most severely affected, while B cells are usually normal. In most of the autosomal recessive forms, both T and B cells are deficient, but NK cells are normal. Some autosomal recessive SCIDs are deficient in red cell adenine deaminase (ADA). Patients with SCID are generally identified early in life as the result of multiple opportunistic infections, and with-

out bone marrow transplantation or ADA gene therapy or replacement they die within a few years. In addition to infectious complications, most of these children fail to grow normally. The clinical manifestations of SCID are very similar to neonatal HIV-1 disease.

The neonate and the aged are susceptible to infection due to organisms for which T cells are the major mechanism of defense (Table 24–5). This explains the increased susceptibility of these populations to toxoplasmosis, listeriosis, and infections with the herpes viruses. Depressed cellular immune responses are also found in a number of neoplastic diseases. Hodgkin's disease represents an example of such an acquired T-lymphocyte dysfunction. Depression of T-cell function due to enhanced suppressor-cell activity and alteration of lymphocyte traffic to lymph nodes has also been noted in certain intracellular infections, such as lepromatous leprosy, disseminated tuberculosis, coccidioidomycosis, and histoplasmosis. Measles is the classic example of a viral illness that transiently depresses cell-mediated immunity. Long before the mechanisms of cellular immunity were delineated it was recognized that a measles epidemic among children with quiescent tuberculosis led to exacerbations of the mycobacterial disease. Depression of cell-mediated immune responses has been noted following influenza, rubella, infectious mononucleosis, cytomegalovirus infection, severe bacterial infections, sepsis, and immunization with live viral vaccines.

### TABLE 24–5.  COMMON PATHOGENS ASSOCIATED WITH CELLULAR IMMUNE DYSFUNCTION

Bacteria
  *Legionella pneumophila*
  *Listeria monocytogenes*
  *Mycobacterium* sp.
  *Nocardia asteroides*
  *Salmonella* sp.
Fungi
  *Coccidioides immitis*
  *Cryptococcus neoformans*
  *Histoplasma capsulatum*
Viruses
  Cytomegalovirus
  Herpes simplex
  Varicella-zoster virus
  Parvovirus B19
Protozoa
  *Pneumocystis carinii*
  *Cryptosporidium*
  *Toxoplasma gondii*

Immunodeficiency is also commonly observed secondary to medications. The most commonly used drugs that suppress the immune system are corticosteroids. Their effect on immune regulation is due to blocking of lymphocyte and macrophage activation. Cyclosporine, OKT3, and FK-506 (tacrolimus) are three potent immunosuppressants used to prevent rejection following transplantation. These agents block T-cell activation and inhibit production of IL-2 and IFN-gamma. Because these medications profoundly inhibit T-cell function, an increased risk of B-cell lymphomas is observed in patients taking them. Other immunosuppressive medications include azathioprine, cyclophosphamide, chlorambucil, and methotrexate.

Depressed *in vitro* lymphocyte responsiveness and skin-test reactivity are also found in patients with protein-calorie malnutrition. In these patients, the number of circulating T cells is diminished as are antigen-specific responses. Despite defects in cell-mediated immunity, B-cell function is relatively well preserved.

In the late 1970s and early 1980s, infections due to *Pneumocystis carinii*, endemic mycoses, cytomegalovirus (CMV), and nontuberculosis mycobacteria were noted in gay men, injection drug users, and hemophiliacs. Profound defects in cell-mediated immunity and increased occurrence of Kaposi's sarcoma, as well as lymphoproliferative tumors, were also reported. The cause of this alteration in immune regulation is a depletion of helper T cells as a consequence of infection with HIV-1. The details of this important infectious cause of immunodeficiency are discussed in detail in Chapter 23.

## DEFICIENCIES IN MONONUCLEAR PHAGOCYTE FUNCTION

The third cell involved in host defense against microorganisms is the phagocytic monocyte, or macrophage. These cells, which are derived from bone marrow, are located in the peripheral blood (monocytes) or in specific organs, including liver, spleen, and pulmonary alveoli (histiocytes, or macrophages). Monocytes can leave the vascular compartment, enter tissues and organs, and participate in cell-mediated reactions. With appropriate stimulation, the number of mononuclear phagocytic cells in the liver (Kupffer's cells) can increase greatly due to both local proliferation and recruitment from blood.

Macrophages have receptors for IgG and complement that enhance their adherence to and facilitate their ingestion of opsonized particles. They also are capable of non–immune-mediated phagocytosis. Phagocytosis and digestion of antigen by macrophages play an important role in processing and presentation of antigen to lymphocytes — a precondition for T- and B-cell immune responses. In addition, macrophage factors such as IL-1 or cell-to-cell contact between macrophages and lymphocytes facilitate lymphocyte responses to antigens and mitogens.

Mononuclear phagocytes demonstrate a metabolic burst that is critical to activation of the hexose monophosphate shunt following ingestion of bacteria. Killing bacteria requires the production of $H_2O_2$ and the fixation of halide, as happens in neutrophils. Enzymes within macrophages aid in the digestion of macromolecules. However, cationic proteins, necessary for bacterial killing by neutrophils, are lacking in these cells. Some microorganisms have evolved the ability to survive within macrophages. *Mycobacterium tuberculosis* survives and replicates within nonactivated macrophages. Other organisms such as *Toxoplasma gondii* also resist killing unless coated with antibody.

Dysfunction of macrophages has been demonstrated in chronic granulomatous disease, in certain hematologic malignancies, in systemic lupus erythematosus, in HIV-1 infection, and during corticosteroid therapy. Disseminated infections due to intracellular pathogens may represent examples of intrinsic dysfunction of these phagocytes. However, a failure of macrophage–lymphocyte interaction or an inherent lymphocyte defect may be at fault.

## MULTIPLE DEFICIENCIES

It should be noted that patients can have multiple defects in their immune or inflammatory responses. As suggested in the discussion of B-cell deficiencies, a disease such as multiple myeloma typically leads to infection with pneumococci. However, treatment of this hematologic neoplasm often leads to neutropenia secondary to cytotoxic chemotherapy and to subsequent infection with gram-negative bacteria, *S. aureus*, or fungi.

An instructive example of a single patient with multiple defects that occur sequentially is a recipient of an allogeneic bone marrow transplant for the treatment of leukemia. The cytotoxic treatment and/or radiotherapy administered to produce the marrow ablation necessary for transplantation is associated with the usual infections observed in patients with neutropenia. With production of leukocytes by the transplanted marrow, the risk of infection markedly diminishes. However, complications such as graft-versus-host disease can lead to disruption of skin and mucosal integrity, resulting in infections with cutaneous, oropharyngeal, or intestinal organisms. Cytomegalovirus infections follow as a consequence of the defects in cell-mediated and humoral immunity associated with graft-versus-host disease and increasing immunosuppression. If immune function is successfully restored by the transplant, the patient is often left with deficiencies of IgG subclasses 2 and 4 and with resultant susceptibility to infection by encapsulated bacteria. A good match for histocompatibility antigens between donor and host and use of CMV-negative blood products decreases the risk of both graft-versus-host disease and CMV infection. Finally, administration of immunoglobulin preparations and antibiotics can ameliorate the effect of selective deficiency of IgG subclasses.

## OPPORTUNISTIC PATHOGENS AND CLINICAL INFECTION

### Gram-Positive Bacteria

Both *S. aureus* and the coagulase-negative staphylococci characteristically invade skin and adjacent tissues at cutaneous puncture sites as well as the sites of indwelling intravenous catheters. Within 48–72 h, staphylococci are demonstrable on these foreign bodies. The risk of clinical infection correlates with the length of time the catheter remains in place. The use of long-term central venous access devices and subcutaneous implantable ports have become commonplace in patients with cancer or HIV-1 infection. Additionally, they are used routinely for patients requiring prolonged outpatient management of infections such as endocarditis or osteomyelitis. Infection associated with these devices is relatively common and may manifest as either a local exit site infection, a subcutaneous tunnel infection, or line-related bacteremia. Peripheral intravenous catheters in adults should be changed every 48–72 h to prevent bacteremia; however, replacing central devices is

problematic, especially in patients with life-threatening thrombocytopenia. Recent data suggest that removing these devices is not always necessary in patients with infections. Administering antibiotics through the catheter and rotating the ports is often effective for bacterial infections. Clearance of fungal infections, on the other hand, requires removal of the catheter.

*Streptococcus pneumoniae* infection occurs at a higher frequency in patients with humoral immune deficiencies, and in individuals who have undergone splenectomy. Patients with inadequate antibody production as seen with multiple myeloma or HIV-1 infection are also at risk.

Infections with the gram-positive bacillus *Listeria monocytogenes* occur in patients with hematologic malignancies, as well as in the neonate and elderly. Pregnant women are also at increased risk for listeriosis because of defects in cell-mediated immunity that occur with gestation. In the neonate, infection usually manifests as bacteremia, whereas in adults, meningitis is more common. A Gram's stain of cerebrospinal fluid revealing gram-positive bacilli should alert the clinician to the possibility of listeria infection. In some instances, these bacteria are mistaken for diphtheroids and discarded as contaminants, with disastrous consequences.

### Gram-Negative Bacteria

Neutropenia is the major risk factor associated with aerobic gram-negative infections. Bacteremia or sepsis is the most common clinical manifestation, and in approximately one third of such patients, no other source of infection is identified. The clinical findings range from low-grade fever to life-threatening septic shock (see Chapter 32). The most commonly identified pathogen in these patients is *E. coli*. When the absolute neutrophil count falls below $500/mm^3$, the risk of gram-negative bacteremia increases precipitously. An important organism in this setting is *Pseudomonas aeruginosa*, which invades the endothelial cell lining of the vasculature. The mortality rate for *Pseudomonas* bacteremia in the neutropenic host is quite high.

Empiric therapy directed against gram-negative bacteria, including *P. aeruginosa*, is critical in the treatment of the febrile granulocytopenic host. Prompt initiation of broad-spectrum, usually synergistic combinations of antibiotics (an aminoglycoside plus a beta-lactam antibiotic) is associated with improved outcome in this patient population. The relative proportion of gram-negative infections in neutropenic patients has declined over the past decade with a corresponding increase in gram-positive and fungal infections. Early initiation of empiric antimicrobial therapy in febrile, neutropenic patients and the widespread use of central venous catheters likely contribute to this shift in types of infections.

### Acid-Fast Bacteria

Reactivation of *Mycobacterium tuberculosis* occurs more frequently in patients receiving immunosuppressive therapy, in patients with HIV-1 infection, and in malnourished and alcoholic patients (see Chapter 13). Pulmonary disease and disseminated tuberculosis are the most common clinical manifestations.

Other mycobacterial infections are also likely to occur in the compromised host. In patients with severe underlying chronic lung disease, *Mycobacterium avium* complex (MAC) is associated with an indolent course that may persist for many years. In patients with advanced HIV-1 disease, the clinical manifestations of MAC are quite different in that dissemination is common and cultures of blood and bone marrow are usually positive. Because of their large mycobacterial load, most AIDS patients with MAC infection are symptomatic with fever, chills, malaise, and weight loss. Currently, MAC is responsible for the most common severe bacterial infection seen in patients with AIDS. As patients with HIV-1 disease continue to live longer, there will likely be an increase in the incidence of disseminated infection due to MAC. Recently, rifabutin has been found to be effective for prophylaxis against MAC in AIDS patients with CD4 counts less than $100/\text{mm}^3$. Treatment remains in evolution but generally requires a combination of several antibiotics with activity against mycobacteria to help prevent the development of resistance.

Another nontuberculous mycobacterium that causes infection in immunocompromised hosts is *M. kansasii*. Infection with this organism is commonly encountered in transplant recipients and is manifested by localized disease in the lungs, skin, or bone, or by widespread dissemination. Other less virulent mycobacteria include *M. marinum* and *M. chelonei*. Management of these infections often requires a combination approach of decreasing immunosuppression, surgical débridement, and antimicrobial therapy.

Despite the fact that *Nocardia asteroides* is a true bacterium, its acid-fast staining characteristics and the morphology of the organism has led to its erroneous classification as a fungus. At times, it may be confused with mycobacteria on acid-fast–stained smears; however, *N. asteroides* causes a very different type of disease, consisting of abscess formation, especially in the lung and central nervous system. Nocardiosis typically occurs in immunocompromised patients who have been on long-term corticosteroid therapy. Sulfa drugs are effective therapy for nocardiosis.

### Fungi

*Candida albicans* and *Aspergillus fumigatus* are common fungal pathogens in immunocompromised patients. They occur most frequently in individuals who are neutropenic and/or who have defects in cell-mediated immunity. In granulocytopenic patients, these infections may be life-threatening. A recent study from a major cancer center revealed that mortality in patients with fungemia was nearly 50%. Factors that predispose patients to systemic fungal infections include prolonged broad-spectrum antibiotic therapy, indwelling vascular or bladder catheters, corticosteroids, and hyperalimentation, all common in the severely ill cancer patient (see Chapter 14).

One of the major diagnostic problems with fungal infections in compromised hosts is that isolation of the organism may not indicate clinical infection. Opportunistic fungi tend to colonize mucosal surfaces throughout the body and are ubiquitous in the environment. Documentation of invasive disease is often difficult, especially in patients undergoing bone marrow transplantation. Therefore, a high index of suspicion is necessary and the threshold for treatment must be low. Empiric antifungal therapy with amphotericin B is indicated when no other source of fever can be documented in patients who are neutropenic and already receiving antibiotic therapy.

Infection with *Cryptococcus neoformans* has long been associated with malignant lymphoma, especially Hodgkin's disease. Dissemination of this fungus may occur following exposure to pigeon feces. The organism is initially inhaled, with resulting hematogenous spread from the lungs to a variety of organs. *C. neoformans* has a propensity for the central nervous system, especially in patients with impaired cell-mediated immunity. Unlike bacterial meningitis, the clinical manifestations of cryptococcal meningitis are more chronic.

Symptoms range from mild headache associated with low-grade fever to coma. The cerebrospinal fluid is surprisingly unremarkable, often containing no inflammatory cells. Diagnosis is made by identifying the cryptococcal capsular polysaccharide antigen, as measured by latex agglutination and confirmed by fungal culture.

Infections due to unusual fungal pathogens such as *Fusarium, Trichosporon, Curvularia,* and *Alternaria* have now emerged in immunocompromised patients. Patients with disseminated fusarium infections develop skin lesions associated with subcutaneous nodules, and chronic disseminated trichosporosis may mimic chronic systemic candidiasis. Overall, the prognosis in immunocompromised patients infected with these fungi is poor.

### Pneumocystis Carinii

Although *Pneumocystis carinii* pneumonia (PCP) is a relatively common infection, the taxonomy of the organism remains controversial. *P. carinii* was initially classified as a protozoan based on its clinical characteristics, morphology, and failure to grow in culture. It was then thought to most closely resemble fungi based on an analysis of ribosomal RNA; however, recent studies have led to contradictory results. In addition, the life cycle of *P. carinii* resembles that of protozoa, and it does not respond to antifungal therapy.

*P. carinii* is ubiquitous in nature and infects most children by age 4; however, few if any develop symptomatic pneumonitis. Reactivation of latent *P. carinii* is associated with immune impairment. Most patients with PCP have a defect in cell-mediated immunity due to leukemia, HIV-1 infection, or immunosuppression. PCP has rarely been reported in patients with chronic granulomatous disease, and a recent report identified a cluster of PCP in elderly patients without known risk factors.

The typical clinical presentation of PCP in the compromised host includes fever, nonproductive cough, and dyspnea. Symptoms are usually present for several days to months, especially in AIDS patients. Chest radiographs classically reveal diffuse, bilateral interstitial infiltrates; however, in early cases the x-ray may be normal. Arterial blood gases demonstrate hypoxia. When PCP is suspected, sputum should be obtained for cytologic examination. Direct fluorescent antibody testing has improved the ability to diagnose this infection. An induced sputum, generated after 3% saline mist inhalation, is most appropriate for sampling. In patients unable to produce an adequate sputum sample, fiberoptic bronchoscopy with bronchoalveolar lavage can aid in the diagnosis. Rarely, an open lung biopsy may be considered if bronchoscopy is negative and the diagnosis remains uncertain.

PCP is fatal if left untreated, and when it is suspected empiric therapy with either trimethoprim-sulfamethoxazole or pentamidine is indicated until the diagnosis can be confirmed. In AIDS patients with moderate to severe PCP, the addition of adjuvant corticosteroids has resulted in improved outcome. Significant adverse effects are associated with standard therapy for PCP. In patients who fail or are intolerant of trimethoprim-sulfamethoxazole and pentamidine, alternatives include clindamycin-primaquine, dapsone-trimethoprim, trimetrexate, and atovaquone.

Relapse of PCP is common in face of persistent immunodeficiency; however, recurrences can be significantly reduced if prophylaxis with trimethoprim-sulfamethoxazole or inhaled pentamidine is administered. In patients receiving aerosol pentamidine for PCP prophylaxis, the clinical manifestations of pneumonitis may be atypical and extrapulmonary infection may develop.

### Viruses

Four DNA viruses commonly cause infection in immunocompromised patients. They are herpes simplex virus, varicella-zoster virus, cytomegalovirus, and less commonly Epstein-Barr virus (EBV). The first three are capable of producing disseminated disease, and EBV is associated with the development of lymphoma in compromised patients.

Herpes simplex usually presents as an extensive cutaneous infection that may spread locally to involve the gastrointestinal tract, particularly the esophagus and rectum. This represents reactivation of latent infection rather than acute infection. In the presence of persistent immunosuppression, the infection may become chronic.

Varicella-zoster is also associated with extensive local dermatomal eruptions and, in severe cases, involves multiple dermatomal areas. Multidermatomal zoster warrants an evaluation for impaired host defenses in an otherwise healthy individual. Reactivation of varicella-zoster, like herpes simplex, may disseminate widely. Immunocompromised patients who have never experienced childhood varicella are highly susceptible and are at increased risk for disseminated varicella, especially to the lungs. Exposure of an immunocompromised child or susceptible adult to varicella necessitates therapy with varicella-zoster immune globulin (VZIG) to prevent or ameliorate the infection because of the significant morbidity and mortality associated with this disease. Treatment of both herpes simplex and varicella-zoster in the compromised host is with acyclovir. Therapy is most effective if it is administered early in the clinical course. Two new antiviral agents, famciclovir and valacyclovir are under investigation in this patient group.

CMV is the most important virus affecting transplant recipients. Depending on the immunosuppressive regimen, evidence of CMV infection occurs in two thirds of these patients and may involve multiple organ systems. Acute infection may mimic infectious mononucleosis or hepatitis. The indirect effects of CMV have gained a great deal of attention in recent years. This virus plays a prominant role in allograft rejection following kidney, pancreas, liver, and cardiac transplantation. Pneumonia due to CMV results in significant mortality among patients undergoing allogeneic bone marrow transplantation. In AIDS patients, retinitis and gastrointestinal involvement are common presentations, but CMV infections of the central nervous system are increasing in frequency.

The most common clinical presentation of CMV infection in the compromised host is that of a mononucleosis-like syndrome with fever, malaise, and hepatosplenomegaly. The next most common syndrome is pneumonia. Typically, CMV pneumonia is an interstitial process associated with fever and a nonproductive cough. Findings may be indistinguishable from PCP. The onset of CMV infection usually occurs 6–8 weeks following organ transplantation. However, the availability of more potent immunosuppressive agents has resulted in early CMV infections in some organ transplant recipients.

Ganciclovir is the treatment of choice for CMV infections. Because its efficacy in CMV pneumonitis is only 50–60%, the addition of CMV hyperimmune globulin is often included. In AIDS patients with CMV retinitis, following induction therapy, patients receive maintenance treatment indefinitely. Another antiviral agent used to treat CMV infections is foscarnet, which is reserved for patients who fail ganciclovir or whose organism is resistant. CMV prophylaxis with ganciclovir may be warranted in CMV-positive patients undergoing a bone marrow or solid organ transplant to prevent reactivation.

The clinical manifestations of EBV and CMV are very similar (see Chapter 8). Whether EBV plays a role in allograft rejection is unclear, but it does contribute to immunosuppression. The most important role for EBV in transplant recipients is in the development of B-cell malignancies and nonmalignant B-cell proliferative disorders. These occur with greatest frequency in patients treated with FK506 or cyclosporine. In addition, EBV is frequently detected in lymphomas arising in patients with AIDS.

Parvovirus B19 is a DNA virus that is associated with erythema infectiosum (fifth disease) in children and bone marrow failure in immunosuppressed individuals (see Chapter 31). Antibody to this virus is present in about half of the adult population of the United States, and most people develop immunity during childhood. Chronic bone marrow failure due to parvovirus B19 has been documented in HIV-1–infected individuals as well as those with leukemia, sickle cell disease, and congenital immunodeficiencies. In immunodeficient patients with documented infection, treatment with immunoglobulin is recommended.

## Protozoans

Defects in cell-mediated immunity are associated with infections with two major protozoans, *Toxoplasma gondii* and *Cryptosporidium*. Other protozoal infections are discussed in Chapters 18 and 30.

*T. gondii* infects many animals worldwide. The definitive host is the cat, which appears to be responsible for the bulk of transmission to other animals as well as to humans. *T. gondii* infection appears in four clinical settings: (1) an asymptomatic infection of older children and adults from ingestion of contaminated undercooked meat or vegetables; (2) an acute infection in pregnant women in whom transmission to the fetus may occur, resulting in congenital infection of the fetus (see Chapter 26); (3) in persons receiving long-term immunosuppressive drugs, particularly transplant recipients; and (4) in persons infected with HIV-1.

In the immunocompetent host, acute infection with toxoplasma is infrequently associated with symptoms. When present, they usually consist of lymphadenopathy and simulate infectious mononucleosis. The clinical course is self-limited and benign. In the compromised host, the clinical picture is quite different. In this situation, *T. gondii* has a striking propensity to invade and establish persistent infection in the central nervous system. Toxoplasmic encephalitis presents clinically with findings such as cranial nerve abnormalities, focal seizures, mental status changes, or localized headache. Computed tomography (CT) or magnetic resonance imaging (MRI) of the brain usually reveals several space-occupying lesions typical of toxoplasmosis. Cerebrospinal fluid examination is usually normal.

Ocular toxoplasmosis presents as chorioretinitis, mostly as a result of congenital infection. Patients are usually asymptomatic until reaching the second or third decade of life. Relapse of toxoplasmic chorioretinitis may occur during periods of immunosuppression associated with the chemotherapy given for malignancies.

*Cryptosporidium* is a protozoan that infects many animals such as turkeys, cattle, and sheep, as well as humans. In the competent host, this organism results in diarrhea that is self-limited and does not require treatment. However, in individuals with impaired cell-mediated immunity, the diarrhea can be relentless and chronic, resulting in profound malnutrition, dehydration, electrolyte imbalances, and even death. The diagnosis of cryptosporidiosis is made by acid-fast examination of unformed stool showing cryptosporidial oocysts or by intestinal biopsy. Unfortunately, no antimicrobial treatment is uniformly effective against *Cryptosporidium*. Limited experience with spiramycin, diclazuril, and azithromycin has not been promising. Therefore, appropriate fluid and electrolyte management is essential. In patients receiving immunosuppressive medications, diarrhea often resolves when these medications are stopped.

*Isospora belli* is another protozoan that induces severe diarrhea in immunocompromised hosts. This organism is widely distributed throughout the world and is endemic in the United States. The clinical manifestations of isosporiasis are indistinguishable from those of cryptosporidiosis. Immunocompetent patients generally have self-limited diarrhea, while immunocompromised hosts, especially HIV-1-infected persons, have chronic and relapsing symptoms. Diagnosis is made by identification of the oocysts in stool samples. These organisms are also acid-fast, but are larger than *Cryptosporidium*. Isosporiasis responds to therapy with trimethoprim-sulfamethoxazole. In AIDS patients, chronic suppressive therapy may be necessary to prevent relapses.

*Microsporidia* represent a large group of spore-forming protozoa that consist of over 1000 species. These organisms are unique and should not be confused with the more familiar *Cryptosporidium* and *Isospora*. Microsporidiosis is most commonly recognized in HIV-1-infected individuals and in most cases in those with severe immunosuppression. Infection with *Microsporidia* generally results in chronic diarrhea and weight loss. Diagnosis is made by identification of the organism in tissue or stool. Because of their small size (1–2.5 $\mu$m), demonstration of this protozoan is difficult and requires a skilled pathologist. There is no standard therapy for microsporidiosis. The two agents with the best success in small clinical trials are metronidazole and albendazole.

## PREVENTION OF INFECTION

Infections result in significant morbidity and mortality in the compromised host. Several factors contribute to predispose these patients to infection. The most important is granulocytopenia followed by immunosuppression associated with malignancies, medications, or congenital defects. Most of the approaches to prevent infection have been developed for patients with neutropenia and HIV-1 infection, although they may be applicable to other immunodeficiency states.

One of the early approaches to prevent infection which remains in place today is the use of a protected environment. This can be accomplished with the use of laminar-flow rooms in which the air pressure within the room is higher than pressure in the hallways; therefore only filtered air enters the patients room and then flows to the general hospital environment. Another environmental maneuver is to place a high-efficiency particulate air (HEPA) filter in the rooms of compromised patients. This also reduces the risk of infection, especially with fungal pathogens.

Several measures are useful in decreasing the risk of acquisition of new infections, the most important of which is *hand washing*. More than any other intervention, proper hand washing significantly reduces the risk of infection in the compromised host. Most institutions prohibit flowers, fresh fruits, and vegetables in the rooms of neutropenic patients, because these are often heavily contaminated with bacteria.

Selected use of prophylactic antibiotics has become critical in the prevention of infection in patients with impaired host defenses, particularly in patients with HIV-1 infection. Trimethoprim-sulfamethoxazole, dapsone, and aerosolized pentamidine are widely used to prevent PCP. Rifabutin and clarithromycin are somewhat effective in preventing disseminated infection due to MAC. Clinical trials indicate that fluconazole and ganciclovir can be used to prevent fungal infections and CMV retinitis, respectively, in this population.

In patients with leukemia or undergoing bone marrow transplantation, prevention of infection requires several different agents. Trimethoprim-sulfamethoxazole is widely used to prevent PCP and other bacterial infections. Several studies have evaluated the use of fluoroquinolones as prophylaxis against infection in neutropenic patients. Although these agents are effective in preventing infection, they are associated with an unacceptably high rate of resistant organisms and are not routinely used for this purpose in the United States. Because of difficulty in diagnosis and the high mortality associated with systemic fungal infections, several approaches to prevent these infections have met with variable success. Fluconazole is used as prophylaxis against candidal infections, but it has no activity against *Aspergillus* species. While very effective in preventing infections due to *Candida albicans*, patients receiving this medication may be predisposed to infection with *C. krusei*, which is resistant to fluconazole. Itraconazole has the advantage of activity against *Aspergillus*, but this antifungal agent requires gastric acidity for absorption and many immunocompromised patients are functionally achlorhydric or receiving $H_2$-blockers. Low-dose amphotericin B (10 mg/day) or inhaled amphotericin B has had moderate success in preventing fungal infections, but is limited by toxicities. Acyclovir, either orally or intravenously, can be used to prevent herpes simplex virus infections in patients undergoing solid organ or bone marrow transplantation. Acyclovir has also been used to prevent CMV infections in renal transplant recipients, although it is largely ineffective for treatment of CMV.

## CASE HISTORIES

### Case History 1

A 20-year-old male restaurant worker presented to his local emergency room complaining of shortness of breath and increasing edema of his lower extremities. His past medical history was remark-

able for aplastic anemia at age 7 while living in St. Louis. He had a partial remission and was able to complete high school and work full-time. During the past 3 years, he required periodic blood product transfusions. He also underwent several investigational therapies at various medical centers throughout the United States. He was considering a bone marrow transplant at the time of his current hospitalization.

Physical examination revealed a grossly edematous 20-year-old male who appeared older than his stated age and who was in mild respiratory distress. His temperature was 102.1°F, pulse 120/min and regular, respiratory rate 28/min, and blood pressure 100/60 mm Hg. Palatal and conjunctival petechiae were present. The lung examination was remarkable for bilateral crackles halfway up both fields. The cardiac examination was remarkable for sinus tachycardia and a grade III/VI systolic murmur. There was 2+ pitting edema of both lower extremities and in the sacral area. There were two tender, swollen areas on the right lateral thigh measuring $4 \times 6$ cm. The overlying skin was normal.

Laboratory evaluation was significant for a hemoglobin of 3.9 g/dL; WBC was 1100/mm³ with an absolute neutrophil count of 120/mm³. Platelets were 12,000/mm³. The serum aminotransferases were three times the upper limit of normal. Chest radiograph revealed bilateral alveolar and interstitial infiltrates, predominantly in the lower lobes. An electrocardiogram was normal.

Blood cultures on admission grew *Staphylococcus aureus*. A sputum culture also grew *S. aureus* plus normal respiratory flora. On the fifth hospital day, one of the tender nodules on his leg was aspirated. The Gram's stain revealed gram-positive cocci in clusters; however, the culture was negative for growth.

The patient was initially treated with an aminoglycoside and an antipseudomonal penicillin. He was transfused with packed red blood cells and platelets. Diuretics were administered for his volume overload. When culture results became available, vancomycin was added to his regimen. Despite significant clinical improvement he remained febrile and dependent on multiple blood products. During his hospital course, he developed multiple additional nodules in other areas of his body. Several of the nodules developed into frank abscesses and required surgical drainage. He was treated with parenteral antibiotics for 2 months and was discharged home to continue an oral antistaphylococcal antibiotic. He was evaluated for a bone marrow transplant but was rejected because his infection was never completely controlled. One month following discharge from the hospital, he developed high spiking fever associated with rigors and died as a consequence of septic shock.

### Case 1 Discussion

This young man had a chronic illness characterized by an inability to produce significant quantities of blood components. For the last 3 years of his life, he was able to function surprisingly well despite severe pancytopenia. On his final hospital admission, he had a widely disseminated staphylococcal infection and high-output cardiac failure. Most likely he did not have bacterial pneumonia, but his rather rapid clinical response to diuretics was more likely related to congestive heart failure.

He had a relentless bacterial infection that disseminated throughout his body. He was unable to form abscesses except in a few areas because of chronic granulocytopenia. It is somewhat surprising that he never developed a gram-negative or fungal infection in light of his profound neutropenia. He ultimately died because his underlying disease, aplastic anemia, never improved. His only hope for remission or cure was a bone marrow transplant, but this was not feasible because of his ongoing infection.

## CASE HISTORY 2

A 12-year-old girl was referred to the hospital with fever of 8 weeks' duration associated with weight loss and night sweats. A thorough history revealed that the child's pet monkey had died 12 weeks earlier while the girl was recovering from measles. When the fever began, the physician, recognizing the risk of tuberculosis in monkeys, placed an intradermal purified protein derivative (PPD) skin test on the child. The test was negative. The physical examination was unrevealing except for a temperature of 38.5°C. The initial laboratory studies, including a chest radiograph, were unrevealing. A consultant noted several exudative lesions upon careful examination of the retina. A presumptive diagnosis of miliary tuberculosis was made and therapy initiated. A repeat skin test using intermediate strength PPD (5 TU) resulted in erythematous induration of 22 mm in diameter. A repeat chest x-ray 14 days later demonstrated multiple nodular densities consistent with miliary tuberculosis. The child responded to initiation of antituberculous therapy and had complete recovery.

## CASE 2 DISCUSSION

This case illustrates the effects of a viral infection (measles) upon cellular resistance to tuberculosis and the ability to react to skin test antigens. The physician correctly entertained tuberculosis in this clinical setting, but skin tested the child only once and did not determine whether or not she was anergic. Testing with several intradermal antigens would have demonstrated cutaneous anergy and should have prompted a search for tuberculosis. The recognition of the eye lesions after referral led to the correct diagnosis and initiation of appropriate therapy. In addition, it should be recognized that for up to 6 weeks after initial infec-

tion with *Mycobacterium tuberculosis*, PPD skin test can remain negative and that miliary disease itself can result in anergy.

## REFERENCES

### Books

Brown, A. E., and White, M. H., eds. *Controversies in the Management of Infections in Immunocompromised Patients.* In: *Clin. Infect. Dis.* (Suppl. 2), 1993.

Mandell, G. L., Bennett, J. E., Dolin, R., eds. *Principles and Practices of Infectious Diseases.* 4th ed. New York: Churchill Livingstone, 1995.

Rubin, R. H., and Young, L. S., eds. *Clinical Approach to Infection in the Compromised Host.* 3rd ed. New York: Plenum Press, 1994.

### Articles

Bodey G. P., Buckley, M., Sathe, Y. S., et al. Quantitative relationships between circulating leukocytes and infection in patients with acute leukemia. *Ann. Intern. Med.* 64:328–340, 1966.

Buckley, R. H. Immunodeficiency diseases. *JAMA 268*: 2797–2806, 1992.

Fisher, A. Severe combined immunodeficiencies. *Immunodef. Rev. 3*:83–100, 1992.

Hughes, W. T., Armstrong, D., Bodey, G. P., et al. Guidelines for the use of antimicrobial agents in neutropenic patients with unexplained fever. *J. Infect. Dis. 161*:381–396, 1990.

Hughes, W. T., Rivera, G. K., Schell, M. J., et al. Successful intermittent prophylaxis for *Pneumocystis carinii* pneumonitis. *N. Engl. J. Med. 316*:1627–1632, 1987.

Kaufmann, S. H. E. Immunity to intracellular bacteria. *Annu. Rev. Immunol. 11*:129–164, 1993.

Murray, H. W. Interferon-gamma, the activated macrophage, and host defenses against microbial challenge. *Ann. Intern. Med. 108*:595–608, 1988.

Pizzo, P. A. Management of fever in patients with cancer and treatment-induced neutropenia. *N. Engl. J. Med. 328*:1323–1332, 1993.

Puck, J. M. Molecular and genetic basis of X-linked immunodeficiency disorders. *J. Clin. Immunol. 14*:81–89, 1994.

Rose, R. M. The role of colony-stimulating factors in infectious disease: Current status, future challenges. *Semin. Oncol. 19*:415–421, 1992.

Schimpff, S. C., Hahn, D. M., Brouillet, M. D., et al. Infection prevention in acute leukemia. Comparison of basic infection prevention techniques, with standard room reverse isolation or with reverse isolation plus added air filtration. *Leuk. Res. 2*:231–240, 1978.

Walsh, T. J., Lee, J., Lecciones, J., et al. Empiric therapy with amphotericin B in febrile granulocytopenic patients. *Rev. Infect. Dis. 13*:496–503, 1991.

Whitley, R. J., and Gnamm, J. W., Jr. Acyclovir: A decade later. *N. Engl. J. Med. 327*:782–789, 1992.

Wingard, J. R., Merz, W. G., Rinaldi, M. G., et al. Increase in *Candida krusei* infection among patients with bone marrow transplantation and neutropenia treated prophylactically with fluconazole. *N. Engl. J. Med. 325*: 1274–1277, 1991.

# 25

# NOSOCOMIAL INFECTIONS

GARY A. NOSKIN, M.D.

Hospital-acquired, or nosocomial, infections represent an increasing problem in the United States and are a major source of morbidity and mortality. The changing composition of hospitalized individuals has resulted in patients who are more acutely ill, are immunocompromised, require more medical and surgical intervention, and are at increased risk for developing infection. Hospitalized patients are generally at increased risk of infection because of their underlying disease as well as breeches in the natural protective barriers that result from invasive procedures (Table 25–1). In addition, in immunocompromised patients, organisms encountered in the health care setting that do not normally cause infections can have devastating consequences. Finally, the hospital environment selects for multi–drug-resistant organisms because of the widespread use of antimicrobial agents.

The risk of developing an infection while hospitalized in the United States is approximately 5%. The annual cost of treating these infections is more than $5 billion and significantly increases length of stay, morbidity, and mortality. For example, nosocomial bacteremia results in an average increase in hospitalization by 7.4 days at a cost of over $5000 per episode. The death rate related to nosocomial bloodstream infections is 13.1%. This chapter reviews the definitions, epidemiology, etiology, management, and prevention of nosocomial infections.

## DEFINITIONS

Simply stated, a *nosocomial infection* is one for which there is no evidence that the infection was present or incubating at the time of hospitalization. In general, an infection is considered nosocomial if it occurs greater than 48 h after admission to the hospital or occurs in association with frequent outpatient visits to a hospital clinic. With more surgical procedures being performed on an outpatient basis, it will be increasingly difficult to accurately identify these infections. Therefore, an infection present on admission may be considered nosocomial if it was directly related to a previous hospitalization. In addition, as the severity of illness increases among hospitalized patients, the nosocomial infection rate in acute-care hospitals, especially tertiary care hospitals, can be expected to increase.

For an infection to be considered nosocomial, the patient must have clinical evidence of disease, not merely colonization with an organism often associated with nosocomial infection. For example, a patient who is admitted for abdominal surgery and receives broad-spectrum antibiotics and total parenteral nutrition, has an indwelling bladder catheter, and who then has a sputum culture positive for *Candida albicans* but a normal chest radiograph is colonized. However, if he becomes febrile and *C. albicans* is cultured from his blood, he has developed a nosocomial fungemia. A hospital-acquired infection

## TABLE 25–1.   RISK FACTORS ASSOCIATED WITH NOSOCOMIAL INFECTIONS

| Infection Type | Risk Factors |
| --- | --- |
| Bacteremia | Age <1 or >60 years<br>Immunosupressive chemotherapy<br>Breeches in skin integrity<br>Intravenous lines<br>Severe underlying illness |
| Pneumonia | Intubation<br>Surgery (especially abdominal or thoracic)<br>Congestive heart failure<br>Advanced age<br>Depressed cough reflex<br>Immunosuppression |
| Skin and soft tissue | Immobilization<br>Obesity<br>Malnutrition<br>Invasive procedures<br>Burns<br>Loss of skin integrity<br>Diabetes mellitus<br>Trauma |
| Urinary tract | Duration of catheterization<br>Female gender<br>Bacterial colonization of collection bag<br>Genitourinary manipulation<br>Abnormal renal function<br>Improper catheter care<br>Advanced age<br>Severe underlying illness |

generally exists if pathogenic microorganisms are recovered from normally sterile body sites (e.g., blood, cerebrospinal fluid, peritoneal fluid) from cultures obtained at least 48 h after hospital admission.

Nosocomial urinary tract infections are defined as more than $10^5$ colonies of bacteria per milliliter of urine acquired while hospitalized. Lower counts may be considered significant if associated with pyuria or symptoms such as dysuria, frequency, or urgency. These infections are most frequently associated with the use of indwelling bladder catheters.

In adults, hospital-acquired pneumonia requires the presence of a new infiltrate on chest radiograph in association with purulent sputum production. In addition, the clinical picture should be consistent with a lower res-

piratory tract infection. In immunocompromised patients, especially those with neutropenia, diagnosis may be difficult.

Skin and soft tissue infections are defined by the presence of purulent drainage. The presence of pus is important to distinguish infection from colonization. Surgical procedures are classified by their risk of infection and are categorized as clean, contaminated, or dirty.

Nosocomial bacteremia is defined as a clinically significant organism in a blood culture that is obtained more than 48 h following hospitalization. When there are no clinical signs or symptoms of infection or when only one of many sets of cultures is positive, this usually represents contamination. This is particularly true of coagulase-negative staphylococci. Nosocomial bloodstream infections are *primary* if there is no other focus of infection and *secondary* if the same organism is identified at another site. For example, a patient with a central venous catheter site that appears erythematous and tender and who has a positive blood culture for *Staphylococcus aureus* is considered to have a secondary bacteremia due to infection of the central line site.

Vascular catheter-related infections can be divided into local infections, such as an exit site or tunnel infection, or systemic infections. An exit site infection is characterized by purulence around the site where the catheter exits the skin or inflammation consisting of erythema, warmth, tenderness, or edema. A tunnel infection is observed with catheters that are placed subcutaneously, such as the Hickman catheter. These consist of an area of cellulitis around the subcutaneous tunnel tract.

## EPIDEMIOLOGY

The most common nosocomial infection involves the urinary tract, followed by pneumonias, skin and soft tissue infections, and invasive bloodstream infections (BSIs). Over the last 20 years, there has been a change in the distribution of these infections. There has been a gradual decline in urinary tract infections (UTIs) but an increase in bacteremias. The overall incidence of infections is dependent on the hospital size and the specific clinical service. For small community hospitals (<200 beds), 35.9% of nosocomial infections are UTIs, while 9.6% are bacteremias. On the other hand, for large teaching hospitals (>500 beds) the rates for UTI and BSI are 31.5% and 16.9%, respectively. Nosocomial bacteremia is the second most common hospital-acquired infection in large, medical-school–affiliated teaching hospitals, a characteristic presumably related to the more complex patients cared for in those hospitals.

Not surprisingly, the incidence of infection differs by services within an institution, reflecting the degree of exposure to high-risk devices or procedures (Table 25–1). This explains why patients on the surgical service have a higher skin and soft tissue infection rate compared to the medical service. Similarly, the relatively low nosocomial urinary tract infection rate on pediatric services is due to limited use of bladder catheters.

Nosocomial infection involving the urinary tract usually occurs following urologic manipulation. Approximately 80% are associated with the use of indwelling bladder catheters and another 5–10% occur following genitourinary instrumentation. Insertion of the catheter may result in the introduction of bacteria into the bladder. Once this occurs, the catheter itself serves as a nidus for infection. This foreign body also leads to urethral inflammation, which may impair local immune responses. In patients with chronic indwelling catheters, urease-splitting organisms such as *Proteus* can result in catheter obstruction, urinary calculi, and pyelonephritis. Few nosocomial urinary tract infections result in bacteremia except in the presence of obstruction. Although elderly women are frequently infected, elderly men with prostate abnormalities more commonly develop bacteremia.

Pneumonia represents an especially troublesome form of nosocomial infection, and the elderly and the very young are at greatest risk. Other determinants that predispose patients to pulmonary infection include an altered mental status and endotracheal intubation. During the postoperative period, patients are extremely vulnerable to pulmonary infections. This occurs because patients are often immobile (which favors aspiration), not ventilating fully, and receiving pain medication that impairs coughing and swallowing. Thoracic and upper abdominal incisions, antecedent respiratory infections, and obesity add to the risk. Few pneumonias occur on obstetric, surgical specialty, orthopedic, or pediatric services unless the patients are in the intensive care unit. Finally, therapeutic reduction of gastric acidity with $H_2$-blockers has increased the risk of nosocomial pneumonia.

The lower respiratory tract accounts for approximately 15% of all nosocomial infections, and they are associated with a mortality of 20–50%. Hospital-acquired pneumonia is the most lethal of all nosocomial infections. Consequently, any interventions that can prevent this infection would have a significant impact on mortality in hospitalized patients. Only 10% of nosocomial pneumonia is associated with bacteremia, but the mortality in this group is threefold higher than in patients bacteremic without pneumonia. More importantly, adverse outcome is more commonly associated with pneumonia due to gram-negative bacilli than with gram-positive organisms or viruses. For example, nosocomial pneumonia due to *Pseudomonas aeruginosa* is associated with a mortality rate of nearly 70%.

Pneumonia in postoperative patients is common, with 74% of all nosocomial pneumonias occurring in patients who have undergone surgery. Other exogenous factors may also predispose patients to this infection. Many investigators have implicated the use of broad-spectrum antibiotics in the pathogenesis of hospital-acquired pneumonia. Antibiotics that are active against gram-positive bacteria, especially streptococci, and bowel anaerobes are frequently associated with gram-negative bacilli colonization of the respiratory tract. The hospital environment itself may, in part, be responsible for this infection. Favorable conditions exist for the propagation of staphylococci (especially oxacillin-resistant), gram-negative bacilli, and fungi (especially *Aspergillus*).

Skin and soft tissue infections occur in hospitalized patients as the result of immobilization and the development of pressure sores (decubitus ulcers) or invasive procedures that breech the natural protective barriers of the skin. Decubitus ulcers and wound infections are rarely associated with bacteremia. Patients at highest risk for these infections are the immobile elderly and those who have just had bowel, rectal, or urologic surgery.

The organisms causing the great majority of postoperative wound infections are acquired at the time of surgery. In general, organisms are present in the operating room and are transmitted to the patient. The source for these infections may be hospital personnel, other patients, or the hospital environment. Hands have rarely been implicated in nosocomial wound infections because of surgical scrubs and the use of sterile gloves. However, several outbreaks of group A streptococcal infections have been found to be related to asymptomatic carriage in the rectum or vagina of health care workers. The majority of surgical wound infections are caused by bacteria that are normal skin flora. This usually occurs if the skin is not properly sterilized prior to surgery or in a patient who is persistently colonized with *S. aureus.* In addition, normal gastrointestinal flora can cause infection if the bowel is perforated during the operation. Finally, the hospital environment may serve as a reservoir for nosocomial skin and soft tissue infections. *Clostridium perfringens* has been associated with contaminated surgical instruments, *Pseudomonas* species have been reported on occlusive dressings, and *Rhizopus* has been implicated due to contaminated tape.

Primary bacteremia generally occurs in hospitalized patients with indwelling vascular catheters. More than any other nosocomial infection, bacteremia is hospital service dependent. In the most recent National Nosocomial Infection System (NNIS) survey, BSI occurred in 13.1% of patients. However, among newborns and pediatric patients, 36.1% and 29.7% of nosocomial infections were bacteremias, respectively. Among these two group, primary BSI occurred more than twice as frequently as any other infection.

Nosocomial BSI are usually due to skin flora. Patients in critical care units are at particularly high risk for nosocomial bacteremia related to the multiple lines that are required for hemodynamic monitoring. Any procedure that breeches the protective barrier of the skin can result in bacteremia. This may occur as the result of direct inoculation of bacteria into the bloodstream during venipuncture (extremely rare) or by contamination of the vascular device, delivery apparatus, tubing, transducer, or intravenous fluid. Furthermore, the introduction of vascular catheters facilitates infection because of irregularities of the luminal surface that attract platelets, fibrin, and clotting factors.

An emerging problem in patients with nosocomial BSI is *Candida albicans,* which is now the fourth most commonly identified nosocomial organism. The risk factors for invasive fungal infections are detailed in Chapter 14. Not surprisingly, many of the medical illnesses that predispose patients to these infections require the use of central venous catheters. Therefore, the incidence of these BSIs can be anticipated to increase as the use of these devices grows.

Vascular catheters are the most frequently used indwelling medical devices and are commonly associated with infection. Central venous catheters are associated with a significantly higher rate of bacteremia and fungemia than are peripheral intravenous catheters. It is estimated that 3 million central venous catheters are inserted every year in the United States and that the infection rate ranges from 3–14%. As expected, the most commonly isolated organisms are staphylococci and *Candida.* The most important risk factors for catheter-related infection are prolonged catheterization, frequent manipulation, improper insertion techniques, and number of catheter lumens. The risk of infection can be diminished by the use of topical disinfectants, silver-impregnated cuffs, and maintenance of catheter by dedicated personnel experienced in catheter management.

## ETIOLOGY

Shortly after penicillin became widely available, penicillin-resistant *S. aureus* was noted to be a cause of infection in hospitalized patients. By the mid 1950s, nosocomial *S. aureus* infection due to the specific phage type 80/81 was a worldwide problem that resulted in the closure of some surgical and neonatal units and the development of infection control programs. Coincident with the introduction of penicillinase-resistant penicillins, the frequency of these infections decreased, and nosocomial infections due to aerobic gram-negative bacilli became a major problem. This has resulted in a vicious cycle of antibiotic discovery, increased clinical use, and the development of resistance. While aerobic gram-negative bacilli predominated as the nosocomial pathogens of the 1970s and 1980s, the etiology of nosocomial infections has now changed, and gram-positive bacilli are most frequently implicated in the 1990s.

The increasing number of antibiotic-resistant gram-positive organisms has reached epidemic proportions in some hospitals. Among teaching hospitals that reported data to the NNIS in 1991, 40% of staphylococci were methicillin resistant (oxacillin resistant). Among all hospitals, regardless of size, the incidence of methicillin-resistant *S. aureus* (MRSA) rose from 2.4% in 1975 to 29% in 1991. In many nursing homes and chronic care facilities, the rate of MRSA colonization exceeds 50%.

Coagulase-negative staphylococci are now recognized as important pathogens. Until recently, many patients from whom these organisms were cultured were thought to be colonized rather than infected. Hence, the reporting of coagulase-negative staphylococci has increased dramatically. From 1980 to 1990, the percentage of nosocomial BSIs due to coagulase-negative staphylococci increased more than threefold, from 9% to 31%. More than half of these bacteria are methicillin resistant, necessitating the use of vancomycin to treat these infections. The rise in coagulase-negative staphylococci has occurred in hospitals regardless of size.

The most disturbing recent trend in nosocomial infections has been the emergence of vancomycin-resistant enterococci (VRE). These bacteria were nonexistent in the United States until 1989 and now account for nearly 10% of enterococci isolated from hospitalized patients. In all likelihood, the increased incidence of MRSA and methicillin-resistant coagulase-negative staphylococci resulted in greater empiric usage of vancomycin, which selected for these multi–drug-resistant bacteria. For many isolates of VRE there is no effective antibiotic therapy. Vancomycin-resistant enterococci can be spread from patient to patient and have the propensity to survive for prolonged periods on hands and environmental surfaces. In our institution, approximately half of the *Enterococcus faecium* are vancomycin resistant.

Vancomycin resistance has also been reported in coagulase-negative staphylococci, and these organisms may be responsible for the transmission of resistance genes to other gram-positive bacteria. Although there have been no documented clinical isolates of vancomycin-resistant *S. aureus*, this phenotype has been created in the lab, confirming the feasibility of natural acquisition of vancomycin resistance. Obviously, if vancomycin resistance were to be transferred to *S. aureus*, the public health consequences would be devastating.

The aerobic gram-negative bacilli associated with nosocomial infection include enteric bacilli, such as *Escherichia coli*, *Proteus mirabilis*, *Serratia marcescens*, *Klebsiella*, and *Enterobacter* species. In addition, *Stenotrophomonas* (*Xanthomonas*) *maltophilia*, *Acinetobacter*, and *Pseudomonas* species are frequently encountered nosocomial pathogens, especially in critical care units. Similar to the gram-positive bacteria, these bacteria have developed increased degrees of antimicrobial resistance over the last decade.

In the 1970s and 1980s, infections with aminoglycoside-resistant gram-negative bacilli be-

gan to increase, but varied by institution. However, after the introduction of the extended-spectrum penicillins, third-generation cephalosporins, monobactams, and fluoroquinolones, the 1990s have been characterized by organisms with emerging resistance to multiple classes of antimicrobial agents, with aminoglycoside resistance rates remaining rather constant over the last decade. Because of concerns of increasing gram-negative resistance, restriction of antibiotics known to promote resistance has been implemented at many medical centers. This has occurred because selective pressures from the overuse of antibiotics, especially cephalosporins, has promoted induction of beta-lactamases, a major mechanism by which gram-negative bacilli develop resistance to beta-lactam antibiotics. Beta-lactam antibiotics kill bacteria by binding to penicillin-binding proteins, the enzymes responsible for cell-wall synthesis of these bacteria. Beta-lactamases hydrolyze the beta-lactam ring of many penicillins and cephalosporins, rendering them inactive.

To date more than 50 different beta-lactamases have been identified among gram-negative bacilli. A major problem among gram-negative bacilli that frequently causes nosocomial infections is their rapid exchange of genetic information encoding these enzymes. Most of the resistance genes are carried on plasmids which are readily transferable among bacterial species. An example of this is an enzyme that encodes for an extended-spectrum beta-lactamase that results in ceftazidime-resistant *K. pneumoniae*. This enzyme also inactivates cefotaxime and aztreonam, antibiotics originally thought to be beta-lactamase stable. The resistant phenotype of *K. pneumoniae* has resulted in nosocomial pneumonias, is difficult to detect in the laboratory, is associated with a high mortality rate, and is costly to treat.

The etiology of a nosocomial infection often can be suspected based on the site of the infection and the patient's underlying disease. *E. coli* remains the most commonly identified nosocomial pathogen and accounts for 25% of all UTIs. Other organisms that are associated with nosocomial UTIs, in order of decreasing frequency, are enterococci, *P. aeruginosa*, *Candida albicans*, *Klebsiella pneumoniae*, *Proteus mirabilis*, and *Enterobacter* species. Nosocomial pneumonias are most frequently due to *P. aeruginosa* and *S. aureus*. Other organisms that have been implicated in the etiology of pneumonia include *Enterobacter* species, *K. pneumoniae, Haemophilus influenzae,* and *Acinetobacter* species. As expected, nearly half of nosocomial skin and soft tissue infections are due to staphylococci, both *S. aureus* and coagulase-negative staphylococci. Other less common organisms include enterococci, *P. aeruginosa, Enterobacter* species, and *E. coli.* The etiology of bloodstream infections has markedly changed over the past decade, in part due to the recognition of coagulase-negative staphylococci as pathogens rather than contaminants. Hence, coagulase-negative staphylococci are now the most common cause of primary nosocomial bacteremia followed by *S. aureus,* enterococci, and *C. albicans.* The changing etiology of bloodstream infections from gram-negative bacilli to gram-positive cocci and fungi is related to the widespread use of broad-spectrum antibiotics and the increased use of indwelling vascular catheters.

The etiology of nosocomial infections is also influenced by underlying host factors. Examples include the association of staphylococci with intravascular devices; *P. aeruginosa* in patients with severe burns, neutropenia, cystic fibrosis, or allergic bronchopulmonary aspergillosis (ABPA); and *Enterococcus faecium,* which commonly infects patients receiving second- and third-generation cephalosporins. *S. maltophilia* has recently been recognized as an important nosocomial pathogen in patients receiving imipenem who have had prolonged hospitalizations. Another well-recognized association is the development of candidal infections in patients who are receiving multiple antibiotics, hyperalimentation, and who have undergone gastrointestinal surgery.

At least nine nosocomial outbreaks of tuberculosis have occurred in recent years, primarily in New York and Florida. A cluster of tuberculosis was reported among human immunodeficiency virus (HIV)–infected men within weeks of exposure to a patient with smear-negative pulmonary tuberculosis. This report suggested that HIV-infected individuals were both highly susceptible to tuberculous infection and that when infected they were prone to rapid evolution of active disease (see Chapter 13). Molecular epidemiologic studies, in this and in other outbreaks, documented that the organisms were genetically identical, confirming nosocomial transmission. A major factor in the severity of these infections was delay in diagnosis. Other factors contributing to hospital spread of tuberculosis are drug-resistant strains, and multiple lapses in engineering and infection control

practices. These included isolation rooms with positive pressure or with doors left open, improper recirculation of air, and inadequate use of masks by health care workers. The HIV-1 epidemic has also contributed to the nosocomial transmission of multi–drug-resistant tuberculosis in hospital and long-term housing facilities. Clearly, the problem of HIV-tuberculosis co-infection presents an extraordinary challenge to tuberculosis treatment and control programs worldwide.

Pseudomembranous colitis due to *Clostridium difficile,* an anaerobic spore-forming organism that produces an enterotoxin, occurs in patients receiving antibiotics, especially clindamycin, penicillins, or cephalosporins, and chemotherapy for neoplastic disease. It is felt that the majority of cases are due to overgrowth of endogenous *C. difficile,* but there have been documented nosocomial outbreaks due to transmission by hospital personnel. Diarrheal diseases are very common infections among children in pediatric hospitals, and nosocomial outbreaks of enteric pathogens such as rotavirus, *Campylobacter jejuni,* and *Salmonella* species have been documented. Rotavirus has been recovered from the hands of hospital staff and a variety of environmental surfaces encountered in the health care setting. The spread of rotavirus among hospitalized children or to children admitted to a room previously occupied by a child with this virus confirms environmental dissemination.

A recent phenomenon is the development of infections with more resistant candidal strains, such as *C. krusei,* in patients who have received fluconazole for antifungal prophylaxis. Furthermore, the nosocomial transmission of C. *albicans* has been well documented, sometimes including isolates that are fluconazole resistant. Another very important nosocomial fungal infection in immunocompromised patients is aspergillosis. This organism is ubiquitous in the environment and can cause pulmonary as well as rhinocerebral infections in patients with impaired host defenses (see Chapter 14). Nosocomial outbreaks have been reported following major construction projects.

Viral infections can also occur during hospitalization. In the past, transfusion-related infections due to hepatitis C and HIV-1 were a major cause of nosocomial viral infections; however, since the blood supply is now screened for both of these viruses, transmission via this route has become rare. Currently, nearly all cases of nosocomial transmission of

HIV-1 occur as a consequence of needle-stick injuries or the inadvertent infusion of HIV-infected blood. The occupational risk to health care workers following percutaneous exposure to HIV-infected blood is directly proportional to the depth of penetration by the needle and to the volume of blood injected. Other important factors may include the immune status of the patient and previous antiviral therapy. Although well-controlled trials are lacking, the estimated risk of HIV-1 seroconversion following a needle-stick injury is 0.4%. The ability of postexposure prophylaxis with zidovudine (AZT) to prevent transmission following percutaneous exposure is unproven.

Cytomegalovirus, which causes a mononucleosis-like syndrome in normal hosts and severe pneumonitis or hepatitis in immunocompromised patients, can be transmitted by blood or blood products (i.e., platelets, fresh frozen plasma) (see Chapter 8). The majority of nosocomial viral infections occur in pediatric patients and are primarily caused by respiratory agents, including respiratory syncytial virus (RSV), influenza, parainfluenza, adenovirus, rhinovirus, as well as varicella and measles. Recently, a nosocomial outbreak of parainfluenza infection was reported in patients following bone marrow transplantation. Hospital outbreaks of these infections reflect their presence in the community and are the result of patient contact with infected hospital staff or visitors or of transmission from infected to noninfected patients by health care workers. Children at risk are those who lack specific immunity to these agents, rather than individuals predisposed to infection by therapy or underlying disease. Nosocomial varicella-zoster virus infection, however, may produce very severe infection in nonimmune immunocompromised children or adults. It is highly contagious, producing infection in about 80% of susceptible individuals. Outbreaks can occur as a result of contact with patients or staff with unrecognized chickenpox or herpes zoster.

A major advance in determining whether a cluster of apparent nosocomial infections is actually due to a single organism has resulted from the use of molecular techniques to characterize the causative agent. In the past, hospital epidemiologists used antibiotic susceptibility profiles, phage typing of *S. aureus*, and other phenotypic characteristics of the microbe to demonstrate that an outbreak was due to a single strain of the bacteria. Typing systems based on biochemical properties or antibiotic susceptibility profiles are generally limited because epidemiologically diverse bacteria may have identical biotypes or susceptibility patterns. However, molecular techniques can identify the genetic or enzymatic characteristics of isolates, enabling investigators to document that an outbreak was actually due to spread of a single clone from patient to patient or from staff to patient. A number of molecular epidemiologic techniques have been developed to investigate nosocomial outbreaks including restriction enzyme analysis (REA), ribotyping, pulsed-field gel electrophoresis (PFGE), polymerase chain reaction (PCR), and DNA-DNA hybridization (for more details see Willey, et al.).

## PATHOGENESIS

Nosocomial infections generally occur when natural barriers to microbial invasion are violated or when the patient is debilitated. The skin and the mucous membranes of the gastrointestinal tract, urinary tract, and upper airway act as natural barriers to the establishment of infection. Much of modern medical therapy—including surgery and utilization of techniques to support life such as intubation and mechanical ventilation, or intravascular and bladder catheters—violates these barriers. Nasogastric tubes and the reduction of gastric acidity through the use of $H_2$-blockers or antacids also decrease the efficiency of important defense barriers. In addition, the normal flora of the oropharynx and the lower intestinal tract are altered through elimination of oral intake or use of antibiotics, enhancing colonization of these locations by potential pathogens.

Control of the majority of bacterial infections depends upon an adequate number of normally functioning polymorphonuclear neutrophils (PMNs) and the effective interaction of these phagocytes with the serum opsonins, cytokines, complement, and antibody. A number of diseases and therapies interfere with this primary systemic mechanism of host response to microbial invasion (see Chapter 4).

Neonates and the elderly are at increased risk for nosocomial infections. A specific age-related defect in the inflammatory response, however, has been difficult to identify. One reasonable explanation for the association of age and nosocomial infection is the prevalence of such conditions as cancer, diabetes, malnutrition, and cerebrovascular disease in the elderly. All of these diseases require use of therapy that alters neutrophil number, are associated with altered neutrophil function, or result in the use of support systems that bypass natural protective barriers. For instance, hematologic malignancies are treated with cytotoxic chemotherapy that results in granulocytopenia or hypogammaglobulinemia. In addition, the introduction of colony-stimulating factors has allowed higher doses of chemotherapy to be administered and to patients who previously were not appropriate candidates. Solid tumors may obstruct organs, resulting in undrained secretions that, when infected, result in abscess formation or bacteremia. This is most evident in patients with malignancies of the respiratory or gastrointestinal tract. Specific tumors, such as bronchogenic carcinoma and Hodgkin's disease, are associated with serum inhibitors of neutrophil chemotaxis and cytokines which are important components of the inflammatory response.

Corticosteroid therapy used to treat a number of neoplastic and allergic diseases also interferes with neutrophil adherence to endothelial cells, resulting in poor delivery of the phagocytes to the locus of infection in tissue. Diabetes is associated with defective chemotaxis and, in association with ketoacidosis, deficient intracellular killing of bacteria, such as S. aureus. Although it is difficult to document that infections occur with greater frequency in diabetics, the infections that do occur clearly result in increased morbidity and mortality.

Patients infected with HIV-1 have defects in both the cellular and humoral components of the immune system (see Chapter 23). Although traditionally thought of as a T-cell deficiency, these patients also manifest B-cell dysfunction and alterations in cytokine production with disease progression. This complex process, which has not been completely elucidated, ultimately results in quantitative and functional abnormalities in immunity. Regulatory cytokines such as interleukins, interferons, colony-stimulating factors, and tumor necrosis factor (TNF) all play a role in the pathogenesis of HIV-1.

Nosocomial pneumonia with aerobic gram-negative bacilli is associated with endotracheal intubation, use of antibiotics, reduction of gastric acidity, and augmented acuity of illness, all of which are associated with colonization of the upper airway or endotracheal tube with these organisms. Decreased gag and cough reflexes enhance the possibility of aspiration of these organisms and ultimate development of pneumonia. The changing ecology of critical care units due to the use of cephalosporins has resulted in more patients becoming colonized with *Acinetobacter* and *Enterobacter* species. A specific nosocomial pneumonia that occurs in normal as well as in individuals with an altered immune response is that due to *Legionella* species. Legionella pneumonia occurring in hospitalized patients has been especially troublesome in oncology and transplant units. This organism is capable of surviving and replicating in any standing water and is aerosolized from water taps and shower heads. Patients with hairy cell leukemia are at particularly high risk for this infection.

The pathogenesis of catheter-related infections has recently been elucidated. It appears that the initial event is adherence of bacteria to the catheter surface. A biofilm, rich in fibrin and fibronectin, forms on the foreign body. Both coagulase-negative staphylococci and *Candida* species adhere tightly to this biofilm. The organisms also produce a fibrous glycocalyx that serves as a barrier to protect bacteria and fungi from antibiotics, macrophages, and neutrophils. Finally, certain organisms, especially staphylococci and *Candida* species, adhere well to polyvinylchloride, the material used in most catheters. With better knowledge of the pathogenesis of catheter-related infection, it is hoped that strategies can be developed to prevent them.

## MANAGEMENT

Nosocomial infections are often difficult to diagnose because the classic signs of infection, fever, tachycardia, and tachypnea can be muted by therapy or attributed to the underlying illness of the patient. Therefore, the diagnosis requires that the physician have a high clinical index of suspicion for patients at greatest risk of acquiring infection. All postoperative patients, those who are intubated, and those in whom an intravascular device or urinary catheter is placed should be considered susceptible. Additions to this high-risk group of patients are those receiving cytotoxic chemotherapy, intravenous infusions that can be contaminated in manufacture or preparation, broad-spectrum antibiotics, or glucocorticoids.

As mentioned, clinical signs and symptoms of infection may be subtle or absent. Unexplained fever or hypothermia, change in respiratory status, and development of hypotension should stimulate a search for infection. Laboratory findings in association with these signs include either leukocytosis or leukopenia, thrombocytopenia, or evidence of disseminated intravascular coagulation. These clinical or laboratory alterations can occur together or alone in both bacteremic and nonbacteremic patients.

When a hospital-acquired infection is suspected, two sets of blood cultures separated by at least 15 min should be obtained. A thorough review of the hospital course, therapy, and invasive procedures plus a complete physical examination should be performed. If possible, Gram's stain and culture of urine, sputum, draining secretions, or pus should be performed. A chest radiograph should be performed on all immunocompromised patients and those suspected of having a lower respiratory tract infection. Additional radiologic tests such as ultrasonography or computed tomography (CT) can be helpful in specific situations. If a focus of infection can be readily identified, it should be removed or drained expeditiously. In patients in whom there is a suspicion of central nervous system involvement, including those having undergone recent neurosurgery, a lumbar puncture to evaluate the cerebrospinal fluid is mandatory. In these cases, it may be necessary to perform a CT scan of the brain to determine if there is an intracerebral mass producing increased intracranial pressure before performing a lumbar puncture. In the neutropenic patient, empiric antibiotics should be started immediately after obtaining the appropriate cultures. Patients with evidence of sepsis with hypotension should receive antibiotics immediately and transferred to an intensive care unit, where hemodynamic monitoring is available. In addition, insertion of a pulmonary artery catheter may facilitate reconstitution of intravascular volume during fluid replacement. In less critically ill patients, therapy can be delayed until the evaluation is complete and they can be safely managed on the floor.

The choice of empiric antibiotics can be based on the organisms frequently isolated in a specific institution or unit within the hospital. Susceptibility patterns and bacteria may actually vary within an institution. For example, there may be an outbreak of VRE in the surgical intensive care unit, but not in the medical intensive care unit. Alternatively, in the burn unit there may be a high incidence of ciprofloxacin-resistant *P. aeruginosa* that is not present on the general medical floors.

In oncology units, infections due to *P. aeruginosa*, viridans streptococci, and staphylococci are seen related to neutropenia and the widespread use of central venous catheters. Therefore, initial empiric coverage should include agents active against these organisms; an antipseudomonal penicillin or cephalosporin in combination with an aminoglycoside is often selected. Institutional resistance patterns should be reviewed to determine the most appropriate agents in each class. In patients with intraabdominal infections, therapy should include antibiotics with activity against anaerobes including *Bacteroides fragilis* in addition to the aerobic, enteric, gram-negative bacilli. Methicillin-resistant staphylococci should be suspected in patients with indwelling catheter infections, and vancomycin is appropriate in this setting.

The dose and interval of antibiotic therapy is determined by the physiologic state of the patient. Thus, in patients with renal insufficiency, the interval between doses of aminoglycosides is prolonged. The same strategy is required for all agents that are excreted by the kidneys, such as vancomycin, quinolones, penicillins, and cephalosporins. It is important to remember that some decrease in renal dysfunction is present in the majority of elderly patients, even those with a normal serum creatinine. If empiric antibiotic therapy is initiated, results of culture and sensitivity should be used to select the most narrow spectrum, least toxic, and cost-effective antibiotic to complete the treatment. See Chapters 37 and 38 for a complete discussion of antimicrobial therapy.

The duration of treatment is dependent upon the course of the nosocomial infection, the clinical condition of the patient, and the response to therapy. Bacteremia due to *S. aureus* associated with the use of an intravenous catheter usually requires 2 weeks of an effective parenteral antibiotic if the catheter is removed, the patient responds, has no defect in resistance to infection, and has normal cardiac valves. Four to six weeks of antistaphylococcal antibiotic therapy is generally necessary if the patient has a complicated infection, has a metastatic infection, or is immunocompromised. Nonbacteremic urinary tract infection can be effectively treated with 1 week of orally administered antibiotics in the absence of obstruction to urine flow. Nosocomial pneumonia is usually treated for 14 days, unless due to *Legionella* or *Pseudomonas*, when 21 days of therapy is required. Pseudomembranous colitis due to *C. difficile* is managed by discontinuation of the offending antibiotic (if possible) and administration of metronidazole (see Chapter 17). In patients who fail or are intolerant of metronidazole, oral vancomycin is an alternative. This antibiotic should be used with caution because it has been implicated in selecting for vancomycin-resistant enterococci and is significantly more expensive than metronidazole.

## PREVENTION

The prevention of infection in hospitalized patients requires a commitment by physicians, nurses, and administrators to institute policies and procedures designed to reduce the prevalence of this major cause of morbidity and mortality. The Joint Commission on the Accreditation of Healthcare Organizations (JCAHO) mandates that each institution establish a committee to supervise this effort. This committee must be empowered to implement any programs that are necessary to reduce the risk of nosocomial infection within the medical center. The infection control department is responsible for educating the medical and nursing staffs about hospital-acquired infections and performing surveillance to ensure the safety of all hospital personnel and patients. They also have the authority to remove hospital employees who can be linked epidemiologically to the nosocomial transmission of infection or are contagious because of infections such as chickenpox. Although uncommon, the infection control team can take dramatic steps such as closing a hospital unit to control an epidemic.

Effective infection control requires a multidisciplinary approach to be successful. In general, the program is coordinated by a physician with training in infectious diseases and/or hospital epidemiology. Representatives from other important hospital services should be included such as clinical microbiology, pharmacy, nursing, central supply, engineering, environmental services, dietary, employee health services, administration, and risk management. Since virtually every aspect of the hospital plays an important role in infection control, appropriate representation is necessary. A strong working relationship between infection control and the clinical microbiology laboratory is critical. Specific criteria should be developed that allow the microbiology laboratory to report organisms of epidemiologic importance (i.e., MRSA, VRE) to the infection control department in a timely fashion. The microbiology laboratory also plays an important role in epidemiologic surveillance, as they can identify trends in antimicrobial resistance. Organisms of epidemiologic significance or associated with outbreaks should be saved for molecular epidemiologic studies that may need to be performed at a later date. Sufficient resources must be available to both the infection control department and the clinical microbiology laboratory to perform these essential duties.

The most common vectors of transmission of the majority of organisms causing nosocomial infection are the hands of medical personnel. VRE can survive on hands and on gloved fingertips for up to 60 min, implying that not only is hand washing essential, but so is the removal of gloves following every patient encounter. Handwashing remains one of the simplest and most important interventions to prevent the transmission of nosocomial infections, yet despite its simplicity compliance is generally poor. For routine patient care activities, hands should be thoroughly covered with soap and water and vigorously rubbed together for 15 sec. In high-risk areas such as intensive care units or oncology floors, an antibacterial soap is preferred. Studies have shown that as much as 20% of experimentally inoculated hepatitis A virus remains on hands after routine washing. For VRE, a 30-sec hand wash is necessary for complete removal. Gloves have been recommended in many circumstances in an attempt to prevent the nosocomial transmission of bacteria. Both latex and vinyl gloves provide substantial protection; however, leaks can occur. In one study, hand contamination with gram-negative bacilli or enterococci occurred in 13% of the procedures when gloves were worn. This again emphasizes the importance of glove removal and routine hand washing following patient contact.

Environmental surfaces frequently encountered in the health care setting can serve as reservoirs for hospital-acquired infections. During nosocomial outbreaks, various organisms of clinical significance have been cultured from countertops, bedrails, stethoscopes, telephones, blood pressure cuffs, tourniquets, electrocardiogram monitors, and infusion pumps. During a nosocomial outbreak of *Acinetobacter calcoaceticus* in a pediatric intensive care unit, investigators found the infecting strain persisting on countertops for 10.2 days. This same organism was also cultured from the hands of two nurses, a respiratory therapist, a pediatric resident, a telephone, and a coffee pot. Control of the outbreak occurred after educating the staff about the importance of hand washing and proper disinfection of environmental surfaces. Vancomycin-resistant enterococci are also known to persist for prolonged periods of time on inanimate objects and can also survive for at least 1 week on countertops and for days on bedrails. While investigating a nosocomial outbreak of VRE, a tourniquet left in a patient room yielded the epidemic strain when cultured 4 days after the patient had been discharged.

Another major technique to reduce infection is the cautious use of therapies or support devices that enhance the risk of infection. Thus, the use of antibiotics should be limited to situations where these agents have been proved to be necessary and effective. This is particularly true for cephalosporins, which increase the risk of enterococcal colonization and infection.

Intravascular lines should be left in place only as long as absolutely necessary. The use of a specialized team to insert and care for intravascular catheters has been shown in several studies to help guard against infection. In medical centers with a high rate of catheter-related infections, this approach can be cost effective. Proper preparation of the insertion site is critical to prevent infection. The use of alcohol and povidone-iodine are clearly superior to chlorhexidine. Attachable, silver-impregnated cuffs have also been shown to decrease the risk of infection in patients with central lines inserted for short-term use; however, they are of no benefit for long-term catheters. An area of controversy is the practice of changing central venous catheters over a guidewire at routine intervals. If the line site appears infected, then a new insertion site should be chosen, but changing over a guidewire has not been shown conclusively to diminish the risk of infection.

Urinary catheters, similar to central venous catheters, should be used only when absolutely necessary. They should not be used routinely for monitoring urine output or for nursing convenience. The most significant factor to prevent indwelling bladder catheter infection is the use of a closed drainage system. In addition, catheterization must be performed in a sterile manner by individuals properly trained in insertion. The risk of infection increases significantly if the drainage system is open. The catheter and drainage bag do not require routine changing unless obviously infected. Urinary catheters frequently become colonized with nosocomial organisms; however, in order to diagnose a nosocomial UTI, both bacteruria and pyuria should be present.

There is increasing evidence that in specific surgical situations the judicious use of prophylactic antibiotics reduces the prevalence of postoperative infection. Surgery conducted in contaminated sites, such as the head and neck or colorectal or pelvic areas, is associated with high rates of wound infection in the absence of prophylactic antibiotics. The antibiotics must be initiated shortly before or during surgery with the aim of providing effective blood and tissue levels during and immediately after the procedure. Prolonged preoperative antibiotic administration or continuation beyond 8–12 h postoperatively, however, does not enhance the efficacy of prophylaxis and is clearly associated with the subsequent carriage of antibiotic-resistant bacteria and adverse reactions. Placement of a prosthetic device, such as a cardiac valve or a prosthetic joint, requires prophylaxis to prevent a devastating infection of the prosthesis. Surgical prophylaxis should be directed against the most common organisms that cause infection at the site of surgery. For routine surgical prophylaxis, coverage against staphylococci and streptococci is all that is necessary.

There is increasing evidence that antimicrobial prophylaxis reduces the infection rate in neutropenic patients and those undergoing bone marrow transplantation. However, routine antibacterial prophylaxis is associated with increased colonic carriage of antibiotic-resistant bacteria. This has been well documented in European trials when the fluoroquinolone ciprofloxacin was used. Antifungal prophylaxis with fluconazole has been shown to decrease the risk of superficial and systemic fungal infections in patients with leukemia or those undergoing bone marrow transplantation. Not surprisingly, this has resulted in an increase in infections due to *Candida krusei* and other fluconazole-resistant fungi. Prophylaxis against *Pneumocystis carinii* pneumonia in transplant patients and those infected with HIV-1 remains cost effective and is encouraged.

## ISOLATION

When a patient is admitted to the hospital with a virulent, highly contagious infection, develops an infection with a multi–antibiotic-resistant organism while hospitalized, or has a draining infected wound, appropriate isolation techniques should be instituted to prevent spread of infection. The Centers for Disease Control and Prevention (CDC) have classified diseases into one of six isolation categories based on their mode of transmission. *Strict isolation* requires the wearing of mask, gown, and gloves when entering a patient's room and is reserved for infections that can be spread by both personal contact and by inhalation. These patients must be placed in a private room and whenever possible a room with negative air flow. A common infection that requires strict isolation is varicella. *Contact isolation* is used to prevent the spread of organisms whose mode of transmission is close contact. For these patients, gloves must be worn for all patient care activities and mask or gown if significant soiling is likely. Patients colonized with multi–drug-resistant organisms such as MRSA or VRE are placed in contact isolation. However, a recently published study demonstrated that wearing gloves alone failed to curtail an outbreak of VRE and that both gloves and gowns were required. It is unclear whether the gowns (1) had a protective effect or (2) made hospital staff more aware of resistant enterococci and decreased traffic within these rooms. *Respiratory isolation* is used for patients with infections that are spread by respiratory secretions. Masks are required for these patients, but not gowns or gloves. Patients with suspected tuberculosis are placed in respiratory isolation. If the index of suspicion is high or tuberculosis is documented, then the rooms should have negative air flow with an anteroom. *Enteric precautions* are designed for diseases that are spread by contact with feces. Gowns should be worn if soiling of clothes is likely and gloves must be worn when handling stool. The most frequent indication for this isolation is infectious diarrhea. *Drainage/secretion precautions* are used to prevent the spread of infections due to infected wounds. Gloves are to be worn for contact with purulent material and gowns if soiling is likely to occur. Minor wounds fall into this category of isolation.

*Universal precautions* were developed by the CDC to protect health care workers against blood-borne pathogens and are now mandated by the Occupational Safety and Health Administration (OSHA). These were initially developed to prevent the transmission of HIV-1 and hepatitis B in the health care setting. Currently, these guidelines have been expanded to include protection against any bodily fluid that can transmit infection or is contaminated with visible blood. It is important to remember that these guidelines were developed to protect health care workers, *not* patients, and that compliance with universal precautions does not obviate the need for proper infection control practices.

## EMPLOYEE HEALTH

The prevention of nosocomial infections also requires that hospital employees are free from communicable diseases. All new staff should have a complete history and physical examination performed prior to beginning patient care activities. Care should be taken to avoid placing immunocompromised staff in high-risk areas. New employees are often screened for evidence of past infection or immunity to varicella, rubella, and measles. In individuals without documented immunity or written evidence of prior infection, vaccination should be offered. All staff involved in direct patient care activities should be screened for immunity to hepatitis B. For those without antibody to hepatitis B, vaccination should be strongly encouraged. A tuberculin skin test should be part of preemployment screening and repeated on a yearly basis or after exposure to a patient with tuberculosis. A history of bacille Calmette-Guérin (BCG) vaccination should not prevent the use of tuberculin skin testing. A positive skin test should be followed up with a chest x-ray to rule out active disease (see Chapter 13). Routine testing of women of childbearing age for cytomegalovirus (CMV) is not recommended because the risk of acquiring CMV in the health care setting is minimal. It is critical that any health care worker who is exposed to potentially contagious diseases report the exposure to employee health service so that proper treatment and follow-up is provided.

Nosocomial outbreaks frequently result in confusion and anxiety among both the medical and nursing staff. It is the responsibility of the infection control department to handle outbreaks in a professional and timely fashion. Reinforcement of infection control procedures including hand washing and proper isolation generally controls most outbreaks. If an outbreak occurs, a specific unit may have to be closed to new admissions. Those patients are all assumed to be potentially infected and kept in that area until ready for discharge. The infection control team then reviews current practices, assesses compliance, and then corrects any apparent problems. Investigation of the reason for spread of the infection should be undertaken, and only when secondary cases cease can the unit be allowed to admit new patients. The investigation of the outbreak can involve obtaining cultures from personnel and the environment, and a search for possible vectors such as infected intravenous solutions or a break in sterilization techniques of critical care equipment. Further details describing the epidemiologic investigation of nosocomial outbreaks can be found in the references.

## CASE HISTORIES

### CASE HISTORY 1

A 55-year-old man was admitted to the hospital with substernal chest pain and hypotension. A diagnosis of acute myocardial infarction was established. His hemodynamic status was rapidly stabilized after emergent placement of a pulmonary artery catheter and an intraaortic balloon pump. On the fourth hospital day, while making good recovery in the intensive care unit, the patient developed a fever of 101.5°F associated with chills. He denied headache, sore throat, cough, chest pain, shortness of breath, dysuria, abdominal discomfort, or diarrhea. Physical examination revealed a supple neck, a clear chest, no cardiac murmur, and a soft, nontender abdomen with normoactive bowel sounds. There was moderate erythema surrounding the site of the intravenous catheter, which had not been changed since arrival in the emergency room. Suspecting bacteremia due to an infected venous catheter, his physician obtained two sets of blood cultures using blood obtained from each antecubital vein, and a third set was drawn from the venous catheter; other tests included urine for analysis and culture, a complete blood count, and a portable chest x-ray. The pulmonary artery catheter and aortic balloon were removed and cultured, and venous access was maintained with a peripheral intravenous line.

The white cell count was 18,900/mm$^3$ with 40% segmented neutrophils and 35% band forms. The urine contained no leukocytes or bacteria, and the chest x-ray was normal. Vancomycin, 1 g intravenously every 12 h, was begun empirically for possible line-related bacteremia due to staphylococci.

The patient's temperature gradually improved, and he was afebrile within 48 h. All blood cultures and the pulmonary artery catheter tip grew methicillin-resistant *S. aureus*. Repeat blood cultures at 5 days were sterile. After 14 days of therapy, there was no evidence of metastatic infection or cardiac murmur. Vancomycin was discontinued and the patient underwent coronary angiography and an uncomplicated percutaneous transluminal coronary angioplasty.

### CASE 1 DISCUSSION

The emergent placement of an intravenous catheter and inatraaortic balloon pump to treat cardiogenic shock following an acute myocardial infarction are common occurrences. However, the situation described above often prevents complete asepsis during placement of the catheter. The intravenous catheter was left in place for 4 days rather than being replaced within 48 h, and bacteremia secondary to *S. aureus* resulted. This oversight complicated this patient's recovery, delaying evaluation of the coronary arteries and prolonging hospitalization. In similar patients who do not have the complication of infection, angiography and angioplasty could have been carried out and the patient discharged much earlier.

The use of empiric vancomycin for treatment of a suspected line-related bacteremia was appropriate because the most likely organisms are *S. aureus* or coagulase-negative staphylococci. The majority of nosocomial infections due to these staphylococci are resistant to oxacillin. However, if the organism was oxacillin susceptible, therapy should be changed to this agent or another appropriate beta-lactam antibiotic. The duration of therapy in the absence of metastatic infection is 14 days. If infection is detected in bones or joints, on a cardiac valve, or of the pericardium, then 6 weeks of antibiotics is necessary.

### CASE HISTORY 2

A 23-year-old woman with acute myelogenous leukemia was admitted to the hospital for induction chemotherapy. Following chemotherapy, she became profoundly neutropenic, requiring broad-spectrum antibiotics and amphotericin B. Three weeks into her hospital course she had a rectal swab positive for vancomycin-resistant *Enterococcus faecium*. Her neutropenia resolved, the remainder of her course was unremarkable, and she was discharged after 27 days. Two months later she was readmitted for an allogeneic bone marrow transplant. Once again, she became febrile and neutropenic, requiring a prolonged course of antimicrobial therapy. Ten days into this admission, a catheterized urine culture grew 40,000 vancomycin-resistant *E. faecium*. This organism was resistant to all currently approved antibiotics and she was placed in strict isolation while awaiting resolution of neutropenia. Her bone marrow transplant was successful, and she was discharged. Four months later, she presented to the emergency room with recurrence of her leukemia and sepsis. Two sets of blood cultures obtained on admission were positive for vancomycin-resistant *E. faecium*. She was transferred to the medical intensive care unit where despite mechanical ventilation and pressor support she expired 3 days later.

## CASE 2 DISCUSSION

This unfortunate case exemplifies the emerging problem of multi–drug-resistant enterococci. This patient initially became colonized with this organism either because of nosocomial transmission or antimicrobial selection. Once colonized, she remained persistently colonized until she developed sepsis when her leukemia relapsed. Unfortunately, this organism was of the VanA phenotype, that is, highly resistant to vancomycin and teicoplanin. In addition, it was also highly beta-lactam and aminoglycoside resistant, making this infection untreatable. Restriction endonuclease analysis of genomic DNA revealed that all three isolates were genetically identical, confirming that the initial colonizing strain resulted in her fatal bacteremia. An important point is that patients with multi–drug-resistant bacteria should be placed in strict isolation. All health care workers must wear gowns and gloves prior to patient contact and thoroughly wash hands following contact. As there are no effective antibiotics for many strains of vancomycin-resistant enterococci and patients are generally immunocompromised, the mortality rate is high.

## REFERENCES

### Books

Bennett, J., and Brachman, P., eds. *Hospital Infections.* 3rd ed. Boston: Little, Brown & Co., 1992.

Wenzel, R. P. *Prevention and Control of Nosocomial Infections.* 2nd ed. Baltimore: Williams & Wilkins, 1993.

### Articles

Cox, C. Nosocomial urinary tract infections. *Urology 32*: 210–215, 1988.

Centers for Disease Control. Update: Universal precautions for prevention of transmission of human immunodeficiency virus, hepatitis B virus, and other blood-borne pathogens in health-care settings. *MMWR 37*: 377–382, 387–388, 1988.

Dooley, S. W., Villarino, M. E., Lawrence, L., et al. Nosocomial transmission of tuberculosis in a hospital unit for HIV-infected patients. *JAMA 267*:2632–2635, 1992.

Emori, T. G., and Gaynes, R. P. An overview of nosocomial infections, including the role of the microbiology laboratory. *Clin. Microbiol. Rev. 6*:428–442, 1993.

Georghiou, P. R., Hamill, R. J., Wright, C. E., et al. Molecular epidemiology of infections due to *Enterobacter aerogenes*: Identification of hospital outbreak-associated strains by molecular techniques. *Clin. Infect. Dis. 20*: 84–94, 1995.

Goldman, D. A. Nosocomial infection control in the United States of America. *J. Hosp. Infect. 8*:116–119, 1986.

Holmberg, S. D., Solomon, S. L., and Blake, P. A. Health and economic impacts of antimicrobial resistance. *Rev. Infect. Dis. 9*:1065–1079, 1987.

Kislak, J. W., Eickhoff, T. C., and Finland, M. Hospital-acquired infections and antibiotic usage in the Boston City Hospital. *N. Engl. J. Med. 271*:834–835, 1964.

Maki, D. G. Nosocomial bacteremia: An epidemiologic overview. *Am. J. Med. 70*:719–732, 1981.

Miller, J. M. Molecular technology for hospital epidemiology. *Diagn. Microbiol. Infect. Dis. 16*:153–158, 1993.

Noskin, G. A., Peterson, L. R., and Warren, J. R. *Enterococcus faecium* and *Enterococcus faecalis* bacteremia: Acquisition and outcome. *Clin. Infect. Dis. 20*:296–301, 1995.

Schaberg, D. R., Culver, D. H., and Gaynes, R. P. Major trends in the microbial etiology of nosocomial infection. *Am. J. Med. 91*(Suppl. 3B):72S–75S, 1991.

Sepkowitz, K. A. AIDS, tuberculosis and the health care worker. *Clin. Infect. Dis. 20*:232–242, 1995.

Steere, A. C., and Mallison, G. F. Handwashing practices for the prevention of nosocomial infections. *Ann. Intern. Med. 83*:683–690, 1975.

Raad, I. I., and Bodey, G. P. Infectious complications of indwelling vascular catheters. *Clin. Infect. Dis. 15*:197–210, 1992.

Willey, B. M., McGeer, A. J., et al. The use of molecular typing techniques in the epidemiologic investigation of resistant enterococci. *Infect. Control Hosp. Epidemiol. 15*:548–556, 1994.

# 26
# INFECTIONS AT THE EXTREMES OF LIFE

TINA Q. TAN, M.D. and JOHN R. WARREN, M.D.

Infections in the very young or very old present special challenges to physicians caring for these patients. At one extreme the host's defense systems are not fully developed, and at the other extreme the systems are senescent. Specific microbial flora associated with distinctive areas of skin and mucosal sites are influenced by the age of the host, the environment, diet, temperature, and moisture. The most common pathogens seen in these extremes of life are somewhat unique, especially in the neonate, and the disease processes they cause often present in different ways than in other hosts.

## HOST AND PATHOGEN INTERACTIONS

The immune response of the host differs depending on the type of infecting agent (viruses, pyogenic bacteria, fungi, and nonviral intracellular pathogens). Viruses enter the host in several different ways, but there are two major types of immune responses the host uses to defend itself: (1) humoral immunity, in which antibodies present in secretions or in the circulation act to neutralize the infectivity of viruses; and (2) lymphocyte-mediated cytotoxic cellular immunity, in which CD8+ cytotoxic lymphocytes or natural killer (NK) cells destroy infected host cells that express virus-specific antigens on their surface. In the neonate, especially in the premature infant, the cytotoxic activity of mononuclear cells and NK cells is impaired, and their ability to destroy infected host cells is deficient. The development of a specific T-cell–mediated immune response against various viruses is diminished and/or delayed in the neonate. The diminished number of antigen-specific memory T cells is thought to be the primary cause for the deficient production of various cytokines by neonatal T cells. This may be the critical factor in the increased susceptibility of neonates to pathogens against which these defense mechanisms play an important role. Antibody-mediated protection passively provided from the mother adds to the protective immune response, but if the mother lacks IgG antibody or if the infection occurs at a point in gestation (first half) when the fetus has few or no detectable T or B cells, these deficits also add to the increased susceptibility to infection.

Host defense mechanisms against pyogenic bacteria include nonspecific protective barriers such as the intact skin, mucus, antibacterial agents in secretions, gastric acid, and gastrointestinal motility. However, the most important host immune defense mechanisms against pyogenic bacteria involve the process of phagocytosis, coupled with opsonization and the complement system. Ingestion of microorganisms by polymorphonuclear leukocytes and monocytes/macrophages triggers oxidative and nonoxidative bactericidal mechanisms (oxygen radicals and proteolytic enzymes), leading to death of the microorganism. Specific opsonic antibodies recognize and bind to bacterial surface structures, facilitating the phagocytosis of the microorganism. The presence of immunoglobulin opsonins on the bacterial surface may also lead to activation of the complement cascade, resulting in deposition of both opsonic complement factors and the terminal lytic complex. In the neonate, the major deficits in host defense leading to increased susceptibility to bacterial infection include lack of secretory IgA in secretions, the absence of maternally derived and endogenous type-specific antibody, a deficiency of opsonins, and a limited ability to mobilize neutrophils to sites of infection (impaired chemotaxis).

The most important host defense mechanism against fungi is the killing mechanisms of phagocytic cells. Systemic fungal infections are most often associated with neutropenia or functional neutropenia and immunosuppression, both of which are characteristic in the neonate.

The principal mechanisms of host defense against nonviral intracellular pathogens appear to be the close interaction between NK cells and macrophages, followed by the actions of antigen-specific T lymphocytes and cytokines produced by T cells. In the neonate, the immaturity in NK cell function, the slower immigration of neonatal monocytes to sites of infection, the deficient production of various cytokines (tumor necrosis factor–alpha [TNF-alpha], interferon-gamma [IFN-gamma]), and the delay in development of memory T cells all contribute to the neonate's increased susceptibility to infection.

At the other extreme of life, aged individuals also demonstrate defective immunity. The number of immature T lymphocytes is increased, both in the thymus and the peripheral blood, suggesting that the aging thymus gland loses its capacity to promote the differentiation of immature lymphocytes. In addition, T lymphocytes show a decreased proliferative response both to nonspecific mitogens and to specific microbial antigens, and the production of interleukin-2 (IL-2) (T-cell growth factor) and IFN-gamma by senescent T lymphocytes is diminished. The age-dependent decrement in T-lymphocyte activity is pivotal for the immunodeficiency that accompanies

aging, as the overall number and function of macrophages and neutrophils are unchanged with age. The loss of T-cell function with age adversely affects both cell-mediated and humoral immunity. Aged individuals show decreased delayed cutaneous hypersensitivity to common microbial antigens, and decreased antibody responses to pneumococcal, influenza, and hepatitis B vaccines. Most importantly, the elderly host is unusually susceptible to infection by a wide variety of viral, facultative intracellular bacterial, and encapsulated extracellular bacterial parasites.

## PATHOGENESIS OF NEONATAL INFECTION

Infections in the neonate may be acquired (1) *in utero*, (2) during birth, or (3) soon after birth. *In utero* infections may result in abortion, stillbirths, intrauterine growth retardation, malformations, and other sequelae of chronic infection. Infections acquired during the birth process or soon after birth may result in severe systemic disease, persistent postnatal infection, or death. Late-onset disease may occur with *in utero* infection or infection acquired during birth, in which the infection may present with signs and symptoms weeks to even years later.

The fetus *in utero* is protected from infections that the mother may contract in the community, through the efficient function of the maternal immune system. Most maternal infections involve the upper respiratory and gastrointestinal tracts and are either self-limited and resolve spontaneously or are easily treated with antimicrobial agents. However, if the infecting organism invades the maternal bloodstream, this can lead to infection of the fetus. Transplacental spread after maternal infection and bacteremia is the most common route by which the fetus becomes infected. The fetus may also become infected by extension of infection from adjacent tissues (infections of the urogenital tract), or as a result of invasive methods for the diagnosis and therapy of fetal disorders, but these are less frequent routes.

The efficiency of transplacental transmission of a microorganism from the infected mother to the fetus varies depending on the agent and the trimester of pregnancy. The most common microorganisms that utilize this route include those that are identified in the acronym TORCH: *toxoplasma gondii*, rubella virus, cytomegalovirus (CMV), and herpes simplex virus (HSV). The other organisms not included in this acronym but which are well known causes of *in utero* infection include *Treponema pallidum* (syphilis), enteroviruses, varicella-zoster virus, and human immunodeficiency virus (HIV).

The results of infection following hematogenous transplacental spread are variable, and range from an infant with no detectable abnormalities to abortion and stillbirth of the fetus, or the live birth of a severely damaged infant with multiple developmental and growth anomalies. Infection may persist after birth and may be apparent soon after birth, or may not be recognized for months or years, resulting in significant anomalies in growth and development.

During the birth process, the newborn and placenta often become colonized by the flora of the maternal genital tract. If there is premature rupture of the fetal membranes or if delivery is delayed after membrane rupture, the fetus may acquire an infection when the vaginal microflora ascend in the genital tract and in certain instances produce inflammation of the fetal membranes, umbilical cord, or placenta. The fetus may also become infected following the aspiration of infected amniotic fluid. A large variety of microorganisms may be present in the maternal birth canal, including gram-positive cocci (staphylococci and streptococci), gram-negative cocci (*Neisseria meningitidis* and *Neisseria gonorrhoeae*), gram-negative enteric bacilli (*Escherichia coli*, *Klebsiella*, *Salmonella*, *Shigella*, *Proteus*, and *Pseudomonas*), anaerobic bacteria, viruses (CMV, HSV, and HIV), chlamydiae, mycoplasmas, fungi, and protozoa (*Toxoplasma gondii* and *Trichomonas vaginalis*). Some of these organisms may cause severe disease in the newborn infant, while others rarely affect the neonate.

The newborn is initially colonized on the skin and mucosal surfaces, and the organisms present usually proliferate without causing illness. However, infants may become infected by direct extension from sites of colonization or through invasion of the bloodstream. Risk factors that have been associated with the development of bacterial sepsis include low birth weight, premature or prolonged rupture of maternal membranes, fetal anoxia, septic or traumatic delivery, and maternal peripartum infections. However, the greatest risk factor for the neonate's increased susceptibility to infection is the immaturity of the newborn's immune system.

## Clinical Manifestations

Typical manifestations that may be present in a neonate with an infection acquired *in utero* or at delivery include underweight for gestational age, jaundice, chorioretinitis, hepatosplenomegaly, purpura/petechiae, pneumonia, meningoencephalitis, eye and cardiac defects, bone lesions, intracranial calcifications, microcephaly, or hydrocephalus. Some of these are more prevalent in various diseases than others (Table 26–1).

Other nonspecific signs and symptoms that may indicate that the infant is infected include hypothermia, poor appetite and feeding, decrease in activity, tachypnea and grunting respirations, apnea, and increased irritability, among others. Many of the manifestations may be very subtle and nonspecific, and close monitoring coupled with a high level of suspicion may be necessary to make the diagnosis.

## Etiologies

### Bacteria

The bacterial organisms that are most important as causative agents of neonatal sepsis include group B streptococcus (most prevalent), *E. coli* and other gram-negative enteric organisms, *Treponema pallidum*, *Staphylococcus aureus*, and *Listeria monocytogenes*. Group B streptococci (*S. agalactiae* or GBS) and *Listeria monocytogenes* classically cause both early- and late-onset sepsis. Table 26–2 illustrates the features of early- and late-onset sepsis due to these organisms.

GBS is found in the genital and lower gastrointestinal tracts of colonized men and women. More than 20% of women of child-bearing age are colonized with GBS. Recognized risk factors for GBS colonization include use of an intrauterine device, sexual activity, low parity (<4), and younger age (<21 years). During pregnancy, GBS may cause maternal infection by ascending the genitourinary tract, by entering the bloodstream, or by causing local infection. Other manifestations of maternal disease include preterm labor, premature rupture of membranes, chorioamnionitis, endometritis, postpartum fever, and urinary tract infection. Infants may acquire the organism by aspiration of infected amniotic fluid or by colonization during the birth process. Of infants born to women who are colonized with GBS, 30–50% will become colonized at anorectal, umbilical, or oral sites, and 1–2% of these infants may manifest in-

**TABLE 26–1.   CLINICAL MANIFESTATIONS OF NEONATAL INFECTIONS ACQUIRED IN UTERO OR AT DELIVERY**

| Clinical Signs | *Toxoplasma gondii* | Rubella Virus | Cytomegalovirus | Herpes Simplex Virus | *Treponema pallidum* | Enteroviruses | Group B Streptococcus or *Escherichia coli* |
|---|---|---|---|---|---|---|---|
| Hepatosplenomegaly | + | + | + | + | + | + | + |
| Jaundice | + | + | + | + | + | + | + |
| Adenopathy | + | + | − | − | − | − | − |
| Pneumonitis | + | + | + | + | + | + | + |
| Petechiae or purpura | + | − | + | ++ | + | − | + |
| Vesicles | − | − | − | ++ | + | + | − |
| Maculopapular lesions | + | − | + | + | ++ | + | − |
| Meningoencephalitis | + | + | ++ | ++ | + | + | + |
| Microcephaly | + | − | ++ | + | − | − | − |
| Intracranial calcifications | ++ | − | ++ | − | − | − |  |
| Hydrocephalus | ++ | + | ++ | + | − | − | − |
| Hearing loss | ++ | ++ | ++ | − | − | − | − |
| Chorioretinitis | − | ++ | + | + | ++ | − | − |
| Cataracts | ++ | ++ | + | + | + | − | − |
| Myocarditis | + | ++ | − | + | − | − | − |
| Bone lesions | + | ++ | − | − | ++ | ++ | − |

+, Frequency of finding; −, not present.

**TABLE 26–2. CHARACTERISTICS OF NEONATAL INFECTION WITH GROUP B STREPTOCOCCUS AND *LISTERIA MONOCYTOGENES***

| ORGANISM | GROUP B STREPTOCOCCUS | | LISTERIA MONOCYTOGENES | |
|---|---|---|---|---|
| Features | Early-onset | Late-onset | Early-onset | Late-onset |
| Mean age at onset | 8 h after birth | 7 days after birth | At birth | 4 weeks after birth |
| Birthweight | Preterm or low birthweight | Term | Low birthweight | Term |
| Obstetric complications | Common | Unusual | Common | Unusual |
| Manifestations | Pneumonia (40%) Bacteremia (45%) Meningitis (15%) | Bacteremia (50%) Meningitis (35%) | Bacteremia (73%) | Meningitis (87%) |
| Serotypes | All | Primarily type III | 1a, 1b, 4b | 4b |
| Fatality rate | 8–16% | 2–10% | 25% | 5% |

fection. Low levels of maternal antibody to the GBS type III capsular polysaccharide have a high correlation with increased neonatal susceptibility to disease caused by GBS capsular type III. This maternal antibody deficiency also leads to increased susceptibility to disease caused by GBS capsular types Ia, Ib, and II. Other factors found to play a role in increasing the risk of early-onset neonatal GBS infection include heavy maternal genitourinary tract colonization, gestational age less than 37 weeks, prolonged rupture of membranes (>18–24 h), maternal GBS bacteremia, multiple births, black race, previous delivery of a child with GBS disease, and maternal fever during labor. Many of these factors also play a role in the development of late-onset neonatal GBS disease.

Neonatal *Listeria monocytogenes* infection presents very similarly to GBS disease. The organisms may be acquired from maternal ingestion of contaminated food, may colonize the urogenital tract, and can cause symptomatic maternal disease. Development of infection during the early part of pregnancy (<16 weeks) may lead to abortion or stillbirth. Maternal illness often presents as a febrile influenza-like illness 2–14 days prior to delivery, with chorioamnionitis being the most common manifestation. The infant is usually infected through ascending intrauterine infection or transplacentally.

*Treponema pallidum* is the causative organism of syphilis (see Chapter 16). Infection in the fetus occurs by transplacental hematogenous acquisition during the early stages of maternal infection. This infection may cause preterm labor and delivery, stillbirth, congenital infection, or fetal demise, depending on the stage of maternal infection and the duration of fetal infection before delivery. Infants born to mothers with primary or secondary syphilis are at greatest risk for acquiring the infection because of a large systemic spirochete load. The large majority of these infants become congenitally infected, and up to 50% present with clinical symptoms. However, the more latent the stage of syphilis in the mother, the lower the incidence of infection in the fetus. The manifestations of congenital syphilis in the neonate are mostly systemic, including immune hydrops, jaundice, hepatosplenomegaly, maculopapular or vesiculobullous lesions, osteochondritis, snuffles, lymphadenopathy, pseudoparalysis, pneumonitis, myocarditis, nephrosis, and signs of central nervous system (CNS) infection. Up to 65% of infants with congenital syphilis are asymptomatic at birth, and symptoms may not become apparent for years. Table 26–1 illustrates other manifestations of the disease.

### Viruses

The predominant viral organisms that cause most cases of congenital infection in the newborn are CMV, rubella virus, HSV, enteroviruses, and HIV. Cytomegalovirus is the most common cause of congenital infection and disease in the United States. The incidence of congenital infection ranges from 0.25–2.5%, and maternal infection can be transmitted to up to 50% of fetuses whose mothers had no antibody prior to pregnancy. The transmission of primary maternal CMV infection to the fetus results in disease in about 20% of infants. Prior maternal infection that is reactivated during pregnancy is transmitted to the fetus in 0.2–1.5% of cases. The course of disease in infants of mothers with recurrent or reactivation infection is most often benign, probably due to the beneficial effect of pre-existing maternal antibody. Mortality in symptomatic newborns ranges from 20–30%. CMV infection transmitted to the fetus in the first 6 months of pregnancy is more likely to affect the fetus severely. CMV may also be transmitted postnatally to the infant from the mother's cervicovaginal secretions, urine, saliva, and breast milk. More than 50% of mothers shedding virus from these sites are likely to transmit the infection to their infants, with the genital tract and breast milk the predominant sites of transmission. These infants are usually asymptomatic, but can spread virus to other children and adults.

Fetuses may become infected with the rubella virus after their mothers become viremic. The virus seeds the placenta, leading to fetal viremia and infection of fetal organs. The classic triad of congenital rubella syndrome is cataracts, sensorineural deafness, and congenital heart disease (patent ductus arteriosus or malformations of the pulmonary arterial system), but many other features of this syndrome are recognized, as illustrated in Tables 26–1 and 26–3. Infection during the first trimester more commonly causes spontaneous abortion or fetal infection with significant defects and neonatal sequelae compared to infection occurring later in gestation.

Herpes simplex infection of the newborn can be acquired *in utero*, intrapartum, or after birth, with the majority of infections acquired from the maternal genital tract either through ascending infection or during the birth process. Both HSV-1 and HSV-2 can cause clinical illness in the neonate, although HSV-2 is the primary etiologic agent, causing about 70% of the cases. The risk of HSV infection in an infant born to a mother with primary infection is 40–50%; this drops to 3–4% for the infant born to a mother with recurrent infection, indicating that transplacental antibodies possibly have a protective role. *In utero* infection is characterized by disease at birth ranging from skin vesicles and keratoconjunctivitis to much more severe manifestations such as microcephaly and chorioretinitis. The predominant risk factor for *in utero* HSV transmission is primary maternal infection. Circumstances that favor intrapartum transmission of infection include primary maternal infection with a large viral burden excreted for prolonged periods, prolonged rupture of membranes, and vaginal delivery. Therefore, it is recommended that women with active genital lesions at onset of labor be delivered by cesarean section to decrease the risk of transmission of infection to the newborn. Postnatally acquired HSV infection may be a consequence of nursing on an infected breast, or through contact with persons who have orolabial herpes.

The clinical presentation of the infant with neonatal HSV infection is a direct reflection of the site of viral replication. Neonatal infection may manifest as a local infection limited to the portal of entry—namely, the skin, eye, or mouth (SEM); as CNS disease; or as disseminated disease. SEM infection most often presents at around 10 days of life. Infection involving the eyes may present as keratoconjunctivitis or chorioretinitis. Skin manifestations include the presence of discrete vesicles on an erythematous base that are the hallmark of the disease. Clusters of vesicles often appear initially on the presenting body part that was in direct contact with virus during the birth process. These vesicles occur in 90% of infants with SEM disease, and recurrences are common during the first 6 months of life.

### TABLE 26–3.    SYNDROMES OF CONGENITAL INFECTIONS

| MICROORGANISMS | SIGNS |
| --- | --- |
| *Toxoplasma gondii* | Diffuse intracranial calcifications, hydrocephalus, chorioretinitis |
| Rubella virus | Cataracts, sensorineural hearing loss, cardiac defects, chorioretinitis |
| Cytomegalovirus (CMV) | Periventricular calcifications, microcephalus, hearing loss, chorioretinitus |
| Herpes simplex virus (HSV) | Vesicular lesions, keratoconjunctivitis |
| *Treponema pallidum* | Skin lesions involving the palms and soles, rhinorrhea, signs of osteochrondritis and periostitis |
| Human immunodeficiency virus (HIV) | Failure to thrive, severe thrush, calcification of the basal ganglia, recurrent bacterial infections |

Central nervous system involvement alone or in combination with disseminated disease presents classically with findings of encephalitis. This form of the disease is usually seen at around 15–17 days of life. About 70% of infants with neonatal herpes have evidence of acute brain infection, and this is the most common manifestation of the disease. Clinical manifestations include seizures, irritability, thermal instability, poor feeding, and bulging fontanel. Examination of the cerebrospinal fluid (CSF) usually reveals pleocytosis and elevated protein. Electroencephalography (EEG) combined with computed tomography (CT) or magnetic resonance imaging (MRI) of the brain is useful in defining the presence and location of CNS abnormalities. The long-term prognosis is poor, and up to 75% of children have some degree of psychomotor retardation associated with microcephaly, porencephalic cysts, spasticity, blindness, or learning disabilities. Disseminated disease may occur with or without CNS involvement, and usually appears around 9–11 days of life. Signs and symptoms of this form of infection include seizures, irritability, respiratory distress, jaundice, bleeding diathesis, shock, and a vesicular exanthem. Prognosis is poor, with most survivors impaired. The most common cause of death is either HSV pneumonitis or disseminated intravascular coagulopathy. There is an 80% mortality rate in untreated cases.

The transmission of HIV from an infected mother to the fetus can occur *in utero*, or intrapartum during labor and delivery where there is contact with maternal blood, but the exact route and timing of transmission during pregnancy are not known (see Chapter 23). Maternal factors that may increase the rate of transmission include advanced HIV disease in the mother represented by high viral burden, p24 antigenemia, low CD4 count, clinical acquired immunodeficiency syndrome (AIDS), and seroconversion during pregnancy. Without maternal and neonatal antiviral therapy, the rate of transmission from an infected mother to her infant varies from 10–55%. Postpartum transmission of HIV to the infant has been associated with breast-feeding. Manifestations of disease may not be apparent at birth and may not become apparent for months to years.

### Fungi

Candida species are the most common fungal pathogens seen in the neonate. The spectrum of disease ranges from thrush (oral candidiasis) to disseminated candidiasis with frank sepsis and shock. The risk factors for development of a systemic candidal infection in the neonate include low birth weight, prematurity, fungal colonization, the presence and prolonged use of intravascular catheters, use of intravenous hyperalimentation, administration of multiple or prolonged courses of broad-spectrum antimicrobial drugs, gastrointestinal surgery or disease, the use of corticosteroids, and prolonged endotracheal intubation. Infants with systemic candidiasis most often present with signs and symptoms that suggest bacterial sepsis.

### Nonviral Intracellular Organisms

*Toxoplasma gondii* is the causative agent of toxoplasmosis, which represents the "T" of the TORCH acronym. It is an intracellular protozoan parasite that is a cause of congenital infection. The fetus appears to acquire the infection through transplacental transmission from an infected parasitemic mother. The usual route by which the mother becomes infected is ingestion of oocysts present in cat feces or ingestion of undercooked meat containing live tissue cysts. The parasites first infect the placenta, which subsequently leads to fetal parasitemia and organ infection. The extent of fetal infection depends on the time in gestation when the maternal infection occurs. Maternal infections late in gestation are more likely to cause infection of the fetus. Infections early in gestation tend to produce a more severely affected infant. Infants with congenital toxoplasmosis classically present with intrauterine growth retardation, microcephaly, intracranial calcifications, chorioretinitis and significant CNS disease, and other systemic manifestations illustrated in Table 26–1. Signs and symptoms of congenital infection may not be apparent at birth and may take years to develop.

### Diagnosis

The diagnosis of infection in the pregnant woman and in the newborn is based primarily on a thorough maternal history and assessment of clinical signs and symptoms. Infants with congenital infections may present with one or more signs that may indicate a specific diagnosis (Table 26–3). The diagnosis of many infectious diseases that may have serious consequences for the fetus is difficult in the mother based only on clinical signs and symptoms. The most direct method of diagnosis is isolation of the microorganism from maternal tissues and body fluids, including blood, CSF, or urine. The proper technique of isolation is based on the organism's epidemiology and its natural history and pathogenesis in the host. Examination of histologic sections of tissue and cytology may provide a presumptive diagnosis in certain infections, such as varicella-zoster virus, herpes simplex virus, and cytomegalovirus. The serologic diagnosis of infection in the pregnant woman requires the demonstration of a significant rise in antibody titer against the specific agent suspected to be causing the illness. Difficulties arise when antibody levels rise rapidly initially, so that demonstration of a significant rise in titer in patients tested more than 7 days after the onset of suspected illness is precluded. Diagnosis can be made by measuring antibody levels that increase more slowly over a period of several weeks.

The clinical diagnosis of systemic infection in the newborn infant is difficult, because signs of infection may be nonspecific and subtle, and they may be associated with a variety of noninfectious causes. Also, many of the signs of congenital infection may not be present immediately after birth but manifest days to months later. Laboratory methods that may assist in the diagnosis of infections in the newborn include complete blood count with platelet and differential count, serologic titers (especially IgM) for specific infectious agents obtained at the appropriate times, histopathologic examination of the placenta and umbilical cord for signs of inflammation, and Gram's stain or other stains of various body fluids to look for the presence of microorganisms and polymorphonuclear leukocytes. The isolation of microorganisms by culture from a specific or systemic focus, however, remains the most valid method for the diagnosis of a systemic neonatal infection. Other methods that may be helpful include antigen identification for group B streptococci, *Pneumocystis carinii*, and *Toxoplasma gondii*; and electron microscopic examination of tissue specimens for inclusion bodies or viral particles. Further studies may be necessary to determine the extent of infection in neonates with suspected systemic fungal disease, including echocardiogram; abdominal ultrasound for liver, spleen, and kidney lesions; and ophthalmologic examination.

### Treatment

The early diagnosis and timely initiation of appropriate antimicrobial therapy and supportive measures often leads to the successful management and outcome of neonatal bacterial sepsis. If a neonate is suspected to be septic, the appropriate cultures should be obtained and antimicrobial therapy started promptly. Initial empiric therapy should include antimicrobial agents that are effective against gram-positive cocci (especially group B streptococci) and gram-negative enteric bacilli as well as listeria; this usually includes a penicillin and an aminoglycoside. Most experts recommend ampicillin with gentamicin for presumed non-CNS sepsis and ampicillin with cefotaxime or ceftriaxone for presumptive neonatal bacterial meningitis. Antibiotic therapy is tailored when the culture results and susceptibility test results are available. The duration of therapy depends largely upon the clinical response of the patient. For focal or systemic sepsis not involving the CNS, the usual duration of antimicrobial therapy is 10–14 days, while the duration of therapy for meningitis caused by group B streptococci or gram-negative enteric bacilli is 14–21 days (preferably 21 days). For infants treated for congenital syphilis, penicillin G is the drug of choice (see Chapter 16). Infants should be treated if maternal treatment did not occur or was inadequate, if it is unknown whether the mother received treatment, or if the mother was treated with drugs other than penicillin. If the infant has no signs of CNS involvement and is asymptomatic, a single 50,000-unit/kg intramuscular dose of benzathine penicillin G is sufficient. However, if the infant is symptomatic or if there is indication of CNS involvement, the infant should receive a 10-day course of procaine penicillin G at a dose of 50,000 units/kg every 12 h.

Various antiviral agents are available for treatment of newborns infected with specific viruses. Herpes simplex virus is treated with acyclovir, varicella-zoster virus may be treated with acyclovir, respiratory syncytial virus with ribavirin, cytomegalovirus with gancyclovir or foscarnet, and zidovudine may be used in the infant born to the mother with HIV.

Amphotericin B is the drug of choice for systemic fungal infections in the neonate, with the duration of therapy based upon the extent and source of the infection. Serum electrolyte concentrations (especially potassium) and kidney function are closely monitored during the course of therapy to look for any possible developing toxicity. The drugs of choice for treating congenital toxoplasmosis are pyrimethamine 1 mg/kg/day and sulfadiazine 100 mg/kg/day divided every 6 h for 6 months.

Various immune globulins are effective in preventing certain infections that occur during the neonatal period and are administered to neonates who are at high risk of developing these infections. These include immune globulins against varicella-zoster and hepatitis B virus (see Chapter 40).

Intrapartum chemoprophylaxis of pregnant women known to be colonized with group B streptococci who have an additional risk factor has been shown to be effective in reducing the incidence of early-onset neonatal infection. Intravenous ampicillin or penicillin is administered beginning at least 4 h before delivery and continued until delivery. The initial loading dose of ampicillin is 2 g followed by 1–2 g every 4–6 h, while the dose of penicillin is 5 million units every 6 h. Clindamycin and erythromycin are alternative agents for penicillin allergic patients.

## PATHOGENESIS OF INFECTION IN THE AGED

As discussed previously, an age-dependent decline in T-lymphocyte function impairs both humoral and cell-mediated immunity. The increased susceptibility of the aged host results from interaction of this immunodeficiency with a number of other factors, particularly degenerative changes in cutaneous surfaces, loss of primary defense mechanisms of the urinary and respiratory tracts, alteration in the endogenous microflora, inability to mount a febrile response, environmental factors, and underlying disease. The skin is an important primary barrier to bacterial infection. The arterial and venous obstructive diseases of aging cause chronic ischemic skin ulcers that become infected and can serve as portals of entry for disseminated infection. Elderly people are often confined to bed and thus may develop decubitus ulcers, most frequently in the lumbosacral region. Prostatic enlargement in elderly men obstructs urine outflow and results in urinary stasis and loss of the normal washing action of micturition. Combined with indwelling urinary catheters that are frequently used in older individuals, this leads to a high rate of urinary tract infection. Pulmonary function declines with age because of (1) degeneration of elastin fibers around alveoli and alveolar ducts causing diminished outflow of air due to loss of elastic recoil, (2) an increase in the anterior-posterior diameter of the chest with decreased respiratory excursion, and (3) weakening of the respiratory muscles with loss of the ability to cough up debris and secretions from the airways of the lung. The inability of the aged host with declining pulmonary function to clear the lung of bacteria-laden secretions and tissue debris aspirated from the oropharynx sets the stage for bacterial pneumonia. Unlike younger individuals for whom the normal oropharyngeal flora consists of gram-positive commensal organisms such as diphtheroids and coagulase-negative staphylococci, aged humans often develop an oropharyngeal flora comprised of gram-negative bacilli and *Staphylococcus aureus*, with a concomitant increase in the incidence of gram-negative and *Staphylococcus aureus* pneumonia. The febrile response is host-protective by its ability to potentiate both humoral and cell-mediated immunity, and the febrile response decreases with age. Environmental factors that predispose the elderly to infectious diseases are tragically common and include institutionalized living, economic deprivation, and undernutrition. Also, advanced age brings a high prevalence of malignant disease, atherosclerosis, cerebrovascular diseases, and diabetes mellitus. Infections in the elderly are almost always inextricably linked in their development to these and other conditions of aging.

### Etiologies

#### Encapsulated Extracellular Bacteria

Although there is an increase in the susceptibility of all organ systems to infection with extracellular bacteria in the elderly, there is a particularly large increase in hospital-acquired (nosocomial) bacterial pneumonia due to gram-negative bacteria (especially *Klebsiella pneumoniae* and *Pseudomonas aeruginosa*) and the gram-positive organism *Staphylococcus aureus*. Starting with the seventh decade of life, there is also a sharp increase in urinary tract infection, especially for men. The most frequent infection is *asymptomatic bacteriuria* (presence of bacteria in the urine without signs or symptoms of infection), but symptomatic urinary tract infection also occurs. Unlike younger individuals in whom the gram-negative bacillus *Escherichia coli* is the dominant cause, urinary tract infection in older debilitated individuals is due to a variety of gram-negative bacteria, including *E. coli*, urea-splitting *Proteus*, *Klebsiella*, and *P. aeruginosa*.

Among the elderly, bloodstream infections

are associated with increased mortality. Bacteremia secondary to urinary tract infection (urosepsis) is usually caused by gram-negative bacilli or the enterococci; bacteremia secondary to respiratory tract infection by gram-negative enterics, *Haemophilus influenzae*, or *Streptococcus pneumoniae*; and bacteremia secondary to skin infections *Staphylococcus aureus*, *Staphylococcus epidermidis*, or obligate anaerobes. The prevalence of degenerative cardiovascular disease in the elderly and frequent hospitalization with use of intravenous catheters and monitoring devices have made infective endocarditis an important infectious disease in individuals 60 years or older. Enterococcal endocarditis in the elderly is usually due to urinary tract infection and/or manipulation. Malignant and inflammatory diseases of the colon in the elderly predispose to bacteremia and endocarditis due to the nonenterococcal group D streptococcus, *Streptococcus bovis*.

### Facultative Intracellular Bacteria

The incidence and mortality of reactivation tuberculosis increase greatly beyond the age of 60 years. Until the recent AIDS epidemic, tuberculosis had become largely a disease of the aged in the United States. The decrement of T-cell–dependent immunity with aging allows latent infection by the facultative intracellular parasite *Mycobacterium tuberculosis* to "flare up" with development of pulmonary tuberculosis, and even hematogenous dissemination of the tubercle bacillus with generalized (pulmonary and extrapulmonary) tuberculosis. Other diseases due to facultative intracellular bacteria that show an increased incidence with aging include infectious diarrhea caused by *Salmonella*, and meningitis caused by *Listeria monocytogenes*.

### Viruses

Varicella-zoster virus (VZV), like other herpesviruses, causes latent infection of the host that persists for many years, most often following the occurrence of chickenpox during childhood. In the elderly individual, age-related loss of cytotoxic T-cell and NK cell activity results in reactivation of this latent infection, especially when combined with emotional or physical stress, or underlying malignant disease. VZV primarily infects satellite cells around neurons in dorsal root ganglia of the spinal cord, and with reactivation VZV infects one or more sensory nerves, which carry the virus to skin dermatomes supplied by the sensory nerves. *Shingles* results,

with formation of cutaneous vesicular lesions distributed over the region of the infected dermatomes, which intensely itch, burn, and/or are sharply painful.

### Clinical Manifestations and Diagnosis

A high level of suspicion must be maintained for the diagnosis of infection in the elderly person. Urinary tract infection is often asymptomatic. Fever and cough are frequently absent in pneumonia, chest x-ray changes can be minimal or absent, and leukocytosis may not be present. Mental changes and neck stiffness in meningitis are often attributed to dementia and degenerative joint disease, and frequently there is no spinal fluid pleocytosis. Bacteremia in the elderly can be difficult to recognize, since "afebrile bacteremia" is common in this age group. Elderly patients with pulmonary tuberculosis are significantly less likely to be initially suspected of having the disease than younger patients, perhaps due to the less frequent occurrence of cough as a presenting symptom in the elderly. The initial diagnosis of the elderly person with tuberculosis is frequently cancer or bacterial pneumonia. Thus, rigorous adherence to accepted standards of clinical laboratory testing and careful interpretation of results are particularly important for the diagnosis of infection in the aged. It is especially critical that the laboratory evaluation of bacterial pneumonia include sputum examination by Gram's stain and culture, blood culture, and Gram's stain and culture of pleural effusions (if present). Bacteremia and endocarditis require submission of two and preferably three separate sets of blood cultures obtained at different times. Optimal diagnosis of tuberculosis is achieved by submission of at least three early-morning sputum specimens (and not more than five) for acid-fast smear and mycobacterial culture.

### CASE HISTORIES

#### CASE HISTORY 1

A 2600-g male is born to a 17-year-old $G_2P_2$ mother at 36 weeks' gestation by precipitous vaginal delivery in the hospital hallway after the mother was taken to the hospital for fever and abdominal cramping. A vaginal culture at 26 weeks' gestation was positive for group B streptococcus. Presumed rupture of membranes occurred approximately 20 h prior to delivery while the mother was taking a shower. A small amount of light greenish fluid was noted by her at that time. The mother had been ill with a flu-like illness for the last several days and had a temperature of 102.3°F at the time of delivery. The infant seemed vigorous at delivery with Apgar scores of 8 and 9 at 1 and 5 min, respectively, but 10 h later he developed tachypnea with grunting respirations. Physical examination revealed a small infant in moderate respiratory distress with acrocyanosis of the hands and feet. Vital signs were temperature of 96.8°F; pulse, 130/min; respiration, 100/min; blood pressure, 90/40 mm Hg; and $O_2$ saturation on room air of 90%. Nasal flaring was present and chest examination revealed moderate subcostal and substernal retractions with use of the abdominal muscles. Coarse breath sounds were present diffusely, and the liver was palpable 1–2 cm below the right costal margin. The infant was placed in 40% $O_2$ giving a saturation of 100%. A sepsis work-up was performed, and the infant was empirically begun on ampicillin 30 mg/kg/day divided into 4 doses administered every 6 h, and gentamicin 2.5 mg/kg/dose given every 12 h.

Significant laboratory findings included a white blood cell (WBC) count of 3000/mm³ with a differential of 45% neutrophils, 30% band forms, 22% lymphocytes, and 3% monocytes, and a platelet count of 90,000/mm³. Lumbar puncture showed a WBC count of 250/mm³ with a differential of 85% neutrophils and 15% mononuclear cells, red blood cell (RBC) count of 10/mm³, glucose concentration of 30 mg/dL, and protein concentration of 80 mg/dL. No organisms were seen on the Gram's stain. Chest radiograph revealed a diffuse pneumonic process. Urine and CSF antigen detection tests for group B streptococcus were positive.

The infant responded very well to his antibiotic therapy. Blood and CSF cultures were subsequently positive for group B streptococcus that was highly susceptible to penicillin. On day 5, the infant's antibiotic therapy was changed to penicillin G, 400,000 units/kg/day divided every 4 h. Cultures from a repeat lumbar puncture performed on day 3 of life were sterile. The infant completed a 21-day course of antibiotics without any problems. Computed tomographic scan of the head and auditory brainstem-evoked response were normal.

## CASE 1 DISCUSSION

The case illustrates the major clinical findings in neonatal early-onset group B streptococcal disease. The important points worth emphasizing are the infant is born to a young mother with a positive culture for GBS; the infant is premature; the mother had premature rupture of membranes for more than 18 h; the mother had a prior illness and was febrile at the time of delivery; and the mother had not received prophylactic antibiotics during labor. The significant findings pertaining to the in-

fant are his being small for gestational age, and he developed signs of infection shortly after birth. These clinical findings coupled with the laboratory data support the diagnosis of early-onset GBS infection. This clinical presentation also is consistent with early-onset listeria infection, which is difficult to differentiate from early-onset GBS infection prior to return of the culture results and must be considered in the differential diagnosis.

## CASE HISTORY 2

A 72-year-old man fell at home and, when discovered, had been on the floor for 6 h. During the fall, he bruised his left hip, but did not lose consciousness. He had been well until 9 months prior to falling, when he was hospitalized with a left-sided cerebrovascular accident and residual right hemiparesis. During this previous hospital stay, gross hematuria was noted, and cystoscopy revealed a focus of transitional cell carcinoma of his bladder, as well as marked enlargement of his prostate gland due to benign hyperplasia. Transurethral resection of the bladder tumor was performed, following which a continuous indwelling catheter was required for incontinence. He was treated with ampicillin for recurrent urinary tract infection due to enterococcus.

Because of his fall, he was taken to the hospital, where physical examination revealed a frail elderly man with a temperature of 37.7°C, heart rate of 90/min, respiratory rate of 16/min, and blood pressure of 130/76 mm Hg. His lungs were clear to auscultation, but a grade 4/6 holosystolic murmur was present at the lower left sternal border. Neurologic examination revealed mildly dysarthric speech, approximately 50% of normal motor strength in his right upper and lower extremities, and normal motor strength on the left. Laboratory values included a hemoglobin of 6.7 mg/dL, a WBC count of 5800/mm³ with 78% neutrophils, 18% lymphocytes, and 4% monocytes, and a platelet count of 62,000/mm³. Microscopic urinalysis was remarkable for pyuria (>50 white cells per high-power field), hematuria (30–35 RBCs per high-power field), and bacteriuria (presence of numerous gram-positive cocci). An echocardiogram showed thickening of the mitral valve leaflets with a 1- to 2-cm vegetation on the posterior leaflet of the mitral valve. The left atrium was enlarged with a diameter of 5.5 cm, and moderate mitral regurgitation was present. Urine culture was positive for *Enterococcus faecalis* (>100,000 organisms per milliliter of urine), and all four blood culture sets were positive for the same organism. The *E. faecalis* was susceptible to ampicillin and vancomycin by microbroth dilution testing, and was negative for both beta-lactamase production and high-level resistance to the aminoglycosides gentamicin and streptomycin. Intravenous therapy was initiated with a combination of ampicillin and gentamicin.

## CASE 2 DISCUSSION

The vicissitudes of aging and their contribution to a high prevalence of serious infectious disease in the elderly are clearly seen with this man. He suffered both cerebrovascular and malignant disease, and developed recurrent urinary tract infection as a complication of an obstructive uropathy (benign prostatic hyperplasia) and chronic placement of an indwelling bladder catheter following an invasive procedure (cystoscopy) for removal of a focus of bladder cancer. His urinary tract infection with *Enterococcus faecalis* provided a source for bacteremic seeding of his mitral valve with the development of infective endocarditis. Urinary tract infection with enterococcus is common in older men with an obstructive uropathy, and the urinary tract is frequently a source of infection in the elderly for enterococcal endocarditis. The atypical response to invasive infection of the elderly including absence of both fever and neutrophilic leukocytosis are also apparent with this case. The presence of a heart murmur combined with echocardiographic data and a history of chronic urinary tract infection by enterococcus prompted the appropriate use of blood cultures to obtain a specific etiologic diagnosis for the endocarditis. The antimicrobial susceptibility results allowed the use of ampicillin in treatment of endocarditis, in preference to the use of vancomycin, which should be utilized only when no other antimicrobial drug is available based on susceptibility results. The restricted use of vancomycin is mandated by the recent emergence of enterococcal resistance toward this glycopeptide antibiotic. Also, combination treatment with two antimicrobials was implemented in this case to ensure bactericidal chemotherapy with sterilization of the cardiac vegetation.

## REFERENCES

### Books

Feigin, R. D., and Cherry, J. D. *Textbook of Pediatric Infectious Diseases.* 3rd ed. Philadelphia: W. B. Saunders Co., 1992.

Remington, J. S., and Klein, J. O. *Infectious Diseases of the Fetus and Newborn Infant.* Philadelphia: W. B. Saunders Co., 1995.

### Review Articles

Ciccimarra, F. Fetal and neonatal immunology. *J. Perinat. Med. 22*(Suppl. 1): 84–87, 1994.

Edwards, M. S. Complement in neonatal infections: An overview. *Pediatr. Infect. Dis. 5*:S168–S170, 1986.

Evans, H. E., and Frenkel, L. D. Congenital syphilis. *Clin. Perinatol. 21*:149–162, 1994.

Gardner, I. D. The effect of aging on susceptibility to infection. *Rev. Infect. Dis. 2*:801–810, 1980.

Haft, R. F., and Kasper, D. L. Group B streptococcus infection in mother and child. *Hosp. Pract. 26*:111–134, 1991.

Hanshaw, J. D. Cytomegalovirus infections. *Pediatr. Rev. 16*:43–48, 1995.

Kohl, S. Herpes simplex virus infection—the neonate to the adolescent. *Isr. J. Med. Sci. 30*:392–398, 1994.

Krause, P. J., Herson, V. C., Eisenfeld, L., and Johnson, G. M. Enhancement of neutrophil function for treatment of neonatal infections. *Pediatr. Infect. Dis. J. 8*: 382–389, 1989.

Peakman, H., Senaldi, G., Liosis, G., Gamsu, H. R., and Vergani, D. Complement activation in neonatal infection. *Arch. Dis. Child. 67*:802–807, 1992.

Prober, C. G., Corey, L., Brown, Z. A., Hensleigh, P. A., Frenkel, L. M., and Bryson, Y. J. The management of pregnancies complicated by genital infections with herpes simplex virus. *Clin. Infect. Dis. 15*:1031–1038, 1992.

Quie, P. G. Antimicrobial defenses in the neonate. *Semin. Perinatol. 14*(Suppl. 1):2–9, 1990.

Saltzman, R. L., and Peterson, P. K. Immunodeficiency of the elderly. *Rev. Infect. Dis. 9*:1127–1139, 1987.

Starling, S. P. Syphilis in infants and young children. *Pediatr. Ann. 23*:334–340, 1994.

Stoll, B. J. Congenital syphilis: Evaluation and management of neonates born to mothers with reactive serologic tests for syphilis. *Pediatr. Infect. Dis. J. 13*:845–852, 1994.

Tarlow, M. J. Epidemiology of neonatal infections. *J. Antimicrob. Chemother. 34*(Suppl. A): 43–52, 1994.

Wendel, G. D. Gestational and congenital syphilis. *Clin. Perinatol. 15*:287–303, 1988.

Wilson, C. B. Immunologic basis for increased susceptibility of the neonate to infection. *J. Pediatr. 108*:1–12, 1986.

Wolach, B., Carmi, D., Gilboa, S., Satar, M., Segal, S., Dolfin, T., et al. Some aspects of the humoral immunity and the phagocytic function in newborn infants. *Isr. J. Med. Sci. 30*:331–335, 1994.

Zeichner, S. L., and Plotkin, S. A. Mechanisms and pathways of congenital infections. *Clin. Perinatol. 15*:163–188, 1988.

### Original Articles

Araneo, B. A., Woods, M. L., II, and Daynes, R. A. Reversal of the immunosenescent phenotype by dehydroepidandrosterone: Hormone treatment provides an adjuvant effect on the immunization of aged mice with recombinant hepatitis B surface antigen. *J. Infec. Dis. 167*:830–840, 1993.

Counsell, S. R., Tan, J. J., Dittus, R. S. Unsuspected pulmonary tuberculosis in a community teaching hospital. *Arch. Intern. Med. 149*:1274–1275,1989.

Matur, P., Sacks, L., Auten, G., et al. Delayed diagnosis of pulmonary tuberculosis in city hospitals. *Arch. Intern. Med. 154*:306–310, 1994.

Rytel, M. W., Larratt, K. S., Turner, P. A., and Kalbfleisch, J. H. Interferon response to mitogens and viral antigens in elderly and young adult subjects. *J. Infect. Dis. 153*:984–987, 1986.

# VIII ADDITIONAL INFECTIONS

# 27

# INFECTIONS CAUSED BY ANAEROBIC BACTERIA

## DALE N. GERDING, M.D. and LANCE R. PETERSON, M.D.

Anaerobes are a major part of the usual flora of man. They outnumber the aerobic bacteria and facultatives in many parts of the body including throughout the oral cavity and gastrointestinal tract. They may not cause disease and can even be protective when they remain in their usual habitats. Because of the sites they normally colonize, anaerobic bacterial infections often arise from and involve cutaneous and mucosal surfaces. In some in

stances infections are also due to exogenous anaerobic organisms that are ingested or contaminate wounds. The most common infections caused by anaerobic bacteria are listed in Table 27–1. Examples of the endogenous infections are dental abscesses, tonsillar abscesses, perirectal abscesses, and infected ulcers in diabetic patients. Botulism, tetanus, gas gangrene, and antibiotic-associated diarrhea (due to *Clostridium difficile*) are examples

### TABLE 27-1.    INFECTIONS CAUSED BY ANAEROBIC BACTERIA

| ANATOMIC SITE | INFECTION |
| --- | --- |
| Skin and skin structure | Bite wounds |
| | Crepitant cellulitis |
| | Decubitus/diabetic foot ulcer infection |
| | Myonecrosis (gangrene) |
| | Necrotizing fasciitis |
| | Tetanus |
| Head and Neck | Brain abscess |
| | Chronic sinusitis |
| | Gingivitis |
| | Odontogenic and oropharyngeal abscess |
| Respiratory | Aspiration pneumonia |
| | Empyema in adults |
| | Lung abscess |
| | Necrotizing pneumonia |
| Gastrointestinal | Antibiotic-associated diarrhea and colitis |
| | Intraabdominal abscess |
| | Liver abscess |
| | Peritonitis (not spontaneous bacterial peritonitis) |
| | Botulism |
| Genital tract (female) | Bacterial vaginosis |
| | Bartholin's gland abscess |
| | Salpingitis |
| | Septic abortion and endometritis |
| | Tuboovarian abscess |

of exogenous infections. It is not surprising that anaerobes colonize the colon and vagina where oxygen tensions are low, but they are also found in high numbers on the skin, teeth, nose, and tonsils, areas of relatively high oxygen tension. Facultative anaerobic bacteria (those bacteria that can grow in either the presence or the absence of oxygen), such as Enterobacteriaceae, staphylococci, and streptococci, are postulated to utilize oxygen, providing the low-oxygen environment necessary for the survival of the obligate anaerobic organisms. The anaerobes are also able to survive in the relatively anaerobic microenvironments in the dental crevices, tonsillar crypts, and hair follicles. Areas of the body harboring large numbers of endogenous anaerobic flora typically occupy sites on the body's surface or interface with the external environment, sites such as the lumen of the colon or the vagina, and the oral cavity. In the colon they surpass the other bacteria by 300:1 to 1000:1. Other regions where anaerobic bacteria are found in high concentration include the skin pores and tonsillar crypts—areas of the body where the microorganisms are kept warm and moist and are protected from oxygen concentrations that would inhibit or prevent growth.

The widespread anaerobic bacterial colonization has been underappreciated, perhaps because of the technical difficulty encountered in the sampling, specimen transport, isolation, and identification of anaerobic bacteria. Once the importance of maintaining anaerobic conditions was recognized as essential to clinical anaerobic bacteriology, the high prevalence of anaerobic bacteria causing infections previously thought to be "sterile" was understood. The development and general application of improved procedures for the recovery and isolation of anaerobic bacteria have shown anaerobes to be more widely involved with disease at all sites in the body than had previously been recognized.

## ELEMENTS OF AN ANAEROBIC INFECTION—ANAEROBIOSIS

### Definition of an Anaerobe

Anaerobes are those bacteria that cannot grow in the presence of an atmosphere containing 18–20% oxygen that may be enriched with up to 10% $CO_2$. Most anaerobes do not contain catalase so they cannot degrade the peroxides formed when oxygen is present. They also cannot destroy superoxide radicals, and most of the clinically important anaerobic bacteria have little superoxide dismutase, an enzyme whose level of production generally correlates with the degree of aerotolerance of the anaerobe. Strict anaerobes are defined as those that must be in an atmosphere containing <0.5% $O_2$ in order to grow on an agar surface.

## Oxidation–Reduction Potential ($E_h$)

The concept of infection by bacteria that cannot tolerate oxygen relates to their survival in environments with a low oxidation–reduction potential ($E_h$) and reduced concentrations of oxygen. Infections by anaerobic bacteria are produced by growth of the organism in tissues that have lost their oxygen (blood) supply and thus have a local environment with a low oxidation–reduction potential. The $E_h$, like the hydrogen ion concentration (pH), can be measured and expressed in terms of defined units. Oxidation is defined as a reaction in which electrons are lost, and reduction as a reaction in which electrons are gained. Any compound with a tendency to be oxidized can be thought of as possessing a corresponding measure of electrons available for donation. If a solution of such a compound is arranged to form a half cell in a circuit with a different half cell of known potential, a potential difference is set up whose magnitude is related to the oxidizing (or reducing) power of the compound and can be expressed in volts. Oxidation–reduction potential is expressed by the positive or negative electric potential across a calomel half cell and can be measured either *in vivo* or *in vitro*.

The oxidation–reduction potential at any site in the body is usually but not necessarily related to the distance of that site from oxygen-carrying red blood cells, the integrity of the vascular capillary network, and the metabolic activity occurring at the site. The $E_h$ of the blood depends on the oxygen saturation of hemoglobin in red blood cells and, to a lesser but significant extent, on the dissolved oxygen content of the serum. The $E_h$ in most tissues in the body varies between $+0.126$ V and $+0.246$ V, depending on blood supply and whether the measurement is taken near sites of high (arterial) or low (venous) oxygen saturation. Strict anaerobic bacteria generally cannot survive in the presence of $O_2$ greater than 0.5% and therefore will not grow in tissues with these $E_h$ values. For example, the highest $E_h$ recorded for germination of *Clostridium tetani* is $+0.110$ V, whereas other clostridial spores usually need an $E_h$ less than $-0.100$ V for germination and growth. The majority of anaerobic bacteria require an $E_h$ of $-0.100$ V to $-0.250$ V for growth *in vitro*. Body areas like periodontal pockets have $E_h$

values of $-0.48$ to $-0.300$ V and harbor large numbers of anaerobic flora. The oxidation–reduction potential of many normal tissues prevents growth of anaerobic bacteria unless blood flow is reduced and the $E_h$ falls. Infection by other bacteria can markedly increase local metabolism and oxygen consumption, permitting aerobic bacteria to grow with only modest reduction of normal circulation to the infection site.

## Effect of Tissue Injury on $E_h$

Anaerobic bacteria are normally present in well-delineated sites throughout the body, and situations that predispose to disease can be anticipated. This is particularly true at sites adjacent to mucous membranes, where large numbers of anaerobic bacteria are part of the indigenous microbiota. An injury that interrupts the capillary blood flow, with a resulting decrease in tissue $E_h$ at that site, predisposes to anaerobic bacterial replication. If a toxin-producing organism is present, such as some clostridia, toxin production will also occur. Injury may result from surgery, trauma, arteriosclerosis, growth of a malignant tumor with ischemic necrosis, or even another infection. The importance of the reduction of blood flow and its subsequent effect on the decrease in the tissue $E_h$ are illustrated by experimental clostridial infections in animals. Production of vascular spasm and ischemia by injecting epinephrine into the hind leg of a guinea pig reduces by 1000-fold the number of *Clostridium perfringens* required to initiate infection at that site. Disruption of blood flow also halts delivery of oxygen to the site, leading to rapid development of anoxia. Experimental abscess models show that infection with a facultative bacterium in a closed space can render the area anaerobic in less than 1 h. Therefore, it is easy to see why anaerobic bacteria can produce serious infections, particularly when the setting is an abscess or other necrotic, devitalized tissue.

## Variability of Anaerobic Bacterial Requirements

Some anaerobic bacteria are more fastidious than others in their need for a low-oxygen environment. *C. perfringens*, the microorganism most frequently associated with gas gangrene, grows with only a slight reduction of oxygen tension, 70–80 mm Hg (normal, $\approx$150 mm Hg), whereas *C. tetani* has been reported to be intolerant of oxygen concentrations greater than 2 mm Hg (<0.5% $O_2$). This variety of oxygen sensitivity also indicates why the isolation of microorganisms by the clinical laboratory depends on protection of the specimen from exposure to air or oxygenated media. Since most anaerobic bacteria cannot tolerate more than 30 min of exposure to atmospheric oxygen, speed of delivery of the culture to the laboratory can be critical.

Most species of anaerobic bacteria require conditions necessary for growth before they can cause disease. Frequently, these conditions are met most rapidly in company with other anaerobic or facultative anaerobic bacteria. *In vitro* dilute suspensions of anaerobes, incapable of growth when widely dispersed in a fresh broth culture medium, grow rapidly when centrifuged to pellet them in a smaller volume of medium. The change from a stationary to a rapidly growing bacterial population is thought to be due to the ability of bacteria to reduce the immediate microenvironment by metabolism of residual oxygen, thus making rapid growth possible. This same principle of rapid utilization and depletion of available oxygen facilitates the development of anaerobic infection. Facultative anaerobic bacteria, such as *Escherichia coli* or *Klebsiella pneumoniae*, metabolize available oxygen, thereby reducing the oxygen atmosphere of the microenvironment to a level at which clinically important anaerobic bacteria can grow. With reduction of tissue $O_2$, anaerobes start to grow, producing a deepening anaerobic environment along with necrosis, toxins, or other virulence factors. The ability of mixed bacterial microcolonies to alter their immediate environment helps to explain the otherwise confusing findings that large numbers of anaerobic bacteria can be cultured from the mouth, nasal sinuses, and lower respiratory tract, areas that are usually considered continuously exposed to air and unlikely sites for colonization with anaerobic bacteria.

## POLYMICROBIC NATURE OF ANAEROBIC DISEASE

Infection with non–spore-forming anaerobic bacteria is commonly found in a necrotizing abscess and may yield as many as 20 different strains of bacteria. Because of the multiple microbial species that can be isolated, *polymicrobic* infection is sometimes used to refer to anaerobic bacterial abscesses. For this reason, diseases caused by anaerobic bacteria

sharply contrast to the "one microorganism–one disease" concept that characterizes many infections, such as streptococcal pharyngitis, typhoid fever, cholera, tetanus, and diphtheria. Anaerobic infections commonly result from the extension of the indigenous microflora to adjacent submucosal tissues. Improved isolation and identification techniques for anaerobic bacteria have reemphasized the need for a better understanding of the interactions among microorganisms.

The most clinically important anaerobic bacteria are listed in Table 27–2, organized on the basis of Gram's-strain reactivity and morphologic appearance. Those most commonly found are the *Bacteroides fragilis* group (especially *B. fragilis*), those previously denoted as the pigmented *Bacteroides* species (*Prevotella* species and *Porphyromonas* species), *Peptostreptococcus*, *Clostridium difficile*, *C. perfringens*, *C. ramosum*, and *Fusobacterium nucleatum*. Although additional genera and species exist, they are only rarely associated with disease. Within genera, there may be a large number of different species; this is particularly true for the clostridia and the organisms comprising the former *Bacteroides* species.

Clinically, the significance of each organism in a "polymicrobic" infection can be difficult to evaluate. The interaction among different species of bacteria may be antagonistic, synergistic, or indifferent. Several examples serve to underline this point. A classic example of a synergistic infection involves organisms that together cause a serious, necrotizing infection of the oral mucous membranes of an animal model. Individually, none of the four can cause the infection. One of the organisms, a diphtheroid, secretes vitamin K, a growth factor needed by *Prevotella melaninogenica*, another of the organisms in this synergistic infection. *Prevotella melaninogenica* in turn secretes numerous proteolytic enzymes toxic to the host and leading to local tissue necrosis. Another form of interaction between two bacterial species can be detrimental to the host unexpectedly. This is the protection of one species by another from the action of an antibiotic. In experimental animals, penicillinase-producing *Bacteroides fragilis* can prevent the successful treatment of infection by penicillin-susceptible *Fusobacterium necrophorum*. Protection occurs even with only small numbers of *B. fragilis* injected as long as 24 h after the infecting dose of *F. necrophorum*. The reason for this is that *B. fragilis* produces beta-lactamase, an enzyme that destroys penicillin, and when

## TABLE 27–2. MAJOR CLINICALLY IMPORTANT ANAEROBIC BACTERIA

**GRAM-POSITIVE COCCI:**
  *Peptostreptococcus* sp. (*P. anaerobius, P. intermedius, P. micros, P. magnus, P. asaccharolyticus, P. prevotii*)
**GRAM-NEGATIVE COCCI:**
  *Veillonella*
**GRAM-POSITIVE BACILLI:**
  Spore-forming
    *Clostridium* sp. (*C. perfringens, C. difficile, C. titani, C. botulinum, C. ramosum, C. innocuum, C. septicum, C. novyi, C. sporogenes, C. sordellii, C. bifermentans*)
  Non–Spore-forming
    *Actinomyces* sp. (*A. israelii, A. naeslundii, A. odontolyticus, A. viscosus*)
    *Lactobacillus* sp.
    *Proprionibacterium* sp. (*P. propionicum, P. acnes*)
    *Bifidobacterium dentium*
**GRAM-NEGATIVE BACILLI:**
  *Bacteroides* sp. (*B. fragilis* group, *B. thetaiotaomicron, B. distasonis, B. ovatus, B. vulgatus*)
  *Porphyromonas* sp. (*P. asaccharolytica*)
  *Prevotella* sp. (*P. corporis, P. denticola, P. intermedia, P. melaninogenica, P. oris, P. buccae, P. oralis* group, *P. bivia, P. disiens*)
  *Fusobacterium* sp. (*F. nucleatum, F. necrophorum, F. mortiferum, F. varium*)
  *Bilophila wadsworthia*

---

these two organisms cause a mixed infection, treatment with penicillin is ineffective.

However, the best example of bacteria acting together to harm the host is perhaps in intraabdominal abscesses. Most Enterobacteriaceae are susceptible to the aminoglycoside antibiotics and resistant to clindamycin. In contrast, anaerobic bacteria are susceptible to clindamycin but are nearly uniformly resistant to the aminoglycosides. In a classic experiment, gelatin capsules containing colonic contents were placed intraperitoneally in rats. The subsequent infection had two stages. In untreated animals, acute peritonitis occurred first and was associated with a mortality rate of 37%. All untreated animals surviving the initial infection went on to develop chronic intraabdominal abscesses caused by strict anaerobic bacteria. When the rats were treated with gentamicin (active only against Enterobacteriaceae), the initial mortality rate decreased to 4%, but 98% of the survivors had anaerobic intraabdominal abscesses, indicating this potential of the anaerobic organisms. When clindamycin (active only against the anaerobes) was given alone, the early mortality rate was similar to untreated animals (35%) but the incidence of chronic intraabdominal abscesses decreased to 5%, further documenting the lethal potential of the "aerobic" portion of this infection. When both gentamicin and clindamycin were given, the early mortality rate decreased to 7% and the incidence of intraabdominal abscess was reduced

to 6%. For this reason, therapy for "polymicrobic" abdominal infection usually requires antimicrobial agents effective against both the Enterobacteriaceae and anaerobic bacteria.

## CLINICAL SETTINGS SUGGESTING INFECTION WITH ANAEROBIC BACTERIA

Infections at certain anatomic sites suggest a strong possibility of anaerobic infection, including intraabdominal infections, dental and oral infections, pelvic infections in women, and serious foot infections in patients with diabetes. A feculent-smelling discharge, infection (abscess) located in or adjacent to a mucous membrane, or the presence of gangrene or necrotic tissue should suggest the presence of anaerobiosis where these organisms can proliferate. Gas in the tissues may suggest infection by members of the genus *Clostridium*, but facultative organisms can also produce gas in tissues. In fact, gas in tissues is typically a very late sign of infection due to *C. perfringens* but can occur early in a necrotizing, closed space infection with *Escherichia coli*. Infections associated with malignancies or necrotic tissue, or developing during therapy with aminoglycosides, should be suspected to be due to anaerobic bacteria. Patients with septic thrombophlebitis or infected human or animal bites often have primary infections with anaerobic bacteria. Discharges from sinus tracts containing palpable "sulfur granules" (feeling like sand), or bacteremia with jaundice, may also signify serious underlying anaerobic infections.

In the following sections, general principles and predisposing factors associated with anaerobic infections in several organ systems are described. The unusual clinical symptoms associated with the very potent toxins secreted by certain clostridia are also briefly reviewed.

## DISEASES CAUSED BY NON–SPORE-FORMING ANAEROBES

### Upper Respiratory Tract Infections

Chronic infection of the paranasal sinuses or mastoids can be caused by anaerobic bacteria alone or in combination with facultative anaerobic bacteria. Over half of patients with chronic sinusitis and chronic otitis media have anaerobic bacteria either in pure culture or in combination with facultative anaerobic bacteria when appropriate cultures are done. Peptostreptococci, along with penicillin-resistant *Bacteroides fragilis*, and *P. melaninogenica* are among the most commonly isolated bacteria. Conversely, acute sinusitis and otitis media are rarely associated with anaerobes.

Anaerobic bacteria are commonly isolated from the mouth, particularly in the presence of dental caries and infection of the adjacent gingival tissues (see Chapter 9). Almost all periodontal infections are caused by anaerobic bacteria. It is important to note that strains found in the oral cavity, including *P. melaninogenica*, *Prevotella oralis*, *Fusobacterium nucleatum*, and numerous species of *Peptostreptococcus* and *Veillonella* are also among the most commonly isolated anaerobic bacteria associated with pulmonary disease (see Chapter 10).

Peritonsillar abscesses in adults yield anaerobic bacteria in over 70% of cases, usually in mixed culture with facultative (aerobic) bacteria. The most common aerobic bacteria are *Streptococcus pyogenes* and *Streptococcus milleri*. The most common anaerobes are *Fusobacterium necrophorum* and *Prevotella melaninogenica*, followed by *Prevotella intermedia* and *Peptostreptococcus micros*. Nearly 60% of adult patients have at least one beta-lactamase–producing anaerobic isolate, indicating the need to treat with something other than penicillin alone.

### Lower Respiratory Tract Infections

Anaerobic infection of the lung occurs in several forms. It may be an *abscess*, defined in this context as a solitary pulmonary cavity frequently measuring at least 2 cm in diameter. Alternatively, a diffuse pulmonary infiltrate without evidence of cavitation is called *anaerobic pneumonia*, and the term *necrotizing pneumonia* is applied to disease characterized by multiple areas of necrosis and cavitation within one or more pulmonary segments or lobes. Extension of intrapulmonary infection to the surface of the lung with involvement of the pleural space is called *empyema* and may or may not occur as a sequela to pulmonary abscess or anaerobic or necrotizing pneumonia (Fig. 27–1).

The pathogenesis of these different disease processes varies, but the similarity of the bacteria isolated from most patients with anaerobic pulmonary disease to the indigenous flora of the oropharynx (noted earlier) supports the theory that aspiration of oropharyngeal secretions is an important contributing factor. Thromboemboli from abdominal or

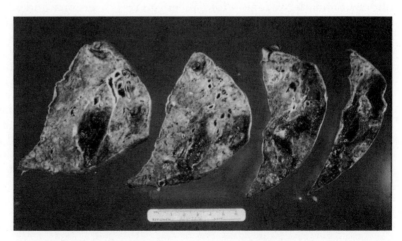

**FIGURE 27–1.** Serpiginous anaerobic bacterial abscess in the lower lobe of a lung. Extension to the pleural surface is seen in the section on the right and was associated with empyema. Culture revealed *Staphylococcus aureus* and four separate anaerobic bacterial species.

pelvic disease associated with thrombophlebitis may contribute to the development of an anaerobic lung abscess, although this association is often difficult to prove. *Staphylococcus aureus* is commonly associated with anaerobic pulmonary abscess formation (particularly in nosocomial infections) and may contribute to this process by production of necrotizing toxins (see Chapter 34). The resulting ischemia and reduced oxygen tension provide a proper environment to facilitate growth of anaerobic bacteria, and they in turn cause further tissue destruction.

The microorganisms found in anaerobic pulmonary disease include *Prevotella melaninogenica, Fusobacterium nucleatum*, peptostreptococci, and *Veillonella*. In contrast to anaerobic abscesses elsewhere, surgical drainage of anaerobic abscesses in the lung is often not necessary, and treatment with clindamycin alone is adequate unless empyema is present. With empyema, drainage with a chest tube is necessary in addition to antimicrobial therapy.

### Intraabdominal Infections

In view of the large numbers of anaerobes indigenous to the gastrointestinal tract (see Chapter 2), it is not surprising that anaerobic infections within or adjacent to the gastrointestinal tract account for a significant proportion of disease due to anaerobes. Ulceration of the gastrointestinal tract, by either inflammatory disease, ischemia, or malignant tumor, can provide a portal of entry, first to the regional lymphatics and later to the intravascular compartment. Septicemia with anaerobic bowel bacteria should suggest the abdominal cavity as a source for the bacteria. Such a site can be an ulcerated tumor of the right colon, or diverticulitis, or mucosal ulceration of the small intestine or colon from leukemia or lymphoma. Similarly, treatment for cancer can result in severe mucositis that can lead to sepsis from bowel organisms.

Anaerobic bacterial disease following intestinal surgery, ruptured appendicitis, or penetrating trauma to the intestinal tract is usually associated with multiple species of aerobic and anaerobic bacteria at the site of infection. Contamination of the peritoneum with large numbers of obligate and facultative anaerobic bacteria results in the rapid lowering of the local oxidation–reduction potential and creates conditions advantageous for worsening infection. Anaerobic bacteria, once established in the peritoneum, can be self-sustaining, with the oxygen and $E_h$ reaching very low levels,

thereby permitting growth of even the most fastidious microorganisms. Abscesses within the peritoneal cavity or beneath the diaphragm are typically difficult to treat unless antimicrobial therapy is accompanied by surgical drainage or drained radiologically by catheter placement.

Abscesses in the liver frequently yield anaerobic bacteria when properly cultured. Inflammatory disease of the bowel (Crohn's disease or ulcerative colitis) or obstruction of the biliary tract are predisposing factors to this infection. The blood supply to the liver is predominantly venous from the intestine, with a lower oxidation–reduction potential compared to other tissues. Thrombophlebitis in mesenteric or portal veins with embolism to the liver can initiate anaerobic seeding and abscess formation. In addition, certain anaerobic bacteria, such as *Bacteroides fragilis* and *Clostridium perfringens*, have a potential advantage over other microbes in causing infection in the liver or biliary tract, since they can grow in high concentrations of bile that inhibit or lyse other bacteria. These pathogens are the most commonly isolated anaerobic bacteria from cultures of the gallbladder at the time of cholecystectomy. The ability to grow in high concentrations of bile may also explain the association of *C. perfringens* with postsurgical biliary tract infection.

### Female Genital Tract Infections

The large majority of female genital infections that are not sexually transmitted diseases (see Chapter 16) are due to anaerobes. Pelvic inflammatory disease (PID), often caused by sexually transmitted gonorrhea or chlamydia infection, is also a mixed polymicrobial infection containing anaerobic bacteria, especially if pelvic abscesses are present. Anaerobic bacteremia and septicemia are complications of pregnancy. Septicemia may also result from induced or spontaneous abortion. Presumably, the anaerobic and facultative aerobic flora of the vagina gain entrance to the endocervical canal when the embryo or fetus and fetal membranes are being expelled. The highly vascularized endometrial surface is particularly susceptible to bacterial invasion during pregnancy, and septicemia may result. Bacteremia associated with abortion, while potentially life threatening, is usually transitory and clears promptly following curettage débridement of the uterus.

In the female pelvis, anaerobic infection not associated with pregnancy may include salpingitis or be a complication of gynecologic surgery. Careful bacteriologic study of pelvic infections yields numerous microorganisms similar to those of the vagina and lower female genitourinary tract. The most commonly isolated bacteria are species of peptostreptococci, *Bacteroides, and Clostridium.*

### Anaerobic Bacteremia

Bacteremia may occur in association with anaerobic infection at any site. Over the past two decades the proportion of bacteremias due to anaerobic bacteria has declined dramatically in comparison to aerobic bacteremias in many medical centers. For example, of all patient blood cultures in a 1991–1992 study, about 12% were positive for any bacteria, and only 4% of the 12% contained anaerobic bacteria. In contrast, a study in 1972 showed 26% of all positive blood cultures to contain anaerobic bacteria. Our recent experience at Northwestern Memorial Hospital confirms this trend, with only 2.5% of all positive blood cultures harboring anaerobic species. The reason for this is unclear, but proposed causes include the more frequent use of effective antibiotics, more rapid and effective surgical drainage and débridement of abdominal infections, and an increased awareness by clinicians of the possibility of anaerobic infection. *Bacteroides fragilis* group organisms, *Fusobacterium nucleatum* and *F. necrophorum, Propionibacterium acnes*, and *Clostridium* species are still the most frequently isolated anaerobic organisms found in blood cultures. As expected, most *B. fragilis* group and *Clostridium species* bacteremias originate from intraabdominal sources, whereas *Fusobacterium* sepsis originates from upper or lower respiratory sources. Mortality from bacteremias due to *Bacteroides fragilis* group is highest, ranging from 24 to 38%. Rarely, patients with anaerobic bacteremia have endocarditis, and they are at high risk of embolization from their lesions.

### Central Nervous System Infections

In the brain, anaerobic infections may be the result of direct extension from the paranasal sinuses or mastoids, causing epidural abscess or meningitis. Anaerobic brain abscess also may be metastatic from an embolus secondary to infection in the lungs or a vegetation on a heart valve. Patients with cyanotic congenital heart disease (with a right-to-left shunt) are at greater risk of developing cerebral abscesses from anaerobic bacteria than are normal persons, possibly because their arterial blood supply has a lowered oxygen saturation and venous organisms bypass the normal pulmonary capillary filter. The association of recent cerebral infarction with anaerobic bacterial abscess has also been noted and is thought to reflect the decreased oxygenation in the ischemic tissue. Brain abscesses are most often polymicrobic, with anaerobic bacteria classically present.

## DISEASES CAUSED BY SPORE-FORMING ANAEROBES (CLOSTRIDIA)

### General Characteristics

The clostridia are gram-positive, spore-forming, anaerobic bacilli. Some species sporulate only under special conditions. Spore formation is a protective mechanism that allows the organism to survive in a harsh (oxygen-containing) environment. Spores are not part of active, normal growth of these anaerobes, so they should not be expected to be visible in histologic slides made from infected material. Although there are more than 50 species of clostridia described and classified, disease in humans is caused by only about 10 species (Table 27–2). Clostridia are commonly found in human feces, the most frequent being *C. ramosum*, present at a density of $10^{10}$ organisms/g of stool. *C. perfringens*, among the most pathogenic of clostridial species, is found in 70% of human feces at densities of $10^9$ organisms/g of stool. Considerable variation exists in the ability of different clostridia to tolerate oxygen. Some are considered to be aerotolerant, whereas others germinate and proliferate only under strictly anaerobic conditions.

Clostridia also vary widely in their ability to utilize carbohydrates and to split proteins. Such characteristics are helpful in the laboratory for purposes of identification and classification, but they also aid in explaining clinical manifestations of diseases caused by individual species. For example, *C. perfringens*, the microorganism most often associated with gas gangrene, produces proteolytic and saccharolytic enzymes that contribute to the spread of infection. Glycogen, present in large amounts in skeletal muscle, is fermented with almost explosive formation of gas, and when coupled with collagenase and other proteolytic enzymes secreted by the microorganism, contributes to the rapid spread of infection. In contrast, *C. tetani*, the microorganism that causes tetanus, has few enzymes for carbohydrate fermentation or protein degradation. Therefore, growth of *C. tetani* with production of toxin can occur without much evidence of an inflammatory reaction.

### Exotoxins

A characteristic of the clostridia that are pathogenic for humans is the production of one or more potent exotoxins that significantly contributes to the ability of these microorganisms to cause disease. Tetanus and botulism are each due to a single toxin having a well-defined mode of action. Table 27–3 lists the medically important, lethal exotoxins produced by selected clostridia. *C. perfringens* produces at least 12 separate exotoxins that facilitate production of disease, even though only four are key to the lethality associated with this infection. Secretion of toxins is a highly specialized function of microorganisms in general, and many of these clostridia are very fastidious, requiring a very low oxygen tension. As the $E_h$ increases, toxin production ceases before death of the bacterium. This concept is important, since any mechanism (including the use of hyperbaric oxygen) that increases the oxidation–reduction potential at the site of the bacterial growth first interrupts toxin formation and then threatens the survival of the microorganism. Toxins of the clostridia are some of the most potent poisons known. Figure 27–2 lists representative toxins from animal and bacterial sources and highlights the very low human lethal doses for botulinus and tetanus toxins.

### Gas Gangrene

The classic disease caused by *Clostridium perfringens* is gas gangrene, which is also pro-duced by *C. novyi* and *C. septicum*. The organism can be isolated from the skin of many noninfected hospitalized patients. These patients are at risk of developing gas gangrene postoperatively under appropriate conditions. In World War I, gas gangrene associated with traumatic wounds from shell fragments was responsible for a great number of fatalities. In most cases, the wounds were contaminated with soil that had been fertilized with animal or human fecal material. The presence of multiple species of clostridial spores in the soil frequently resulted in infections with more than one species, including *C. novyi* and *C. septicum*, as well as *C. perfringens*.

Clinical manifestations of gas gangrene are due to the vigorous utilization of glycogen and other fermentable carbohydrates by the organism, resulting in the rapid production of lactic acid and gas. Increased tissue tension from gas formation caused decreased blood flow, a lowered tissue oxygenation, and more favorable conditions for growth of anaerobic bacteria producing toxins. The alpha-toxin is composed of two domains. The N-terminal domain has phospholipase C activity splitting lecithin to phosphoryl choline and diglyceride, whereas the C-terminal domain confers cytolytic properties. Control of this disease can usually be achieved by a combination of surgical excision of accessible tissue and the prompt administration of antibiotics (penicillin G). In more severe infections, hyperbaric oxygen therapy is sometimes used in some centers. *Hyperbaric oxygen therapy* is the exposure of the patient to increased atmospheric pressure of oxygen for short periods. This exposure does not significantly change the oxygen-carrying capacity or saturation of the red

### TABLE 27–3. MEDICALLY IMPORTANT EXOTOXINS PRODUCED BY PRINCIPAL TOXIGENIC CLOSTRIDIA

| BACTERIAL SPECIES | DISEASE | TOXIN | ACTION |
|---|---|---|---|
| *Clostridium botulinum* | Botulism | Seven strain-specific toxins (toxin types A through G) | Paralytic |
| *C. tetani* | Tetanus | Tetanospasmin | Spastic |
| *C. perfringens* | Gas gangrene | Alpha-toxin | Lecithinase: necrotizing, hemolytic |
| | | Beta-toxin, | Necrotizing |
| | | Epsilon-toxin | Permease |
| | | Iota-toxin | Dermonecrotizing |
| *C. septicum* | Gas gangrene | Alpha-toxin | Hemolytic |
| *C. novyi* | Gas gangrene | Alpha-toxin | Lecithinase: necrotizing, hemolytic |
| | | Beta-toxin | Necrotizing |
| | | Epsilon-toxin | Permease |

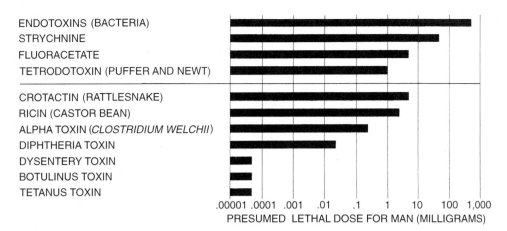

**FIGURE 27-2.** Toxicity of the bacterial toxins, including tetanus, as compared with that of other poisons. Crotactin and ricin, like the bacterial exotoxins, are simple proteins. The scale is logarithmic. The dosage figures are theoretical and they assume that the toxin is injected. (From van Heyningen, W. E. Tetanus. *Sci. Am. 218*:69, 1968. Copyright © 1968 by Scientific American, Inc. All rights reserved.)

blood cells, but does result in a small increase in the oxygen tension of the serum and the interstitial tissues. The increase in interstitial oxygen tension resulting from 1–2 h in a hyperbaric chamber is postulated to be sufficient to interrupt toxin formation and microbial replication. Normal phagocytic and host defense mechanisms may then be able to control the infection.

Although gas gangrene has been an infection classically associated with trauma and devitalized tissue, it is occasionally seen in hospitalized patients in situations in which necrosis, vascular insufficiency, and possible microbial contamination occur. Invasion of the bloodstream by *C. perfringens* may result from ulcerating lesions of the gastrointestinal tract. Recovery of *C. septicum* by blood culture is correlated with the presence of neutropenia and with malignant tumor in the gastrointestinal tract. *C. septicum* is the most common cause of spontaneous or nontraumatic gangrene. Isolation of *C. perfringens* from skin wounds or cultures from the female genital tract in asymptomatic patients should be neither viewed with alarm nor dismissed as contaminants. Such patients should be observed carefully and treated with surgical débridement and appropriate antimicrobial therapy only if signs of infection are present.

Disease due to *C. perfringens* also occurs at several other sites in the body. As noted above, *C. perfringens* may play a role in cases of cholecystitis, particularly postoperatively. Other gas-forming bacteria, such as species of Enterobacteriaceae and peptostreptococci, may also cause gas production. Gas gangrene may occur as a postoperative complication in patients; this can be a rare but lethal complication in patients with diabetes following amputation of an extremity for lower extremity gangrene or infection. Disease under these circumstances results from decreased blood flow, decreased tissue oxygenation, and necrosis from the surgical procedure. The microorganism presumably is present on the skin, possibly as a result of being the normal flora of the large bowel in the patient at risk.

Infectious complications of spontaneous or induced abortion are well known to involve *C. perfringens*. Retained nonviable fetal material, endometrial necrosis, and bacterial contamination from the vagina contribute to the infection. Alpha-toxin produced by *C. perfringens* is a lecithinase, causing necrosis and hemolysis. Under optimal conditions (for the bacteria), large amounts of alpha-toxin are secreted that can result in massive intravascular hemolysis in the infected patient.

### Tetanus

Tetanus, or "lockjaw," is a disease caused by *Clostridium tetani*, a spore-forming, gram-positive, anaerobic bacillus widely distributed in soil that is fecally contaminated by humans or animals. Cases of tetanus result from contamination of wounds by soil. Injection drug users may acquire tetanus through the practice of subcutaneous drug injection ("skin popping"). The incidence of tetanus in the

United States has dropped dramatically in the past four decades with the use of tetanus toxoid immunization; however, cases may still occur in the elderly, particularly among elderly women who were never immunized (older men were often immunized as a part of prior military service), or in immunized older adults whose immunity has waned because of failure to receive booster immunizations.

*C. tetani* is considered to be part of the indigenous intestinal microbial flora of humans and domestic animals. The spores are resistant to wide temperature changes and may remain viable in the environment for years. In contrast to *C. perfringens*, *C. tetani* requires a very strict anaerobic environment for toxin production. Wounds are usually the site of infection, owing to the interruption of blood flow in traumatized tissue, which results in deceased tissue oxygen. A further decrease in the $E_h$ can occur if there is microbial contamination and growth of facultative anaerobic bacteria. Clinical tetanus from spores germinating long after likely exposure, presumably introduced into wounds months or years previously, has also been reported. The lack of significant numbers of proteolytic and saccharolytic enzymes in *C. tetani* tends to minimize any inflammatory reaction that may develop from bacterial replication with resultant toxin formation. This means that in rare cases the site of infection in patients with tetanus may not be apparent (cryptogenic tetanus).

The gene for tetanospasmin, the paralytic toxin of tetanus, is encoded on a plasmid. Tetanus toxin, like botulinus toxin, enters the neuron at the neuromuscular junction but acts by blocking transmission of inhibitory impulses of the internuncial neurons located in the spinal cord. The result is production of prolonged muscular spasms of both the flexor and extensor muscle groups. Studies have shown that the toxin moves by retrograde axonal transport from the site of infection across synapses in the central nervous system (Fig. 27–3). Inasmuch as the flexor muscles are usually dominant, the patient with advanced tetanus shows generalized flexion contractures. Severe, prolonged spasm of the masseter muscle may restrict opening of the mouth and has led to the condition commonly known as *lockjaw*. Progression of the disease to include the muscles of respiration may result in respiratory failure. In less severe cases, loss of control of pharyngeal musculature can lead to tracheobronchial aspiration resulting in severe pneumonia.

Not well known in the United States is the considerable worldwide mortality rate from neonatal tetanus. Although the incidence of neonatal tetanus is very low in the United States with only rare cases occurring each year, it is common elsewhere in the world

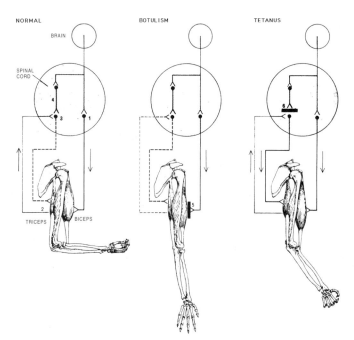

**FIGURE 27–3.** Nervous control of muscles that raise and lower the forearm is diagrammed schematically. In a normal individual (*left*), impulses from the brain can excite a motoneuron (1) to cause the biceps to contract, stretching the triceps. A stretch-sensitive receptor (2) in the triceps would then cause a triceps motor neuron (3) to fire and oppose the stretching —except that this firing is inhibited by impulses from an inhibitory nerve (4). In botulism (*center*), the neuromuscular junction is blocked (5), causing flaccid paralysis. In tetanus (*right*), the inhibitory impulses to the triceps motoneuron are blocked (6); both muscles contract, causing a spasm. (From van Heyningen, W. E. Tetanus. *Sci. Am. 218*:69, 1968. Copyright © 1968 by Scientific American, Inc. All rights reserved.)

where there is poverty, crowded living conditions, and lack of even minimal medical care. Neonatal tetanus usually results from contamination of the umbilical cord of newborns with tetanus spores. In India, it has been associated with packing of the birth canal with cattle dung, a practice in some regions where religious significance is assigned to cows. This results in contamination of both the umbilical cord and the endometrial surface with tetanus spores.

Tetanus is a disease produced by an exotoxin that can be inactivated by an antitoxin vaccine. Therefore, clinical tetanus is *preventable*. Tetanus toxin can be made nontoxic by the addition of small amounts of formalin, thereby forming a toxoid. This modification does not change the antigenicity of the toxin. Preparations of toxoid are made with alum to facilitate slow absorption and prolonged antigenic exposure (see Chapter 40). Current recommendations are for primary immunization at 2, 4, and 6 months of age, followed by a "booster" dose 12 months and 4 years later. Such a schedule will produce active immunity to the toxin; this immunity is reported to be protective for 10–20 years. Booster immunizations are recommended at 10-year intervals to maintain immunity. Patients who recover from clinical tetanus should undergo a primary immunization series with toxoid because, by getting tetanus once, these patients have demonstrated that they live and work in a manner that predisposes them to future exposure. It is important to remember that *recovery from tetanus does not confer immunity*.

Passive protection in patients not previously actively immunized with toxoid can be provided temporarily by the use of antitoxin. Hyperimmune human gamma globulin is now used for this purpose. Experience with human globulin has shown it to be at least as effective as the previously used equine antiserum in treating and preventing tetanus, but it has the important advantage of eliminating serum sickness and allergic reactions to the animal sera. Benzathine penicillin, released over a 28-day period, is useful for treating active infection.

## Botulism

Botulism should more properly be called an intoxication than an infectious disease. In most cases of botulism, preformed toxin in food is ingested with the tainted food. In addition to classic botulism, cases of botulism that result from wounds contaminated with *Clostridium botulinum* have been recognized. In these patients there is usually a history of a traumatic injury with contamination by soil. Pathogenesis of the infection is presumed to be similar to that of tetanus, with growth of the organism in depths of the wound and subsequent production of the toxin. Systemic absorption of the toxin readily occurs at the wound site.

The toxin of botulism acts at the neuromuscular junction of skeletal muscle, preventing acetylcholine release and blocking neural transmission (Fig. 27–3). Symptoms of botulism are due to a progressive decrease of skeletal muscle function, which eventually results in paralysis. The first muscles to become affected are the small muscles of the eye, larynx, and pharynx; consequently, diplopia and dysphonia develop early. Later, weakness of the extremities may appear, and impairment of the muscles of respiration occurs. Death usually is caused by cardiac arrest due to respiratory failure.

*C. botulinum* organisms are separated into groups I through IV, and produce seven known types of toxin, types A–G, with types A, B, and E most often seen in humans. Group I makes toxin types A, B, or F; group II type B, E, or F; group III toxin types C or D; and group IV type G. Only type G is plasmid mediated. A single bacterial strain rarely produces more than one type of toxin. Improperly canned foods, smoked uncooked foods, and fermented foods are usually implicated as the source for botulism toxin. Toxin types A and B are associated with the growth of the microorganism in home-prepared vegetables and meats (the word *botulus* is Latin, meaning "sausage"), including such exotic delicacies as fermented beaver tail. Curiously, in the United States strains producing type A toxin most commonly occur in the west and type B in the east. *C. botulinum* toxin type C causes limberneck in fowl, and type D causes botulism in cattle but not in humans. Type E toxin is most frequently acquired from fish or marine animals, whereas type F has caused disease in several outbreaks, one from home-canned mushrooms and a second from home-prepared venison jerky. Type F from *C. botulinum* has also been isolated from salmon and soil. Toxin type G has not been associated with human disease. Spores from all types of *C. botulinum* are in the soil and may be present on plants and vegetables. They are resistant to heat, and if contaminated food is not thoroughly heated during preparation, anaerobic conditions resulting from the canning procedure may allow germination, growth, and production of toxin. This is particularly dangerous in home-canned foods, when canning temperatures are not always carefully controlled.

Although spores of *C. botulinum* are resistant to heating, the toxin is susceptible to increased temperatures and may be inactivated by heating at a temperature as low as 60°C for 30 min. Type A *C. botulinum* toxin is apparently more lethal than type B, as the mortality rate in patients ingesting type A toxin is 60%; in those with type B toxin it is slightly less (48%). Several outbreaks of botulism caused by *C. botulinum* type E toxin involving smoked whitefish from the Great Lakes prompted investigation of the incidence of spores in fish taken from Lake Michigan. These studies showed that *C. botulinum* spores could be recovered from up to 13% of whitefish being transferred from brine vats to smoking rooms, with the presence of the spores resulting from cross-contamination by infected fish. This would indicate that the potential for clinical botulism would be considerably greater than documented cases indicate. One interesting characteristic differentiating toxin types A and E *C. botulinum* is the minimal proteolytic activity of type E toxin (from group II organisms) compared with type A toxin (from group I strains). Patients who had ingested food contaminated with type A toxin usually remember that the food tasted spoiled, but few patients complain of the bad taste or evidence of spoilage with toxin type E from group II *C. botulinum*. The fewer proteolytic enzymes in group II organisms presumably produce less offensive end products that cause food to taste "spoiled."

The diagnosis of botulism is best established by culture of the organism and demonstration of toxin in the serum of the sick patient and in the suspected food. Even minute quantities of toxin may be detected by injecting mice with serum from patients ill with the disease or with extracts of the suspected food. However, enzyme-linked immunosorbent assay (ELISA) testing is now more widely used to detect and type the clostridial toxins. The treatment of botulism should be directed toward ventilatory support of the patient and, in severe cases, removing unbound toxin from the circulation with either specific or polyvalent equine type A, B, and E antitoxin. Because progressive disease usually causes death by paralysis of the muscles of respiration, patients with botulism must be watched carefully for need for respiratory assistance. With the exception of wound-associated botulism and infant botulism, the toxin is not produced within the body and antibiotics are not helpful. As noted earlier, heat lability of the toxin suggests that the best therapy is prevention.

### Infant Botulism

Infant botulism is caused by *C. botulinum* that produces either type A, B, or F toxin. In 1976, several pediatricians in central California recognized a syndrome in infants suggesting botulism. They noticed several infants between 5 and 13 weeks of age who had constipation and muscle weakness as manifested by less vigorous sucking from breast to bottle, a weak cry, and loss of neck and limb strength, creating a "floppy" appearance. Although serum specimens were negative for toxin, the stools of all infants were positive for both *C. botulinum* organisms and toxin. In contrast to food-borne botulism, the disease appeared to result from the ingestion of *C. botulinum* spores with intracolonic growth and toxin formation. Presumably, the colon is less permeable to the toxin than is the small intestine, and thus there is decreased absorption of toxin with low or undetectable levels in the serum of most affected infants. This is correlated with a less severe form of disease. In some infants the organism and toxin can be found in the stools for as long as 100 days following discharge from the hospital for the acute illness. Antitoxin has not been considered necessary in treatment, and therapy is based on general supportive measures. The clinical symptoms include constipation followed by signs of weakness. The illness may progress for 1–2 weeks before stabilizing, and recovery may not begin for another 2–3 weeks.

Because of the paralytic effects of botulism toxin on skeletal muscles, there was a possibility that infant botulism might be a contributing factor to the sudden infant death syndrome (SIDS). This syndrome is characterized by the unexpected death of an infant, usually at less than 6 months of age. Most SIDS victims are found dead in their cribs without signs or symptoms of antecedent illness or an adequate explanation for their death on autopsy examination. The overlapping epidemiologic curves for SIDS and infant botulism cases are of interest, but infant botulism has not been implicated as a cause.

## *C. difficile*–Associated (Antimicrobial Agent) Diarrhea and Colitis

Development of diarrhea as a side effect of taking antimicrobial agents is a common complication. An infectious cause of this problem, *C. difficile*–associated diarrhea (CDAD) occurs almost uniquely in patients in hospitals and other long-term care institutions (e.g., nursing homes). Most antimicrobial agents have been incriminated, including penicillin G, ampicillin, cephalosporins, tetracyclines, trimethoprim-sulfamethoxazole, and clindamycin. The most serious of the gastrointestinal complications associated with antibiotics is pseudomembranous colitis. Pseudomembranous colitis is characterized clinically by abdominal pain, leukocytosis, fever, and profuse diarrhea. Mortality rates as high as 60% were reported initially in untreated patients. The changes noted in the colon include the presence of yellow, plaque-like mucosal lesions with diffuse infiltration of neutrophils; disruption of the villus tips; and the presence of fibrin, bacteria, and inflammatory cells (pseudomembrane) on the surface of the intestinal epithelium (Fig. 27–4). Following increasing use of clindamycin for anaerobic bacterial infections, pseudomembranous "clindamycin" colitis began to occur sporadically, with wide variation in its incidence following the use of clindamycin. In some hospitals the incidence was as high as 10%, whereas other large centers had no reported cases. The presence of a cytotoxic substance in the stools suggested the presence of a bacterial toxin. *C. difficile* eventually was identified as the source of the bacterial toxin and as the cause of pseudo-membranous colitis as well as some antibiotic-related diarrhea without the presence of pseudomembranes. The wide variation in the rate of pseudomembranous colitis related to clindamycin use is now explained by the epidemic nature of the disease that requires not only antibiotic treatment (which alters the normal bowel flora) but also acquisition of toxigenic *C. difficile* to cause the disease. Studies of humans developing pseudomembranous colitis after clindamycin, ampicillin, or a cephalosporin have shown the cytotoxin of *C. difficile* to be present in stools in high titer in most patients. In contrast, patients with simple antibiotic-associated diarrhea do not have colitis or cytotoxin in their stools.

*Clostridium difficile* is considered to be a member of the normal flora of the colon in less than 5% of free-living adults. *C. difficile* produces the two largest bacterial toxins known, toxin A (308,000 D), which is a weak cytotoxin and a potent enterotoxin, and toxin B (270,000 D), which is a potent cytotoxin. Both toxins cause cytotoxic cell "rounding" by disorganizing the cell cytoskeleton via interference with Rho proteins. The activities of the toxins appear to potentiate each other in producing CDAD, with the enterotoxin (toxin A) acting first on the intact mucosa, and later the cytotoxin (toxin B) exerting its cytotoxic activity after the normal colonic mucosa is disrupted.

The diagnosis of pseudomembranous colitis is made by the sigmoidoscopic visualization of pseudomembranes in a patient who has diarrhea following antibiotics. The diagnosis of CDAD is made by demonstrating toxin in the

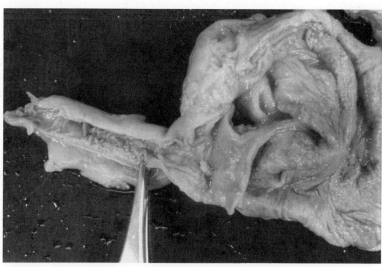

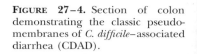
**FIGURE 27–4.** Section of colon demonstrating the classic pseudomembranes of *C. difficile*–associated diarrhea (CDAD).

stool by cytopathic effect in tissue cell culture systems, and the neutralization of the toxin by specific antitoxin. Alternatively, an antigen–antibody (EIA) test to detect toxin A can be used. The diagnosis of CDAD can also be made by culture of toxin-producing *C. difficile* from the stool of a patient who has diarrhea following antibiotic administration. The clinical picture of CDAD requires that a patient have at least three loose stools daily for at least 2 days, has received antimicrobial agent therapy within the previous 2 months, and has no other obvious reason for diarrhea. In this setting, laboratory confirmation of the presence of *C. difficile* toxin, or of a toxin-producing organism in the stool, can be diagnostic. CDAD and pseudomembranous colitis are treated with oral vancomycin or metronidazole for 10 days. They are equally efficacious, but the latter is much less expensive. Recurrence of pseudomembranous colitis and CDAD follows cessation of therapy in 7% and 20% of patients, respectively, and can be managed in the majority of patients by a second course of treatment. Giving less than 10 days of therapy increases the risk of relapse. Since 15% of patients may be stool-positive for *C. difficile* after successful treatment, it is inappropriate and costly to evaluate outcome of therapy with follow-up laboratory testing. Clinical resolution of diarrhea is sufficient.

CDAD is the most common identified cause of hospital-acquired diarrhea in adults. Disease rates vary from less than 1 to 30–40 cases per 1000 discharges. Rates are influenced by antimicrobial usage in the institution, particularly use of clindamycin, penicillins, and cephalosporins, and by the presence of specific epidemic strains of *C. difficile*. Morbidity with prolongation of hospitalization is a major clinical problem, and mortality ranges from 0.5 to 4%. Use of gloves when handling body substances, elimination of electronic thermometers, and control of clindamycin use have all been effective in reducing case rates.

## CULTIVATION AND IDENTIFICATION OF ANAEROBIC BACTERIA

Most anaerobic bacteria have two cardinal requirements for growth—a low oxidation–reduction potential (a reducing environment), and the absence of oxygen. The critical factors necessary for a low $E_h$ are not clearly understood. Peroxides formed during aerobic metabolism may be toxic and are usually inactivated by catalase, an enzyme that many anaerobes lack. Most anaerobes cannot tolerate more than a 30-min exposure to these compounds. Exposure to oxygen and oxygen radicals is rapidly lethal to a large number of anaerobes. However, exposure to oxygen is not the only factor involved, since it is known that oxygen can be bubbled through a culture medium containing growing anaerobes if a low oxidation–reduction potential is maintained by strong chemical-reducing agents. Conversely, studies with *Bacteroides fragilis* have shown that chemical changes in $E_h$ do not impair growth if no oxygen is introduced, but that growth stops abruptly when oxygen is provided; these results suggest a direct toxic effect of oxygen. The presence of large amounts of the enzyme superoxide dismutase in aerobic and facultative anaerobic bacteria but not in many of the fastidious anaerobic bacteria also plays a role. Superoxide $(O_2^-)$ is a highly reactive (free radical) compound produced when oxygen is reduced by a single electron, and it is generated during the normal catalytic action of a number of enzymes. Superoxide dismutase catalyzes the conversion of two molecules of superoxide to one molecule of oxygen and one molecule of hydrogen peroxide. The absence of superoxide dismutase in obligate anaerobic bacteria creates obvious disadvantages to survival. The ability to produce this enzyme may provide varying degrees of protection to individual bacteria upon exposure to different amounts of oxygen.

Many, but not all, anaerobic bacteria grow more slowly in culture than do facultative anaerobic bacteria and usually require 48 h for colony formation. In addition, multiple anaerobic and aerobic bacterial species are usually present in anaerobic infections. This means that the isolation, separation, and complete characterization of individual species may take 4–10 days.

## Collection and Transport of Specimens

For the optimal recovery of anaerobic bacteria, cultures should be taken in a manner that minimizes exposure to air. When cultures for anaerobes are to be obtained, oxygen-free tubes or vials should be used (Fig. 27–5). A variety of methods for taking cultures are available, but most are based on the use of containers with an atmosphere free of oxygen and with incorporation of a reducing agent into media or broth to diminish the effect of

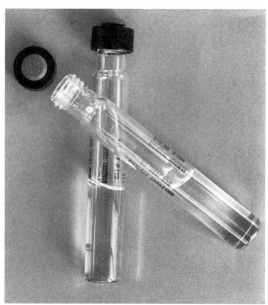

**FIGURE 27–5.** A collection tube with semisolid agar for transporting specimens for anaerobic culture. The tube contains an oxygen-free atmosphere and a small quantity of a reducing agent along with agar to maintain viability of the specimen contents. Material can be inoculated through the rubber port at the top of the tube, or the cap can be unscrewed for inoculation of larger tissues.

residual air. Collection of aspirated fluid, pus, or tissue is preferable to collection of specimens by swabs, even when transported in anaerobic containers. Cotton or Dacron swabs are often toxic to many bacteria, and if not specially prepared for anaerobic specimen collection, they will be filled with oxygen when placed into the anaerobic transport collection container, killing any anaerobes present during transport to the laboratory. Precautions should be taken to reduce contamination by the indigenous microbial flora from contiguous sites of infection, such as oropharyngeal or vaginal secretions. Prompt delivery to the laboratory and inoculation to reduced culture media greatly improves recovery of fastidious anaerobic bacteria. Direct examination of Gram's-stained material from the original specimen should be done to correlate the bacterial morphology with organisms later identified by culture.

### Methods for Culture

The standard procedure for isolation of anaerobic bacteria in many clinical laboratories includes the use of anaerobic jars and pouches, an anaerobic chamber (glove box), or a prereduced anaerobically sterilized (PRAS) media system (see Chapter 36). Culture plates are placed in a plastic or glass jar, and hydrogen is added by evacuation and replacement with a mixture of 80% $N_2$, 10% $CO_2$ and 10% $H_2$, or by a disposable $H_2$–$CO_2$ generating system. Another technique is the use of an anaerobic glove box, a closed chamber of rigid or flexible plastic with transfer ports in which cultures can be handled in a completely controlled, oxygen-free atmosphere. These chambers may be heated and may serve as both an incubator and a work area. Since most aerobic organisms also grow anaerobically, aerobic cultures must be done in parallel with the anaerobic ones in order to determine rapidly which organisms grow both aerobically and anaerobically, and which ones grow anaerobically with no aerobic growth on agar plates.

### Culture Media for Anaerobes

Most culture media for anaerobic bacteria require components not found in standard media. Reducing agents may be necessary to keep the $E_h$ in the $-0.010$ V range or less. Anaerobic environmental systems (jars, chambers, and incubators) contain a quality control indicator showing when the oxygen tension of the environment is above a certain level. The most commonly used indicator is resazurin, which is colorless when reduced and pink when oxidized. Recovery of different bacterial species may be enhanced if different additives are incorporated, such as bile for the inhibition of growth of anaerobes other than the *Bacteroides fragilis* group, hemin to enhance growth of the *Bacteroides fragilis* group and other *Bacteroides* and *Prevotella* species, and menadione (vitamin $K_1$) for the growth of pigmented *Prevotella* and *Porphyromonas* species. Antibiotics inactive against anaerobes, such as gentamicin and kanamycin, are frequently added to anaerobic isolation media to inhibit growth of aerobic organisms that might otherwise overgrow the slower growing anaerobes. The best results for the isolation and identification of anaerobic bacteria are reportedly obtained by the use of PRAS culture media. These are prepared under an oxygen-free gas, usually nitrogen, reducing exposure to air or oxygen during preparation. Culture media exposed to air and oxygen during preparation may form "toxic peroxides," which will inhibit growth of fastidious microorganisms. One such microorganism, *Clostridium haemolyticum*, usually does not grow on a blood agar plate exposed to atmospheric air for longer than 3 h.

## ADVANTAGES OF ANAEROBIC BACTERIAL IDENTIFICATION

Understanding the host–parasite interaction first requires the accurate identification of all participating parasites. One example of why such identification is advantageous is illustrated by the clinical information provided by the identification of certain members of the genus *Bacteroides*. Of the many species that make up this genus, one, *Bacteroides fragilis*, is more frequently isolated than others from abscesses and other sites of infection, even though it is present in the colon in considerably smaller numbers than other species of *Bacteroides*. In contrast to other species in this genus, *B. fragilis* has a polysaccharide capsule that confers the ability to incite abscess formation either by live or by heat-killed bacteria, a finding not shared by unencapsulated strains. The capsular polysaccharide of *B. fragilis* also stimulates circulating serum antibody, and this is one of the more important virulence factors of this organism. *B. fragilis* is also frequently resistant to antibiotics. For these reasons, identification of *B. fragilis* indicates to the clinician that active therapeutic measures should be taken, including selection of appropriate antimicrobial treatment. Identification of different species of anaerobic bacteria is accomplished by combining gross and microscopic appearance of the organism with results of biochemical tests, antibiotic susceptibility tests, and serologic tests. Gas-liquid chromatography (GLC) for the detection and semiquantitation of volatile fatty acids produced by different bacterial species is also used to assist in some identifications. The strong and offensive odor often associated with anaerobic disease is in part related to the release of volatile fatty acids and the formation of strongly aliphatic amines, such as cadaverine and putrescine, by biosynthetic and biodegradative decarboxylases.

Other anaerobic organisms for which specific identification is critical include *Clostridium septicum* (associated with gastrointestinal and hematologic malignancies), *C. ramosum*, *C. innocuum*, and *C. clostridiiforme* (resistant to antibiotics), and *C. perfringens* (a cause of potentially life-threatening infection). *C. difficile* also warrants specific identification from stool.

## ANTIMICROBIAL AGENT SUSCEPTIBILITY TESTING

Detecting drug resistance in microbial pathogens is a major service offered by microbiology laboratories. However, determining susceptibility of anaerobic bacteria to antimicrobial agents has posed a technical problem for a number of years. A frequently used procedure, that of measuring a zone of growth inhibition around a paper disc impregnated with a known amount of antibiotic, does not have the same validity for the slowly growing anaerobic bacteria that has been shown for rapidly growing bacteria. The use of an agar growth medium containing varying dilutions of antimicrobial drugs has given results more uniform than those produced by disc diffusion and has been recommended for anaerobe susceptibility by the National Committee for Clinical Laboratory Standards. Because the procedure is costly, only large reference laboratories employ the agar dilution method routinely, and because of the lack of a simple widely accepted and inexpensive method for susceptibility testing, many laboratories do not perform the procedure.

Susceptibility testing of anaerobes should be performed to determine the activity of new antimicrobials, to monitor susceptibility profiles in major geographic areas, to monitor susceptibility profiles periodically in certain hospitals, and to provide assistance in the clinical treatment of selected patients with anaerobic infections. The latter group usually includes patients who have severe infections such as bacteremia or endocarditis in which antimicrobial treatment is critical, those who have infections with organisms for which the susceptibility is not predictable, or those who have infections that fail to respond to empiric antimicrobial treatment. Laboratories that offer testing for anaerobic bacteria will often routinely do this testing when the isolate is recovered from a normally sterile body site (other than urine) such as blood or a brain abscess, or upon request.

Anaerobic bacteria have become more resistant to antimicrobials over the past decade, and many traditional agents such as penicillin can no longer be relied upon for treatment of infections such as anaerobic lung abscess. Thus, there is the clinical dilemma of increasing resistance that makes empiric therapy more difficult, and reluctance to do routine susceptibility testing on all anaerobic isolates because of the large cost required. Fortunately, a number of antimicrobials such as metronidazole, imipenem, and the beta-lactam–beta-lactamase inhibitor combinations remain highly effective. This allows a policy of selective testing of anaerobic isolates for susceptibility to be cost effective and clinically efficacious.

## ANTIMICROBIAL AGENT THERAPY

Because anaerobic infection predisposes to abscess and localized collections of pus in a closed space, the primary treatment is often a surgical or radiologic drainage procedure. In addition to drainage procedures, it may be necessary to surgically resect necrotic and gangrenous tissue. Therapy with an appropriate antimicrobial agent is always employed in addition to drainage, and in many instances treatment can be successful without drainage. Initial antimicrobial agents selected should have a spectrum of activity against both aerobic and anaerobic bacteria because of the polymicrobial nature of most anaerobic infections. Identification and susceptibility testing results can then be used to adjust the initial agents selected.

Agents previously considered effective in treating anaerobic infection, penicillin and tetracycline, are no longer useful because of the development of widespread resistance. Chloramphenicol, which continues to retain activity against anaerobic bacteria, is rarely used because of its toxicity (bone marrow suppression and aplastic anemia). Agents that are almost always active (including against *B. fragilis*) and are widely used to treat anaerobic infection include metronidazole, ampicillin-sulbactam, amoxicillin-clavulanic acid, ticarcillin-clavulanic acid, piperacillin-tazobactam, and imipenem-cilastatin (Table 27–4). The

beta-lactam–beta-lactamase inhibitor combinations and imipenem-cilastatin are particularly suited to treatment of mixed aerobic and anaerobic infection because they are active against many aerobic organisms as well as anaerobes. Other agents that are somewhat less active but are frequently used to treat anaerobic infections include clindamycin, cefoxitin, ceftizoxime, cefotetan, ticarcillin, piperacillin, and mezlocillin. Characterisitics of these agents are reviewed in Chapters 37 and 38.

## CASE HISTORIES

### CASE HISTORY 1

A 72-year-old woman was admitted to the hospital complaining of polydipsia, nocturia, fever, and increasing shortness of breath of 10 days' duration. She had noted poor appetite for the preceding 8 months and had shown a 60-lb weight loss. The patient lived by herself but had moved to her daughter's apartment 8 days before she was hospitalized. While living with her daughter, the patient was found to have a temperature of 101°F, for which her physician prescribed cephalexin. During this period, the patient complained to her daughter about symptoms of hemorrhoids and described some vague discomfort in the perineal region.

Physical examination at the time of hospitalization revealed an elderly white female who appeared dehydrated and lethargic. Her blood pressure was 146/90 mm Hg, and the pulse rate was 126/min and regular. Examination of the optic fundi revealed venous congestion and hyperemia of the discs. The heart had a rapid but regular rate, and no murmurs were heard. The right lung was resonant, and the left revealed coarse rales. The abdomen was soft and scaphoid with no masses. The skin was rough and dry, although warm to the touch. Deep tendon reflexes were present and normal.

The white blood cell (WBC) count was 44,000/mm$^3$, with 76% segmented neutrophils. The blood glucose was 900 mg/dL, and the urine was strongly positive for ketones. A chest roentgenogram showed patchy infiltrates in the left lower lung field. The patient was started on insulin management for what was presumed to be diabetes mellitus. On the morning of the third hospital day, she was found in a coma and had a fever of 102°F. Four blood cultures at that time were subsequently reported to be negative for bacteria. Because of the fever, gentamicin was added and cephalexin was changed to intravenous cephalothin. Control of the diabetes proved difficult, and on the eleventh hospital day two decubitus (pressure) ulcers were noted over the sacrococcygeal region. By the 13th hospital day, the decubiti were associated with a

**TABLE 27–4. ANTIMICROBIAL SUSCEPTIBILITY (LISTED AS % SUSCEPTIBLE IN THE TABLE) OF SELECTED ANAEROBES AT NMH\* DURING 1994**

| Drug | Microorganism [No. of Strains] | | | | | | | |
|---|---|---|---|---|---|---|---|---|
| | *B. FRAGILIS* [44] | *B. VULGATUS* [12] | *B. DISTASONIS* [8] | *B. OVATUS* [12] | *VEILLONELLA* [7] | *PEPTOSTREPTOCOCCUS* [79] | *C. PERFRINGENS* [17] | OTHER CLOSTRIDIA [19] |
| Metronidazole | 100% | 100% | 100% | 100% | 100% | 96% | 100% | 89% |
| Clindamycin | 89% | 58% | 88% | 63% | 100% | 90% | 100% | 84% |
| Penicillin | 2% | 0% | 13% | 0% | 86% | 94% | 100% | 95% |
| Ampicillin-sulbactam | 100% | 92% | 100% | 100% | 100% | 97% | 100% | 100% |
| Imipenem | 95% | 92% | 100% | 100% | 86% | 91% | 76% | 100% |
| Cefoxitin | 93% | 67% | 75% | 100% | 100% | 96% | 100% | 84% |
| Ceftizoxime | 80% | 42% | 63% | 100% | 100% | 90% | 100% | 63% |
| Piperacillin | 84% | 75% | 63% | 100% | 86% | 99% | 100% | 95% |
| Chloramphenicol | 100% | 100% | 100% | 100% | 100% | 99% | 100% | 100% |

\*Northwestern Memorial Hospital, Chicago.

fluctuant mass. This mass was surgically incised, releasing a large amount of foul-smelling, clay-colored material. Culture of the material was reported to yield beta-hemolytic streptococci. Following the incision and drainage, the patient appeared to improve, although blood glucose levels continued to fluctuate. Because of a continued decline in her clinical course, the patient was transferred to a second hospital on the 16th hospital day.

At the time of admission to the second hospital, the patient was lethargic and responded poorly to questioning. Her temperature was still 101°F; blood pressure, 85/50 mm Hg; pulse 140/min; and respirations, 48/min. The chest was clear to auscultation and percussion. The abdomen was distended, with voluntary guarding and diffuse tenderness to palpation. Examination of the gluteal region revealed a large fluctuant mass extending from the sacrococcygeal region laterally through the left gluteus maximus to the left femoral trochanter. The skin had a brownish discoloration over the area. Arterial blood gases were $PO_2$, 108 mm Hg; $PCO_2$, 12 mm Hg; and pH, 7.05. The WBC count was 45,000/mm³; the blood glucose, 183 mg/dL; and the blood urea nitrogen, 141 mg/dL. The patient was continued on insulin management of diabetes, which included vigorous fluid replacement and intravenous sodium bicarbonate. Clindamycin was started in preparation for surgery to drain the abscess. Cultures were obtained from the abscess. Attempts to probe the extent of the abscess cavity were only partially successful, and the patient was scheduled for a complete incision and drainage of the gluteal region the following morning. Approximately 4 h after admission, the patient had a cardiac arrest. Resuscitation procedures were not successful. Blood cultures taken shortly after death failed to grow bacteria, although a blood culture taken from the right ventricle at the time of autopsy grew *Clostridium perfringens*. At autopsy, a large, necrotic abscess cavity was found extending from the sacrococcyx laterally through the left gluteus maximus to the region of the left greater trochanter. The abscess culture taken shortly before death revealed the following: *Clostridium perfringens, Bacteroides vulgatus, Bacteroides thetaiotaomicron, Bacteroides* species #1, *Bacteroides* species #2, *Prevotella melaninogenica, Bifidobacterium adolescentis* var. B., *Peptostreptococcus anaerobius, Peptostreptococcus prevotii, Enterococcus faecalis, Escherichia coli, Pseudomonas aeruginosa,* and *Candida albicans.*

## CASE 1 DISCUSSION

The patient was hospitalized initially with uncontrolled diabetes mellitus. This was evident by the history of polydipsia, nocturia, weight loss, and increasing shortness of breath. Whether she had an infection in the sacrococcygeal region at the time of admission to the first hospital is not clear, but the history of vague pain or discomfort mentioned to her daughter would suggest the possibility. It is likely that the sacrococcygeal infection precipitated diabetic coma on the third day. Severe infection in the diabetic may lead to uncontrolled hyperglycemia and coma. In reviewing the bacteria isolated from the sacral abscess, it is difficult to decide which of the 12 strains were responsible for septic shock that probably resulted in the patient's death. *Clostridium perfringens* is associated with severe infection and septicemia, but there was no evidence either before or after death of gas production. Each of the other microorganisms isolated can also be associated with severe infection, but what role individual ones played or how they may have interacted cannot be determined. None of the anaerobic bacteria present would be expected to be susceptible to either gentamicin or cephalothin, her empiric antibiotic therapy.

Furthermore, the setting of an anaerobic abscess means both a low oxygen tension and lowered pH existed within the abscess, making the aminoglycoside essentially inactive against any facultative (aerobic) bacteria present. Similarly, the beta-lactamases of the gram-negative anaerobes in the abscess would have destroyed the cephalothin, so that it too would be ineffective against the original beta-hemolytic streptococci or the *E. coli* recovered from the infection. In retrospect, if cultures for anaerobic bacteria had been obtained in the first hospital, the difficulty in bringing the patient's diabetes under control could have alerted her physicians to the significance of the underlying infection. The recognition of a polymicrobic abscess with anaerobic bacteria should have prompted more careful attention to an appropriate antimicrobial agent. Gentamicin, although a very good agent against many gram-negative bacteria, is ineffective against anaerobic bacteria. In this instance, early treatment with either clindamycin, metronidazole, imipenem, or a beta-lactam–beta-lactamase inhibitor combination would have been a better selection.

Treatment of anaerobic bacterial infections with antimicrobial agents ineffective against anaerobic bacteria results in a greatly decreased survival rate of seriously ill patients. When facultative anaerobic and strict anaerobic bacteria are present in the same infection, survival is significantly aided if agents are employed that are selected for use against the anaerobic bacteria. This patient had an anaerobic bacterial infection of the skin and subcutaneous tissue called necrotizing fasciitis. This is often due to mixed anaerobic bacteria and is frequently associated with some underlying host defect, such as diabetes mellitus. Adequate control usually requires aggressive surgical incision and drainage as well as an effective antimicrobial agent.

## CASE HISTORY 2*

Four hours after a lunch including home-canned gefilte fish that had been stored in a re-

---

*Adapted from Armstrong, R. W., Stenn, F., Dowell, V. R., Jr., et al. Type E botulism from home-canned gefilte fish. *JAMA 210*:303, 1969.

frigerator for 7 weeks, a 57-year-old woman with mild hypertension complained of headache, blurred vision, epigastric distress, hoarseness, and mild dyspnea. She vomited repeatedly and experienced dryness of the mouth, weakness, constipation, and urinary retention. Examination that evening revealed an anxious, moderately obese woman with a respiratory rate of 26/min, blood pressure of 80/58 mm Hg, and a pulse rate of 110/min. Her pupils were equal in size and dilated but were reactive to light. Extraocular movements were normal, and no facial weakness was noted. The patient's mouth and throat were dry, and her voice was hoarse. Bowel sounds were decreased, but her abdominal examination was otherwise normal. Examination of the chest and heart was normal. Because of hypotension and epigastric distress, the patient was hospitalized on the suspicion of myocardial infarction.

On admission, hemoglobin, hematocrit, and WBC count and differential were normal, as was urinalysis. The next morning serum electrolytes, bilirubin, amylase, and serum protein were normal, as were chest and abdominal roentgenograms and electrocardiogram. The patient was treated symptomatically with antacids, and with oral plus intravenous fluids. Thirty-six hours later the patient had a cardiopulmonary arrest and was resuscitated. Spontaneous respiration did not recur, and breathing was maintained on a mechanical respirator. The following day no apparent benefit resulted from the administration of 80,000 units of bivalent (types A and B) botulism antitoxin and 10,000 units of type E botulism antitoxin, which were given intravenously. One day later the patient died.

At autopsy the patient had generalized ischemic changes in the central nervous system, moderate arteriosclerosis of the coronary arteries, and mild hypertrophy of the left ventricle. The liver and spleen were enlarged and hyperemic. The lungs showed pulmonary edema and focal acute bronchopneumonia. Sera from the first, second, and third days after eating the gefilte fish had type E botulinum toxin detected. The fish contained 10 mouse intraperitoneal 50% lethal doses (IP $LD_{50}$) of type E botulinum toxin per gram. Trypsinization of the food extract increased the toxin activity to 780 mouse IP $LD_{50}$/g. Cultures of the gefilte fish yielded group II *C. botulinum* producing type E toxin. Type E antitoxin had been given to the patient 10 h before her death, and serum obtained at autopsy neutralized type E toxin.

## CASE 2 DISCUSSION

Botulism due to type E toxin can present a confusing clinical picture in that neurologic signs may be less prominent than the acute, severe gastrointestinal symptoms. The clinical illness of the patient illustrates how the prominence of gastrointestinal symptoms with type E toxin can be confused with symptoms of bowel obstruction or myocardial infarction, thus delaying specific treatment of the intoxication. Hypotension, epigastric distress, and tachycardia suggested myocardial ischemia and possible myocardial infarction. This case is noteworthy because of the lack of classic ocular and facial muscle manifestations, although transitory blurring of vision was reported in the patient, and she had dilated, but not fixed pupils.

*Clostridium botulinum* that produces toxin type E is widely distributed. Spores of this organism have been demonstrated in sediment and in fish from all northern oceans and from waterways and soils of all northern continents, including the Great Lakes and the Atlantic, Gulf, and Pacific coasts of North America. The greatest concentration of spores is in the sediments of shallow offshore waters, especially near the mouth of rivers. Smoking or light cooking may not be sufficient to inactivate all spores. In contrast to other varieties of *C. botulinum*, group II spores can germinate and produce toxin at refrigerator temperatures, with optimal growth at room temperature (25°–30°C). Therefore, in fresh or processed fish, lethal accumulations of botulinum toxin may develop when a lightly contaminated fish is held at low temperatures under anaerobic or nearly anaerobic conditions.

## REFERENCES

### Books and Symposia

Baron, E. J., Peterson, L. R., and Finegold, S. M. *Bailey and Scott's Diagnostic Microbiology*. 9th ed. St. Louis: Mosby-Year Book Inc., 1994:474–550.

Mandell, G. L., Bennett, J. E., and Dolin, R. *Mandell, Douglas and Bennett's Principles and Practice of Infectious Diseases*. 4th ed. New York: Churchill Livingstone, 1995:221–224.

Finegold, S. M., Baron, E. J., and Wexler, H. M. *A Clinical Guide to Anaerobic Infections*. Belmont, CA: Star Publishing Co., 1992.

Finegold, S. M., Goldstein, E. J. C., and Mulligan, M. E. Proceedings of the 1994 Meeting of the Anaerobe Society of the Americas. *Clin. Infect. Dis.* 20(Suppl. 2): S111–S383, 1995.

Nord, C. E., and Phillips, I. Anaerobic bacteria and infections. *Clin. Microbiol. Infect. Dis.* 11:997–1104, 1992.

### Review Articles

Bartlett, J. G. Anaerobic bacterial infections of the lung and pleural space. *Clin. Infect. Dis.* 16(Suppl. 4):S248–S255, 1993.

Gerding, D. N., Johnson, S., Peterson, L. R., Mulligan, M. E., and Silva, J., Jr. Society for Healthcare Epidemiology of America position paper on *Clostridium difficile*–associated diarrhea and colitis. *Infect. Control Hosp. Epidemiol.* 16:459–477, 1995.

Styrt, B., and Gorbach, S. L. Recent developments in the understanding of the pathogenesis and treatment of anaerobic infections. *N. Engl. J. Med. 321*:240–298, 1989.

## Original Articles

Bartlett, J. G., Chang, T. W., Gurwirth, M., et al. Antibiotic-associated pseudomembranous colitis due to toxin-producing clostridia. *N. Engl. J. Med. 298*:531, 1978.

Bartlett, J. G., Gorbach, S. L., Tally, F. P., et al. Bacteriology and treatment of primary lung abscess. *Am. Rev. Respir. Dis. 109*:510, 1974.

Clabots, C. R., Peterson, L. R., and Gerding, D. N. Characterization of nosocomial *Clostridium difficile* outbreak by using plasmid profile typing and clindamycin susceptibility testing. *J. Infect. Dis. 158*:731, 1988.

Gerding, D. N. Foot infections in diabetic patients: The role of anaerobes. *Clin. Infect. Dis. 20*(Suppl. 2):S242–S249, 1995.

Weinstein, W. M., Onderdonk, A. B., Bartlett, J. G., et al. Antimicrobial therapy of experimental intraabdominal sepsis. *J. Infect. Dis. 132*:282, 1975.

Boschman, C. R., Tucker, L. J., Dressel, D. C., Novak, C. C., Hayden, R. T., and Peterson, L. R. Optimizing detection of microbial sepsis: A comparison of culture systems using packaged sets with directions for blood collection. *Diagn. Microbiol. Infect. Dis. 23*:1–9, 1995.

# 28

# RICKETTSIAL DISEASES

STANFORD T. SHULMAN, M.D.

The rickettsioses are caused by a group of small coccobacilli (rickettsiae) that share certain features of viruses and bacteria, but more closely resemble bacteria. Although like viruses they grow only intracellularly, they resemble bacteria by multiplying by transverse binary fission; by containing both DNA and RNA; by possessing Krebs's cycle (tricarboxylic acid cycle), electron transport, and protein synthetic enzymes; and by being susceptible to several antibacterial agents. Rickettsiae were named to honor Dr. Howard Taylor Ricketts, who in studies from 1906–1909 elucidated the etiology of Rocky Mountain spotted fever and who died of typhus in 1910 while working to determine the etiology of that disorder. Ricketts, a graduate of Northwestern University Medical School, clearly established the importance of ticks and lice as vectors for these disorders.

For all major rickettsioses except louse-borne typhus, man is only an incidental and accidental host, with the reservoir of rickettsial infection existing in lower animals or in the vectors. Rapid changes in the classification of these agents have occurred in recent years and likely will continue. At present, the rickettsiae include four genera, *Rickettsia, Coxiella, Ehrlichia*, and *Bartonella* (*Rochalimaea*), that are grouped together because they share certain characteristics:

1. They are of similar size ($0.3 \times 1–2 \ \mu$m)

and shape, appearing as nonmotile, gram-negative, pleomorphic coccobacilli (Figs. 28–1 and 28–2).

2. Most occur naturally in insects (lice and fleas) or in arachnids (ticks and mites) that, except for *C. burnetii* and some bartonella, serve as the major mode of transmission to humans.

3. They multiply within certain host cells, many particularly within endothelial cells.

4. They characteristically produce a widespread vasculitis of small blood vessels.

5. Most result in an acute infection characterized by fever, headache, and rash, with the exception of Q fever, which produces no rash.

6. They are all inhibited by certain antibiotics, particularly chloramphenicol and tetracyclines.

7. Except for Q fever and rickettsialpox, rickettsial infections induce agglutinins to *Proteus vulgaris* OX-19, OX-2, or OX-K antigens (Weil-Felix reaction).

Clinical and epidemiologic features facilitate presumptive diagnosis of the rickettsioses, with laboratory support provided by Weil-Felix reaction and confirmation by specific complement-fixing antibody responses (Table 28–1). Because antibiotic therapy must be instituted early in the course of rickettsial infection to be effective, clinical suspicion must be high to consider these diagnoses prior to

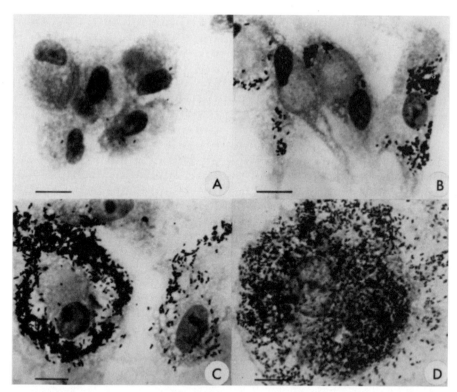

**FIGURE 28–1.** Photomicrographs of growth of *Rickettsia mooseri* in macrophages in cell culture containing normal human serum (Gimenez stain). (*Solid bars*, 10 μm.) *A*, After 2 h of exposure to *R. mooseri* suspension (× 1480). *B*, Day 3 after infection (× 1400). *C*, Day 6 after infection (× 1400). *D*, Day 6 after infection. Destruction of *R. mooseri*–infected macrophage (day 6) with release of microorganisms (× 1560). (From Gambrill, M. R., and Wisseman, C. L., Jr. Mechanisms of immunity in typhus infections. I. Multiplication of typhus rickettsiae in human macrophage cultures in the nonimmune system: Influence of virulence of rickettsial strains and of chloramphenicol. *Infect. Immun. 8*: 519, 1973. With permission.)

serologic confirmation. Except for scrub typhus, long-lived immunity results from rickettsial infection.

The rickettsial genome is composed of a single circular chromosome of $1.0–1.5 \times 10^9$ D. Although physiologically similar to bacteria, with multiple enzymatic systems, including oxidative phosphorylation and glutamate oxidation for energy production, rickettsiae appear to require certain cofactors provided by the host cell. Except for *C. burnetii* and bartonellae, the rickettsiae quickly lose viability outside host cells. Polychromatic stains such as Giemsa stain are superior to Gram's stain for identification of intracellular rickettsiae.

## PATHOGENESIS

After the bite of an infected vector, rickettsiae invade endothelial cells of small blood vessels and are demonstrable in both the nucleus and cytoplasm. They then multiply within those cells and are widely disseminated by the bloodstream. Focal areas of endothelial cell damage and proliferation with perivascular mononuclear cell infiltration result in local areas of hemorrhage and thrombosis. Postulated mechanisms of cell damage include (1) toxic rickettsial metabolic products, (2) competition for vital substrates, (3) adenosine triphosphate (ATP) depletion by rickettsiae leading to sodium pump failure and influx of water, and (4) cell-membrane damage related to multiple rickettsial penetration and later to massive rickettsial release. Vascular lesions are most prominent in small vessels of skin, myocardium, and brain and appear to account for the most common clinical manifestations, including rash. In contrast to other rickettsioses, *C. burnetii* is transmitted most frequently by inhalation of dust or aerosols contaminated by rickettsia-infected body fluids of infected animals, leading to prominent respira-

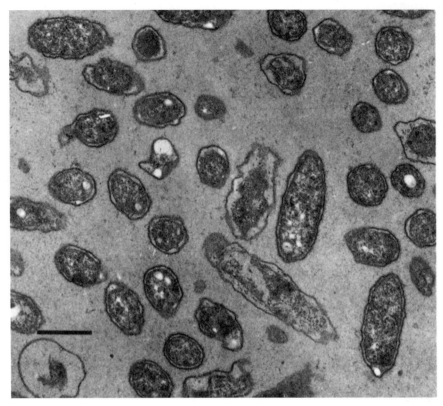

**FIGURE 28–2.** Ultrathin section through cells of *Rickettsia prowazekii* typical of those seen in the lumen of the louse midgut (*bar*, 0.5 μm). (From Silverman, D. J., Boese, J. L., and Wisseman, C. L., Jr. Ultrastructural studies of *Rickettsia prowazekii* from louse midgut cells to feces: Search for "dormant" forms. *Infect. Immun. 10:*257, 1974. With permission.)

tory tract manifestations. Rocky Mountain spotted fever has also been acquired via aerosol, particularly in laboratory settings.

The host response to rickettsiae is complex. Host defenses including antibody do not impair rickettsial replication within endothelial cells, and when released from endothelial cells rickettsiae are phagocytosed by macrophages. In the absence of antibody, rickettsiae replicate well within macrophages (Fig. 28–1), passing from the phagolysosome into the cytoplasm, where replication occurs. However, in the presence of antibody, rickettsiae remain within the phagolysosome, perhaps because of neutralization of a rickettsial product or substrate, and are killed and degraded within that structure. In contrast, the killing of rickettsiae within endothelial or other target cells is antibody independent and is most likely due to acquired T-cell immunity. Additionally, it can be shown *in vitro* and in animal models that rickettsia-stimulated lymphocytes release lymphokines that can kill rickettsiae within phagocytic or endothelial cells.

## CLINICAL DISORDERS

The rickettsioses are divided into several groups, including spotted fevers, typhus-like fevers, scrub typhus group, Q fever, ehrlichiosis, and the infections caused by bartonella organisms (trench fever, cat-scratch disease, bacillary angiomatosis, and bartonellosis) (Table 28–1).

### Spotted Fevers

#### Rocky Mountain spotted fever

Rocky Mountain spotted fever (RMSF) is by far the most important and the most severe of the spotted fevers which, except for rickettsialpox, are all tick-transmitted. RMSF has a fatality rate of 20–25% without specific therapy (5% overall), and although early treatment is important to lower the mortality, diagnosis in the early stages is frequently very difficult. RMSF is caused by *R. rickettsii*, which is antigenetically and genetically closely related to other members of the spotted fever

**TABLE 28–1.  CLINICAL FEATURES OF RICKETTSIAL DISEASES**

| | AGENT | VECTOR | RESERVOIR | GEOGRAPHY | SEVERITY | ESCHAR | UNIQUE FEATURES |
|---|---|---|---|---|---|---|---|
| Spotted fever group RMSF | *Rickettsia rickettsii* | Tick | Tick/rodents | Western Hemisphere | Severe | 0 | Most important in U.S. |
| Tick typhuses Boutonneuse | *R. conorii* | Tick | Ticks/rodents/ dogs | Mediterranean, Africa, India | Moderate | + | |
| Queensland | *R. australis* | Tick | Marsupials | Queensland, Australia | Moderate | + | |
| Siberian | *R. sibirica* | Tick | Long-tailed suslik | China, Mongolia, Pakistan, USSR | Moderate | + | |
| Rickettsialpox | *R. akari* | Mite | Mites/mice | U.S., USSR, Korea | Mild | + | Vesicular rash |
| Typhus group Epidemic typhus | *R. prowazekii* | Louse | Man/flying squirrel | Worldwide | Severe | 0 | Rash spares hands, feet |
| Brill-Zinsser disease | *R. prowazekii* | (Reactivation) | Humans | Worldwide | Mild | 0 | Occurs years after infection |
| Murine typhus | *R. typhi (mooseri)* | Flea | Rodents | Scattered foci worldwide | Moderate | 0 | |
| Scrub typhus | *R. tsutsugamushi* | Chigger (mite larva) | Mites/rodents | Japan, southeast Asia, southwestern Pacific | Variable (strain-dependent) | + | General adenopathy; immunity doesn't follow illness |
| Q Fever | *C. burnetii* | Ticks possibly | Ticks/mammals | Worldwide | Mild (usually) | 0 | Inhalation transmission; no rash; hardy organism; reticuloendothelial system target |
| Ehrlichiosis | *E. sennetsu* | Unknown | Humans | Far East | Mild | 0 | Intraleukocytic parasites |
| | *E. canis* | Dog tick | Dogs | Worldwide | Not defined | 0 | Few cases documented to date |
| | *E. equi*-like | Deer tick | Unclear | Upper Mid-West U.S. | Severe | 0 | Affects homeless, can cause endocarditis |
| Trench fever | *Bartonella quintana* | Louse | Humans | Eastern Europe, North Africa, Mexico | Mild | 0 | |
| Cat scratch disease | *B. henselae* | None | Kittens, cats | U.S., etc. | Mild-moderate | 0 | Lymphadenopathy |
| Bartonellosis | *B. bacilliformis* | Sandfly | Humans | South America | Severe | 0 | Resembles malaria |
| Bacillary Angiomatosis | *B. quintana* or *henselae* | — | ? | — | Severe | 0 | Immunocompromised hosts |

group. RMSF was first described in Idaho and Montana in the late 1800s but since the mid-1940s has almost completely disappeared from the Rocky Mountain region. Since 1931, RMSF has been recognized in the southeastern United States, and the vast majority of U.S. cases now occur in the region from Virginia to Georgia, the Ohio River Valley, Tennessee, Arkansas, and Oklahoma (Figs. 28–3 and 28–4). At present, RMSF occurs to some degree throughout the Western Hemisphere.

The epidemiologic characteristics of RMSF are directly related to the ixodid ticks that serve as reservoir and vector (the dog tick, *Dermacentor variabilis,* in the southern and eastern United States; the wood tick, *D. andersoni,* in the west; the Lone Star tick, *Amblyomma americanum,* in the south central United States; and others in Mexico and South America). *R. rickettsii* in ticks are passed transovarially to subsequent generations of ticks, and the ticks require a blood meal, usually from a dog, horse, or sheep, to proceed through their stages of development (eggs, larvae, nymphs, adults) to maturity. Most cases occur from April to September, coinciding with tick prevalence. Humans are incidental hosts, with rickettsial transmission occurring from salivary secretions when an infected adult tick remains attached to humans for at least several hours. The rickettsiae disseminate widely and establish infection within vascular endothelial and smooth muscle cells, resulting in vascular damage.

The major clinical features of RMSF are high fever, headache, rash, toxicity, nausea, confusion, and myalgia. On average, RMSF is a fairly serious illness. The course is highly variable, with some patients manifesting only mild nonspecific symptoms but others with a fulminant course leading to death within a few days. The mean incubation period is 5–7 days (range is 2–14 days) after an infected tick bite, with the earliest symptoms being nonspecific. The classic triad of fever, rash, and history of tick bite is present in only 3% of patients by the third day of illness. Rash develops as late as the sixth day but is usually present on the third or fourth day, first appearing as macules and papules on the wrists and ankles and spreading within hours up the extremities to the trunk (Fig. 28–5). Rash on the palms and soles is highly characteristic. The rash initially consists of small red macules that blanch with pressure and that then progress to macular–papular, and ultimately, to petechial–purpuric lesions. Intense, persis-

tent headache is common, and patients appear toxic. Signs of meningoencephalitis, such as lethargy, confusion, delirium, stupor, ataxia, coma, seizures, and focal neurologic findings, may develop, with central nervous system (CNS) damage being a major factor in RMSF mortality. Fatality rates increase with age and are higher in males, blacks, those older than 30 years, those without history of tick bite, and those treated more than 3 days after onset. The diagnosis of early RMSF is difficult, especially prior to development of the skin rash, and must be suspected on the basis of symptoms, signs, and epidemiologic features in order to institute specific therapy sufficiently early to affect favorably the course of the illness.

Early nonspecific laboratory features include leukopenia, thrombocytopenia, and hyponatremia. *R. rickettsii* often can be demonstrated by immunofluorescence in biopsies of skin lesions, but this is not widely available. Culture of rickettsiae is difficult and generally impractical. Polymerase chain reaction (PCR) diagnosis should be possible in the future. Serologic tests are not useful early in the disease, but are very valuable for diagnosis in retrospect (Table 28–2). Rising titers to *Proteus* OX-19 or OX-2 are usually seen in the second week of illness, but sera of some healthy individuals are positive for these Weil-Felix reactions. More specific antirickettsial antibodies can be detected in convalescent sera by 7–10 days after onset by complement-fixation (CF), indirect immunofluorescence, or other methods, but again, they are only useful in retrospect and cannot be relied upon to facilitate early treatment decisions. Considerable cross-reactivity exists among rickettsiae.

The differential diagnosis of RMSF includes meningococcal infection, measles, enteroviral exanthems, toxic shock syndrome, leptospirosis, disseminated gonococcal infection, secondary syphilis, systemic lupus, thrombotic thrombocytopenic purpura, immune thrombocytopenia, and other rickettsioses.

Within the first week of illness, antibiotic therapy is highly effective in RMSF, but therapy instituted later may have little effect on the course of this potentially fatal disease. Effective agents are chloramphenicol, 50–100 mg/kg/day orally or intravenously divided into four doses, or tetracycline, 25–50 mg/kg/day orally or 15–25 mg/kg/day intravenously divided into four doses. Therapy is continued until the patient is completely afebrile for at least 48 h, usually about a 1-week

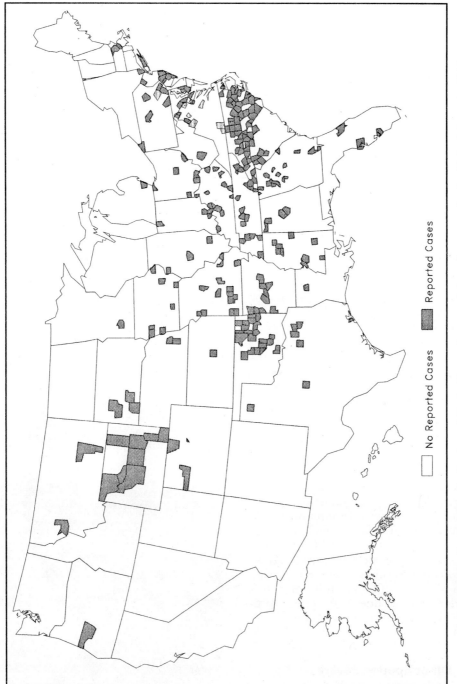

**FIGURE 28–3.** Geographic distribution of Rocky Mountain spotted fever, by county in the United States in 1993. (From *Morbidity and Mortality Weekly Report,* October 21, 1994. p. 48.)

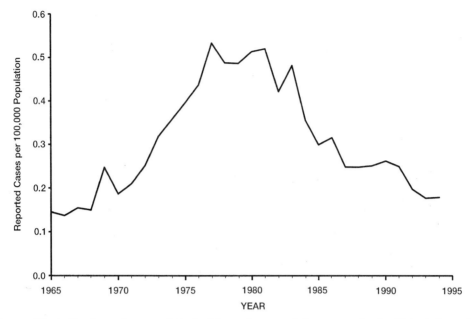

**FIGURE 28-4.** Number of reported Rocky Mountain spotted fever cases in the United States for 1965–1994, by year. (From *Morbidity and Mortality Weekly Report,* October 21, 1995, p. 49.)

course. Tetracycline is avoided in pregnancy and generally for children younger than 9 years old, although some consider tetracycline the drug of choice at all ages. Both chloramphenicol and tetracyclines are rickettsiostatic, not rickettsiocidal. The value of corticosteroids in severe RMSF has been suggested but not proved. The overall mortality from RMSF in the United States is 5–7%, primarily occurring in patients undiagnosed until the second week of illness. Death is usually related to vascular collapse, cardiac or renal failure, encephalitis, or thrombocytopenia. Solid immunity develops in those who recover. Prevention requires avoidance or reduction of tick exposure in endemic areas. Frequent deticking is useful, since ticks must remain attached for at least 4–6 h to transmit RMSF. Although an RMSF vaccine was prepared as early as 1924, no effective vaccine is currently available. Prophylactic antibiotic following tick bite in endemic areas does not appear justified, since only a small proportion of ticks in these areas are actually infected with *R. rickettsii.*

## Other Spotted Fevers

### Rickettsialpox

The second most common rickettsiosis of the spotted fever group in the United States is rickettsialpox, caused by *R. akari.* This benign infection was first recognized in New

York City in 1946 and is seen primarily there and in other cities in the northeastern United States. Occasional cases are seen in other parts of the United States, Ukraine, Croatia, and Korea. This disease is the result of dis-

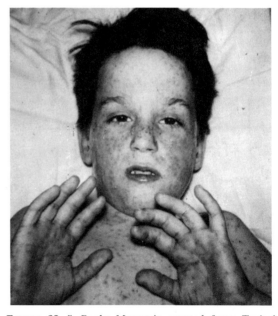

**FIGURE 28-5.** Rocky Mountain spotted fever. Typical rash occurring on the face and the palms. (From Hazard, G. W., et al. Rocky Mountain spotted fever in the eastern United States. *N. Engl. J. Med. 280:*57, 1969. Reprinted by permission.)

**TABLE 28–2.    SEROLOGIC RESPONSES IN RICKETTSIAL INFECTIONS**

| | WEIL-FELIX REACTIONS | | | COMPLEMENT-FIXATION TESTS | | |
|---|---|---|---|---|---|---|
| | OX-19 | OX-2 | OX-K | Typhus | Spotted Fever | Q Fever |
| Spotted Fevers | | | | | | |
|   RMSF | + + + | + + + | 0 | 0 | + + + | 0 |
|   Tick typhuses | + + + | + + + | 0 | 0 | + + + | 0 |
|   Rickettsialpox | 0 | 0 | 0 | 0 | + + + | 0 |
| Typhus Fevers | | | | | | |
|   Epidemic louse-borne | + + + | + | 0 | + + + | 0 | 0 |
|   Brill-Zinsser disease | + + +/0 | 0 | 0 | + + + | 0 | 0 |
|   Murine typhus | + + + | + | 0 | + + + | 0 | 0 |
| Scrub Typhus | 0 | 0 | + + + | 0 | 0 | 0 |
| Q Fever | 0 | 0 | 0 | 0 | 0 | + + + |

ruption of the natural cycle between the mite vector (*Liponyssoides sanguineus*) and the house mouse (*Mus musculus)*, with humans infected when a paucity of mouse hosts leads mites to seek humans as alternative hosts. After an incubation period of 9–14 days, a red papule develops at the mite bite site and evolves to a papulovesicle and then to a black eschar. Concomitantly, regional lymph glands become enlarged and moderate fever (100°–103°F) occurs, lasting up to 1 week, along with headache, malaise, and myalgia. A remarkable rash develops within a few days of the onset of fever, consisting of 5–40 scattered macules that rapidly become firm maculopapules and then papulo vesicles. Lesions develop over the face, trunk, and extremities, and the rash is very similar to chickenpox; hence the name rickettsialpox. Weil-Felix reactions are negative. Diagnosis can be established by direct immunofluorescence of biopsy of the eschar or by serologic response to *R. akari* over 3–8 weeks. The illness is benign and self-limited. Therapy is not necessary, although chloramphenicol and tetracycline have been used.

### Tick-Borne spotted fevers

Three additional tick-borne spotted fevers (also called *tick typhuses*) are widely distributed in Europe, Asia, Africa, and Australia and are caused by rickettsiae that share the same group antigen as *R. rickettsii* but have different type-specific antigens. These species include *R. conorii* complex, causing boutonneuse fever in India, Pakistan, Israel (Israeli spotted fever), Ethiopia, Kenya, South Africa, Morocco, and southern Europe; *R. australis*, causing Queensland tick typhus in Australia; and *R. sibirica*, causing Siberian tick typhus in China, Mongolia, Pakistan, and the former Soviet Union. Several newly identified spotted fever rickettsiae have been described in Africa, Japan, and Brazil.

### Typhus Fevers

These are three illnesses that are caused by two rickettsial species, *R. prowazekii* and *R. typhi* (formerly *R. mooseri*). Although they are similar clinically and pathologically, these illnesses differ epidemiologically and in severity.

### Classic epidemic typhus (Louse-Borne)

Classic epidemic typhus is an acute infection by *R. prowazekii* transmitted by the body louse (*Pediculus humanus corporis*). Its existence has been well documented for at least five centuries. Lice are essential for typhus fever, and therefore it occurs in epidemics during famine, war, and other catastrophes associated with louse proliferation. For example, more than 30 million cases occurred in eastern Europe following World War I, causing about 3 million deaths. Cases occur in Mexico, central Africa (Rwanda, Burundi, Ethiopia). and western South America. In the small number of sporadic cases in the United States, the flying squirrel serves as the reservoir.

*R. prowazekii* is antigenically distinct from the spotted fever rickettsial agents and is more closely related to *R. typhi*. Clinically, 1–2 weeks after the bite of an infected louse, high fever (40°C), chills, rash, myalgia, arthralgia, and severe headache appear abruptly. Untreated epidemic louse-borne typhus has a reported fatality rate of 60–70% in those older than 50 and about 10% in young adults. Small vessel vasculitis leads to protean clinical manifestations that may include renal failure, myocardial disease, CNS dysfunction, pneumonia, and gastrointestinal involvement, in addition to the fairly characteristic rash. Rash begins on the trunk and spreads in 1–2 days to the extremities (the opposite of RMSF), usually sparing the face, palms, and soles (unlike RMSF). The rash progresses from macules to papules to hemorrhagic or even necrotic lesions. Without treatment, the illness lasts about 2 weeks. Early diagnosis depends on clinical and epidemiologic features. Serologic tests are useful for confirmation of the diagnosis: *Proteus* OX-19 reactivity is generally positive by the seventh day of illness and more specific CF and enzyme-linked immunosorbent assay (ELISA) tests are now available. Therapy is the same as for RMSF (chloramphenicol, tetracycline or doxycycline), and complete recovery is the rule when therapy is begun early. Premature discontinuation of therapy (before 5 days) is associated with recrudescence many years later (Brill-Zinsser disease, see below). Prevention is achieved by louse control; vaccines are under investigation.

### Brill-Zinsser disease

Brill-Zinsser disease is a relapse or recrudescence of louse-borne typhus years after the initial attack, first noted by Nathan Brill in 1898 in Russian and Polish immigrants living in New York. *R. prowazekii* lie dormant, probably in the reticuloendothelial system, until reactivation occurs. Clinical manifestations are similar to epidemic louse-borne typhus noted above. Probably because of partial immunity as a result of the initial infection, recrudescent disease is milder and of short duration.

Tetracycline or chloramphenicol is the recommended therapy. Frequently, history of a previous episode of epidemic typhus can be elicited from patients with Brill-Zinsser disease. As predicted, an IgG (secondary) rather than IgM (primary) immune response can be demonstrated.

### Murine (endemic) typhus

Murine typhus is a flea-borne disease caused by *R. typhi* (previously known as *R. mooseri*) and is transmitted worldwide from its rat reservoir by the oriental rat flea *(Xenopsylla cheopis)*. Humans are incidentally infected from the bite of an infected flea. Once the flea is infected asymptomatically with *R. typhi* after feeding on an acutely ill rat, the organism multiplies in the flea gut and is excreted in feces. When feeding on humans, the flea defecates and rickettsia-contaminated feces can be inoculated into skin abrasions or bites, leading to human infection. As recently as the 1940s, 2000–5000 cases of murine typhus occurred yearly in the United States, particularly in the southeastern and Gulf Coast areas. More recently, with rat-control programs, only 40–80 cases have been reported yearly, mostly in Texas (Fig. 28–6).

The clinical features are similar to those for louse-borne typhus but are milder and of shorter duration. Fever is up to 39°C and regresses after about 10 days. Headache and rash are less severe and of shorter duration than in louse-borne typhus. Complications are rare and mortality is less than 1%. The serologic responses in murine typhus are very similar to those in louse-borne typhus, al-

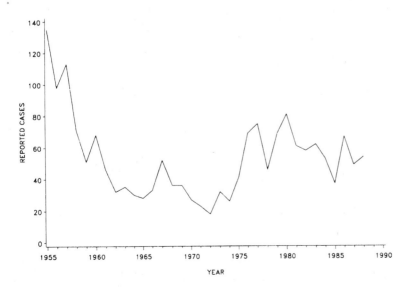

**FIGURE 28–6.** Incidence of flea-borne typhus fever (endemic, murine) from 1955–1988 (by year) in the United States. (From *Morbidity and Mortality Weekly Report.* Summary of notifiable disease. October 6, 1989, p. 45.)

though *R. typhi* antigens should be used for specific CF and ELISA tests. Therapy is as outlined for other rickettsioses. Prevention obviously depends upon rat- and flea-control measures.

### Scrub Typhus

Scrub typhus is a mite-borne rickettsiosis indigenous to Southeast Asia, Japan, and the southwestern Pacific. The etiologic agent is *R. tsutsugamushi*; the illness is also known as tsutsugamushi fever. There is marked antigenic heterogenicity among strains of *R. tsutsugamushi* that appear to correlate with striking differences in severity. This disease was first described in Japan by Hashimoto in 1810. It was noted early that this illness was confined to farmers in river valleys in July and August and that they developed a characteristic eschar at the site of the bite of a mite. Trombiculid mites, such as the red mite, serve as both vector and reservoir, with transmission occurring transovarially; there is a wild field rodent reservoir as well. Humans that intrude upon the low vegetation or scrub areas may become infected incidentally from larval mite bites. Clinically, scrub typhus is a potentially very serious disease, although its severity is quite variable. A necrotic eschar develops in 50% of individuals during the 6- to 21-day incubation period. High fever, headache, maculopapular rash, and (unlike any other rickettsiosis) generalized adenopathy develop. Splenomegaly and conjunctivitis are common. Scrub typhus among western troops in endemic areas during World War II was associated with pneumonitis, myocarditis, shock, seizures, and hemorrhagic phenomena. Preantibiotic era mortality ranged from 1–60%, but fatalities are rare in the antibiotic era. Diagnosis is facilitated by *Proteus* OX-K agglutinins in about 50% of patients and by specific CF or immunofluorescent assays. The latter are difficult because of the great degree of strain variability. Treatment is the same as for other rickettsioses. Reinfections are relatively common in scrub typhus, in contrast to other rickettsial infections.

### Q Fever

Q (or query) fever is a worldwide acute rickettsiosis caused by *Coxiella burnetii* that is unique in that it is transmitted to humans primarily by inhalation rather than by an arthropod bite. Q fever was first recognized in the 1930s by MacFarlane Burnet in Australia and Cox and Davis in the United States. Although still considered a rickettsiosis, the organism is actually more closely related to legionella. Cattle, sheep, goats, and ticks are the major reservoirs for *C. burnetii*, and infection is usually subclinical in animals, with transmission occurring as a result of excretion of rickettsiae in milk, urine, and feces. *C. burnetii* is uniquely highly resistant to desiccation, heat, and physical and chemical agents, and is extremely infectious for humans and from animals such as cattle, goats, and sheep.

Q fever is unique among the rickettsioses in that it is most often acquired by inhalation of contaminated aerosols, arthropods are unimportant in spread, and the clinical illness is not associated with rash. In domestic livestock the infection is usually inapparent until an event like parturition leads to reactivation, with contamination of soil with infected milk, urine, feces, placental tissues, and fluids. Dried dust particles containing *C. burnetii* remain potential sources of infection for many months. The incubation period averages 20 days (range is 14–39 days), and the illness most often begins abruptly with rigors, high fever, severe headache, retrobulbar pain, and myalgia, but no rash. Respiratory symptoms (cough, chest pain) are common, with multiple round lesions or patchy pulmonary infiltrates seen in about 50%. Hepatosplenomegaly is frequent, with only minimal liver dysfunction and only occasional icterus. Gastroenteritis and hemolytic anemia are also seen. The most frequent form of chronic Q fever is Q fever endocarditis, a rare but severe and often fatal complication in patients with preexisting valvular heart disease or who are immunocompromised. Otherwise, Q fever is generally a mild, self-limited disease lasting only 1–2 weeks and associated with less than 1% mortality. No Weil-Felix reaction develops in Q fever, but highly specific ELISA, CF, and immunofluorescence assays allow confirmation of the diagnosis from convalescent sera. Attempts to isolate the organism may be dangerous and should be avoided if possible. Q fever responds promptly to tetracyclines (doxycycline for 15–21 days) or chloramphenicol, and relapses are rare. Treated patients appear to recover somewhat more quickly than those who do not receive treatment. Endocarditis requires very prolonged therapy (12 months or more), probably because the effective agents are rickettsiostatic rather than rickettsiocidal. Attempted preventive measures include development of a vaccine (not yet available) and control of infected herds and of aerosol in laboratories.

## Ehrlichiosis

*Ehrlichia,* a genus of the family Rickettsiaceae, are intraleukocytic parasites that infect humans and a variety of animals. The oldest known human pathogen is *E. sennetsu,* which causes an infectious mononucleosis-like illness in the Far East, particularly in southeast Kyushu, Japan, probably after the bite of an unknown vector. Patients manifest fever, myalgia, headache, sore throat, and generalized lymphadenopathy; rash and eschar are very rare.

*E. chaffeensis* is a newly described human pathogen that was isolated in 1991 from a patient suspected to have human ehrlichiosis, a disorder recognized in the United States in 1986. More than 300 cases have been identified in 21 states but primarily in the south central and southeastern United States. Leukopenia and recent tick exposure are hallmarks of this disease, and thrombocytopenia and hepatitis are very common. Fever, headache, nausea and myalgias occur early, with cough, confusion, pharyngitis, and diarrhea later. Rash is present in 36% of cases; one fifth of the rashes are petechial, the remainder maculopapular. Bone marrow exam reveals hypercellularity despite peripheral leukopenia, lymphopenia, neutropenia, and thrombocytopenia. Granulomas and hemophagocytosis have been seen in the marrow. When analyzed, cerebrospinal fluid (CSF) is abnormal with cells and elevated protein. *E. chaffeensis* has been seen within macrophages in the bone marrow and sometimes on peripheral smears. Cases range from the asymptomatic to fatal illnesses, the latter particularly in those over 60 years old. Sixty-two percent of cases have been hospitalized, and 1.3% have died. Two percent have developed coma or seizures. Cases have occurred opportunistically in a few acquired immunodeficiency syndrome (AIDS) patients. Tetracycline and chloramphenicol appear to be beneficial.

Human infection by *E. canis,* the worldwide agent of tropical canine pancytopenia, has been reported, although some of these may have actually represented infection with *E. chaffeensis* with serologic cross-reactivity. The vector is the brown dog tick, and a few humans with illnesses resembling RMSF but without rash have been thought to have *E. canis* infection.

Recent reports indicate another ehrliosis in the United States, human granulocytic ehrlichiosis. Patients from the upper Midwest (Wisconsin and Minnesota) and Northeast United States have fever, chills, severe headache, and myalgias associated with granulocytic cytoplasmic inclusions. More than 32 patients have now been identified. Patients have various combinations of leukopenia, anemia, hepatitis, and thrombocytopenia, and the illness is potentially fatal. These patients appeared to be infected with an ehrlichia related to *E. equi* and *E. phagocytophilia,* the former causing infections in horses and the latter in sheep, deer, bison, and cattle. These infections in man appeared to respond well to doxycycline. The tick agent appears to be *Ixodes scapularis,* the deer tick.

Erhlichiosis should be suspected in those with seronegative RMSF-like illnesses and perhaps in some with pancytopenias. Confirmation includes identifying intraleukocytic inclusions and observing a specific serologic response.

## Bartonella infections

The organisms now classified as the genus *Bartonella* were until recently designated *Rochalimaea.* These agents are associated with several infectious diseases: *B. quintana* causes trench fever; *B. henselae* is the agent of cat-scratch disease; and *B. bacilliformis* is the cause of Carrión's disease, Oroya fever, and verruga peruana (these are classsically known as bartonellosis). Both *B. henselae* and *B. quintana* have been associated with bacillary angiomatosis, bacteremia, and endocarditis.

### Trench fever

This illness is caused by *B. quintana* transmitted to man by the body louse (*Pediculus humanus corporis*) and affected more than 1 million World War I soldiers. The incubation period is 5–20 days, and there may be insidious onset of nonspecific flu-like symtpoms or sudden onset of fever, malaise, headache, bone pain, and a transient macular rash. Recurrent febrile episodes every 4–5 days also have been reported, and recurrent or chronic bacteremia appears common. Recent reports of *B. quintana* bacteremia or endocarditis primarily in homeless, alcoholic urban men in the United States and France have focused new attention on this old disorder. It is endemic in Mexico, North Africa, and Eastern Europe. Humans are thought to be the reservoir, and this infection emerges when louse-infected humans are gathered in unhygienic circumstances (e.g., prisons, refugee camps). Tetracycline is a highly effective treatment.

### Cat-Scratch disease

This rather common pediatric infection is characterized by local adenopathy (usually axillary or cervical) in a normal host sometimes associated with fever and systemic symptoms. The agent is now thought to be *B. henselae*, most commonly transmitted by scratch or bite of a kitten or cat. Although healthy, the implicated animal is likely chronically bacteremic with this organism. Following a scratch, a papule often develops within 7–12 days at site and regional adenopathy develops 1–3 weeks later. Rare manifestations include Parinaud's oculoglandular syndrome, encephalitis, erythema nodosum, osteolytic lesions, thrombocytopenia, and hepatitis. Histologic features of cat-scratch nodes include granuloma formation as well as suppuration. Warthin-Starry stain may demonstrate clusters of bacteria, and most patients have a positive serologic test for antibody to *B. henselae*. Therapy is supportive, although aspiration or incision and drainage is often useful in managing suppurating lesions.

### Bartonellosis

This infection caused by *B. bacilliformis* (known as Carrión's disease, Oroya fever, or verruga peruana) occurs exclusively in Andean valleys in northwest South America. The vector is the sandfly (*Phlebotomus*), and the major reservoir appears to be asymptomatic humans. *B. bacilliformis* invades red blood cells, in which it multiplies and leads to brisk intravascular hemolysis, as well as reticuloendothelial cells. Clinical manifestations resemble malaria (fever, hemolysis, hepatosplenomegaly), with mortality rates as high as 40% without treatment with chloramphenicol or tetracylines.

### Bacilliary Angiomatosis

This relatively newly recognized disorder is seen primarily in immunocompromised patients including those who are human immunodeficiency virus (HIV) infected and organ recipients and is characterized by cutaneous and visceral vascular lesions containing bacilli that stain by the Warthin-Starry silver stain. Many organ systems have been involved, with the term "peliosis hepatis" used when there is hepatic involvement. No granulomatous changes occur. Bacillary angiomatosis is due to infection with *B. quintana* or *B.*

*henselae*, and patients appear to respond to therapy with erythromycin or doxycycline.

## CASE HISTORY

### CASE HISTORY 1

An 11-year-old boy from North Carolina was admitted to the hospital in June with severe headache, fever, and rash. Three days earlier he had complained of not feeling well. The next day a rash appeared on his wrists and ankles and his temperature was 103.5°F (39.7°C). The next day, rash had spread to the arms and was noted on the soles and palms. His temperature remained high, a severe frontal headache developed, and marked tenderness of the calves and swelling of the ankles appeared. Headache was not relieved by aspirin. At this time he was brought to the hospital.

Upon admission the boy appeared acutely ill, with temperature of 103.6°F (39.8°C), pulse 115/min, respirations 34/min, and blood pressure 128/66 mm Hg. Confluent erythematous macular lesions were present on the palms and soles and over the distal parts of all four extremities. The lesions extended to the proximal part of the extremities, with a few lesions on the abdomen and chest. In some areas, the lesions were papular, but none blanched upon pressure. Lymphadenopathy and nuchal rigidity were not noted. There was marked tenderness when pressure was exerted on both gastrocnemius muscles.

Examination of the urine revealed no abnormalities. The white blood cell (WBC) count was 11,500/mm³, with 65% segmented neutrophils, 5% band forms, 20% lymphocytes, and 10% monocytes. A chest roentgenogram and an electrocardiogram revealed normal findings. Spinal fluid obtained by lumbar puncture was clear; the pressure was 300 mm Hg. The spinal fluid contained 20 WBCs/mm³, mostly mononuclear cells. No microorganisms were seen.

Because of the typical distribution and appearance of the rash, the severe frontal headache, and the muscle tenderness, Rocky Mountain spotted fever was suspected. It was learned that on the previous weekend the patient had taken an overnight camping trip with several friends in an area known to be infested with ticks. Three campers, including the patient, had tick bites. Because of the high probability that the patient had Rocky Mountain spotted fever, tetracycline was started immediately. Symptoms promptly abated and the patient made an uneventful recovery. He was discharged on the fifth hospital day.

Serum collected on the first hospital day (3 days after the onset of illness) was negative in both the Weil-Felix and complement-fixation tests for Rocky Mountain spotted fever. However, a second serum 2 weeks later had an OX-19 titer of 1:640. The specific complement-fixation test was strongly positive.

Thus, the diagnosis of Rocky Mountain spotted fever was confirmed.

# REFERENCES

## Books

Manson-Bahr, P. E. C., and Bell, D. R., eds. *Manson's Tropical Diseases.* 19th ed. London: Bailliere Tindall, 1988: 213–245.

Walker, D. H., ed. *Biology of Rickettsial Diseases.* Boca Raton, FL: CRC Press, 1988.

Zinsser, H., ed. *Rats, Lice and History.* Boston: Little, Brown & Co., 1935.

## Review Articles

Font-Creus, B., Bella-Cueto, F., Espejo-Arenas, E., et al. Mediterranean spotted fever. *Rev. Infect. Dis. 7:*635–643, 1985.

Hase, T. Developmental sequence and surface membrane assembly of rickettsiae. *Annu. Rev. Microbiol. 39:*69–88, 1985.

Helmick, C. G., Bernard, K. W., and D'Angelo, L. J. Rocky Mountain spotted fever: Clinical, laboratory and epidemiological features of 262 cases. *J. Infect. Dis. 150:*480–488, 1984.

McDade, J. E., and Newhouse, V. F. Natural history of *Rickettsia rickettsii. Annu. Rev. Microbiol. 40:*287–309, 1986.

Raoult, D., and Marrie T. Q fever. *Clin. Infect. Dis. 20:*489–496, 1995.

Sawyer, L. A., Fishbein, D. B., and McDade, J. E. Q fever: Current concepts. *Rev. Infect. Dis. 9:*935–946, 1987.

## Original Articles

Bakken, J. S., Dumler, J. S., Chen, S-M., et al. Human granulocytic ehrlichiosis in the upper Midwest United States. A new species emerging? *JAMA 272:*212–218, 1994.

Brill, N. E. An acute infectious disease. A clinical study based on 221 cases of unknown origin. *Am. J. Med. Sci. 139:*484, 1910.

Fishbein, D. B., Dawson, J. E., and Robinson, L. E. Human ehrlichiosis in the United States, 1985 to 1990. *Ann. Intern. Med. 120:*736–743, 1994.

Huebner, R. J., and Armstrong, C. Rickettsialpox—A newly recognized rickettsial disease. I. Isolation of the etiologic agent. *Public Health Rep. 61:*1605–1614, 1946.

Kass, E. M., Szaniawski, W. K., Levy, H., et al. Rickettsialpox in a New York City Hospital, 1980 to 1989. *N. Engl. J. Med. 331:*1612–1617, 1994.

Maeda, K., Markowitz, N., Hawley, R. C., et al. Human infection with *Ehrlichia canis,* a leukocytic rickettsia. *N. Engl. J. Med. 316:*853–856, 1987.

Perine, P. L., Chandler, B. P., Krause, D. K., et al. A clinico-epidemiological study of epidemic typhus in Africa. *Clin. Infect. Dis. 14:*1149–1158, 1992.

Relman, D. A., et al. The organism causing bacillary angiomatosis, peliosis hepatis, and fever and bacteremia in immunocompromised hosts. *N. Engl. J. Med. 324:*1514, 1991.

Ricketts, H. T. The study of Rocky Mountain spotted fever (tick fever?) by means of animal inoculations: A preliminary communication. *JAMA 47:*33–36, 1906.

Salgo, M. P., Telzak, E. E., Currie, B., et al. A focus of Rocky Mountain spotted fever within New York City. *N. Engl. J. Med. 318:*1345–1348, 1988.

Woodward, T. E. A historical account of the rickettsial diseases with a discussion of unresolved problems. *J. Infect. Dis. 127:*583–594, 1973.

Woodward, T. E.: Rocky Mountain spotted fever: Epidemiological and early clinical signs are keys to treatment and reduced mortality. *J. Infect. Dis. 150:*465–468, 1984.

Yagupsky, P., and Wolach, B. Fatal Israeli spotted fever in children. *Clin. Infect. Dis. 17:*850–853, 1992.

Zinsser, H. Varieties of typhus virus and epidemiology of American form of European typhus fever (Brill's disease). *Am. J. Hyg. 20:*513–532, 1934.

# 29
# ZOONOSES

## A TODD DAVIS, M.D.

Zoonoses are infectious diseases that occur principally in animals but which may spread to humans. Table 29–1 lists some, but certainly not all, of the diseases that fall under this category. Viruses, bacteria, fungi, and protozoans are all represented in zoonotic diseases. Given the large number of infectious agents and the animal hosts they infect, it is not surprising that the skin, digestive tract, and respiratory tract may serve as portals of entry for these diseases. For example, tularemia may be acquired transcutaneously by contact with infected animal tissue. Trichinosis is acquired by ingestion of infected meat. Psittacosis and plague may be acquired by the airborne route.

Control of zoonoses rests on diminishing the incidence of disease in the animal reservoir; animal vaccination when possible; preventing the importation of infected birds or animals; changing hygienic practices, such as preventing pigs from eating raw sewage; pasteurization of milk to reduce the likelihood of brucellosis or listeriosis; and control of vectors, such as eradication of fleas, which may transmit plague from animal to animal.

## BRUCELLOSIS

Sir David Bruce discovered the etiology of brucellosis while investigating an outbreak of Malta fever in the early part of the 20th century. Brucellosis, named after him, is caused by a fastidious, gram-negative, aerobic bacterium found throughout the world.

The animal reservoirs for this disease include cattle (*Brucella abortus*), dogs (*B. canis*), pigs (*B. suis*), goats (*B. melitensis*), and sheep (*B. ovis*). Patterns of transmission include handling of infected carcasses during the slaughtering process in abattoirs, handling of infected animals or touching their secretions, or consuming contaminated and unpasteurized milk and milk products such as cheese.

The organism gains entry to the human host through broken skin, the conjunctivae, the lungs, and the gastrointestinal tract. Humans are terminal hosts, unable to transmit the infection to other humans. Adults, because of occupational exposure, are much more frequently infected than are children.

After gaining entry, the organisms are phagocytized by polymorphonuclear leukocytes (PMNs), but they are not effectively killed in the intraphagocytic vacuoles. As infected PMNs burst, macrophages and reticuloendothelial cells ingest the organisms, which then may persist for weeks or months; this is the biologic basis for chronic human infections.

Clinical manifestations, whether in children or adults, may be acute or gradual in onset. Fever, shaking chills, weakness, lethargy, and weight loss occur. The nonspecific nature of the symptoms mimics other diseases such as

## TABLE 29-1.  SELECTED ZOONOSES

| Disease | Etiology | Usual Reservoir | Usual Mode of Transmission | Disease in Nonhuman Host | Disease in Human | Human-Human Transmission |
|---|---|---|---|---|---|---|
| Anthrax | *Bacillus anthracis* | Cattle, sheep, goats | Infected animals or their products | Systemic illness, GI problems | Pneumonitis, malignant pustule | No |
| Brucellosis | *Brucella* sp. | Cattle, swine, goats | Milk or infected carcasses | Abortion, mastitis, lameness, abscesses | Fever, nodes, bacteremia, etc. | No |
| Campylobacteriosis | *Campylobacter fetus, C. jejuni* | Cattle, sheep, pets, wild mammals | Contaminated food and water | Usually none | Gastroenteritis | Yes (fecal-oral) |
| Leptospirosis | *Leptospira* sp. | Cattle, rodents, other mammals | Water contaminated by urine | Usually none | Nephritis, hepatitis, systemic disease | No |
| Tularemia | *Francisella tularensis* | Rabbits, other small mammals | Bite of fleas, deer flies, mosquitoes | Usually none | Pneumonia, skin lesion, adenitis | No |
| Psittacosis | *Chlamydia psittaci* | Birds (especially imported) | Contact with birds | Usually none | Pneumonia | No |
| Plague | *Yersinia pestis* | Rats and other rodents | Flea bite | Usually none | Bubonic, pneumonic, septicemic plague | Yes (respiratory droplet) |
| Listeriosis | *Listeria monocytogenes* | Mammals, birds | Ingestion of contaminated food (cheese, etc.) | Usually none | Meningitis, abortion | No |
| Relapsing fever | *Borrelia* sp. | Rodents | Tick bite | Usually none | Relapsing fevers, hemorrhage | Yes (body louse) |
| Salmonellosis | *Salmonella* sp. | Poultry, cattle | Ingestion of contaminated food | Usually none | Gastroenteritis, sepsis | Yes (fecal-oral) |
| Pasteurellosis | *Pasteurella multocida* | Animal oral cavities | Animal bites or scratches | Usually none | Wound infection | No |
| Orf | Parapoxvirus | Sheep, goats | Animal contact | Pustular lesions | Papulovesicular granulomatous skin lesions | No |

| Rabies | Rabiesvirus | Small mammals | Animal bite | None, or death with paralysis | Hydrophobia, excitation, paralysis, death | No |
|---|---|---|---|---|---|---|
| Yellow fever | Yellow fever virus | Nonhuman primates | Mosquito bites | Usually none | Hepatitis | Rare |
| Melioidosis | Pseudomonas pseudomallei | Rats, mice, rabbits, ruminants, primates | Inhalation or direct inoculation | Usually none | Lung abscess, septicemia | Very Rare |
| Sleeping sickness | Trypanosoma brucei | Wild ungulates, humans | Tsetse fly | Usually none | Meningoencephalitis | Yes |
| Lyme disease | Borrelia burgdorferi | White-footed mouse | Bite of deer tick (Ixodes) nymphs | Usually none | Erythema chronicum migrans, arthritis, carditis, neuropathy | No |

influenza, malaria, typhoid fever, tularemia, and miliary tuberculosis. On occasion, brucellosis has been confused with lymphoma. Physical findings are often limited to such reticuloendothelial signs as hepatosplenomegaly or lymphadenopathy. However, splenomegaly occurs less than 50% of the time and hepatomegaly in about 25% of bacteremic patients. Serum liver enzyme tests are usually normal.

The diagnosis is largely dependent on clinical suspicion, particularly if there is no clearcut history of exposure to a known source of brucellosis. Although the definitive diagnosis is made by recovering the organism from blood cultures, a strongly presumptive diagnosis can be made by obtaining a positive febrile agglutinin response (i.e., demonstrating high titer of specific brucella agglutinins).

The principle underlying therapy is the use of at least one appropriate antibiotic for a sufficient time. Very low rates of relapse are associated with treatment with intramuscular gentamicin for the first 5 days and oral trimethoprim-sulfamethoxazole or, in those older than 8 years, oral tetracycline for 3 weeks.

## TULAREMIA

Tularemia is a bacterial disease caused by *Francisella tularensis*, a pleomorphic, gram-negative, aerobic coccobacillus. The illness was first detected in Tulare County, California, hence the species name *tularensis*. The genus name, *Francisella*, is in honor of Dr. Edward Francis, who extensively studied the disease in the early part of the 20th century.

Rabbits, particularly snowshoe rabbits but also jackrabbits, muskrats, and occasionally beavers, can harbor the organism for a long time without becoming demonstrably ill. Fleas, deer flies, and ticks serve as vectors for transmitting the disease to other rodents and to human beings. Given the nature of the animal and insect reservoirs and the environments in which they live, there are a variety of ways in which humans become infected. The most frequent route may be through the bite of an insect, although the bite of an animal can transmit the organism if the animal has recently consumed infected flesh. Handlers of wild game such as rabbits are occasionally infected through undetected or visible breaks in the skin. Occasionally, when water becomes contaminated by beavers, the

organism can enter through the conjunctivae. Air-borne transmissions occur following harvesting in fields contaminated by small animals or in laboratory workers handling infected material or cultures.

All strains of *F. tularensis* appear to be antigenically identical. However, there are biologic strain differences: the so-called Jellison type A strain causes severe and fulminant illness, whereas Jellison type B causes much milder disease in humans.

The typical infection begins after an incubation period of only 1–3 days. A maculoerythematous lesion develops at the inoculation site and soon evolves into a papule. As the papule continues to develop, the overlying skin becomes thinned and taut, ulcerating within 1–2 days. As the papule enlarges, fever, systemic symptoms, and regional lymphadenopathy develop. If the infection remains unrecognized, it may linger for 2–4 weeks. If infection occurs by air-borne transmission, organisms may deposit anywhere along the respiratory tract, causing tracheitis, bronchitis, or pneumonia. The last is an extremely serious disease, with a mortality rate approaching 30%. As organisms escape the lung parenchyma, they may temporarily lodge in the hilar lymph nodes on their way to the bloodstream. As bloodstream invasion occurs, a typhoid-like septic illness develops. Ironically, *F. tularensis* seems unable to infect the gut as a prelude to sepsis.

Streptomycin or gentamicin remains the drug of choice for managing tularemia. The local lesion, systemic symptoms, and regional lymphadenopathy usually resolve within a few days of treatment. With adequate therapy, mortality is less than 1%, except in cases of pneumonic or typhoidal tularemia.

## PLAGUE

*Yersinia pestis*, the causative agent of plague, is a small, pleomorphic, nonmotile, gram-negative bacillus. Staining with Wayson or Giemsa stains gives the cell a bipolar or "safety pin" morphology. Plague has caused large-scale epidemics throughout history, thereby altering history itself. Indeed, one third of the population of Europe died of plague during the 14th century. *Y. pestis* apparently entered the United States from shipboard rats in San Francisco in the early part of the 20th century.

Reservoirs include infected rodents and

their fleas. Persistence of plague over the centuries probably depends on the organisms' surviving in hibernating animals over the winter, and on fleas, which may harbor the organisms for 12–15 months after becoming infected from a rodent. In addition, *Y. pestis* may be able to survive in soil.

Humans invariably become infected by either the bite of a flea, inhalation, or handling an infected animal. Within 3–4 days, there is an abrupt onset of illness characterized by fever, malaise, weakness, and headache. The fever is frequently high and hectic. The organisms move from the initial site of inoculation to the regional lymph nodes, causing extremely tender and painful lymph glands—buboes (thus, bubonic plague). The nodes are typically large, fixed, edematous, and exquisitely tender. The most frequent site is in the groin, although the axillary or cervical glands may be involved. Usually only one set of regional glands is involved.

As the local defenses in regional nodes are overcome, the organisms quickly spread throughout the body. Many of the fulminant manifestations of the illness, such as coagulation disturbances, shock, and death, appear related to the release of endotoxin by the organisms.

Pulmonary involvement, either by direct inhalation of organisms or secondary to septicemic spread, results in rapidly progressive, highly fatal pneumonic plague. Plague should be considered in the face of a rapidly progressive febrile illness in the rural southwestern part of the United States where plague is endemic—an average of 18 cases per year have been documented in that region.

Rapid treatment is mandatory. A number of antibiotics are effective, including tetracycline, streptomycin, and chloramphenicol. Even with prompt, effective therapy, death still occurs in about 5% of cases. However, this rate is vastly different from the almost universal mortality for untreated pulmonic plague and the 40–70% mortality rate seen in other forms in the preantibiotic era.

## BORRELIOSIS (RELAPSING FEVER)

Relapsing fever is caused by a gram-negative motile spirochete of which there are several species. Each species is associated with a particular vector. Louse-borne disease, which is seen in parts of the world other than the United States, is caused by *Borrelia recurrentis*.

The organism can also be transmitted by ticks, with different species of the spirochete closely linked with a unique tick species.

The disease is characterized by sudden onset of high fever, chills, headache, myalgia, and symptoms that are nonspecific and similar in nature to influenza. There may be a fleeting rash present on the trunk. Some patients develop hepatosplenomegaly. Other symptoms include arthralgias, eye pain, cough, chest pain, and sore throat. The signs and symptoms generally abate after 3–6 days. However, a second febrile episode may recur 5–10 days later. Subsequent relapses may occur, particularly with tick-borne disease.

Louse-borne disease is typically seen during periods of social unrest such as war, crowding, and mass migrations. Louse-borne disease has not been seen in the United States since the early 1900s. On the other hand, tick-borne disease is occasionally seen in the warmer months in the United States, generally in the western states in people staying in and around tick-infested log cabins.

Despite occasional complications such as iridocyclitis and myocarditis, complete resolution of symptoms without therapy is to be expected. However, a number of antibiotics such as tetracycline, penicillin, and erythromycin are effective in preventing relapses.

## TICK PARALYSIS

Tick paralysis is occasionally seen in the United States. The disease is transmitted only by female ticks. It is more prevalent in children than in adults. The classic case is an ascending flaccid paralysis. Before the modern era of superb respiratory support, death often ensued once bulbar involvement occurred, a consequence of a neurotoxin elaborated by the attached tick.

While it is sometimes thought that the tick must adhere at the base of the skull to cause disease, in fact, the tick may adhere anywhere. One of the most gratifying experiences in medicine is the prompt resolution of symptoms over 3–5 days once the tick is removed.

Poliomyelitis, polyneuritis, myelitis, and Guillain-Barré syndrome are other entities that should be considered when confronting a patient with ascending paralysis.

## YELLOW FEVER

Yellow fever is caused by an arbovirus that belongs to the Flaviviridiae family in the genus *Flavivirus*. Yellow fever is rare in the United States, the last outbreak occurring in the early 1900s. However, yellow fever continues to be a problem in tropical and semitropical areas. Fortunately, yellow fever vaccine is extraordinarily effective. Accordingly, U.S. tourists going to yellow fever–infected areas should be immunized.

The incubation period is 3–6 days. Transmission occurs by mosquitoes biting humans, nonhuman primates, or other vertebra hosts. The spectrum of illness ranges from asymptomatic infection to fulminant illness consisting of jaundice and coagulation abnormalities. Inapparent illness resolves without difficulty. However, in fulminant cases, death may ensue within days of onset. Unfortunately, many cases in the third world occur far from medical facilities, where there is little possibility to successfully intervene.

When traveling, tourists should check with the Centers for Disease Control (CDC) about the advisability of receiving yellow fever vaccine.

## TRICHINOSIS

Trichinosis differs in four ways from those diseases discussed previously in this chapter. First, it is not a bacterial disease; rather, the causative agent is a nematode parasite, *Trichinella spiralis*. Second, only occasionally does the illness have distinctive enough clinical features to allow a clinical diagnosis. Third, the disease is self-limiting and rarely fatal. Fourth, therapy is of uncertain benefit.

*Trichinella spiralis* is transmitted directly to wild carnivorous animals and to domesticated pigs through ingestion of infected meat. The latter occurred in the past when pigs were fed raw garbage that contained infected table scraps.

The disease in humans begins with the ingestion of raw or undercooked meat containing trichinella cysts. Upon reaching the small intestine, encysted organisms become sexually mature within 24–48 h. Larvae are produced within 5 days, and invasion across the mucosa occurs within another day or two. Accompanying symptoms consist of fever, diarrhea, and abdominal pain during the intestinal phase of the illness. Dissemination occurs during the second week following ingestion as parasites are carried throughout the body via the blood and lymphatic systems. Striated muscles, including those of the arms, legs,

chest, and diaphragm, are the principal targets. The fourth week after ingestion, larval migration from the intestine to peripheral tissues diminishes, and the larvae already in the muscles begin to encyst. Symptoms during this phase include periorbital edema and muscle pain. Eosinophilia may be present in the peripheral blood.

It should be emphasized that infections are often mild in the United States and frequently remain undiagnosed. When trichinosis is suspected on the basis of ingestion of food, the aforementioned symptoms, the history of ingesting undercooked meat, in addition to eosinophilia and results from several tests may be helpful in diagnosing the disease. Serum levels of muscle enzymes, such as aldolase and creatine phosphokinase, may be elevated. A variety of serologic tests are available, with bentonite flocculation being the usual first test. It may take 3 or more weeks before sufficient antibodies are present for detection. Other methods include complement-fixation, fluorescent antibody, latex agglutination, and immunoelectrophoresis. Because of insufficient sensitivity of any of these tests, two or more tests may be necessary to obtain a positive result.

The most definitive diagnostic technique is muscle biopsy. However, even this may be negative when the infestation is light. Fortunately, the overall prognosis is good in the majority of cases. However, occasionally myocarditis or meningitis may occur.

Treatment with an antihelmintic agent, thiabendazole, is often recommended, but its efficacy is unproven.

## PSITTACOSIS

Psittacosis is caused by *Chlamydia psittaci*. Birds, particularly imported birds, are the major reservoir for this organism in the United States. The organisms may be excreted intermittently in fecal matter for long periods by either ill or healthy birds. Persons in close proximity to infected birds, such as pet shop employees and poultry workers, are at particular risk for inhaling *C. psittaci*. This infection is quite uncommon in children.

The incubation period ranges from 7–14 days. The illness is characterized by high fever, chills, and pronounced cough. Initially, the cough may be dry, later becoming more productive. Auscultation often reveals a disproportionately slow heart rate, tachypnea, and diffuse fine rales. The patient may have constitutional symptoms similar to those of other illnesses discussed in this chapter, such as fatigue, malaise, anorexia, and myalgia. As expected, most patients with psittacosis demonstrate pulmonary infiltrates on chest roentgenograms. The diagnosis depends on eliciting a history of bird exposure in the patient with fever, chills, and pneumonia. Because laboratory workers are at unusually high risk, isolation of the organism should *not* be attempted in most laboratories. Rather, a rising complement-fixation antibody titer is the preferred diagnostic test.

Tetracycline is the drug of choice and should be continued for at least 3 weeks.

## TOXOPLASMOSIS

Toxoplasmosis is a parasitic disease caused by a coccidian parasite, *Toxoplasma gondii*. The disease is worldwide in distribution, although more common in warmer climates than in cold ones. *Toxoplasma gondii* exists in three forms, leading to a variety of ways in which the disease is transmitted and varying pathogenesis. The tachyzoite form is a proliferative form seen during acute infections. The organism produces an enzyme that alters the host membrane, allowing entry into the cell. Subsequently, the bradyzoite form exists in tissue cysts. There is usually little inflammatory reaction surrounding the cysts, but organisms persist for a prolonged time. This characteristic allows for occasional reactivation of infection in body tissues. Finally, the oocyst form is found exclusively in the intestinal tract of cats. Oocysts become infectious after undergoing sporulation, which occurs from 1 to 21 days after defecation. Ingestion of the sporulated oocyst is probably the most frequent way in which humans become infected. However, some infections occur by the ingestion of undercooked meat or milk products containing encysted bradyzoites.

The vast majority of acquired toxoplasmosis is asymptomatic. Only about 10% of infected individuals develop signs or symptoms. Commonly, the patient develops lymphadenopathy, frequently around the head and neck, without fever (see Chapter 8). Occasionally, lymphadenopathy may be accompanied by fever, malaise, fatigue, sore throat, and myalgia, mimicking infectious mononucleosis. On occasion, toxoplasmosis has also been confused with lymphoma.

In immunocompromised adults and children, disseminated infection may develop, involving any body tissue including lungs, myocardium, liver, and central nervous system (CNS). In adult patients with acquired immunodeficiency syndrome (AIDS), cerebral toxoplasmosis is a particular problem (see Chapter 24). Toxoplasmosis in pregnancy is particularly important because of the risk of fetal infection (see Chapter 26).

Ocular toxoplasmosis is a troublesome, recurrent problem following congenital disease and occasionally after acquired infection. For example, chorioretinitis may occur unilaterally or bilaterally. From time to time, these white or yellowish elevated foci may activate, presumably on the basis of reactivation of infection. Hypersensitivity accompanies reactivation, which may be a prominent cause of inflammation and sequelae. Following treatment of a reactivation, there often is some permanent loss of vision, which is particularly worrisome because of the perimacular location of many of these lesions.

Although the organisms can sometimes be seen in tissue, the diagnosis of acute toxoplasmosis is usually made on the basis of rising antibody titers. Indirect immunofluorescent antibody (IFA) test is the most widely available. Reference laboratories continue to provide the Sabin-Feldman dye test, which is the most reliable test. Other tests that are sometimes used include complement-fixation and enzyme-linked immunosorbent assay (ELISA). The presence of either cysts in tissue or a high titer cannot date the age or activity of a toxoplasma infection.

Treatment is not required for the vast majority of infections. In symptomatic patients, a combination of pyrimethamine and sulfadiazine is usually used. Other agents are sometimes used, including spiramycin, which is preferred in the treatment of pregnant women.

## ANTHRAX

Anthrax is caused by *Bacillus anthracis*, a sporulating, non-motile, aerobic, gram-positive rod. The disease was first described in 1850 by Rayer.

The pathogenesis of anthrax has been particularly well worked out. Production of the antiphagocytic capsule, which is an important virulence factor, is phage mediated. Another important virulence factor is a three-component protein exotoxin comprised of edema factor, lethal factor, and protective antigen (protective antigen is so-named because, when modified, it plays an important role in producing an efficacious vaccine). The protective antigen is thought to bind to specific receptors on the host cell surface. After cleavage of a small part of the protective antigen protein, a binding site is provided for edema factor and lethal factor, which then undergo endocytosis into the cytosol. Once internalized, the edema factor and lethal factor work their devastation on the cellular machinery.

There are essentially three sources of *B. anthracis*, namely, spores in soil, infected animals or their products, and infected humans. *B. anthracis* spores can survive in the soil for prolonged periods of time. In one example, viable spores were found 20 years after deliberate inoculation of the soil.

Anthrax is extraordinarily uncommon in the United States. Imported fibers (i.e., goat hair used in garment manufacture) constitute one known reservoir.

There are several clinical entities, depending on the route of exposure. Anthrax causes pharyngitis if the inhaled spores are greater than 5 $\mu$m in size. Spores between 2 and 5 $\mu$m in size travel farther down the respiratory tract to infect the alveoli. Once the infection is established in the lungs, the infection can move to the mediastinal lymph nodes, and from there to the bloodstream, causing bacteremia and meningitis.

Gastrointestinal anthrax occurs following the ingestion of heavily contaminated meat. Symptoms of this entity begin to occur after the *B. anthracis* has been transported to the mesenteric lymph nodes followed by hemorrhagic adenitis and septicemia. Untreated, the organism can multiply extraordinarily rapidly in the bloodstream, leading to death.

Cutaneous anthrax begins as a small, painless but itchy papule. Within 2 days of its formation, the papule begins to ulcerate and form an eschar. Viable bacteria can usually be cultured from the papule, accompanied by an occasional PMN. The combination of a painless papule, rare PMNs on Gram's stain, and the presence of disproportionate edema around the papule point to the diagnosis. Most of the cutaneous lesions occur on the face, neck, arms, or hands.

A variety of antibiotics work well for cutaneous anthrax. These include penicillin, ciprofloxacin, erythromycin, tetracycline, and chloramphenicol. With the prompt institution of antimicrobial therapy, fatalities from cutaneous anthrax are rare, even though antibiotics do not stop progression of the papule to eschar formation. On the other hand, inhalation, gastrointestinal, and meningeal anthrax are associated with high mortality.

## CAT-SCRATCH DISEASE

The etiology of cat-scratch disease had long eluded medical scientists. But beginning in the 1980s, elegant histologic, bacteriologic, serologic, and epidemiologic studies have demonstrated that two principal bacterial species are responsible for cat-scratch fever. *Bartonella henselae* and *Afipia felils* can both cause the illness, although *B. henselae* seems to be the far more prevalent pathogen (see Chapter 26).

## HANTAVIRUS INFECTION

In the summer of 1993, an epizootic of a previously unknown viral illness occurred in the Four Corners area of the southwestern United States. The causative agent was quickly identified as a hantavirus genus of the Bunyaviridae family. Other viruses in this family have been known for decades throughout Asia and Europe as the cause of hemorrhagic fever with renal syndrome.

In retrospect, occasional isolated cases of hantavirus infection have previously occurred in the United States but never as a recognized epidemic. Subsequent to the outbreak in the Four Corners area, sporadic hantavirus infections have occurred in 19 of the United States, causing a total of 100 cases by the end of 1994.

Rodents appear to be the reservoir for hantaviruses. In the case of the outbreak in the southwest United States, the deer mouse was the responsible reservoir. As is often the case in epizootics, a confluence of events occurred to trigger the expansion of the reservoir. In the Four Corners outbreak, 6 years of drought were followed by heavy rains and snow in 1993, producing large amounts of forage for deer mice. At the same time, for unknown reasons, the bull snake population of the area decreased markedly. That event further contributed to the expansion of the deer mouse population. Close proximity of rodents to the Navajo population permitted the transmission of the virus from mice to man.

The cotton rat was the reservoir harboring a Black Creek Canal hantavirus causing a case of disease in Florida. The Norway rat and the meadow vole have served as reservoirs in other places.

Clinically, the illness begins as a nonspecific constitutional illness not dissimilar from influenza. Fever, myalgia, headache, cough, nausea, vomiting, chills, malaise, and diarrhea are all common. Dizziness is present less than half the time, as are arthralgia, back pain, and chest pain. A cardinal feature is the rapid development of shortness of breath within 2–3 days of onset. The mortality rate, which is in excess of 50%, is caused predominantly by pulmonary failure.

The pathogenesis of the profound respiratory insufficiency seems to lie in the increased permeability of the pulmonary capillaries. It is unclear whether the lung pathology in hantavirus illness is due to a direct cellular effect of the virus or mediated by immune mechanisms. Unfortunately, respiratory insufficiency tends to worsen rapidly in many patients despite all available medical efforts.

## LYME DISEASE

Lyme disease (LD) is a multisystemic disease caused by the spirochete, *Borrelia burgdorferi*, transmitted to humans by *Ixodes* ticks, in the nymphal stage. LD occurs primarily in the northeastern United States and Wisconsin, Minnesota, and California. Adult *Ixodes* mate on deer in the fall and winter and deposit eggs in the spring. In summer larvae obtain a blood meal from the white-footed mouse, the main reservoir of *B. burgdorferi*, and ingested spirochetes persist in the tick. The nymphal tick obtains a blood meal from a vertebrate such as a human the following spring or summer and thus may transmit *B. burgdorferi*. Engorged nymphs mature into adult ticks and complete their 2-year life cycle by parasitizing deer. LD does not occur in areas not inhabited by deer. Many other mammals (e.g., dogs) can be infected with *B. burgdorferi*. Infection usually occurs from May to September and is most common in children. LD demonstrates three illness stages. The primary stage includes flu-like symptoms of fever, muscle and joint aches, and headache or mild meningeal irritation; there is also a characteristic rash, *erythema chronicum migrans* (ECM). ECM begins as a small macule or papule at the tick bite site within 3–14 days and then expands to an annular lesion with a raised red border and central clearing. This slowly expands, and adjacent rings may form. Without treatment, ECM disappears after several weeks and constitutional symptoms appear after several months.

Weeks or months after resolution of ECM, the second stage may develop, involving the nervous system and/or the heart. Symptoms involving the nervous system include peripheral neuropathy, facial palsy, and fluctuating meningitis. Cardiac involvement includes atrioventricular block and/or acute myocarditis. These features may subside spontaneously within several months. The third stage of LD involves fluctuating arthritis of the large joints (i.e., the knees) weeks to years after infection. In some patients, chronic erosive arthritis develops. Because spirochetes are only rarely demonstrated in tissues after the first stage of LD, host immune responses are probably responsible for the cardiac, arthritic, and neurologic manifestations of the second and third stages.

Diagnosis of LD generally requires serologic evidence of infection, that is, identification of IgG and/or IgM antibodies to *B. burgdorferi*, particularly by Western blot test. Standardization of assays is a serious problem. Demonstration or culture of spirochetes from tissues is very difficult.

Treatment of early LD is oral tetracycline or doxycycline for those older than 8 years and oral penicillin V or amoxicillin for those younger than 8 years for 10–30 days. Isolated Bell's palsy, arthritis, or mild cardiac disease is treated with these same agents for 30 days. More serious neurologic or cardiac disease is treated with parenteral ceftriaxone or penicillin for 14–21 days. Measures to prevent LD include minimizing skin exposure in endemic areas, spraying of clothes with permethrin, and daily inspection and removal of ticks. Prophylactic antibiotics following tick bites are not warranted.

## CASE HISTORIES

### CASE HISTORY 1

A female mammalogist, after collecting small mammals near La Paz, Bolivia, had the sudden onset of chills, fever, sweating, severe headache, pain and swelling of the right axilla, muscle pains in the lower back and hip, and anorexia. She was initially treated with amoxicillin without benefit. The pain and swelling in the axilla continued to increase.

Within a day or two, she developed a dry cough. Upon her return to the United States a few days after the onset of her illness, her temperature was 101.3°F and she had a fluctuant 2.5-cm lymph node in the right axilla. These findings led to a presumptive diagnosis of bubonic plague. The diagnosis was subsequently confirmed by isolation of *Y. pestis* organisms from the node. She responded well to streptomycin.

## CASE 1 DISCUSSION

During the collection of specimens in Bolivia, she had used pentobarbital to euthanize the animals rather than chloroform. Chloroform kills fleas, but pentobarbital does not. She had noted fleas on the animals, and had crushed some between her fingers. This was the probable mechanism of infection. The initial symptoms were nonspecific—that is, chills, fever, and headache, all of which can be seen in a variety of conditions such as influenza, brucellosis, malaria, typhoid fever, tularemia, miliary tuberculosis, among others. The epidemiologic setting in which the nonspecific symptoms and signs developed are helpful in pruning a diagnostic list. For example, during the winter in much of the United States, such symptoms would most likely be caused by influenza B. In a family eating imported cheese from Mexico, the cause of the illness might be brucellosis, but more probably listeriosis. Thus, the careful physician considers all of the relevant information in formulating a diagnosis. This is particularly true now that worldwide travel has become easy, inexpensive, and frequent.

There was no compelling reason to treat this person with amoxicillin. The pain in the right axilla followed by enlargement of the lymph nodes, along with a history of working with mammals in a third world country, pointed to the correct diagnosis. There are clearly systemic effects, either from the liberation of endotoxin or invasion of the bloodstream. She was fortunate in not developing fulminant disease, which would have included coagulation defects and possibly pneumonia, both of which might have been a prelude to death.

## CASE HISTORY 2

An 8-year-old child in Tulare County, California, presents to your office with a history of a lump in the left axilla. In taking the history, you learn that the child is afebrile, has no pain in the left axilla, and has had no sweats, chills, weight loss, headache, or myalgia.

The family lives in a semirural area. The father's principal business is raising rabbits for slaughter and for the Easter pet trade. As is often the case on farms and ranches, there are a number of cats that breed frequently, and there are 10–15 kittens at any one time. This 8-year-old has a particular fondness for kittens, frequently plays with them,

and is often scratched and bitten. He also was caught inside a rabbit pen 2 days previously.

On examination, you see a healthy appearing boy in no acute distress. There is a 3-cm firm, non tender, nonfluctuant node in the left axilla. You notice a small papule on the left hand that the parents had not noted before. The question confronting you is, Does this child have cat scratch disease, tularemia, or something else?

## CASE 2 DISCUSSION

While it's possible that the child has tularemia, it is highly improbable, since tularemia is found primarily in wild rabbits. Therefore, you can safely exclude the diagnosis of tularemia even though the child had entered one of the domesticated rabbit pens.

Accordingly, you turn your attention to the possibility of cat-scratch fever. Kittens are a more likely reservoir for the infection than are adult cats. This patient clearly has had frequent contact with kittens and apparently has been scratched and bitten quite often. Like many patients with cat-scratch disease, there is a small papule at the site of the lesion that is painless, and not surrounded by the erythema or swelling typical for tularemia. The lymph nodes are localized to one anatomic area, and are not reddened or inflamed. All of this leads to the conclusion that this child most likely has cat-scratch disease.

The possibility of toxoplasmosis should also be entertained. While cat feces are certainly the major source of toxoplasmosis in the United States, we have no knowledge about whether the child changes a cat litter box or in fact if he has any contact with cat feces. Parenthetically, the major way to prevent toxoplasmosis during pregnancy is for the pregnant woman *never* to empty a cat litter box unless wearing gloves and using strict hygenic technique. Axillary lymphadenopathy is an unusual location for lymphadenitis secondary to toxoplasmosis, which generally is not localized to one anatomic area of the extremities. Bilateral cervical adenopathy or generalized adenopathy is more typical.

# REFERENCES

**Books**

Gould, S. E., ed. *Trichinosis in Man and Animals.* Springfield, IL: Charles C Thomas, 1970.

Hoeprich, P. D., and Jordan, M. C., eds. *Infectious Diseases: A Modern Treatise of Infectious Processes.* 5th ed. Philadelphia: J. B. Lippincott Co., 1994.

Mandell, G. L., Douglas, R. G., Jr., and Bennett, J. E., eds. *Principles and Practice of Infectious Diseases.* 4th ed. New York: Churchill Livingstone, 1994.

Manson-Bahr, P. E. C., and Bell, D. R. *Manson's Tropical Diseases.* 19th ed. London: Ballière Tindall, 1988.

Spink, W. W. *The Nature of Brucellosis.* Minneapolis: University of Minnesota Press, 1956.

### Review Articles

Adal, K. A., Cockerell, C. J., and Petri, W. A., Jr. Cat scratch disease, bacillary angiomatosis, and other infections due to *Rochalimaea. N. Engl. J. Med. 330*(21): 1509–1515, 1994.

Butler, T. Yersinia infections: Centennial of the discovery of the plague bacillus. *Clin. Infect. Dis. 19*:655–663, 1994.

Christie, A. B. The clinical aspects of anthrax. *Postgrad. Med. J. 49*:565–570, 1973.

Foshay, L. Tularemia. *Annu. Rev. Microbiol. 4*:313–330, 1950.

Francis, E. A summary of the present knowledge of tularemia. *Medicine 7*:411–432, 1928.

Holliman, R. E. J. Toxoplasmosis and AIDS. *Infection 16*: 121–128, 1988.

LaForce, F. M. Anthrax. *Clin. Infect. Dis. 19*:1009–1014, 1994.

Margileth, A.M. Cat scratch disease. *Adv. Pediatr. Infect. Dis.*, Vol. 8, Mosby-Year Book, Inc., 1993.

Yung, A. P., and Grayson, M. L. Psittacosis—a review of 135 cases. *Med. J. Aust. 148*:228–233, 1988.

### Original Articles

Human plague—India, 1994. *MMWR 43*(38):689–691, September 30, 1994.

Kaufmann, A. F., Boyce, J. M., and Martone, W. J. Trends in human plague in the United States. *J. Infect. Dis. 141*:522–524, 1980.

Webster, G. F., Cockerell, C. J., and Fridman-Kien, A. E. The clinical spectrum of bacillary angiomatosis. *Br. J. Dermatol. 126*:535–541, 1992.

Zangwill, K. M., Hamilton, D. H., Perkins, B. A., et al. Cat scratch disease in Connecticut: Epidemiology, risk factors, and evaluation of a new diagnostic test. *N. Engl. J. Med. 329*:8–13, 1993.

# 30
# MALARIA

## BORIS REISBERG, M.D.

Malaria is a parasitic infection produced by one of four species of the genus *Plasmodium*: *P. vivax, P. falciparum, P. ovale,* and *P. malariae.* Humans become infected with one of these strains of *Plasmodium* following the bite of an infected female *Anopheles* mosquito. Rarely, infection may occur via other means: following transfusion of blood or blood components, *in utero* as a result of malaria complicating pregnancy, or through the use of shared needles by drug addicts. Humans are the intermediate host of the malarial parasites in which the asexual forms develop. The *Anopheles* mosquito is the definitive host in which the sexual reproductive phase of the cycle takes place.

Malaria remains the most common serious infection of humankind. Approximately 2 billion people live in areas of the world where malaria is endemic. It is estimated that 250–300 million people are currently infected and that there are between 1 and 2.5 million deaths per year. The vast majority of deaths from malaria are in children.

In the United States malaria is an episodic illness occurring mostly in travelers returning from endemic areas or in foreign citizens who become ill while in residence in the United States. Over 1000 cases of malaria are reported annually to the Centers for Disease Control (CDC). Anopheline species capable of transmitting malaria are present in southeastern and western sections of the United States. In fact, an outbreak of 30 cases of *P. vivax* malaria occurred in San Diego County, California, in 1988 and was the largest outbreak of introduced malaria in the United States since 1952, when 35 *P. vivax* infections were reported in members of a girls' club in California.

## LIFE CYCLE

Infection in humans is initiated by the bite of the female *Anopheles* mosquito. In the process of feeding, sporozoites present in the saliva of the mosquito are injected into the blood of the human host. The sporozoites are cleared from the blood by the liver within 60 min. The mechanism by which the sporozoites bind to and penetrate the liver cells is poorly understood. The initial development of the malarial parasites occurs within the liver. This exoerythrocytic phase usually takes 6–16 days, depending upon the species of *Plasmodium* involved. Growth of the malarial parasite within the hepatocytes is not associated with symptoms of infection. During the exoerythrocytic phase, the parasite undergoes growth and several nuclear divisions leading to the formation of tissue merozoites. The number of merozoites produced from a single sporozoite varies considerably with the infecting species. A single *P. falciparum* sporozoite may form as many as 40,000 merozoites, whereas sporozoites from the other species of *Plasmodium* produce only 2000–15,000 merozoites. Once formed, the tissue merozoites rupture the hepatocyte and enter the circulation. Many of the merozoites are quickly destroyed, but a significant number attach to specific receptor sites on the red blood cell (RBC). The merozoites then penetrate the red cell membrane, and development of the asexual, erythrocytic cycle begins (Fig. 30–1).

The earliest recognizable form of the parasite within the erythrocyte is the ring-stage trophozoite, which appears as a ring of blue cytoplasm with a dot-like nucleus of red chromatin as seen on Giemsa stain of the peripheral blood smear. With time, the trophozoites enlarge and appear ameboid or band-like in shape. The nucleus of the trophozoite divides and, with nuclear division, the schizont stage is reached. Successive nuclear divisions occur, and each nucleus is surrounded by a small amount of cytoplasm. The merozoites thus produced rupture the erythrocyte and attach to unparasitized erythrocytes, starting the cycle again. The duration of the erythrocytic cycle is constant for each species of malaria. For *P. falciparum*, *P. vivax*, and *P. ovale*, the cycle length (ring trophozoite to blood merozoite) is 48 h. In *P. malariae* infection, the erythrocyte cycle requires 72 h for completion (Table 30–1); this translates to longer periods between cyclic recurrences of fever and can be helpful in differential diagnosis.

In *P. vivax* and *P. ovale* infection, not all of the sporozoites that enter the liver develop into mature schizonts; some remain dormant, hypnozoites (sleeping forms) for up to several years. At any point in this period of dormancy stimulation of growth can occur, producing relapse of infection. Relapse may thus occur months to years after the primary infection. There is no persistent exoerythrocytic stage of *P. falciparum* and *P. malariae*. Thus, no true relapse of infection occurs with these malarial species. In patients who acquire their infection because of blood or blood component transfusion, no exoerythrocytic stage develops because only the sporozoites that develop in the mosquito are capable of hepatic invasion.

A small number of merozoites that enter the red blood cell develop into male and female gametocytes. The gametocytes do not rupture the red blood cells but have to be ingested by the *Anopheles* mosquito for further development. Fertilization of the gametocytes occurs within the stomach of the mosquito. Further maturation leads to the production of sporozoites that migrate through the body cavity of the mosquito to reach the salivary glands. When such a mosquito bites a person, a new cycle is initiated.

## PATHOGENESIS OF INFECTION IN HUMANS

### Erythrocyte Age and Susceptibility to Infection

There are a number of factors that govern the ability of the malarial parasite to invade the red blood cell. The age of the erythrocyte is a major determinant of its susceptibility to parasitism by all species of malaria except *P. falciparum*. Infection by *P. vivax* or *P. ovale* is limited to the reticulocyte or very young erythrocyte. *P. malariae* merozoites parasitize senescent erythrocytes. The selection of specific red blood cells for parasitism accounts in large part for the low percentage of erythrocytes parasitized by *P. vivax*, *P. ovale*, and *P. malariae*, a number that rarely exceeds 2%. *P. falciparum* merozoites are capable of invading red cells of all ages, although recent experimental evidence indicates that the rate of parasitic invasion is higher in young compared with old erythrocytes. The resulting parasitemia may approach 60% of the circulating erythrocytes. When infection of 5% or greater of the circulating erythrocytes occurs, especially in travelers to endemic areas, serious, life-threatening disease may occur, a condition that has been termed *malignant tertian malaria*.

### Erythrocyte Receptor Sites

It was discovered recently that the merozoite attaches to a specific receptor site on the surface of the red blood cell. It has been known for many years that the majority of Africans and African-Americans are resistant to *P. vivax* infection. This inherent resistance is related to blood types. The majority of people of African ancestry are Duffy blood group–negative; that is, they are *FyFy* and lack both the Fy$^a$ and Fy$^b$ alleles. When such individuals are deliberately exposed to the bite of a vivax-infected mosquito, infection does not occur.

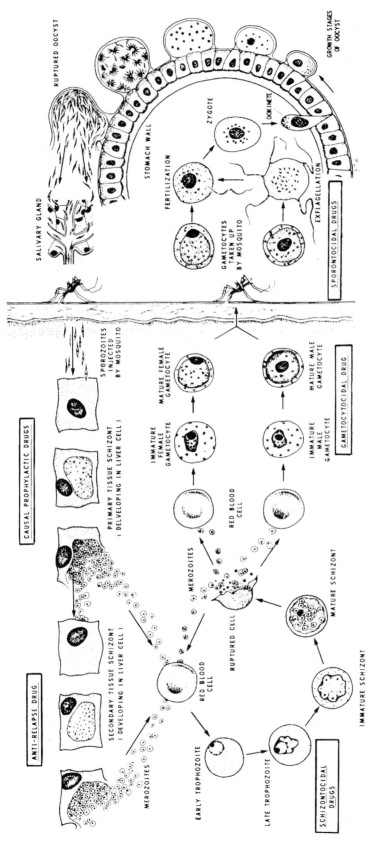

## CYCLE IN MOSQUITO

## CYCLE IN MAN

**FIGURE 30–1.** Life cycle of *Plasmodium*. (Modified from Bruce-Chwatt and Alvarado. Courtesy of the University of Florida College of Medicine, Gainesville. From Hunter, G. W., III, Swartzwelder, J. C., and Clyde, D. F. *Tropical Medicine.* 5th ed. Philadelphia, W. B. Saunders Co., 1976. With permission.)

**TABLE 30–1.   COMPARISON OF THE LIFE CYCLES OF MALARIAL SPECIES THAT INFECT HUMANS**

|  | P. FALCIPARUM | P. VIVAX | P. OVALE | P. MALARIAE |
|---|---|---|---|---|
| Incubation period (days) | 10–14 | 12–15 | 12–15 | 18–30 |
| Persistence of exoerythrocytic parasites | No | Yes | Yes | Probably not |
| Stage of erythrocyte parasitized | All | Reticulocyte | Reticulocyte | Senescent |
| Duration (hours) of erythrocytic cycle | 48 | 48 | 48 | 72 |
| Magnitude of RBC parasitemia | High (Up to 60%) | Low (<2%) | Low (<2%) | Low (<1%) |

People of African heritage who are Duffy blood group–positive and who are exposed in a similar manner do develop infection. This specificity of the merozoite–RBC antigen binding is highly suggestive of a classic receptor–ligand interaction.

Determinants other than blood types per se influence the capacity of erythrocytes of persons of diverse racial backgrounds to be invaded by plasmodia. For example, the receptor for *P. falciparum* attachment appears to be glycophorin A, the principal membrane sialoglycoprotein of red cells. Red blood cells that are blood group En (a−) are resistant to invasion of *P. falciparum* merozoites. En (a−) cells are totally deficient in glycophorin A. In addition, antibody against glycophorin A blocks invasion of normal En (a+) erythrocytes. Even though there is marked resistance to invasion by *P. falciparum* merozoites, once inside a susceptible cell, parasitic maturation occurs normally. The specific receptor sites for *P. ovale* and *P. malariae* have not yet been determined.

### Invasion

The merozoites attach themselves to the red cell membrane at their apical pole, which contains specialized organelles. Next, there are waves of marked deformation of the erythrocyte surface, producing a small invagination at the site of attachment. The invagination deepens, encasing the entire merozoite in an erythrocyte membrane-lined vacuole. At the end of this process, the red cell membrane is resealed. This process of interiorization is rapid, taking about 20 sec, and requires major alterations in the surface structure of the erythrocyte.

### Intracellular Growth of the Malarial Parasite and Cellular Adherence

Once inside the erythrocyte, the developing malarial parasite ingests 25–75% of the red blood cell hemoglobin content by endocytosis. In the process of growth and development, the malarial parasite also alters the structure of the parasitized red cell and its biologic properties. Schüffner's dots, or granules, found on the cell wall of red cells parasitized by *P. vivax* or *P. ovale* have been shown by electron microscopy to be small invaginations surrounded by vesicles. Red cells parasitized by *P. falciparum* and *P. malariae* develop small electron-dense protrusions at the cell surface, called knobs. The knobs found on the surface of *P. falciparum*–infected red cells have been found to promote the adherence of these cells to the surface of endothelial cells of the postcapillary venular bed.

Adherence is probably mediated by a number of different receptor molecules on the endothelial surface that bind specifically with ligands associated with the knobs of the *P. falciparum*–infected erythrocyte. Some of the suggested receptor molecules as determined by *in vitro* studies have included CD36, platelet glycoprotein thrombospondin, intercellular adhesion molecule 1 (ICAM-1), E-selectin, and vascular cell adhesion molecule-1 (VCAM-1). It has been shown that in severe malaria tumor necrosis factor alpha (TNF-alpha) is markedly increased. TNF-alpha has the ability to up-regulate the expression of ICAM-1 on the endothelial cell surface, which then increases the sequestration of parasitized cells in the microvasculature with resulting tissue anoxia and potential organ failure. Interleukin-1 (IL-1) and interferon-beta (IFN-beta) may also play a role in up-regulating the expression of ICAM-1, CD36, and thrombospondin. The increased production of these cytokines is felt to play a significant role in the pathophysiology of cerebral malaria. It is also possible that two or more of the above-described receptor molecules work in concert to bind infected cells.

Certain variant hemoglobins affect the growth and development of malarial parasites. Red cells that contain fetal hemoglobin (Hb

F) retard the intracellular growth of *P. falciparum*. Interestingly, attachment and invasion of the erythrocyte are not inhibited, but because of the retardation in intracellular growth, clinical infection in the first 6 months of life is extremely uncommon.

Under aerobic conditions, erythrocytes from persons with sickle cell trait (AS) support the normal development and maturation of *P. falciparum* parasites. Under reduced oxygen tension, however, the intracellular parasites are damaged. Electron-microscopic studies of these reduced Hb S–containing cells reveal needle-like aggregates of deoxyhemoglobin S, producing disruption of the parasites. Reduced oxygen tension also leads to intracellular loss of potassium, and this may lead to the death of the parasite. Hemoglobin C also retards invasion and intracellular growth of malarial parasites. Heterozygotic (AC) red cells reduce invasion and growth only minimally. Less clear is the effect of red cells that are deficient in glucose-6-phosphate dehydrogenase (G6PD) and those containing thalassemia ($A_2$) hemoglobin.

## EPIDEMIOLOGY

Malaria occurs mostly in the tropical areas of the world, where the climate is warm and moist. This region includes parts of Mexico, Haiti, Central America, South America, Africa, the Middle East, the Indian subcontinent, Southeast Asia, Korea, Indonesia, and Oceania (Fig. 30–2). More than 2 billion people live in these areas. In the United States, malaria was endemic until the early 1950s.

Much has been done to eradicate malaria in many parts of the world, but any hope of total elimination of the disease is still in the distant future. Eradication has been impeded by the emergence of mosquitos resistant to residual insecticides, expecially DDT. A more pressing clinical problem, however, has been the emergence of strains of *P. falciparum* that are resistant to chemotherapeutic agents. There have also been social and political impediments to the implementation of eradication procedures.

Of the four species of malarial parasites that infect humans, *P. vivax* and *P. falciparum* are the species most frequently responsible for producing disease. *P. falciparum* infection predominates in Africa where the tropical climate permits the *Anopheles* mosquito to exist throughout the year. Vivax malaria is rare because of the high prevalence of native African population lacking the erythrocyte receptor site of *P. vivax* infection. Infection with *P. malariae* is uncommon, and *P. ovale* infection, which is confined to Africa, is quite rare.

Very rarely, malaria is acquired through blood transfusion. During the period 1927–1981, 26 cases of transfusion-acquired malaria were reported to the CDC in Atlanta, Georgia. Nine patients developed malaria with *P. malariae*; eight developed infection with *P. falciparum* and eight with *P. vivax*; and one case was due to *P. ovale*. The estimated risk was one case of malaria for every 4 million units of blood collected.

## CLINICAL MANIFESTATIONS

The initial symptoms of malaria often are nonspecific and are similar to those occurring in patients with systemic viral illness. Thus, arthralgias, myalgias, headache, back or abdominal pain, and low-grade fever are frequently the first symptoms experienced by patients. With time, typical paroxysms of chills and fever commonly develop.

The typical paroxysm of malaria is initiated by a violent rigor that lasts from a few minutes to an hour. At times the associated vasoconstriction is so intense that the patient appears cyanotic. The rigor is followed by a rapidly rising temperature that reaches 104–106°F (40°–41°C). The fever usually lasts 3–8 h, and with defervescence, marked sweating occurs. At this point, the patient usually feels drained and exhausted and may even fall asleep. These successive stages have been respectively referred to as the cold phase, hot phase, and wet phase of the typical malarial paroxysm. The patient experiencing periodic fevers may feel fairly well between paroxysms. The paroxysm of chills and fever is related to the synchronization of the erythrocytic cycle and is initiated by the liberation of merozoites from the erythrocyte.

Thus, *P. falciparum*, *P. vivax*, and *P. ovale* malarias classically produce fever every 48 h, and *P. malariae* malaria produces fever every 72 h. Early in the course of most cases of malaria, erythrocytic schizogony does not occur in a synchronized fashion, and the fever tends to remain elevated or to be more than one spike per day. This pattern is especially true of *P. falciparum* malaria, which may never exhibit periodicity.

Gastrointestinal symptoms of nausea, vom-

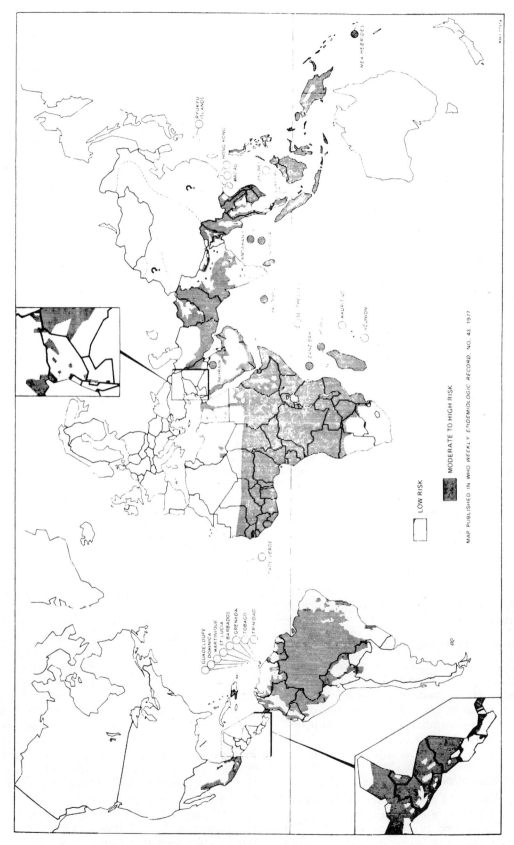

**FIGURE 30–2.** Areas of risk for malaria transmission, December 1976. (From Centers for Disease Control, U.S. Public Health Sevice, Annual Summary 1977, July 1978. With permission.)

iting, and diarrhea are fairly common in malaria. These symptoms, in association with high fever and chills, may be confused with bacillary dysentery or typhoid fever. Patients also frequently complain of headache, low back pain, arthralgia, and myalgia (Table 30–2).

Physical examination usually shows an elevated pulse rate and normal blood pressure. In patients with *P. falciparum* malaria, orthostatic hypotension and periorbital and facial edema are not uncommon. Herpes labialis is commonly present in patients with malaria. The lungs are usually clear to auscultation, but in severe *P. falciparum* malaria with pulmonary involvement, scattered rhonchi and rales may be heard. The spleen is palpable in 50% of patients with acute malaria and is often tender to palpation. The liver is less commonly enlarged.

Routine laboratory examination usually reveals a normal to low white blood cell (WBC) count and a normal hematocrit and hemoglobin. In *P. falciparum* malaria, anemia is often seen, reflecting the severe hemolysis. Thrombocytopenia is not uncommon, but again is most frequently seen with falciparum malaria. Hypoglycemia and increased lactic acid levels frequently occur in *P. falciparum* infections, especially in children and pregnant women. Hypoglycemia may be secondary to increased consumption by a heavy parasite burden, to the effects of increased production of TNF-alpha, and to the release of insulin from pancreatic beta cells in patients treated with quinine or quinidine. In approximately one third of patients, routine urinalysis demonstrates proteinuria and an increased number of white cells in the sediment. Liver studies reveal mild elevations of transaminases, and in patients with brisk hemolysis, the bilirubin level is elevated. Clinical jaundice is uncommon.

### Plasmodium falciparum Malaria

The severity of falciparum malaria is directly related to the net mass of the parasitized red cells. As mentioned above, the net effect of adherent parasitized erythrocytes in the venular and capillary microvasculature is stasis of blood flow, tissue hypoxemia, lactic acidosis, and potential organ dysfunction.

### Renal Dysfunction

Renal failure is a result of decreased microcirculation within the kidney. In those patients who have died, postmortem examination reveals acute tubular necrosis and hemoglo-

---

**TABLE 30–2. MALARIA: COMMON SYMPTOMS**

| |
| --- |
| Fever |
| Chills |
| Headache |
| Nausea, vomiting |
| Diarrhea |
| Low back pain |
| Arthralgia, myalgia |
| Anorexia |
| Fatigue |

---

bin casts within the renal tubules. Dehydration and hypotension also play a role in promoting acute tubular necrosis in a significant number of patients.

Glomerular damage may also develop in falciparum malaria. The glomerulonephritis and nephrotic syndrome that occur after the first week of infection in some patients are thought to be produced by immunologic mechanisms. Kidney biopsies in such patients demonstrate deposition of immunoglobulins, mostly IgM, and complement at the glomerular basement membrane and within the mesangium. Malarial antigen is also found, though less often, in a similar distribution. These findings indicate immune complex–mediated glomerular injury. In patients with acute renal failure, peritoneal dialysis or hemodialysis may be a life-saving measure.

### Cerebral Malaria

Clinical manifestations of central nervous system (CNS) dysfunction in acute falciparum malaria are uncommon, occurring in only 1–2.5% of all cases. Although rare, cerebral malaria is often life threatening, with mortality rates of 15–20% despite antimalarial therapy in modern medical facilities. Disturbances in consciousness, ranging from lethargy and stupor to frank coma, are the most frequently observed signs of cerebral malaria. Patients may also develop focal neurologic signs, such as disturbances in movement (myoclonus and chorea), acute changes in personality, and seizures. Lumbar puncture most frequently reveals an elevated opening pressure and clear cerebrospinal fluid (CSF). The CSF protein level ranges from normal to elevated, and the glucose concentration is normal. Usually there is no increase in inflammatory cells in the CSF. The basic pathologic process is anoxic damage secondary to capillary and venular occlusion by red blood cells containing mature pigmented trophozoites and schizonts. This process leads to the development of cerebral edema, ring (perivascular) hemorrhages, and necrosis around central veins. If the patient survives, there is usually no residual neurologic disability.

### Respiratory Failure

In a small number of patients with falciparum malaria, noncardiac pulmonary edema may develop in the absence of fluid overload. These patients exhibit marked impairment of gas exchange and become hypoxic and cyanotic. Chest roentgenograms usually reveal bilateral, diffuse pulmonary infiltrates. Pulmonary involvement is a grave complication of falciparum malaria, since it does not respond to the therapy that is effective in clearing parasitemia.

### Hepatic and Cardiac Involvement

In some patients with falciparum malaria, centrilobular necrosis of the liver is found. Usually, liver dysfunction is not severe. Involvement of the heart, including cardiac failure, has been observed in cases of fatal falciparum malaria. At autopsy, plugging of myocardial capillaries and venules by parasitized erythrocytes has been observed, as well as petechial hemorrhages and edema of cardiac muscle.

### Bacterial Gastrointestinal Infections

There appears to be an increased incidence of bacterial infection of gastrointestinal origin, especially salmonella, in patients with severe malaria. Salmonella infections are known to be more common in patients with hemolytic anemia of other causes (e.g., sickle cell disease). Decreased splenic clearance may also account for a higher incidence of bacteremia.

### Plasmodium vivax and Plasmodium ovale Malaria

In untreated vivax malaria, the primary attack lasts from 3 weeks to 2 months. Similar to falciparum infection, the initial febrile period for *P. vivax* and *P. ovale* infection is often irregular and the fever sustained. Early in the course of vivax malaria there may be two groups of parasites maturing on alternate days. When this occurs, the patient has a daily temperature spike (quotidian fever). Usually by the end of the first week, one of the two groups of parasites drops out, and the typical malarial paroxysms occur every 42–47 h (tertian fever). Complications are uncommon, and the prognosis, even without therapy, is good. Because of the persistence of parasites in the liver, relapse may occur as long as 3–5 years after the initial attack. Ovale malaria is similar to vivax infection but tends to be even milder.

### Plasmodium malariae Malaria

Malaria produced by *P. malariae* (quartan malaria) is very similar to vivax infection except that the febrile period occurs every 72 h. The periodicity of the fever tends to be established early and may even be present from the onset of the infection. Recurrent infection with *P. malariae* has been implicated in the development of the nephrotic syndrome. It is thought that repeated antigenic stimulation by recurrent episodes of malariae malaria leads to the deposition of immune complexes at the glomerular capillary basement membrane. Renal biopsy in patients with malariae malaria who have the nephrotic syndrome has demonstrated the presence of IgG and IgM in 96% of the specimens examined. The third component of complement (C3) was present in over half the specimens, and *P. malariae* antigen was found in one quarter of the kidney biopsies studied. The resulting nephrotic syndrome unfortunately does not respond to corticosteroid therapy, and even aggressive antimalarial therapy has little effect on the clinical course.

## HOST FACTORS IN MALARIAL INFECTION

Both humoral and cellular immunity serve to limit the extent and duration of malarial infection. In individuals living in highly endemic areas of malaria, a relative immunity to symptomatic infection develops. This immunity is associated with the development of tolerance to erythrocyte parasitemia. It is not unusual to find children living in holoendemic areas of Africa to be asymptomatic in spite of erythrocyte parasitemias as high as 20%.

Human beings and experimental animals can also be protected from malarial infection by the passive administration of immunoglobulin derived from individuals or animals who have recovered from malarial infection. Antibody may protect the red cell from invasion and prevent intracellular development of the malarial parasite. Red cells with parasitic antigen on their surfaces may also be opsonized by antibody, leading to accelerated destruction of the erythrocytes by the monocyte/macrophage reticuloendothelial system.

Malarial infection may be associated with generalized immunosuppression of the host. Infected children tend to have lower antibody responses to certain antigens, including tetanus toxoid and certain bacterial vaccines. Immunosuppression may also account for greater susceptibility to and severity of intercurrent viral infections.

Pregnant women, especially primigravidas, appear to be especially susceptible to malarial infection. In geographic areas endemic for *P. falciparum*, attack rates 4–12 times greater than those found in nonpregnant women have been observed. The higher attack rate in pregnant women may be due in part to a loss of acquired immunity during pregnancy. Not only is the woman's health jeopardized by malaria but the fetus may also become infected via the transplacental route. Infections during pregnancy have been associated with spontaneous abortion, stillbirth, intrauterine growth retardation, and prematurity.

Recently, soluble monocyte mediators, such as TNF-alpha and IL-1, have been shown to play a role in the host response to malarial infection. In a recent study by Kern et al., 31 of 32 patients with severe falciparum malaria had elevated serum levels of TNF-alpha. TNF-alpha levels were proportional to the number of parasitized red blood cells, with the highest concentrations being found in patients with cerebral malaria and hypotension.

## DIAGNOSIS

Malaria should be considered in any patient who develops fever and chills and who has visited, or is a citizen of, a country where malaria is known to exist (see Fig. 30–2). Malaria should also be considered in the differential diagnosis of patients who present with fever of undetermined origin and a history of transfusions of blood or blood components or of intravenous (IV) drug abuse.

The vast majority of travelers who develop malaria in the United States after having visited an endemic area become clinically ill within the first month of their return to the United States. A smaller number of patients develop symptoms 1–6 months after their return. Only rarely do patients (usually those with vivax or malariae infections) develop clinical illness as long as 1 year after their visit to a malarious area.

The definitive diagnosis of malaria is made by demonstrating the presence of parasites within the red blood cell. To do this, both thick and thin blood smears are stained with either Giemsa's or Wright's stain. If the initial smears are negative, additional smears should be obtained every 8–12 h for an additional 72 h. The thick smear is most useful when there is low-grade parasitemia, since in these cases parasites may be impossible to find in the thin smears. However, when parasites are present in sufficient numbers, as in most cases of malaria, they are most easily recognized by inexperienced personnal in the thin smear. The thin smear is also used for speciation of the infection.

Monitoring of serial thick and thin smears is also useful in following the disappearance of parasitemia after the institution of chemotherapy.

There are several serologic tests that are useful in detecting the presence of malarial antibody. These include agar gel diffusion, passive hemagglutination, immunofluorescence, and the enzyme-linked immunosorbent assay (ELISA) technique. Antibody is usually not detectable within the first week of a primary infection, and, therefore, attempting to determine its presence is not helpful when the patient first presents. A nonimmune person with a primary infection may develop only low antibody titers that persist only a few weeks to months if rapid and adequate chemotherapy is administered. On the other hand, individuals living in endemic areas with minimal or no treatment develop high levels of antibody with a broad spectrum of reactivity. These antibodies may persist for years even after the person has left an endemic area.

When blood smears are negative, serologic testing can establish a diagnosis of malaria in individuals returning from an endemic area with a fever of undetermined origin. The smears may be negative as a result of suppressive chemoprophylaxis taken by the patient, or they can be negative if obtained at the wrong time. Serologic testing has been useful for detecting individuals responsible for transmitting transfusion-related malaria. Such individuals, usually carriers of *P. vivax* or *P. malariae*, have such low-grade parasitemia that blood smears are often negative.

## TREATMENT

In areas where malaria is known to exist, the traveler should take precautions to reduce exposure to mosquito bites. Since the *Anopheles* mosquito feeds primarily from dusk to dawn, the traveler should limit outdoor exposure at these times, especially when traveling in forested areas away from large population centers. Insect repellent containing DEET should be applied to exposed skin and long-sleeved shirts and pants worn. At night, beds should be screened with mosquito netting inpregnated with pyrethrin insecticide. Living areas can be sprayed with knock-down insecticides.

### Acute Infections

Patients with malaria generally should be treated initially in the hospital, with attention being given to fluid and electrolyte therapy; serious complications of falciparum malaria should be anticipated. Those patients with organ dysfunction or with 5% or greater of their erythrocytes parasitized should be managed and monitored in an intensive care unit.

In many institutions, medical personnel are not capable of making a species-specific diagnosis. In such cases, patients should be considered to have falciparum malaria and treated accordingly. This procedure should be followed especially when only ring trophozoites are seen in the thin smear and red cell parasitemias approach 5% or greater. Treat-

ment of falciparum malaria must take into account the possibility of chloroquine resistance. At present, chloroquine-resistant strains of *P. falciparum* are found in Southeast Asia, South America, Africa, and India (Fig. 30–3).

In patients who have, or are suspected of having, chloroquine-resistant falciparum malaria, treatment should begin with oral quinine sulfate, 650 mg three times a day for 7 days. (For all medications listed, adult dosages are provided.) Quinine therapy frequently produces nausea, vomiting, tinnitus, and vertigo. The presence of these side effects (cinchonism), although distressing, should not deter continuation of therapy. Patients who are seriously ill or who cannot tolerate oral medication can be given intravenous quinidine by continuous infusion. The initial dose of quinidine gluconate is 10 mg/kg over 1–4 h followed by a maintenance dose of 0.02 mg/kg/min. When the patient can tolerate oral medication, quinine is given to complete a 7-day course. An additive effect is achieved if doxycycline 100 mg every 12 h is given along with quinine. The combination tablet sulfadoxine and pyrimethamine (Fansidar) can be substituted for doxycyline. Alternative agents that have proved useful in treating chloroquine-resistant *P. falciparum* are mefloquine at 15–25 mg/kg as a single dose or as

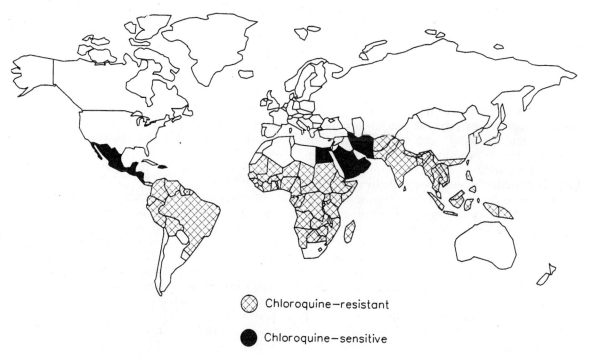

◈ Chloroquine—resistant

● Chloroquine—sensitive

**FIGURE 30–3.** Malarious areas with *Plasmodium falciparum* resistant and sensitive to chloroquine, 1990. (From *Morbidity and Mortality Weekly Report*, March 9, 1990, 39, pp. 140–142. With permission.)

a split dose 12–24 h apart to reduce the incidence of vomiting. Newer agents available in Europe and Asia include halofantrine 8 mg/kg three times a day on day 1 of treatment and repeated on day 7 and an agent produced by China—artemesinin, which seems very promising in treating multi–drug-resistant *P. falciparum.* All patients treated for malaria should be followed by thick and thin blood smears twice daily to follow the effectiveness of therapy. A 75% reduction in the number of parasitized red blood cells should be seen within 48 h of effective treatment. Failure to achieve this reduction in parasitemia may be secondary to a resistant organism or inadequate absorption of oral chemotherapeutic agents.

Chloroquine phosphate is given to patients with *P. vivax, P. ovale, P. malariae,* and chloroquine-sensitive *P. falciparum* infections for the suppression of symptoms and the elimination of etythrocytic parasites. The initial adult dose for chloroquine phosphate (a 4-aminoquinoline) is 1000 mg orally, followed by an additional 500 mg in 6 h and a third dose of 500 mg 24 h after the initial dose. A final dose of 500 mg of chloroquine phosphate is given 48 h after the initial dose. In seriously ill patients who cannot tolerate oral medication, chloroquine can be given intramuscularly (IM) or IV. When given parenterally, 250 mg of chloroquine hydrochloride dissolved in normal saline is administered every 6 h until oral therapy is possible.

In infections caused by *P. vivax* and *P. ovale,* it is necessary to eliminate hepatic parasites to prevent future relapses. This can be accomplished by administration of primaquine phosphate, 26.3 mg (15 mg of the base) orally once a day for 14 days. Primaquine may be given concomitantly with chloroquine or started after chloroquine has been discontinued. The combination of chemotherapeutic agents effective against both erythrocytic and exoerythrocytic parasites is frequently referred to as a *radical cure.* Primaquine phosphate (an 8-aminoquinoline) can produce hemolysis in patients whose red blood cells lack G6PD. The anemia produced is of major consequence, primarily in Caucasians with the Mediterranean type of G6PD deficiency. It is imperative, therefore, to assay the patient's red blood cells for the presence of G6PD deficiency before primaquine is started. Persons of African ancestry who are G6PD-deficient usually experience only mild hemolysis.

## Prophylaxis

Individuals who are traveling to areas where malaria is endemic should receive chemoprophylactic treatment. Travelers to Africa are at the highest risk of developing malaria since, in most rural and many urban areas, infected anopheline mosquitoes are present. From 1980 to 1988, over 1500 cases of *P. falciparum* malaria occurred in U.S. travelers. Of these, 80% of the infections were acquired in sub-Saharan Africa. Travelers to South America and Asia are at less risk for developing malaria, since most urban and resort areas have limited if any risk of exposure.

In areas where chloroquine-resistant *P. falciparum* is not a consideration, chloroquine phosphate, 500 mg (one tablet) once a week, starting 1 or 2 weeks before departure and continued for 4 weeks after return, is the drug of choice. Chloroquine is capable of suppressing the clinical symptoms of the disease and eliminating the erythrocytic parasites of all four forms of human malaria (except chloroquine-resistant *P. falciparum*).

Mefloquine is now considered the most effective prophylactic agent for travelers to areas endemic for chloroquine-resistant *P. falciparum* malaria. Mefloquine is recommended at a dosage of 250 mg started 1 week before departure, then one 250-mg tablet weekly while in an endemic area, and an additional weekly tablet for 4 weeks after returning to a malaria-free area. Mefloquine should not be given to travelers who have cardiac conduction defects or who are taking beta blockers. Because confusion, depression, anxiety, and psychotic manifestations have been reported rarely, patients with psychiatric disorders and individuals involved in tasks requiring fine coordination and spatial discrimination, such as airline pilots and operators of heavy machinery, should not take mefloquine prophylaxis.

Alternative prophylaxis for chloroquine-resistant *P. falciparum* is doxycycline, 100 mg by mouth once a day starting 1–2 days prior to departure, then taken daily while in an endemic area, and continued for 4 weeks after returning to a malaria-free area. Because of the potential for photosensitivity resulting in a severe sunburn reaction, persons taking doxycycline are advised to use an efficient sunscreen that absorbs ultraviolet light. Doxycycline, like all tetracyclines, cannot be given to pregnant women and young children under 8 years old.

A second alternative is chloroquine 500 mg weekly along with proquanil 200 mg daily. This regimen is recommended for pregnant women traveling in an endemic area. Chloroquine-proquanil chemoprophylaxis is less effective than mefloquine. Every effort should be made to dissuade pregnant women from traveling in a malarious area, since no prophylactic regimen is 100% effective.

Many physicians also give travelers three tablets of Fansidar as back-up treatment to be taken all at once should they be in an area where medical attention is not readily available and an illness suggestive of malaria occurs. Three tablets of Fansidar may be curative and, if not, will at least blunt the attack of falciparum malaria until the individual can return to a population center where medical attention is available.

The CDC has set up a malaria hotline where detailed recommendations for the prevention of malaria may be obtained 24 h a day. The CDC Malaria Hotline number is (404) 332-4555.

## Vaccine Development

Unlike the life-long immunity that is induced by many viral infections, such as mumps and measles, the immunity that results from malaria is partial and transient. An individual living in an area endemic for malaria typically is infected multiple times over many years, and benefits only by having milder courses of disease than if he had not been infected. Therefore, in order to induce effective, sterile immunity, vaccination must result in the generation of immune responses that are actually *better* than those that result from natural infection. Unfortunately, to date there is no malaria vaccine that induces sterile immunity and is applicable to widespread use. However, experimental animals and human volunteers vaccinated with irradiated sporozoites become resistant to the natural challenge of being bitten multiple times by *P. falciparum*– or *P. vivax*–infected mosquitoes, suggesting that effective vaccination is possible.

The problem with this approach, and the use of other live or live-attenuated vaccines, is that the methods for culturing plasmodium do not produce significant numbers of organisms for large-scale immunization programs. Further complicating the problem is the fact that plasmodium has several life cycle stages, each of which has some stage-specific antigens. Finally, there are parasite species- and strain-specific antigenic determinants on some blood-stage antigens, and a vaccine that may be useful for preventing infection by one plasmodial species or strain may not be protective against another. In theory, it should be feasible to target any of the life cycle stages for vaccine development, since destruction of (1) sporozoites, (2) hepatic merozoites, (3) blood-stage organisms, or (4) gametocytes would either prevent clinical malaria or prevent transmission of parasites to the mosquito and thereby disrupt the parasite's life cycle.

For all these reasons and others, researchers have concentrated on the use of parasite proteins produced by recombinant DNA technology for vaccine development. Once the gene encoding a malarial surface antigen has been molecularly cloned, it can be introduced into bacteria and expressed in large amounts, much as the hepatitis B vaccine and the new varicella vaccine are produced. The first such gene to be tested is that encoding the circumsporozoite (CS) protein, which is found on the surface of the infective sporozoite stage of the parasite and is the parasite protein that engages a specific receptor on the hypatocyte to permit invasion. The immunodominant B-cell epitope of the CS protein consists of repeats of the tetrapeptide asparagine-alanine-asparagine-proline (NANP), and the initial antigen tested consisted of three of these NANP repeats linked to tetanus toxoid. This molecule was only partially effective in preventing infection, but additional vaccines based upon this epitope, plus other immunodominant B-cell and T-cell epitopes of the CS protein are currently being tested.

Many other recombinant parasite proteins are being studied, most of which are derived from blood stages such as the merozoite. To date, the most promising of these is the SPf66 protein, which initially was found to protect monkeys from infection with blood stages of the parasite. Recently, a recombinant SPf66 vaccine was tested in adults and children, and a double-blind, placebo-controlled trial showed that vaccination led to a 39% reduction in clinical episodes of malaria. It is believed by most that a safe, effective malaria vaccine will contain a combination of key antigens or epitopes from different developmental stages of the parasite and induce both humoral and cell-mediated immunity in the recipient. Many research groups around the world are working feverishly toward this goal and are hopeful that it can be achieved before the end of the decade.

# CASE HISTORY

## CASE HISTORY 1

After graduating from college, L. R., a 22-year-old woman, traveled to Southeast Asia including Thailand and Cambodia, with excursions to rural areas. Because of nausea and mild anorexia after taking her second weekly dose of mefloquine, she discontinued this medication prescribed for malaria prophylaxis. While traveling in the rural areas the patient noted bites by mosquitoes on several occasions. The day before returning to the United States, headache, muscle pains, nausea, low-grade fever, and mild diarrhea developed.

When seen by her internist on the day she returned, a presumptive diagnosis of gastroenteritis was made. Stool was obtained for culture and parasitic examination, and ciprofloxacin was started. The next day (third day of illness), the patient reported that her fever had risen to almost 104°F, preceded by a severe, whole-body shaking chill. Because of this, the patient was admitted to the hospital.

On admission she appeared acutely ill. The temperature was 103°F, blood pressure 110/70 mm Hg, pulse 92/min. The physical examination was essentially normal. Specifically, the abdomen was nontender and the liver and spleen were not palpable.

Laboratory studies revealed a WBC count of 4300/mm$^3$ with 70% polymorphonuclear leukocytes (PMNs). The platelet count was 88,000/mm$^3$ and the hemoglobin and hematocrit were normal. The technician performing the manual differential WBC count noted several ring-shaped trophozoites in the red blood cells. This was confirmed by the supervising pathologist, and a diagnosis of *P. falciparum* malaria was made. The patient was treated with oral quinidine and doxycycline and made an uneventful recovery.

## CASE 1 DISCUSSION

This is not an unusual case. Not infrequently, persons traveling in areas of the world where malaria is endemic fail to take their prophylactic medicine. Most often the onset of malaria is nonspecific, with symptoms suggestive of gastroenteritis or the "flu." More often than not, the physical examination is unremarkable.

All patients returning from a malarious area of the world who develop a febrile illness should have a blood smear examined for intraerythrocytic parasites. This should be repeated if the cause of the febrile illness is not established with initial efforts.

# REFERENCES

**Book**

Wyler, D. J. Plasmodium and babesia. In: Gorbach, S. L., Bartlett, J. G., and Blacklow, N. R., eds. *Infectious Diseases.* Philadelphia: W. B. Saunders Co., 1992.

**Original Articles**

Berendt, A. R., Ferguson, D. J. P., Gardner, J., et al. Molecular mechanisms of sequestration in malaria. *Parasitology 108*:519–528, 1994.

Centers for Disease Control. Recommendations for the prevention of malaria among travelers. *MMWR 39*: (RR-3): 1990.

Gopanath, R., Keystone, J. S., and Kevin, K. C. Concurrent falciparum malaria and salmonella bacteremia in travelers: Report of two cases. *Clin. Infect. Dis. 20*: 706–708, 1995.

Hoffman, S. L. Diagnosis, treatment, and prevention of malaria. *Med. Clin. North Am. 76*:1327–1355, 1992.

Kern, P., Hemmer, C. J., Damme, J. V., Gruss, H. J., and Dietrich, M. Elevated tumor necrosis factor alpha and interleukin-6 serum levels as markers for complicated *Plasmodium falciparum* malaria. *Am. J. Med. 87*:139–143, 1989.

Miller, L. H., Good, M. F., and Genevieve, M. Malaria pathogenesis. *Science 264*:1878–1893, 1994.

Nussenzweig, R. S., and Long, C. A. Malaria vaccines: Multiple targets. *Science 265*:1381–1383, 1994.

White, N. J., and Pukrittayakamee, S. Clinical malaria in the tropics. *Med. J. Aust. 159*:197–203, 1993.

Wyler, D. J. Malaria: Overview and update. *Clin. Infect. Dis. 16*:449–456, 1993.

# 31
# EXANTHEMATOUS DISEASES

## A TODD DAVIS, M.D.

RUBEOLA (MEASLES)
RUBELLA

CHICKENPOX (VARICELLA)
ERYTHEMA INFECTIOSUM (FIFTH DISEASE)
ROSEOLA (EXANTHEM SUBITUM)

KAWASAKI DISEASE
CASE HISTORIES
REFERENCES

Viral exanthems, cutaneous manifestations of viral infection, have long fascinated physicians. Exanthems often challenge diagnostic acumen because they are associated with infections caused by herpes, pox, enteric, respiratory, and other viruses. Some viral exanthems such as roseola (exanthem subitum) and erythema infectiosum (fifth disease) are benign and self-limited in the normal host. In contrast, rubeola (measles), rubella (German measles), and varicella (chickenpox), although usually self-limited, may be associated with serious disease. Measles virus can produce acute encephalitis, subacute sclerosing panencephalitis, and may be etiologically linked to multiple sclerosis. Worldwide, measles is the most frequent cause of demyelinating brain disease. Rubella has been a major contributor to congenital defects, and chickenpox is a potentially life-threatening illness in immunocompromised patients.

There are hundreds of diseases with cutaneous manifestations. Only a few are discussed here; they have been chosen because of their occurrence in the United States and for the lessons they teach about immunology, epidemiology, and immunization practices. Excellent color photographs illustrating the features of the exanthematous diseases discussed here can be found in the color atlas by Lambert and Farrar (see References).

## RUBEOLA (MEASLES)

Measles virus is currently included in the genus *Morbillivirus* and the family Paramyxo-viridae. This is a relatively large virus, 150–300 nm in diameter, having helical capsid symmetry and containing ribonucleic acid (see Chapter 5 for overview and comparison with other viruses).

Measles can be thought of as a serious respiratory illness that happens to have an associated skin rash. The measles virus gains access to the respiratory tract, invades the lymphatic tissue, and then spills over into the bloodstream. As this occurs, respiratory symptoms and fever become manifest 2–3 days prior to the development of the skin rash. The early phase of the illness, the prodrome, consists of fever (with the temperature gradually rising to 103°–104°F), cough, coryza, and conjunctivitis. Within 2–3 days, a pathognomonic enanthem consisting of Koplik's spots begins on the buccal mucosa opposite the first and second molars, followed by an exanthem beginning on the head and neck. Koplik's spots are tiny white lesions on an erythematous base, whereas the exanthem consists of small, reddish, flat macules and papules. Within 24 h Koplik's spots disappear and the rash begins to spread onto the arms, upper trunk, and back. Over the next 2–3 days, the fever remains elevated as the rash continues to spread caudally, ultimately involving the legs. Within a day or two of the appearance of the rash on any body site, the discrete maculopapular lesions begin to coalesce, forming large, reddish areas. The rash during the convalescent phase is called morbilliform. This term is often used to describe nonmeasles coalescent rashes. During the healing phase of the exanthem, there may be a brownish discoloration of the skin.

While most children recover uneventfully from measles, some suffer complications or death. Croup or pneumonia often require hospitalization. The absence of good medical care may lead to death. Worldwide, 1 to $1^1/_2$ million children die each year from measles, largely from respiratory complications. Because vitamin A deficiency contributes to morbidity and mortality, vitamin A supplementation is recommended for affected children in the United States and abroad.

In the United States during the prevaccine era, encephalitis was the major, albeit rare, complication. Approximately 1 in every 1000–2000 children with measles develops acute encephalitis; half of those so afflicted die and at least half of the survivors suffer serious neurologic impairments. Worldwide, measles encephalitis is the most common initiating cause of demyelinating inflammatory disease in human beings. In some other children with measles, subacute sclerosing panencephalitis develops months to years later. Fortunately, this occurs rarely, in approximately 1 per 100,000 cases.

A search was begun in the early 1960s for an effective immunizing agent to prevent these serious sequelae (see Chapter 40). Initial efforts focused on a *killed*-virus vaccine. It was soon appreciated, however, that the vaccine was not highly protective and that some immunized children, upon contracting the wild virus, developed very serious measles. This same paradoxic situation (i.e., recipients of killed vaccine contracting disease more severe than that occurring in susceptible children) also occurred in recipients of a killed respiratory syncytial virus vaccine.

The first *live* measles virus vaccine, the Edmonston B vaccine, was highly protective but frequently caused side effects such as fever, which necessitated concomitant administration of gamma globulin. The gamma globulin dosage was carefully titrated to decrease the incidence of serious complications, while not impairing antigenic potency. By 1967, this burdensome procedure was supplanted by a further attenuated vaccine that could be used without gamma globulin. The Schwarz vaccine, which is in current use, produces seroconversion in 95% of vaccinees and has few side effects.

The effectiveness of any vaccine can be tested in numerous ways. Seroconversion rates to the Schwarz vaccine are about 95%.

This means that 95% of subjects who receive the vaccine at 15 months of age or older can be expected to produce a fourfold or higher rise in antibody titer. The effectiveness of measles vaccine, or vaccine efficacy, also has been measured in various studies in which a population sustaining a measles outbreak is thoroughly investigated. Attack rates are calculated for those children who have been vaccinated and for those who are susceptible. It is assumed that the attack rate among the members of the vaccinated group, had they not been immunized, would have been the same as the attack rate among those in the susceptible group. Accordingly, an equation can be generated to show the number of cases observed versus the number expected in the vaccinated group. This reduction in cases experienced by the vaccinees is mathematically converted to a percentage called the vaccine efficacy. Multiple studies have revealed an efficacy of about 95% for measles vaccine.

The marked reduction in the number of children with measles in the United States further attests to the effectiveness of this vaccine. In the prevaccine era, about 500,000 cases of measles were reported annually. In 1994, about 1000 cases were reported, representing a reduction of 99.7%. This impressive control effort stemmed from two key immunization strategies: (1) the achievement and maintenance of high immunization levels; and (2) the rapid detection of new cases of measles with immunization of susceptible contacts as quickly as possible. This latter strategy was borrowed from the program that resulted in eradication of smallpox from the world in the late 1970s.

Unfortunately, the United States may never be totally free of measles. Indeed, several large American cities including Chicago, Los Angeles, Houston, New York, and others experienced extensive outbreaks during the late 1980s and early 1990s. In 1989, for example, 17,850 measles cases were recorded in the United States. Unimmunized preschool children, most from impoverished neighborhoods, served as major reservoirs for propagation of the outbreaks.

Occasional outbreaks will probably continue to occur in the United States. First, there will likely continue to be occasional pockets of endemic spread among certain social and ethnic groups with low vaccination rates in American cities. Second, measles continues to be highly epidemic and endemic throughout the world. Accordingly, periodic importations can be expected into the continental United States.

There are a number of interesting immunologic and biologic questions that remain unanswered with respect to measles. What produces the rash? Why does the rash invariably begin on the head and spread downward in the susceptible host? Why does the rash go through a fixed progression—macules, confluence, and fading?

Immunofluorescence and electron-microscopy studies have demonstrated both measles antigen and viral particles in the exanthematous lesions. However, the precise mechanism or mechanisms directly leading to the individual cutaneous lesions that constitute the rash of rubeola are unknown. Possibilities include (1) host cell injury caused by the virus; (2) acute inflammation in response to the presence of the virus or injury caused by the virus, or both; (3) *in situ* binding of measles antibody to, or interaction of sensitized lymphocytes with, intact virus or residual viral antigens, with resulting immune injury; and (4) a combination of two or more of these pathogenetic sequences of events.

The fixed sequential body site distribution of the rash is probably caused by immunologic mechanisms. Evidence for this is derived from two clinical conditions. When gamma globulin is administered to an exposed susceptible host, the intensity of the illness may be attenuated, but the same general features are present as in fully susceptible subjects. Atypical measles stands in marked contrast. This entity occurs in previously, but only partially, immunized children who lack measurable antibody titers. However, the cellular immune system was primed, as determined by *in vitro* T-lymphocyte studies that show a lymphoblast response upon exposure to measles antigen. In atypical measles, there is no prodrome, Koplik's spots are absent, the rash begins on the ankles and wrists and spreads towards the trunk, and the rash may assume many different forms. These two examples suggest that the site, distribution, and characteristics of the rash are determined more by the cellular immune system than by the humoral system.

The preceding examples also illustrate the important role of antibodies in protection against measles. *Protection* is highly correlated with the presence of serum antibodies. Administration of serum globulin can modify the severity of naturally acquired infection. In atypical measles, serum antibody is unmeasur-

able at the beginning of the illness, thus permitting wild virus to proliferate and cause illness. Although the role (if any) of the cellular immune system in protection against acquisition of measles is unclear, cellular immunity seems to be of key importance in *eradicating* measles virus from the host. Children who have hypogammaglobulinemia but intact cellular immunity recover from measles. In contrast, children with impaired cellular immunity do poorly.

## RUBELLA

Rubella virus is a member of the *Rubivirus* genus of the family Togaviridae. This virus is spherical, has a diameter of 50–60 nm, and contains single-stranded RNA.

In contrast to measles, rubella is usually a mild disease. Young children rarely have prodromal symptoms. Adolescents and adults may have a variety of prodromal symptoms such as eye pain, headache, fever, and myalgia. When a rash occurs, discrete, pinkish maculopapular lesions begin on the head and spread downward over a 2- to 3-day period and then disappear. The rash does not coalesce, in contrast to measles. Accordingly, exanthems consisting of discrete macules and papules are called rubelliform. However, the distribution, appearance, and extent of the rash are highly variable in rubella. Indeed, one third to one half of patients with rubella never develop a rash. The absence of the characteristic rash in many individuals makes the clinical diagnosis of an isolated case quite difficult. When present, occipital adenopathy and joint pain suggest the diagnosis but are not pathognomonic. Accurate diagnosis depends on a significant rubella antibody titer rise between acute and convalescent sera.

The majority of children with rubella have a mild illness and suffer no sequelae. When questioned, as many as 25% of children report mild joint pain. Rubella is a more serious illness in adults, with 25–40% complaining of short-lived joint pain. Permanent joint sequelae are quite rare. The most serious effects of rubella occur in the fetus whose susceptible mother becomes infected during the first trimester. Severely affected infants may have cataracts, sensorineural deafness, congenital heart disease, mental retardation, and other features (see Chapter 26).

Rubella vaccine was developed to interrupt or eliminate the usual 6- to 9-year cycle of major epidemics in the United States that had been observed in the first half of the 20th century and thereby to reduce the large number of resulting rubella-related congenital defects in affected infants. In the 1964 outbreak, it was estimated that about 20,000 infants were born with severe congenital rubella syndrome.

Live attenuated rubella vaccine became commercially available in the United States in 1969. Since that time, efforts have been directed toward immunization of school-aged children. There were two major reasons for choosing this strategy. First, rubella usually began in school-aged populations (horizontal transmission) and spread to infect preschool children, older adolescents, and young adults (vertical transmission). Thus, it was postulated that creation of a large "immune herd" of school-aged children would effectively disrupt the traditional patterns of transmission. Second, there were concerns about the possible teratogenic effects that could occur if the vaccine virus was inadvertently administered to a woman during the first trimester of pregnancy.

This strategy has effectively prevented any large-scale outbreak since introduction of the vaccine. As expected, there also has been a marked reduction in the number of children born with congenital rubella syndrome in the United States (<5 in 1994). However, there continue to be small outbreaks of rubella in adolescents and young adults that occasionally involve susceptible pregnant women, resulting in infants with congenital rubella syndrome.

In contrast to the United States, Great Britain chose to immunize preadolescent girls. This strategy was based on administration of the vaccine to the population at risk (each preadolescent female is assumed to be susceptible and about to become fertile). In addition, the risk of pregnancy was considered to be essentially nonexistent in prepubertal females. As one might expect, rubella continued to be an endemic and epidemic problem in Great Britain; the incidence of congenital rubella syndrome decreased, but not as markedly as in the United States.

Evidence accumulated since the 1970s shows that inadvertent administration of rubella virus to women in the first trimester rarely results in fetal damage. In fact, the risk to the fetus is so small that official advisory committees suggest that abortion is *not* indicated in such situations. This new knowledge about the extremely low risk of inadvertent vaccine immunization during early pregnancy may lead to additional public health measures in the United States. In particular, women of childbearing age (15–45 years) who have not been previously immunized should be strongly considered for immunization as long as they are reasonably sure that they are not pregnant or will not become pregnant around the time administration of the vaccine is planned. In the past, such women were immunized only when effective contraception for the 3 months subsequent to the vaccination could be ensured. In addition, there may be immunization programs specifically aimed at girls who are just entering puberty.

Rubella vaccine markedly diminishes the risk of infection in persons subsequently challenged experimentally with wild rubella virus. Like measles vaccine, rubella vaccine results in seroconversion rates of at least 95%. Efficacy rates for rubella vaccine are thought to be approximately 95%, although remarkably few studies have been done.

## CHICKENPOX (VARICELLA)

Chickenpox is usually a benign disease in normal children, caused by the varicella-zoster virus, which belongs to the herpes virus family. This is not true, however, in children with compromised immune defenses from diseases such as acquired immunodeficiency syndrome (AIDS), leukemia, lymphoma, or receiving immunosuppression therapy. Fully one third of immune-suppressed children will have dissemination to visceral organs resulting in substantial morbidity and mortality. In one study, 7% (4 of 77) of such children died. This has led to both passive and active immunization strategies. In the spring of 1995, a live attenuated vaccine was licensed for use in the United States.

There is no prodrome in chickenpox. Rather, the first sign of the illness is the presence of small, fluid-filled, clear vesicles, often dimpled in the middle. The child may have fever as well as mild constitutional symptoms such as myalgia, irritability, and some fussiness. The first lesions may occur anywhere on the body. Subsequent vesicles occur without any discernible pattern of progression from one body area to another. During the first 3–4 days, vesicular lesions continue to appear on various body sites. New lesions are uncommon after 6 or 7 days. Some but not all of the vesicles progress to pustular lesions, resulting in dry, crusted lesions. All three kinds of lesions are usually present after the first or second day. Although the diagnosis is usually obvious on clinical grounds, a smear of epithelial cells from the base of a vesicle invariably demonstrates multinucleated cells and intranuclear inclusion bodies, suggesting the diagnosis. This test, in conjunction with electron-microscopic studies, may be essential for rapid differentiation of chickenpox from smallpox and rickettsialpox (see Chapter 28).

The appearance and distribution of chickenpox, which so markedly differs from measles and rubella, suggests different mechanisms for cutaneous manifestations of these viral diseases. In chickenpox, the skin lesions, heavily laden with virus, are almost certainly caused either by the virus itself, by an acute inflammatory reaction to the virus, or by both. The evolution from vesicle to pustule to crusted lesion is primarily due to an acute inflammatory reaction and not to a cellular immune response.

As with measles and rubella, the role of the immune system in protection against subsequent challenge by chickenpox is better understood than its role in controlling an established infection. Specific antibody seems to be of crucial importance in protection against disease. Newborn babies whose mothers had chickenpox are immune for the first few months of life. There is no reason to believe that such infants have received sensitized lymphocytes from their mothers. As maternally acquired antibody wanes, the child becomes fully susceptible to chickenpox. Further evidence suggesting the importance of antibody for protection is seen in the efficacy of varicella-zoster hyperimmune globulin (VZIG) in protection of immunocompromised hosts (see Chapter 40). This regimen works very well either to prevent entirely or to significantly attenuate the severity of chickenpox. The role of the cellular immune system in terminating the disease process can be extremely important, as evidenced by the lethality of chickenpox in immunosuppressed patients.

The virus has an uncanny propensity for establishing latent or persistent infection of spinal cord ganglia, as do other herpesviruses. Decades later, in association with dwindling cell-mediated immune defense or subtle onset of an underlying malignant disorder, the virus may become activated and produce vesicular lesions. These lesions are essentially identical to those of varicella except that zoster lesions are ordinarily restricted to the region of skin over the dermatome innervated by the peripheral nerves originating from the ganglia that harbor the virus. This disease, called herpes zoster, or shingles, was once thought to be caused by a virus different from the varicella virus. It is now clear, however, that the same virus is responsible for both entities. If cellular immunity is profoundly and persistently impaired, the localized form of herpes zoster may become disseminated and life threatening (see Chapter 24).

## ERYTHEMA INFECTIOSUM (FIFTH DISEASE)

Similar-appearing childhood rashes were numbered as they were described and differentiated. Thus, erythema infectiosum was named "fifth disease" because it was described after scarlet fever, rubeola, rubella, and epidemic pseudoscarlatina. Erythema infectiosum is caused by the parvovirus B19.

Erythema infectiosum is a benign childhood disease whose principal feature is an exanthem, with mild or absent systemic toxicity and fever. The condition is easily diagnosed when the child has the classic presentation that includes very red cheeks ("slapped cheeks") and an erythematous rash in a lacy distribution over the extensor surfaces of the arms and legs. The rash may recur for several weeks upon exposure to sunlight or changes in temperature.

A variety of other rashes have been found during documented outbreaks of erythema infectiosum including vesicular, purpuric, and rubella-like rashes. None of these is sufficiently characteristic to make a clinical diagnosis.

Erythema infectiosum is a benign disease in the normal host. However, the propensity of the virus to affect red cell precursors in the bone marrow causes serious illness in two groups: the developing fetus and individuals with hemoglobinopathies. On occasion, *in utero* infections occur. Evidence from Great Britain suggests that overall risk of fetal loss associated with parvovirus B-19 is no greater than in a non–B-19 infected cohort, except during the second trimester when severe anemia may occur resulting in hydrops fetalis secondary to heart failure. As a result of inadequate myocardial function, death of the fetus is not uncommon. Fortunately, fetal infections occur infrequently. There are no known congenital anomalies associated with fetal B19 infection.

Children with hemoglobinopathies, such as sickle cell anemia, have circulating red cells with shortened lifespans. The transient interruption of red cell production by parvovirus B19 leads to a clinically significant anemia, the so-called aplastic crisis. Parvovirus B19 infection has occasionally caused long-lasting chronic anemia in individuals whose bone marrow has been damaged by chemotherapeutic agents or who have T-cell defects.

A variety of disease manifestations have been noted in adults. Approximately one fourth to one third may remain asymptomatic. One half to two thirds may have influenza-like illness, 50% a rash, and of particular concern, acute-onset polyarthropathy, which is more common in women than in men. The joint symptoms may persist from days to months, and may recur. Hands, feet, and knees, in a symmetric distribution, are the most frequently involved joints.

## ROSEOLA (EXANTHEM SUBITUM)

Until the etiology of this exanthem was discovered—human herpesvirus-6 (HHV-6)—roseola, was often described as a benign, although frightening, febrile disease of young children. The work of Hall and co-workers has markedly amplified our understanding of this common illness.

Only about 17% of children develop the classic illness with several days of fever, usually in excess of 39°C with no physical findings, culminating in rapid defervescence with the onset of a macular rash lasting 24–48 h. As a result of Hall's work, the spectrum of illness enlarged. While most newborns acquire anti–HHV-6 from the mother, nonetheless, infections occur in the first 4 months of life, suggesting that maternal antibody may not be present in sufficient amounts to prevent infection. Roseola, on the other hand, is infrequently seen after age 2, most children having acquired antibodies and hence, protection.

In Hall's study, HHV-6 accounted for approximately 10% of all emergency department visits for infants and young children with fever. Of particular note is the frequent association of HHV-6 infection with first febrile seizures, with about 12% of all children with HHV-6 infection manifesting a seizure. One third of all first-time febrile seizures presenting for care in an emergency department

were caused by this viral infection. While febrile seizures associated with seizure are frightening to parents, they rarely result in any permanent neurologic damage. However, more than one third of children with febrile seizures may have another seizure with a febrile illness.

Because cerebrospinal fluid (CSF) findings are normal in children with HHV-6 associated febrile seizures, one surmises that the seizure is indeed triggered by temperature elevation rather than by the virus invading or otherwise directly perturbing the central nervous system.

## KAWASAKI DISEASE

This illness was described by Dr. Tomisaku Kawasaki in 1967. He noted the appearance of a previously unrecognized febrile, exanthematous disease in Japanese children. Subsequently, this disease has been found throughout the world.

Were it not for the complication of coronary artery disease, Kawasaki syndrome would be but another curious viral exanthem. However, 20–25% of untreated patients develop aneurysms and some progress to subsequent stenosis of the coronary arteries, which may lead to significant coronary ischemia or even death if left untreated. Accordingly, the early recognition and treatment of this entity is mandatory to prevent fatal myocardial infarction, which occurs in about 0.2% of untreated children.

Typically, the illness begins with the onset of a high fever for several days. Initially, there may be no associated findings, although soon bulbar conjunctival injection without discharge begins, mucous membranes of the mouth become inflamed, and the lips may become fissured and cracked. The dorsa of the hands and feet often become swollen and a rash with pleomorphic features may occur over a variety of body surfaces. Urticarial lesions on erythematous plaques, and morbilliform and scarlatiniform erythroderma have all been described. The above features are each present in about 90% of children with Kawasaki disease. Enlargement of one or more cervical lymph nodes (≥1.5 cm) is seen in about 50% of affected children.

If left untreated, a subacute phase of the disease supervenes, characterized by anorexia, extreme irritability, persistent conjunctival injection, and desquamation of the fingers and toes. The desquamation typically begins in the periungal regions, usually involving only the distal parts of the fingers and toes, although on occasion more extensive desquamation of the hands and feet may occur. This phase of the illness lasts from about day 10 to day 25 after onset of the acute manifestations.

The third stage of the illness (convalescence) begins after all clinical signs of illness have abated, but an elevated erythrocyte sedimentation rate and thrombocytosis persist. It often takes 6–10 weeks for the sedimentation rate and platelet count to return to normal.

The fever of untreated Kawasaki disease frequently lasts 7–14 days. However, with the onset of the other clinical features mentioned above, the skillful physician will consider this diagnosis and institute intravenous gamma globulin and high-dose aspirin therapy. Although its mechanism of action is unknown, this treatment, when begun within 10 days of the onset of the fever, is highly effective in reducing coronary artery disease to fewer than 3% of recipients.

The etiology of this condition is presently unknown. The epidemic characteristics, which lead to outbreaks with little intervening endemic spread, suggest an infectious etiology. However, the search for the agent has been frustratingly difficult. Common bacterial and viral pathogens have been studied and excluded as possibilities. Similarly, retroviruses have been extensively looked for but not found. The search for the agent causing this entity is currently one of the most fascinating challenges in pediatric infectious disease.

## CASE HISTORIES

### CASE HISTORY 1

A mother brings a 4-year-old child to the office with a history of 4–5 days of fever to 104°F–105.6°F. The child has had red eyes, with no runny nose, but dry cracked lips. His hands and feet were not swollen. The rash, noticed a few days after the onset of fever, started on the head and spread caudally. The groin and diaper area were not particularly involved. The child's mother was concerned about the high fever causing brain damage. His brother had a similar illness starting 10 days ago. At the time that this disease was occurring, there was both an outbreak of Kawasaki disease and of measles in the community.

### CASE 1 DISCUSSION

One of the key questions to ask is if this child had been immunized against measles. If so, the likelihood is that he is immune. However, several other factors need to be taken into consideration. If the child was immunized prior to 1 year of age, the vaccine may not have been entirely effective because of persistence of maternal antibody interfering with the child's immune mechanism. If the child had been immunized prior to 1988 or 1989, when the vaccine was not stabilized as well as it is today, he may not have had an adequate immune response. If he had been immunized in 1990 or later, when the vaccine was stabilized, and if he were older than 12–15 months of age at the time of immunization, he has at least a 95% chance of being immune.

In both Kawasaki disease and measles, fever can occur before the onset of a rash. The measles rash typically begins on the head and spreads distally, while the rash for Kawasaki disease does not follow any particular progression. However, the rash in Kawasaki disease is often markedly worse in the groin than elsewhere. The child had conjunctivitis, which can be seen in both conditions, but the presence of conjunctival discharge strongly favors Kawasaki disease. He lacked the rhinorrhea that is typically seen in measles. He had dried, cracked lips, which can be seen in both Kawasaki's and measles, and he lacked swelling of the hands and feet, frequently seen in Kawasaki disease.

Given the presence of a measles outbreak and the progression of the rash, this illness is much more likely to be measles than Kawasaki disease. In support of this, outbreaks of Kawasaki disease may occur, but the cases are generally limited in number, and there is little spread to family members or close contacts. In contrast, during an outbreak of measles, there are hundreds to thousands of cases, and multiple cases in a household are common. This child's brother had been ill 10 days previously with a similar illness. The virus is highly contagious, and susceptibles in the presence of an active case are highly likely to develop measles. All things considered, the diagnosis is much more likely measles than Kawasaki disease.

### CASE HISTORY 2

A 4-year-old child with sickle cell disease has been noticed to become pale, somewhat lethargic, and short of breath on exertion. The mother comes to you frightened that something is terribly wrong with her child.

On examination, the child is indeed pale, and his conjunctivae are pale. He is alert and cooperative, but indicates that he doesn't have "much energy." Examination reveals a pulse rate of 120/min which is elevated for a 4-year-old who is afebrile. He also is noted to have an enlarged spleen.

Complete blood count (CBC) shows a hemoglobin of 4 g/dL with an elevated white count, and normal differential. He has no reticulocytes present in the peripheral smear. What infectious disease is likely?

## CASE 2 DISCUSSION

Children with sickle cell anemia have increased splenic destruction of their red blood cells and have palpable splenomegaly at least early in life. The life span of his red blood cells is likely 7–9 days once they are in the periphery. Thus, interruption of erythrogenesis for a few days will cause a rapid decline in the hemoglobin concentration. The fact that the child had no reticulocytes present in the peripheral smear is dramatic evidence that no erythrocytes are being produced from the bone marrow. One should be able to document that this child has acute parvovirus B19 by detecting antigen using polymerase chain reaction (PCR). Alternatively, one could make a retrospective diagnosis by showing a four-fold or greater rise in antibody titer to B19 in acute and convalescent sera.

# REFERENCES

## Books

Feigin, R. D., and Cherry, J. D., eds. *Textbook of Pediatric Infectious Diseases.* 3rd ed. Philadelphia: W. B. Saunders Co., 1992.

Krugman, S., Katz, S. L., Gershon, A. A., and Wilfert, C. M., eds. *Infectious Diseases of Children.* 9th ed. St. Louis: C. V. Mosby Co., 1992.

Lambert, H. P., and Farrar, W. E. *Infectious Diseases Illustrated. An Integrated Text and Color Atlas.* 2nd ed. Philadelphia: W. B. Saunders Co., 1992.

American Academy of Pediatrics. *1994 Red Book: Report of the Committee on Infectious Diseases.* 23rd ed. Elk Grove, IL: American Academy of Pediatrics, 1994.

## Review Articles

American Academy of Pediatrics, Committee on Infectious Diseases. Measles: Reassessment of the current immunization policy. *Pediatrics 84*:1110–1113, 1989.

Cherry, J. D. The "new" epidemiology of measles and rubella. *Hosp. Pract. 15*:49–57, 1980.

Fawzi, W. W., Chalmers, T. C., Herrera, M. G., and Mosteller, F. Vitamin A supplementation and child mortality. A meta-analysis. *JAMA 269*(7):898–903, 1993.

Lindegren, M. L., Fehrs, L. J., Hadler, S. C., and Hinman, A. R. Update: Rubella and congenital rubella syndrome, 1980–1990. *Epidemiol. Rev. 13*:341–348, 1991.

Rowley, A. H., Gonzalez-Crussi, F., and Shulman, S. T. Kawasaki syndrome. In: Barness, L. A., ed. *Adv. Pediatr.* 1991:51–74.

Ware, R. Human parvovirus infection. *J. Pediatr. 114*: 343–348, 1989.

## Original Articles

Asano, Y., Yoshikawa, T., Suga, S., et al. Viremia and neutralizing antibody response in infants with exanthem subitum. *J. Pediatr. 114*:535–539, 1989.

Breese Hall, C., Long, C. E., Schnabel, K. C., et al. Human herpesvirus-6 infection in children. A prospective study of complications and reactivation. *N. Engl. J. Med. 331*(7):432–438, 1994.

Brodsky, A. L. Atypical measles. Severe illness in recipients of killed measles virus vaccine upon exposure to natural infection. *JAMA 222*:1415–1416, 1972.

Centers for Disease Control. Current trends: Update: Childhood vaccine-preventable diseases—United States, 1994. *MMWR 43*(39):718–720, October 7, 1994.

Centers for Disease Control. Current trends: Rubella vaccination during pregnancy—United States, 1971–1982. *MMWR 32*:429, August 26, 1983.

Centers for Disease Control. Rubella and congenital rubella—United States, 1984–1986. *MMWR 36*:664, October 16, 1987.

Centers for Disease Control. Risks associated with human parvovirus B19 infection. *MMWR 38*:81, February 17, 1989.

Cherry, J. D., Feigin, R. D., Lobes, L. A., Jr., et al. Atypical measles in children previously immunized with attenuated measles virus vaccines. *Pediatrics 50*:712–717, 1972.

Clark, M., Boustred, J., Schild, G. C., et al. Effect of rubella vaccination programme on serological status of young adults in United Kingdom. *Lancet 1*:1224–1226, 1979.

Feldman, S., Hughes, W. T., and Daniel, C. B. Varicella in children with cancer: Seventy-seven cases. *Pediatrics 56*(3):388–397, 1975.

Frank, J. A., Jr., Orenstein, W. A., Bart, K. J., et al. Major impediments to measles elimination. The modern epidemiology of an ancient disease. *Am. J. Dis. Child. 139*: 881–888, 1985.

Hinman, A. R. Measles and rubella in adolescents and young adults. *Hosp. Pract. 17*:137–146, 1982.

Hinman, A. R., Orenstein, W. A., Bart, K., et al. Rational strategy for rubella vaccination. *Lancet 1*:39–41, 1983.

Kipps, A., Dick, G., and Moddie, J. W. Measles and the central nervous system. *Lancet 2*:1406–1410, 1983.

Marks, J. S., Halpin, T. J., and Orenstein, W. A. Measles vaccine efficacy in children previously vaccinated at 12 months of age. *Pediatrics 62*:955–960, 1978.

Public Health Laboratory Service Working Party on Fifth Disease. Prospective study of human parvovirus (B19) infection in pregnancy. *Br. Med. J. 300*:1166–1170, 1990.

Suringa, D. W. R., Bank, L. J., and Ackerman, A. B. Role of measles virus in skin lesions and Koplik's spots. *N. Engl. J. Med. 283*:1139–1142, 1970.

Woolf, A. D., Campion, G. V., Chishick, A., et al. Clinical manifestations of human parvovirus B19 in adults. *Arch. Intern. Med. 149*:1153–1165, 1989.

Yamanishi, K., Shiraki, K., Kondo, T., et al. Identification of human herpesvirus-6 as a causal agent for exanthem subitum. *Lancet 1*:1065–1067, 1988.

# 32

# SEPSIS

## JOHN R. WARREN, M.D.

The presence of bacteria or fungi in blood (*bacteremia* or *fungemia*) is transient, intermittent, or continuous. *Transient bacteremia* clears within a few minutes, and occurs as a result of instrument probing of colonized mucosal surfaces, especially dental procedures or cystoscopy, and as a consequence of surgery involving infected tissue, such as drainage of an abscess. Transient bacteremia is not significant except in patients with underlying valvular heart disease, for whom bacterial seeding of thrombi present on diseased cardiac valves can cause infective endocarditis (see Chapter 33). *Intermittent bacteremia* is associated primarily with an extravascular source of infection in tissue, most notably pneumonia, meningitis, pyelonephritis, osteomyelitis, peritonitis, pyogenic arthritis, subcutaneous soft tissue infection, and undrained abscesses. This form of bacteremia results from failure of the host to contain tissue infection, with intermittent escape of bacteria or fungi into the circulation via lymphatic vessels. For patients with intermittent bacteremia, approximately 75–80% of blood cultures obtained in a series of several cultures are positive (Fig. 32–1). *Continuous bacteremia* is a cardinal feature of intravascular foci of infection, especially infective endocarditis and contaminated intravenous catheters, but also infected arteriovenous fistulae and vascular aneurysms (*mycotic aneurysms*). When one blood culture from a patient with infective endocarditis is positive, the probability that subsequent blood cultures will be positive is 95–100% (Fig. 32–1).

The signs and symptoms of bacteremia and fungemia (*sepsis*) include hyperventilation, altered mental status, fever, chills, and occasionally hypothermia. The earliest clinical findings in bacteremia are hyperventilation with respiratory alkalosis and apprehension. Fever and chills generally follow, but in markedly debilitated patients, or in the very young or the very old, euthermia (normal body temperature) or hypothermia may be present. The mortality due to bacteremia and fungemia shows an inverse relationship with body temperature, with an increased risk of death among patients whose body temperature is low or normal during sepsis (Fig. 32–2). A serious complication of sepsis is the development of hypotension (*septic shock*), which can progress to hypoperfusion of tissues and organ failure with oliguria, jaundice, congestive heart failure, and metabolic lactic acidosis. Once shock occurs in bacteremic patients, the mortality rate increases severalfold. To

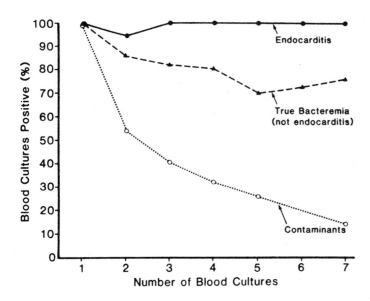

**FIGURE 32–1.** Patterns of positivity with successive blood cultures from patients with endocarditis, with nonendocarditis bacteremia, or with an initial culture contaminated by a skin commensal. The continuous bacteremia of endocarditis and the intermittent bacteremia secondary to tissue infection are indicated by the two top curves. With skin contaminants, the probability that subsequent blood cultures will be positive is very low. Also, if skin contaminants are detected in subsequent cultures, they are generally different from the contaminants detected in the initial culture (e.g., diphtheroids in the initial culture, followed by coagulase-negative staphylococci in a subsequent culture). (From Weinstein, M. P., Reller, L. B., Murphy, J. R., et al. *Rev. Infect. Dis.* 5:35, 1983. With permission.)

prevent septic shock, the bacterial or fungal cause of sepsis must be identified promptly using blood culture, and appropriate therapy initiated. Other complications of sepsis include adult respiratory distress syndrome (ARDS), bleeding due to disseminated intravascular coagulation (DIC), precipitous neutropenia, thrombocytopenia, and hemorrhagic (petechiae, purpura, ecchymoses) and ulcerative skin lesions.

Most septic patients demonstrate a focus of tissue infection as the source of their bacteremia, either intravascular or extravascular. This type of bacteremia is known as *secondary bacteremia*, and occurs most frequently in association with urinary and respiratory tract infection. Other important sources include intraabdominal infection (biliary tract, abscess, enteritis, peritonitis), and infections of wounds, the central nervous system (CNS), bone, soft tissue of skin, and intravascular catheters or heart valves. In a significant number of septic episodes, however, tissue or vascular sources of bacteremia are not identified, a circumstance designated as *primary bacteremia*. Bacterial flora of the intestinal tract are recognized as major pathogens in primary bacteremia. It has been postulated that motile phagocytes ingest intestinal bacteria, fail to achieve intracellular killing, transport the phagocytosed bacteria to extraintestinal sites *(translocation)*, and liberate the bacteria to cause bacteremia. Primary bacteremia can also be caused by direct invasion of intestinal microorganisms across ulcers and necrotic tumors of the gastrointestinal tract. Etiologic

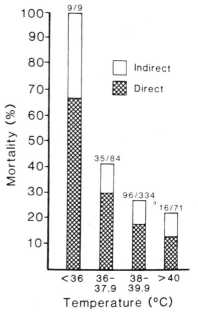

**FIGURE 32–2.** Outcome of bacteremia and fungemia in relation to body temperature. Two thirds of the hypothermic (<36°C) and about one third of the euthermic (36°–37.9°C) patients died as a direct result of sepsis. The lowest mortality was observed among patients with moderate (38–39.9°C) or marked (>40°C) fever. The total number of patients who died (numerator) and the total number of patients with the indicated temperature response (denominator) are reported at the top of each data bar. (From Weinstein, M. P., Murphy, J. R., Reller, L. B., et al. *Rev. Infect. Dis.* 5:54, 1983. With permission.)

agents in both primary and secondary sepsis include gram-negative bacteria, gram-positive bacteria, obligately anaerobic bacteria, and fungi, and sepsis can be due to a single organism *(monomicrobial)* or to multiple organisms *(polymicrobial).*

## GRAM-NEGATIVE BACTEREMIA

Highly virulent gram-negative bacteria, especially *Neisseria meningitidis, Yersinia pestis,* and *Salmonella typhi,* can cause fulminant or persistent bacteremia in the normal host. However, most bacteremic episodes due to gram-negative organisms occur in individuals with an underlying debilitating disease, are acquired in the hospital, and are often caused by microorganisms present in the endogenous flora. Cytokines and inflammatory mediators released in the bacteremic patient can result in life-threatening hemodynamic instability or pulmonary insufficiency.

### Clinical Aspects

The development of septic shock and/or ARDS is of paramount importance in gram-negative bacteremia. Shock is observed in 20–35% of patients with gram-negative bacteremia. In previously normotensive adults shock is clinically defined as systolic blood pressure less than 90 mm Hg and diastolic pressure less than 60 mm Hg. Peripheral vasodilatation with warm dry skin ("warm shock") is present initially, but if shock persists, skin and splanchnic vasoconstriction develops in an attempt to maintain blood flow to vital organs (brain, heart, kidneys), and the skin becomes pale and cool ("cold shock"). A moribund phase of shock with anuria reflects inability of compensatory mechanisms to maintain arterial perfusion of vital organs. A greatly increased mortality results from the development of shock in gram-negative bacteremia. ARDS is characterized by severe dyspnea, tachypnea, hypoxemia, and diffuse bilateral infiltrates on chest radiograph. The occurrence of ARDS reflects diffuse damage to both alveolar septal capillaries and alveolar lining epithelium of the lung, with fulminant interstitial and intraalveolar fibrinous exudation. ARDS usually occurs when shock has already complicated bacteremia. The mortality of ARDS due to gram-negative bacteremia is high (50–80%).

A fulminant variant of gram-negative bacteremia is caused by the gram-negative diplococcus *Neisseria meningitidis* (meningococcus). Hematogenous dissemination follows nasopharyngeal colonization with *N. meningitidis.* Meningococcemia is accompanied by activation of the blood coagulation system, with coagulation proteins and platelets being consumed (and depleted). The consumption coagulopathy, in turn, results in hemorrhage with dramatic development of skin petechiae and ecchymoses. Bilateral adrenal gland hemorrhage (Fig. 32–3), shock, and meningococ-

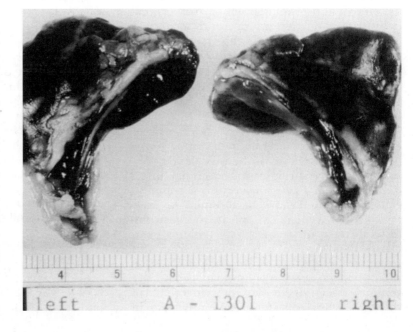

**FIGURE 32–3.** Adrenal gland hemorrhage in bacteremia due to *Neisseria meningitidis* (Waterhouse-Friderichsen syndrome). Endotoxic lipopolysaccharide activates factor XII (Hageman factor), which in turn activates the intrinsic coagulation system with formation of fibrin microthrombi. In fulminant meningococcemia (or other forms of gram-negative bacteremia), disseminated intravascular coagulation (DIC) can develop, resulting in tissue hemorrhage. DIC is a secondary reflection of severe gram-negative bacteremia and is not a primary cause of lethal shock. (From Warren, J. R., Scarpelli, D. G., Reddy, J. K., et al. *Essentials of General Pathology.* New York: Macmillan Publishing Company, 1987. With permission.)

cemia were first described as a syndrome by Waterhouse and Friderichsen. Another fulminant variant of gram-negative bacteremia is *plague*, a bacteremic infection due to *Yersinia pestis* in which mortality in untreated cases is greater than 50%. *Y. pestis* is a gram-negative coccobacillus transmitted to humans by contact with rodent fleas. A distinctive feature of plague is marked inflammatory enlargement of infected lymph nodes *(acute lymphadenitis)*, with large (1–10 cm) ovoid lymph node swellings *(buboes)* visible in the femoral, inguinal, axillary, and cervical regions. Patients with bubonic plague are typically febrile and hypotensive due to the *Y. pestis* bacteremia.

The sepsis of typhoid fever is a severe and prolonged disease, and *Salmonella typhi* is recovered from blood cultures in over 80% of patients during the first week of illness. The portal of entry for *S. typhi* is the small intestine. Following ingestion of organisms in contaminated food, the typhoid bacilli multiply in the small intestine, penetrate the mucosal barrier, infect mesenteric lymph nodes, and eventually enter the bloodstream through the thoracic duct to cause sepsis. The onset of typhoid fever is insidious. Fever is prominent, but the pulse is typically slow *(bradycardia)* relative to body temperature. Neutropenia due to bone marrow depression is almost uniformly present, following early transient leukocytosis. Bradycardia and neutropenia in a febrile septic patient strongly suggest *Salmonella* bacteremia. Complications of typhoid fever include toxic myocarditis, persistent and disseminated infection with *S. typhi* (arthritis, endocarditis, meningitis), gastrointestinal hemorrhage or perforation, and secondary bacterial pneumonia with an organism other than *S. typhi*. The mortality of untreated cases is 12–16%.

## Microbiologic Aspects

### Enterobacteriaceae

The most frequently observed organism in gram-negative bacteremia is *Escherichia coli* (Table 32–1) because of the prevalence of *E. coli* in pyelonephritis and abdominal infections. *Klebsiella pneumoniae* is also a common cause of gram-negative bacteremia. *K. pneumoniae* often replaces *E. coli* in the gastrointestinal tract of seriously ill patients, and causes life-threatening bacteremia from this reservoir. In addition, *K. pneumoniae* is a common etiologic agent of both urinary and respiratory tract infections. Other members of the family Enterobacteriaceae implicated in

gram-negative bacteremia (although not as frequently) are *Enterobacter* and *Serratia* species, as well as *Proteus* and *Providencia* species. As is true for *E. coli* and *K. pneumoniae*, bacteremia due to these organisms is frequently hospital acquired (nosocomial). *Proteus* and *Providencia* bacteremia is especially associated with urinary tract infection. *Salmonella* bacteremia, which often occurs in the normal host with enteric infection, is made worse by impairment of T-lymphocyte function, particularly in the acquired immunodeficiency syndrome (AIDS).

### Nonfermentative and Oxidase-Positive Fermentative Gram-Negative Rods

The *nonfermentative gram-negative rods*, most notably the oxidative organism *Pseudomonas aeruginosa*, closely follow the Enterobacteriaceae as a frequent cause of bacteremia (Table 32–1). Infection with *P. aeruginosa* is nearly always nosocomial, and generally occurs among severely ill, neutropenic, or burn patients. Other nonfermentative gram-negative organisms that cause nosocomial bacteremia are *Stenotrophomonas (Xanthomonas) maltophilia* and *Acinetobacter baumannii*. *S. maltophilia* is a motile, oxidative bacillus closely related to *Pseudomonas* but lacks cytochrome oxidase. *A. baumannii* is a nonmotile bacillus that also does not produce cytochrome oxidase. As with *P. aeruginosa*, resistance to multiple antimicrobial agents is an important aspect of bacteremia due to S. *maltophilia* and *A. baumannii*. Yet a third group of gram-negative rods is emerging as an important cause of sepsis in debilitated individuals, the *oxidase-positive fermenters*, particularly *Aeromonas hydrophila* and *Vibrio vulnificus* (Table 32–1). The natural habitat of *A. hydrophila* is water, and soft tissue (wound) or gastrointestinal tract infection related to exposure to fresh or salt water can result in bacteremia, particularly among patients with cirrhosis or malignancy. *V. vulnificus* bacteremia characteristically occurs among individuals with underlying liver disease who have recently ingested raw oysters. However, as with *A. hydrophila,* wound infection related to water exposure can also serve as a portal of entry.

### Fastidious Gram-Negative Bacteria

The fastidious gram-negative bacteria cause sepsis in a variety of clinical settings (Table 32–1). *Neisseria meningitidis* can cause fulminant sepsis in normal individuals but can also

## TABLE 32–1. ETIOLOGIC AGENTS OF GRAM-NEGATIVE BACTEREMIA

| GROUP | MICROORGANISMS |
| --- | --- |
| Oxidase-negative fermenters (Enterobacteriaceae)* | Escherichia coli<br>Klebsiella<br>Enterobacter<br>Serratia<br>Proteus<br>Providencia<br>Salmonella<br>Yersinia |
| Oxidase-positive nonfermenters[†] | Pseudomonas aeruginosa |
| Oxidase-negative nonfermenters[‡] | Stenotrophomonas (Xanthomonas) maltophilia<br>Acinetobacter baumannii |
| Oxidase-positive fermenters[§] | Aeromonas hydrophilia<br>Vibrio vulnificus |
| Fastidious species[‖] | Neisseria meningitidis and N. gonorrhoeae<br>Haemophilus influenzae, H. parainfluenzae, H. aphrophilus, and H. paraphrophilus<br>Cardiobacterium hominis<br>Actinobacillus actinomycetemcomitans |

*Fermentation is an oxidation–reduction process that utilizes a carbohydrate to produce ATP, and for which an organic acid serves as the final electron acceptor. Fermentation generates strong acids and $CO_2$, and is easily measured. Members of the family Enterobacteriaceae metabolize glucose fermentatively and lack the electron-transport enzyme of aerobic respiration, cytochrome oxidase.

[†]P. aeruginosa is an oxidative organism that produces the respiratory enzyme, cytochrome oxidase, and is incapable of glucose fermentation.

[‡]S. maltophilia and A. baumannii are aerobic organisms that are cytochrome oxidase–negative. S. maltophilia oxidizes maltose, hence its species designation.

[§]These organisms metabolize glucose fermentatively, but also produce cytochrome oxidase.

[‖]Fastidious bacteria require special nutritional media and ambient gases for their growth. Both Neisseria and Haemophilus species grow best on chocolate agar in the presence of $CO_2$. Likewise, increased $CO_2$ tension promotes the growth of Cardiobacterium hominis and Actinobacillus actinomycetemcomitans.

cause chronic and repeated episodes of bloodstream infection in individuals deficient in the fifth, sixth, seventh, or eighth component of complement (as can Neisseria gonorrhoeae). Bacteremia due to Haemophilus influenzae type b was a scourge of children between ages 3 months and 6 years, after the disappearance of maternal H. influenzae antibody and before the appearance of the child's own protective antibody. This has largely disappeared since the H.influenzae type b vaccine has been used (see Chapter 21). Finally, some infrequently occurring, fastidious, and slow-growing gram-negative species can be associated with endocarditis and systemic embolization, including several Haemophilus species (H. parainfluenzae, H. aphrophilus, H. paraphrophilus), Cardiobacterium hominis, and Actinobacillus actinomycetemcomitans (see Chapter 33).

## Pathophysiologic Mechanisms

Mechanisms of gram-negative sepsis operate in the dynamic context of host–parasite interaction and include both host defense factors and invasive and toxic properties of bacteria. On the host side of the equation, the nature and severity of underlying disease, the source of bacteremia, and the age of the host are critical determinants of outcome. The risk of death increases with age (older than 40 years), especially in individuals with neoplastic disease, asplenia, cirrhosis, granulocytopenia, renal failure, diabetes mellitus, or corticosteroid therapy. Mortality is high for bacteremic patients with a primary infected focus in the respiratory tract, a surgical wound, or an abscess. Properties of bacteria that promote host invasion include adherence to mucosal surfaces via specific adhesin molecules in surface pili (Fig. 32–4), resistance to complement-dependent lysis in the absence of antibody, resistance to neutrophil phagocytosis due to surface encapsulation, and production by bacteria of protein enzymes and toxins that cause tissue necrosis and thereby facilitate spread of infection. Pseudomonas aeruginosa produces elastases, which degrade extracellular connective tissue matrix and blood vessel walls, and exotoxin A, which inhibits tissue protein synthesis by a mechanism analogous to that of diphtheria toxin (ADP-ribosylation of elongation factor 2) (see Chapter 4).

The outer membrane antigens of gram-negative bacteria are of fundamental importance in determining host responses to bacteremia. Polysaccharide O antigens of the outer membrane are composed of long chains of repeating carbohydrate units exposed on the surface of bacterial cells (Fig. 32–4). The carbohydrate composition of O antigens shows strain variation within individual gram-negative species. For example, there are more than 160 different strains of Escherichia coli, each with a unique O antigen. O-antigen chains are linked to a core region, which consists of an acidic oligosaccharide of N-acetyl-glucosamine, glucose, galactose, heptose phosphate, and 2-keto-3-deoxyoctonate (KDO). The KDO residues link the core polysaccharide to an acylated glucosamine disaccharide termed lipid A

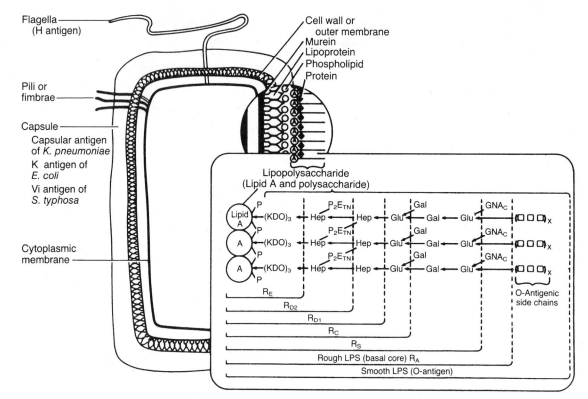

**FIGURE 32–4.** Schematic depiction of endotoxic lipopolysaccharide (LPS) and its position in the gram-negative bacterial cell wall. Lipid A anchors LPS in the outer membrane, and core and O-antigen arise from lipid A as linear polysaccharides. The chemical structure of smooth wild-type (S) and rough (R) mutant strains of *Salmonella* is shown in the insert. The R mutants $R_A$, $R_B$, $R_C$, $R_{D1}$, $R_{D2}$, and $R_E$ are shown in order of increasing roughness, resulting from deletion of O-antigen and core polysaccharide. The core polysaccharide includes *N*-acetylglucosamine ($GNA_C$), glucose (Glu), galactose (Gal), heptose (Hep), ethanolamine ($E_{TN}$), and phosphate (P). Lipid A is present in all pathogenic gram-negative bacteria, and the carbohydrate 2-keto-3-deoxyoctonate (KDO), which links lipid A to core antigen, is present in most, except for a few obligate anaerobes. Also depicted are the pili (or fimbriae), which contain adhesins, the antiphagocytic capsule, and the cytoplasmic membrane of the bacterial cell. The periplasmic space is located between the cytoplasmic membrane and the murein (peptidoglycan) layer. (From McCabe, W. R. Endotoxin: Microbiological, chemical, pathophysiologic and clinical correlations. In: Weinstein, L., and Fields, B. N., eds. *Seminars in Infectious Disease.* Vol. 3. New York: Thieme-Stratton, 1980:38–88. With permission.)

(Fig. 32–5). Lipid A is amphipathic (both hydrophilic and lipophilic) because of the simultaneous presence of both a hydrophilic structure (phosphorylated glucosamine disaccharide) and lipophilic structures (long-chain fatty acids). This molecular composition is unique to lipid A and is highly conserved among diverse species of gram-negative bacteria. The macromolecular complex composed of O antigen, core oligosaccharide, and lipid A is called *endotoxic lipopolysaccharide* (LPS). Endotoxic LPS is the dominant structure present in the gram-negative outer membrane and is held within the outer membrane by a combination of noncovalent hydrophobic and electrostatic bonds. Endotoxic LPS in-

duces tissue inflammation, fever, and shock in the infected host, and lipid A structures carry the toxic conformations of LPS responsible for these host reactions. Highly ordered and rigidly packed structures of fatty acid chains and the charged functional groups of the phosphorylated diglucosamine are essential for induction of host reactions. The hydrophilic polysaccharides of O and core-region antigen are needed to make lipid A soluble, thereby facilitating delivery of lipid A to cellular and plasma protein targets, but these hydrophilic polysaccharides do not play a direct role in LPS toxicity.

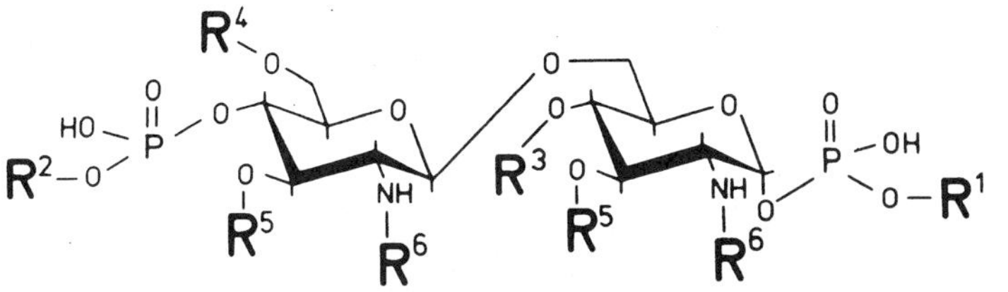

**FIGURE 32–5.** Structure of lipid A. The phosphorylated diglucosamine backbone possesses O-linked (at position $R^5$) and *N*-linked (at position $R^6$) 3-hydroxy long-chain fatty acids. Frequently, a second long-chain fatty acid is esterified to the 3-hydroxy group of the primary fatty acid chain. A variety of constituents can be linked to the phosphate groups at positions $R^1$ and $R^2$, including another phosphate group, phosphoryl ethanolamine, D-glucosamine, or furanosidic D-arabinose. Linkage to KDO occurs at position $R^4$ to the primary 6'-hydroxyl group. (From Rietschel, E. Th., Wollenweber, H-W., Russa, R., et al. Concepts of the chemical structure of lipid A. *Rev. Infect. Dis.* 6:432, 1984. With permission.)

## Paracrine and Systemic Mechanisms

Endotoxic LPS initiates the pathophysiologic reactions of gram-negative sepsis, as demonstrated by the following observations:

1. LPS injection in humans and experimental animals induces chills, fever, and shock.
2. High plasma levels of LPS correlate with high mortality in septic patients.
3. Mortality due to shock can be reduced by LPS antibodies.

However, LPS is not directly toxic. Rather, the lipid A moiety of LPS binds to an acute-phase plasma protein called *LPS-binding protein* (LBP), and the LPS/LBP complex in turn binds with high affinity to monocytes and macrophages. Another plasma protein, *septin*, also binds LPS and, like LBP, enhances presentation of low LPS concentrations to monocytes and macrophages. Binding of LPS/LBP occurs to the monocyte differentiation protein *CD14*, and induces the synthesis and secretion by monocytes and macrophages of the polypeptide cytokines *tumor necrosis factor* (TNF) (cachectin) and *interleukin 1* (IL-1). The biologic effects of TNF and IL-1 are expressed both locally in tissue *(paracrine effects)* and systemically. Paracrine effects are directed primarily to the vascular endothelium. Both cytokines induce the synthesis and surface expression of endothelial adhesion molecules, including *E-selectin, intercellular adhesion molecule 1* (ICAM-1), and *vascular cell adhesion molecule 1* (VCAM-1), thereby enhancing adherence of neutrophils to the vascular endothelium (Fig. 32–6). Also, endothelial membrane cyclooxygenase activity is stimulated, producing potent prostaglandin vasodilators. Vasodilatation with increased blood flow, and neutrophil adherence to vascular endothelium, strongly promote inflammation with plasma exudation of antibody and complement, and emigration of phagocytic cells into infected tissue. The paracrine effects of TNF and IL-1 are enhanced by the ability of LPS to activate the alternative complement pathway and Hageman factor (factor XII). Complement activation generates the anaphylatoxins, C3a and C5a, which increase blood vessel permeability by stimulation of histamine release from tissue mast cells and blood basophils. C5a is also a strong chemoattractant (chemotaxin) and activator of blood neutrophils. Factor XII activation leads to generation of the vasodilatory nonapeptide bradykinin.

These inflammatory mechanisms promote the clearance of gram-negative bacteria from infected tissue. However, in sepsis tissue clearance mechanisms are overwhelmed, and bacteremia ensues from the release of organisms into the systemic circulation. Free LPS also escapes from dead bacteria in tissue abscesses and enters the bloodstream via draining lymphatics. Failure of the septic patient to prevent bacterial dissemination results in circulating LPS and cytokines, especially TNF, resulting in "systemic activation" of vascular endothelium. Clinical studies reveal that plasma levels of TNF are high and sustained in patients who do not survive septic shock. In addition to TNF actions on endothelial cells, circulating soluble CD14 also mediates LPS activation of endothelial cells. Generalized vasodilatation and increased blood vessel permeability lead to reduction in the effective blood volume and hypovolemic shock. Pulmonary leukostasis (Fig. 32–6), with its accompanying local neutrophilic release of oxygen radicals (especially hydroxyl radicals) and neutral proteases (especially elastase), causes endothelial and alveolar epithelial damage, effecting the development of ARDS. Excessive complement activation with C3a and (especially) C5a, and markedly accelerated factor XII activation with bradykinin production also both contribute to septic shock and ARDS. An increased concentration of activated complement has been associated with fatal outcome in septic shock, and bradykinin antagonists show protection in animal models of sepsis.

### Fever

Both TNF and IL-1 induce fever through their ability to stimulate hypothalamic synthesis of prostaglandins $E_1$ and $E_2$, which stimulate the firing of thermosensitive neurons. Elevated body temperature reduces the replication of many bacteria and also augments helper T-cell activation and antibody synthesis by B cells. Consequently, fever as an acute-phase systemic reaction is beneficial to the host (see Fig. 32–2).

### LPS and Cytokine Inhibitors

Bactericidal/permeability-increasing protein (BPI) is a cationic protein stored in cytoplasmic azurophilic granules of neutrophils. BPI has 45% sequence homology with LBP, but unlike LBP which enhances LPS actions, BPI neutralizes the biologic effects of LPS by binding the lipid A moiety of LPS, including cytokine production. Thus, BPI released from neutrophils during tissue inflammation would inhibit LPS toxicity. Circulating *soluble TNF re-ceptor* (sTNFR) has been detected in the serum of septic patients. By competitive binding, sTNFR functions as a TNF antagonist, thereby protecting against endotoxic shock. Also, a small protein *IL-1 receptor antagonist* (IL-1ra), has been isolated from the urine of febrile patients as well as from culture supernatants of activated macrophages. BPI, sTNFR, and IL-1ra acting together serve to inhibit both the LPS-induced production and direct actions of cytokines in gram-negative sepsis.

## GRAM-POSITIVE BACTEREMIA

Gram-positive bacteremia has become more frequent in recent years. This increase is due primarily to growing utilization of intravascular catheters, CNS ventricular shunts, and surgical placement of prosthetic devices, all of which disrupt natural mucocutaneous barriers and introduce foreign bodies into tissue. Many blood isolates of gram-positive bacteria demonstrate resistance to multiple antibiotics. Consequently, prompt recognition of gram-positive bacteremia is necessary to ensure effective antimicrobial therapy.

### Clinical Aspects

Although shock and ARDS may develop, these complications are not as common as in gram-negative bacteremia. Patients typically present with signs and symptoms of local infection, such as pneumonia, meningitis,

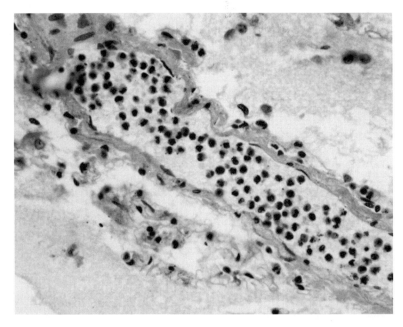

**FIGURE 32–6.** Leukostasis in ARDS caused by increased adherence of polymorphonuclear neutrophils to endothelium of pulmonary blood vessels. (Photomicrograph courtesy of Dr. Kenneth Haines, Department of Pathology, Northwestern University Medical School.)

wound infection, skin abscess, or endocarditis. Two major concerns arise in gram-positive bacteremia. First, metastatic dissemination of infection is common. For example, during *Staphylococcus aureus* bacteremia, organisms can directly seed the kidneys from the bloodstream, causing acute pyelonephritis and numerous cortical abscesses. The recovery of *S. aureus* from urine culture is an important clue that the patient is bacteremic with *S. aureus*, as this organism rarely causes primary urinary tract infection. Second, many gram-positive bacteria can directly infect heart valves. Thus, patients bacteremic with these organisms must be carefully evaluated for endocarditis (see Chapter 33).

## Microbiologic Aspects

### Gram-Positive Cocci

Among the gram-positive cocci, the staphylococci, enterococci, and streptococci are important causes of bacteremia (Table 32–2). Bacteremia with *Staphylococcus aureus* (coagu-

**TABLE 32–2. ETIOLOGIC AGENTS OF GRAM-POSITIVE BACTEREMIA**

| GROUP | MICROORGANISMS |
|---|---|
| Gram-positive | |
| Catalase-positive* | *Staphylococcus aureus* (coagulase-positive) *Staphylococcus epidermidis* (coagulase-negative) |
| Catalase-negative | *Enterococcus faecalis*[†] *Streptococcus pneumoniae*[‡] *Streptococcus viridans*[‡] |
| Gram-positive rods[§] | |
| Nonhemolytic | *Corynebacterium jeikeium* |
| Hemolytic | *Listeria monocytogenes* |

*Catalase is an intracellular enzyme that decomposes hydrogen peroxide to water and $O_2$, and is uniformly present in staphylococci. Coagulase is a thrombin-like substance that causes visible clotting of plasma, and its presence identifies catalase-positive, gram-positive cocci as *Staphylococcus aureus*. Among the coagulase-negative species, *S. epidermidis* is most common, but *S. hominis*, *S. haemolyticus*, *S. simulans*, and others can cause bloodstream infection.

[†]Enterococcus was previously classified as a group D streptococcus, but nucleic acid hybridization measurements reveal little genetic relatedness of enterococci to the genus *Streptococcus*. *E. faecalis* is responsible for about 90% of enterococcal bloodstream infections, with occasional infections caused by *E. faecium*.

[‡]*S. pneumoniae* is an alpha-hemolytic *Streptococcus* that is bile-soluble and susceptible to lysis by the detergent optochin. The viridans streptococci are alpha-hemolytic (or rarely, nonhemolytic) and lack both bile solubility and optochin sensitivity. *S. mitior* and *S. sanguis* are the viridans streptococci most often associated with endocarditis.

[§]*Corynebacterium jeikeium* grows as a nonhemolytic, penicillin-resistant, gram-positive bacillus on blood agar, whereas colonies of *L. monocytogenes* demonstrate distinct zones of beta-(clear) hemolysis on blood agar.

lase-positive staphylococci) most often occurs in older hospitalized patients with underlying disease, children, patients with vascular access infections, or young adults who acquire their infection in the community by intravenous drug abuse. The overall incidence of endocarditis in adult *S. aureus* bacteremia is 5–20%. The coagulase-negative staphylococci have also been implicated in nosocomial bloodstream infections, especially *Staphylococcus epidermidis*. Emergence of coagulase-negative staphylococci as blood pathogens is due to their great numbers on the skin and their ability to adhere to surfaces of vascular catheters and prosthetic implants. Although endocarditis involving native heart valves is not often caused by *S. epidermidis*, coagulase-negative staphylococci frequently produce prosthetic valve endocarditis.

The enterococci (Table 32–2) are normally found in the feces, and bacteremia due to these organisms is very frequently hospital-acquired. Prolonged hospitalization and the use of cephalosporins, which have little or no activity against the enterococci, are important risk factors for the development of enterococcal bacteremia. *Enterococcus* is unusual in that, unlike other gram-positive bacteria, bacteremia with this organism is associated with a high overall mortality (~40%). Around 2–8% of patients with enterococcal bacteremia have endocarditis. The *viridans streptococci* (alpha-hemolytic, or green, streptococci) continue to account for the majority of cases of endocarditis (Table 32–2). Finally, the isolation of *Streptococcus pneumoniae* in blood culture always indicates bacteremia, which occurs most often in association with pneumococcal pneumonia or meningitis. Certain groups of patients are at increased risk of pneumococcal bacteremia, including *asplenic individuals* (autosplenectomy in sickle cell anemia, congenital, traumatic, surgical removal), patients with B-cell lymphoma or leukemia, and individuals with multiple myeloma. This increased risk reflects the importance of opsonizing antibody and splenic clearance in host defense against heavily encapsulated pneumococci.

### Gram-Positive Rods

A number of gram-positive rods also produce bacteremia, most notably the diphtheroid *Corynebacterium jeikeium* (JK), and *Listeria monocytogenes*. Although diphtheroids are most often normal skin commensals, *Corynebacterium jeikeium* causes nosocomial bacteremia in patients with indwelling catheters, in those with extended periods of granulocytopenia due to hematologic malignancy, or in those who have undergone bone marrow transplantation. As many as 20% of blood isolates of *Corynebacterium jeikeium* are associated with serious nosocomial infection. *Corynebacterium jeikeium* has also been isolated from patients with prosthetic valve endocarditis. *L. monocytogenes* is a facultative intracellular parasite whose dissemination is favored by immaturity or impairment of T-lymphocyte function. Meningitis is often present in listeriosis, and endocarditis can occur.

### Pathophysiologic Mechanisms

Shock and ARDS occur in gram-positive sepsis, primarily as a result of excessive cytokine and inflammatory mediator production. Cell-free supernatants from cultures of gram-positive bacteria induce TNF release from monocytes, and TNF concentrations in the serum of patients with gram-positive sepsis are as high as serum TNF levels for patients with gram-negative sepsis. But in contrast to gram-negative bacteria, a unique, highly conserved, and toxic cell-wall antigen analogous to LPS has not been discovered. Metastatic infection and a propensity to produce tissue abscesses are the dominant pathophysiologic determinants in gram-positive bacteremia.

## ANAEROBIC BACTEREMIA

The obligately anaerobic bacteria fail to multiply when exposed to the oxygen tension of air. Many indigenous anaerobic bacteria grow on mucosal surfaces where local oxygen tension is sufficiently low. Large concentrations of anaerobic bacteria are thus found in gingival crevices of the oral cavity, the distal ileum and colon, and the endocervix and vagina. Anaerobic bacteremia in most instances represents infection related to these indigenous organisms.

### Clinical Aspects

Anaerobic bacteremia is most often associated with intraabdominal abscess, infection of the female genital tract, or aspiration pneumonia. The development of hypotension is relatively common, especially with gram-negative species.

### Microbiologic Aspects

The bacteriology of anaerobic bacteremia depends on the portal of entry. *Bacteroides fragilis,* an anaerobic, gram-negative bacillus, is the dominant isolate in intraabdominal sepsis. *Bacteroides* organisms, including *B. bivius* and other *Bacteroides* species, are commonly associated with bacteremic genital tract infections, along with the anaerobic, gram-positive *Peptostreptococcus. Bacteroides, Peptostreptococcus,* and anaerobic gram-negative *Fusobacterium nucleatum* are frequently recovered in patients with bacteremic aspiration pneumonia. The variable bacteriology reflects the indigenous flora at the different portals of entry.

### Pathophysiologic Mechanisms

Isolation of anaerobic bacteria from blood cultures suggests a breach in a normal mucocutaneous barrier, such as occurs in colon carcinoma with obstruction or perforation, in inflammatory bowel disease, and in gynecologic surgery or obstetric procedures. Compromised consciousness is a predisposing factor in the aspiration of colonized or infected material from the oral cavity, which leads to pleuropulmonary infection.

A number of virulence factors have been identified for anaerobic organisms. *Bacteroides fragilis* possesses a polysaccharide capsule that impedes phagocytosis and promotes abscess formation. Also, many anaerobic organisms produce succinic acid, which inhibits phagocytic killing at the low pH of abscesses. Anaerobic gram-negative bacteria contain LPS, but *Bacteroides* LPS lacks KDO and beta-hydroxymyristic acid and is without toxicity when injected into primates. However, *Fusobacterium* contains a biologically active LPS.

## POLYMICROBIAL BACTEREMIA

Polymicrobial bacteremia is the isolation of more than one microorganism from blood culture in a single episode of sepsis. Polymicrobial bacteremia is detected in around 10% of bacteremic patients and in the vast majority of cases is hospital acquired. Polymicrobial bacteremia most often arises from infections in sites contiguous to body surfaces normally colonized with bacteria, including the gastrointestinal and female genital tracts and the skin. Thus, intraabdominal infections (abscesses, cholangitis), pelvic abscesses, necrotizing fasciitis, decubitus ulcers, and subcutaneous soft tissue infections are common sources for polymicrobial bacteremia. The Enterobacteriaceae, enterococci, and anaerobic bacteria are disproportionately frequent in polymicrobial bacteremia, which reflects intestinal and genital tract colonization with these organisms. Polymicrobial bacteremia is often detected among patients with underlying malignant disease, especially acute leukemia, who have undergone immunosuppressive therapy and invasive procedures. Shock and death directly related to sepsis are more frequent in polymicrobial than in monomicrobial bacteremia.

## FUNGEMIA

The presence of fungi in the bloodstream is known as *fungemia*. The incidence of fungemia has risen in recent years, especially fungemia due to yeast forms. *Candida* species are the most common fungi isolated from blood. Ulceration of the normal gastrointestinal mucosa, usually due to a carcinoma or therapy for malignant disease with cytotoxic drugs, and overgrowth of the gastrointestinal flora with *Candida* after treatment with broad-spectrum antibiotics facilitate invasion of the bloodstream by gut *Candida*. Additionally, disruption of the skin by catheters and wounds predisposes to candidemia. Phagocytic neutrophils and T lymphocytes constitute major host defense mechanisms against invasion by *Candida*. As a consequence, illnesses or treatment modalities that cause neutropenia or loss of T lymphocytes are frequently complicated by candidemia. The clinical presentation of candidemia resembles bacteremia, with fever that can progress to hypotension, metabolic acidosis, and ARDS.

*Cryptococcus neoformans* is an encapsulated yeast that produces meningitis and fungemia. Appearance of cryptococci in the blood indicates suppression of host T-lymphocyte function, and cryptococcal infection occurs in approximately 10% of AIDS patients. CNS signs in cryptococcal meningitis are highly variable and may be minimal. Consequently, detection of *C. neoformans* in blood culture is often the first sign of cryptococcosis in an AIDS patient.

## LABORATORY DIAGNOSIS OF SEPSIS

Most bacteremias and fungemias in adults are of a low order of magnitude, that is, relatively few organisms are present per milliliter of blood. Adult patients septic with Enterobacteriaceae, *Pseudomonas*, *Staphylococcus*, *Strepto-*

*coccus,* anaerobic bacteria, or yeast are generally culture-positive for 10 or fewer organisms per milliliter of blood, and frequently fewer than one organism is detected per milliliter of blood. Detection of bacteremia or fungemia requires at least one viable microorganism in the sample of blood cultured. Consequently, a blood specimen smaller than 10 mL will miss many bacteremic episodes in adults, and at least 10 mL and preferably 20–30 mL of blood should be obtained for each blood culture. In infants and children, the magnitude of bacteremia is usually far greater, so that smaller volumes of blood (1–5 mL) are sufficient.

In addition to low intensity, most bacteremias are intermittent. To increase the probability of detecting bacteremia, two or three blood cultures should be obtained to evaluate each episode of sepsis, and if possible each blood culture should be obtained at 1-h intervals. The diagnosis of bacteremia can be established in 99% of patients with three separate blood cultures (Fig. 32–7). In most instances it is not necessary to submit more than three cultures to the clinical microbiol-

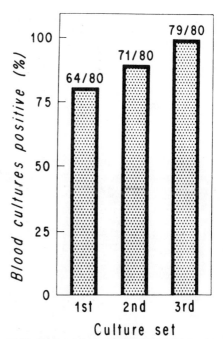

**FIGURE 32–7.** Cumulative rates of positivity in three blood culture sets obtained from bacteremic patients. A broth culture system was utilized in this study of 80 patients. The number of positive patients with one, two, and three culture sets is reported at the top of each data bar. (From Washington, J. A., II. Blood cultures: Principles and techniques. *Mayo Clin. Proc. 50*:91, 1975. With permission.)

ogy laboratory. However, occasional patients have received antibiotics prior to admission, and concern may arise that the antibiotics might suppress growth of organisms in blood culture. In this setting, it is reasonable to obtain another two blood cultures on each of three successive days, if cultures from the previous days are negative.

### Discrimination between Bacteremia and Contamination

The skin is heavily colonized with coagulase-negative staphylococci, *Corynebacterium* species, alpha-hemolytic streptococci, and the lipophilic anaerobic organism *Propionibacterium acnes*. Despite rigorous aseptic technique in the collection of blood, 2–3% of blood cultures are contaminated with these skin commensals. Because patients can develop bona fide sepsis with these organisms, it is necessary to discriminate true bacteremia from contamination. If only one of multiple blood cultures is positive for coagulase-negative staphylococci, *Corynebacterium*, or alpha-hemolytic streptococci, the isolate is probably a skin contaminant (see Fig. 32–1). However, if the same organism is recovered from two or more blood cultures, the isolate is a likely cause of a septic episode. Thus, not only are multiple blood cultures important for the detection of intermittent bacteremia, but they are needed to document true bacteremia due to gram-positive organisms generally regarded as skin contaminants. Presence of gram-negative bacteria or yeast in a single blood culture generally indicates true bacteremia or fungemia.

### Diagnostic Methods

The laboratory diagnosis of bacteremia and fungemia is accomplished using broth, lysis-concentration, and biphasic culture methods (Table 32–3). The responsibility of the clinical microbiology laboratory is to identify the species of bacteria and fungi responsible for sepsis and to assess the antibiotic susceptibility of bacterial isolates. Direct communication between the clinical microbiology laboratory and the patient's physician is ideal, since bacteremia is acute and life threatening and the

**TABLE 32–3   BLOOD CULTURE METHODS FOR THE LABORATORY DIAGNOSIS OF BACTEREMIA AND FUNGEMIA**

| BLOOD CULTURE METHOD | PRINCIPLE |
| --- | --- |
| Broth | Culture bottles containing nutrient broth (tryptic or trypticase soy, supplemented peptone, Columbia) are inoculated with blood. Each blood culture consists of at least two culture bottles, one of which is incubated under aerobic conditions and the other under anaerobic conditions. Blood cultures are monitored for bacterial and fungal growth by turbidity, gas, colony formation, hemolysis, and Gram's stains of broth smears. Gas production is detected by appearance of bubbles in the broth. Automated blood culture systems detect growth by monitoring change in pH, $CO_2$ production, or consumption of $O_2$. |
| Lysis-centrifugation | Following lysis of red and white cells in blood, bacteria or fungi present are concentrated into a pellet by centrifugation. The pellet is then inoculated to solid growth media for recovery of microorganisms. |
| Biphasic | Culture bottles are designed to permit immersion of solid growth media in nutrient broth inoculated with blood by tilting or inverting the bottles. Microorganisms in blood can thus be recovered by growth in broth or on solid media. |

physician must have accurate and comprehensive information for effective therapy.

Endotoxic LPS induces coagulation of extracts obtained from the pluripotential hematologic cell (amebocyte) of the horseshoe crab, *Limulus polyphemus*. This property forms the basis of the *in vitro Limulus gelation assay* (LGA), which is sensitive to trace quantities (0.1 pg/mL) of LPS. The LGA has found application in the screening of parenteral fluids for absence of LPS contamination and also in the laboratory testing of cerebrospinal fluid (CSF) for the rapid diagnosis of gram-negative meningitis. High plasma LPS levels measured by LGA correlate with development of severe septic shock in systemic meningococcal disease. Also, plasma levels of free LPS are elevated after administration of bactericidal antibiotics to patients with gram-negative bacteremia. Often, the clinical condition of such patients worsens despite bactericidal antibiotic therapy, perhaps due to free LPS released by antibiotic-induced bacterial cell lysis. The inflammatory mediators TNF and IL-1 can be detected by immunoassay in the blood of bacteremic patients. Laboratory measurement of plasma LPS and inflammatory mediators is not generally available, but it holds promise for use in the future to assess patient prognosis.

## THERAPY OF BACTEREMIA AND FUNGEMIA

Removal of infected catheters or other intravascular devices and drainage of infected tissue are necessary for the effective treatment of bloodstream infection. Sepsis generally begins with proliferation of microorganisms at sites of tissue infection. Thus, identification of the infecting microorganism and characterization of its antibiotic susceptibility are important. Early initiation of appropriate antibiotic therapy is associated with improved survival. In patients who develop septic shock, supportive therapy with fluid replacement and vasopressor amines is necessary.

Perfusion of vital organs, especially the brain and heart, must be maintained in the patient with septic shock. The first goal is volume replacement with crystalloid solutions, in order to expand intravascular fluid volume. If aggressive volume replacement fails to maintain blood pressure, sympathomimetic amines should be considered, especially dopamine. At low doses dopamine exerts a positive ino-

tropic effect on the myocardium while reducing regional arterial resistance in the kidneys, heart, and brain. The end result is an increase in systolic blood pressure and heart rate and an increased flow of blood to these vital organs. The administration of corticosteroids or anticoagulants is, in general, not indicated. Adjunctive treatments are currently being developed that either block the production of cytokines in sepsis, or inhibit their actions. Candidate therapies include monoclonal antibodies to LPS, recombinant BPI, and nontoxic lipid A analogues which block LPS actions, and monoclonal antibodies to TNF, chimeric sTNFR, and recombinant Il-1ra which inhibit cytokines. In addition, a number of drugs are being studied that block inflammatory mediators involved in the vasodilation and increased vascular permeability of septic shock. Important examples of this group include antagonists of the potent inflammatory mediator *platelet activating factor* (PAF), and inhibitors of nitric oxide (NO) synthesis by vascular endothelium. Synthesis of NO by endothelium is stimulated by LPS and cytokines, and NO is an important mediator of the profound vasodilation in septic shock. The multifactorial nature of septic shock requires use of antibiotics, fluid replacement, and vasopressor therapy as necessary for the individual patient. It is hoped that adjunctive therapy based on pathophysiologic actions of bacterial cell-wall components, cytokines, and inflammatory mediators will soon be available for general clinical use.

## CASE HISTORY

### CASE HISTORY 1

A 65-year-old man complained of abdominal pain, nausea, and vomiting. The patient had recently been diagnosed as having type II (non–insulin-dependent) diabetes mellitus. Physical examination revealed a temperature of 100.2°F, pulse rate of 86/min, respiration of 20/min, and blood pressure of 132/88 mm Hg. The abdomen was tender to palpation in the epigastric to right upper quadrant, but rebound tenderness or guarding was not evident. On the second hospital day, jaundice became apparent, and abdominal ultrasound revealed gallstones with dilatation of the hepatic ducts and gallbladder. Three sets of blood cultures were positive for *Klebsiella pneumoniae* and *Enterococcus faecalis*. Treatment was begun with intravenous ampicillin-sulbactam and gentamicin, and by the sixth hospital day the patient was afebrile, blood cultures were negative, and antimicrobial chemotherapy was discontinued. The patient underwent a cholecystectomy, and bile and peritoneal cultures obtained at the time of surgery were negative. However, a few days following surgery the patient again became febrile, and was found to have a white blood cell (WBC) count of 22,000/mm³ with 50% polymorphonuclear leukocytes (PMNs) and 34% immature band forms. Laboratory evaluation showed elevated serum amylase and lipase levels, and three blood culture sets were positive for *Klebsiella pneumoniae*. Antimicrobial therapy was instituted with ampicillin-sulbactam, but the patient progressed to severe respiratory distress and hypoxemia, and developed refractory hypotension. Resuscitation efforts were unsuccessful.

At autopsy, the right ventricular cavity of the heart was filled with coils of an embolus, which extended into the large pulmonary arteries near the hilum of both lungs. Thus, the immediate cause of death in this patient was acute pulmonary embolism. Microscopic examination of the lung showed marked leukostasis in pulmonary blood vessels and severe intraalveolar edema. Sections through the pancreas revealed a large intrapancreatic abscess in the junction between the head and body, and another abscess cavity immediately adjacent to the pancreatic tail. The peripancreatic fat demonstrated numerous gray to tan plaques of acute enzymic fat necrosis, and eight loculated abscesses were present in the retroperitoneal adipose tissue adjacent to the pancreas. Gram's staining of smears prepared from the pancreatic and peripancreatic abscesses revealed gram-negative rods and many neutrophils, and culture of aspirated pus was positive for *Klebsiella pneumoniae*. Enteric bacteria can reach the pancreas by reflux of contaminated bile, particularly in patients with biliary obstruction. It is likely that reflux of bacteria into the pancreas of this patient occurred secondary to cholelithiasis, with accompanying development of pancreatic and retroperitoneal abscesses; gram-negative bacteremia was a complication of the abscesses. The presence of leukostasis and edema in the lung suggest early vascular injury due to gram-negative bacteremia.

# REFERENCES

## Review Articles

Bryan, C. S. Clinical implications of positive blood cultures. *Clin. Microbiol. Rev.* 2:329–353, 1989.

Dinarello, C. A. The proinflammatory cytokines interleukin-1 and tumor necrosis factor and treatment of the septic shock syndrome. *J. Infect. Dis. 163*:1177–1184, 1991.

Glauser, M. P. Heumann, D., Baumgartner, J. D., and Cohen, J. Pathogenesis and potential strategies for prevention and treatment of septic shock. *Clin. Infect. Dis. 18*:S205–S216, 1994.

Lynn, W. A., and Cohen, J. Adjunctive therapy for septic shock: A review of experimental approaches. *Clin. Infect. Dis. 20*:143–158, 1995.

Nowotny, A. Review of the molecular requirements of endotoxic actions. *Rev. Infect. Dis. 9*:S503–S511, 1987.

Parrillo, J. E. Pathogenetic mechanisms of septic shock. *N. Engl. J. Med. 328*:1471–1477, 1993.

Reuben, A. G., Musher, D. M., Hamill, R. J., et al. Polymicrobial bacteremia: Clinical and microbiologic patterns. *Rev. Infect. Dis. 11*:161–183, 1989.

Rietschel, E. Th., Wollenweber, H-W., Russa, R., et al. Concepts of the chemical structure of lipid A. *Rev. Infect. Dis. 6*:432–438, 1984.

Washington, J. A., II, and Ilstrup, D. M. Blood cultures: Issues and controversies. *Rev. Infect. Dis. 8*:792–802, 1986.

Wells, C. L., Maddaus, M. A., and Simmons, R. L. Proposed mechanisms for translocation of intestinal bacteria. *Rev. Infect. Dis. 10*:958–979, 1988.

## Original Articles

Beutler, B., Milsark, I. W., and Cerami, A. C. Passive immunization against cachectin/tumor necrosis factor protects mice from lethal effect of endotoxin. *Science 229*:869–871, 1985.

Brandtzaeg, P., Kierulf, P., Gaustad, P., et al. Plasma endotoxin as a predictor of multiple organ failure and death in systemic meningococcal disease. *J. Infect. Dis. 159*:195–204, 1989.

Calandra, T., Baumgartner, J-D., Grau, G. E., et al. Prognostic values of tumor necrosis factor/cachectin, interleukin-1, interferon-alpha, and interferon-gamma in the serum of patients with septic shock. *J. Infect. Dis. 161*:982–987, 1990.

Cannon, J. G., Tompkins, R. G., Gelfand, J. A., et al. Circulating interleukin-1 and tumor necrosis factor in septic shock and experimental endotoxin fever. *J. Infect. Dis. 161*:79–84, 1990.

Heumann, D., Gallay, P., Betz-Corradin, S., et al. Competition between bactericidal permeability-increasing protein and lipopolysaccharide-binding protein for lipopolysaccharide binding to monocytes. *J. Infect. Dis. 167*:1351–1357, 1993.

Kreger, B. E., Craven, D. E., Carling, P. C., et al. Gram-negative bacteremia. III. Reassessment of etiology, epidemiology and ecology in 612 patients. *Am. J. Med. 68*:332–343, 1980.

Kreger, B. E., Craven, D. E., and McCabe, W. R. Gram-negative bacteremia. IV. Re-evaluation of clinical features and treatment in 612 patients. *Am. J. Med. 68*:344–355, 1980.

Miller, P. J., and Wenzel, R. P. Etiologic organisms as independent predictors of death and morbidity associated with bloodstream infections. *J. Infect. Dis. 156*:471–477, 1987.

Noskin, G. A., Peterson, L. R., and Warren, J. R. *Enterococcus faecium* and *Enterococcus faecalis* bacteremia: Acquisition and outcome. *Clin. Infect. Dis. 20*:296–301, 1995.

Opal, S. M., Cross, A. S., Kelly, N. M., et al. Efficacy of a monoclonal antibody directed against tumor necrosis factor in protecting neutropenic rats from lethal infection with *Pseudomonas aeruginosa*. *J. Infect. Dis. 161*:1148–1152, 1990.

Russell, D., Tucker, K. K., Chinookoswong, N., et al. Combined inhibition of interleukin-1 and tumor necrosis factor in rodent endotoxemia: Improved survival and organ function. *J. Infect. Dis. 171:*1528–1538, 1995.

Shenep, J. L., Flynn, P. M., Barrett, F. F., et al. Serial quantitation of endotoxemia and bacteremia during therapy for gram-negative bacterial sepsis. *J. Infect. Dis. 157:*565–568, 1988.

Schumann, R. R., Leong, S. R., Flaggs, G. W., et al. Structure and function of lipopolysaccharide binding protein. *Science 249:*1429–1431, 1990.

Tracey, K. J., Fong, Y., Hesse, D. G., et al. Anti-cachectin/ TNF monoclonal antibodies prevent septic shock during lethal bacteraemia. *Nature 330:*662–664, 1987.

Waage, A., Halstensen, A., and Espevik, T. Association between tumor necrosis factor in serum and fatal outcome in patients with meningococcal disease. *Lancet 1:*355–357, 1987.

Weinstein, M. P., Murphy, J. R., Reller, L. B., et al. The clinical significance of positive blood cultures: A comprehensive analysis of 500 episodes of bacteremia and fungemia in adults. II. Clinical observations, with special reference to factors influencing prognosis. *Rev. Infect. Dis. 5:*54–70, 1983.

Weinstein, M. P., Reller, L. B., Murphy, J. R., et al. The clinical significance of positive blood cultures: A comprehensive analysis of 500 episodes of bacteremia and fungemia in adults. I. Laboratory and epidemiologic observations. *Rev. Infect. Dis. 5:*35–53, 1983.

Wright, S. D., Ramos, R. A., Tobias, P. S., et al. CD14, a receptor for complexes of lipopolysaccharide (LPS) and LPS binding proteins. *Science 249:*1431–1433, 1990.

# 33

# INFECTIVE ENDOCARDITIS

## STANFORD T. SHULMAN, M.D. and JOHN P. PHAIR, M.D.

The treatment of infective endocarditis (IE), a universally fatal disease before the introduction of antibiotics, represents a major triumph of "modern medicine" and a continuing challenge. Ninety-five percent of cases of endocarditis due to penicillin-susceptible streptococci can be bacteriologically cured. In contrast, management of fungal endocarditis is still inadequate. Other remaining concerns include effective prophylaxis, appropriate timing of surgical intervention, and management of endocarditis in persons using intravenous drugs, a major source of patients of IE in urban centers.

Malignant endocarditis due to infection was not clearly distinguished from endocarditis secondary to rheumatic fever until the early 1900s, even though Sir William Osler had recognized in the 1880s that "cocci" were sometimes present in the vegetations of endocarditis. By the late 1930s, the potential of antibiotics for cure was beginning to be appreciated. Work since then has delineated the clinical forms; pathogenesis; principles of therapy; and hemodynamic, infectious, and immunologic complications of IE.

## CLINICAL DESCRIPTION

Two basic forms of IE were formerly distinguished: acute and subacute, and this distinction remains useful clinically (Table 33–1).

Many patients present typically, although features of acute and subacute disease may be combined. Thus, patients with valvular infection due to viridans (alpha-hemolytic) streptococci may lack classic features of subacute endocarditis. In contrast, patients infected with *Enterococcus faecalis* are often acutely ill with a fulminant infection that rapidly destroys the infected valve, mimicking acute endocarditis.

### Acute Endocarditis

The patient with acute IE usually presents with signs and symptoms of severe fulminant infection (e.g., high fever, rigors, prostration, and significant leukocytosis) without history of chronic illness. Staphylococci are the most frequent etiologic agents. Commonly, there is no evidence of significant preexisting cardiac disease on a rheumatic or congenital basis; the organisms usually associated with acute IE can infect a normal valve. Acute staphylococcal endocarditis is rising in frequency among the elderly, who often have calcific sclerosis of the aortic or mitral valve, and is frequent in patients with prosthetic valves and in intravenous drug users (IDUs).

Initially, the patient with acute IE may have few signs to indicate a cardiac focus of infection. Murmurs may be absent and attention drawn to other organs, the sites of metastatic infection or immune-mediated vascular disease, that is, *hypersensitivity angiitis.* These or-

## TABLE 33–1.    CLINICAL–ETIOLOGIC CLASSIFICATION OF ACUTE AND SUBACUTE FORMS OF INFECTIVE ENDOCARDITIS

| FEATURES | ACUTE FORM OF DISEASE | SUBACUTE FORM OF DISEASE |
|---|---|---|
| Duration of disease | Less than 6 weeks | 6 weeks or longer |
| Cardiovascular status | Normal heart valve or prosthetic valve implant | Rheumatic or congenital heart disease; prosthetic valve implant |
| Most important causative microorganisms | *Staphylococcus aureus* and *S. epidermidis*<br>*Streptococcus pneumoniae*<br>Lancefield group A beta-hemolytic streptococci (*Streptococcus pyogenes*)<br>*Neisseria gonorrhoeae*<br>*Pseudomonas aeruginosa* | *Viridans (alpha-hemolytic) streptococci*<br>*Lancefield group D enterococci (Enterococcus faecalis)*<br>Anaerobic or microaerophilic streptococci |
| Therapy | Penicillin class drug (plus an aminoglycoside for *P. aeruginosa* infections)<br>Antifungal agents<br>Surgery | Penicillin class drug plus aminoglycoside in combination |

gans are typically the central nervous system (CNS), joints, long bones, and kidneys. The skin may show evidence of embolic pustules or hemorrhage secondary to an intravascular co-agulopathy. Occasionally, Janeway lesions—flat, painless, erythematous areas—are seen on the palms and soles. The typical patient with acute staphylococcal endocarditis is ill for 7 days or less before seeking medical at-tention. Mitral and aortic valves are most com-monly involved, and a murmur is often of re-cent onset or develops under observation. In the preantibiotic era, acute gonococcal and pneumococcal endocarditis were common but are now only rarely seen. Acute IE due to gram-negative bacilli and fungi is increasing in frequency.

### Subacute Endocarditis

In contrast to acute IE, subacute disease presents either as a vague wasting illness, sug-gesting a malignancy, or as a fever of un-known origin. The patient feels unwell and often has anorexia and weight loss. The du-ration of the illness is unclear, or the patient may state that an episode of "flu" never com-pletely resolved. A heart murmur, splenomeg-aly, and petechiae (usually restricted to the conjunctivae, head, neck, and upper thorax) represent typical physical findings. The classic findings of Osler's nodes (red painful nodules on the fingertips) and Roth spots (pale le-sions on an erythematous base in the retina) are uncommon in subacute IE in the antibi-otic era. Splinter hemorrhages are common. Although a changing murmur is often cited as a major finding in IE, it usually occurs if an infected valve perforates or a papillary muscle ruptures. Laboratory evaluation may reveal a normal white cell count or slight leukocytosis, and normochromic normocytic anemia. Microscopic hematuria is frequent.

### Culture-Negative (Abacteremic) Endocarditis

In older series, the frequency of blood culture–negative endocarditis ranged from 10–20%. Today, abacteremic endocarditis ac-counts for about 2%, if patients who received antibiotics prior to culture are excluded. Causes of abacteremic endocarditis include IE due to chlamydia, rickettsiae (Q fever), *Bar-tonella quintana* and certain fungi, notably *As-pergillus*. Occasionally, gram-positive cocci are demonstrated in vegetations at surgery or au-topsy despite sterile blood cultures. Fastidi-ous, nutritionally deficient streptococci that

require supplementation with specific nutri-ents such as pyridoxine may account for such cases.

Culture-negative endocarditis should be suspected in any patient with signs of IE and an elevated sedimentation rate. Transesopha-geal echocardiography is a very sensitive method of detecting vegetations in a patient with suspected abacteremic IE. Established atrial fibrillation and congestive heart failure are uncommon antecedents for IE.

The differential diagnosis of a patient with suspected culture-negative IE includes those illnesses that cause prolonged and perplexing fevers including lymphoproliferative diseases, collagen vascular diseases, recurrent pulmo-nary emboli, hepatic disease, valvular myx-oma, and neoplastic tumors. Following a neg-ative investigation, a trial of antibiotic therapy for abacteremic IE may be warranted if no alternative diagnosis has been established.

### Fungal Endocarditis

In contrast to abacteremic endocarditis, fungal endocarditis is increasing in frequency. Responsible factors include:

1. Use of central venous and arterial lines for therapy and for monitoring.
2. Increasing numbers of immunocom-promised patients who survive for extended periods.
3. Increasing numbers of patients under-going valve replacement.
4. The increasing prevalence of intrave-nous drug use.

Fungal endocarditis represents a difficult diagnostic and therapeutic dilemma. Organ-isms such as aspergillus are infrequently iso-lated from blood cultures even when IE is present, and currently available medical ther-apy is ineffective. Treatment includes antifun-gal agents and surgery, but cures are uncom-mon. Patients with fungal endocarditis usually present with acute IE as described above. A characteristic of fungal endocarditis is the presence of large vegetations that commonly embolize and occlude large arteries.

### Endocarditis and Injection Drug Abuse

Endocarditis as a result of injection drug use (IDU) is increasingly diagnosed in urban centers. Patients may develop acute aortic or mitral valve infection; however, 30–40% of IDU-associated endocarditis involves the tri-cuspid valve. Because right-sided endocarditis is otherwise uncommon, tricuspid endocarditis should suggest IDU and infection of this valve should be suspected with fever, sustained bacteremia, and multiple septic pulmonary emboli. The murmurs of the tricuspid valve lesions are often inaudible, and echocardiography can be helpful in establishing this diagnosis.

IE most frequently associated with IDU involves *Staphylococcus aureus, Pseudomonas aeruginosa, Serratia marcescens,* and *Candida* species. Methicillin-resistant staphylococci are increasingly found in IDU-associated IE, although staphylococci are not readily cultured from street drugs or apparatus. Users of intravenous drugs have heavy skin carriage of *S. aureus,* and the organisms infecting cardiac valves are of the same phage type as those colonizing the noses, axillae, and groins of these patients.

### Prosthetic Valve Endocarditis

Infection of prosthetic cardiac valves is common and carries substantially greater mortality than other forms of IE. Two distinct forms of prosthetic valve endocarditis (PVE) are discernible: early (occurring within 60 days of valve implantation), and late (developing after the 60-day postoperative period). Early PVE must be differentiated from the postpericardiotomy syndrome, an immunologically mediated disease resulting from injury to the pericardium or myocardium. Fever is common to PVE and postpericardiotomy syndrome, and both may occur 2–3 weeks after surgery. Blood cultures are often positive in PVE and not in the latter illness. The postpericardiotomy syndrome commonly presents with signs and symptoms of pericarditis or pleuritis. It is usually self-limited or responds to antiinflammatory agents. When present, embolic events strongly suggest PVE. Arterial lines used in cardiac surgery may be associated with petechiae or splinter hemorrhages.

Other causes of fever in the immediate postoperative period include urinary tract infection, postoperative pneumonia or atelectasis, and phlebitis or arteritis secondary to intravascular monitoring. Sternotomy wound infections are uncommon but can cause diagnostic difficulties.

Four to six weeks after surgery, fever due to cytomegalovirus mononucleosis transmitted by infected blood can be confused with PVE. This infection lacks many features of mononucleosis due to Epstein-Barr virus, such as pharyngitis and adenopathy, but it is associated with fever, splenomegaly, and occasionally hepatitis. Rarely, retinitis may be noted. Atypical lymphocytosis, which is not present with PVE, is common (see Chapter 8).

Although PVE may be obscured by prophylactic perioperative antibiotics, diagnosis is established by demonstrating sustained bacteremia. Staphylococcal species are the most common isolates. Coagulase-negative staphylococci like *S. epidermidis* in blood cultures in this clinical setting should not be dismissed as contaminants. Gram-negative bacilli, diphtheroids, and fungi are also causes of early PVE. Late PVE is usually due to staphylococci; *S. aureus* predominates, but infection with coagulase-negative staphylococci still occurs. Organisms associated with acute and subacute IE on natural valves are commonly isolated in the late form of PVE.

Specific signs of PVE include obstruction by a vegetation, which is associated with changing sounds of valve closure and a narrowing pulse pressure if the aortic valve is involved, or valve ring dehiscence, demonstrated by the development of a regurgitant murmur or by echocardiography. Finally, evidence of intravascular hemolysis is not uncommon in patients with PVE. Surgical therapy is commonly required (see below).

## ETIOLOGY

The majority of cases of IE are due to infection with streptococci or staphylococci. Many other organisms, however, can produce IE. In community hospitals where IDU is less common, the classic causative agent of IE (i.e., viridans streptococci) accounts for 70–80% of cases. Viridans streptococci are particularly associated with IE in patients with poor dental hygiene, especially following dental manipulation, and in those with preexisting heart disease. *Enterococcus faecalis* endocarditis most often results from bacteremia due to manipulation of the genitourinary or gastrointestinal tracts. IE due to *Streptococcus bovis,* another group D streptococcal organism, is associated with colonic lesions. The prevalence of this organism in stool of patients with colonic carcinoma is five times greater than in patients without colon lesions. Other bacteria associated typically with IE include the HACEK group of gram-negative organisms: haemophilus species. *Actinobacillus actinomycetemcomitans, Cardiobacterium hominis, Eikenella* species, and *Kingella kingae.*

The association of specific organisms with

IE appears to be due to specific bacterial–valvular interaction resembling bacterial adherence (see Chapter 3). Streptococci that convert sucrose to dextran adhere better to the platelet–fibrin mesh produced by blood flow disturbances or endothelial damage, the primary lesion required for the development of IE. Staphylococci readily cause platelet aggregation and consequently also adhere well to this nidus. The most common overall blood culture isolates in modern hospitals, aerobic gram-negative bacilli, cause endocarditis only infrequently and adhere poorly to endothelial cells *in vitro*. Anaerobic gram-negative bacilli are also uncommon causes of IE. Viruses have not been proved to cause IE despite intensive efforts to implicate them as causes of abacteremic endocarditis.

## PATHOGENESIS

Infective endocarditis requires bloodstream invasion with an organism capable of colonizing an intravascular site, most commonly a previously damaged valve, a prosthetic valve, or an intracardiac shunt. Bacteremia with mouth organisms occurs following brushing of teeth, chewing hard candy, or dental manipulation. Positive blood cultures may also be found after certain endoscopic procedures or biopsies. These bacteremias are transient; rarely are bacteria demonstrable in blood 5 min after the procedure; and the number of colony-forming units per milliliter of blood is low.

The importance of the fibrin–platelet mesh as the nidus of intravascular infection was established in Freedman's rabbit model of IE. Microscopic deposition of fibrin and platelets was established with placement of a plastic cannula across a valve, producing endothelial damage. Following catheter removal, intravenous inoculation of organisms, such as *Staphylococcus aureus, Enterococcus faecalis,* or *Streptococcus sanguis,* resulted in colonization and valvular infection. Earlier clinical studies showed that vegetations occurred in areas of turbulence, which favor fibrin–platelet deposition. Thus, in a child with a ventricular septal defect and a left-to-right shunt, the vegetation occurs at the site where the jet stream hits the right ventricular wall or on the right ventricular side of the septum where maximum turbulence exists.

A unique feature of intravascular infection is that the platelet—fibrin mesh excludes neutrophils, the major host defense against most microorganisms associated with IE. In addition, antibody is not bactericidal for the usual organisms that cause IE. In contrast to streptococci and staphylococci, many aerobic gram-negative bacilli are lysed by complement. When *Pseudomonas* species and *Escherichia coli* cause IE, however, they are serum-resistant and produce experimental endocarditis easily in rabbits. Thus, it has been stated that IE is an opportunistic infection occurring at an immunocompromised site. The importance of the platelet–fibrin mesh in the pathogenesis of IE is perhaps best illustrated by the clinical observation that endocarditis is uncommon in thrombocytopenic leukemic patients, although bacteremia with pyogenic organisms occurs frequently in this setting.

## PATHOLOGY

The majority of the clinical manifestations of IE are due to valvular infection, valve destruction or dysfunction, arrhythmias resulting from myocardial abscesses, metastatic infection, and embolic phenomena. Valvular destruction and myocardial involvement occur in acute endocarditis and can be fatal despite bacteriologic cure. Metastatic infection is also usually the consequence of infection by organisms causing the acute form of IE. Brain abscess; meningitis; infection of long bones or joints; and hepatic, renal, and splenic abscesses are frequent sequelae of staphylococcal endocarditis.

Mycotic aneurysms are vasculitic lesions resulting from intramural infection arising in the vaso vasorum; they occur in both acute and subacute IE. These aneurysms can result in arterial insufficiency or can rupture.

Embolic phenomena can be trivial, resulting in splinter hemorrhages, or devastating if a large piece of vegetation reaches the central nervous system or a major artery. Emboli occur in both the subacute and acute forms of IE and occasionally occur even after sterilization of the blood. Fungal endocarditis is frequently associated with large and friable vegetations that can occlude major arteries. Janeway lesions probably result from emboli. Microscopic evaluation and culture sometimes demonstrate the infecting organism in peripheral lesions. The few histologic studies of retinal lesions indicate that they are due to embolic disease rather than to immune vasculitis.

## IMMUNOPATHOLOGY

Persistent bacteremia, the hallmark of IE, has a profound impact on the immune system, including marked production of immunoglobulins, which are only partially directed at the infecting organism. This polyclonal hyper gammaglobulinemia results in high titers of non–cross-reacting antigen, rendering inaccurate a diagnosis of the infecting organism that is based solely on serologic evaluation. Circulating immune complexes also are demonstrable. The components of these circulating complexes have not been well defined and may represent bacterial antigens plus antibody and/or complement components plus antibody directed against a wide range of endogenous or exogenous antigens.

Glomerulonephritis due to immune complex deposition represents a serious consequence of the immune response to endocardial infection. In untreated patients, uremia accounts for 10% of the deaths due to valvular infection. Antibiotic therapy renders IE a reversible cause of renal insufficiency. A second much less common syndrome associated with circulating immune complexes is a form of thrombotic thrombocytopenic purpura. Thrombocytopenia and intravascular hemolysis are reversible with antibiotic treatment.

Among the well-studied serologic responses in IE is the development of antiglobulins—rheumatoid factors. Antiglobulins develop in about 50% of patients with IE of at least 6 weeks' duration, occur in people with no familial tendency toward collagen vascular disease, are independent of the infecting microorganism, and disappear following cure of IE. The role, if any, of antiglobulins in the clinical picture of IE is not defined. These antiantibodies are not associated with glomerulonephritis. Antiglobulins bind to the Fc fragment of IgG and can block complement fixation, which could be deleterious to the defenses against bacterial infection. There is no evidence, however, that antiglobulin-positive patients have a poorer prognosis. Other autoantibodies are frequently noted in IE, including antimyocardial antibodies, but there is no evidence to indicate that they alter cardiac function during or following recovery from IE.

## DIAGNOSIS

The diagnosis of IE is established in the appropriate clinical setting by documentation of sustained bacteremia or fungemia and a valvular endocardial or myocardial lesion. Other laboratory tests may be helpful. The erythrocyte sedimentation rate is usually elevated. Leukocytosis is usually present, and anemia is frequent. Antiglobulins are present in 50% of people with subacute disease, usually with polyclonal hypergammaglobulinemia.

Three blood cultures per day for 2 days in subacute IE, and three cultures over 1–2 h before initiation of therapy in acute IE, establish the presence of sustained bacteremia. In proven IE the first culture is positive in 95% of patients; fewer than 5% of patients require more than three cultures for confirmation of the diagnosis.

Bacteremia in endocarditis is continuous, and there is no need to wait for a chill or rising temperature to obtain blood cultures. Skin preparation is important in reducing the risk of contamination of the culture with skin flora. The skin should be cleaned with 70% alcohol and 1–2% iodine or povidone-iodine, which should be allowed to dry. Arterial blood provides no higher yield. Separate venipunctures must be used to document sustained bacteremia.

The two-dimensional sector echocardiogram is often helpful in the diagnosis and treatment of patients with IE, although the transesophageal echocardiogram is more sensitive (at least in adults) and can detect a myocardial abscess and unsuspected vegetations. In addition, echocardiography can detect signs of acute left-ventricular strain, such as early closure of the mitral valve, which accompany destruction of the aortic valve. Such findings represent indications for early surgical intervention. Echocardiography can determine the size of a vegetation, and larger vegetations may be associated with more frequent emboli, hemodynamic alterations, and difficulty in achieving bacteriologic cure.

The diagnosis of IE can be difficult, and criteria have been established recently in an attempt to provide a more rational basis for initiating therapy in patients suspected of having this diagnosis. Durack and his colleagues at Duke University defined three diagnostic categories: definite, possible, and rejected. They further defined two major criteria and six minor criteria (including echocardiographic features) to be used in categorizing patients with suspected IE (Table 33–2). Patients with definite IE include those with pathologic findings at autopsy or surgery consistent with endocarditis or myocardial abscess,

## TABLE 33–2. DUKE CRITERIA FOR INFECTIVE ENDOCARDITIS (IE)*

*Major criteria*

1. Positive blood culture
   a) Typical endocarditis organism from 2 separate blood cultures

   *OR*

   b) Persistently positive blood cultures (>12 h apart, or all of 3, or majority of ≥4 cultures)
2. Evidence of endocardial involvement
   a) Positive echocardiogram (oscillating intracardiac mass, abscess, or new partial dehiscence of prosthetic valve)

   *OR*

   b) New valvular regurgitation

*Minor criteria*

1. *Predisposition:* heart condition or intravenous drug use
2. *Fever:* ≥38.0°C.
3. *Vascular phenomena:* arterial emboli, septic pulmonary infarct, mycotic aneurysm, intracranial hemorrhage, subconjunctival hemorrhage, Janeway lesions
4. *Immune phenomena:* nephritis, Osler's nodes, Roth spots, rheumatoid factor
5. *Echocardiogram:* consistent with IE but not meeting major criterion noted above
6. *Microbiologic evidence:* positive blood culture not meeting major criterion above *OR* serologic evidence of active infection with organism consistent with IE

I. **Definite infective endocarditis**
   A. Pathologic criteria
      1. Demonstrable microorganisms by culture or histology in a vegetation or an embolized vegetation

      *OR*

      2. Histologic evidence of acute endocarditis

      *OR*

   B. Clinical criteria (from above major and minor criteria list)
      1. 2 major criteria

      *OR*

      2. 1 major + 3 minor criteria

      *OR*

      3. 5 minor criteria

II. **Possible infective endocarditis:** Findings consistent with IE that fall short of definite, but not rejected

III. **Infective endocarditis rejected**
   1. Firm alternate diagnosis is established

   *OR*

   2. Resolution of syndrome with ≤4 days of antibiotic therapy

   *OR*

   3. No pathologic evidence at surgery or autopsy after ≤4 days of antibiotic therapy

*Adapted from Durack, D. T., et al. *Am. J. Med.* 96:200–209, 1994. Copyright 1994 by Excerpta Medica Inc. With permission.

those with two major criteria, those with one major plus three minor criteria, or those with five minor criteria. Rejected diagnoses include patients with a firm diagnosis of an alternate condition, resolution of signs and symptoms suggestive of IE with less than 4 days of antibiotics, or no pathologic evidence of IE with less than 4 days of antibiotic treatment. Possible cases are those not rejected but falling short of definite clinical or pathologic evidence of IE.

## PRINCIPLES OF THERAPY

Rational therapy of IE is predicated on isolation, identification, and determination of the antibiotic susceptibility of the infecting microorganism. Cure requires effective high-dose (usually intravenous) antibiotic therapy and, in carefully selected situations, surgical intervention. The antibiotics chosen must be rapidly bactericidal. With certain infections such as those due to enterococci, two antibiotics are necessary to achieve the synergistic killing of the infecting organisms required for cure. After antibiotics have been chosen, treatment should be monitored closely. Blood cultures should be obtained after approximately 3 and 6 days of therapy to confirm sterilization of the bloodstream. In addition, peak and trough serum specimens should be assayed for bactericidal effect against the patient's own infecting organism (see Chapter 39). Peak serum bactericidal titers should be maintained at 1:16 or greater. It may be difficult with some infections to maintain this titer without producing antibiotic toxicity. To be useful, the serum bactericidal assay must be carefully standardized (see Chapter 39).

One of the more vexing problems of endocarditis therapy relates to the optimal duration of treatment. A number of factors are relevant to the sterilization of a vegetation. First, the organism is a major determinant: highly penicillin-sensitive viridans streptococcal IE can be cured with 2 weeks of penicillin plus an aminoglycoside such as gentamicin or streptomycin; in contrast, 6 weeks of ticarcillin plus an aminoglycoside rarely cures aortic valve infection due to *Pseudomonas aeruginosa*. Second, the duration of disease influences results of therapy. Patients infected with penicillin-susceptible streptococci for less than 2 months are easily cured with 2 weeks of therapy, but IE of longer duration caused by the same organism often requires 4 weeks of treatment. Finally, prolonged disease results in larger vegetations that contain metabolically inactive organisms deep within the fibrin–platelet mesh. Such organisms divide slowly and are less susceptible to penicillin, thus necessitating prolonged therapy for eradication of bacteria.

Right-sided IE is more easily cured than left-sided endocarditis in humans and in experimental animals. The IDU with staphylococcal tricuspid endocarditis often will not remain in the hospital to complete an optimal course of therapy (4 weeks); bacteriologic cure is achieved in most such patients with 3 weeks or less of therapy. In contrast, the presence of an intravascular prosthesis such as a prosthetic valve necessitates prolonged antibiotics, even for late-onset IE. Early PVE often requires surgical replacement in addition to antibiotics, with higher mortality rates associated with less aggressive approaches.

IE has provided one of the clearest examples of the value of antibacterial synergism. *Enterococcus faecalis* is much less susceptible to penicillin than other streptococci, with minimum inhibitory concentration (MIC) ranging from 0.8–25 $\mu$g/mL. In contrast, viridans streptococci typically are inhibited by 0.02 $\mu$g/mL penicillin or less. *Enterococcus faecalis* and the other group D enterococci, *E. faecium* and *E. durans*, also are resistant to cephalosporins and other cell-wall–active agents. Penicillin G or ampicillin alone is not successful in curing IE due to *E. faecalis*. Thus, treatment has required either penicillin G or ampicillin plus an aminoglycoside to achieve synergy. The American Heart Association's recommended treatment regimens for streptococcal, enterococcal, and staphylococcal endocarditis are shown in Tables 33–3 through 33–5.

Penicillin-aminoglycoside synergism against enterococci is based on increased uptake of aminoglycoside by the organism in the presence of a cell-wall–active agent (Fig. 33–1). The actual killing of the organisms is due to the action of the aminoglycoside. Not all enterococci are killed synergistically by all penicillin-aminoglycoside combinations. Thus, *E. faecalis* with its high level of resistance to streptomycin (MIC >2000 $\mu$g/mL) is killed synergistically only by the combination of penicillin and gentamicin. Because high-level streptomycin resistance is very common among blood isolates of *E. faecalis*, penicillin and gentamicin is the treatment of choice unless susceptibility to streptomycin is determined. High-level gentamicin resistance has also been

**TABLE 33–3. TREATMENT OF NATIVE-VALVE STREPTOCOCCAL INFECTIVE ENDOCARDITIS (NON–PENICILLIN-ALLERGIC)\***

**Highly penicillin-sensitive streptococci (MIC ≤ 0.1 µg/mL)**
Penicillin G, IV 12–18 × 10⁶ units/day for 4 weeks
*OR*

Penicillin G, IV 12–18 × 10⁶ units/day for 2 weeks
*plus* gentamicin, 1.0 mg/kg/dose IM or IV (up to 80 mg) every 8 h for 2 weeks
*OR*

Ceftriaxone, IV or IM 2 g once daily for 4 weeks

**Relatively penicillin-resistant streptococci (MIC > 0.1 µg/mL, < 0.5 µg/mL)**
Penicillin G, IV 18 × 10⁶ units day for 4 weeks
*plus* gentamicin, 1.0 mg/kg/dose IM or IV (up to 80 mg) every 8 h for 2 weeks

**Enterococci, or streptococci with penicillin MIC ≥ 0.5 µg/mL, or nutritionally variant streptococci, or prosthetic valve endocarditis due to viridans streptococci or S. bovis**
Penicillin, IV 18–30 × 10⁶ units/day for 4–6 weeks
*plus* gentamicin, 1.0 mg/kg/dose IM or IV (up to 80 mg) every 8 h for 4–6 weeks
*OR*

Ampicillin, 12 g/day IV for 4–6 weeks
*plus* gentamicin 1.0 mg/kg/dose IM or IV (up to 80 mg) every 8 h for 4–6 weeks

\*Adapted from Wilson, W., Karchmer, A. W., Bisno, A. L., et al. Antibiotic treatment of adults with infective endocarditis due to streptococci, enterococci, staphylococci, and HACEK microorganisms. *JAMA* 274:1706–1713, 1995. Copyright 1995, American Medical Association. With permission. Adult dosages are provided.

## TABLE 33–4.    TREATMENT OF NATIVE-VALVE STREPTOCOCCAL INFECTIVE ENDOCARDITIS (PENICILLIN-ALLERGIC)*

**Highly penicillin-sensitive streptococci (MIC ≤ 0.1 μg/mL)**
Ceftriaxone, 2 g IV once daily for 4 weeks (not in patients with anaphylactic or immediate-type penicillin hypersensitivity)

*OR*

Vancomycin, 30 mg/kg/day IV in two divided doses (up to 2 g/day) for 4 weeks

**Relatively penicillin-resistant streptococci ( MIC > 0.1 mg/mL, <0.5 μg/mL)**
Cephalothin, 2 g IV every 4 h for 4 weeks (not in patients with immediate-type penicillin hypersensitivity)
*plus* gentamicin, 1.0 mg/≤g/dose IM or IV (up to 80 mg) every 8 h for 2 weeks

*OR*

Vancomycin, 30 mg/kg/day IV in two divided doses (up to 2 g/day) for 4 weeks

**Enterococci, or streptococci with penicillin MIC ≥ 0.5 μg/mL**
**Vancomycin, 30 mg/kg/day IV in two divided doses (up to 2 g/day) for 4–6 weeks**
*plus* gentamicin, 1.0 mg/kg/dose IM or IV (up to 80 mg) every 8 h for 4–6 weeks

*Adapted from Wilson, W., Karchmer, A. W., Bisno, A. L., et al. Antibiotic treatment of adults with infective endocarditis due to streptococci, enterococci, staphylococci, and ḨACEK microorganisms. *JAMA* 274:1706–1713, 1995. Copyright 1995, American Medical Association. With permission. Adult dosages are proviced.

### TABLE 33–5. TREATMENT OF STAPHYLOCOCCAL INFECTIVE ENDOCARDITIS*

**Methicillin-susceptible staphylococci in absence of prosthetic valve or material**

 Nafcillin or oxacillin, 2 g IV every 4 h for 4–6 weeks *with or without* gentamicin, 1.0 mg/kg IV (up to 80 mg) every 8 h for 3–5 days

   *OR* (for penicillin-allergic patients)

 Cefazolin or cephalothin, 2 g IV every 8 h for 4–6 weeks (not in patients with immediate-type penicillin hypersensitivity) *with or without* gentamicin, 1.0 mg/kg IV (up to 80 mg) every 8 h for 3–5 days

   *OR* (for penicillin-allergic patients)

 Vancomycin, 30 mg/kg/day IV in two divided doses (up to 2 g/day) for 4–6 weeks

**Methicillin-resistant staphylococci in absence of prosthetic valve or material**

 Vancomycin, 30 mg/kg/day IV in two divided doses (up to 2 g/day) for 4–6 weeks

**Methicillin-susceptible staphylococci in presence of prosthetic valve or material**

 Nafcillin or oxacillin, 2 g IV every 4 h for at least 6 weeks *plus* rifampin, 300 mg every 8 h orally for at least 6 weeks *plus* gentamicin, 1.0 mg/kg IV (up to 80 mg) every 8 h for 2 weeks

   *OR* (for penicillin-allergic patients)

 Vancomycin, 30 mg/kg/day IV in two divided doses (up to 2 g/day) for at least 6 weeks *plus* rifampin, 300 mg every 8 h orally for at least 6 weeks *plus* gentamicin, 1.0 mg/kg IV (up to 80 mg) every 8 h for 2 weeks

**Methicillin-resistant staphylococci in presence of prosthetic valve or material**

 Vancomycin, 30 mg/kg/day IV in two or four divided doses (up to 2 g/day) for at least 6 weeks *plus* rifampin, 300 mg every 8 h orally for at least 6 weeks *plus* gentamicin, 1.0 mg/kg IV (up to 80 mg) every 8 h for 2 weeks

*Adapted from Wilson, W., Karchmer, A. W., Bisno, A. L., et al. Antibiotic treatment of adults with infective endocarditis due to streptococci, enterococci, other streptococci, staphylococci, and HACEK microorganisms. *JAMA* 274:1706–1713, 1995. Copyright 1995, American Medical Association. With permission. Adult dosages are provided.

reported recently. In patients allergic to penicillin, vancomycin-aminoglycoside combinations are the treatment of choice. Unfortunately, *E. faecalis* and especially *E. faecium* strains resistant to vancomycin have been isolated with increasing frequency. Van B resistant organisms retain susceptibility to high concentrations of ampicillin and often streptomycin or gentamicin. On the other hand, Van A resistance is mediated by a plasmid, and these organisms are resistant to most treatment regimens used for enterococcal infection, making it difficult or impossible to treat such infections.

 Enhanced killing of viridans streptococci in vegetations in the rabbit model of endocarditis by penicillin plus streptomycin confirms clinical results with this combination. This regimen has allowed shortening of therapy to 2 weeks in specific low-risk cases caused by a penicillin-susceptible organism. Similar synergism both *in vitro* and in animal models has been demonstrated for *S. aureus* and *P. aeruginosa*. Clinical results in staphylococcal endocarditis with a beta-lactam antibiotic plus gentamicin, however, are generally disappointing. Treatment of pseudomonas endocarditis requires the combination of carbenicillin or ticarcillin plus an aminoglycoside.

 One unresolved issue is the problem of antibiotic tolerance of *S. aureus*. Tolerant staphylococci are inhibited by the usual concentrations of beta-lactam antibiotics but require at least 32 times higher concentrations for killing. Although tolerant staphylococci have been isolated from blood of patients with IE, the clinical relevance of this phenomenon is not clear. The disparity between inhibitory and bactericidal antibiotic concentrations is affected by a number of methodologic variables, and bacteriologic cure of rabbits with experimental endocarditis caused by tolerant organisms is achieved with usual therapy. However, in patients with persistent bacteremia with tolerant staphylococci, combination of a penicillin and an aminoglycoside or rifampin is advocated.

 Since the 1970s, surgery has become an increasingly important therapeutic modality for IE. If necessary, an infected native or prosthetic valve can be replaced safely before the vegetation is sterilized by antibiotic therapy.

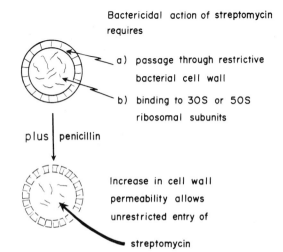

**FIGURE 33–1.** Schematic representation of postulated synergistic bactericidal activity of penicillin plus streptomycin or other aminoglycoside for enterococci.

Indications for surgical intervention include failure to clear the bloodstream of the infecting microorganism with appropriate antibiotics. This frequently occurs with infection due to *Pseudomonas* species, fungi, or aerobic gram-negative bacilli when a large vegetation is present, and in some cases of staphylococcal endocarditis. Another indication for valve replacement is destruction of the valve, with resultant congestive heart failure. PVE occurring within 2 months of placement of the valve usually requires reoperation for bacteriologic cure. Dysfunction of a prosthetic valve, loosening of the ring, and obstruction of blood flow are all indication for surgical replacement. Embolization is the last major indication for surgical intervention because emboli remain major causes of morbidity and mortality despite the introduction of effective antimicrobial therapy. Emboli to the brain, coronary arteries, the eye, and the kidney can result in long-term disability or in death. A second major embolic event is a clear indication for the removal of the vegetation or replacement of the valve, but controversy continues as to whether a single major embolus or demonstration of a large mobile vegetation by echocardiography represents an indication for prompt surgery.

Finally, it is imperative to monitor IE patients after completion of antibiotic therapy. The majority of relapses of IE occur during the first 3 months of convalescence. Blood cultures may become positive prior to significant constitutional signs or symptoms. Therefore, a patient should be seen at least monthly for 3 months, at 6 months, and at 1 year following therapy. Occasionally, emboli occur after completion of antibiotic treatment. This does not necessarily indicate a bacteriologic relapse but requires thorough evaluation including blood cultures to ensure that infection has not recurred.

One of the major problems encountered in designing antibiotic therapy for IE is penicillin allergy. Penicillin G or a semisynthetic analog is the mainstay of treatment of most forms of endocarditis. Cephalosporins are adequate substitutes for penicillin for viridans streptococcal and staphylococcal but not for enterococcal endocarditis. Vancomycin can be substituted for penicillin in cases of endocarditis due to these three organisms. With endocarditis due to *Pseudomonas* species, ceftazidime and an aminoglycoside is probably adequate, but penicillin desensitization and treatment with either ticarcillin or piperacillin plus an aminoglycoside should be considered.

## PROGNOSIS AND COMPLICATIONS

The prognosis of endocarditis patients infected with viridans streptococci is generally good except in the presence of valve destruction or perforation. Major complications include cerebral emboli and relapse. The latter event is most common in patients who have a prolonged illness, and retreatment usually results in cure. Infection with enterococci is associated with a higher frequency of relapse. With relapse, enterococcal susceptibility to the combinations of penicillin plus the various aminoglycosides again should be investigated. The results of therapy of staphylococcal IE in patients who are not IDU can be poor. The majority of non-IDU patients with staphylococcal IE are older, with a high rate of failure of medical therapy, sometimes associated with significant metastatic infection, such as meningitis.

Death during treatment is most common in patients with high fever that persists for more than 7 days into therapy and who have CNS involvement, gross hematuria, and marked leukocytosis. The long-term prognosis among survivors of such infection is poorer than that of the general population, with increased mortality due to heart failure related to the degree of valvular damage consequent to IE. Thus, cardiovascular surgery should be strongly considered with the development of congestive failure related to valvular incompetence. Another long-term complication is the development of reinfection, with a 5–10% reinfection rate in patients who have recovered from one episode of IE. The majority of these recurrences are due to penicillin-susceptible streptococci and require no more intensive therapy than did the initial infection.

## PROPHYLAXIS

Attempts to prevent IE represent one of the most traditional forms of antibiotic prophylaxis. Principles of prophylaxis are based on recognition of the common causes of bacteremia and the identification of patients at risk (e.g., those with rheumatic valve disease, congenital heart disease, mitral valve prolapse with regurgitation, or prosthetic valves). Antibiotics should be administered to achieve adequate blood and tissue levels before, during, and for 8 h after the potential bacteremic episode. There are no controlled studies to prove that antibiotics prevent IE and a number of failures of prophylaxis have been reported. Despite these limitations, attempts to prevent this potentially fatal illness are justified. The American Heart Association periodically publishes guidelines for use of prophylactic antibiotics that should be followed (Table 33–6). Rheumatic heart disease patients receiving long-term oral penicillin to prevent recurrences harbor penicillin-resistant organisms in the oropharynx, and therefore endocarditis prophylaxis for these patients relies on antibiotics other than penicillin.

### TABLE 33–6.   PREVENTION OF INFECTIVE ENDOCARDITIS*

**Standard regimen for dental, oral, esophageal, or upper respiratory tract procedures in patients at risk**
　Amoxicillin, 2 g orally 1 h before procedure
　For amoxicillin- or penicillin-allergic patients: cephalexin or cefadroxil, 2 g orally 1 h before procedure (not in patients with immediate-type hypersensitivity)
*OR*
Clindamycin, 600 mg orally 1 h before procedure
*OR*
Azithromycin or clarithromycin 500 mg orally 1 h before procedure
**Alternative regimes for dental, oral, esophageal or upper respiratory tract procedures**
　For patients unable to take oral medications:
　　Ampicillin, 2 g IV or IM within 30 minutes of procedure
　For ampicillin- or penicillin-allergic patients:
　　Clindamycin, 600 mg IV 30 min before procedure
　For patients considered at high risk:
　　Half the dose can be repeated 6 h after the initial dose (except for azithromycin)
**Regimes for genitourinary or gastrointestinal procedures (excluding esophageal)**
　High risk patients:
　　Ampicillin, 2 g IV or IM *plus* gentamicin 1.5 mg/kg IV or IM (up to 120 mg) within 30 minutes of procedure. Ampicillin 1 g IV orIM or amoxicillin 1 g orally 6 h later
　High risk patients (penicillin-allergic):
　　Vancomycin 1 g IV over 1–2 h plus gentamicin 1.5 mg/kg IV or IM (up to 120 mg).
　Medium risk patients:
　　Amoxicilin 2 g orally 1 hr before procedure.
　Medium risk patients (penicillin-allergic):
　　Vancomycin 1 g IV over 1–2h.
**Pediatric initial doses (not to exceed adult doses)**

| | |
|---|---|
| Amoxicillin or ampicillin | 50 mg/kg |
| Cephalexin or cephadroxil | 50 mg/kg |
| Clindamycin | 20 mg/kg |
| Cefaxolin | 25 mg/kg |
| Azithromycin or clarithromycin | 15 mg/kg |
| Gentamicin | 1.5 mg/kg |
| Vancomycin | 20 mg/kg |

*Adapted from Dajani, A. S. Prevention of bacterial endocarditis. In press. With permission.

Monthly injections of benzathine penicillin for rheumatic prophylaxis obviates this problem: resistant oral organisms are less common in patients receiving this form of penicillin.

## CASE HISTORIES

### CASE HISTORY 1

A 10-year-old boy with surgically corrected tetralogy of Fallot was admitted to the hospital with a 12-day history of fever and loss of appetite. Examination in his physician's office failed to document the cause of fever. At admission, the temperature was 38°C, the pulse 120/min, respirations normal, and blood pressure 120/80 mm Hg. Examination revealed a murmur that was unchanged from previous examinations, splenomegaly, and petechiae over the thorax. The white blood cell (WBC) count was 11,500/mm$^3$ with 70% polymorphonuclear neutrophils and 20% band forms. The hemoglobin was 11 g/dL. The urine contained four to six erythrocytes per high-power field. Six of six blood cultures grew viridans streptococci after 24 h of incubation. The concentration of penicillin required to inhibit growth was 0.01 $\mu$g/mL. Therapy was begun with penicillin at 9.0 × 10$^6$ units/day and gentamicin 80 mg every 8 h. The patient was afebrile within 36 h, his appetite returned, and he stated that he had not realized he had been feeling so poorly before coming to the hospital. The peak-and-trough serum bactericidal assay revealed killing of the infecting organism by patient sera at dilutions of 1:512 and 1:256, respectively. Therapy was continued for 2 weeks. The patient was discharged and was well 1 year later. Close questioning during hospitalization revealed that the patient had been to the dentist for a gingival procedure 1 week before the onset of the febrile illness, but no antibiotic prophylaxis had been administered. The patient's mother was informed that prophylaxis would be necessary for any future dental treatments with risk of inducing bleeding.

### CASE HISTORY 2

A 65-year-old woman was admitted with a 2-day history of chills and fever. When she became confused and developed widespread bruising, she was brought to the emergency room. Purpura fulminans probably due to meningococcemia was suspected. Lumbar puncture revealed cloudy cerebrospinal fluid (CSF); the Gram's stain was nondiagnostic. Penicillin was begun, 2.0 × 10$^6$ units every 2 h. There was no improvement during the initial 24 h of hospitalization. The laboratory reported that all three blood cultures and the CSF were growing *Staphylococcus aureus*.

Intravenous oxacillin (3 g every 6 h) and gentamicin (80 g every 8 h) were substituted for penicillin. Coagulation studies revealed prolonged prothrombin time and partial thromboplastin time, increased fibrin split products, and low fibrinogen. The WBC count was 20,000/mm$^3$ with 50% neutrophils, and 40% band forms. The platelet count was 80,000/mm$^3$. The patient gradually awakened. An apical systolic murmur with radiation to the axilla was first noted on the third hospital day. Coagulation studies returned to normal. Serum bactericidal titers were 1:32, peak, and 1:16, trough. After the first week, gentamicin was discontinued. Oxacillin was continued for a total of 42 days. The patient's recovery was uneventful.

## CASE HISTORY 3

A 24-year-old man attending a methadone clinic was admitted to an outside hospital with fever. No cause of the fever was ascertained upon admission, but four of four blood cultures grew *Pseudomonas aeruginosa*. Pseudomonas endocarditis was diagnosed, and intravenous ticarcillin and tobramycin begun. A blowing diastolic murmur was heard along the left side of the sternum on the second hospital day. Despite serum bactericidal titers of 1:8 or greater throughout a 6-week course of therapy, blood cultures remained positive. Therefore, the patient was transferred to another hospital for valve replacement. On admission to the second hospital, the patient had a low-grade fever, leukocytosis, anemia, an aortic regurgitant murmur, and splenomegaly. Blood cultures were positive, and the aortic valve was replaced with a porcine prosthesis. Following surgery, blood cultures became sterile. Ticarcillin and tobramycin were continued for 1 month. Following discharge the patient was afebrile for 2 weeks, but fever recurred, and he was readmitted. Blood cultures grew *Pseudomonas aeruginosa* with the same antibiotic susceptibilities as the original isolate. Following reinstitution of antibiotics, the patient had a grand mal seizure, became comatose, and died. Postmortem examination revealed a ruptured intracerebral mycotic aneurysm. Cultures of the prosthesis and the aneurysm grew *Pseudomonas aeruginosa*.

## DISCUSSION OF CASE HISTORIES

The first patient is a classic example of subacute infective endocarditis. The child has a surgically corrected congenital cardiac lesion, received dental care without antibiotic prophylaxis, and presented with a febrile illness characterized by sustained bacteremia and peripheral stigmata of endocarditis. The infecting organism, a viridans streptococcus, was very susceptible to penicillin G. Diagnosis was established and appropriate treatment begun within a month of the onset of the illness. Two weeks of therapy with a combination of penicillin and an aminoglycoside resulted in eradication of the valvular infection.

The clinical presentation of acute infective endocarditis, as illustrated by the second patient, can mimic many other serious infections. The rapid onset of illness associated with disseminated intravascular coagulation, widespread bruising, and meningitis led to an initial diagnosis of meningococcemia. The cultures of blood and CSF established the diagnosis, led to an appropriate alteration in antibiotic therapy and, with prolonged (6 weeks) treatment, cure of both the valvular and metastatic meningeal infection. This form of endocarditis is occurring with increasing frequency in older individuals with atherosclerotic valvular lesions. Often murmurs are not appreciated at initial evaluation. The use of a semisynthetic penicillinase-resistant penicillin plus an aminoglycoside for the first weeks of treatment is associated with more rapid sterilization of the blood but does not allow for shortening of the length of therapy.

The difficulty in curing endocarditis due to *Pseudomonas aeruginosa* is demonstrated by the course of the third patient. This gentleman, an IDU, was treated with an appropriate combination of antimicrobial agents that did not eradicate the valvular infection after 6 weeks of treatment. The failure to sterilize the peripheral blood is an indication for surgical intervention under intense antibiotic coverage. Following surgery, antibiotics were continued for another 4 weeks, during which time blood cultures remained sterile. Two weeks after completing the course of treatment the patient relapsed; at postmortem, the prosthetic valve was infected. The cause of death was a ruptured mycotic aneurysm in the central nervous system, a well recognized complication of endocarditis. Surgical replacement of infected valves results in bacteriologic cure of streptococcal and staphylococcal endocarditis. Cure of endocarditis due to *Pseudomonas aeruginosa* or fungi even with aggressive antibiotic management combined with surgery is more problematic.

## REFERENCES

### Books

Bisno, A. L., ed. *Treatment of Infective Endocarditis*. New York: Grune & Stratton, 1981.

Freedman, L. R. *Infective Endocarditis and Other Intravascular Infections*. New York: Plenum, 1982.

Finch, R. G., ed. *Infective Endocarditis*. New York: Academic Press. 1988.

Kaye, D., ed. *Infective Endocarditis*, 2nd ed. New York: Raven Press, 1992.

Bisno, A. L., and Waldvogel, F. G., ed. *Infections Associated with Indwelling Devices*, 2nd ed. American Society of Microbiology, 1994.

### Original Articles

Bayer, A. S. Infective endocarditis. *Clin. Infect. Dis. 17*: 13–22, 1993.

Beeson, P. B., Brannon, E. S., and Warren, J. V. Observations on the sites of removal of bacteria from the blood in patients with bacterial endocarditis. *J. Exp. Med. 81*:9–23, 1945.

Birmingham, G. D., Rahko, P. S., and Ballantyne, F., III. Improved detection of infective endocarditis with transesophageal echocardiography. *Am. Heart. J. 123*:774–781, 1992.

Dajani, A. S., Bisno, A. L., Chung, K. J., et al. Prevention of bacterial endocarditis. *JAMA 264*:2919–2933, 1990.

Durack, D. T., Lukes, A. S., and Bright, D. K. New criteria for diagnosis of infective endocarditis. *Am. J. Med. 96*: 200–209, 1994.

Klein, R. S., Recco, R. A., Cotalona, M. T., et al. Association of *Streptococcus bovis* with carcinoma of the colon. *N. Engl. J. Med. 297*:800–802, 1977.

Mansur, A. J., Grinberg, M., Lemos da Luz, P., and Bel-lotti, G. The complications of infective endocarditis. *Arch. Intern. Med. 152*:2428–2432, 1992.

Okell, C. C., and Elliott, S. D. Bacteremia and oral sepsis with special reference to the etiology of subacute endocarditis. *Lancet 2*:869–872, 1935.

Osler, W. The Gulstonian lectures on malignant endocarditis. *Br. Med. J. 7*:467, 1885.

Vuille, C., Nidorf, M., Weyman, A. E., and Picard, M. H. Natural history of vegetations during successful medical treatment of endocarditis. *Am. Heart. J. 128*:1200–1209, 1994.

Wilson, W., Karchmer, A. W., Bisno, A. L., et al. Antibiotic treatment of infective endocarditis due to viridans streptococci, enterococci, other streptococci, staphylococci, and HACEK microorganisms. *JAMA 274*:1706–1713, 1995.

# 34

# STAPHYLOCOCCI, STAPHYLOCOCCAL DISEASE, AND TOXIC SHOCK SYNDROME

STANFORD T. SHULMAN, M.D.

Staphylococci are very important bacterial causes of human disease. They normally inhabit the human upper respiratory tract, skin, intestinal tract, and vagina and are particularly likely to produce infection when host resistance is lowered, such as by an antecedent viral infection or a foreign body. These microorganisms are remarkable for the production of many exotoxins and other extracellular substances. Precisely how these extracellular products are involved in disease production remains somewhat obscure.

## CLASSIFICATION

Staphylococci are nonflagellate, nonmotile, gram-positive, catalase-positive cocci, approximately 0.5–1.5 $\mu$m in diameter. Cells divide in more than one plane and as a result form irregular masses resembling clusters of grapes.

Only a minority of the 12 species in the genus *Staphylococcus* that colonize humans are of major medical importance. These are conveniently divided into coagulase-positive *(S. aureus)* and coagulase-negative (all others, including *S. epidermidis* and *S. saprophyticus*) staphylococci (Table 34–1), which differ very substantially in their disease-producing capac-

ity. *S. aureus* is highly pathogenic, producing serious infections in previously healthy individuals and the immunocompromised, whereas coagulase-negative species generally produce infection in those whose host defenses are compromised or in those with an implanted foreign body.

## GROWTH

Staphylococci are aerobes and facultative anaerobes that grow well on ordinary media. Colonies are fairly large, smooth, and glistening after 24–48 h of incubation on agar plates. *S. aureus* colonies are usually pigmented, from a light yellow to a deep orange or lemon yellow color, resulting from carotenoid pigments elaborated by the microorganism. *Aureus* means "gold" in Greek. Colonies of coagulase-negative staphylococci are white, lacking carotenoid pigments. Because *S. aureus* produces hemolysins, colonies are usually surrounded by a variable zone of beta hemolysis on blood agar. Colonies of staphylococci on blood agar plates are much larger than those of *Streptococcus, Neisseria,* or *Haemophilus* species and are easily recognized.

Staphylococcal cells grow over a wide range

**505**

## TABLE 34–1. DIFFERENTIAL CHARACTERISTICS OF SPECIES OF STAPHYLOCOCCI

| CHARACTERISTIC | S. AUREUS | COAGULASE-NEGATIVE STAPHYLOCOCCI |
|---|---|---|
| Coagulase | + | − |
| Mannitol | | |
| Acid aerobically | + | + or − |
| Acid anaerobically | + | − |
| Alpha toxin | + | − |
| Heat-resistant endonucleases | + | − |
| Biotin for growth | − | + |
| Cell wall | | |
| Ribitol | + | − |
| Glycerol | − | + |
| Protein A | + | − |
| Salt resistance | + | − |

+: 90% or more strains positive.
−: 90% or more strains negative.

of temperatures, from 5°–46°C, with the optimum temperature for growth between 30° and 37°C. Two other growth characteristics are of importance. Most strains of *S. aureus*, but not coagulase-negative staphylococci, grow in high concentrations of sodium chloride (10–15%) and are resistant to the action of bile salts, growing well in up to 40% bile.

## HABITAT

Because *S. aureus* and coagulase-negative staphylococci are members of the indigenous microbial flora of humans (see Chapter 2), many persons are asymptomatic carriers of staphylococci and thus may serve as a source of infection for themselves as well as for others. This situation is analogous to that for infections with *S. pyogenes*, *S. pneumoniae*, *H. influenzae*, and *N. meningitidis*. Epidemics of staphylococcal disease may occur, especially with so-called epidemic types of *S. aureus* in hospitals or other institutions, but more often staphylococcal disease occurs sporadically in the community.

In contrast to the microorganisms mentioned above, which colonize primarily the upper respiratory tract, staphylococci are also found in other regions of the body. Skin is frequently inhabited, and staphylococci are commonly found in the umbilicus, axilla, perineum, face, hands, hair, and vagina. In the upper respiratory tract, staphylococci colonize the oropharynx and nasopharynx, but they occur in greatest numbers in the anterior nares. Colonization of the anterior nares by *S. aureus* provides a source for colonization of the skin, and assessment of cultures of this site serves to indicate colonization.

It is estimated that 20–75% of all persons at any given time harbor *S. aureus* in or on one of the sites referred to above. Hospital employees demonstrate rates at the higher end of this range. Asymptomatic carriers of *S. aureus* can be divided into several types: *persistent carriers*, who harbor a specific strain of *S. aureus* for prolonged periods; *occasional carriers*, who sporadically harbor pathogenic staphylococci; and *intermittent* or *transient carriers*, who harbor one staphylococcal type for a period and then a different type.

When outbreaks of *S. aureus* infections occur, it is essential to identify the responsible strain in order to characterize those who have been infected or colonized by that strain. Determination of the antibiogram (pattern of antibiotic resistance) and phage typing are important epidemiologic tools. Phage typing assesses the pattern of susceptibility of a strain of *S. aureus* to lysis by an international set of more than 20 bacteriophages after overnight incubation. Molecular assessment of strains, usually by examination of electrophoretic patterns of nucleic acid fragments after restriction enzyme digestion, is being utilized increasingly for epidemiologic studies.

## DISSEMINATION

Figure 34–1 indicates the epidemiologic cycle of staphylococci in the hospital and in the community. Staphylococci harbored by either asymptomatic carriers or by a person with an infection can be disseminated in a number of ways to others or to the environment. Staphylococci may be expelled from the upper respiratory tract during sneezing. Inanimate objects and even the dust on the floors and walls of rooms may be contaminated in this manner and then may serve as sources of spread to others. Staphylococci can also be transmitted to others by the hands of an asymptomatic carrier. Hands are readily contaminated by staphylococci that have colonized the anterior nares, and *S. aureus*, therefore, can be transmitted directly to others. Hospital personnel are particularly apt to spread staphylococci in this manner; thus, handwashing between patients is very important in preventing transmission. The asymptomatic carrier can also transmit staphylococci to his or her own skin

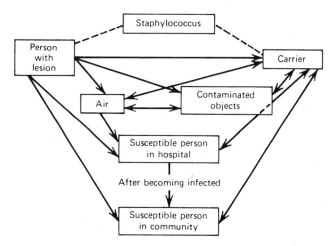

**FIGURE 34–1.** Epidemiologic cycle of staphylococci in the hospital and in the community. (From Nahmias, A. J., and Schulman, J. A. Epidemiologic aspects and control methods. In: Cohen, J. O., ed. *The Staphylococci.* New York: John Wiley & Sons, 1972. With permission.)

and clothing by sneezing or by contaminated hands.

A number of studies have examined the spread of strains of *S. aureus* in neonatal nurseries. The upper respiratory tract and skin of newborns become colonized with staphylococci within a few hours after birth. Impetigo, conjunctivitis, omphalitis (infection of the umbilical stump), and even pneumonia or septicemia may develop. The staphylococcal strain may originate from another colonized infant in the nursery or from carriers among the nurses or other hospital personnel or parents. The major mode of transmission to the newborn is by the hands of health care professionals who handle the infants. Fomites such as diapers, undershirts, sheets, and blankets, if heavily contaminated with staphylococci, may also serve as vectors rarely.

Staphylococcal disease occurs more frequently in patients in hospitals (nosocomially) than in individuals in the nonhospital population. The major reason for this higher incidence is that staphylococcal infection occurs more commonly in persons with lowered host resistance. Asymptomatic carriers of pathogenic staphylococci only rarely develop staphylococcal disease while their resistance to this microorganism is high; however, if there is a reduction in host resistance (e.g., influenza infection, foreign body), resident staphylococci may cause infection. Table 34–2 lists factors known to predispose to disease by *S. aureus*, readily explaining why *S. aureus* infections are more common in hospital patients.

## TABLE 34–2.   FACTORS PREDISPOSING TO STAPHYLOCOCCUS AUREUS INFECTION*

Injury to normal skin (e.g., traumatic abrasions and wounds, surgical incisions, burns, primary skin diseases)
Prior viral infections (e.g., influenza, measles)
Leukocyte defects
   Decreased numbers of leukocytes (e.g., congenital or acquired leukopenia, immunosuppressive drugs)
   Defects in chemotaxis
   Defects in phagocytosis or facilitation of this process by serum opsonins or other serum factors
   Defects in intracellular killing (e.g., Chronic Granulomatous Disease)
Deficiencies in humoral immunity
Presence of foreign bodies (e.g., intravenous catheters, sutures, prosthetic cardiac valves, tampons)
Prior prophylacic or therapeutic use of antibiotics to which the infecting *S. aureus* is not susceptible
Miscellaneous illnesses with less well understood defects in host resistance (e.g., diabetes mellitus, alcoholism, cystic fibrosis, coronary artery disease, various malignant tumors, uremia)

*From Schulman, J. A., and Nahmias, A. J. Staphylococcal infections: Clinical aspects. In: Cohen, J. O., ed. *The Staphylococci.* New York: John Wiley & Sons, 1972. With permission.

## PATHOGENESIS

Staphylococci may produce disease in almost every organ and tissue. The skin is particularly prone to infection, and staphylococcal skin infections are probably among the most common of infectious diseases. For example, over 1.5 million cases of furunculosis occur in the United States each year. The spread of staphylococcal infection and the major organs and tissues in which infections occur are shown in Figure 34–2. This figure demonstrates that *S. aureus* infections may spread by direct extension to contiguous tissues or by way of lymphatics and then hematogenously. Metastatic infections in a wide variety of tissues may result.

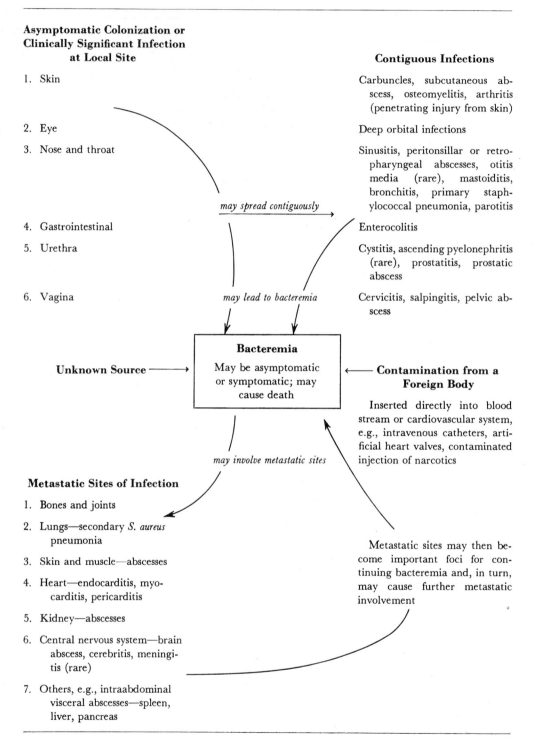

**Asymptomatic Colonization or
Clinically Significant Infection
at Local Site**

1. Skin

2. Eye

3. Nose and throat

4. Gastrointestinal

5. Urethra

6. Vagina

*may spread contiguously*

*may lead to bacteremia*

**Contiguous Infections**

Carbuncles, subcutaneous abscess, osteomyelitis, arthritis (penetrating injury from skin)

Deep orbital infections

Sinusitis, peritonsillar or retropharyngeal abscesses, otitis media (rare), mastoiditis, bronchitis, primary staphylococcal pneumonia, parotitis

Enterocolitis

Cystitis, ascending pyelonephritis (rare), prostatitis, prostatic abscess

Cervicitis, salpingitis, pelvic abscess

**Unknown Source** ⟶

**Bacteremia**

May be asymptomatic or symptomatic; may cause death

⟵ **Contamination from a Foreign Body**

Inserted directly into blood stream or cardiovascular system, e.g., intravenous catheters, artificial heart valves, contaminated injection of narcotics

*may involve metastatic sites*

**Metastatic Sites of Infection**

1. Bones and joints

2. Lungs—secondary *S. aureus* pneumonia

3. Skin and muscle—abscesses

4. Heart—endocarditis, myocarditis, pericarditis

5. Kidney—abscesses

6. Central nervous system—brain abscess, cerebritis, meningitis (rare)

7. Others, e.g., intraabdominal visceral abscesses—spleen, liver, pancreas

Metastatic sites may then become important foci for continuing bacteremia and, in turn, may cause further metastatic involvement

**FIGURE 34–2.** Pathogenic sequence of *Staphylococcus aureus* infection. (From Schulman, J. A., and Nahmias, A. J. Staphylococcal infections: Clinical aspects. In: Cohen, J. O., ed. *The Staphylococci.* New York: John Wiley & Sons, 1972. With permission.)

The disease process is initially localized with an acute inflammatory response and the local accumulation of enormous numbers of segmented neutrophils. Lesions tend to become walled off as a result of the deposition of fibrin. Subsequently, central necrosis and liquefaction may develop and an abscess is formed. Clinically, suppuration or liquefaction of the contents within the infected area often appears fluctuant and can drain spontaneously through the skin. Thus, the hallmark of local staphylococcal infections is abscess formation. Dissemination as outlined in Figure 34–2 may occur from an initial abscess, appearing most often in compromised hosts.

The enormous influence of foreign bodies on susceptibility to staphylococcal infection was shown dramatically by the classic studies of Elek and Conan. These investigators found that it was necessary to inject $5 \times 10^6$ viable *S. aureus* into the skin of human volunteers in order to produce infection. However, as few as 100 viable *S. aureus* were required if the microorganisms were impregnated on a silk suture and tied into the skin. This phenomenon helps explain why cardiac prostheses, indwelling venous catheters, and other surgically implanted foreign bodies are so frequently colonized by staphylococci, even by low-virulence, coagulase-negative staphylococci.

## VIRULENCE FACTORS

*S. aureus* probably elaborates more extracellular toxins, hemolysins, enzymes, and cellular components than any other medically significant bacterium, and all of these factors at one time or another have been thought to be responsible for virulence. Table 34–3 shows a partial list of these bacterial constituents and products. At present, it is not clear that any one or any combination of these factors accounts completely for the virulence of *S. aureus*. It is likely that many of them play some role in the pathogenesis of staphylococcal disease, but it is more likely that no one factor is essential for pathogenicity.

Some of these substances are, however, of particular interest. *Coagulase,* a protein that promotes the clotting of plasma, is thought by some to be largely responsible for the virulence of *S. aureus*. There is a high correlation between the presence of coagulase and virulence, because most strains isolated from infectious processes in previously healthy humans are coagulase-positive (see Table 34–1). A simple procedure, the slide coagulase test, has been developed for detecting the presence of coagulase.

The hemolysins of *S. aureus* are of interest, particularly the *alpha hemolysin*, or alpha toxin. This was the first staphylococcal hemolysin to be investigated. It is a chromosomally encoded protein exotoxin that not only lyses red cells and destroys other cells but also kills rabbits when injected intravenously in sufficient amount. If injected into the skin of rabbits or guinea pigs, alpha toxin also produces acute inflammation and necrosis (dermonecrosis). On sheep blood agar plates, colonies of *S. aureus* are surrounded by a large zone of beta hemolysis due to the lysis of the red cells by this and other hemolysins.

Although alpha hemolysin may play some role in the pathogenesis of staphylococcal disease (since it may be responsible for some of the resulting necrosis), it does not appear to be the major factor in disease production. Antitoxin directed against alpha hemolysin has no protective effect against staphylococcal infection, even though the toxin is effectively neutralized in this manner. None of the other hemolysins appears to play an important role in virulence.

The enterotoxins of *S. aureus* are clearly re-

**TABLE 34–3.  POTENTIAL VIRULENCE FACTORS**

| |
|---|
| Enzymes |
|    Coagulase |
|    Hyaluronidase |
|    Phosphatase |
|    DNAse |
|    Penicillinase |
|    Proteases |
|    Lipases |
|    Lysozyme |
|    Lactate dehydrogenase |
| Hemolysins |
|    Alpha toxin |
|    Beta toxin |
|    Gamma toxin |
|    Delta toxin |
| Enterotoxins |
|    Leukocidin |
|    Exfoliatin |
| Cellular Antigens |
|    Polysaccharide A |
|    Polysaccharide 263 |
|    Protein A |
|    Protein B |
|    Antigen D |
|    Capsular antigen (SSA, SPA) |
|    Teichoic acids |

sponsible for the syndrome known as *staphylococcal food poisoning*. There are four antigenically distinct enterotoxins (A, B, C, and D). Staphylococcal food poisoning occurs when food has become contaminated with an enterotoxin-producing strain of *S. aureus*. If such food remains at room temperature, staphylococci multiply rapidly and produce toxin, which is excreted into the food; when the food is ingested, acute gastroenteritis results. Rather than acting directly on the gastrointestinal tract, the toxin is absorbed and reaches the central nervous system (CNS) via the systemic circulation. The action of the toxin on selected areas of the nervous system results in the often violent gastrointestinal tract manifestations of this disease. Not infrequently, there is marked malaise and sometimes prostration. Normally, the acute phase is self-limited, lasting no longer than 24 h. Rarely, prostration and dehydration are severe enough to warrant hospitalization.

*S. aureus* is the most common cause of food poisoning in the Western world. The disease frequently occurs in epidemics, when contaminated food is ingested by large groups of people. (An example of such an epidemic is given at the end of this chapter.) The disease can also occur sporadically and be limited to members of a household.

Food is usually contaminated by an infected person or by an asymptomatic carrier. A person with a staphylococcal lesion on the hand may infect food directly. Food may also be contaminated by the hands of a noninfected person if he or she is carrying an enterotoxin-producing strain of staphylococci on the skin. Regardless of the manner in which the food is contaminated, all staphylococcal food poisoning cases have one common characteristic. Following staphylococcal contamination, there must be a period of several hours in which the food is maintained at a temperature high enough to permit multiplication of staphylococci and elaboration of enterotoxin. Therefore, staphylococcal food poisoning is best prevented by refrigerating prepared foods at all times. Ham is a very common source of staphylococcal enterotoxin. Because of the use of a high salt concentration for curing ham, the meat does not readily support most bacterial growth. However, since staphylococci grow readily in high concentrations of sodium chloride, ham is an excellent medium for the growth of these particular microorganisms. It is wise to avoid ingestion of ham and other foods preserved in this manner when it

cannot be ascertained that the food has been kept refrigerated until served.

*S. aureus* strains produce *exfoliatins*, two distinct exotoxins (one chromosome-mediated and the other plasmid-mediated). Exfoliatin produces separation and loss of the most superficial layers of the epidermis, apparently by selectively destroying cells of the stratum granulosum of the epidermis. Exfoliatin produced locally can cause marked exfoliation at distant sites, resulting in Ritter's disease in neonates and staphylococcal scalded skin syndrome (SSSS) in older individuals. Circulating antiexfoliatin confers protection.

The polysaccharide capsular antigens of only certain strains of *S. aureus* are antiphagocytic and thus are definite virulence factors. Antibody against these antiphagocytic capsular antigens serves as opsonin. The exact role of capsular antigens in the virulence of these strains for humans has not been ascertained, but in experimental animals they act as antiphagocytic factors and their antiphagocytic action is neutralized by specific antibody.

Penicillinase production results in resistance of almost all staphylococcal strains to penicillin. Resistant strains began to appear rapidly after the introduction of penicillin therapy. Now both community-acquired and hospital-acquired staphylococci must be considered to be penicillin-resistant unless proved otherwise. Plasmid-encoded penicillinase (beta-lactamase) production is the basis of this penicillin resistance. Antibiotics such as methicillin, oxacillin, cephalosporins, and vancomycin are not susceptible to the degradative action of staphylococcal penicillinase. However, staphylococci can rapidly develop resistance to these beta-lactamase–resistant penicillins by means of transduction between *S. aureus* strains, or conjugative transfer of plasmids from other *S. aureus*, coagulase-negative staphylococci, or enterococci. An exception is vancomycin, to which staphylococcal resistance fortunately is very rare.

Recent epidemics of hospital-acquired infections have called attention to the increasing occurrence of multiresistant staphylococcal strains that are also resistant to the penicillinase-resistant penicillins and cephalosporins. These are commonly termed *methicillin-resistant S. aureus* (MRSA). They are considered to be *heteroresistant* in that most staphylococcal cells are fairly sensitive to penicillinase-resistant antibiotics such as methicillin, but a small fraction are quite resistant to even high concentrations of these agents. This resistance is chromosomally mediated and involves production of penicillin-binding protein PBP-2′, a peptidoglycan transpeptidase with low affinity for beta-lactams. MRSA strains are very important clinically and should be considered resistant to all penicillinase-resistant penicillins and cephalosporins. Fortunately, vancomycin remains effective against these organisms.

Penicillinase-producing strains of staphylococci have been found in the absence of known exposure to penicillin. Some staphylococcal isolates collected in late 1951–1952 from natives of the interior of Borneo, where medical care including penicillin therapy had never existed, proved to be highly resistant to penicillin. These strains may have been induced to produce penicillinase by contact in nature with *Penicillium notatum.*

## IMMUNITY

There is remarkably little information not only on the role of specific products of *S. aureus* in the genesis of staphylococcal disease but also on the host factors that work specifically to prevent staphylococcal infection. *S. aureus* is an extracellular parasite and therefore is killed ordinarily following phagocytosis, which appears to be primarily responsible for resolution of infection. Although most humans, particularly adults, have fairly high levels of circulating antibody to staphylococci, the relative roles of humoral and cellular immunity are unclear. Efforts to induce specific antistaphylococcal immunity have been unsuccessful.

## LABORATORY DIAGNOSIS

The definitive diagnosis of staphylococcal disease is made by isolation and identification of the species of staphylococcus involved. Material such as sputum or purulent drainage can be plated on appropriate media, and the size and the pigmentation of colonies of *S. aureus* surrounded by a zone of beta hemolysis usually make recognition of staphylococci on the plate fairly easy. Once a staphylococcus has been identified, *S. aureus* must be differentiated from coagulase-negative staphylococci. The latter frequently show little pigmentation, but the most important differential characteristic is the presence or absence of coagulase production. There is a high degree of correlation between production of coagulase and pathogenicity. Coagulase-negative staphylococci rarely produce alpha toxin (see Table 34–1).

Coagulase-positive strains can be differentiated into groups and types by bacteriophage typing or by molecular methods (see above). Phage typing for coagulase-negative strains is not fully developed.

Antibody to cell-wall teichoic acid antigens in serum has been studied for usefulness as a diagnostic test for staphylococcal infection. However, these assays are insufficiently specific to be of much use clinically.

## PREVENTION

No specific prevention for staphylococcal disease is available. Immunization with products of the staphylococcus, although producing some increase in resistance in experimental animals, has not been proved useful in humans.

In those with recurrent staphylococcal infection, prevention is directed toward controlling reinfection and, if possible, eradicating carriage. Use of chlorhexidine soaps and high-temperature laundering may be useful in reducing risk of reinfection. Application of creams containing antistaphylococcal antibiotics (neomycin, bacitracin, mupirocin) to the anterior nares, with or without oral agents such as rifampin or ciprofloxacin, may be helpful. To prevent infection of surgical implants (e.g., prosthetic valves or joints), short-term administration of a systemic perioperative antistaphylococcal antibiotic is used.

The most important prevention of nosocomial staphylococcal infections is *careful handwashing* by hospital personnel between patients.

## TOXIC SHOCK SYNDROME

It has long been known that *S. aureus* infections rarely could be accompanied by a scarlatiniform rash that desquamated—a clinical syndrome known as *staphylococcal scarlet fever.* This infection was thought to reflect production of an erythrogenic toxin by *S. aureus,* which was biologically similar to the extracellular product of group A streptococci responsible for the classic form of scarlet fever (see Chapter 7). In 1978, Todd and co-workers reported a group of children with an acute multisystemic illness that they designated as *toxic shock syndrome* (TSS). This syndrome is characterized by high fever, rash, vomiting, diarrhea, myalgia, hypotension (shock), and eventual desquamation. By 1980, it was realized that the persons at greatest risk of developing TSS were young menstruating women who used highly absorbent tampons.

*S. aureus* was isolated from these cases and is now established as the etiologic agent responsible for TSS. TSS may develop in persons of any age, race, or sex who have staphylococcal infection or colonization with a strain that elaborates toxic shock syndrome toxin-1 (TSST-1). Regardless of the type of infection, the clinical and laboratory findings are the same as those found in menstruating women. Unless recognized and treated vigorously, the case fatality rate of TSS may be as high as 10–15%.

In tampon-associated TSS, *S. aureus* grows in large numbers adjacent to the tampon and releases TSST-1. Toxin release seems to be facilitated by binding of magnesium to fibers of certain high-absorbency tampons. Magnesium deficiency slows bacterial growth and increases toxin release. The toxin is absorbed from the site of infection or colonization and acts upon distant tissues and organs in individuals who lack antibody to TSST-1. Thus, the classic pattern seen in diphtheria, tetanus, and some other infectious diseases is followed. Repeated attacks of TSS have occurred, reflecting the fact that many affected individuals do not develop antibody to TSST-1 after infection. Since the removal of certain high-absorbency tampons, such as Rely, from the market, the incidence of TSS has fallen sharply.

The pathologic manifestations of TSS are numerous and widespread; many tissues and organs may be involved, including disseminated intravascular coagulation, inflammation and desquamation of the skin, periportal inflammation in the liver, hyaline membrane formation in the lung, and acute tubular necrosis in the kidney. Late sequelae may include chronic renal failure, prolonged neuromuscular disorders, late-onset rash, cyanotic extremities, and neuropsychologic abnormalities. The diagnosis of TSS must be made on clinical grounds, relying on major manifestations of the clinical setting; there are few laboratory tests of diagnostic help, other than documenting multi–organ system involvement. Criteria have been established for the

**TABLE 34–4.   CLINICAL CRITERIA FOR TOXIC SHOCK SYNDROME***

I. Fever >38.9°C (102°F)
II. Rash:
  1. Diffuse macular erythrodema
  2. Desquamation after 1–2 weeks, especially on palms and soles
III. Hypotension:
  1. Systolic < 90 mm Hg in adults or below fifth percentile in children <16 years
  2. Orthostatic drop >15 mm Hg in diastolic blood pressure from lying to sitting: orthostatic syncope or dizziness
IV. Multisystem involvement (≥3):
  1. *GI:* Vomiting or diarrhea at onset
  2. *Muscular:* Severe myalgias or CPK more than twice upper normal limit
  3. *Mucosae:* Vaginal, oropharyngeal, or conjunctival hyperemia
  4. *Renal:* BUN or creatinine more than twice upper normal limits or urine sediment with >5 WBC per high-power field (without infection)
  5. *Hepatic:* Total bilirubin, and/or alanine or aspartate transaminase values more than twice upper limit of normal
  6. *Hematologic:* Platelets <100,000/mm$^3$
  7. *CNS:* Disorientation or altered consciousness without focality when fever and hypertension are absent
V. 1. Normal laboratory results (if tests performed):
    1. Rocky Mountain spotted fever, leptoospirosis, measles titer
  2. Blood (may be positive for *S. aureus*), throat, CSF cultures

*All criteria are necessary for a definite diagnosis.

diagnosis of TSS, with the most characteristic features hypotension and multi–organ system involvement (Table 34–4).

Treatment of TSS should be prompt and vigorous, including removal or reduction of the nidus of infection. The need for removal of tampons when present is obvious. Other sites of focal infection may require drainage. Intravenous high-dose antistaphylococcal therapy is essential. Fluids, electrolytes, and drugs to combat shock are part of the overall supportive treatment of patients with TSS.

TSST-1–producing *S. aureus* has been suggested to be causally related to disorders other than TSS, including Kawasaki disease (a febrile vasculitic disorder of childhood), but attempts to confirm this have failed.

## CASE HISTORY

CASE HISTORY 1

This previously healthy 10-year-old male presented to an emergency room with fever to 102°F and vomiting. He was treated symptomatically but returned 2 days later because of continued high fever, muscle aches, inability to walk, and loss of appetite. He was found to have a painfully swollen right knee and hepatomegaly. There was a 1-cm pustular lesion on the right back that had had small amounts of intermittent bloody drainage for 2 weeks. His mother, a nurse, had been cleaning and dressing this lesion daily. During this hospitalization, pain in the right knee persisted and extended to involve the thigh and the hip. Aspiration of the right knee yielded pus and cultured MRSA. Blood culture also yielded MRSA. Serum liver enzyme levels were elevated. Therapy with intravenous vancomycin and clindamycin was instituted, and he was transferred to a large children's hospital on the third hospital day.

At that time, he was febrile and intermittently mildly hypotensive. He appeared extremely tired and in discomfort. The sclerae were mildly icteric, and the chest and cardiac examinations were unremarkable. The abdomen was very distended and slightly tender diffusely, with mild hepatomegaly but no splenomegaly. A denuded 1-cm pustule was noted over the right lower back with granulation tissue and no drainage. The right thigh was nearly twice the size of the left and was very painful, with the skin tense and taut. There was significant swelling and tenderness of the right knee with an effusion. He was unable to bend either the knee or hip. No neurologic deficits were detected.

Laboratory tests included a white blood cell (WBC) count of 21,300/mm$^3$ with 49% polymorphonuclear neutrophils, 22% bands, 23% lymphocytes, 5% monocytes, and 1% eosinophils. Hemoglobin was 9.8 g/dL, hematocrit was 28.6%, platelet count was 185,000/mm$^3$, electrolytes were normal, blood urea nitrogen (BUN) was 15, creatinine was 1.1 mg/dL, and total bilirubin was 5.1 mg/dL (4.0 mg/dL direct). Creatine kinase was 393 (normal, <150). SGPT (ALT) and SGOT (AST) were moderately elevated. Serum albumin was 1.7 g/dL. Coagulation studies were normal. Chest x-ray showed small peripheral nodular infiltrates throughout both lungs. Computed tomography (CT) of the right leg showed a fluid collection in the thigh adjacent to the iliopsoas, with diffuse muscle edema of the entire right leg. The hip was normal. Blood culture and repeat knee aspiration again yielded MRSA. Two days after transfer, persistent painful right leg swelling prompted drilling several holes in the right femoral shaft, which yielded pus, and aspiration of the right knee again demonstrated septic arthritis. Cultures of bone and joint material yielded MRSA. Several additional needle aspirations of the thigh muscles were performed under CT guidance, yielding purulent material.

Epidemiologic history was of interest in that the patient's mother had had a finger infection 3 weeks earlier for which she had been hospitalized and from which MRSA had been cultured. She was treated with vancomycin and clindamycin. The MRSA isolated from the boy and that isolated from the mother's finger lesion were identical by DNA fragment electrophoretic analysis after restriction enzyme digestion.

He continued to be highly febrile despite intravenous vancomycin and oral rifampin. Echocardiogram demonstrated no evidence of endocarditis. An abdominal CT scan demonstrated bilateral small renal abscesses. Seventeen days after transfer a subperiosteal fluid collection over the distal right femur was drained under CT guidance, yielding 40 mL of sterile pus. Subsequently a chest x-ray demonstrated cavitary lung lesions and resolving pleural effusion. He finally ceased spiking high fevers after 3 weeks of appropriate antibiotic therapy. The child received a total of 12 weeks of intravenous vancomycin and an additional 3 months of clindamycin and rifampin orally. Immunologic evaluation was unremarkable, demonstrating no defects in B- or T-cell number, phagocytic function, complement levels, or immunoglobulin concentrations. The patient ultimately recovered and is without residua.

## CASE 1 DISCUSSION

This immunologically normal youngster had a very extensive infection involving knee, femur, lung, muscle, kidney, and possibly liver. The organism responsible for this widespread infection was methicillin-resistant *Staphylococcus aureus,* an organism that is almost always hospital-acquired. In this case, molecular epidemiologic study strongly suggested the patient's mother (a nurse) to be the source of her son's infection with transmission likely during manipulation of his back lesion. The child failed to improve despite appropriate antibiotic therapy until most infected foci were surgically drained. This is often the case with well-localized abscesses. Staphylococcal infections occasionally disseminate hematogenously to multiple sites, even in the presence of apparently normal immune function. Children are particularly susceptible to hematogenous bone and joint infections. On the other hand, adults, but much less frequently children, are found to have endocarditis with staphylococcal bacteremia. Infections such as the one described here indicate the need to continue to respect *S. aureus* as a potentially very serious pathogen, even in the immunocompetent.

## STAPHYLOCOCCAL FOOD POISONING (A TYPICAL OUTBREAK)

Staphylococcal food poisoning is an intoxication rather than an infection: as noted above, it results from ingestion of food that contains preformed staphylococcal enterotoxin at the time of ingestion. Typically, the food is moist, most often potato salad or other creamy dishes. After the food has been contaminated with toxin-producing *S. aureus* by an infected (or rarely by a carrier) food preparer and has been inadequately refrigerated, *S. aureus* can multiply to greater than $10^5$ organisms per gram with enterotoxin elaboration. Since the toxins are heat-resistant, toxicity persists even if the food is subsequently heated to boiling. After ingestion of the contaminated food, acute vomiting and diarrhea without fever develop within 1–10 h. Except in the elderly or in debilitated individuals, recovery occurs rapidly. A description of a typical epidemic follows.

On July 26–27, approximately 725 incoming freshmen, 475 parents, and 150 faculty and staff members attended summer preregistration activities at a large state university. On July 27, several hours after a box lunch was served between 12:00 and 1:00 P.M., an estimated 300 persons experienced the onset of vomiting and diarrhea, and 84 were subsequently evaluated at a nearby emergency room. Two adults and one student had documented hypotension responsive to intravenous fluids. All but four patients were released the same evening.

A sample of 198 of the students (27%) and their families was randomly chosen for a telephone survey; 22 students and 45 parents reported gastrointestinal symptoms. For those who ate the box lunch, the attack rate was 27.5% for students and 50.6% for parents. For those not eating the box lunch, the attack rate was 0%. Symptoms included nausea (76%), cramps (71%), diarrhea (67%), vomiting (44%), chills (25%), fever (25%), and collapse (9%). The incubation period in 98% of cases was between 1 and 10 h; the median was 4.5 h. Those whose symptoms included nausea and vomiting had shorter incubation periods than those with only diarrhea. Forty percent of those ill sought medical attention. The median duration of illness was 5 h for students and 7.5 h for parents. Of the 150 faculty members who were given free tickets for the box lunch, 84 ate the lunch; 47.7% of those (but none who did not eat the lunch) became ill.

Food-specific attack rates implicated the macaroni salad. Chicken could not be excluded as a vehicle of transmission, because all but one of the individuals also ate chicken. No other foods were significantly associated with illness.

The macaroni was cooked and rinsed on July 25 and refrigerated overnight. On July 26, between 10 A.M. and 2 P.M., celery, fresh green peppers, onions, and canned red peppers were hand sliced, chopped mechanically, and hand mixed with the macaroni and commercial dressing, which did not contain egg. The salad was placed into 30-lb closed plastic containers in a walk-in cellar overnight. At 6:00 A.M. on July 27, it was taken out of storage, and from 6:30 A.M. to 12:20 P.M. individual portions were put into Styrofoam boxes, which were transported in large groups to eating areas. The lunches were kept at room temperature during this time.

Examination of the macaroni salad from unused trays left at room temperature until 7 or 8 P.M. revealed $10^4$–$10^5$ coagulase-positive staphylococci per gram and $10^6$–$10^9$ enterococci per gram and contained staphylococcal enterotoxin C. The chicken contained small numbers of coagulase-positive staphylococci. The staphylococci isolated from these foods were nontypable.

Twenty-four kitchen workers were interviewed, and cultures from anterior nares, back of wrist, and rectum were obtained on August 2. Four workers had nontypable staphylococci isolated from wrists or nares. Antibiotic sensitivity testing of nontypable organisms from two workers and from the macaroni salad revealed them to be identical. One of the workers was directly involved in the preparation and serving of the macaroni salad and was the probable source of contamination.

# REFERENCES

## Review Articles

Arbuthnott, J., and Bergdoll, M. S., eds. Toxic shock syndrome. *Rev. Infect. Dis. 11*(Suppl. 1):S1–S333, 1989.

Bhakdi, S., and Tranum-Jensen, J. Alpha-toxin of *Staphylococcus aureus*. *Microbiol. Rev. 55*:733–751, 1991.

Hedberg, C. W., MacDonald, K. L., and Osterholm, M. T. Changing epidemiology of food-borne disease: A Minnesota perspective. *Clin. Infect. Dis. 18*:671–680, 1994.

Lyon, B. R., and Skurray, R. Antimicrobial resistance of *Staphylococcus aureus*: Genetic basis. *Microbiol. Rev. 51*: 88–134, 1987.

## Original Articles

Davis, J. P., Chesney, P. J., Wand, P. J., et al. Toxic shock syndrome: Epidemiologic features, recurrence, risk factors, and prevention. *N. Engl. J. Med. 303*:1429–1435, 1980.

Elek, S. D., and Conan, P. E. The virulence of *Staphylococcus pyogenes* for man. A study of the problems of wound infections. *Br. J. Exp. Pathol. 38*:573–577, 1957.

Melish, M. E., Glasgow, L. A., and Turner, M. D. The staphylococcal scalded-skin syndrome. Isolation and partial characterization of the exfoliative agent. *J. Infect. Dis. 125*:129–140, 1972.

Peters, G. New considerations in the pathogenesis of coagulase-negative staphylococcal foreign body infections. *J. Antimicrob. Chemother. 21*(Suppl. C):139–148, 1988.

Pfaller, M. A., and Herwaldt, L. A. Laboratory, clinical and epidemological aspects of coagulase-negative staphylococci. *Clin. Microbiol. Rev. 1*:281–290, 1988.

Tenover, T. C., Arbeit, R., Archer, G., et al. Comparison of traditional and molecular methods of typing isolates of *Staphylococcus aureus*. *J. Clin. Microbiol. 32*:407–415, 1994.

Todd, J., and Fishaut, M. Toxic shock syndrome associated with phage-group-I staphylococci. *Lancet 2*:1116–1118, 1978.

# 35

# BONE AND JOINT INFECTIONS: SEPTIC ARTHRITIS AND OSTEOMYELITIS

JOHN T. CLARKE, M.D. and TINA Q. TAN, M.D.

Septic arthritis and osteomyelitis are significant infections of joints and bones, respectively, that have many features in common. *Staphylococcus aureus* is the most common cause of each in both adults and children. Bacteria may reach either site by three basic routes: (1) hematogenous spread from a primary focus; (2) spread of infection from adjacent tissues; or (3) direct inoculation into the site. Early diagnosis and treatment usually lead to complete resolution of infection. Late recognition or inappropriate therapy may lead to chronic infection that can persist for decades, with accompanying loss of normal structure and function, and the development of significant disability or need for amputation. This can be especially devastating in a child; complications and sequelae of bone and joint infections may not become apparent for months to years after the initial insult because of the dynamic state of growth of their skeletal system.

## SEPTIC ARTHRITIS

### Clinical Description

A healthy adult patient may present with chills, fever, and pain in one or more joints.

Classic findings of warmth, redness, swelling, and pain are commonly found. An uncomplicated case in a previously healthy adult usually poses little diagnostic difficulty.

The clinical manifestations of septic arthritis in children are age dependent. In infants less than 1 year of age, the disease is usually monoarticular and involves the large joints, primarily the knees, hips, and shoulders. The clinical findings may be subtle and include swelling, tenderness, and erythema of the skin overlying the joint, with guarding and limitation of motion of the affected extremity. In the neonate and young infant pseudoparalysis may be the only clinical manifestation. Children over a year of age usually present with fever and the classic findings of warmth, redness, swelling, and tenderness of the involved joint. Infections in the shoulder and particularly in the hip may be difficult to diagnose because of the overlying muscle tissue, or referral of pain to the knee. A careful history should be obtained to look for a primary cutaneous, sinopulmonary, ear, or genitourinary focus of infection or evidence of injection drug use. One should also ascertain if there was any antecedent infection or previous trauma involving the involved joint. Physi-

515

cal examination in the adult should demonstrate the presence of an effusion in the index joint, and other joints should also be screened for less prominent involvement. Physical examination in the child yields two major findings: tenderness over a bone or joint, and limitation of range of motion (passive or active). Infants with involvement of the hip joint may position the involved leg so that it is abducted and externally rotated (''frog-leg'' position).

## Etiology

Septic arthritis acquired through the hematogenous route arises from bacteremia; hence, the offending organism is directly related to the most common organisms causing bacteremia in a specific age or other identifiable risk group (Table 35–1). The bacteriology is itself a reflection of the host's age-related microbial flora, immunologic status, acquired immunity, biopsychosocial risks, and acquired disease.

In children, a microbial etiology is identified in about two thirds of the cases of bacterial arthritis. *S. aureus* is the most common cause of septic arthritis overall; in children under 2 years of age *Haemophilus influenzae* type b was recognized as the predominant pathogen until the introduction of the *H. influenzae* type b conjugate vaccine for use at 2 months of age (see Chapter 40). The actual frequency of *H. influenzae* type b as the etiologic agent for septic arthritis in this age group is unknown but appears to have decreased dramatically. Other gram-negative bacilli cause 10–15% of the cases of septic arthritis and this figure is relatively constant. *Neisseria gonorrhoeae* is the dominant organism during the period of greatest high-risk sexual activity and also occurs in the neonate occasionally. Although the specific streptococcal species change with age (group B streptococ-

cus in neonates and young infants, group A and pneumococci in older infants and children, and group D in adults), overall the proportion of cases of septic arthritis that they cause is relatively stable.

In all age groups *Staphylococcus aureus* is the dominant pathogen that colonizes normal epithelium and produces more extracellular substances than any other bacterium. These are discussed in further detail in Chapter 34. These substances facilitate the microorganism's ability to enter the bloodstream, to resist humoral immunity and phagocytosis, to penetrate into the joint space, and to bind to sialoprotein receptors located on the synovial membrane.

## Pathogenesis and Pathology

In children, the pathogenesis of hematogenous septic arthritis is poorly understood. The rich synovial blood supply and the presence of membrane receptors for bacterial structures and products may allow insignificant trauma to play a role in the pathogenesis of septic arthritis. In infants under 18 months of age there is a communication between the arterial supply of the metaphysis and the epiphysis by transepiphyseal vessels. Venous channels perforate the cartilaginous growth plate, so there is no anatomic barrier to extension of infection from the metaphysis to the epiphysis. The consequence of this communication is that extension of infection to the epiphysis can easily lead to secondary involvement of the adjacent joint. In both adults and children the articular capillaries lack a basement membrane, and *S. aureus* and other organisms in the bloodstream may gain access to the articular space by passing through the walls of these capillaries. Organisms reaching the joint space encounter an environment rich in nutrients. Bacterial replication pro-

## TABLE 35–1.    AGE-RELATED ETIOLOGY OF SEPTIC ARTHRITIS (PERCENTAGE BY AGE)

| Gram's Stain | Organism | Age (Years) | | | |
|---|---|---|---|---|---|
| | | 0–2 | 2–14 | 15–34 | ≥35 |
| Gram-positive cocci | *S. aureus* | 25–30 | 40–60 | 20–40 | >50 |
| | Streptococci | 10–20 | 10–20 | 10–20 | 10–20 |
| Gram-negative cocci | *Neisseria* | <10 | <10 | 40–70 | Rare |
| Gram-negative bacilli | *H. influenzae* type b | * | <10 | Rare | Rare |
| | Enterobacteriaceae and *Pseudomonas aeruginosa* | 10–15 | 10–15 | 10–15 | 10–15 |
| All other bacteria | | <10 | <10 | <10 | <10 |

*Actual frequency not known since introduction of *H. influenzae* type b conjugate vaccine.

vides the stimulus that elicits a brisk host inflammatory response consisting of a rapid influx of polymorphonuclear neutrophils (PMNs) and the release of lytic enzymes. This results in an increase in synovial fluid protein concentrations with a concomitant decrease in the pH and glucose concentrations. The resultant inflammation leads to synovial thinning, infiltration of polymorphonuclear leukocytes, and fibrin deposition within the joint space. Prompt and effective therapy can lead to complete reversal and resolution of these changes; however, delayed antibiotic treatment, or the presence of an extremely virulent organism (i.e., *S. pyogenes*), can irreversibly destroy articular cartilage within 1–2 days. If the infection is incompletely or inappropriately treated, the fibrin deposition in the joint space can make effective antibiotic therapy difficult and osteomyelitis may develop beginning on the articular surfaces. These events may lead to irreversible changes in joint anatomy and function, with ankylosis common in this setting.

### Diagnosis

The diagnosis of septic arthritis requires a high index of suspicion, especially in children in whom physical examination findings may be confusing. Aspiration of synovial fluid provides the specimens necessary to make a tentative diagnosis and to initiate therapy. This is very important, since the primary criterion for the diagnosis of septic arthritis is the isolation of an organism from the joint fluid. Once the specimen is obtained it should be sent for Gram's stain, cultures, and analysis of cellular and protein/glucose concentrations. Gram's stain smear of the fluid demonstrates a presumptive organism in about 50% of cases. Normal synovial fluid usually is clear and nearly colorless, but when infected appears turbid and cloudy. Analysis of the fluid reveals the presence of a large number of white blood cells (WBCs), usually over 70,000/mm$^3$ with greater than 80% of these being PMNs. The protein concentration is elevated and glucose concentration is depressed. Synovial fluid cultures are positive only in about 50–70% of the cases, but the yield can be enhanced if one drop of the fluid is inoculated into a blood culture bottle to dilute out the antibacterial substances present. Cultures of the blood and other relevant tests should also be obtained. Blood cultures in children are positive in about 40% of patients. If gonococcal arthritis is a considera-

tion, cultures should be obtained from the cervix, urethra, pharynx, and rectum. Various collagen vascular and rheumatologic disorders can mimic septic arthritis in their presentation, and specific tests should be performed to differentiate these disorders. Crystalline arthritis (gout and pseudogout) can produce very high WBC counts in the synovial fluid, and polarizing microscopy should be performed in adults to look for crystals if doubt exists concerning the diagnosis.

In general, the higher the WBC count in synovial fluid with a predominance of PMNs, the greater the probability of a bacterial infection. The age of the patient is a strong indicator as to the most likely pathogen(s), and predictably organisms are commonly found in specific settings (Table 35–2).

Radiographic studies add very little to the diagnosis of septic arthritis in those joints that are readily accessible to physical examination. In the pediatric population, the joint for which radiographic evaluation is a valuable adjunct to diagnosis is the hip joint. The radiographs should be taken with the child in the frog-leg position, as well as with the legs extended at the knee and slightly internally rotated. The early radiologic signs of septic arthritis are due to swelling of the capsule, which displaces the fat lines. Findings on a plain radiograph that are consistent with a septic hip joint include the obturator sign and obliteration or lateral displacement of the gluteal fat lines.

### Principles of Therapy and Prognosis

Most cases of septic arthritis can be managed medically. The major role of surgical intervention occurs during the initial diagnosis when synovial fluid is obtained for studies, and in the treatment of septic arthritis of the hip or shoulder (in infants), where drainage is best achieved by surgical incision and decompression of the joint to preserve the blood supply to the epiphysis. Open drainage is especially crucial with septic arthritis of the hip because the increased intraarticular pressure compromises the blood supply to the joint and may result in avascular necrosis of the femoral head and destruction of the joint space.

The goal of therapy is to provide adequate concentrations of an antimicrobial agent to the inflamed synovial space in order to eradicate the infection. This, however, does not require direct instillation of antibiotic into the joint space, since parenteral administration of

## TABLE 35–2.  EPIDEMIOLOGIC SETTINGS IN WHICH SPECIFIC ORGANISMS ARE FOUND

| | Organisms Commonly Found In | |
|---|---|---|
| Epidemiologic setting | Septic Arthritis | Osteomyelitis |
| Injection drug use | S. aureus | S. aureus |
| | P. aeruginosa | P. aeruginosa |
| | Enterobacteriaceae (sternoclavicular) | Enterobacteriaceae (vertebral, ribs) |
| Hemodialysis | | S. aureus |
| | | S. epidermidis |
| Rheumatoid arthritis | S. aureus | S. aureus |
| Prosthetic materials | S. aureus | S. aureus |
| | P. aeruginosa and Enterobacteriaceae | S. epidermidis Pseudomonas species |
| Tennis shoe nail puncture | | P. aeruginosa |
| | | S. aureus |
| Sickle cell disease | Salmonella | S. aureus |
| | | S. pneumoniae |
| | | Salmonella |
| | | Shigella |
| | | Klebsiella |
| | | Gram-negative enterics |
| Animal bites | Pasteurella multocida | P. multocida |
| Tick exposure | Borrelia burgdorferi | |

antibiotics results in excellent penetration into the joint space. Initial systemic antimicrobial therapy of septic arthritis is directed toward the most common pathogen(s) at various ages, guided by the results of the Gram's stain smear of aspirated material, other special considerations, and culture results (Table 35–3).

In the neonate, a combination of intravenous (IV) nafcillin and an aminoglycoside provides adequate initial antibiotic coverage. Cefuroxime covers the most common organisms causing septic arthritis in normal children between 2 months and 10 years of age (i.e., *S. aureus* and *H. influenzae* type b) and may be used as empiric initial therapy until an organism is isolated. Cefotaxime or ceftriaxone plus an antistaphylococcal penicillin

such as nafcillin is an excellent alternative choice for empiric therapy of hematogenous septic arthritis. Once an organism is isolated, antibiotic therapy may be tailored based on the antimicrobial susceptibility of the isolate. In children over 10 years of age, *S. aureus* is the most common pathogen causing septic arthritis, and monotherapy with a penicillinase-resistant antistaphylococcal penicillin may be used as empiric initial therapy. The duration of therapy varies from 2 weeks for *N. gonorrhoeae* to 4 weeks for *S. aureus* infection. Comments on antibiotic dosage and duration are seen in Table 35–4. All treatment should be initally administered intravenously.

The results of therapy must be closely monitored. Systemic symptoms and local joint findings should largely resolve within the first

## TABLE 35–3.  ANTIBIOTIC SELECTION BASED ON THE PATIENT AGE AND GRAM'S STAIN FINDINGS

| Age (Years) | Gram-Positive Cocci | Gram-Negative Bacilli | Gram-Negative Cocci | No Organism Seen |
|---|---|---|---|---|
| 0–2 | Oxacillin (staphylococci) (streptococci) | Cefotaxime or ceftriaxone (*H. influenzae*, Enterobacteriaceae, *P. aeruginosa*) | Cefotaxime or ceftriaxone (*N. gonorrhoeae*) | Oxacillin and a third-generation cephalosporin |
| 2–14 | As above | As above | As above | As above |
| >15 | As above | Ciprofloxacin | As above | Oxacillin and ciprofloxacin |

**TABLE 35–4. ANTIBIOTIC THERAPY FOR SEPTIC ARTHRITIS**

| ORGANISM (FROM TABLE 35–3 OR CULTURES | FIRST CHOICE | ALTERNATE CHOICE | DURATION AND COMMENTS |
|---|---|---|---|
| S. aureus | Oxacillin or nafcillin IV 150 mg/kg/day in 4–6 doses | Vancomycin or cefazolin, or clindamycin | 3–4 weeks, consider addition of rifampin in refractory cases |
| S. epidermidis | Vancomycin 30 mg/kg/day in 2 doses | Oxacillin | Oxacillin only if confirmed sensitive; major pathogen with prosthetic joints, sensitivities vary with species; penicillin only if confirmed sensitive |
| S. pneumoniae | Cefuroxime 150 mg/kg/day, cefotaxime or ceftriaxone | Penicillin or vancomycin | |
| S. pyogenes | Penicillin 250,000 units/kg/day in 4 doses | Clindamycin | 2 weeks of therapy |
| H. influenzae | Cefuroxime IV 150 mg/kg/day Cefotaxime IV 150 mg/kg/day in 3 doses or Ceftriaxone IV 100 mg/kg/day | | 2–3 weeks of therapy |
| Enterobacteriaceae: includes E. coli, Enterobacter, Klebsiella, Proteus, and Salmonella | Ciprofloxacin 20 mg/kg/day in 2 doses | Third-generation cephalosporin, ticarcillin-clavulanate, ampicillin-sulbactam, or piperacillin | 3 weeks of therapy; ciprofloxacin should not be used in children <18 years or during pregnancy |
| P. aeruginosa | Pipercillin 250 mg/kg/day in 4–6 doses plus an aminoglycoside, or ceftazidime | Ciprofloxacin or antibiotics above as for Enterobacteriaceae | 2 weeks of therapy |
| Neisseria gonorrhoeae | Cefotaxime 90 mg/kg/day in 3 doses | Ceftriaxone Spectinomycin | 2 weeks of therapy |

week after initiation of therapy. Repeated aspirations of joint fluid should be performed until it is certain that the WBC count in the joint fluid is falling, and that Gram's stain and cultures are negative. Parenteral therapy with the appropriate antibiotic allows therapeutic levels to be achieved in the joint fluid for the eradication of susceptible organisms. The instillation of antibiotics directly into the joints is not necessary, and open drainage is not indicated with the definite exception of the hip and possibly the shoulder joint.

Several points must be reexamined if clinical improvement is not satisfactory: accuracy of diagnosis; sensitivity of the organism; correct antimicrobial dose and interval; or the presence of undrained infection, necrotic tissue, or foreign body. Orthopedic consultation should be obtained if the latter are suspected.

After 1 week of therapy, if all clinical and laboratory parameters indicate a successful course, compliance with an oral regimen can be guaranteed, an oral antibiotic exists with

adequate antimicrobial activity against the patient's isolate, and serum bactericidal titers indicate a peak equal to or greater than 1:8 with a trough level equal to or greater than 1:2, a switch to oral therapy may be considered in children, however, parenteral therapy remains the "gold standard." Home IV therapy is another option to consider for completion of the antimicrobial course; it is a more cost-effective step and allows the patient extra freedom compared to keeping the patient in the hospital for the duration of therapy.

The duration of therapy varies depending on the organism isolated. In general, arthritis caused by S. aureus or gram-negative bacilli should be treated a minimum of 3 weeks, while infections caused by H. influenzae type b should be treated for at least 2 weeks and arthritis caused by N. gonorrhoeae should be treated for at least 7 days.

The prognosis of adequately treated septic arthritis is very good, with no sequelae and the return of complete function and mobility of the involved joint. The most important variables predicting adverse outcome in children are the duration of symptoms prior to initiation of specific therapy and infants who are younger than 1 year of age. The longer the symptoms are present prior to starting appropriate therapy and the younger the age of the child, the higher the incidence of adverse sequelae, such as progression of disease to osteomyelitis, permanent dislocation of the joint, and decreased function and mobility of the joint. Studies suggest that infections caused by the Enterobacteriaceae and *S. aureus* are associated with a higher incidence of sequelae.

## OSTEOMYELITIS

### Clinical Description

There are three major pathogenic routes by which osteomyelitis is produced: (1) hematogenous, which is responsible for about 90% of the cases in children under the age of 16; (2) spread from a contiguous focus, which includes direct inoculation of the bone primarily by trauma; and (3) that due to vascular insufficiency or peripheral vascular disease. These forms differ with respect to the population at risk, the bones involved, the bacteriologic agents, the therapeutic management (both medical and surgical), and the prognosis. Each type may present in an acute or a chronic phase.

Acute hematogenous osteomyelitis occurs as a complication of bacteremia and shares many characteristics with septic arthritis. In children, the clinical findings in osteomyelitis differ with the age of the patient. In newborns and infants, because of the thin cortex, presence of transepiphyseal vessels, and extension of the joint capsule, the infection may progress rapidly and rupture through the bone to cause infection within contiguous joint or muscle. Classic findings include an irritable infant with an edematous, red, and warm extremity who may become more irritable when the infected extremity is moved or touched; pseudoparalysis may also be present. About 50% of neonates have multifocal bone involvement.

In the older child, symptoms of an acute bacterial infection predominate with fever, chills, malaise, anorexia, muscle aches, nausea, and vomiting; edema, erythema, warmth, and tenderness are present over the involved bone. Frequently, signs of a preceding focus

of infection are present, and a history of preceding trauma may be found in about 50% of children. The patient may refuse to bear weight on the affected extremity and may limp and complain of pain on palpation. The long bones of the legs and arms are the most common sites of involvement, usually affecting the metaphysis of the bones (the region adjacent to the epiphyseal growth centers). Preferential involvement of the metaphysis involves areas adjacent to the most active growth centers (e.g., distal femur and proximal tibia around the knee, the proximal humerus, and the distal radius and ulna). Boys are 2.5 times more likely to develop osteomyelitis than are girls, perhaps related to an increased incidence of minor trauma. Blood cultures are documented to be positive in about 60% of the patients.

Hematogenous vertebral osteomyelitis is a similar disease occurring with a peak incidence in the sixth and seventh decades of life. The major symptoms are fever, back pain, and stiffness. Children with vertebral osteomyelitis may complain of abdominal pain that is poorly localized. The presentation of this disease is often subacute, and the patient may have been ill for weeks prior to the time of diagnosis. Infection in males is also more common.

The diagnosis of pelvic osteomyelitis is difficult to establish, since it can mimic appendicitis and urinary tract infections; therefore, most patients have subacute disease by the time the correct diagnosis is made. Point tenderness at the site of the lesion can be elicited in only half of the patients, and most children with pelvic osteomyelitis present with poorly localized abdominal pain or hip pain and tenderness over the buttock or the sciatic notch.

Contiguous-focus osteomyelitis occurs when infection spreads to bone from adjoining infected tissue or prosthetic material. The femur and tibia are the most common sites of involvement. The organisms are often introduced during a traumatic injury that results in a fracture, or during open reduction and internal fixation of the fractures. Infections in the pelvis, hands (from bite wounds), sinuses, periodontal area, and other tissues may also serve as the primary focus and the source of the initial symptoms. Acutely, symptoms of swelling, redness, warmth, and pain predominate; during recurrences these symptoms are less prominent. Intermittent seropurulent or serosanguinous drainage from a small aperture (often over a surgical scar) and the presence of a sinus tract are the hallmark findings in chronic infection. It is paradoxical that this infection, which may persist throughout a patient's lifetime and lead to decades of intermittent drainage and therapy, often has a benign presentation.

Osteomyelitis due to vascular insufficiency or peripheral vascular disease is related to longstanding diabetes mellitus in the great majority of cases, with peripheral neuropathy being the most common accompanying complication. It also may be seen in pediatric patients with myelomeningoceles who have sensory and motor deficits. It is a disease almost exclusively of the feet, usually presenting with evidence of local infection and/or ulceration. By history the patient may recall having problems with the affected foot for weeks or months prior to presentation, and x-rays may reveal the presence of ulceration or a foreign body. Occasionally, cases may be related to severe atherosclerosis or radiation damage.

Iatrogenic osteomyelitis is made up of infections at several distinct sites that are associated with particular medical procedures. In neonates, bone infections of the heel have occurred following repeated heel puncture, and infections in the hip and pelvis may develop after femoral vessel phlebotomy or cannulation of femoral or umbilical vessels. Osteomyelitis of the sternum is a complication that may be seen following median sternotomy for coronary artery bypass grafting or in the repair of congenital heart defects.

### Etiology

*Staphylococcus aureus* is by far the most common organism responsible for acute hematogenous osteomyelitis in both children and adults. In children it accounts for about 80–85% of all cases. Other organisms that less frequently cause osteomyelitis include group A streptococcus, *Haemophilus influenzae* type b (in children <2 years of age), and *Streptococcus pneumoniae*. In infants less than 2 months of age, group B streptococcus (especially serotype III) and coagulase-negative staphylococci (especially in premature infants), are frequent causes of osteomyelitis. In children with hemoglobinopathies such as sickle cell anemia, unusual organisms such as *Salmonella* species, *Escherichia coli*, *Shigella*, and *Klebsiella* may be the etiologic agent of osteomyelitis.

*S. aureus* and group A streptococcus are the most commonly isolated organisms in contiguous-focus osteomyelitis, but mixed infections may be seen. *Pseudomonas aeruginosa* is com-

monly associated with puncture wounds of the calcaneus, and enteric organisms are common in the neonatal period as a cause of contiguous-focus osteomyelitis.

In osteomyelitis due to vascular insufficiency, cultures frequently reveal multiple organisms including staphylococci, streptococci, enterococci, Enterobacteriaceae, *Pseudomonas aeruginosa*, and anaerobes. Anaerobic organisms may also cause osteomyelitis in patients with predisposing conditions including paranasal sinusitis, peridontal disease, and trauma.

Osteomyelitis due to fungi such as *Candida* species and *Aspergillus* most frequently occurs in the immunocompromised host or in the premature infant who requires a central venous catheter or prolonged antimicrobial therapy.

### Pathogenesis and Pathology

Microorganisms are introduced into the long bones at the metaphysis, which is the broad cancellous end of the bone shaft adjacent to the epiphyseal growth centers. The nutrient artery that supplies the bones divides into branches and then into a narrow plexus of capillaries that make sharp loops in the vicinity of the epiphyseal plate and then enter a system of large sinusoidal vessels, in which there is sluggish blood flow and the absence of lining reticuloendothelial cells. Thrombosis of slow-flowing vessels secondary to trauma or embolization provides a site for the localization of infection. Blood-borne bacteria can lodge in this relatively avascular area and proliferate, relatively protected from the host's defense system.

As bacteria proliferate in this area, there is accumulation of bacterial products, which stimulate an acute inflammatory response; this leads to a change in pH and an influx of polymorphonuclear neutrophils. This influx of leukocytes and other humoral factors accumulate under increased pressure, leading to vascular thrombosis, pressure necrosis of bone, and death of small islands of bone. As the process continues, parts of the epiphyseal growth plate may become involved and larger islands of dead bone (sequestrum) accumulate and become recognizable by plain roentgenograms and other imaging studies, or at surgery. In children, in the absence of therapy, the expanding infection may cause necrosis of cortical bone and marrow and as the pressure continues to increase, the exudate is forced through the haversian systems and Volkmann's canal into the cortex. The pressure may be released by dissection of the periosteum from the cortex, creating a subperiosteal abscess. The infection may spread further along the marrow cavity and the periosteum into a joint space, causing septic arthritis, or rupture through the periosteum into adjacent muscle leading to soft tissue infection (which is frequently seen in neonates), with eventual sinus tract formation in some cases. Dead bone tissue presents a major therapeutic problem because it is underperfused and inaccessible to phagocytes and antibiotics; it can serve as a reservoir for infection despite prolonged course(s) of high-dose antibiotics. The histologic appearance of chronic osteomyelitis shows dead osteocytes, with areas of increased osteoclastic and osteoblastic activity, and evidence of chronic inflammation.

## Diagnosis

Precise bacteriologic diagnosis is critical for selection of optimal antibiotic therapy for this type of infection. Open bone biopsy of the affected bone provides the gold standard for histologic diagnosis and bacterial identification. Specimens obtained from subperiosteal abscesses and associated septic joints by needle biopsy and/or aspiration also provide material for culture and Gram's stain and are positive in approximately 70–80% of patients with osteomyelitis. The yield may be enhanced if some of this material is also inoculated into a blood culture bottle to dilute out the antibacterial substances present. Blood cultures should be obtained and are positive in about 50–60% of the patients with acute hematogenous osteomyelitis. Drainage material from sinus tracts is easily cultured, but frequently provides misleading information because of skin flora contamination, unless a pure culture of one organism is recovered, especially if it is *S. aureus*. In contiguous-focus osteomyelitis, because blood cultures are usually negative and sinus tract cultures are often confusing, open biopsies are the most effective means of obtaining material for culture and histologic examination. The erythrocyte sedimentation rate (ESR) is generally elevated in osteomyelitis. Although it is a nonspecific finding, it has been shown to be useful in following the progress of proven osteomyelitis and determining the duration of therapy.

Plain roentgenograms of the affected area obtained early in osteomyelitis commonly show soft tissue swelling with obliteration of the tissue planes. Frequently, especially in adults, plain roentgenograms in acute osteomyelitis are completely normal, or show only the fracture and evidence of surgical intervention (in the case of contiguous-focus osteomyelitis). In general, destruction of bone is not apparent on plain roentgenograms until about 40–50% of the bone mineral has been destroyed; therefore, at least 10 days to 3 weeks are required before bony changes (i.e., destruction and periosteal new bone formation) are visible on plain roentgenograms. Changes are usually seen earlier in small bones (digits) and in younger patients. Plain roentgenograms taken several weeks or months after the initial infection may show an area of decreased radiodensity at the site of the acute infection, at a time when the patient has already shown a remarkable response to therapy. Thus, there is often a major discrepancy between a patient's physical examination findings (representing the current status of the disease), and the radiographic findings (representing the events that occurred weeks earlier). Infections in the most dense bones (femur, sacrum, and the lumbar vertebrae) may not be visible on plain roentgenograms for several weeks or months. Areas of hypodense bone (representing remodeling by osteoclasts) may be seen adjacent to hyperdense bone (representing osteoblastic activity). Details of the soft tissues, especially marrow, muscle, articular cartilage, fibrin deposits, as well as sinus tracts, may be seen in their precise anatomic relation to healthy and diseased bone using magnetic resonance imaging (MRI).

Bone scans with technetium-99 pyrophosphate or technetium-99 methylene diphosphate are more sensitive early in the infection and may be helpful in diagnosing osteomyelitis early in the course of illness, especially in children, at a time before bone changes are apparent on plain roentgenogram. However, bone scans in neonates and young infants are likely to be nondiagnostic, probably due to the limited amount of mineralization in the bones. There may be destruction of cortical bone and periosteal new bone formation on plain radiographs of bones with a normal bone scan. The inflammation associated with cellulitis and fractures may also cause difficulty in interpreting these scans. Scanning techniques using gallium-67, and more recently indium, utilize the property of these substances to label neutrophils *in vivo*, and thus, to indicate a site where there is aggregation of these cells. These scans provide greater specificity in complex clinical cases; however, they are not a useful way to follow the progress of a patient with osteomyelitis, because they continue to be positive in many patients despite clinical and laboratory indications of disease resolution.

## Principles of Therapy

The optimal management of skeletal infections involves a combination of adequate surgical drainage of purulent material (sequestrum, dead bone, and pus) and antimicrobial therapy. The microscopic clearance of dead bone and eradication of organisms embedded in extracellular products (slime) require the activity of phagocytic cells and osteoclasts and occurs over a prolonged period of time. Antimicrobial therapy should be guided by the Gram's stain result and antimicrobial susceptibility of the organism(s) recovered from blood cultures or bone aspirates. Empiric therapy should include an antistaphylococcal antibiotic, since *S. aureus* is the single leading cause of osteomyelitis in both adults and children. Thereafter, antibiotic therapy should be tailored based on the antibiotic susceptibility of the organism isolated. Duration of therapy is critical as seen in Table 35–5.

Most authorities agree that high-dose parenteral antibiotics should be administered for at least 4 weeks to decrease the chance of progression of acute osteomyelitis to chronic osteomyelitis. Retrospective studies in adults have demonstrated that high-dose parenteral therapy for less than 4 weeks leads to an unacceptably high failure rate (>50%) for both acute hematogenous osteomyelitis and vertebral osteomyelitis. Because specific, prolonged parenteral antibiotic therapy is mandatory (and not without its own potential complications), it is essential that all efforts be made to obtain clinical specimens that allow for the precise identification of the pathogenic microbe and its antimicrobial sensitivity. For most patients with acute hematogenous osteomyelitis, 4–6 weeks of precisely targeted, high-dose parenteral therapy is generally accepted as the standard, and has a success rate of over 90% in uncomplicated patients. In these patients, no additional oral therapy is indicated after completion of their parenteral antibiotic course.

Because of the highly diverse nature of patients with contiguous-focus osteomyelitis (age of the patient, nature of trauma, type of surgery, complexity of microbial isolates), the optimal duration of therapy has not been established. A prolonged course of parenteral therapy (4–6 weeks) followed by an additional course of oral antibiotic therapy may be indicated in order to treat the infection adequately, and/or to suppress it sufficiently to allow for bone healing to occur. A team approach is essential in optimizing the care of complex patients with contiguous-focus osteomyelitis. An orthopedic surgeon should be intimately involved in providing stability of the bone so that nonessential hardware, old cement, and other foreign bodies are removed. If healing is delayed secondary to the presence of internal fixation hardware and/or if large portions of the bone are infected and unstable, external fixation devices may be necessary to facilitate healing. The Ilizarov technique allows long segments of infected bone to be removed while bone stability is maintained by an Ilizarov external fixator, giving the patient's proximal bone a chance to

**TABLE 35–5.  THE RELATIONSHIP OF LENGTH OF THERAPY TO OUTCOME IN PATIENTS WITH OSTEOMYELITIS**

| AUTHOR (YEAR) | TYPE OF OSTEOMYELITIS | DEFINITION OF OPTIMAL Rx | PATIENT OUTCOME | TOTAL PATIENTS | OPTIMAL Rx | SUBOPTIMAL Rx |
|---|---|---|---|---|---|---|
| Waldvogel (1970) | AHO* first episode | 4 weeks IV | Good | 27 | 26 | 1 |
| | | | Failure | 6 | 1 | 5 |
| Waldvogel (1970) | CHO† | 4 weeks IV | Good | 4 | 4 | 0 |
| | | | Failure | 13 | 4 | 9 |
| Sapico (1979) | PVO‡ | 4 weeks IV | Sucess | 29 | 25 | 4 |
| | | | Failure | 4 | 1 | 3 |
| Bamberger (1987) | Diabetic foot | 4 weeks IV or combined IV plus PO for at least 10 weeks | Good | 22 | 20 | 2 |
| | | | Poor | 29 | 7 | 22 |

*AHO, acute hematogenous osteomyelitis.
†CHO, chronic hematogenous osteomyelitis.
‡PVO, peripheral vascular insufficiency osteomyelitis.

grow and fill in the void created by the removal of the infected segment.

In patients with osteomyelitis due to vascular insufficiency, a therapeutic regimen combining a prolonged course of parenteral therapy followed by an additional prolonged course of oral antibiotics generally has shown good results.

For all types of osteomyelitis, participation of specialists in vascular catheter insertion, home care, chemical dependence, psychiatry, physical therapy, and nutrition as part of the team are frequently necessary in order to optimize patient compliance with therapy and to allow healing to occur.

### Prognosis and Complications

The prognosis for a complete cure in acute hematogenous osteomyelitis is excellent, occurring in about 90–95% of all cases. Complications are infrequent in both adults and children, but include prolonged bacteremia, septic arthritis, and the progression of disease to a more chronic form. Adverse reactions to the antibiotic therapy and line-associated infections are not uncommon; surveillance is required in order to prevent these complications from occurring and progressing. Over 60% of patients with contiguous-focus osteomyelitis are cured after completing their first course of therapy, with the most common complication being recurrence of the disease. Bacteremia is very rare.

The most common and serious complication of all forms of osteomyelitis is chronicity and nonunion. This is characterized by the formation of sinus tracts that intermittently drain to the skin surface; bacteremia is very rare. Squamous cell carcinoma and amyloidosis have been reported in cases of chronic osteomyelitis that have persisted for decades. Other potentially devastating complications, especially in children, include pathologic fractures, damage to the epiphyseal growth centers, and growth abnormalities (either undergrowth or overgrowth) of the affected bone and adjacent joint. This disease and its complications remain a major source of personal suffering, physical disability, and financial burden costing millions of dollars each year.

### CASE HISTORIES

#### Case History 1

A 14-year-old high school student presented to his physician because of fever and left forearm swelling and pain 2 weeks after being hit in the arm with a baseball during batting practice. An erythematous area was noted, and ice was placed on the arm immediately. The student was able to move his arm without problems, and no medical attention was obtained. During the week prior to presentation he had developed left forearm swelling with progressive tenderness and pain in the area where he had been hit.

Physical examination revealed a moderately swollen area on the ulnar side of his left distal forearm with a 2 × 2–cm area of overlying induration, warmth and erythema, and marked point tenderness at the center of this area. Wrist examination was normal. The temperature was 101.5°F; the remainder of his physical examination was within normal limits.

Laboratory studies indicated that his ESR was 85 mm/h (uncorrected); WBC count was 10,500/mm$^3$ with 55% PMNs, 15% band forms, 30% lymphocytes; and plain roentgenograms revealed an osteolytic lesion in the distal ulna with overlying soft tissue swelling. The patient was taken to the operating room for incision and drainage with bone aspiration. Purulent material was aspirated from the cortical region. Gram's stain demonstrated gram-positive cocci in clusters. He was treated with intravenous oxacillin. Cultures taken in the operating room were positive for *Staphylococcus aureus*, resistant to penicillin but susceptible to oxacillin and clindamycin.

He was discharged from the hospital 5 days after surgery to complete the remainder of his IV therapy at home. He received a 4-week course of IV oxacillin therapy with rapid improvement in his condition. He had a progressive decline in serial ESR measurements, and follow-up plain roentgenograms of his left arm showed operative changes with findings consistent with healing.

#### Case 1 Discussion

This patient's presentation is typical for acute hematogenous osteomyelitis in an older child. The preceding history of trauma (present in up to 50% of patients) with the subsequent development of swelling, warmth, erythema, and point tenderness are classic findings. The high normal peripheral WBC count (most patients with acute osteomyelitis have WBC counts <15,000/mm$^3$) and elevated ESR are further nonspecific indicators supporting the diagnosis of osteomyelitis in this clinical setting. Plain roentgenograms obtained early in the course of osteomyelitis usually only demonstrate soft tissue swelling with no bony changes. A period of 10–20 days from the time of injury is required before destructive lesions and periosteal new bone formation are apparent on plain roentgenograms, as in this case. The osteolytic lesion on plain roentgenogram of his left forearm is indicative of a destructive process, further supporting the diagnosis of osteomyelitis.

*Staphylococcus aureus* is the organism responsible for over 80% of the cases of osteomyelitis in children. Other less frequent bacteriologic causes include group A streptococcus, *Haemophilus influenzae* type b (usually occurs in children <6 years), and *Streptococcus pneumoniae*. Knowledge of the bacteriologic cause of osteomyelitis is essential for optimal management of the infection. Operative intervention to débride the area and obtain material for culture is one of the best ways to determine the causative agent of the osteomyelitis, and drainage of this abscess within bone helps to hasten recovery.

Initial empiric antibiotic therapy of osteomyelitis in children is based primarily on a knowledge of the most likely bacterial pathogens in a specific age group, the results of the Gram's stain of aspirated material, and any other special circumstances that may exist. In the case of this patient, the most likely etiologic agent for his osteomyelitis are gram-positive cocci, so an antistaphylococcal antibiotic such as oxacillin, nafcillin, or clindamycin can be used for therapy. Once the pathogen has been identified, antibiotic therapy is tailored to cover the organism based on its antimicrobial susceptibilities. Duration of intravenous therapy is usually 3–4 weeks, and serial ESR measurements are used as a nonspecific indicator of the response of the infection to therapy. Repeat plain roentgenograms may be obtained to monitor the healing process.

## CASE HISTORY 2

An 18-month-old toddler was seen in the emergency room of a children's hospital with a 3-day history of fever to 102°F; several episodes of emesis, cough, and rhinorrhea; and a 1-day history of a swollen right knee with refusal to walk or bear weight. One day earlier he was seen by his private doctor, who diagnosed bilateral otitis media and started cefaclor. That evening he was noted by his mother to be "walking funny," but as the evening progressed he refused to walk, preferring to scoot along on his buttocks, and was found to have a swollen right knee. According to his mother there was no history of trauma or recent injury to the area. Immunizations were not up to date; he had received three doses of DPT, an MMR, two doses of OPV, and a single *Haemophilus influenzae* type b vaccine.

Physical examination revealed a playful toddler sitting on his mother's lap. He had a temperature of 101.5°F and his tympanic membranes bilaterally were erythematous and dull with decreased mobility. His right knee was swollen and warm with overlying erythema of the skin. There was marked limitation to flexion of the knee and, when placed in a standing position, the child immediately sat, refusing to bear weight or walk on his right leg. The remainder of his examination was within normal limits.

An orthopedic consultant performed a needle aspiration of his right knee joint. The joint fluid was mildly xanthochromic and cloudy in appearance. Gram's stain revealed a few gram-negative pleomorphic bacilli, a moderate number of red blood cells (RBCs), and many WBCs. Analysis of the fluid showed a WBC count of 120,000/mm$^3$ with a differential of 87% PMNs and 13% mononuclear cells, RBCs of 80,000/mm$^3$, a glucose concentration of 40 mg/dL, and a protein concentration of 3.4 g/dL. Bacterial antigen detection assay on the synovial fluid was positive for *Haemophilus influenzae* type b. Cultures of synovial fluid and blood were obtained, and empirically cefuroxime 150 mg/kg daily divided into three doses was begun. The child rapidly improved within the next 48 h, with a marked decrease in the swelling and the erythema of his right knee and the ability to bear weight and walk. Cultures of the joint fluid and a blood culture subsequently grew *Haemophilus influenzae* type b.

The patient received a 21-day course of IV antibiotic therapy with no complications and continued to show improvement in his condition. Serial follow-up examinations of his right knee all demonstrated full range of motion with complete resolution of the swelling and erythema.

## CASE 2 DISCUSSION

This child's presentation is very common in younger children with septic arthritis, and several points of this case are worth emphasizing. First, by history the child has had several days of upper respiratory infection type symptoms and was found to have a focus of infection on physical examination prior to the development of the septic knee. He also had no history of trauma to the knee. In one series of such children, a history of upper respiratory infection or otitis media during the 2 weeks prior to the development of septic arthritis was noted in up to 45% of the cases. Second, the patient's immunizations were not up to date by history. He had only received a single dose of *Haemophilus influenzae* type b vaccine; studies have shown that completion of the three-dose primary series is almost 100% efficacious in preventing invasive *H. influenzae* type b disease. Third, the clinical presentation of the child is typical—he was nontoxic appearing but febrile, with the typical clinical findings of a septic arthritis: a swollen, warm, erythematous, tender joint with refusal to bear weight. Fourth, aspiration made the diagnosis of a septic joint. The Gram's stain results and other parameters of the fluid are typical findings in a bacterial pyoarthritis. Fifth, empiric antibiotic therapy is begun based on the Gram's stain findings and a knowledge of the most likely etiologic agents for a particular age group. *Staphylococcus aureus* is the most common organism isolated, but in children under 2 years of age one also needs to consider *Haemophilus influenzae* type b (particularly if the child is not fully immunized). Cefuroxime is a second-generation cephalosporin that provides excellent coverage for each of the above organisms as well as for other organisms that cause septic arthritis in children. Antibiotic coverage can be tailored once the culture results are known. Follow-up examination of the infected joint is important to ensure that antibiotic therapy is effective and that sequelae of infection have not developed.

# REFERENCES

## Books

Feigin, R. D., and Cherry, J. D., eds. *Textbook of Pediatric Infectious Diseases.* 3rd ed. Philadelphia: W. B. Saunders Co., 1992.

Hoeprich, P., Jordan, M. C., and Ronald, A. *Infectious Diseases: A Treatise of Infectious Processes.* 5th ed. Philadelphia: J. B. Lippincott Co., 1994.

Kaplan, S. L., ed. *Current Therapy in Pediatric Infectious Diseases.* 3rd ed. St. Louis: Mosby-Year Book, Inc., 1993.

Mandell, G. L., Bennett, J. E., and Dolin, R. *Principles and Practice of Infectious Diseases.* 4th ed. New York: Churchill Livingstone, Inc., 1995.

Sanford, J. P., Gilbert, D. N., Gerberding, J. L., and Sande, M. A. *The Sanford Guide to Antimicrobial Therapy 1994.* Antimicrobial Therapy Inc., 1994.

## Review Articles

Bengtson, S. Prosthetic osteomyelitis with special reference to the knee: Risks, treatment, and costs. *Ann. Med. 25*:523–529, 1993.

Correa, A. G., Edwards, M. S., and Baker, C. J. Vertebral osteomyelitis in children. *Pediatr. Infect. Dis. J. 12*:228–233, 1993.

Dagan, R. Management of acute hematogenous osteomyelitis and septic arthritis in the pediatric patient. *Pediatr. Infect. Dis. J. 12*:88–92, 1993.

Dirschl, D. R. Acute pyogenic osteomyelitis in children. *Orthop. Rev. 23*:305–312, 1994.

Esterhai, J. L., Jr., and Gelb, I. Adult septic arthritis. *Orthop. Clin. North Am. 22*:503–514, 1991.

Goldenberg, D. L., Brandt, K. D., Cathcart, E. S., et al. Acute arthritis caused by gram-negative bacilli: A clinical characterization. *Medicine (Balt.) 53*:197–208, 1974.

Green, S. A. Osteomyelitis. The Ilizarov perspective. *Orthop. Clin. North Am. 22*:515–521, 1991.

Gutman, L. T. Acute, subacute, and chronic osteomyelitis and pyogenic arthritis in children. *Curr. Probl. Pediatr. 15*:1–56, 1985.

Ho, G., Jr. Bacterial arthritis. *Curr. Opin. Rheumatol. 13*: 603–609, 1991.

Ingram, C. W., Nichole, B., Martinez, S., and Corey, G. R. Gonococcal osteomyelitis. Case report and review of the literature. *Arch. Intern. Med. 151*:177–179, 1991.

Kaplan, S. L. Osteomyelitis in children. *Compr. Ther. 8*: 69–75, 1982.

Laing, P. Diabetic foot ulcers. *Am. J. Surg. 167*(1A):31S–36S, 1994.

Mader, J. T., and Calhoun, J. Long-bone osteomyelitis diagnosis and management. *Hosp. Pract. 29*:71–76, 1994.

Morrissy, R. T., and Shore, S. L. Bone and joint sepsis. *Pediatr. Clin. North Am. 33*:1551–1565, 1986.

Nelson, J. D. Acute osteomyelitis in children. *Infect. Dis. Clin. North Am. 4*:513–522, 1990.

Nelson, J. D. Skeletal infections in children. *Adv. Pediatr. Infect. Dis. 6*:59–78, 1991.

Oestreich, A. E. Imaging of the skeleton and soft tissue in children. *Curr. Opin. Radiol. 3*:889–894, 1991.

Rodriguez, A. F., and Kaplan, S. L. Outpatient management of skeletal infections in children. *Semin. Pediatr. Infect. Dis. 1*:365–370, 1990.

Sapico, F. L., and Montgomorie, J. Z. Pyogenic vertebral osteomyelitis: Report of nine cases and review of the literature. *Rev. Infect. Dis. 1*:754–776, 1979.

Smith, J. W., and Piercy, E. A. Infectious arthritis. *Clin. Infect. Dis. 20*:225–231, 1995.

Waldvogel, F. A., and Vasey, H. Osteomyelitis: The past decade. *N. Engl. J. Med. 303*:360–370, 1980.

## Original Articles

Bamberger, D. M., Daus, G. P., and Gerding, D. M. Osteomyelitis in the feet of diabetic patients. *Am. J. Med. 83*:653–660, 1987.

Dich, Q., Nelson, J. D., and Haltalin, K. C. Osteomyelitis in infants and children. *Am. J. Dis. Child. 129*:1273–1278, 1975.

Emslio, K. R., and Nade, S. Pathogenesis and treatment of acute hematogenous osteomyelitis: Evaluation of current views with reference to an animal model. *Rev. Infect. Dis. 8*:841–849, 1986.

Jacobs, R. F., McCarthy, R. E., and Elser, J. M. *Pseudomonas* osteochondritis complicating puncture wounds of the foot in children: A 10-year evaluation. *J. Infect. Dis. 160*:657–661, 1989.

Kunnamo, I., Kallio, P., Pelkonen, P., and Hovi, T. Clinical signs and laboratory tests in the differential diagnosis of arthritis in children. *Am. J. Dis. Child. 141*:34–40, 1987.

Lewis, R., Gorbach, S., and Altner, P. Spinal *Pseudomonas* chondroosteomyelitis in heroin users. *N. Engl. J. Med. 286*:1303, 1972.

Mackowiak, P. A., Jones, S. R., and Smith, J. W. Diagnostic value of sinus-tract cultures in chronic osteomyelitis. *JAMA 239*:2772–2775, 1978.

Nelson, J. D. The bacterial etiology and antibiotic management of septic arthritis in infants and children. *Pediatrics 50*:437–440, 1972.

Tetzlaff, T. R., McCracken, G. H., Jr., and Nelson, J. D. Oral antibiotic therapy for skeletal infections of children. *J. Pediatr. 92*:485–490, 1978.

# IX TREATMENT AND PREVENTION OF INFECTIOUS DISEASES

# 36

## LABORATORY EVALUATION OF INFECTIOUS DISEASES

### KRISTIN A. ENGLUND, M.D. and LANCE R. PETERSON, M.D.

## WHY HAVE A LABORATORY?

Clinical acumen is very important for patient care. A particular rash or a predictable fever pattern may point strongly in the direction of one specific infectious disease or another. Patients, however, can have very similar clinical responses to infections from very dissimilar organisms. Careful questioning may ascertain a history of work exposure, presence of household pets, recent travel, new food or medication ingestion, sexual preference, or other clues to a particular infection-related syndrome. Unfortunately, a careful history and physical examination is not always accurate or diagnostic. For a definitive diagnosis to be made regarding a disease process and its causative agent, the microbiology laboratory is important. Making a definitive diagnosis helps the patient by eliminating the need for further tests, by providing an explanation for symptoms, and by being able to offer specific treatment directed against the disease-producing organism. Physicians benefit by learning which organisms can produce the various clinical syndromes. In addition, the general population benefits when infectious outbreaks are prevented because the spread of the disease can be halted.

A recent example of a clinical syndrome that needed laboratory diagnosis was an outbreak of young, otherwise healthy people dying of a severe respiratory illness in the southwest United States recognized during 1993. Physicians in the area were alarmed. The patients' symptoms were nonspecific and could have been caused by a variety of organisms or toxins. Patient histories were not helpful, except that they all lived in the same geographic area. In order to treat these patients and to prevent any further illness, an accurate etiology had to be found. The Centers for Disease Control and Prevention (CDC) was able to establish that this pulmonary syndrome was due to a rodent hantavirus by a study of patient samples in their laboratory in Atlanta, Georgia. A field mouse was identified as the animal vector, thereby enabling control of further spread of the disease.

## HOW TO USE THE LABORATORY— QUESTIONS TO CONSIDER

In order for the laboratory personnel to be able to identify an organism, they must receive appropriate clinical specimens. *Good specimens are the key* to accurate and cost-effective laboratory-assisted diagnosis. The process begins with the physician asking him or herself a few questions:

"**What do I think are the possible diseases present?**"
"**What specimen(s) can give me the diagnosis?**"
"**What tests do I need to order on this specimen?**"

It is important to *answer these questions before you collect a specimen* in order to ensure that the specimen obtained will accurately either rule in or rule out the diagnosis. This is especially important if the procedure needed to obtain the specimen is an invasive one. For example, if a human immunodeficiency virus (HIV)–infected patient presents with fever and headache, and you suspect meningitis, a lumbar puncture is an appropriate test. This patient, however, could have a wide variety of organisms causing the infection. If you request bacterial cultures only, you will miss fungal, viral, parasitic, or tuberculous meningitis.

Also, because fungal and tuberculous meningitis are usually associated with very few organisms in the lumbar fluid (because they cause a basilar meningitis), if you do not submit sufficient fluid for testing (3–5 mL each for fungus and tuberculosis) the result may well be falsely negative. To avoid repeating tests, know what you suspect in advance, what samples and specimen volumes are needed, and have all appropriate collection containers ready. If there is uncertainty, it is good practice to call the laboratory prior to specimen acquisition.

### "When should I collect the sample?"

Whenever possible, *obtain specimens before the patient receives antimicrobial therapy.* Even one dose of antibiotics can prevent bacterial growth in some cultures, and this can make eventual diagnosis very difficult. Sometimes starting therapy is unavoidable. If the microbiology laboaotry is notified of this, they may be able to modify testing to deal with the drugs' effect. Another important indicator of when to obtain a sample is fever. Early in the temperature spike is the ideal time to obtain blood cultures or samples for a malaria smear, as this is when bacteria or parasites are most likely to be found in the bloodstream.

### "How do I handle the specimen?"

Regardless of the specimen source and the organism you are seeking, *each specimen must be collected and transported properly.* In the following sections basic aseptic techniques, collection materials, media for transportation, and any special considerations are described for specific types of cultures. When in doubt, consult the microbiology laboratory about proper specimen collection and handling.

### "What does it mean when the laboratory calls?"

Laboratory technologists call the physician for three basic reasons. *One,* the specimen needs to be re-collected. To be useful this should occur promptly, and this call can be avoided by advance planning. *Two,* a very important result is found and the laboratory wants to ensure that the patient's physician is aware of the test finding. An example of this is a positive blood or a spinal fluid culture or Gram's stain. *Three,* the laboratory has a culture that requires clinical information in order to proceed correctly. Typically this occurs when multiple organisms are present that may represent contamination by mouth, skin, or even bowel flora. If the patient is well, the laboratory can curtail an expensive work-up of a clinically unnecessary specimen. Full identification and susceptibility testing of all microbes should only be done in this setting if the patient is clinically failing the empiric treatment that was selected. Doing otherwise adds unnecessarily to medical care costs.

## SPECIMENS FROM SPECIFIC SITES

### Blood Cultures

In an inpatient setting, this is one of the most common and important cultures. For proper collection, the patient's skin must be thoroughly prepared with an antiseptic solution. Begin cleaning at the point of the anticipated venipuncture site and move in enlarging circles to the periphery. Do not go back over areas already cleaned with the used antiseptic pad or swab. With a new pad, repeat the procedure for a total of three times. Often 70% alcohol is used alone, but a full 2 min of contact time with the skin is needed. Some people choose to use an iodophor such as Betadine. These are very effective but they must dry on the skin completely before the venipuncture in order to be effective. With iodophors, alcohol should not be used as a second cleansing agent, as it may deactivate the iodophor. It can be used after the culture is collected to remove the residual iodophor so as to avoid sensitizing the patient to the Betadine. Also, always wear gloves as part of universal precautions—they do not have to be sterile unless you plan to touch (palpate) the disinfected area.

A typical blood culture "set" consists of two or three components, as depicted in Figure 36–1. This includes two bottles, one for aerobic and facultative anaerobic bacteria, and one for strictly anaerobic bacteria. Often an Isolator tube to optimize detection of yeast is also included. Between 5 and 10 mL of blood should be inoculated into each blood culture set component in adults. Needles should *not* be changed to inoculate the bottles or tubes. Obtaining less than 10 mL of blood per culture set will result in a significant decrease in recovery of certain bacteria, especially the Enterobacteriaceae and *Pseudomonas aeruginosa*— 10 mL per bottle or tube is optimal. Each additional 1 mL cultured over 10 mL adds 3% to the expected recovery of pathogenic microbes per set collected; 60 mL of blood cultured per day, divided in two or three sets, in

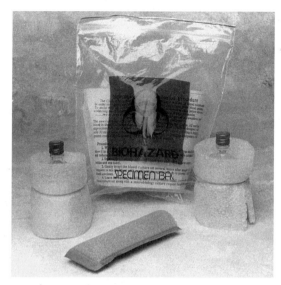

**FIGURE 36–1.** Photograph of the packaged blood culture set consisting of two broth bottles and a lysis centrifugation tube with brief instructions.

several studies provided the optimal amount for detection of bacteremia in septic-appearing adults. False-negative cultures can result from collecting too little blood, since there may be fewer than one organism per 10 mL of blood in up to 20% of adult patients who are clinically bacteremic. Less can be taken from children, but two or three separate sets from distinct blood draws should still be collected. The media contained in the blood culture bottles is a broth that can support the growth of a small number of organisms. In most instances, bacteria and yeasts grow promptly, allowing rapid detection. Unfortunately, even a few colonies of bacteria not properly cleaned from the skin can also grow in these cultures. These contaminants can be difficult to distinguish from a true bloodstream infection.

If a patient has been treated with antimicrobial agents prior to obtaining the blood cultures, the antimicrobial(s) present may inhibit growth. Agents can be added to the culture media to bind or deactivate the drug(s). More commonly now, media are prepared that contain resins to nonselectively adsorb antibiotics to their surface. Dilution of the blood by the culture media also diminishes the effect of antimicrobials present. Therefore, it is important to list the drugs the patient is receiving so the laboratory can properly process the blood culture.

Many clinical microbiology laboratories now use an automated detection instrument for at least part of their blood culture processing. Common automated blood culture systems, such as BACTEC, ESP, and BacT/Alert, detect bacterial growth by measuring microbial metabolic processes. These metabolic products are read by computers that signal the technologists when a sample is positive, thereby eliminating the need for visual examination of each bottle, and allowing many more specimens to be processed by the staff. In a visually inspected, nonautomated system, a blood culture shows signs of bacterial growth by producing turbidity of broth, gas bubbles, hemolysis of red blood cells, or colonies on a plate. Once a blood culture shows signs of bacterial growth, a sample is removed, Gram's stained, and inoculated onto several different solid media for growth. This is discussed more in the bacteriology section.

Lysis-centrifugation is the typical method of culturing blood on solid agar. An inoculated Isolator tube contains reagents that lyse all blood cells. The tube is then centrifuged, trapping bacteria present against a chemical cushion in the bottom of the tube, and the sediment is plated onto solid media. Lysis-centrifugation is an excellent method for detecting fungi and mycobacteria in the blood. The major problems with this system are frequent recovery of contaminants on the plated media, and poor performance in growing some fastidious organisms like *Streptococcus pneumoniae*, *Listeria monocytogenes*, and *Haemophilus influenzae*.

### Sputum Cultures

Saliva and oropharyngeal secretions normally contain a large amount of bacteria. These microbes do not reflect an infectious process in the lower respiratory tract. Unless a sputum sample is properly collected, it will be contaminated with oral epithelial cells and bacteria, making diagnosis impossible. Many laboratories have criteria for accepting sputum specimens based upon the number of epithelial cells and/or white blood cells (WBCs) seen on initial Gram's staining. If too many epithelial cells and/or too few white blood cells are present, the specimen is assumed to be contaminated and rejected for culture. To avoid this, the following methods are recommended for collecting culture material from the lower respiratory tract:

1. If the patient is able to cough up frankly purulent material, a good sample can be obtained simply by instructing the patient to produce secretions from a deep cough and not hold the specimen in the mouth before depositing it in the container.

2. The patient may inhale ultrasonically nebulized, sterile saline that coats the lower respiratory tract and enables thick secretions to be expectorated.

3. Hypertonic saline is inhaled when sputum is *induced* to identify *Pneumocystis carinii*. Patients must be instructed to thoroughly brush their teeth and rinse their mouth prior to the induction. Induction of sputum for *Mycobacterium tuberculosis* must be done in a respiratory isolation room, and everyone but the patient must wear a mask specifically designed for tuberculosis prevention. Three consecutive specimens are necessary to rule out tuberculosis. A single specimen appears sufficient for *P. carinii*.

4. Bronchoscopy specimens are generally less contaminated than expectorated specimens, but there is still a potential for significant oropharyngeal contamination. This is an invasive procedure that may be necessary if the patient is unable to cough up an adequate specimen. Specimens for quantitative culture are best collected by a "protected" catheter or brush.

### Urine Cultures

Roughly 10–20% of the female population have a symptomatic urinary tract infection, or UTI, at some time during their life. The incidence of bacteriuria is lower in men, but increases with age due to the development of prostatic hypertrophy. Urinary tract infection broadly refers to infections of the kidneys, ureters, bladder, or urethra. Diagnosis of urinary infections is generally made by urine chemistry, microscopy, and urine culture. The urine chemistry measures protein, glucose, nitrites, leukocyte esterase, and blood in the urine. Microscopic examination looks for crystals, white blood cells, red blood cells, yeast and bacteria.

Collection of urine for culture requires careful counseling of patients. The perineum of the female is colonized with bacteria. If this area is not properly cleaned the urine culture may be contaminated with several organisms. Females must clean the labia and external urethral meatus, hold the labia apart while urinating, and collect the urine for culture in a sample container. For men, collection of the midstream urine involves starting the urine stream to wash out bacterial growth that may have developed in the urethra since last voiding. Five to 10 mL are then collected in a urine container. Urine should not be colleced during the end of voiding because prostatic secretions or urethral sphincter contractions may dislodge small clumps of bacteria and artificially increase the bacterial count.

Specimens of urine can be obtained through temporary or indwelling catheters, especially if the patient is unable to cooperate with collection. Suprapubic puncture of the bladder is a method that minimizes contamination the most, but this procedure is usually neither necessary nor desired when testing adults. Bacteria can replicate in urine rapidly, making small amounts of contaminating bacteria appear significant. This can be slowed with refrigeration, but the best procedure is to transport the urine sample immediately to the laboratory or to use a special urine transport tube.

### Cerebrospinal Fluid Cultures

Cerebrospinal fluid (CSF) must be collected using aseptic technique. The volume of CSF collected for culture is important, especially for fungi or mycobacteria. At least 3–5 mL is required for a meaningful negative result with either fungal or mycobacterial infection, since these are typically basilar meningitides associated with small numbers of organisms. Meningococci do not tolerate room temperatures well, so immediate transport of the specimen to the laboratory is essential. Immediate Gram's staining and antigen testing of the CSF should be requested if meningitis is suspected and results should be communicated promptly.

### Genital Cultures

When dealing with genital infections, there is typically only a small amount of material to examine. Any vaginal discharge can be collected using a swab and can then be placed on a glass slide with a drop of sterile saline to look for trichomonas, white blood cells, or bacteria. It should also be examined on a glass slide with a drop of potassium hydroxide (KOH) to look for yeast. A cervical discharge can also be collected with a sterile swab to look for *Neisseria gonorrhoeae* (GC) or *Chlamydia trachomatis*. GC can be visualized directly in inflammatory leukocytes. The swab is first used to inoculate a plate of Thayer-Martin media for GC culture, and then rolled on a glass slide to be Gram's stained. This culture must be specially handled because GC, a facultative

anaerobic organism, requires low oxygen tension.

Routine cultures for chlamydia are not often available and the organism cannot be visualized directly with light microscopy. A swab of endocervical material can be placed in special transport media and sent for PCR, genetic probing or fluorescent antibody analysis. These methods are both highly specific and sensitive. The same sample can also be genetically probed for GC, but this is very expensive and does not provide an organism for sensitivity testing. For males, the specimen is collected from the urethra, using either the swab included in the genetic probe kit, or a "calgi swab." The calgi swab is slightly thinner, and can be used to inoculate a Thayer-Martin plate if GC culturing is desired.

Herpes cultures require a stabilizing medium for collection and transport. The base of a broken blistered lesion should be cleaned and swabbed for culture, and a second lesion should be scraped for cells and then smeared on a glass slide for direct fluorescent antibody (DFA) staining. Scraped material from the base of a lesion smeared on a glass slide for specific DFA screening to detect either Herpes simplex or varicella-zoster virus (VZV) can provide results within a few hours. Vesicles can also be aspirated and the material sent to the laboratory for culture.

Syphilis is not cultured, but instead requires direct visualization of the *Treponema pallidum* with a darkfield microscope for rapid diagnosis. An alternative approach in settings where the prevalence of syphilis is low is to use serum antibody (Venereal Disease Research Laboratory [VDRL] and fluorescent treponemal antibody absorption [FTA-ABS]) testing to replace darkfield evaluation. This approach is both highly sensitive and specific (see Chapter 16).

### Wound Cultures

Cultures from wounds may require special media, collection materials, and transportation guidelines. Here, a few important principles are discussed.

A sample of infected tissue is optimal for culture but obtaining tissue is not always feasible. Culture of purulent material from the wound is the next best option. As much purulent material as possible should be aspirated into a syringe to allow culturing of both aerobic and anaerobic organisms. The collected material can be directly injected into a sterile transport tube or cup. The syringe also can be sent to the laboratory directly but without a needle attached, as transporting syringes with needles in place puts transporters and lab workers at unnecessary risk for needle stick injuries.

Small amounts of purulence can be collected using a sterile swab, but this method often results in poor isolation of organisms, since some adhere to the swab material. Swabs are also very poor to use when anaerobic infection is suspected. If a swab is used, the best method is to use a sterile cotton, calcium alginate, or Dacron-tipped swab, preferably on a plastic shaft. Some commercially available culture systems provide a sterile swab with a plastic transport tube that contains transport medium in a glass ampule. After the inoculated swab is placed into the transport tube, the glass ampule is squeezed and broken, releasing the liquid transport medium. This protects the specimen from desiccation and provides a reduced (anaerobic) environment. Operative specimens should *not* be sent to the microbiology lab in preservative (formalin), since this rapidly kills any microbes present. Biopsies or swabs from wounds for viral culture should be transported in viral transport media.

## Stool Cultures

Stool can be cultured for a wide variety of pathogens. Microbes can be isolated from patients with recent travel to endemic areas, suspected food exposures, or immunocompromising illness. *Clostridium difficile* can be cultured from diarrheal stool from patients with recent antibiotic use. Bacterial cultures can reveal *Salmonella*, toxigenic *Escherichia coli*, and other pathogens capable of producing diarrhea. In the HIV-infected patient, the protozoa *Cryptosporidium* and *Isospora* must be considered (see Chapter 23).

Fecal specimens should be collected before any barium studies of the gastrointestinal (GI) tract are performed. Barium makes visualization of parasites difficult for up to 1 week. The sample should be collected in a clean (not necessarily sterile) wide-mouthed container, and should not be contaminated with urine or toilet water. Multiple samples over several days are often necessary for diagnosis, as organisms may not be shed continuously in the stool. Stool samples should be taken to the laboratory for immediate evaluation. If this is not possible, special transport media for cultures or a fixative for parasites are available. Helminths (worms) passed in the stool

should be placed into a clean cup and transported to the laboratory for identification.

## SPECIMEN EVALUATION

After the specimen reaches the laboratory, the evaluation process begins. An overview of basic laboratory procedures is provided.

### Direct Smear Analysis

#### Gram's Stain

One of the most useful and rapid procedures in the diagnosis of infections is the Gram's stain of appropriate clinical material. This can be performed quickly and easily on exudates, fluids, aspirates, and tissue impressions. The entire staining technique takes about 15 min, including making the smear, drying, fixing, and staining, but requires training and experience. Proper staining includes fixing the specimen, followed by a crystal violet stain, tap water rinse, iodine stain, rinse, decolorizer (ethyl alcohol or acetone), rinse, safranin counterstain, and a final rinse. Gram-positive bacteria are organisms that hold on to the crystal violet stain and resist decolorization. This is due to their thick peptidoglycan cell wall with extensive teichoic acid cross-linking. Because they retain crystal violet, they appear purple under the light microscope. Gram-negative bacteria have a thin peptidoglycan layer with a thick surrounding lipopolysaccharide coating; they are decolorized easily and take up the counterstain, safranin, appearing pink. If the decolorizer is left on too long, then some gram-positive bacteria will appear gram-negative. With too thick a smear, gram-negative bacteria may not be fully decolorized and can then appear gram-positive. A good check on the quality of the stain is to look at the cell nuclei present. Mammalian cell nuclei should always stain gram-negative. Microscopic examination of the Gram's stain permits the morphology of the organism, whether it is round (a coccus), or long and narrow (a rod or bacillus), to be determined.

The value of the smear result depends upon forms seen on the smear and the clinical setting of the patient. For example, the presence and types of inflammatory cells should be noted. Segmented neutrophils in large numbers commonly signify an acute bacterial infection. Figure 36–2 demonstrates degenerating neutrophils with a cluster of gram-positive cocci consistent with *Staphylococcus*

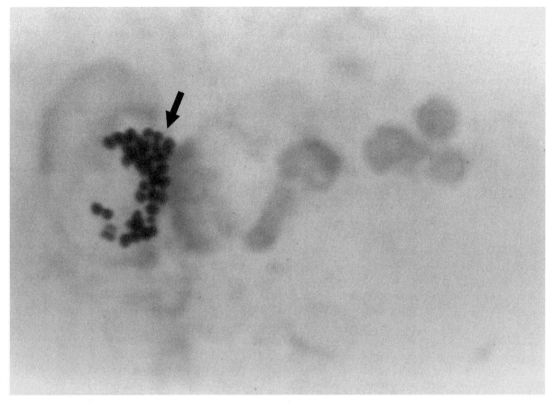

**FIGURE 36-2.** Degenerating neutrophils with a large cluster of gram-positive cocci (*S. aureus*).

*aureus.* Smears from clinical specimens showing bacteria without inflammatory cells should be interpreted with caution, since this may simply indicate colonization or contamination except in the neutropenic patient unable to mount an inflammatory response. Another example relates to the evaluation of gonorrhea. A urethral swab should show intracellular gram-negative diplococci in order to conclude that it is positive for gonorrhea. An organism seen on Gram's stain that does not grow on routine culture indicates an anaerobe or nonviable organisms related to antimicrobials prior to specimen collection.

### Direct Wet Mount

This simple procedure involves placing a small amount of culture material on a slide with a drop of sterile saline to dilute the specimen. A coverslip is then placed over the specimen before evaluating it with the microscope. This procedure is often used on genital secretions to look for *Trichomonas vaginalis* or *Gardnerella vaginalis*. This is also used with fresh stool to look for motile protozoa, like *Giardia lamblia* (Fig. 36-3) and *Entamoeba histolytica*.

### Peripheral Blood Smear

Organisms such as *Plasmodium* species (the etiologic agents of malaria) or fungi such as *Histoplasma capsulatum* in HIV-infected patients (Fig. 36-4) can be seen with the light microscope and routine (hematoxylin-eosin, or Giemsa) staining. Direct visualization of the organism saves much time in making the diagnosis. This is the method for speciation of malaria; correct identification requires considerable technical skill. This is generally performed in either the microbiology or the hematology laboratory.

### Definitive Specimen Analysis

### Bacteriology

This is the major activity of any microbiology laboratory. After the initial Gram's stain, specimens are plated on media that allow the bacteria to grow for identification. The type(s) of media used depends on the source of the specimen and the organisms being sought. Some media such as sheep blood agar are general purpose; some are enriched with nutrients to help fastidious organisms grow, such as chocolate agar (for *Neisseria* species); some

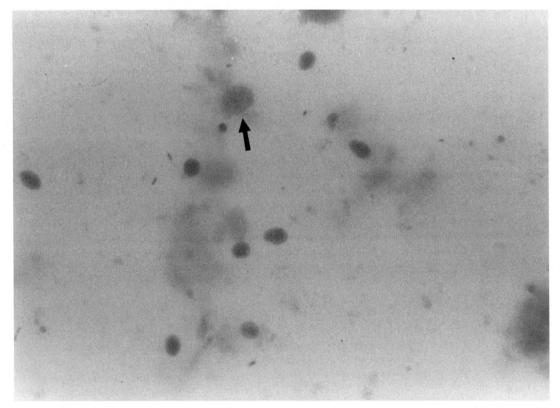

**FIGURE 36–3.** *Giardia lamblia* cysts seen in a "wet prep" of a fresh stool specimen.

are selective because they contain agents to suppress the growth of organisms except those to be identified (i.e., Salmonella-Shigella agar); and others are termed differential media because they allow specific identifying biochemical reactions, such as MacConkey agar, upon which lactose fermenting bacteria yield pink colonies and lactose nonfermenters clear colonies. Each specimen is inoculated onto several agar plates and incubated. For specimens from a normally sterile site, most often only one organism grows when an infection is present. If the specimen is from a throat culture, genital tract, or stool sample, many different bacterial organisms may be isolated, and the normal flora must be differentiated from the potentially pathogenic organisms. Figure 36–5 compares the laboratory recovery of *S. aureus* on a blood plate from a bacteremic patient to multiple colony types encountered when stool specimens are cultured.

Identification begins once growth occurs. The appearance of the colony on the agar (color, size, texture, and even the smell) can be suggestive of a *family* of organisms. Isolated colonies are then Gram's stained and a series of biochemical tests performed. Identification to the *genus* and *species* levels may require from 3–25 tests, depending on the organism. Rarely, an organism does not match a pattern of tests, and requires the resources of a reference lab for full identification. The general time for most bacterial identification is 48 h.

Apart from the routine culturing, bacteria can also be detected by other tests. When bacterial meningitis is suspected, a rapid diagnosis is critical. If the Gram's stain has been nondiagnostic, latex agglutination using specific antibodies can be performed to identify bacterial antigens. *Neisseria meningitidis*, *Streptococcus pneumoniae*, and *Haemophilus influenzae* all have soluble polysaccharide capsules that act as strong antigens. Antigen testing has become less important in many microbiology laboratories with the use of cytocentrifugation to prepare a 1000-fold concentrated smear for Gram's stain analysis. These concentrated smears are usually positive when infection is present.

## Anaerobes

Special care must be used when handling specimens for anaerobic culture, as these or-

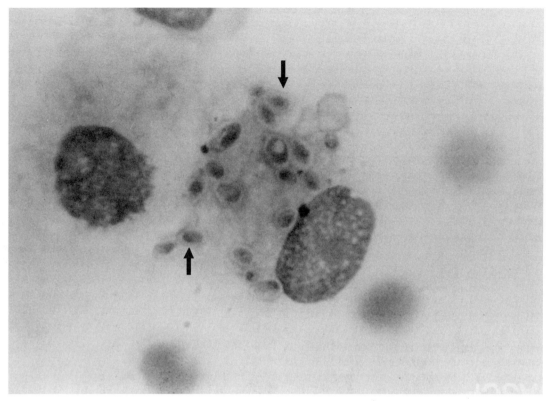

**FIGURE 36–4.** Giemsa stain of *Histoplasma capsulatum.*

ganisms cannot resist the peroxides formed with air exposure. Even short periods (30 min) in room air oxygen kills many organisms. Thus, standard anaerobic incubators contain an atmosphere composed of 85% nitrogen, 10% hydrogen, and 5% carbon dioxide. Culturing is often done in special anaerobic chambers using a process that requires special media. If an anaerobic incubator (chamber, Fig. 36–6) is not available, culture plates are kept in jars or individual anaerobic environmental pouches. Once growth is apparent, the organism is identified using Gram's stain morphology and a series of biochemical tests. Important organisms for identification include *Bacteroides fragilis, Peptostreptococcus* species, and *Fusobacterium* species. *Clostridium difficile* can also be cultured, but since this organism may be a common colonizer of the GI tract in some long-term hospitalized patients, only those with diarrhea should be investigated for this pathogen. A test for toxin must be performed to determine if the isolated strain is likely pathogenic. Toxin is detected either immunologically or by inoculating tissue culture tubes containing a monolayer of cells with cell-free stool fil-

trate; any toxin present will cause cell death, or a cytopathogenic effect (CPE). Confirming that the CPE is due to specific *C. difficile* toxin is accomplished by demonstrating that CPE is neutralized by *C. difficile* antitoxin.

Gas-liquid chromatography (GLC) is the standard method of identifying anaerobes, utilizing the fact that certain anaerobic bacteria produce specific short-chain volatile organic acids. For example, *Propionibacterium* produces propionic acid and lactobacilli produce lactic acid. This type of testing is generally only available in larger clinical laboratories (see Chapter 27).

### Acid-Fast Bacilli (AFB)

All specimens suspected of containing acid-fast microorganisms, such as *Mycobacterium tuberculosis*, are processed using special biosafety precautions because of the infectious nature of these organisms if aerosolized (see Chapter 13). Virtually any specimen can be tested for this group of organisms. They are termed acid-fast because of their ability to retain certain stains even after exposure to strong acids. The stain is captured by the cell wall that contains long-chain mycolic acids. The best

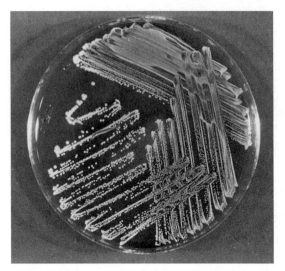
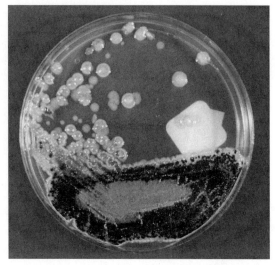

**FIGURE 36–5.** Pure growth of *S. aureus* from a bacteremic patient (*left*) compared to multiple colony types recovered from culture of stool (*right*).

known acid-fast stain is the Ziehl-Neelsen, which requires carbolfuchsin be applied to the smear or tissue section over a steaming bath. A similar stain, the Kinyoun stain, also uses carbolfuchsin, but phenol replaces the steam and it is therefore referred to as a "cold" stain. With both techniques, acid-fast organisms appear red and thus over the years these bacteria have come to be termed "red snappers" (Fig. 36–7). Since the early 1960s, fluorochrome stains for mycobacteria have gained popularity. Auramine, often prepared in combination with rhodamine, is the most commonly used fluorochrome stain. Most laboratories that employ auramine for identifying mycobacteria within tissues and smears find it to be slightly more sensitive for less experienced readers, and faster than the car-

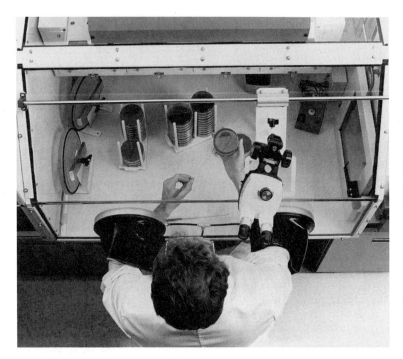

**FIGURE 36–6.** Picture of an anaerobic chamber used for processing and incubation of specimens submitted for recovery of anaerobic bacteria.

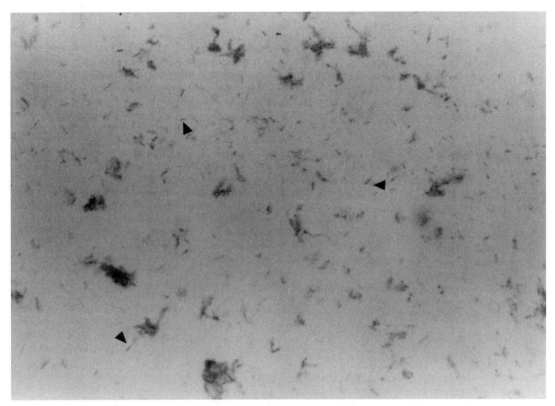

**FIGURE 36–7.** Photograph of many acid-fast bacilli ("red snappers") consistent with tuberculosis.

bolfuchsin stains. The organisms are more easily seen with use of auramine because it stains them bright yellow or gold against a contrasting dark background.

After the staining process, all specimens are inoculated onto special media such as the egg-based Löwenstein-Jensen (LJ) agar. This medium must provide enough moisture and enrichment to allow the cultures to be kept up to 8 weeks. Some acid-fast bacilli, like *Mycobacterium fortuitum*, grow within 1 week and are termed rapid growers. Others grow very slowly and can take up to 8 weeks to grow. Organisms may be differentiated by their ability to produce pigment in the light only, in the light and the dark, or not at all. They are termed photochromogenic, scotochromogenic, and nonchromogenic, respectively (Fig. 36–8). Once sufficient growth has occurred, the organism can be identified using biochemical testing, specific DNA-RNA probes, GLC, or high-pressure liquid chromatography (HPLC).

Another (now preferred) method of culturing mycobacteria is a broth-based system such as the BACTEC or ESP culture method. The BACTEC automated system detects radiolabeled $CO_2$ produced by the microorganisms as they are replicating, while the ESP system detects consumption of gas by the growing mycobacteria that lowers the head-space pressure in the culture bottle. Automated instruments detect these "signals" typically before visible growth can be recognized. As a result, cultures may be positive more rapidly than with traditional agar methods. Genetic probing can be used directly with these systems, making identification even more rapid, but adequate growth still must be achieved before antimicrobial susceptibility testing can be performed. Recently, polymerase chain reaction (PCR) has been used as an aid to reduce the time to diagnosis of mycobacteria. This technique is relatively insensitive in smear-negative specimens, and is expensive when compared with more traditional growth-based testing. It is most helpful in rapid diagnosis of smear-positive *M. tuberculosis*, but culture is still necessary to test the antimicrobial susceptibility of the infecting organism.

## Fungi

These are yeasts, molds, and dimorphic fungi (those that are in yeast form at one tem-

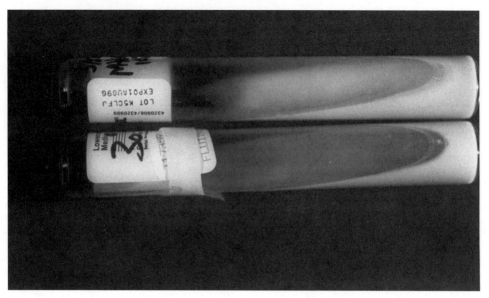

**FIGURE 36–8.** Two strains of mycobacteria, one showing pigment (a scotochromogenic strain) and one without (*M. tuberculosis*).

perature and mold form at another). Yeast refers to growth that appears "creamy" in consistency whereas mold refers to growth that looks "white and cottony" on the agar surface. Some yeasts grow relatively rapidly, in less than 48 h; however, the dimorphic fungi, *Histoplasma capsulatum*, *Coccidioides immitis*, and *Blastomyces dermatitidis*, can take several weeks to grow. Many molds also grow slowly. Virtually any specimen can be cultured for fungi, but the significance of some positive cultures may not be clear. For example, *Candida albicans* normally colonizes the oropharynx and GI tract of humans, and strains of *Aspergillus* are ubiquitous in the environment (see Chapter 14).

Some fungal organisms can be detected directly by microscopy using 10% potassium KOH. This is especially useful for oral, genital, nail, or skin specimens. The fungal forms can be easily visualized because most of the other material is lysed by KOH. Other stains for fungal specimens include periodic acid–Schiff (PAS), methenamine silver, Giemsa, and calcofluor white. Specimens are inoculated onto several agar plates and observed for 4 weeks for growth. Some of the agar plates contain general nutrient-rich growth media, such as brain heart infusion agar, while others are selective, such as the inhibitory mold agar that contains chloramphenicol to inhibit bacterial growth. Once growth is achieved, the organisms are examined under the microscope for

hyphae, budding, spores, and other distinct morphologic features that will distinguish the family (Fig. 36–9). Biochemical or antigen testing is used for definitive identification at the genus and species levels.

An important pathogen, *Cryptococcus neoformans*, can be detected in the CSF and serum by immunologic antigen detection. Latex beads coated with specific antibodies are mixed with a specimen and agglutinate in the presence of cryptococcal polysaccharide antigen. This is commonly used in place of the "India ink" preparation. This older method used a negative staining technique to visualize the organism's capsule. Diagnosis with antigen detection can be made in less than 1 h, is twice as sensitive, and requires only a fraction of the specimen needed for India ink testing. Dilutions of CSF or serum are tested, and the result is reported as a titer. During therapy, repeat testing should show a decrease in the titer of the antigen.

### Parasitology

Parasitology covers a wide range of infections, from malaria to intestinal worms. A typical request of the laboratory is for identification of ova and parasites in stool specimens. This is accomplished by microscopic evaluation of a wet mount specimen (described above), or a preserved, stained stool specimen. To prepare a stained specimen, the stool sample is concentrated, fixed, permanently

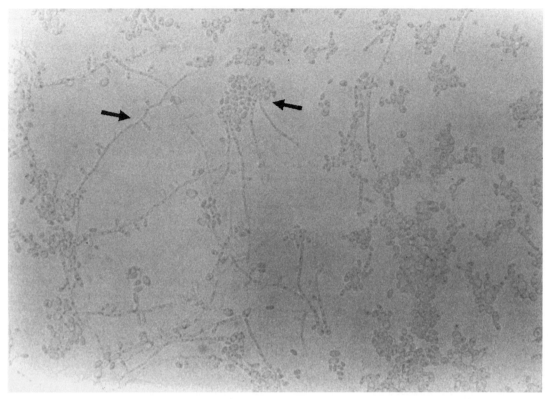

**FIGURE 36–9.** Slide showing the various typical morphologic forms associated with *Candida tropicalis* grown on corn meal agar.

stained on a slide using a trichrome or iron-hematoxylin stain, and examined for any characteristic organisms. Figure 36–10 shows three cysts of *Entamoeba histolytica* in a row, one with a large central clear area of glycogen, visualized by a trichrome stain. Cryptosporidia can be identified using a modified acid-fast stain, or a very sensitive fluorescent monoclonal antibody method.

When malaria is being considered in the disease differential, the diagnosis is best made by blood smears. Finger-stick blood collected just prior to or during a fever spike is optimal, and is prepared as thick and thin smears on glass slides. The thin smear is similar to a peripheral blood smear used in hematology. A thick smear is several cell layers in thickness and concentrates the parasites to make them more easily seen. The slides are stained with a modified Wright-Giemsa stain and carefully examined for parasites. Because of the low level of parasitemia often present, samples often need to be obtained over several days to evaluate the patient fully for malaria (Fig. 36–11) (see Chapter 30).

Another organism of major clinical impor-

tance, especially since the beginning of the HIV epidemic, is *Pneumocystis carinii*. Induced sputum samples can be stained with methenamine silver stain (as used in the fungal lab), but the procedure is time-consuming and requires careful microscopic examination. Toluidine blue O is another stain used. A more rapid and easily performed test now widely used is DFA staining for *P. carinii*. A specific fluorescent-tagged antibody is used to stain the specimen and binds to any *P. carinii* organisms present. The fluorescent stain is easily visualized and the diagnosis can be made quickly. Sensitivity and specificity approach 95% when performed on even a single properly collected induced sputum specimen (Fig. 36–12).

### Virology

Viruses cannot be visualized using light microscopy, and several approaches are used for diagnosis of viral infection:

1. *Tissue biopsy or cytology.* Some viruses produce characteristic changes in these cells, called viral inclusions, that can be seen by a

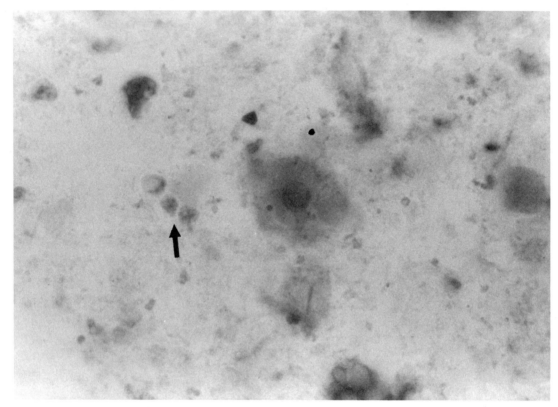

**FIGURE 36–10.** Three cysts of *Entamoeba histolytica* in a row using a trichrome stain of stool.

light microscopy. Viral inclusions may be aggregates of viral particles or cellular material that aggregates in the presence of the virus. For example, in a cervical Papanicolaou's smear, inclusions can indicate infection with the human papillomavirus (HPV). Other viruses cause several cells to fuse together. An example of this is herpes simplex virus (HSV) that causes the formation of distinctive multinucleated epithelioid giant cells. Cytomegalovirus (CMV) produces a typical "owls eye" intranuclear inclusion seen in the bone marrow biopsy in Figure 36–13.

2. *Immunofluorescent staining.* Both direct and indirect fluorescent antibody stains are used for detection of a variety of viruses. Direct staining involves exposing the specimen to antiviral antibody that is tagged with a fluorescent label. The specimen is then examined under a fluorescence microscope. This process is rapid and highly specific. The indirect method uses a two-step process. Unlabeled antiviral antibody is first applied to the specimen, and then a fluorescein-labeled antibody to human immunoglobulin is applied. This method also offers high sensitivity, but may require more time.

3. *Viral culture.* After infecting cells, viruses leave the host cell to infect others by one of two mechanisms. They can simply lyse the host cell, thereby killing the host cell, or virus can bud from the host cell, using part of the host's outer membrane for its own without destroying the host. Viruses that lyse cells can be detected easily after infecting a monolayer of cultured cells and observing them by light microscopy for cell death, referred to as CPE. Typical CPE from HSV and CMV are shown in Figure 36–14. Viruses that do not produce CPE may instead induce receptors on the host cell membranes to which red blood cells attach. When guinea pig red blood cells are added to the culture, they are then adsorbed to the infected cells (hemadsorption). To determine which specific virus is present, immunofluorescent tagging is often used, as described above.

Shell vial culture is a faster method of culturing viruses. Viruses in regular culture may take several days to cause enough CPE to be recognizable. To enhance the process, a specimen is placed in a vial containing a monolayer of cells on a coverslip. The vial is then centrifuged to pellet the virus against the

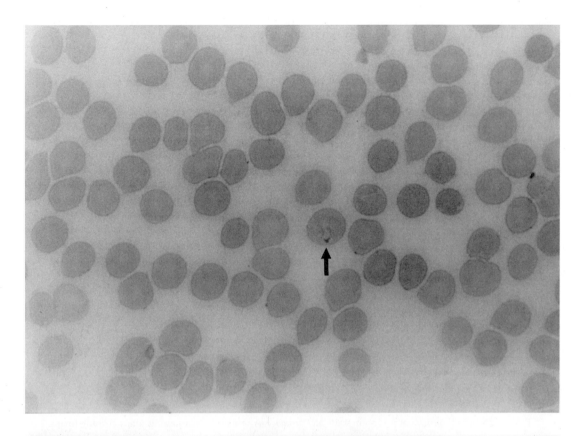

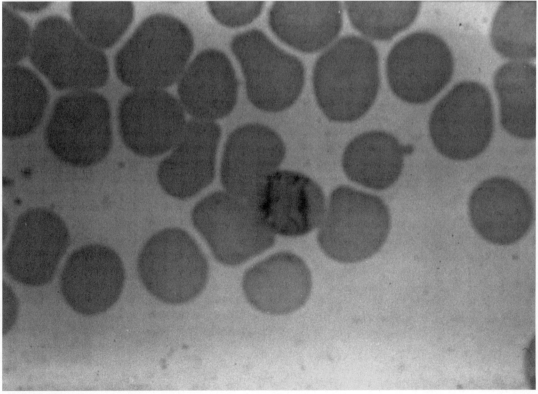

**FIGURE 36–11.** Peripheral smears of malaria. On the *top* is a ring trophozoite form of *Plasmodium falciparum.* On the *bottom* is a band trophozoite form of *P. malariae.*

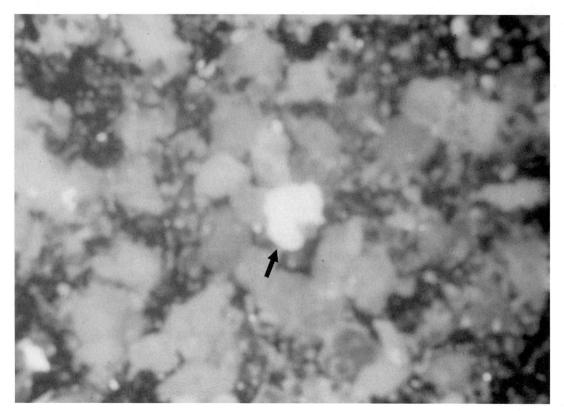

**FIGURE 36–12.** Fluorescent antibody stain of *Pneumocystis carinii* cyst containing many trophic forms.

monolayer. This process speeds the cytopathic effect, and with immunofluorescent staining, many herpes group viruses (HSV, VZV, and CMV) can be detected within about 24 h.

4. *Polymerase chain reaction.* This method amplifies relatively few copies of viral DNA to detectable levels. PCR is being investigated as a method of diagnosis for virtually every group of organisms, including viruses. It can be particularly useful for detecting virus in sites where few cells are present but free virus particles are found (like CSF for the herpes group viruses). This is discussed below.

5. *Nucleic acid probes.* This procedure uses short segments of specifically labeled DNA that are designed to hybridize with a complementary segment on the viral genome. This procedure is less sensitive than other methods described but has been used for the detection of HPV in cervical Papanicolaou's specimens, for example.

6. *Serology.* In the later stages of infection, when viruses are no longer present, serologic methods of identification are used. Some agents, like Epstein-Barr virus (EBV) cannot be cultured easily and serology remains the basis of diagnosis. Viruses, like other foreign agents, elicit measurable antibody responses in the host. Complement-fixing (CF) antibodies appear early in the disease, increase in titer during the acute phase of illness, and decline within 6 months of clinical recovery. A high titer of CF antibody to a specific virus in a single serum specimen suggests recent infection with that virus. A fourfold or greater increase in serum titer in a specimen drawn 2–3 weeks after an initial specimen (called a convalescent specimen) is necessary for confirmation of the viral infection. The drawback to serologic testing is that it is not very rapid, and it is not as definitively diagnostic as actual detection of an infecting organism.

### Molecular Biology

The molecular biology laboratory is playing an increasingly important role in today's diagnostic process. Rapid diagnosis of organisms that are slow or difficult to grow in culture is being accomplished through PCR. This procedure uses short DNA sequence (oligonucleotide) primers that correspond to specific sequences on the DNA or RNA that is to be reproduced. A unique polymerase then

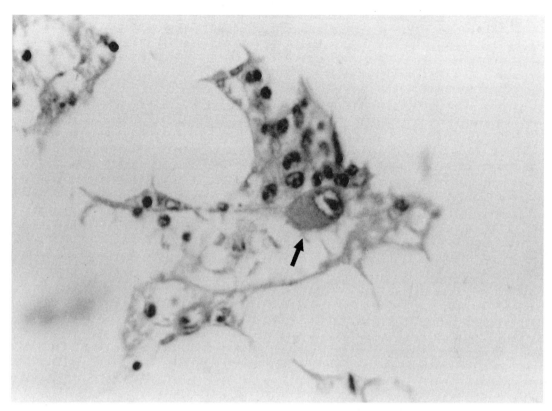

**FIGURE 36–13.** Typical cytomegalovirus-infected cell with "owl's eye" intranuclear inclusion seen in biopsy material.

catalyzes the process within a specially designed heater (thermocycler, Fig. 36–15) and produces a complementary nucleotide sequence by reading the target genome. This procedure is repeated through 20–30 exponential cycles until millions of times the original amount of DNA sequences is produced. PCR can detect tiny amounts of infectious particles present in specimens and has been used to detect viral, mycobacterial, fungal, and bacterial isolates. It is still expensive, requiring considerable skill and equipment, and is not likely to replace routine procedures for organisms that are rapidly and easily cultured.

Another important field is molecular epidemiology for identification of clonal strains of microbes through comparison of gel electrophoresis patterns. This procedure provides a distinct fingerprint of the organism's DNA (Fig. 36–16). As increasing numbers of resistant organisms are encountered, understanding the epidemiology of these infections becomes crucial in preventing spread from patient to patient through application of targeted infection control practices. For example, in an apparent outbreak of vancomycin-resistant *Enterococcus faecalis*, it is important to know if the strains are genetically identical. When strains are identical, nosocomial spread is likely from person to person and strategies to enhance infection control practices must be identified to keep additional patients from being infected. When they are not identical, other causes of increased numbers of resistant microbes, such as antibiotic pressure, need to be investigated and drug usage altered to prevent increased number of infections with resistant strains.

## OTHER LABORATORY ISSUES

### Negative Results

Negative cultures or stains are potentially less helpful than positive cultures. They are often interpreted by the clinician as meaning infection is not present. As discussed above, many factors may contribute to the inability to isolate an organism. These include insufficient sample size, improper collection and

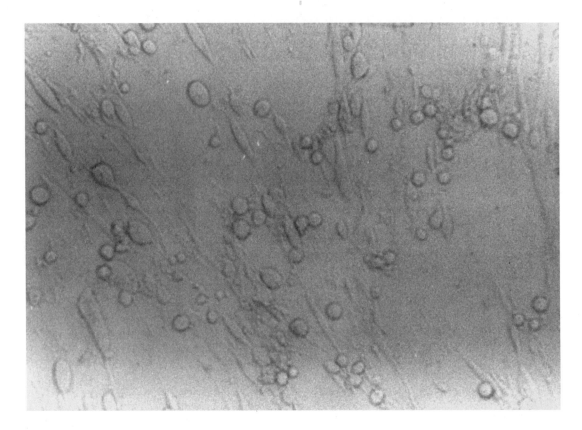

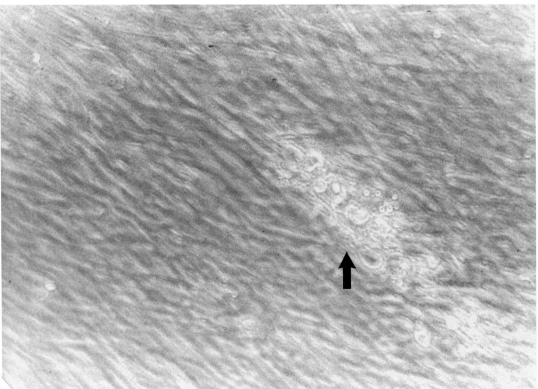

**FIGURE 36–14.** Examples of CPE caused by HSV (*top*) with extensive destruction of the cell monolayer, and of CMV (*bottom*) where only focal areas of the tissue culture cells are initially infected.

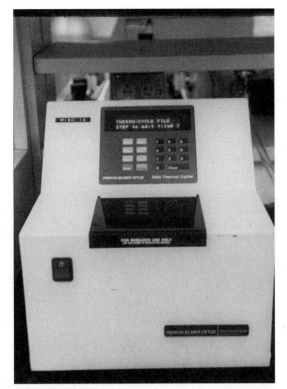

**FIGURE 36–15.** A specially designed hot water bath (thermocycler) for repeated amplifications of target DNA strands during the PCR process.

transport, improper inoculation or incubation in the laboratory, or simply the limitations of the test itself. For example, understanding the sensitivity of the blood cultures helps the clinician to understand that one negative blood culture set does not rule out endocarditis. Two or three blood culture sets, however, will detect organisms in over 95% of patients with endocarditis. A negative test in the face of a strongly suggestive clinical picture warrants further investigation. Alerting the laboratory may insure maximal detection of the infectious pathogens under consideration.

### Automated Systems and Kits

Not all laboratories can employ highly experienced personnel to perform every task. In many smaller laboratories, automation may reduce testing times, and even enhance accuracy. Problems can arise with using automated systems for detection of new resistance determinants, since they are not very flexible in adapting to changes in microbial characteristics. For example, most automated systems have difficulty in detecting penicillin re-

sistance in pneumococci, extended-spectrum beta-lactamase resistance in gram-negative bacilli, and vancomycin resistance in enterococci. It is useful to have familiarity with the methods used in the laboratory and their limitations.

### Susceptibility Testing of Pathogens other than Bacteria

Major functions of clinical microbiology are to detect the presence or absence of an infection rapidly, and to guide therapy by detection of antimicrobial agent resistance. As hospitalized patients become more complex and resistant pathogens increasingly prevalent, there is a need to have available susceptibility testing on such diverse pathogens as fungi, viruses, *Mycobacterium* species, and even parasites (malaria). There are now no standardized methods for performance and interpretation of susceptibility results for other than rapidly growing bacteria. However, work is ongoing in all these necessary testing areas, and highly specialized susceptibility testing is available in some academic centers and reference laboratories. Such testing should be accompanied by expert interpretation of the reported results, since the test performance is very dependent on the precise methods used, and results from one laboratory may not be directly applicable to those from another laboratory. Communication between clinician and laboratory personnel leads to improved patient care and service.

### CASE HISTORIES

#### CASE HISTORY 1

A 67-year-old homeless male alcohol abuser is admitted to your hospital service. He was seen today in a primary medical doctor's office for productive cough, fevers, night sweats, and weight loss over the past 3 weeks. A chest x-ray reveals a right upper lobe infiltrate with a possible cavity. A sputum sample sent today from the office to the laboratory for tuberculosis culture is negative on acid-fast bacilli smear. Do you need to admit this patient to a negative-airflow room until tuberculosis is ruled out?

#### CASE 1 DISCUSSION

This case illustrates the important point that often it is difficult to assess the meaning of a negative result in the face of compelling clinical signs and symptoms. First, you want to be sure the sample

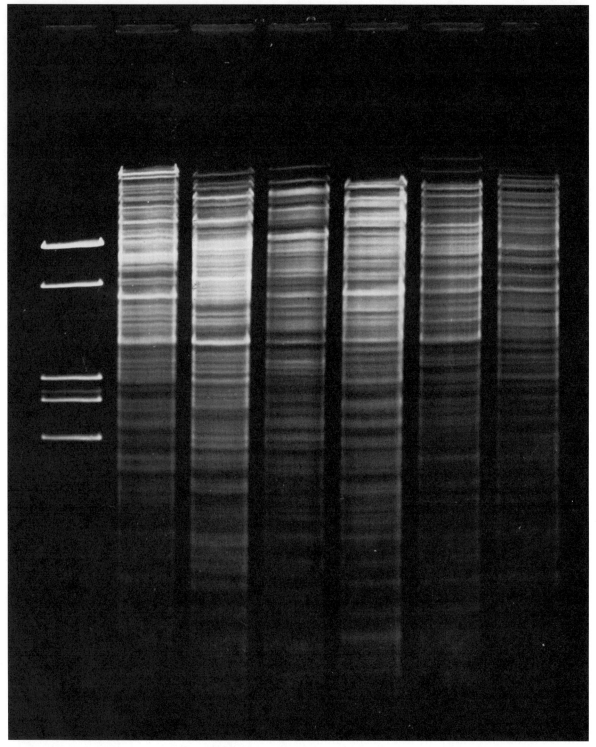

**FIGURE 36-16.** DNA electrophoresis used to demonstrate the "fingerprints" of several microbial isolates possibly causing a nosocomial outbreak. Here the strains each show several distinct banding patterns suggesting they are polyclonal and *not* epidemiologically linked.

was appropriately collected. Also, one negative specimen does not completely rule out an infectious process such as tuberculosis. With the strong clinical history presented here, it is necessary to isolate this patient until three adequate samples are smear-negative for AFB. A repeat (induced) sputum was obtained and found positive for moderate amounts of AFB. At this time. an HIV result also came back as negative. We must decide whether to start empiric antituberculous therapy and to consider what drugs to use.

At this point we have several useful clues from the clinical and laboratory evaluation. First, we know the patient likely has an infection with mycobacteria. Since the patient does not have acquired immunodeficiency syndrome (AIDS) and the lesion is in the upper lung fields, this is very likely typical reactivation *M. tuberculosis*. With reactivation disease in this patient, the organism should be sensitive to most antimycobacterial agents. A complicating factor, however, is the fact that the patient is homeless, which increases his potential for a new infection with a multi–drug-resistant strain of *M. tuberculosis*. The laboratory can again help by providing data on the overall susceptibility of local mycobacterial isolates over the last several years. If the diagnosis were in doubt, PCR testing could also be performed on the sputum from this smear-positive patient to confirm the diagnosis of *M. tuberculosis*.

## Case History 2

A 71-year-old woman presents with a week of fevers. Prior to this she had been well with only moderately severe degenerative arthritis relieved by aspirin. Physical examination did not reveal any localizing findings. Her hemoglobin was 12.6 g/dL, WBC count $12,200^3$ with a normal differential, and a chest x-ray was unchanged from 3 years earlier. Her temperature on admission was 101.8°F. As part of her initial evaluation two sets of blood cultures were drawn. The patient's fever gradually resolved over 48 h without any antimicrobial therapy and she was discharged. Three days later the laboratory calls to report one of two blood culture sets is positive for *Staphylococcus epidermidis* resistant to methicillin. You need to decide if antibiotic therapy must be started now, what should be used, and for how long.

## Case 2 Discussion

This is an example where a simple call to the laboratory can save you and your patient unnecessary testing and therapy. The laboratory should know the performance characteristics of its culture systems, and often can suggest the likelihood that a certain pattern of growth in a series of samples represents a possibly contaminated specimen or true infection. Newer blood culture systems are extremely efficient in recovering staphylococci so that knowing what parts of a blood culture system demonstrated growth can be helpful. In this patient only one of six bottles drawn (two sets of three components each) is positive for *Staphylococcus epidermidis* resistant to methicillin, which is consistent with a skin contaminant being introduced at the time of specimen collection. If this fits with the patient's clinical condition, as in this example, the physician and patient can safely interpret the culture result as a "false-positive" test. If any question as to the significance of this result remained, it would be prudent to draw an additional two sets, using meticulous technique for skin disinfection, and await the culture results before considering treatment.

## REFERENCES

### Books

Baron, E. J., Peterson, L. R., and Finegold, S. M., eds. *Bailey and Scott's Diagnostic Microbiology.* 9th ed. St. Louis: Mosby-Year Book Company, Inc., 1994.

Mandell, G. L., Bennett, J. E., and Dolin, R., eds. *Mandell, Douglas and Bennett's Principles and Practice of Infectious Diseases.* 4th ed. New York: Churchill Livingstone, Inc., 1995.

Murray, P. R, Baron, E. J., Pfaller, M. A., Tenover, F. C., and Yolken, R. H., eds. *Manual of Clinical Microbiology.* 6th ed. Washington, DC: American Society for Microbiology, 1995.

### Review Article

Tenover, F. C., Swenson, J. M., O'Hara, C. M., and Stocker, S. A. Ability of commercial and reference antimicrobial susceptibility testing methods to detect vancomycin resistance in enterococci. *J. Clin. Microbiol. 33*: 1524–1527, 1995.

### Original Articles

Englund, K., Noskin, G. A., Trakas, K., and Peterson, L. R. Antifungal susceptibility testing. In: Program. Thirty-second annual meeting of the Infectious Disease Society of America, Orlando, Florida, October, 1994.

Gerna, G., Sarasini, A., Percivalle, E., Zavattoni, M., Baldanti, F., and Revello, M. G. Rapid screening for resistance to gancyclovir and foscarnet of primary isolates of human cytomegalovirus from culture-positive blood samples. *J. Clin. Microbiol. 33*:738–741, 1995.

Hacek, D. M., Noskin, G. A., Trakas, K., and Peterson, L. R. Initial use of a broth microdilution method suitable for in vitro testing of fungal isolates in a clinical microbiology laboratory. *J. Clin. Microbiol. 33*:1884–1889, 1995.

Hoon, A. H., Lam, C. K., and Wah, M. J. Quantitative assessment of antimalarial activities from Malaysian *Plasmodium falciparum* isolates by a modified in vitro microtechnique. *Antimicrob. Agents Chemother. 39*:626–628, 1995.

# 37

# MECHANISMS OF MICROBIAL SUSCEPTIBILITY AND RESISTANCE TO ANTIMICROBIAL AGENTS

ROBERT J. POOLEY, Jr., M.D. and
LANCE R. PETERSON, M.D.

One of the primary reasons biologists study microorganisms is to learn about the "simple" biochemical systems of prokaryotes and expand that knowledge to the more complex eukaryotic organisms. The primary reason physicians are concerned with microorganisms is to find methods of defeating them when they cause illness in their patients. The discovery of antibiotics, somewhat by accident, has progressed from recovering crude penicillin in a patient's urine for recycling to the development of worldwide efforts for the efficient production of, distribution of, and search for new antimicrobial agents.

This chapter provides an overview of the 'asses of antimicrobial agents, their action, and the primary known (s) of microbial resistance. Similar texts organize antimicrobial agents on the basis of their site of action (e.g., cell-wall inhibitor, protein synthesis inhibitor). In this chapter, the organization will be based more on clinical use, and hinge upon whether the drug has bactericidal or bacteriostatic effects. Also, rather than list every possible organism an agent may inhibit, an effort is made to give functional "clinical" spectra of activity. We refer to the organisms or clinical situations that are typically thought of when considering use of the agent being discussed. For example, although a drug may have anti–gram-negative bacterial activity, the frequent presence of resistance or low overall effectiveness among the gram-negative organisms will make it primarily useful only against the gram-positive microbes, and we will refer to it as a gram-positive drug. Mechanisms of resistance are discussed in the first section of the chapter so that the primary resistance mechanisms involved with a particular antimicrobial agent class can be easily referred to in the subsequent relevant sections.

## MICROBIAL RESISTANCE

### General Principles

In simple terms, the susceptibility of an organism to an antimicrobial agent depends on the interaction of the agent with a target site. This target is usually an enzyme and the end result is the disruption of a critical genetic or metabolic pathway with inhibition of the organism's biologic functions. The affected pathway should be different from those of the host so that toxicity is minimal, and it should be common among many bacteria in order to be widely useful.

When we know something of the mode of action of a drug and expect it to be active because of its specificity for a common bacterial pathway, we are dismayed when some microorganisms show resistance to the drug. Although the actual mechanisms that result in resistance are somewhat limited, the acquisition and expression of resistance can be variable and complex (Table 37–1).

One of the mechanisms noted in Table 37–1 is usually the primary means of resistance to an antibiotic or class of antibiotics. Occasionally, more than one is present, producing an additive effect, leading to very high levels of drug resistance.

### TABLE 37–1.   MECHANISMS OF RESISTANCE

1. *Decreased access of the antibiotic to the target site* may occur from changes in membrane permeability or from active transport of the drug out of the organism.
2. *Enzymatic alteration of the drug* can reduce or eliminate its effectiveness. The breakage of important covalent bonds in the molecule or the addition of chemical groups to the antibiotic prevents its interaction with the target site.
3. *Target site alteration* refers to change(s) in amino acid sequence of a protein or production of a new target site with low affinity for the antibiotic.
4. *Increased synthesis of an essential metabolite that is antagonistic to the antimicrobial.* This prevents the agent from binding effectively to the target site.

### Genetic Basis for Antibiotic Resistance

All resistance is ultimately determined by a change in the genetic composition of an organism. This can be the acquisition of new nucleic acid from other organisms (transduction, plasmid transfer) or from the environment (transformation), or it can be the mutation of genetic material already present in the organism. There are also some cases where resistance is due to the expression of genes that are naturally repressed and then induced to be transcribed in the presence of the antimicrobial (induction). At this point it is important to define some commonly used terms dealing with drug resistance.

### Mutation

Mutation is a change in a DNA or RNA sequence that occurs either spontaneously or as a result of exposure to an environmental agent (usually a mutagenic compound that reacts with DNA and causes changes in base pair sequences, or some form of electromagnetic radiation that does the same). Such permanent changes in DNA are not very common, occurring maximally about once in every $10^5$–$10^7$ cell divisions, and they are not the most typical means of acquiring drug resistance. There are corrective mechanisms to prevent such DNA changes, and a modest probability that such mutations will be "silent" and not expressed phenotypically. Mutations that do confer some degree of resistance are often "genetically recessive" and may not be passed to other organisms. They result in some change or loss of function that is often deleterious in the absence of the antibiotic because the change means competition with other bacterial flora will be poor.

### Transformation

This is a passive means of DNA acquisition by bacteria. Transformation occurs by exposure to DNA from a genetically similar organism and the uptake of this DNA with insertion into the genome of the exposed organism. It is generally not of clinical importance outside of the research laboratory.

### Transduction

Bacteriophages are virus-like particles capable of infecting bacteria. After infection, the bacterial metabolic processes are taken over and directed toward production of more phage particles. The end result, like viral infection of eukaryotic cells, is often cell lysis and death with release of phage progeny. In some instances, the phage enters a latent cycle and the phage DNA is incorporated into the bacterial genome. It remains in this state, replicating with the bacterial genome, until circumstances promote separation and procession through phage replication with or without cell lysis. This movement in and out of bacterial genomes provides a means by which resistance genes can be transferred from one organism to another. A resistance gene in close proximity to the phage DNA may inadvertently be removed with the phage when it enters the lytic cycle. When the phage later infects a new cell, the resistance gene is inserted into the new genome with the phage DNA and can be left behind when it leaves. This kind of DNA shuffling requires that the donor and recipient bacteria have a significant amount of homology between their DNA sequences. In some instances, resistance genes to different antibiotics are closely linked on the bacterial genome and then multiple antibiotic resistances are transferred by the phage infection.

### Plasmid Transfer

Plasmids are rings of extrachromosomal DNA that can be transferred between different genera and species of bacteria. It was recognized during outbreaks of dysentery in Japan during the 1950s that strains of *Shigella* species responsible for enteritis had very similar resistance patterns to strains of *Escherichia coli* that were present in the same host, but not causing disease. This suggested that the resistance was being transferred from *E. coli* to the *Shigella* species by an unknown mechanism. Resistance genes were later located on circular closed loops of DNA within the bacteria. The loops of DNA were termed *plasmids* that are now also known as *resistance factors* or *R factors*. They can be passed between bacteria by conjugation (passing of R factors between bacteria via cytoplasmic extensions called pili), even spreading resistance from one species to another. Plasmids replicate with the chromosomal DNA and can be passed on to bacterial progeny if selective pressure (i.e., exposure to antibiotics) favors retention of the resistance. If there is no selective pressure, plasmids have been shown to lose resistance genes and decrease in size or can be lost completely. There are two functional components of R factors. The actual genes on the plasmid that confer resistance to antibiotics are called

*r determinants*. The part of the plasmid that initiates and controls conjugation is called the *resistance transfer factor* (RTF). Plasmids are the most important mechanism for spreading (clinical) resistance today. They are variable in size and can acquire new genes, leading to multidrug resistance that are transferable to other bacterial genera. Possible transfer of this resistance from low or moderately pathogenic organisms to highly pathogenic organisms potentially could result in a clinical environment similar to the preantibiotic era, where infectious diseases without antibacterial treatment result in significant morbidity and mortality to patients.

### Induction

In any species, the genome contains many genes that are not expressed either because they are permanently "shut off" due to differentiation or they are waiting for specific environmental stimuli to begin transcription. The latter situation occurs in the process of induction. A particular gene is capable of expression but, because of an effect exerted at its promoter region, no RNA production occurs. Often a regulator protein is bound to the promoter region, or just upstream from it, and inhibits interaction with RNA polymerase. When a bacterium is exposed to an antimicrobial agent, the protein is released from the promoter region and transcription of the gene can proceed. If the gene codes for a resistance mechanism, then resistance to the antibiotic will develop. The concept of induction is important for the understanding of how the expression of resistance genes located on chromosomes or R factors is controlled.

The particular mechanism(s) of resistance for each drug class as well as any known or suspected genetic basis for resistance are addressed in the section for that particular antimicrobial agent found later in this chapter.

### ANTIMICROBIALS THAT ARE LETHAL TO MICROBES

### Penicillins

**Mechanism of action: bactericidal**
**Clinical spectrum of activity: variable**

The penicillins belong to a large family of antibiotics called beta-lactams that collectively have a very wide spectrum of activity. They are generally low in toxic potential and easily achievable blood and tissue concentrations are required for bactericidal action. Although the antibacterial effects of the sulfonamides (which are antimetabolites and not beta-lactams) were known earlier, the discovery of the penicillins is considered to be the dawn of the age of antibiotics, and they have been extensively studied for their mechanism of action. Some discussion of the synthesis of bacterial cell walls is necessary to understand how the penicillins act and to understand a key structural component of bacteria.

The major structural component of bacterial cell walls is peptidoglycan, a heteropolymer of carbohydrates and peptides that confers support and protection to the organism. The gram-positive bacteria have cell walls that are 50–100 molecules of peptidoglycan thick, while the gram-negative organisms have cell walls only one to two molecules thick. This characteristic, along with a high teichoic acid content, is responsible for the retention of crystal violet by gram-positive organisms during the decolorization step of the Gram's stain. The different thicknesses of the cell walls may also account for some differences in susceptibility to the penicillins.

The synthesis of the cell wall occurs in three steps (Figs. 37–1 and 37–2):

1. The formation of the precursors, N-acetylmuramic acid (NMA) and N-acetylglucosamine (NAG), takes place in the cytoplasm. Each of the precursors is bound to a molecule of uridine diphosphate (UDP). Normally, NMA is also linked to a D-alanyl-D-alanine dipeptide and a glycine pentapeptide.

2. The energy from hydrolysis of the UDP bond is used to form dimers of NMA and NAG. The dimers are bound to a membrane phospholipid and "flipped" across the cell membrane. On the exterior of the cell, the dimer is then cleaved from the phospholipid.

3. On the surface of the organism, a membrane-bound transpeptidase catalyzes the hydrolysis of one of the D-alanine molecules and insertion of the dimer into the growing peptidoglycan chain by the remaining D-alanine.

An important step of the process is the site of action of the penicillins and the other beta-lactam antibiotics. They interact with *penicillin-binding proteins* (*PBPs*), which are found on the cytoplasmic membrane as 'bound' proteins. Some of these PBPs are the transpeptidases involved in the chain elongation step above, and others are involved in the maintenance of cell shape or septum formation during cell division. The affinity of the penicillins for the PBPs at this point in the process is due to the beta-lactam ring's structural similarity to the D-alanyl-D-alanine dipeptide. The end result is inhibition of the transpeptidases with loss of ability to form peptidoglycan. Without the ability to form new cell wall, autolysis of the cell occurs from unopposed activity of naturally occurring murein hydrolases that are present in the cell. These are enzymes that normally "nick" the cell wall to expose areas for new cell-wall formation during cell enlargement.

Figure 37–3 is a drawing of penicillins and cephalosporins indicating the points of substitution used to alter properties of these two major classes of beta-lactam compounds.

Resistance to the penicillins occurs by three mechanisms:

1. *Change in affinity of PBPs* for the antibiotic so that peptidoglycan formation can proceed.

2. *Decreased penetration of the antibiotic* into the organism. This mechanism is more prominent in the gram-negative bacteria.

3. *Specific beta-lactamase production*. These enzymes hydrolyze the beta-lactam ring (Fig. 37–3) of the molecule so that it no longer mimics the alanine dipeptide and therefore cannot interact with PBPs. These enzymes are the *primary mode of resistance* to the beta-lactam antibiotics. There is some suggestion that these enzymes are at least related to those involved in the formation of cell wall, and have the additional capability of antibiotic degradation. This concept is supported by the fact that many beta-lactamases are structurally very similar to the membrane-bound PBPs. They are produced by some gram-positive bacteria and excreted extracellularly. They are also produced, at least at low level, by virtually all gram-negative bacteria, and here are concentrated in the periplasmic space between the inner and outer cell membranes. When the beta-lactamase is encoded on the chromosome, it is usually of the inducible type and is produced at high levels in response to antibiotic exposure. In some situations, even when the antibiotic is no longer present, beta-lactamase production still occurs. This is termed *stable derepression*, and beta-lactam antibiotics that are weak inducers tend to select for stable derepressed mutants in microbes such as *Pseudomonas aeruginosa* and *Enterobacter cloacae*. Examples of weak inducers are mezlocillin, cefotaxime, ceftizoxime, and ceftazidime. The beta-lactamases en-

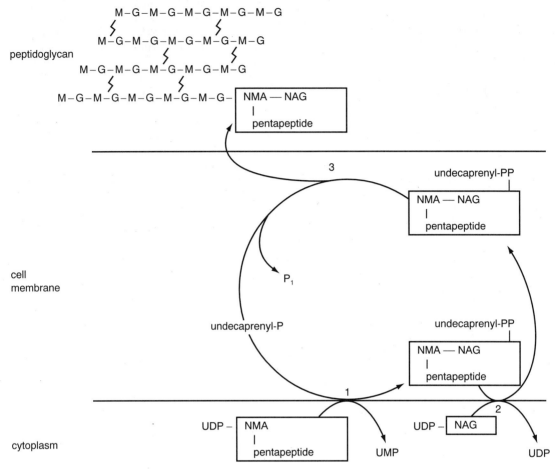

**FIGURE 37–1.** Diagrammatic representation of cell-wall formation. UDP-activated *N*-acetylmuramic acid (NMA; M) is bound to the membrane phospholipid carrier undecaprenyl phosphate. *N*-acetylglucosamine (NAG; G) is transferred to the molecule of NMA and the dimer is flipped across the membrane for incorporation into the growing cell wall. Cross-links between NMA of adjacent peptidoglycan chains are designated by *jagged lines*.

coded by plasmids, in contrast, are usually constitutive and produced even without exposure to antibiotics.

Penicillin G and penicillin V are two of the most widely used penicillins in clinical practice. Penicillin G is the only naturally occurring penicillin (all others are semisynthetic). They both have similar activity against gram-positive organisms. Against gram-negative bacteria, penicillin G has 5–10 times greater activity than penicillin V. In standard practice today they are generally considered as gram-positive drugs only. Penicillin G is administered parenterally, but penicillin V can be given orally due to its greater stability in the acid environment of the stomach. They are of particular use in infections due to *Streptococcus*

*pneumoniae* (pneumococci), *Streptococcus pyogenes* (group A), *Streptococcus agalactiae* (group B), and the viridans group of streptococci. The exception to restriction of penicillin G use for infections due to gram-positive organisms is for the treatment of *Neisseria gonorrhoeae*, the gram-negative organism responsible for gonorrhea, and *N. meningitidis*. It is still very useful in geographic areas where resistance to the antibiotic is not widespread.

Penicillinase-resistant penicillins are semisynthetic drugs designed to avoid deactivation by beta-lactamases and include the compounds methicillin, oxacillin, dicloxacillin, and nafcillin. Because of renal toxicity, methicillin is now of historical interest only. These agents are used in clinical situations where the probable causative organism is a gram-

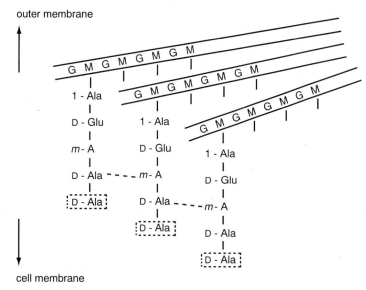

**FIGURE 37–2.** Peptidoglycan cross-link formation. A peptide bond is formed between the fourth amino acid (in this case alanine [Ala]) of a pentapeptide and the third amino acid (a modified alanine [*m*-Ala]) of an adjacent pentapeptide on a different peptidoglycan chain. The fifth amino acid does not participate in the reaction and is cleaved from the pentapeptide. The amino acid sequence of the pentapeptide varies between bacterial species.

positive bacterium like *Staphylococcus aureus* that is likely producing beta-lactamase. Skin infections such as cellulitis or folliculitis that are acquired outside a hospital environment, where staphylococci sensitive to these drugs are found, are common uses. At therapeutic dosage levels they are also very effective clinically against all streptococci with the important exception of enterococci. Resistance to these drugs does occur, but it is independent of beta-lactamase production. Methicillin re-

sistance, for example, is due to the production of an altered PBP-2 (2a) that has lowered affinity for methicillin and the related agents. It is an acquired (via plasmid) chromosomal gene and is regulated by a large plasmid that also codes for beta-lactamase production. Resistance to the semisynthetic penicillins in gram-negative bacilli is largely due to restricted penetration of the antibiotic. Porins in the membrane of gram-negatives can limit diffusion of these beta-lactams and other molecules that have bulky substituents or electrostatic charges.

Extended-spectrum penicillins (the aminopenicillins) are semisynthetic penicillins that still have gram-positive activity against streptococci (including many enterococci) but are modified to exhibit greater activity against gram-negative organisms. They are not resistant to hydrolysis by beta-lactamases. The most often used members of this group are ampicillin and amoxicillin and they are commonly prescribed in cases of otitis media, sinusitis, bronchitis, and urinary tract infections where organisms such as *Haemophilus influenzae*, *Streptococcus pneumoniae*, and susceptible *Escherichia coli* are suspected.

Antipseudomonal penicillins have general gram-negative activity plus antistreptococcal activity (including *Enterococcus faecalis*), but are of special importance because of their activity against the pseudomonads, particularly *Pseudomonas aeruginosa*. They are critical for first-line empiric therapy in situations where extremely ill or immunocompromised patients appear septic and a possible pathogen

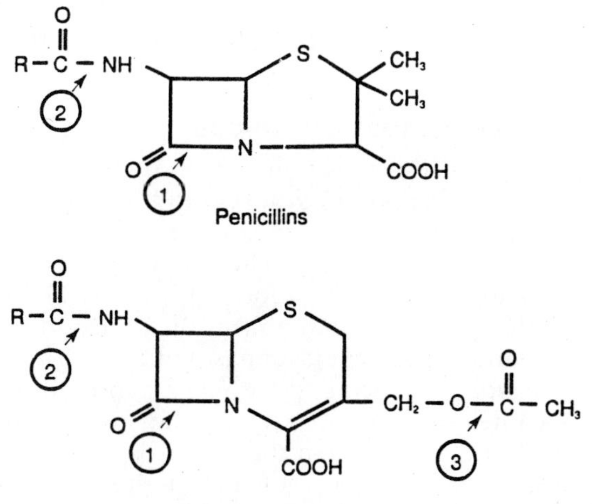

**Penicillins**

**Cephalosporins**

**FIGURE 37–3.** Structure of the penicillins and cephalosporins. The four-member ring (*1*) is the beta-lactam nucleus. *Arrow* (*2*) indicates a side-chain substitution site for both penicillins and cephalosporins, and 3 indicates a second side-chain substitution site available for cephalosporins.

is *P. aeruginosa* or other *Pseudomonas* species. Examples commonly in use are piperacillin, ticarcillin, and mezlocillin.

## Cephalosporins

**Mechanism of action: Bactericidal**
**Clinical spectrum of activity: variable**

The cephalosporins were initially isolated from fungi and exert an antibacterial effect by inhibiting cell-wall formation with a mechanism similar to the penicillins. The cephalosporins are beta-lactam antibiotics that have a core molecule of 7-aminocephalosporinic acid. Modifications have been made by substituting small chemical groups at one or both of two possible sites on the core cephalosporin molecule (Fig. 37–3). Alterations of chemical substitutions at the two sites produce specific changes in drug properties. One site affects antibacterial spectrum and the other alters pharmacokinetics and metabolism of the drug. Researchers continue to explore the numerous possible cephalosporins that can be created from the core molecule. There are many cephalosporins available for use, and they are grouped into "generations" depending on their antibacterial spectrum. As a class, the cephalosporins do not have reliable activity against methicillin-resistant *Staphylococcus aureus* or the genus *Enterococcus*. Overall, the penetration of the cephalosporins into body tissues is good, but only the "third-generation" drugs enter the central nervous system (CNS) efficiently enough to be recommended for treatment of meningitis.

### First-Generation Cephalosporins

Although there are many different drugs belonging to the first generation, they are essentially identical in their antimicrobial activity. Cephalothin is the prototypical member of this group. Cefazolin is closely related to cephalothin but has a longer half-life. Cephalexin is an oral counterpart of these agents. The activity of the first-generation agents is practically confined to the gram-positive organisms and is the best in this regard among all the available cephalosporin generations. The common pathogens methicillin-susceptible *Staphylococcus aureus* (MSSA), *Streptococcus pyogenes* (group A), *Streptococcus agalactiae* (group B), and *Streptococcus pneumoniae* are usually susceptible. Although there is some activity against aerobic gram-negatives like *Escherichia coli*, *Klebsiella pneumoniae*, and *Proteus mirabilis*, the first-generation cephalosporins are not the drugs of choice for these organisms. With the increase of beta-lactamase (cephalosporinase)–producing strains, activity against *Haemophilus influenzae* is not reliable and the use of first-generation drugs for otitis and sinusitis carries a risk of clinical failure.

### Second-Generation Cephalosporins

The alterations made to the second-generation cephalosporins allows retention of gram-positive activity with the addition of better gram-negative activity. They are more resistant to beta-lactamases. Activity is better against *Haemophilus influenzae*, and cefaclor, one of the classic oral members of this group, is often used for this purpose. The second-generation agents are more active against the genera *Escherichia*, *Klebsiella*, *Proteus*, and *Providencia* than first-generation agents, and may be active against *Citrobacter*, *Enterobacter*, *Serratia*, and *Acinetobacter*. None of the second-generation drugs have antipseudomonal activity. There is enough variation in the properties between the members of this group that individual agents may have an advantage over the others in a particular clinical situation. For example, cefoxitin has useful activity against anaerobes like *Bacteroides fragilis*. Cefamandole is the most active member against staphylococci, and sometimes is selected for antibiotic prophylaxis prior to surgical procedures in order to prevent deep wound infections from gram-positive cocci. Cefuroxime is used for empiric therapy in community-acquired pneumonia by some practitioners, and is relatively resistant to many potent beta-lactamases.

### Third-Generation Cephalosporins

The third-generation of cephalosporins have the least potent gram-positive activity but are the most effective of this class against the gram-negative bacteria. They are also the only cephalosporins with good antipseudomonal activity. The third-generation drugs are more resistant to the beta-lactamases of *Haemophilus influenzae*, *Neisseria gonorrhoeae*, and other gram-negative organisms, and they reach suitable concentrations in the cerebrospinal fluid (CSF) for treatment of meningitis due to these pathogens. Some of the agents merit special mention. Ceftriaxone has become the first choice for the empiric treatment of meningitis in many centers due to its safety, excellent CNS penetration, and simple dosing schedule related to its long half-life. Cefixime is now used as single-dose oral therapy for uncomplicated gonorrhea. Ceftazidime provides good antipseudomonal activity when *Pseudomonas aeruginosa* is a suspected pathogen.

## Other Beta-Lactam Antibiotics (Carbapenems and Monobactams)

**Mechanism of action: bactericidal**
**Clinical spectrum of activity: gram-positive and gram-negative aerobes; anaerobes**

The other antibiotics belonging to the beta-lactam class have killing mechanisms similar to penicillin and are also bactericidal. The similarity of all these agents is shown in Figure 37–4. These additional compounds are not generally first-line drugs and are reserved for patients not responding to initial antibiotic regimens and for patients with highly resistant organisms, especially gram-negative aerobic bacilli, and the pseudomonads.

Imipenem is a beta-lactamase–resistant penem antibiotic considered to belong to the

**Penicillins**

**Cephalosporins**

**Monobactams**

**Carbapenems**

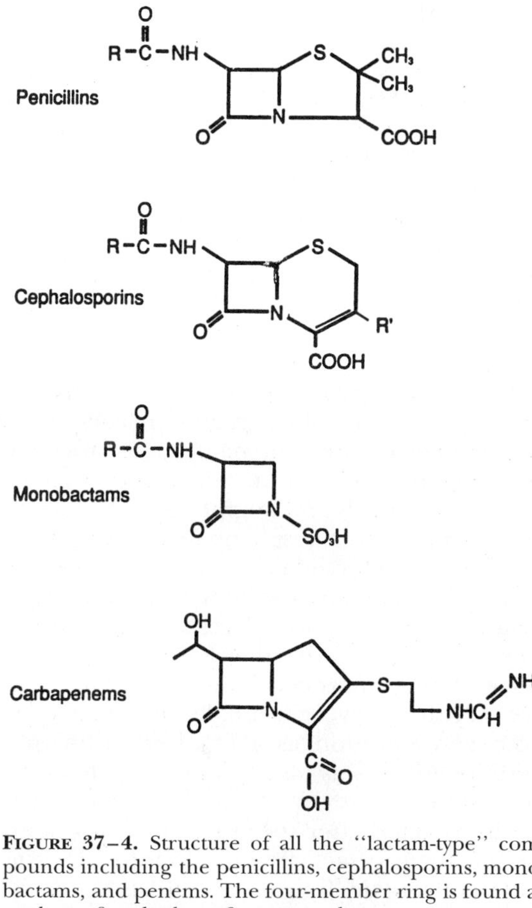

FIGURE 37–4. Structure of all the "lactam-type" compounds including the penicillins, cephalosporins, monobactams, and penems. The four-member ring is found as nucleus of each class of compound.

beta-lactam group that is used in combination with the drug cilastatin. It is the single most broad-spectrum agent available. Imipenem disrupts cell-wall formation like other beta-lactams. Cilastatin inhibits the renal dehydropeptidase that degrades imipenem and therefore prolongs the half-life of imipenem. It also diminishes the renal toxicity of imipenem that is seen when cilastatin is not coadministered with imipenem. This drug combination is given only by the intravenous (IV) route and has potential difficulties, since the kinetics of the two components are very different in the patient with renal impairment. Patients with renal insufficiency are at risk for seizures from toxic levels of cilastatin unless the dosage is reduced. Because of the potential dosing difficulties, and the fact that overuse of this agent can lead to increased nosocomial infections with the multi–drug-resistant pathogen *Stenotrophomonas* (*Xanthomonas*) *maltophilia*, this agent should be used only with the assistance of an expert consultant.

Although imipenem is a strong beta-lactamase inducer, it is generally very stable against most plasmid or chromosomal beta-lactamases. An exception is the chromosomal zinc-containing beta-lactamases found in *Stenotrophomonas maltophilia* and *Bacteroides fragilis*. Resistance in *P. aeruginosa* is probably due to decreased permeability from altered porin proteins in the cell membrane.

Aztreonam is referred to as a "monobactam" and is resistant to many beta-lactamases in a spectrum similar to that of ceftazidime or aminoglycosides. The main advantage of this agent is that there is little or no cross-reaction in patients with known serious allergies, including anaphylaxis, to the penicillins or the cephalosporins. It is an excellent antibiotic against the aerobic gram-negatives, especially *Pseudomonas* species, that is comparable to ceftazidime, but it has essentially no gram-positive or anaerobic activity. It is often used in the setting of a patient with a penicillin allergy that prevents the use of an antipseudomonal penicillin when one is clinically indicated. When organisms are resistant to aztreonam, it is usually because of decreased antibiotic penetration into the cell and not by the production of beta-lactamases. Aztreonam is highly resistant to plasmid beta-lactamases and does not induce chromosomal enzymes.

## Beta-Lactamase Inhibitors

These are beta-lactam molecules that have little direct antimicrobial activity but are used in combination with other drugs to increase bacterial susceptibility. They act as "suicide inhibitors" of beta-lactamases and form covalent products that inactivate the enzymes. This allows the coadministered antibiotic to remain intact and effective. These inhibitors are particularly effective for enhancing the activity of their partner agents against the staphylococci and anaerobic bacteria. Representative structures of these compounds are shown in Figure 37–5.

Clavulanic acid is one of these compounds and when given with amoxicillin the combined drug is known as Augmentin. When given with ticarcillin it is known as Timentin. Because it is a beta-lactam agent, clavulanic acid induces the production of beta-lactamases, the same enzymes that it inhibits. This may be a mechanism by which clavulanic acid can actually antagonize the antibiotic it is meant to protect. Whether such enzyme induction has resulted in any clinical failures using the antibiotic combination is not proven.

Sulbactam and tazobactam are sulfone-type inhibitors. They are combined with ampicillin

(sulbactam) to form the drug Unasyn, and with piperacillin (tazobactam) to form Zosyn. The sulfones are poor beta-lactamase inducers, and this may give them some advantage over clavulanic acid.

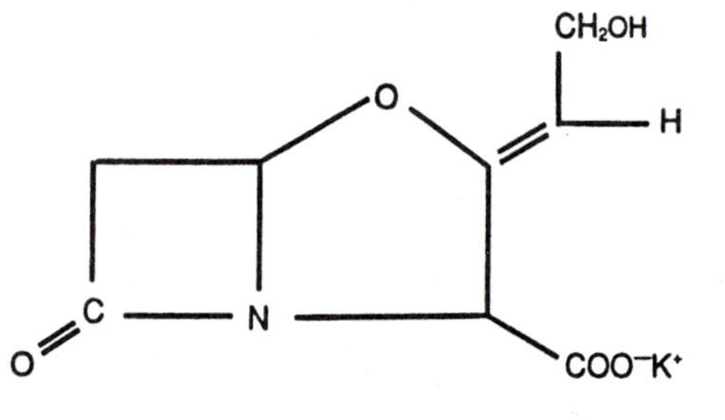

## Aminoglycosides

**Mechanism of action: bactericidal**
**Clinical spectrum of activity: aerobic gram-negative bacilli; many staphylococci; synergy for enterococcal infections**

The aminoglycosides are polycyclic molecules consisting of multiple amino sugars in their structure. They are polycations, and this characteristic contributes to their poor gastrointestinal (GI) absorption, poor CNS penetration, and rapid excretion by the kidney. As a class, they are uniformly nephrotoxic and ototoxic. The degree of toxicity correlates with the level of drug observed in the blood.

Aminoglycosides depend on transport across the inner membrane of gram-negative organisms to exert their effect. This is an energy-dependent process and the organisms generally must use oxidative metabolism with electron transport and have a cell interior with a partially negative charge to allow aminoglycoside accumulation. This transport is inhibited by divalent cations or anaerobic conditions, and it is the rate-limiting step of aminoglycoside activity. Once inside the cell, the aminoglycosides bind to the 30S subunit of the ribosome and interfere with the initiation of protein synthesis. There is also misreading of mRNA as a result of drug interaction with the ribosome. Misreading of mRNA results in synthesis of abnormal proteins, including those that help maintain cell membrane integrity. Loss of membrane integrity facilitates increased diffusion of aminoglycosides into the cell and augments the effect of these agents. As a result of this activity they are rapidly bactericidal.

Streptomycin was the first aminoglycoside isolated. Although initial responses to treatment were good, the development of resistance by the enterococci and the gram-negative aerobes have essentially eliminated it from consideration as a first-line antibiotic. Additionally, it was also found to be toxic to the vestibular system of the inner ear. Neomycin, isolated after streptomycin, has a similar spectrum of activity but is more ototoxic and nephrotoxic. It primarily affects the cochlear function of the ear rather than vestibular

**Clavulanate Potassium**

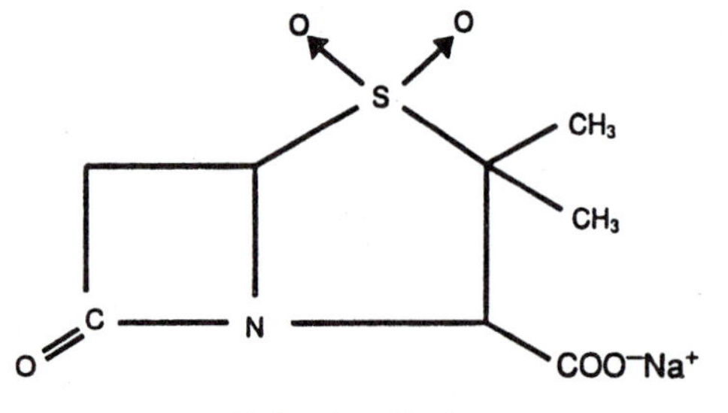

**Sulbactam Sodium**

**FIGURE 37–5.** Structure of the suicide beta-lactamase inhibitors sulbactam, a sulfone, and clavulanate. Formation of an irreversible acyl enzyme link with the target beta-lactamase effectively leads to loss of enzymatic activity preventing destruction of the accompanying antibiotic.

function, and a high-pitched tinnitus may be the first manifestation of toxicity. Its use today is primarily limited to topical treatment of infections, and oral administration to reduce bowel flora in the setting of hepatic encephalopathy or elective bowel surgery. Kanamycin was the third aminoglycoside but, like streptomycin, is now limited in its use because of bacterial resistance and toxicity to the patient. Today, the three most commonly used members of this class are gentamicin, tobramycin, and amikacin. A fourth lesser used agent (due to diminished activity against *P. aeruginosa*) is netilmicin. Like the other aminoglycosides, gentamicin and tobramycin were initially isolated from fungi, while amikacin represents a semisynthetic drug modified from kanamycin.

Resistance to the aminoglycosides is usually by enzymatic modification of the antibiotic. Most of the modifying enzymes are plasmid encoded. There are three types of reactions: acetylation, nucleotidylation, and phosphorylation. A particular enzyme will generally only recognize certain subsets of the aminoglycosides and not the entire class. Amikacin is resistant to most aminoglycoside-modifying enzymes and therefore is the most active of this class of agents. The modifying enzymes are located in the periplasmic space and their concentration is relatively low. However, their affinity for the drug is high, and the aminoglycosides tend to diffuse into the periplasmic space slowly, resulting in an overall efficient rate of inactivation. Some gram-negatives show amikacin resistance, primarily by a nonenzymatic mechanism in which general uptake of the aminoglycosides is markedly decreased. Resistance found in enterococci requires special mention. This genus is naturally somewhat resistant to the aminoglycosides because they are inefficient transporters of the drugs across their membrane. The treatment of enterococcal infections requires concomitant use of ampicillin, penicillin, or vancomycin to facilitate membrane penetration of the aminoglycosides. High-level aminoglycoside resistance is due to plasmid-mediated enzymatic inactivation, and organisms with this level of resistance lack synergy between aminoglycoside and beta-lactams. It is important to remember that *Enterococcus* species resistance may only be present to specific aminoglycosides, and testing for susceptibility to individual drugs (specifically, gentamicin and streptomycin) is necessary.

## Vancomycin

### Mechanism of action: bactericidal
### Clinical spectrum of activity: gram-positive aerobes and anaerobes

Vancomycin belongs to the glycopeptide class of antibiotics. This class has a complex structure of 7 amino acids linked covalently (Fig. 37–6). Five of the seven amino acids are aromatic and are common to all members of the class. The five common aromatic amino acids form a "pocket" that is the binding site of the antibiotic. Teicoplanin is also a member of this class, but it is not licensed for use in the United States. Resistance in some staphylococci develops more rapidly to teicoplanin, so it is uncertain if this agent will be licensed in the United States. Since the early days of its use, vancomycin has represented the final backup for treatment of gram-positive infections, especially those caused by methicillin-resistant *Staphylococcus aureus* (MRSA) and the ampicillin-resistant enterococci.

Vancomycin is used for treatment of infections in penicillin-allergic patients, and for therapy of beta-lactam–resistant gram-positive organisms, especially for ampicillin-resistant enterococci and methicillin-resistant staphylococci, and as an agent for the treatment of pseudomembranous colitis caused by the gram-positive anaerobe *Clostridium difficile*. A unique side effect is the "red man syndrome" that is caused by the release of histamine when vancomycin is infused rapidly. The symptoms are pruritus, erythema (especially of the face), and rarely cardiovascular collapse. Slower infusion rates usually resolve the problem.

The mechanism of action of vancomycin is only now being clearly defined, and the primary action seems to be binding to the D-alanyl-D-alanine portion of *N*-acetylmuramic acid and the inhibition of cross-linking between growing strands of cell-wall peptidoglycan. In recent years, the sudden emergence of vancomycin resistance in the *Enterococcus faecium* has been noted. The infections caused by these enterococci (*E. faecium* and *E. faecalis*) generally occur in patients with multiple medical or surgical problems while in healthy persons the enterococci merely colonize. The concern is that this resistance to vancomycin may be transferred to organisms such as *Staphylococcus aureus* or *C. difficile*, which are of even greater pathogenic potential to less compromised patients. The other issue with vancomycin-resistant enterococci

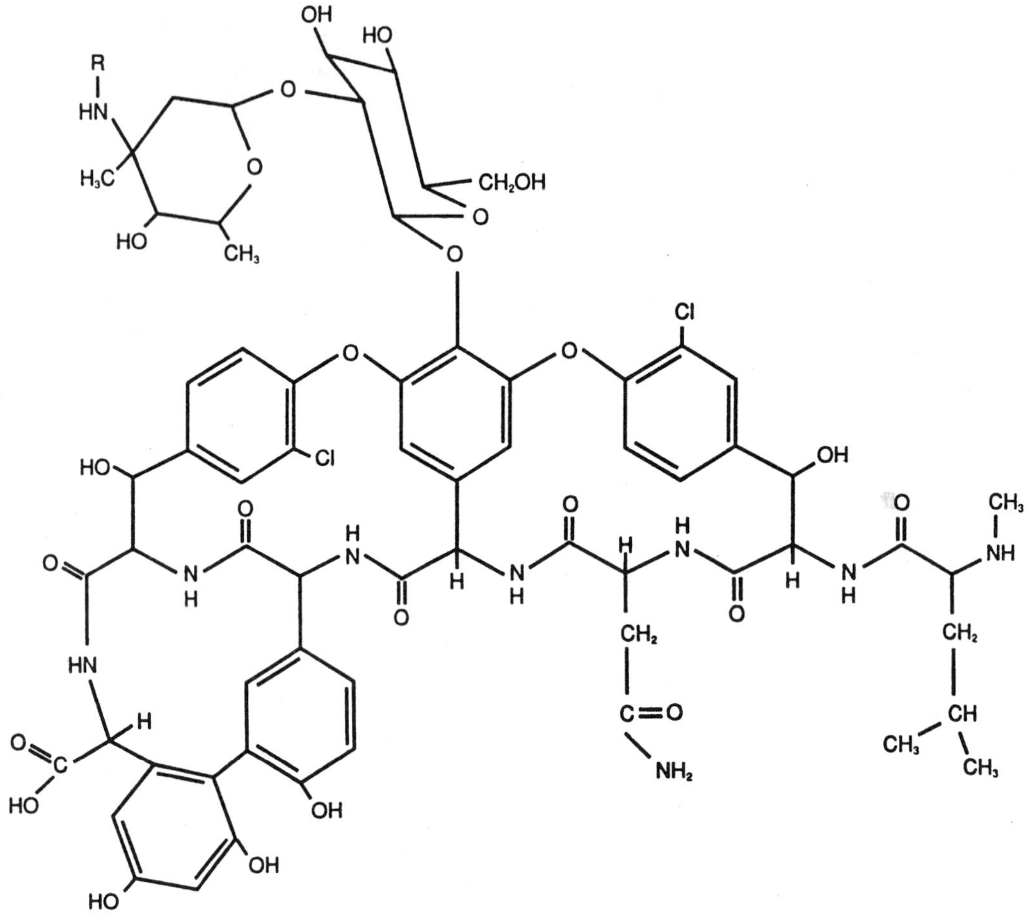

**FIGURE 37–6.** The complex structure of a member of the glycopeptide antibiotic class, vancomycin.

(VRE) is that there is often no other plausible antibiotic regimen for treatment.

Resistance to vancomycin was first noted in 1986, and the mechanisms have been most extensively studied in the enterococci. The rapid dissemination of resistance once it emerged is alarming because there are often no other treatment options. As noted above, the action of vancomycin depends on binding between the antibiotic and the D-alanine dipeptide contained in the peptidoglycan precursors (Fig. 37–2). Resistance to vancomycin results from alteration of the D-alanyl-D-alanine moiety to D-alanyl-D-lactate so that affinity with vancomycin is markedly reduced. Intrinsic resistance to vancomycin occurs in gram-positives that are uncommon pathogens (e.g., *Leuconostoc* species and many *Lactobacillus* species). The external lipid layer of gram-negatives provides a barrier to vancomycin and protects the cell wall, thus providing intrinsic resistance for the gram-negative organisms.

The mechanisms of vancomycin resistance in *Enterococcus* species are of three main phenotypes: Van A, Van B, and Van C.

Van A—high-level vancomycin resistance accompanied by teicoplanin resistance: usually expressed in *Enterococcus faecium* and some *Enterococcus faecalis* isolates

Van B—moderate-level vancomycin resistance accompanied by teicoplanin susceptibility: usually expressed in *E. faecium* and some *E. faecalis* isolates

Van C—low-level vancomycin resistance accompanied by teicoplanin susceptibility: usually expressed in species like *E. gallinarum*

The Van A phenotype is plasmid mediated and easily transferred by conjugation. The plasmid carries five basic genes known as the *van A* gene cluster. Two key proteins encoded on the cluster are Van A and Van H. The Van A product is similar to D-ala-D-ala ligase that forms the D-alanine dipeptide needed for peptidoglycan formation. Instead of joining two alanine molecules, however, Van A links an alanine molecule to a molecule of D-2-hydroxybutyrate and incorporates this into the peptidoglycan precursor NMA. The molecule of D-2-hydroxybutyrate is produced by Van H. This alanine-hydroxybutyrate molecule ultimately takes the place of D-ala-D-ala in the forming peptidoglycan. It confers resistance to vancomycin because it has 1000-fold less affinity for the antibiotic than the usual D-alanine dipeptide and cell-wall formation can proceed unimpeded. Van X (part of the gene cluster) has carboxypeptidase activity and degrades any usual D-ala-D-ala back to the individual amino acids. This decreases the possibility of incorporation into the cell wall and developing a binding site for vancomycin. The mechanism by which the Van B protein confers resistance in the Van B phenotype is not well known. The Van C phenotype is chromosomal and constitutive in *E. gallinarum* and a few related species. It is unrelated to Van A or Van B.

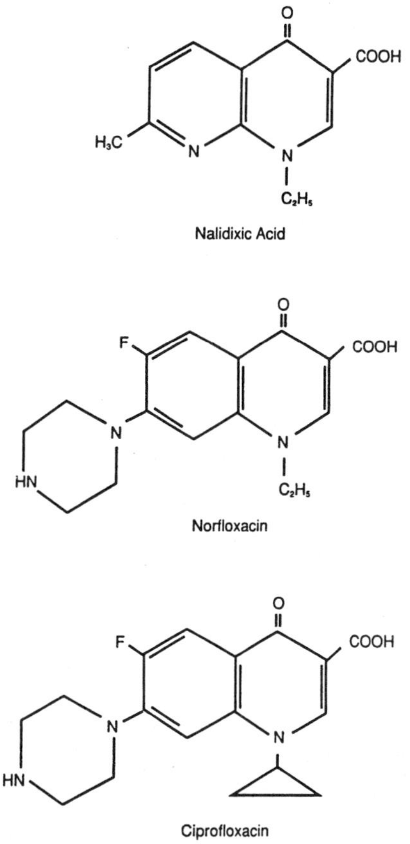

## Quinolones

**Mechanism of action: bactericidal**
**Clinical spectrum of activity: many gram-positive and most gram-negative aerobic bacteria**

Quinolones are totally synthetic compounds and therefore are properly referred to as antimicrobial agents rather than antibiotics (Fig. 37–7). The quinolones are the only agents to date that act at their particular site: the enzyme DNA gyrase. The prototype, nalidixic acid, had limited usefulness because of the rapid development of bacterial resistance to this drug. It was not until the more recent development of the fluorinated quinolones that the real value of the class was apparent. They have a broad spectrum of activity, have oral and intravenous effectiveness, are well-tolerated, and elicit relatively few serious side effects.

DNA gyrase performs the critical function of introducing negative supercoils into DNA. These supercoils relieve the tension placed on upstream portions of the DNA molecule whenever sections of the double helix are unwound for transcription or replication. DNA gyrase is a tetramer of two A subunits and two B subunits. The A subunit performs a "strand-cutting" function necessary for the supercoil formation. The site of interaction or "pocket"

**FIGURE 37–7.** Structures of nalidixic acid, the first clinically available quinolone, and norfloxacin and ciprofloxacin, the early members of the modern fluoroquinolone class of synthetic antimicrobial agents.

between the gyrase A subunit and the chromosomal DNA is currently considered the binding site for the fluoroquinolones. When present at this site the modern quinolones are rapidly bactericidal by preventing reannealing of bacterial DNA. Development of mutations in the A subunit that presumably decrease binding of the drugs are associated with stable, high-level quinolone resistance. Eukaryotic type II topoisomerases perform the same function as DNA gyrase but they are only affected by very high concentrations of the quinolones.

Ciprofloxacin is the prototypic and most frequently used fluoroquinolone, although several are available. It can be administered both IV and orally. Although it has gram-positive activity, it is generally used as a gram-negative drug and is especially useful for patients unable to take antipseudomonal penicillins, or for patients who require empiric two-drug therapy for suspected gram-negative sepsis. It has little anaerobic activity. The use of ciprofloxacin or other quinolones for routine infections, like those arising in the general (nonhospitalized) community, should be done with reservation, since studies already indicate that bacterial resistance to this class is rising and threatens their future utility. Ofloxacin is the other major agent in this class. It is not as active against *Pseudomonas aeruginosa*, but it may be less likely to select for resistance in some gram-positive cocci.

Resistance to the quinolones occurs by two major mechanisms: mutations in DNA gyrase that decrease quinolone-binding affinity, and alterations in permeability. These mechanisms are chromosomal, and no plasmid-mediated, horizontal spread of resistance between either different species or different strains of organisms have been seen yet in clinical practice. Since the fluoroquinolones inhibit conjugative plasmid transfer, it is unlikely plasmid spread of resistance will be a significant contributor to resistance in this agent class. Single point mutations in genes coding for DNA gyrase (*gyr* A) result in stepwise increases in resistance by changing binding between drug and target in an incremental fashion. However, for organisms that are intrinsically less sensitive to the quinolones, such as *S. aureus* and *Pseudomonas aeruginosa*, this single point mutation may alter enzyme-drug binding just enough to extend the minimum inhibitory concentration (MIC) beyond the breakpoint between susceptibility and resistance. When a point mutation occurs in the quinolone resistance determining region (QRDR) of the *gyr* A gene, it typically is associated with high-level, stable resistance. Porin channel alterations also can occur and often result in cross-resistance to other antibiotics such as tetracycline and chloramphenicol. Conversely, the use of tetracycline and chloramphenicol can select for low-level quinolone resistance due to altered porins. Changes seen in porins, or outer membrane proteins, are often associated with expression of an efflux pump mechanism responsible for relatively low but clinically significant levels of bacterial resistance to fluoroquinolones. In summary, low-level resistance to the quinolones can result from either altered DNA gyrase or altered porin. High-level clinical resistance usually only occurs when both mechanisms are present, or when specific mutations are present in the so-called QRDR of *gyr* A.

## Nicotinic Acid Derivatives

**Mechanism of action: bactericidal (tuberculocidal) for dividing organisms; bacteriostatic for resting organisms**
**Clinical spectrum of activity: *Mycobacterium* species**

Isoniazid remains the cornerstone of treatment for infections caused by *Mycobacterium tuberculosis*. It is used in multidrug treatment regimens to avoid the development of resistance. In any microbial population of mycobacteria, spontaneous resistance will occur in at least 1 in $10^6$ organisms. The average number of organisms in a clinical infection ranges from $10^7$–$10^9$. This makes the possibility of resistance high and delineates the need for multiple drug therapy. Of the "non-MTB" *Mycobacterium* species (often called MOTT for "mycobacterium other than tuberculosis"), only *M. kansasii* is typically susceptible to isoniazid (see Chapter 13).

The mechanism of action of isoniazid is not well defined. Hypotheses that are favored suggest isoniazid inhibits the synthesis of mycolic acids, possibly by blocking the formation of the necessary very long fatty acid precursors. Mycolic acids are a component of the mycobacterial cell wall and probably contribute to the organism's ability to cause disease. Isoniazid is effective against both resting and dividing cells but is only tuberculocidal for dividing cells. It is important to note that isoniazid is active against both intracellular and extracellular organisms, since part of the mycobacterial life cycle occurs within macrophages of the host, and this location affects the microbe's susceptibility to some antibiotics. Resistance appears associated with mutations in drug target (*kat*G and *inh*A operon) genes.

While isoniazid is an extremely useful drug, it is not without significant side effects. Foremost among these is the risk of hepatotoxicity, and adult patients may require monitoring of liver enzymes while receiving therapy. Risk of hepatotoxicity increases with age and in those with preexisting liver disease. Another side effect is peripheral neuropathy caused by isoniazid's interference with pyridoxine ($B_6$) metabolism. Postpubertal patients receiving isoniazid therefore often receive oral daily pyridoxine. Seizures are an uncommon but possible adverse effect while on isoniazid.

Pyrazinamide is an analog of nicotinamide and, like isoniazid, is tuberculocidal. The mechanism of action is not known. It is also hepatotoxic. It penetrates well into dead, resting, or active macrophages. However, whether it affects intracellular organisms is still debated.

### Rifampin

**Mechanism of action: bactericidal**
**Clinical spectrum of activity: many gram-positive and selected gram-negative organisms; mycobacteria**

Rifampin inhibits RNA synthesis by inhibiting DNA-dependent RNA polymerase. This agent has several important clinical uses. It is used for the multidrug treatment regimens of mycobacterial infections (but is not used as single-drug therapy). It is essential for treatment of *Mycobacteria kansasii.* It is also used for the prophylaxis of *Neisseria meningitidis* or *H. influenzae* in patients with a history of exposure to these infections. It is occasionally used in synergy with an appropriate antistaphylococcal antibiotic in the treatment of endocarditis or osteomyelitis caused by *Staphylococcus aureus.* Rifampin is highly active against most staphylococci, but resistance rapidly develops if it is administered as a single agent. This resistance may be associated with mutations in rifampin target genes.

A "flu-like syndrome" occurs as an adverse effect more often with intermittent use of rifampin rather than with daily use. This syndrome has rarely been associated with reversible renal failure and hemolysis. Hepatotoxicity may occur.

### ANTIMICROBIAL AGENTS THAT ARE NOT UNIFORMLY LETHAL FOR MICROBES

#### Sulfonamides

**Mechanism of action: bacteriostatic**
**Clinical spectrum of activity: gram-positive aerobes, gram-negative aerobes, Toxoplasmosis, *Pneumocystis carinii***

The sulfa drugs are antimetabolites and act by interfering with the endogenous production of folic acid in prokaryotic cells (eukaryotes require exogenous folic acid and therefore are not affected). They are bacteriostatic, not bactericidal, and require the help of cellular and humoral immune mechanisms to affect a cure. The prototype is Prontosil, that is

an azo dye (benzene ring and an amine group) with a sulfa group that is converted to the active form, sulfanilamide, in the patient.

The sulfonamides are competitive antagonists for the enzyme dihydropteroate synthase. This enzyme converts *para*-aminobenzoic acid (PABA) to dihydropteroate, an intermediate in folate synthesis. Because of their structural similarity to PABA, the sulfonamides inhibit formation of this intermediate and subsequent folate production. Folic acid in the reduced form is required for one-carbon transfer reactions, and a deficiency of folic acid caused by the sulfonamides interferes with many cellular processes.

The sulfa drugs were the first antibiotics used clinically, but the initial treatment successes were eventually tempered by the development of bacterial resistance. They are now only used in a few circumstances such as acute prostatitis, uncomplicated lower urinary tract infections, pyelonephritis in normally healthy adults, acute bronchitis, and an alternative regimen for empiric therapy of community-acquired pneumonia. The combination of sulfamethoxazole plus trimethoprim is very important for the treatment of pneumonia caused by *Pneumocystis carinii* in the setting of human immunmodeficiency virus (HIV) infection. In many infections a sulfonamide is added to another agent because of the rapid development of resistance when they are used as a single agent. The other agent is usually trimethoprim, discussed below. Resistance to sulfonamides can be plasmid or chromosomally mediated. Plasmids carrying sulfonamide-resistant variants of dihydropteroate synthase (DHPS) are responsible for most clinical resistance. Chromosomal resistance is less common and occurs in three ways:

1. Point mutations altering DHPS.
2. Recombination—there is a 10% difference in genome between susceptible and resistant strains of *Neisseria;* research suggests this may be due to recombination in a highly conserved portion of the DHPS enzyme.
3. Mutations resulting in increased production of PABA (compete with sulfonamides).

There is an approximate 5% incidence of side effects to the sulfa drugs, higher in HIV-infected patients. The most common are drug fever and dermatologic reactions. Rare hematologic reactions such as agranulocytosis, hemolytic anemia, and aplastic anemia have

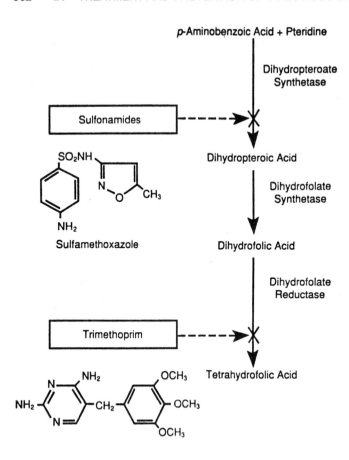

**FIGURE 37–8.** Structures and sites of action of sulfamethoxazole and trimethoprim. This figure illustrates the biosynthesis of tetrahydrofolate in bacteria with an indication of the combined inhibition at separate synthetic steps produced by the two agents.

been reported, but constitute less than 1% of reported side effects.

## Trimethoprim

### Mechanism of action: bacteriostatic
### Clinical spectrum of activity: gram-positive aerobes, gram-negative aerobes

Trimethoprim, when given with sulfamethoxazole (Septra, Bactrim), represents an important concept in antimicrobial chemotherapy. When given alone, resistance to either drug may develop rapidly. Simultaneous dosing, however, theoretically produces a synergistic antibacterial effect by interfering with the same metabolic pathway but at different intermediate steps. A diagram of this is shown in Fig. 37–8. The possibility of resistance is also reduced by giving both drugs at the same time. These findings are supported by *in vitro* studies, but it is unclear whether the combination results in synergy *in vivo*. However, the combination has remained highly effective in clinical practice for many years. The combination of sulfamethoxazole with trimethoprim is used for all of the above-mentioned infections treated with sulfonamides alone

and is the most common combination of a sulfa-type agent in clinical use. It is very inexpensive.

Trimethoprim is a competitive inhibitor of dihydrofolate reductase. This enzyme is necessary for the formation of the final reduced form of folate (tetrahydrofolate) required for the one-carbon transfer reactions mentioned above. The combined drugs not only interfere with folate formation but they also prevent the folate from being converted into its functional form. Resistance to trimethoprim can be plasmid or chromosomally mediated. There are three different mechanisms of chromosomal resistance.

1. Mutational loss of deoxyuridylic acid methylase activity—this loss makes the cell dependent on exogenously produced thymine and relieves cellular DHFR of the major task of regenerating tetrahydrofolate for the thymine-producing methylase reaction.

2. Mutation of DHFR gene resulting in either decreased affinity for trimethoprim or increased production of DHFR.

3. Presence of transposon Tn7—this transposon has a high-frequency transmission rate

and carries a DHFR gene resulting in increased production of an enzyme with low trimethoprim-binding affinity; the transposon recognizes insertion sites on chromosomes of many different bacterial species, facilitating spread of resistance.

Plasmids can carry resistance genes that generally code for DHFR enzymes of various binding affinities for trimethoprim, resulting in diverse MICs.

Reported side effects are dermatologic (75%) but have also included reversible decline of renal function in normal patients and possibly irreversible loss of function in patients with preexisting renal disease. In patients with folate deficiency, megaloblastosis with leukopenia and thrombocytopenia may occur, but it is uncommon. In patients with renal insufficiency the agents can accumulate and exert a sulfonylurea-like effect resulting in reversible hypoglycemia.

## Tetracyclines

**Mechanism of action: bacteriostatic**
**Clinical spectrum of activity: gram-positives and gram-negatives; rickettsia, mycoplasma; chlamydia**

The original "tetracycline," chlortetracycline, was isolated from *Streptomyces aureofaciens* and later altered to form the semisynthetic drug tetracycline. Although not first-line therapy for common infections such as pneumonia and urinary tract infections, it has found usefulness in the treatment of atypical infections caused by diverse organisms and is not restricted in activity to bacteria. For this reason the tetracyclines are often referred to as broad-spectrum agents.

Tetracyclines gain access to the cells by passive diffusion through porins (water filled, channel-forming proteins of gram-negative organisms between the outer membrane and inner membranes), and then by energy-dependent transport across the inner membrane to the cell interior. A one-step process of active transport occurs in the gram-positives. Once inside, tetracyclines bind the 30S ribosomal subunit and prevent access of transfer RNA (tRNA) to the growing polypeptide chain. Protein synthesis is inhibited in this manner. Unfortunately, the tetracyclines are known for numerous side effects. Most notable are dyspepsia, photosensitivity, enamel discoloration in the fetus or young child, and depression of bone growth in the fetus.

Therefore, they should not be used in pregnancy or in children under 8 years old.

Two common examples of the class, tetracycline and doxycycline, can be used for therapy of infections caused by *Rickettsia* species, *Mycoplasma* species, *Chlamydia* species, and *Brucella* species. The class can also be used for uncomplicated gonorrhea, syphilis in penicillin-allergic patients, and acne vulgaris. Resistance to tetracycline is a result of protection of the ribosome that may occur as enzymatic modification of the antibiotic to an inactive form. This type of inactivation causes universal resistance to all members of the class and is plasmid mediated. The other type of resistance relates to rapid efflux of the molecule from the cell and is inducible. Organisms having resistance by the efflux system alone, without enzymatic modification, aren't resistant to some tetracycline formulations, such as minocycline.

## Chloramphenicol

**Mechanism of action: bacteriostatic; bactericidal against some "meningitis" pathogens**
**Clinical spectrum of activity: broad, but use is restricted due to risk of life-threatening side effects**

Chloramphenicol is a unique antibiotic that acts by inhibiting protein synthesis. The antibiotic enters cells well and binds to the 50S subunit of the ribosome. It prevents interaction between the ribosome and the amino acid–containing end of the tRNA molecule and inhibits peptide bond formation. The drug is very well distributed in all tissues including the CNS, and requires glucuronide conjugation in the liver for excretion by the kidney.

Chloramphenicol is effective against many types of organisms but unfortunately has possible side effects that are severe enough to restrict use. Suppression of red blood cell production occurs in a predictable, dose-related, and reversible manner. Most alarming is the possibility of complete marrow aplasia with fatal pancytopenia occurring in approximately 1 in 30,000 patients given the drug. It is idiosyncratic and may present after the first dose or after several doses. Another side effect became known because of chloramphenicol's use in the empiric treatment of neonatal or childhood meningitis. Since premature infants and neonates lack fully functional conjugation pathways in the liver, *gray baby syn-*

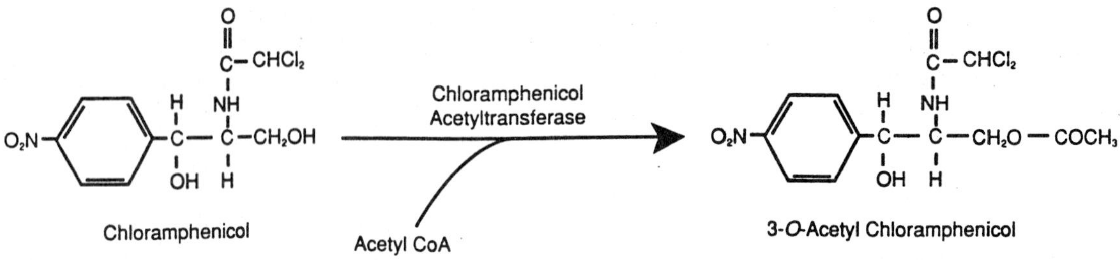

**FIGURE 37–9.** Structure of chloramphenicol and the pathway for enzymatic degradation of this agent.

*drome* can result, and this build-up of drug has a 40% mortality. The use of chloramphenicol for CNS infections is now rare since the development of safer agents like ceftriaxone. Chloramphenicol is generally only used as alternate therapy when other antibiotic choices are significantly limited.

Chloramphenicol is administered either orally or intravenously. It is essentially 100% bioavailable by either route and, since the oral formulation is a free base with a lower molecular weight than the parenteral ester form, it is important to remember that blood levels can actually be higher with oral dosing than those achieved with intravenous administration. Resistance to chloramphenicol is chiefly by enzymatic alteration. This is carried out by an acetyltransferase that is plasmid mediated and inducible. The pathway of this resistance is seen in Fig. 37–9.

### Erythromycin (Macrolides)

**Mechanism of action: bacteriostatic and bactericidal (depending on dose and organism)**
**Clinical spectrum of activity: gram-positive bacteria, chlamydia, mycoplasma, legionella**

Erythromycin, clarithromycin, and azithromycin belong to the macrolide family of antibiotics. Macrolides bind to the 50S ribosomal subunit and inhibit the translocation step in which the ribosome moves on to the next codon for translation. Many chemical forms of erythromycin exist because the base erythromycin molecule must be protected from gastric pH when taken orally. Both erythromycin estolate and erythromycin ethylsuccinate are less acid labile. Erythromycin estolate rarely has been associated with cholestatic hepatitis that mimics acute cholecystitis and is marked by periportal inflammation. Side effects are generally limited to epigastric distress, but occasional auditory impairment has been reported at doses of greater than or equal to 4 g daily needed for the treatment of pneumonia due to *Legionella* species.

Erythromycin is used for empiric therapy of community-acquired pneumonia (at times given with trimethoprim-sulfamethoxazole) to cover *Streptococcus pneumoniae*, *Mycoplasma*, and the unsuspected *Legionella*. Uses also include being the drug of choice in pregnancy for *Chlamydia* or syphilis infections, since it is relatively safe for the fetus. Resistance occurs by one of three mechanisms: decreased permeability into the cell, alterations of the 50S ribosomal target site with decreased drug binding, or enzymatic modification of the antibiotic. Resistance is generally plasmid mediated and most commonly results from an altered ribosomal target site.

### Clindamycin

**Mechanism of action: bacteriostatic**
**Clinical spectrum of activity: aerobic gram-positive cocci; anaerobes**

This antibiotic is similar to erythromycin and belongs to the lincosamide family, acting by inhibiting protein synthesis. It binds the 50S ribosomal subunit at the same site as erythromycin and chloramphenicol and inhibits peptide bond formation between the amino acid and the growing polypeptide chain. It is extremely useful for the treatment of aerobic gram-positive and anaerobic infections in patients who are allergic to penicillin. Clindamycin has been associated classically with a colitis caused by *Clostridium difficile* (see Chapter 27). *C. difficile* proliferates and produces its toxins because its environmental competitors, the normal gastrointestinal flora (particularly anaerobes), are inhibited by clindamycin. *C. difficile*–associated colitis (pseudomembranous colitis) has been shown to be associated with administration of many different types of antibiotics and not just clindamycin.

Resistance to clindamycin occurs primarily by enzymatic drug modification or by alteration of the 50S ribosomal target site. The first clindamycin-resistant strains of *Staphylococcus aureus* seen in the 1950s resulted from an inducible modified 50S ribosome.

## Polymyxins

**Mechanism of action: bacteriostatic**
**Clinical spectrum of activity: gram-negatives**

The clinically useful polymyxins are polymyxin B and colistin (polymyxin E). They are peptides that exert antibacterial effects by acting as detergents and disrupting cell membranes. Polymyxin B binds lipid A of LPS (endotoxin) to exert its effect. They have very poor oral absorption and are only used topically for infections of skin, eyes, or ears. They are rarely given for serious infections in the United States because of the rapid emergence of resistance during use.

## Bacitracin

**Mechanism of action: bacteriostatic**
**Clinical spectrum of activity: gram-positive cocci and bacilli**

This is another detergent-like polypeptide antibiotic, of which bacitracin A is the chief component. It is only used topically because of its nephrotoxicity. It inhibits the transfer of NMA and NAG to the growing cell wall.

## Ethambutol

**Mechanism of action: bacteriostatic**
**Clinical spectrum of activity: mycobacteria**

The mode of action of ethambutol is not known, but it may act by inhibiting the incorporation of mycolic acids into the cell wall. It is used with other antimycobacterial agents for the treatment of tuberculosis or other mycobacterial infections. The primary potential side effect is optic neuritis. Resistance appears to be associated with development of altered (mutated) drug target(s).

## Amphotericin B

**Mechanism of action: fungistatic and fungicidal, depending upon concentration**
**Clinical spectrum of activity: most fungi (both yeast and mold forms)**

Amphotericin is a complex molecule that exerts its effect by having both hydrophilic and lipophilic (cholesterol-like) portions as shown in Figure 37–10. Its infusion intravenously was difficult due to poor water solubility until a colloidal dispersion with the bile acid deoxycholate was developed. Unfortunately, treatment with amphotericin B remains difficult because its therapeutic dose is close to its toxic dose (primarily nephrotoxic). Recent advances in administration may decrease this risk. Amphotericin B acts by binding to ergosterol in fungal membranes. It appears to form pores or channels after this binding that most likely result in leakage of ions across the cell membrane with a resulting disruption of metabolism. Toxicity occurs from incorporation into mammalian membranes with leakage of ions such as potassium. Experimental lipid emulsions have been developed that protect the host membranes by providing an alternate drug binding site. Any amphotericin B not inserted into fungal membranes has a higher affinity for the alternate site than for the mammalian cell membrane, resulting in decreased incorporation into patient cells.

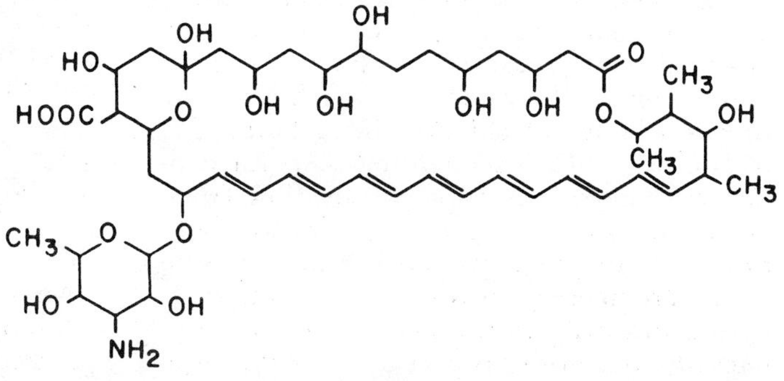

FIGURE 37–10. Structure of amphotericin B with both hydrophilic and lipophilic opposing sides.

Resistance usually results from either a decreased concentration of ergosterol in the membrane or from production of an ergosterol with decreased affinity for amphotericin B. Amphotericin B is an effective drug but is reserved for serious fungal infections because of its toxicity. The following are examples of its use:

- pulmonary histoplasmosis or blastomycosis in immunocompromised hosts
- progressive disseminated histoplasmosis
- meningeal blastomycosis or cryptococcosis
- extrapulmonary coccidioidomycosis in immunocompromised patients
- disseminated aspergillosis in immunocompromised patients

### Imidazoles/Triazoles

**Mechanism of action: fungistatic and fungicidal, depending upon concentration**
**Clinical spectrum of activity: most fungi**

These drugs belong to the azole family of antimicrobial agents and share a common five-membered ring structure that contains either two (imidazoles) or three (triazoles) nitrogen atoms. They have high activity against a broad spectrum of fungal organisms although this can vary with the susceptibility test system used and may correlate poorly with clinical outcome. Standards for susceptibility testing are still being defined. The same mode of action is seen in both classes of drugs. They inhibit sterol 14-alpha-demethylase and impair the synthesis of ergosterol, a critical component of fungal membranes. The result is increased levels of methyl sterol intermediates that are inserted into the fungal membrane, which impairs the function of some membrane-bound enzyme systems. They show different affinities for the mammalian equivalent of the demethylase enzyme, and some of them can inhibit sterol synthesis in humans.

Ketoconazole is the best known imidazole and has many therapeutic uses. It can be given orally but requires an acidic gastric environment for optimal bioavailability. Any functional state of achlorhydria, including use of antacids or $H_2$ histamine blockers for peptic ulcer disease, will impair absorption. Once absorbed, the drug penetrates most tissues well but enters the CNS poorly. Common side effects are nausea, anorexia, and vomiting. As noted, this drug can inhibit sterol synthesis, and 10% of females report menstrual irregu-

larities. A variable number of men report decreased libido, hypospermia or aspermia, and the development of gynecomastia. The cortisol response to adrenocorticotropic hormone (ACTH) stimulation can also be decreased because of impaired cortisol synthesis. Uses include acute, non–life-threatening pulmonary blastomycosis, extrapulmonary blastomycosis, and progressive pulmonary histoplasmosis in immunocompetent patients with underlying pulmonary disease.

Itraconazole is a triazole similar to ketoconazole but without the key requirement for an acid environment to ensure absorption. It is actually better absorbed when administered with food. Itraconazole has good tissue distribution overall but poor CNS penetration. Side effects are similar to ketoconazole. Uses of itraconazole are essentially the same as ketoconazole but with the benefit of better tolerance and less variable absorption. It is also used for oral therapy of disseminated aspergillosis in immunocompromised patients, although most experts consider amphotericin B to be the preferred treatment.

Fluconazole is a triazole that is much more water soluble than the other azole drugs. It is almost completely absorbed, and the majority is free (unbound) in plasma. It has excellent CNS penetration where it may achieve a concentration close to 50–90% that of plasma. It is primarily excreted in the kidney, and the urine concentration may be 10 times that of the plasma. The dose must be decreased when the glomerular filtration rate falls below 50 mL/min. Fluconazole is well tolerated, and although gastrointestinal side effects may occur, they are uncommon. It has very high selectivity for fungal demethylase and thus a lower incidence of endocrine-related side effects.

Uses include serious pulmonary and extrapulmonary coccidioidomycosis in immunocompetent patients, meningeal coccidioidomycosis, and as maintenance therapy after induction therapy with amphotericin B for other serious fungal infections such as cryptococcal meningitis in immunocompromised hosts (especially acquired immunodeficiency syndrome [AIDS]).

### SUMMARY

A new and very dangerous problem faced today by patients and their physicians is the worldwide calamity of emerging multi–drug-resistant microbes. Multi–drug-resistant gram-positive bacteria, especially *Enterococcus faecium*, and *S. pneumoniae*, and gram-negative bacilli like those producing type-I beta-lactamases resistant to the newest and most potent beta-lactam agents are found with increasing frequency. There is also a continued increase in the number of serious nosocomial infections caused by *Stenotrophomonas maltophilia* and methicillin-resistant *Staphylococcus aureus*. Management of these new multi–drug-resistant infections will require increased efforts at interrupting the spread of nosocomial pathogens through sophisticated infection control interventions, as well as a thorough understanding on how to use our currently available antimicrobial agents properly. We may need to avoid use of certain newer agents associated with emergence of these pathogens and possibly return to more use of potent older agents that are associated with a lower frequency of drug-resistant pathogens. While this chapter illustrates there are only a limited number of basic approaches that microbes can take to develop resistance to an antimicrobial compound, it is obvious they possess a multitude of ways to achieve their goal of survival. The future will challenge the ingenuity of all health care practitioners faced with the treatment of patients with infectious diseases.

## CASE HISTORY

### CASE HISTORY 1

The patient is a 46-year-old female who had received a kidney transplant 6 years earlier. She presented to the hospital with a 1-week history of diarrhea and lower abdominal pain. Upon admission, her white blood cell (WBC) count was $14,700/mm^3$ with 87% polymorphonuclear leukocytes. Her temperature was 100.7°F, blood pressure was 100/65 mm Hg, and pulse was 110/min. Her skin turgor was diminished and physical examination revealed a lethargic woman with diffuse abdominal pain. X-ray of the abdomen revealed a small amount of free air under the diaphragm. Urinalysis revealed many leukocytes, and culture grew more than $10^5$ colony-forming units per milliliter of *Enterococcus faecalis* resistant to vancomycin and teicoplanin but susceptible to both ampicillin and synergistic doses of gentamicin.

Because of presumed infection in the abdomen as well as the urine, and knowing that she harbored a high level vancomycin-resistant enterococcus susceptible to ampicillin, she was begun on ampicillin-sulbactam (Unasyn) plus gentamicin, and was taken to surgery. Vancomycin was also added,

since this patient was at risk for an MRSA infection as she had frequent exposures to the hospital related to her underlying disease. At operation, a ruptured colonic diverticulum with purulence throughout the peritoneal cavity was found. The bowel perforation was repaired, the peritoneal cavity cleaned, and she was continued on the antimicrobial agent regimen.

Initially she improved, but at 48 h after surgery her fever recurred and her abdomen again became tender and distended. At this time the microbiology laboratory reported that in addition to the initial vancomycin-resistant *Enterococcus faecalis* (from urine), abdominal fluid cultures from surgery were growing *Enterococcus faecium* resistant to high levels of vancomycin as well as to ampicillin, gentamicin, and streptomycin. The only agent that was active against this new pathogen was the experimental streptogramin antimicrobial agent, Synercid. The antimicrobial regimen was changed to include this new agent in an attempt to treat her vancomycin-resistant enterococcal peritonitis.

### CASE 1 DISCUSSION

Our case demonstrates the possibly fatal consequences of plasmid transfer of antimicrobial resistance between related microbial species. This is very possible when both organisms are found as normal human flora, like *E. faecalis* and *E. faecium*. High-level vancomycin resistance of the Van A phenotype is plasmid mediated and readily transmissible between *E. faecalis* and *E. faecium*. This patient likely carried the resistant *E. faecalis* in her stool when she developed the initial urinary tract infection and diverticulitis. When she was given antimicrobial agents for her bowel perforation, the combination of vancomycin resistance in the *E. faecalis* plus the antimicrobial pressure of her treatment regimen permitted a few vancomycin-resistant *E. faecium* that had acquired resistance from *E. faecalis* to emerge as pathogens.

## REFERENCES

### Books

Gilman, A., Rall, T. W., Nies, A. S., and Taylor, P., eds. *Goodman and Gilman's The Pharmacologic Basis of Therapeutics.* 8th ed. New York: Pergamon Press, Inc., 1990.

Peterson, P. K., and Verhoeff, J., eds. *The Antimicrobial Agents Annual 3.* New York: Elsevier, 1988.

Boyd, R. F., and Hoerl, B.G., eds. *Basic Medical Microbiology.* Boston: Little, Brown & Co., 1991

Hooper, D.C., and Wolfson, J. S., eds. *Quinolone Antimicrobial Agents.* Washington, DC: American Society for Microbiology, 1993.

Lorian, V., ed. *Antibiotics in Laboratory Medicine.* 3rd ed. Baltimore: Williams & Wilkins, 1991.

Gottschalk, G., ed. *Bacterial Metabolism.* 2nd ed. New York: Springer-Verlag, 1986.

**Review Articles**

Dever, L. A., and Dermody, T. S. Mechanisms of bacterial resistance to antibiotics. *Arch. Intern. Med. 151*:886–895, 1991.

Jacoby, G. A., and Archer, G. L. New mechanisms of bacterial resistance to antimicrobial agents. *N. Engl. J. Med. 324*:601–612, 1991.

Huovinen, P., Sundstrom, L., et al. Trimethoprim and sulfonamide resistance. *Antimicrob. Agents Chemother. 39*:279–289, 1995.

Darville, T., and Yamauchi, T. The cephalosporin antibiotics. *Pediatr. Rev. 15*:54–62, 1994.

Gupta, A. K., et al. Antifungal agents: An overview. Part II. *J. Am. Acad. Dermatol. 30*:911–933, 1994.

Sarosi, G. A., and Davies, S. F. Therapy for fungal infections. *Mayo Clin. Proc. 69*:1111–1117, 1994.

**Original Articles**

Saha, V., Gupta, S., and Daum, R. Occurrence and mechanisms of glycopeptide resistance in gram positive cocci. *Infect. Agents Dis. 1*:310–318, 1992.

Silver, L., and Bostian, K. Discovery and development of new antibiotics; the problem of antibiotic resistance. *Antimicrob. Agents Chemother. 37*:377–383, 1993.

Morris, S., Bai, G. H., Suffys, P., Portillo-Gomez, L., Fairchok, M., and Rouse, D. Molecular mechanisms of multiple drug resistance in clinical isolates of *Mycobacterium tuberculosis. J. Infect. Dis. 171*:954–960, 1995.

# 38
# ANTIMICROBIAL THERAPY

DALE N. GERDING, M.D., STANFORD T. SHULMAN, M.D., and JOHN P. PHAIR, M.D.

This chapter is addressed primarily to the treatment of bacterial infections, although drugs used in the systemic treatment of fungal and viral diseases are also discussed.

There are two major indications for the use of antimicrobials: (1) prophylaxis (prevention) of infection, and (2) treatment of an already existing infection. Most of the prophylactic use of antimicrobials is done in association with surgical procedures to prevent wound infections, but there are notable nonsurgical indications as well, such as prevention of malaria in endemic areas, and prevention of endocarditis in patients with heart murmurs who are undergoing dental work.

It is extremely important to emphasize that unnecessary use of antimicrobial agents should be avoided for several reasons, including side effects, allergic reactions, cost, effects upon endogenous normal flora, and induction of antibiotic resistance (relevant to the patient and to society as a whole). The issue of resistance development (possibly due to inappropriate antimicrobial usage) has become such a major problem in many hospitals that enterococci resistant to all available antimicrobials have emerged. As with use of any medication, the risk–benefit ratio to the patient and globally should be favorable to justify use of an antibiotic.

## INITIAL MICROBIOLOGIC EVALUATION

Some infections can be treated without Gram's stain or culture of the site of infection. In these instances the physician makes a diagnosis of infection at a particular site by clinical criteria and institutes *empiric* therapy based upon the most likely bacterial etiology (Table 38–1). Physicians may also initiate empiric therapy while awaiting the results of cultures of specimens that have been submitted to the laboratory.

In contrast to the use of empiric therapy without cultures, efforts to make an accurate microbiologic diagnosis should be driven by the seriousness of the patient's infection and the degree of immunocompromise of the patient. In these situations of severe illness or patient immunocompromise, the infecting organism and its susceptibility pattern cannot be predicted as well and the consequences of missing a diagnosis are more likely to be life threatening. If a clinical specimen (e.g., exudate or cerebrospinal fluid [CSF]) can be examined directly, the correlation between bacteria seen on Gram's stain and the cause of the infection is excellent. When the specimen must pass through a normally colonized area before examination, as with expectorated sputum, the Gram's stain must be evaluated cautiously. Blood cultures should always be obtained when signs and symptoms suggest possible systemic spread of infection.

## INTERPRETATION OF BACTERIAL CULTURE REPORTS

Potential limitations of culture reports include the possible contamination of the specimen with indigenous bacterial flora and consideration of the pathogenic potential of the isolated organism. Positive cultures from normally sterile fluids—such as blood, CSF, synovial fluid—should be assumed to be correct unless there is strong evidence to the contrary. Certain bacteria (e.g., *Streptococcus pneumoniae* and *Haemophilus influenzae*) are almost never contaminants at these sites, and Enterobacteriaceae are rarely contaminants.

However, when normal flora, such as alpha streptococci, *Propionibacterium acnes*, or coagulase-negative staphylococci, are isolated, the clinical significance must be reviewed carefully. Specimens frequently contaminated by normal flora of the sample site or of a contiguous site are more difficult to evaluate, including wound and sputum specimens. Culture results must be correlated with clinical evidence to decide whether the isolated bacteria are indeed pathogens.

## CORRELATION BETWEEN RESULTS OF ANTIBACTERIAL SUSCEPTIBILITY TESTING AND CURE OF INFECTION

The designation of a bacterium as *susceptible* or *resistant* to a particular antibacterial agent relates to an amount of the drug that corresponds to achievable serum concentration with ordinary dosage. The assumption is made that a similar level of antibacterial activity is achievable at the site of infection. Whether this actually occurs depends on dosage level, pharmacologic properties of the individual drug, site of infection, and host factors (see below and Chapter 39).

With these limitations, data correlation between *in vitro* susceptibility and eradication of infection in patients is surprisingly good, although there are exceptions; for example, systemic *Salmonella* infections do not respond uniformly to antibiotics other than chloramphenicol, ampicillin, quinolones, or trimethoprim-sulfamethoxazole, although salmonellae are susceptible *in vitro* to other agents, including aminoglycosides. Because of the critical role of host defenses in recovery, the use of an appropriate antibacterial agent does not always lead to clinical cure. Another way of saying this is that outcome (cure) depends on the bug, the drug, and the host.

The terms *bactericidal* and *bacteristatic* are best defined in terms of the activity of an antibacterial agent *in vitro*, and *in vitro* results cannot be directly translated to clinical effectiveness (see Chapter 39). These terms are also organism specific; for example, chloramphenicol is bacteristatic for *Escherichia coli* but is bactericidal for *H. influenzae*. Similarly, in endocarditis and meningitis bactericidal activity is preferred for eradication of infection because of the relative lack of neutrophils in cardiac vegetations and CSF, but in both diseases bacteristatic agents may be curative as well.

**TABLE 38–1.  MOST FREQUENT CAUSES OF COMMUNITY-ACQUIRED INFECTION AT SELECTED BODY SITES AND SUGGESTED INITIAL ANTIMICROBIAL TREATMENT***

| SITE | MICROORGANISM(S) | ANTIMICROBIAL AGENTS |
|------|------------------|----------------------|
| **Upper Respiratory Tract Infections** | | |
| Tonsillitis and pharyngitis | *Streptococcus pyogenes* | Penicillin |
| Sinusitis and otitis | | |
| Acute | | |
| Adults | *S. pneumoniae, H. influenzae, M. catarrhalis* | Trimethoprim-sulfamethoxazole (TMP/SMX), Amoxicillin-clavulanate |
| Children <12 yr | *S. pneumoniae, H. influenzae, S. pyogenes* | Amoxicillin-clavulanate, erythromycin-sulfa |
| Chronic | Same as acute sinusitis, plus oral anaerobes | Amoxicillin-clavulanate, or add clindamycin or metronidazole to TMP/SMX |
| Epiglottitis | *H. influenzae* | Ceftriaxone, ampicillin-sulbactam, TMP/SMX |
| **Lower Respiratory Tract Infections** | | |
| Acute exacerbation of chronic bronchitis | *H. influenzae, S. pneumoniae, M. catarrhalis* | TMP-SMX, doxycycline |
| Pneumonia | | |
| Age 5–40 yr | *M. pneumoniae, S. pneumoniae, C. pneumoniae, L. pneumophila* | Erythromycin, clarithromycin, azithromycin |
| Age >40 yr | *S. pneumoniae, H. influenzae, S. pyogenes, L. pneumophila* | Ceftriaxone, ampicillin-sulbactam, TMP/SMX, +/− erythromycin |
| **Cardiovascular Infections** | | |
| Endocarditis | | |
| No illicit IV drug use | Viridans streptococci, *S. bovis,* | Penicillin +/− aminoglycoside |
| | *Enterococcus* sp. | Ampicillin + gentamicin |
| Illicit IV drug use | *S. aureus* | Nafcillin or oxacillin +/− gentamicin |
| | Methicillin-resistant *S. aureus* (MRSA) | Vancomycin + gentamicin |
| **Gastrointestinal Infections** | | |
| Diarrhea | | |
| >1 day with fever | *C. jejuni, Shigella* sp., *Salmonella* sp. | Ciprofloxacin, ofloxacin, TMP/SMX |
| After antibiotics | *C. difficile* | Metronidazole, vancomycin |
| Abdominal abscess/ peritonitis | Polymicrobial: Enterobacteriaceae + *Bacteroides* sp. | Aminoglycoside + clindamycin, imipenem, ticarcillin-clavulanate, piperacillin-tazobactam |
| **Genital Infections** | | |
| Urethritis/Cervicitis | *N. gonorrhoeae* | Ceftriaxone, cefixime, ciprofloxacin, ofloxacin |
| | *C. trachomatis* | Doxycycline, azithromycin |
| Genital ulcer | *T. pallidum* | Benzathine penicillin G |
| | *H. ducreyi* | Ceftriaxone, azithromycin |
| Pelvic inflammatory disease | Polymicrobial: *N. gonorrhoea* + *C. trachomatis* + *Bacteroides* sp. + Enterobacteriaceae | Ceftriaxone + doxycycline |
| **Urinary Tract Infections** | | |
| Cystitis | | |
| Woman, Age 12–50 yr | Enterobacteriaceae | TMP/SMX |
| Prostatitis | | |
| Age <35 yr | *N. gonorrhoeae, C. trachomatis* | Ceftriaxone + doxycyline, ofloxacin |
| Age >35 yr | Enterobacteriaceae | TMP/SMX, ciprofloxacin, ofloxacin |
| **Central Nervous System Infections** | | |
| Meningitis | | |
| Adults | *S. pneumoniae, N. meningitidis* | Penicillin G, ceftriaxone, cefotaxime |
| Children, Age 3 mo to 6 yr | Above or *H. influenzae* | Ceftriaxone, cefotaxime |
| Brain abscess | Polymicrobial: viridans streptococci + anaerobes + enterobacteriaceae | Penicillin G + metronidazole +/− ceftriaxone or ceftizoxime |

*Table continued on following page*

**TABLE 38–1.   MOST FREQUENT CAUSES OF COMMUNITY-ACQUIRED INFECTION AT SELECTED BODY SITES AND SUGGESTED INITIAL ANTIMICROBIAL TREATMENT*** *Continued*

| SITE | MICROORGANISM(S) | ANTIMICROBIAL AGENTS |
|---|---|---|
| **Bone and Joint Infections** | | |
| Osteomyelitis | | |
| Hematogenous source | *S. aureus,* Streptococci | Nafcillin, Oxacillin, Cefazolin |
| Foot ulcer; diabetes | Polymicrobial: *S. aureus* + Anaerobes + Enterobacteriaceae | Ciprofloxacin + clindamycin, ampicillin-sulbactam, imipenem |
| Septic arthritis | | |
| Adult, age 12–40 yr | *N. gonorrhoeae* | Ceftriaxone, cefotaxime, ceftizoxime |
| Adult, age >40 yr | *S. aureus, S. pyogenes,* Enterobacteriaceae | Nafcillin or oxacillin + gentamicin |
| Child, age 3 mo to 6 yr | *S. aureus, H. influenzae,* streptococci | Nafcillin or oxacillin + ceftriaxone or cefotaxime |
| **Skin Infections** | | |
| Cellulitis | *S. pyogenes, S. aureus* | Nafcillin or oxacillin, cefazolin |

*Prior antimicrobial therapy or hospital acquisition of infection may alter expected organism or antimicrobial susceptibility or both. The bacterial etiology of infections in newborn infants is not considered here. Drug allergy may necessitate alternative therapy.

## AN ALGORITHM FOR ANTIMICROBIAL SELECTION

The selection of an antimicrobial for the treatment of an infection is dependent upon several factors as outlined in Table 38–2. The patient history and physical findings are used to establish the presence of an infection that is likely to benefit from antimicrobial treatment. Some infections are self-limited and do not benefit from available treatments (e.g., mononucleosis or viral gastroenteritis). The history and physical examination are critical steps to defining the site or organ system involved in the infection. This is the first step toward antimicrobial selection, and is predicated on the association of specific organisms with anatomic infection sites (Table 38–1).

The second step is to use the patient history to establish if the infection is community or hospital acquired. This is an important distinction because of the markedly different pathogens that infect patients inside and outside the hospital. Hospital-acquired organisms are more likely to be antimicrobial resistant and are more likely to be gram-negative bacillary organisms or staphylococci.

The third selection step is to determine if the patient is immunosuppressed or immunocompromised. Immunocompromised patients are more susceptible to infection, and depending upon the part of the immune system compromised, are more susceptible to specific pathogens. Patients with humoral (B-cell) immune deficiency, such as those with multiple myeloma or hypogammaglobuline-

**TABLE 38–2.   AN ALGORITHM FOR THE SELECTION OF ANTIMICROBIAL TREATMENT**

| | |
|---|---|
| I. | From the history and physical examination determine the most likely **site** of infection. |
| II. | Use the history to determine if the infection was acquired in the **community** or in the **hospital**. |
| III. | Use the history to determine if the patient is **immunosuppressed**: |
| | A. Humoral |
| | B. Cell-mediated |
| | C. Phagocyte (PMN) deficiency |
| IV. | Based on the likely site of infection, community vs. hospital acquisition, and the immunocompromise of the patient, determine the most likely **organism(s)**. |
| V. | Select the **antimicrobial(s)** appropriate to the likely organism, site of infection, and host immunocompromise. |
| VI. | Use susceptibility, clinical performance, pharmacokinetics, toxicity, and cost data to refine the antimicrobial choice. |

PMN, polymorphonuclear leukocytes.

mia, are susceptible to infection from encapsulated bacteria such as *Streptococcus pneumoniae* or *Haemophilus influenzae*. Those with a deficiency of polymorphonuclear leukocytes (PMN) (acute leukemia, aplastic anemia) are susceptible to infection with gram-negative bacilli (*E. coli, Klebsiella, Pseudomonas*) and staphylococci. Patients with cellular immune (T-cell) deficiency (Hodgkin's disease, acquired immunodeficiency syndrome [AIDS]) are susceptible to infection with intracellular organisms such as *Pneumocystis carinii, Mycobacterium tuberculosis*, varicella-zoster virus, and *Listeria monocytogenes*.

In the fourth step, the most likely pathogens are determined on the basis of infection site, hospital vs. community acquisition, and immune status of the patient. Examples of typical organisms causing infection at various anatomic sites are given in Table 38–1. To the above data is added any immediate information regarding the causative agent that can be obtained quickly, such as Gram's stain of sputum, urine, wound drainage, chest fluid, spinal fluid, joint fluid, or ascites.

With all this information in hand, an empiric selection of an antimicrobial can be made. The final step is to select the appropriate antimicrobial for the infection site, likely organism(s), and immune status of the patient. At this stage, nuances of antimicrobial spectrum, kinetics, side effects, tissue penetration, and bactericidal vs. bacteristatic action become additional considerations that will be discussed in this chapter.

## CHOICE OF ANTIBACTERIAL AGENT AND TREATMENT COURSE

The optimal spectrum of an antimicrobial treatment is inversely related to the ability of the clinician to identify the specific cause of infection. For example, the optimal antibacterial agent for treatment of an infection for which the organism has been identified and tested for susceptibility is the agent with the narrowest possible spectrum of antibacterial activity (including the infecting bacterium, of course), the fewest side effects, and the lowest toxicity. In contrast, if the infection is serious and little information about site and cause of infection can be obtained (comatose febrile patient in shock with no history available), then the appropriate antibacterial spectrum is very broad, and several antimicrobial agents may be started simultaneously to "cover" the

many possible infectious agents. Such multidrug empiricism is often termed "shotgun" therapy, and whereas it is appropriate for seriously ill patients for whom the cause of infection is unknown, it should not be a substitute for a careful and thorough history and physical examination to localize the site and likely cause of an infection. When therapy for a bacterial infection is begun empirically prior to identification of the causative organism, the choice of an agent is based on the following: (1) the bacteria most likely to cause the particular infection (Table 38–1), (2) the bacteria presumptively identified by Gram's stain of exudate, (3) predicted susceptibility of the organism, (4) pharmacologic and toxicity properties of the antibacterial agent, (5) knowledge that the agent chosen has been successful in treating similar infections, and (6) cost. In all cases, the agent should be administered in a dosage form and by a schedule that achieves an antibacterial level at the site of infection at least equal to (preferably, several times higher than) the level of that agent required to inhibit bacterial growth *in vitro*.

### Allergy to Antibacterial Agents

Although allergic manifestations do not invariably recur on readministration of a drug to which a patient has demonstrated allergy, such history should be considered a contraindication to treatment with an antibiotic. Anaphylactic and immediate hypersensitivity reactions are particularly important drug reactions because of their potential to be fatal. Effective alternative antibiotics are available for virtually all infections (Table 38–3). Rarely, a life-threatening infection that is very difficult to treat with an alternative agent may require administration of an antibacterial agent to which the patient is allergic. One example is enterococcal endocarditis in a patient with penicillin allergy. In this situation the patient may undergo desensitization so that penicillin is tolerated.

### Treatment with More Than One Antibacterial Agent

The indications for using more than one agent in the treatment of a single infection are somewhat limited. The most frequent situations include: (1) treatment of infection due to more than one organism, if the organisms are not susceptible to the same drug; (2) presumptive treatment of life-threatening infection when the causative bacterium is un-

**TABLE 38–3. ALTERNATIVES TO PENICILLIN FOR THE PENICILLIN-ALLERGIC PATIENT**

| BACTERIA | ANTIBACTERIAL AGENT |
|---|---|
| Streptococci, including *S. pneumoniae* | Erythromcyin |
| Enterococci | Vancomycin |
| *Staphylococcus aureus* | Cephalosporin,* clindamycin, vancomycin |
| Anaerobic bacteria | Clindamycin, metronidazole |
| *Neisseria meningitidis* | Chloramphenicol, cephalosporin* |
| *Treponema pallidum* | Erythromycin, tetracycline |

*For non-immediate allergic reactions to penicillin.

known; (3) treatment of difficult-to-treat organisms for which synergism of agents has been demonstrated or is postulated; and (4) prevention of emergence of resistance to antibiotics. This last indication is particularly important in the chemotherapy of tuberculosis. The treatment of *Pseudomonas aeruginosa* bacteremia and pneumonia with a combination of an aminoglycoside and an extended-spectrum penicillin is an example of indication 3, whereas combination therapy for fever and neutropenia relates to indication 2.

### Colonization and Superinfection

Antibiotic therapy leads to alteration in colonizing flora, with antimicrobial-resistant bacteria and fungi becoming more dominant. Gram-positive flora tend to be replaced by gram-negative organisms as the colonizing surface flora. In contrast to this *colonization*, the term *superinfection* refers to a second clinical infection that occurs during or after an earlier course of therapy.

Although colonization with new organisms occurs to some extent in everyone treated with antibiotics, clinical superinfection is unusual in treated outpatients, with the exception of superficial *Candida* infection. In contrast, superinfection is quite frequent in hospitalized patients with severe infections and in patients with granulocytopenia or other host defense impairment.

### Follow-Up Treatment of Infection

Most patients with infection are best followed clinically rather than bacteriologically. Repeated cultures are usually unnecessary if the patient has a good clinical therapeutic response, as in uncomplicated pneumonia. However, if the infection is one for which bacteriologic cure (eradication of the causative agent) is known to be difficult, follow-up cultures are indicated. Examples are the treatment of endocarditis and infections treated with a drug with less than optimal efficacy against the infecting bacterium.

The appropriate duration of antibacterial treatment is defined as the shortest period necessary to prevent bacteriologic or clinical relapse, that is, to produce a cure. The duration of treatment varies with the site and extent of infection, the bacterium, and the host response. A standard duration of treatment is established for reliable cure of some infections, such as streptococcal pharyngitis, but has not been rigorously determined for most other infections. Occasionally, assessing the optimal duration of treatment is complicated by difficulty in determining the exact site of infection by routine means. For example, cystitis requires a shorter course of treatment for bacteriologic cure than do renal infections, but it is often difficult to determine the exact site of a urinary tract infection.

### Failure of Antibacterial Treatment

When a patient appears not to respond to antibacterial treatment, it must be determined whether true antibacterial failure has occurred. Treatment may be considered unsuccessful prematurely if the physician is unfamiliar with the expected rate of clinical and bacteriologic response of a particular infection to effective therapy. A common error is to focus on a single clinical sign, such as fever, rather than to consider the patient's overall response. Bacteriologic failure is the persistence of a bacterium beyond its expected time of clearance and is usually accompanied by clinical failure to respond.

When review of the clinical and bacteriologic findings indicates that the patient has not improved, it is important to determine whether antibacterial treatment was actually indicated for the illness by reexamining the initial diagnosis and subsequent confirmatory data. Of course, antibiotics cannot be expected to affect nonbacterial diseases. If antibacterial therapy had been indicated, details of the regimen should be examined, such as susceptibility of the bacterium, dosage, route of administration, interval between doses, possible drug incompatibilities, and penetration of the drug to the site of infection. When there is a closed collection of inflammatory fluid (e.g., an abscess), drainage is more important than antibacterial treatment in resolving the infection. Among the most common reasons for antibacterial treatment failure, and the most difficult to correct, are deficiencies in specific host defense mechanisms as well as more general host problems, such as poor nutrition, inability to clear respiratory secretions, and poor tissue perfusion. Development of drug resistance by an initially susceptible bacterium during treatment is uncommon.

Occasionally, complications of antibacterial therapy are superimposed on the acute bacterial illness and are difficult to distinguish from antibacterial failure. The antibacterial agent itself may be the cause of symptoms, particularly allergic symptoms or drug fever. Penicillin allergy is more frequent than recurrent infection as a cause of recurrent fever in patients treated for pneumococcal pneumonia. Superinfection with another microbe may cause persistent or recurrent symptoms during antibacterial treatment. In the hospital, the most frequent sites for superinfection are the urinary tract (particularly in catheterized patients), the lower respiratory tract, and intravenous sites (phlebitis) (see Chapter 25).

## Cost of Antibacterial Treatment

In general, newer antimicrobials are more expensive than older agents. Frequently, any of several available agents are appropriate for treatment of a given infection, with approximately the same efficacy and risk. Table 38–4 illustrates the widely differing costs of several oral agents available for oral treatment of acute exacerbations of chronic bronchitis.

In the hospital, the cost of an antibacterial agent is further increased by the cost of drug preparation and administration. A hospital may add a charge of $30 or more per dose for preparation and administration of an intravenous (IV) antibiotic. Such charges may far exceed the purchase cost of the antimicrobial itself. Those agents that require monitoring of serum drug levels or periodic renal or hepatic function testing also have those added costs. Use of the intramuscular (IM) or oral route of administration rather than the IV route, and use of drugs permitting fewer administrations per day, can result in lower costs.

## ANTIMICROBIAL PROPHYLAXIS

Use of antimicrobial agents to prevent infection is termed *antimicrobial prophylaxis*. Prophylaxis is most efficacious when attempting to prevent infection over a relatively brief time period, and it is least effective in attempting to prevent infections in an immunologically compromised host. Penicillin G has been proved to prevent infection by group A strep-

**TABLE 38–4.  COMPARATIVE DRUG COSTS (COST TO THE PHARMACIST) FOR A 10-DAY COURSE OF ORAL THERAPY FOR AN ACUTE EXACERBATION OF CHRONIC BRONCHITIS**

| Antibacterial Agent | Dose | Cost |
| --- | --- | --- |
| Ampicillin | 250 mg q 6 h | $   2.80 |
| Amoxicillin | 250 mg q 8 h | $   2.40 |
| Amoxicillin-clavulanic acid | 250 mg q 8 h | $ 46.50 |
| Cefaclor | 500 mg q 8 h | $112.80 |
| Cefuroxime axetil | 250 mg q 12 h | $ 57.40 |
| Cefixime | 400 mg q 24 h | $ 56.00 |
| Cefprozil | 500 mg q 12 h | $ 99.60 |
| Loracarbef | 200 mg q 12 h | $ 60.40 |
| Cefpodoxime proxetil | 200 mg q 12 h | $ 60.40 |
| Clarithromycin | 500 mg q 12 h | $ 55.00 |
| Azithromycin | 500 mg day 1, 250 mg q 24 h × 4 | $ 48.78 |
| Doxycycline | 100 mg q 12 h | $   2.20 |
| Ciprofloxacin | 500 mg q 12 h | $ 58.40 |
| Trimethoprin/Sulfa | 160/800 mg (1 DS) q 12 h | $   1.60 |

tococci and recurrence of rheumatic fever in persons with history of rheumatic fever (see Chapter 7). Another well-established, but not proven, indication for antibacterial prophylaxis is prevention of infective endocarditis by administration of antibiotics to patients with cardiac valvular disease before specific medical, surgical, or dental procedures (see Chapter 33).

The administration of antibiotics to prevent postoperative wound infections is well accepted for certain surgical procedures. There is good evidence that prophylaxis reduces postoperative wound infection rates following procedures that require incision into sites that are normally heavily colonized with bacteria, such as the oropharynx, vagina, and colon. The evidence that antibiotics prevent wound infections is less compelling for clean procedures that involve only skin incision. Prophylaxis has become accepted for procedures that require placement of a foreign body such as a prosthetic device (hip joint, cardiac valve). In these cases the risk of infection is low, but the consequences of any infection are unacceptably high because the infections often cannot be treated with antimicrobials alone and surgical removal of the prosthesis is required for cure.

When antibacterial prophylaxis is used, a single agent active against the bacteria most frequently isolated from postoperative infections at that site should be employed. The risk of contamination of a wound begins at the time of the initial incision. Therefore, administration of the prophylactic antibacterial agent must be initiated before the operation begins (usually within an hour of the incision), and an effective blood and tissue level must be maintained throughout the procedure. For most operations, a single preoperative intravenous dose of a prophylactic antimicrobial is sufficient, with an additional intraoperative dose if the procedure is a long one. Prolonged administration of prophylactic antimicrobials before or after surgical procedures does not result in lower infection rates and is generally associated with an increased incidence of adverse effects, as well as with colonization and infection due to antibiotic-resistant organisms. In specific situations, such as cardiac surgery or placement of an orthopedic prosthesis, however, prophylactic antibiotics are frequently continued for 2–5 days, using the rationale that postsurgical drains may pose a continued risk for infection.

# CLINICAL PHARMACOLOGY OF ANTIMICROBIAL AGENTS

## Absorption

Many antimicrobial agents are absorbed very well after oral administration. Others are either so poorly absorbed (e.g., vancomycin, aminoglycosides) or so rapidly degraded in the intestinal tract that they must be administered parenterally (intravenously or intramuscularly) to treat systemic infection. With few exceptions, antimicrobial agents are only partially absorbed after oral administration, and serum concentrations are much lower after oral than after identical parenteral dosing. Major exceptions are chloramphenicol, fluoroquinolones (ciprofloxacin, ofloxacin), and metronidazole, which reach serum levels that are as high or higher after oral administration as after intravenous infusion. The serum concentrations achieved by the usual oral doses of such agents as ampicillin, some cephalosporins, and the tetracyclines are generally not high enough to inhibit some of the gram-negative enteric bacilli that are considered susceptible to these drugs. However, oral administration of these agents is useful for treating gram-negative bacillary urinary tract infections because the drugs are concentrated in urine. In hospitalized patients with severe infection, antimicrobial therapy generally should be administered parenterally to avoid the possibility of treatment failure due to poor oral absorption.

## Distribution

After absorption from the intestine or parenteral site, antimicrobial agents are bound by plasma proteins to varying degrees. Initially there is a rapid rise in blood concentration after intravenous administration and a more delayed slow rise after intramuscular or oral administration that is followed by an initial decrease as the drug is distributed to body tissues (the alpha or distribution phase). The subsequent rate of decline (the beta phase) is due to excretion and metabolism. The most frequently used measure of this decline is the serum half-life (the time required for a 50% decrease in serum concentration), a measure of the duration of pharmacologic effect. Serum half-life is an important therapeutic determinant of dosage interval for all patients, and is particularly important for avoidance of toxicity in those patients in whom the half-life is prolonged because of decreased drug excretion or metabolism.

The extravascular concentration of an antibiotic depends on the degree of protein binding, the concentration gradient from blood to tissue fluid, and the drug diffusibility. Diffusibility is affected by molecular size, dissociation constant, and lipid solubility of the drug. Lipid solubility and the dissociation constant of an antimicrobial agent is an important determinant of the ability of the agent to enter cells. Antimicrobials such as clindamycin, the macrolides/azalides (erythromycin, azithromycin, clarithromycin), tetracyclines, rifampin, fluoroquinolones (ciprofloxacin, ofloxacin), and chloramphenicol achieve intracellular concentrations higher than serum concentrations. Most antibiotics penetrate well by passive diffusion into large-volume extravascular sites such as pleural effusions, peritoneal fluid (ascites), pericardial fluid, and joint fluid. Penetration into certain sites is poor because of diffusion barriers or active excretory systems: the brain, CSF, and aqueous and vitreous humor are examples. At still other sites the antimicrobial concentration may be quite variable and is dependent upon active excretion or secretion of the drug by glands or organs: bile, urine, saliva, tears, breast milk, sputum, and prostatic fluid are examples. Drug concentrations in urine are usually very high, whereas in breast milk and prostatic secretions they are very low. In general, penetration of a body compartment increases in the presence of inflammation, at least during the early stages of an infection. For example, penicillin concentration in the CSF is much higher in the inflammatory state (meningitis) than in normal CSF.

### Inactivation and Excretion

Several mechanisms of excretion and inactivation of antimicrobial agents exist. An antibiotic may be metabolized by the liver into biologically active or inactive metabolites, secreted into bile, filtered or actively secreted by the kidney, or inactivated by other, unknown means. It is not unusual for a single agent to undergo more than one of these processes. Inactivation of a few antimicrobials by a secondary means occurs when primary inactivation or excretion does not occur because of organ failure.

Renal excretion is the major means of clearance of most antimicrobials. Chloramphenicol, erythromycin, clarithromycin, azithromycin, clindamycin, doxycycline, and metronidazole are the major exceptions. Some agents are at least partially inactivated by the liver. Renal failure results in accumulation of antimicrobials normally excreted by the kidney, and hepatic failure causes accumulation of drugs inactivated primarily by that organ unless the dose is reduced. Renal function decreases with aging, renal clearance being about one third less in the elderly, a degree of impairment not apparent from serum renal function tests (blood urea nitrogen [BUN] and creatinine). Dosage adjustment is essential for agents such as the aminoglycosides or vancomycin, which have a low therapeutic–toxic ratio (ratio of the concentration of the agent required to inhibit an infecting microorganism and the concentration at which toxic reactions occur) and a completely renal means of excretion or inactivation.

Many antimicrobial agents are secreted into bile, and a few (e.g., erythromycin, tetracycline, piperacillin, ceftriaxone, cefoperazone, metronidazole, clindamycin) reach high concentration relative to serum. However, biliary secretion is generally reduced by the obstructive processes that almost always precede or accompany biliary tract infection.

## CLASSES OF ANTIMICROBIAL AGENTS

The following discussion of antimicrobials is an introduction to their use in the treatment of common infectious diseases, those that an American physician is likely to encounter in practice. Only more frequent and serious side effects and toxicities are noted.

### Penicillins

Penicillin G and its semisynthetic derivatives are one of the most useful classes of antimicrobial agents because of their high therapeutic–toxic ratio. The penicillins are discussed here in groups based on their antibacterial spectra.

#### Penicillin G and Penicillin V

##### Agents to Know in this Group:

*Penicillin G, aqueous, procaine, and benzathine (IV, IM)*
*Penicillin V (oral)*

Penicillin G and V are active against some bacteria at very low concentrations and against others at significantly higher concentrations. The very susceptible group of bacteria includes most aerobic and anaerobic gram-positive streptococci but not staphylococci. *Neisseria meningitidis* (*Treponema pallidum*, and many anaerobic gram-positive and gram-negative bacilli, other than *Bacteroides fragilis* group, *Porphyromonas* species and, *Prevotella* species) are also very susceptible. The less susceptible group of bacteria includes many strains of enterococci, *Listeria monocytogenes*, *Neisseria gonorrhoeae*, *Proteus mirabilis*, and *H. influenzae*. However, because of increasing penicillin resistance in enterococci, *N. gonorrhoeae*, and *H. influenzae*, penicillin is no longer recommended for empiric treatment of infections caused by these organisms.

**Preparations.** The most common parenteral penicillins, in order of increasing half-life and decreasing peak serum concentrations, are aqueous crystalline, aqueous procaine, and benzathine (Bicillin) penicillin G. Oral preparations include potassium penicillin G and penicillin V. Penicillin V is a more acid-stable analogue of penicillin G that is better absorbed orally; its antibacterial activity is similar to that of penicillin G.

The level of penicillin G or V achieved after oral dosage or by intramuscular aqueous procaine penicillin G is adequate for treatment of most infections due to the very susceptible bacteria listed. Benzathine penicillin G is used for treatment of syphilis and treatment and prevention of streptococcal pharyngitis, in which the low but sustained concentration of penicillin achieved by a single injection is sufficient. Certain infections, such as endocarditis and meningitis—as well as most infections caused by the less penicillin-susceptible group of bacteria—require the higher penicillin concentrations attainable by crystalline penicillin G or an unusually high dose of procaine penicillin. Crystalline penicillin G is always combined with an aminoglycoside in treating systemic enterococcal infection.

**Pharmacology and Distribution.** The concentration of penicillins in body fluids and tissues at appropriate dosages are adequate in almost all tissues. The penicillins do not enter the CSF well in the absence of inflammation, but they penetrate well enough in the presence of inflammation that sufficient CSF levels are achieved at high dosages to successfully treat meningitis. Most of a dose of penicillin G is rapidly eliminated by the kidney, primarily by tubular secretion. The serum level is raised and the half-life prolonged by renal failure or by the administration of probenecid (Benemid), which partially blocks tubular secretion of penicillin.

**Side Effects and Toxicity.** Penicillin G is relatively nontoxic; interstitial nephritis occurs rarely. Neurotoxicity (seizures) occurs rarely in patients with renal failure given inappropriately high intravenous doses. Allergy to penicillin is frequent. It is estimated that 5–7% of the general population claims to be allergic to penicillin. A pruritic, erythematous rash occurring after several days of therapy is by far the most frequent allergic manifestation. Other manifestations of hypersensitivity (drug fever, serum sickness, and immediate hypersensitivity reactions such as anaphylaxis, angioedema, and urticaria) occur less frequently. An individual allergic to one penicillin should be presumed to be allergic to other penicillins. Cross-allergenicity between penicillins and cephalosporins is estimated to be less than 5%, but cephalosporin use is not recommended if the allergy to penicillin is immediate (anaphylaxis, angioedema, urticaria). Alternatives to penicillin G for treatment of specific infections are listed in Table 38–3.

**Indications.** Penicillin is the preferred antimicrobial agent for treatment of infections by very susceptible organisms including streptococcal phyaryngitis, cellulitis, and endocarditis; *N. meningitidis* bacteremia and meningitis; syphilis; and pneumococcal pneumonia and meningitis. Resistance in *S. pneumoniae* to penicillin has risen in many areas of the United States and is of concern for future use of penicillin for this organism.

### Penicillinase-Resistant Penicillins

**Agents to Know in this Group:**

*Nafcillin or oxacillin* (*IV, IM*)
*Cloxacillin or dicloxacillin* (*oral*)

These semisynthetic penicillins are active against penicillinase-producing staphylococci. They are also active, although less so than penicillin G, against most other aerobic gram-positive cocci, except enterococci. Penicillinase-resistant penicillins are significantly less active than penicillin G against bacteria other than aerobic gram-positive cocci.

**Preparations.** Several penicillinase-resistant penicillins are available. Despite significant pharmacologic differences, these drugs are of essentially equal efficacy at equivalent dosage. Methicillin (Staphcillin) is not absorbed orally, and is available only parenterally. Nafcillin (Unipen), cloxacillin (Tegopen), and oxacillin (Prostaphlin) are available in both parenteral and oral forms. Dicloxacillin (Dynapen) is available only as an oral preparation. Cloxacillin or dicloxacillin is preferred for oral use because they are better absorbed.

**Pharmacology.** With the exception of methicillin, protein binding of these penicillins is very high (87–97%), but free drug levels are sufficient to be highly active against staphylococci. Metabolism is high for nafcillin (62%) and oxacillin (45%) and, therefore, dosage adjustment for renal failure is not necessary. Half-life is short (30 min), necessitating 4-hourly dosing for serious infections.

**Side Effects and Toxicity.** Mild gastrointestinal symptoms occasionally occur with oral therapy. Abnormal liver function tests and reversible granulocytopenia occur occasionally. Methicillin is associated with a higher rate of interstitial nephritis than the other members of this group and because of this is little used. Allergic reactions are similar to those seen with penicillin G.

**Indications.** The penicillinase-resistant penicillins are preferred for treatment of staphylococcal infections, particularly those due to *S. aureus*, because of their excellent activity, low toxicity, and relatively narrow spectrum.

### Extended-Spectrum Penicillins

**Agents to Know in this Group:**

*Ampicillin (IV, IM, oral)*
*Amoxicillin (oral)*

This class of semisynthetic penicillins includes two penicillins with an extended spectrum of activity against some gram-negative bacteria, but they are not active against penicillinase-producing staphylococci.

Ampicillin and amoxicillin have activity similar to that of penicillin G against streptococci, *L. monocytogenes*, and anaerobic bacteria. They have superior activity against enterococci. These drugs have generally good activity against *N. meningitidis*, most *H. influenzae*, most strains of *P. mirabilis* and *Salmonella*, most strains of *Escherichia coli*, and some strains of *Shigella*. Beta-lactamase–producing *H. influenzae* represent up to 25% of the isolates in many areas, and their recognition has changed the initial presumptive treatment of life-threatening *H. influenzae* infection. These agents have relatively little activity against other common gram-negative bacteria (e.g., *Klebsiella* species, *Enterobacter* species, *Serratia* species, and *P. aeruginosa*). Amoxicillin is somewhat less active *in vitro* than ampicillin against *Shigella*. Its major advantage over ampicillin is better oral absorption and less drug-related diarrhea.

**Preparations.** Ampicillin is available for oral, IV, and IM use. In the United States, amoxicillin is available for oral use only. The concentration of these agents required to inhibit susceptible Enterobacteriaceae, with the possible exception of *P. mirabilis* strains, is generally higher than the peak concentrations achieved by standard oral dosage. Thus, oral use of ampicillin and amoxicillin to treat gram-negative enteric bacilli is primarily for urinary tract infections and diarrhea.

**Pharmacology.** Ampicillin and amoxicillin are primarily excreted unchanged in the urine—about 10% is inactivated in the liver. Their half-lives are just over 1 h.

**Side Effects and Toxicity.** Diarrhea is frequent but does not usually require cessation of treatment. Significant toxicity due to ampicillin and amoxicillin is rare. Reversible hematologic and liver function test abnormalities have been reported. Allergic rashes with ampicillin and amoxicillin are more common than with penicillin.

**Indications.** Ampicillin and amoxicillin are used for the treatment of urinary tract infections and bronchitis. Ampicillin is used with an aminoglycoside to treat enterococcal infections and *L. monocytogenes* infections, including meningitis.

### Antipseudomonal Penicillins

**Agents to Know in this Group:**

*Piperacillin or mezlocillin (IV, IM)*

These penicillins, beginning historically with carbenicillin (Geopen), were developed for their activity against *P. aeruginosa*. Ticarcillin (Ticar), mezlocillin (Mezlin), piperacillin (Pipracil), and azlocillin (Azlin) are more active than carbenicillin against *P. aeruginosa* and a broad range of other gram-negative enteric bacilli. Enterococci are susceptible to mezlocillin, piperacillin, and azlocillin but resistant to carbenicillin and ticarcillin. Penicillinase-producing staphylococci are resistant to all these agents, but streptococci are susceptible. Piperacillin and mezlocillin are active against most strains of *P. aeruginosa, Proteus, Enterobacter, Serratia,* and *Klebsiella*. They are also active against *B. fragilis* as well as against ampicillin-sensitive anaerobes.

**Pharmacology and Preparations.** These penicillins are available as sodium salts to be administered intramuscularly or intravenously, but the high concentration required for inhibition of susceptible gram-negative bacteria, especially *P. aeruginosa*, generally restricts them to the intravenous route at doses ranging from 12–20 g/day.

**Inactivation and Excretion.** These penicillins are excreted primarily unchanged in the urine, less than 15% metabolism occurs in the liver.

**Side Effects and Toxicity.** Administration of these penicillins is occasionally associated with a dose-related bleeding disorder. Reversible neutropenia has been reported rarely. The sodium content of these drugs may contribute to sodium overload in patients receiving large dosages. Similarly, if electrolytes are not monitored, hypokalemia can occur with large dosages, presumably because the penicillin acts as a nonreabsorbable anion, leading to increased excretion of potassium. These electrolyte effects are less common with mezlocillin, piperacillin, and azlocillin because their 1–2 mEq/g sodium content is less than the 5–6 mEq/g sodium content of carbenicillin and ticarcillin. Allergic reactions are similar to those observed with other penicillins.

**Indications.** These penicillins are used for the treatment of *P. aeruginosa* infections, gram-negative enteric infections not susceptible to ampicillin, and infections due to *B. fragilis*. Because *P. aeruginosa*, *E. coli*, and *Klebsiella* sp. cause most of the serious infections in neutropenic patients, these agents have found wide use in combination with an aminoglycoside for the empiric management of the febrile, neutropenic patient.

### Penicillins plus Beta-Lactamase Inhibitor Combinations

#### Agents to Know in this Group:

*Ampicillin-sulbactam (IV, IM)*
*Amoxicillin-clavulanic acid (oral)*
*Ticarcillin-clavulanic acid (IV)*
*Piperacillin-tazobactam (IV)*

Clavulanic acid, sulbactam, and tazobactam are effective inhibitors of beta-lactamases, and have been combined with extended-spectrum or antipseudomonal penicillins to extend the spectrum of these agents by inhibiting the beta-lactamases produced by certain organisms that would otherwise inactivate the penicillin in the combination. Amoxicillin-clavulanic acid (Augmentin) and ampicillin-sulbactam (Unasyn) are similar oral and parenteral extended-spectrum penicillin combinations, and ticarcillin-clavulanic acid (Timentin) and piperacillin-tazobactam (Zosyn) are similar antipseudomonal penicillin plus inhibitor combinations. The major improvement in spectrum

is against staphylococci, aerobic gram-negative bacilli, and anaerobic gram-negatives such as *Bacteroides*. Although plasmid-mediated beta-lactamases are inhibited by these beta-lactamase inhibitors, chromosomally mediated, inducible enzymes, such as those produced by *P. aeruginosa*, are not.

**Pharmacology.** The beta-lactamase inhibitors are prepared in fixed ratios with their penicillin counterpart and should be dosed in a manner similar to the accompanying penicillin if used alone. If Timentin or Zosyn are used to treat *P. aeruginosa* infection, the same high dose must be used as with ticarcillin or piperacillin alone, since addition of the beta-lactamase inhibitor does not add to the antipseudomonal activity of the combination.

**Indications.** Because of the extended spectrum of activity (which includes staphylococci, streptococci, gram-negative aerobic bacilli, and most anaerobic bacteria), Timentin, Unasyn, and Zosyn have been used for serious mixed polymicrobial abdominal and pelvic infections, polymicrobial foot infections in diabetics (Unasyn and Timentin), and in combination with an aminoglycoside for empiric treatment of presumed bacteremia. Unasyn and Augmentin lack sufficient gram-negative bacillary activity to be used alone for treatment of presumed infection by these organisms and should be used in combination with an aminoglycoside for presumptive treatment. At recommended dosages, Zosyn is not adequate alone for treatment of *P. aeruginosa* infections—an aminoglycoside should be added. Augmentin is used for treatment of bronchitis, sinusitis, otitis, community-acquired pneumonia, bite wounds, and urinary tract infections.

### Cephalosporins

The cephalosporins are semisynthetic beta-lactam antibiotics active against gram-positive cocci, including penicillinase-producing *S. aureus* (but not methicillin-resistant *S. aureus*) and against many gram-negative bacilli. Enterococci are not included in the cephalosporin spectrum. Cephalosporin "generations" are a somewhat artificial classification based upon the antibacterial spectrum of the agents.

### First-Generation Cephalosporins

#### Agents to Know in this Group:

*Cefazolin (IV, IM)*
*Cephalexin or cephradine (oral)*

The spectrum of activity of the *first-generation cephalosporins* includes most of the gram-positive bacteria susceptible to penicillin G as well as penicillinase-producing *S. aureus* and *S. epidermidis*. Among gram-negative bacteria, some strains of *E. coli, Klebsiella pneumoniae,* and *P. mirabilis* are susceptible. *P. aeruginosa* is resistant. The parenteral preparations include cephalothin (Keflin), cefazolin (Ancef, Kefzol), and cephapirin (Cefadyl). The oral preparations include cephalexin (Keflex, generic), cephradine (Anspor, Velosef), and cefadroxil (Duricef). The first-generation cephalosporins have better activity against gram-positive bacteria than do other cephalosporins.

## Second-Generation Cephalosporins

### Agents to Know in this Group:

*Cefuroxime (IV, IM, oral)*
*Cefixime and cefpodoxime (oral)*

Cefoxitin (Mefoxin), cefotetan (Cefotan), cefuroxime (Zinacef), cefonicid (Monocid), ceforanide (Precef), cefmetazole (Zefazone), cefamandole (Mandol) and the oral preparations, cefuroxime axetil (Ceftin), cefixime (Suprax), cefprozil (Cefzil), cefpodoxime (Vantin), and cefaclor (Ceclor) are called *second-generation cephalosporins* because they have a somewhat wider range of activity against gram-negative bacteria compared with the first-generation agents. An oral carbacephem agent, loracarbef (Lorabid) is similar in spectrum. The second-generation cephalosporins differ among themselves in pharmacologic properties. They generally have an increased level of activity against the gram-negative enteric bacilli when compared to first-generation cephalosporins. All have good activity against *H. influenzae.* Cefoxitin is often active against *Proteus* species. Gram-positive anaerobes (excluding *Clostridium difficile*) are generally susceptible to the second-generation cephalosporins, but *B. fragilis* is susceptible only to cefoxitin.

## Third-Generation Cephalosporins

### Agents to Know in this Group:

*Ceftriaxone or ceftizoxime (IV, IM)*
*Ceftazidime (IV, IM)*

These cephalosporins have the widest cephalosporin spectrum against gram-negative aerobic bacilli and all have at least some activity against *P. aeruginosa.* The *third-generation cephalosporins* are cefotaxime (Claforan), ceftizoxime (Cefizox), cefoperazone (Cefobid), ceftriaxone (Rocephin), and ceftazidime (Fortaz,

Tazidime, Tazicef). Ceftazidime has the best *in vitro* activity against *P. aeruginosa* and is the only cephalosporin with activity similar to that of the extended-spectrum penicillins against this bacterium. Ceftriaxone and ceftazidime have relatively poor activity against *B. fragilis*; the activity of ceftizoxime against *B. fragilis* is similar to that of cefoxitin and cefotetan, second-generation cephalosporins.

### Pharmacology and Preparations

Half-life and protein binding vary considerably among the cephalosporins. Consequently, the appropriate doses and dosage intervals differ considerably. The parenteral cephalosporins are usually used intravenously because of the large doses required for treatment of systemic infections. Those agents with longer half-lives such as ceftriaxone may be given intramuscularly for relatively susceptible infections. Some of the newer oral second-generation cephalosporins (cefixime, cefprozil, cefuroxime, cefpodoxime) are dosed once or twice daily, an advantage in obtaining patient compliance.

### Distribution, Inactivation, and Excretion

The cephalosporins are widely distributed to body tissues and fluids, but like all beta-lactams, do not enter cells to any great degree. Penetration into the CSF in amounts sufficient for treatment of meningitis occurs only with the third-generation cephalosporins, which have become the treatment agents of choice for gram-negative enteric bacillary meningitis. The cephalosporins are primarily excreted unchanged in the urine. Cephalothin, cephapirin, and cefotaxime also undergo significant inactivation in the liver. Some cephalosporins (ceftriaxone, cefaclor, cefamandole) are secreted into the bile.

### Side Effects and Toxicity

Particularly with the parenteral cephalosporins, eosinophilia is relatively common, as is a positive direct Coombs' test, only rarely associated with hemolytic anemia. Other hematologic and transient liver-function test abnormalities occur rarely. The presence of the thiomethyltetrazole group in cephalosporins has been linked to two undesirable effects: (1) bleeding disorders due to hypoprothrombinemia, and (2) a disulfiram (Antabuse)-like reaction if alcohol is ingested during administration of the antibiotic. Cefamandole, cefoperazone, and cefotetan have this thio-methyltetrazole group, but bleeding disorders are not common.

## Indications

**First-Generation Cephalosporins.** These antibiotics are useful for the treatment of systemic infections and oral treatment of urinary tract infections due to susceptible gram-negative bacilli. They are useful as alternatives to penicillin and to penicillinase-resistant penicillins for gram-positive infections, particularly those due to staphylococci. Cefazolin has become a mainstay of prophylaxis against surgical wound infections, largely because of its long half-life, spectrum, and low cost.

**Second-Generation Cephalosporins.** These antibiotics are indicated for the treatment of infections due to susceptible bacteria that are *not* susceptible to the first-generation cephalosporins. Cefoxitin is used in disease presumed or known to be due to *B. fragilis*. Most are used orally in treating sinusitis, otitis, bronchitis, community-acquired pneumonia, and gonorrhea (cefixime, cefuroxime). All are alternative drugs for the treatment of nonmeningitic *H. influenzae* infections.

**Third-Generation Cephalosporins.** These agents are indicated in the treatment of those gram-negative enteric bacterial infections that are not susceptible to earlier cephalosporins or to broad-spectrum penicillins. Ceftazidime is the most active agent against *P. aeruginosa* infections and is often given with an aminoglycoside in granulocytopenic patients. Because of beta-lactamase–producing *H. influenzae*, one of the third-generation cephalosporins (cefotaxime, ceftazidime, or ceftriaxone) is appropriate for presumptive initial treatment of meningitis in the pediatric (not newborn) age group. A third-generation cephalosporin is indicated in the treatment of gram-negative enteric meningitis in adults or children.

## Other Beta-Lactam Agents

### Monobactams

#### Agent to Know in this Group:

*Aztreonam (IV, IM)*

These beta-lactam agents possess a monocyclic basic structure. The first of these agents is aztreonam (Azactam). The spectrum of aztreonam is limited to aerobic gram-negative bacteria, including neisseria, haemophilus, most Enterobacteriaceae, and *P. aeruginosa*. It is particularly well tolerated by individuals allergic to other beta-lactams.

**Preparations.** Aztreonam must be given parenterally (intramuscularly or intravenously), as it is not absorbed following oral administration.

**Pharmacology.** Aztreonam is widely distributed in tissues, including bone, bile, bronchial secretions, prostate, and CSF, and high concentrations are achieved in urine. About 70% is excreted unchanged in the urine, with only about 7% metabolized and then excreted in urine.

**Side Effects and Toxicity.** This agent, like other beta-lactams, is generally well tolerated. Phlebitis related to the intravenous site occurs occasionally, and rash and gastrointestinal upset are rarely observed. No cross-allergenicity with penicillins or cephalosporins is observed, a very important feature.

**Indications.** Aztreonam appears to be a less toxic alternative to the aminoglycosides for serious aerobic gram-negative infections, particularly in those with renal impairment or at high risk of aminoglycoside toxicity. It is also an alternative agent in patients with penicillin and cephalosporin allergy. Its gram-negative spectrum duplicates that of ceftazidime; therefore, the two should not be used together.

### Carbapenems

#### Agent to Know in this Group:

*Imipenem-Cilastatin (IV)*

This class of beta-lactam agents has the dicyclic ring modified with substitution of carbon for sulfur. The first agent of this class is imipenem-cilastatin (Primaxin). Imipenem has the broadest antibacterial spectrum of all available beta-lactams, with activity against most gram-positives (including some enterococci and Listeria), against most gram-negatives (including *P. aeruginosa*), and against most anaerobes (including *B. fragilis*).

**Preparations.** Imipenem is not absorbed orally and must be given parenterally. It is administered in a 1:1 fixed ratio with cilastatin, a specific inhibitor of dehydropeptidase 1, an enzyme located in the brush border of renal proximal tubular cells that extensively degrades imipenem.

**Pharmacology.** The drug is well distributed into most tissues and body fluids, including CSF. Little drug is excreted in bile, but urinary concentrations are high. When given with cilastatin, about 70% of imipenem is excreted unchanged in urine and the remainder is nonrenally eliminated by metabolic inactivation.

**Side Effects and Toxicity.** Imipenem is generally well tolerated, like other beta-lactams. Rash and gastrointestinal side effects occur occasionally. Cross-allergenicity with other beta-lactams is well-documented. A potentially worrisome toxic effect has been seizure activity, particularly in elderly patients and those with renal insufficiency.

**Indications.** It is useful in treatment of polymicrobial infections, such as peritonitis and foot infection in diabetic patients. It has also been used successfully as empiric therapy for febrile, neutropenic patients. Imipenem alone can often replace several other antimicrobials in mixed polymicrobial infections, thus simplifying treatment.

### Macrolides/Azalides

**Agents to Know in this Group:**

*Erythromycin (IV, oral)*
*Azithromycin or clarithromycin (oral)*

Erythromycin (many trade names), clarithromycin (Biaxin), and azithromycin (Zithromax) are active against many gram-positive bacteria including *S. pneumoniae and S. pyogenes* and against *Chlamydia pneumoniae, Legionella pneumophila,* and *Mycoplasma pneumoniae.* Most strains of *S. aureus* are susceptible initially to erythromycin, but resistance may develop during treatment. Clarithromycin and azithromycin are active against *Mycobacterium avium-intracellulare* (MAI), an opportunistic infectious agent of human immunodeficiency virus (HIV)–infected patients, and against *H. influenzae,* and *Moraxella catarrhalis.*

**Preparations.** Erythromycin is available in oral and intravenous preparations. Among the oral preparations, the parent compound and its stearate and ethyl succinate are less well absorbed than the estolate (Ilosone). Clarithromycin and azithromycin are oral agents.

**Pharmacology.** Erythromycin is widely distributed in tissues, including intracellularly. Most erythromycin is inactivated, probably by the liver, some is secreted in the bile, and relatively little is excreted in the urine. Clarithromycin is also highly concentrated within cells and achieves higher serum levels than erythromycin and can be administered twice a day. Clarithromycin is metabolized to an active 14-hydroxy metabolite that contributes a major portion of the activity against *H. influenzae.* Azithromycin achieves very low serum concentrations, but has tissue (intracellular) levels that are far (10- to 100-fold) in excess of serum concentrations and persist for several days (terminal half-life 60 h) after administration is stopped. This allows azithromycin to be dosed for only 5 days for most infections, and to be used as single-dose treatment for *C. trachomatis* genital infections.

**Side Effects and Toxicity.** Gastrointestinal symptoms, such as abdominal cramping, nausea, vomiting, and diarrhea, occur very frequently with erythromycin, and are related to direct gastrointestinal stimulation by the drug. Erythromycin estolate, but not other forms, is a rare (<1:1000) cause of intrahepatic cholestasis, which occurs much more frequently in adults than in children. This reaction is reversible when the drug is stopped, but promptly returns if the patient is rechallenged. Clarithromycin and azithromycin both have much lower gastrointestinal side effects than erythromycin.

**Indications.** Erythromycin, clarithromycin, and azithromycin are used for the treatment of so-called atypical community-acquired pneumonia that may be caused by *L. pneumophila, M. pneumoniae,* or *C. pneumoniae,* or by the "typical" *S. pneumoniae* organisms. Erythromycin is the first-choice agent because of its long experience and lower cost, but clarithromycin and azithromycin are useful alternatives for patients who have trouble tolerating erythromycin. Erythromycin is also used for treating otitis media, streptococcal pharyngitis, and for penicillin-susceptible infections in penicillin-allergic patients. Although its antibacterial activity against susceptible bacteria is less than that of penicillin G, erythromycin is usually an effective alternative. It should not be used for severe *S. aureus* infections. Clarithromycin or azithromycin are effective for MAI infections and are usually used in combination with other agents.

### Tetracyclines

**Agents to Know in this Group:**

*Tetracycline (IV, oral)*
*Doxycycline (IV, oral)*

Tetracyclines are active against some, but not nearly all, streptococcal and staphylococcal strains, both aerobic and anaerobic. Tetracyclines are active against many *Escherichia, Enterobacter,* and *Klebsiella* strains, as well as many *H. influenzae, N. meningitidis,* and *N. gonorrhoeae* strains. Tetracycline has some gram-negative anaerobic activity and is active against *T. pallidum, M. pneumoniae, Rickettsia,* and *Chlamydia.*

**Preparations.** Numerous tetracycline preparations exist. The newer derivatives—demeclocycline (Declomycin), methacycline (Rondomycin), doxycycline (Vibramycin), and minocycline (Minocin)—are generally better absorbed orally. Peak serum concentrations achieved by recommended dosages of newer tetracycline derivatives are lower. The level of tetracyclines required to inhibit most Enterobacteriaceae exceeds that obtained in serum by ordinary dosage. Thus, for gram-negative enteric infection, tetracyclines are considered useful primarily in the urinary tract.

**Pharmacology.** Tetracyclines are widely distributed, but tissue levels vary with the derivative used. Minocycline, a more lipid-soluble drug, penetrates the subarachnoid space in normal patients better than other tetracyclines, but all penetrate well in the presence of inflammation. Inactivation and excretion of the tetracycline derivatives vary, with all being secreted into bile. About half of a doxycycline dose is inactivated by the liver, and some is excreted by nonrenal mechanisms. There is relatively little inactivation of other tetracyclines, and they are excreted unchanged by the kidney, accumulating in patients with renal failure.

**Side Effects and Toxicity.** Gastrointestinal side effects (nausea, epigastric distress, and occasional vomiting and diarrhea) are relatively common with tetracyclines, but may be less frequent with the newer, better absorbed derivatives. Photosensitivity, manifested by rash on exposed skin, occasionally occurs with doxycycline and is rare with other tetracyclines. All tetracyclines may be deposited in calcifying areas of bones and teeth, causing yellowish discoloration. Although obvious tooth discoloration is usually apparent only after prolonged or repeated usage, tetracyclines should be avoided in pregnant women during the last 24 weeks of pregnancy and in children younger than 8 years of age. Hepatotoxicity (acute fatty liver) was reported after large doses of intravenous tetracycline, particularly in pregnant women, and has also been reported occasionally in individuals with renal insufficiency who were given standard dosages. Further deterioration in abnormal renal function tests may be observed after tetracyclines. Reversible vestibular disturbance, usually with dizziness, weakness, nausea, and vertigo, has been observed with minocycline but not with other tetracyclines.

**Indications.** Tetracyclines are useful in exacerbations of chronic bronchitis and for urinary tract infection due to susceptible bacteria. Doxycycline is the agent of choice because of its once or twice daily administration orally. Tetracyclines are indicated in rickettsial and chlamydial infections and are effective in the treatment of *M. pneumoniae* infections.

## Lincosamides

### Agent to Know in this Group:
*Clindamycin (IV, IM, oral)*

Clindamycin (Cleocin) has replaced its parent drug, lincomycin (Lincocin). Clindamycin is active against aerobic gram-positive cocci, and against most gram-positive and gram-negative anaerobes, including *B. fragilis.*

**Preparations.** Clindamycin is available in parenteral and oral preparations.

**Pharmacology.** Clindamycin is widely distributed to body tissues and achieves a relatively high bone-to-serum ratio whether measured in normal or infected bone. Clindamycin is largely inactivated, probably by the liver. It is secreted in the bile, and a relatively small amount is excreted in the urine.

**Side Effects and Toxicity.** Diarrhea may occur with use of clindamycin, particularly when administered orally. Diarrhea after clindamycin use does not necessarily indicate *C. difficile*–associated diarrhea or pseudomembranous colitis, but the suspicion should be high.

**Indications.** Clindamycin is indicated for the treatment of disease due to anaerobes, including *B. fragilis,* particularly lung abscess and abdominal abscess. It is also useful as an alternative to penicillin and penicillinase-resistant penicillins in the treatment of staphylococcal infections and occasionally other gram-positive infections. This is particularly important in penicillin-allergic individuals.

## Chloramphenicol

Chloramphenicol (Chloromycetin, generic) is active against gram-positive and gram-negative cocci and against *H. influenzae* and *Salmonella.* It is active against *E. coli, K. pneumoniae,* and *P. mirabilis,* and against many anaerobes.

**Preparations.** Chloramphenicol is available as an oral preparation. The sodium succinate salt may be used intravenously or intramuscularly, but absorption from intramuscular sites may be problematic. In marked contrast to other antibacterial agents, oral chloramphenicol achieves higher serum levels than an equivalent intravenous dose.

**Pharmacology.** Chloramphenicol is very widely distributed in tissues, including normal CSF, brain, and eye, which are not well penetrated by many antimicrobial agents. A small amount of chloramphenicol is excreted in an active form in the urine. Most of the drug is inactivated by the liver, and its metabolites are excreted in the urine.

**Side Effects and Toxicity.** Chloramphenicol is associated with bone marrow depression of two distinct types. The first is a common dose-related, reversible depression that is a pharmacologic property of the drug. Bone marrow depression is usual at ordinary dose levels of 2–4 g daily. The second type is a very rare, non–dosage-related (idiosyncratic) aplastic anemia, associated with a high mortality rate, usually occurring weeks to months after completion of therapy. Neonates with immature hepatic glucuronide function can develop the potentially fatal gray baby syndrome unless dosages are reduced.

**Indications.** Because of chloramphenicol's potential for irreversible toxicity, its indications are limited to that of a secondary agent. Chloramphenicol is indicated as an alternative for systemic *Salmonella* infections, and is an alternative agent for treatment of serious *H. influenzae* infections, such as meningitis and bacteremia. Because of its excellent penetration of the blood-brain barrier with or without inflammation, chloramphenicol is also used for treatment of meningitis due to bacteria susceptible to it but not to the penicillins or third-generation cephalosporins, or in penicillin-allergic individuals. Chloramphenicol is also effective in treatment of brain abscess.

## Aminoglycosides and Aminocyclitols

### Agents to Know in this Group:

*Gentamicin (IV, IM)*
*Amikacin (IV, IM)*

The aminoglycosides are active against a wide variety of aerobic and facultatively anaerobic gram-positive and gram-negative bacteria. They are inactive against anaerobes. They are clinically important primarily because of their activity against gram-negative enteric bacilli and *P. aeruginosa*. The aminoglycosides currently in clinical use for systemic disease include streptomycin, gentamicin (Garamycin), tobramycin (Nebcin), netilmycin (Netromycin), and amikacin (Amikin). All

are available as generic preparations. Other aminoglycosides are generally compared with gentamicin, the agent with the most extensive clinical history. Two areas of particular comparative interest are (1) activity against bacteria that have acquired resistance against an aminoglycoside, usually gentamicin, and (2) the frequency of ototoxicity and nephrotoxicity at equivalent dosage levels.

### Gentamicin, Netilmycin, and Tobramycin

Gentamicin, netilmycin, and tobramycin are active against most enteric bacilli and most strains of *P. aeruginosa*. Tobramycin is somewhat more active *in vitro* against many strains of *P. aeruginosa* than is gentamicin or netilmycin, and is slightly less active against some strains of Enterobacteriaceae, particularly *Serratia marcescens*.

### Amikacin

The spectrum of amikacin is similar to that of gentamicin and tobramycin, and although its relative activity against *P. aeruginosa* may be slightly lower, this is more than offset by the much higher serum levels of amikacin. As discussed in Chapter 37, amikacin has the fewest chemical linkages susceptible to bacterial aminoglycoside-inactivating enzymes; therefore, bacteria that produce enzymes inactivating other aminoglycosides are frequently susceptible to amikacin. However, bacteria resistant to aminoglycosides because of failure to transport the antibiotic intracellularly also transport amikacin poorly, and resistance is likely.

### Streptomycin

Streptomycin is no longer used for the treatment of enteric bacterial disease because resistance develops rapidly during treatment and safer agents are available. Streptomycin is used in the treatment of some uncommon infections such as brucellosis and plague, as an adjunct to penicillin in streptococcal endocarditis, and in tuberculosis.

### Kanamycin and Neomycin

Kanamycin and neomycin are active against most enteric bacilli but not against *P. aeruginosa*. Kanamycin is used only infrequently. Neomycin is a poorly absorbed local intestinal antibiotic that can be given orally or used topically, but is far too toxic for parenteral use.

### Spectinomycin

Spectinomycin (Trobicin) is an aminocyclitol antibiotic, active *in vitro* against a number of gram-positive and gram-negative bacteria, but it is used solely as an alternate treatment of *N. gonorrhoeae*. Spectinomycin is administered intramuscularly, and the single dose usually used for gonorrhea is well tolerated.

**Preparations.** Because none of the aminoglycosides is absorbed significantly orally, these drugs are given intramuscularly or intravenously. Oral neomycin and kanamycin are available for their local effect on facultative intestinal bacteria. Gentamicin, netilmycin, and tobramycin are pharmacologically very similar; amikacin has a longer half-life.

**Pharmacology.** The aminoglycosides are well distributed in most tissues and body fluids, but have very low intracellular levels. They do not achieve therapeutic CSF levels in children (except in neonates) or adults, even in the presence of inflammation. All available aminoglycosides are excreted essentially unchanged in the urine. Dosage reduction is essential in patients whose renal function is even mildly impaired.

**Side Effects and Toxicity.** The aminoglycosides have the lowest therapeutic–toxic ratio of the commonly used antimicrobial agents. The eighth cranial nerve and the kidney are the major sites for drug toxicity, with the incidence of toxicity generally related to the intensity and duration of administration. Although any of the aminoglycosides may cause damage to either the auditory or the vestibular portion of the eighth cranial nerve, the auditory portion appears to be the primary site of toxicity from amikacin, kanamycin, and, at a lower order of magnitude, tobramycin and netilmycin. The vestibular portion is the most frequent site for gentamicin and streptomycin toxicity. Improvement in vestibular toxicity may occur, but ototoxicity rarely disappears after discontinuation of therapy. A baseline audiogram should be done in patients anticipated to be receiving long-term aminoglycosides; asymptomatic high-frequency hearing abnormalities unrelated to aminoglycoside usage are fairly common, particularly in the elderly.

Renal function should be monitored at least three times per week during therapy; renal dysfunction is frequent during aminoglycoside therapy, particularly in older people. Renal function abnormalities generally return to baseline level if the antibiotic is discontinued promptly. Clinical studies have not shown consistent differences in nephrotoxicity among the various aminoglycosides currently used. Determination of serum antibiotic concentration is the best way to guide dosage levels. Peak and trough antibiotic levels should be measured on the second full day of therapy and the dosage adjusted. Formulas and nomograms are available to calculate aminoglycoside dosage on the basis of body weight and renal function. Certain diuretics such as furosemide potentiate aminoglycoside ototoxicity, and their concurrent use should be avoided when possible.

**Indications.** Aminoglycosides should be restricted to the treatment of infections not susceptible to other antimicrobial agents and to the initial treatment of serious presumptive gram-negative bacillary infections in which, because of nosocomial acquisition or other circumstances, resistance to other agents is likely. Spectinomycin is indicated as an alternate treatment for genital or disseminated gonorrhea in cephalosporin-allergic patients.

### Vancomycin

Vancomycin (Vancocin, Vancoled) is active against most gram-positive bacteria, including streptococci, methicillin-resistant staphylococci, enterococci, and *C. difficile*, the agent of antibiotic-associated (pseudomembranous) colitis. Vancomycin resistance in enterococci is common in many hospitals, but resistance in *S. aureus* has not been reported. Gram-negative bacteria are generally resistant.

**Preparations.** For systemic use, vancomycin is available only as an intravenous preparation. The drug is not absorbed after oral administration, and the oral preparation is useful only for intraluminal intestinal disease (*C. difficile*).

**Pharmacology.** Vancomycin diffuses readily into most body fluids except CSF, although there is some penetration in the presence of inflammation. A small percentage of the drug is inactivated, but 90% or more is excreted unchanged into the urine.

**Side Effects and Toxicity.** Vancomycin must be administered intravenously over at least 1 h to avoid hypotension or other side effects (*red man syndrome*) of rapid administration. Thrombophlebitis at the administration site is frequent. Auditory nerve toxicity may occur. Measurement of the serum vancomycin concentration is desirable because of the variability in levels achieved after a given dose to different individuals and because of the effect of renal insufficiency on excretion. Allergic reactions to vancomycin are not common.

**Indications.** Vancomycin is the drug of choice for methicillin-resistant *S. aureus*

(MRSA) infections and is useful as an alternative drug to penicillins in the treatment of serious *S. aureus*, *S. epidermidis*, and enterococcal infections when the bacterium is resistant to the penicillins or when allergy precludes their use. When vancomycin is used for enterococcal endocarditis, it should be given in combination with an aminoglycoside. Oral vancomycin is used in the treatment of *C. difficile*–associated diarrhea, but its use has been discouraged in hospitals because of possible increased incidence of vancomycin-resistant enterococci.

## Metronidazole

Metronidazole (Flagyl, generic) is effective in the treatment of trichomoniasis and amoebiasis. More recently, its excellent activity against obligate anaerobic bacteria has been recognized. The drug is effective against gram-negative anaerobic bacilli, including *B. fragilis*, anaerobic gram-positive and gram-negative cocci, and *Clostridia*. Facultative bacteria are resistant.

**Preparations and Pharmacology.** Metronidazole is available in oral and intravenous preparations. It is well absorbed after oral administration, with serum levels similar to those achieved by equivalent intravenous administration. Metronidazole is metabolized in the liver and excreted primarily as an active metabolite in the urine. The drug is minimally protein-bound and is widely distributed in body compartments, including CSF.

**Side Effects and Toxicity.** Anorexia, a metallic taste, and occasionally nausea and vomiting may be observed with metronidazole, which also has an Antabuse-like effect; patients should avoid alcohol while taking metronidazole. Phlebitis after intravenous administration, reversible neutropenia, and rash occur. Peripheral neuropathy and central nervous system (CNS) toxicity have been observed, primarily after high-dose intravenous administration. Long-term administration of metronidazole is carcinogenic in rats and mice, and the drug is mutagenic in bacteria, but follow-up studies in humans have not shown an increased incidence of malignancy.

**Indications.** Metronidazole is indicated for the treatment of trichomoniasis, amoebiasis, and giardiasis. Metronidazole is bactericidal *in vitro* against *B. fragilis*, and thus is preferred for treatment of *B. fragilis* endocarditis. In addition, its excellent penetration into the CSF makes it the primary choice for *B. fragilis* meningitis. It is commonly used for the treatment of brain or liver abscess, and for empiric management of intraabdominal infection in combination with aminoglycosides. Because of metronidazole's lack of activity against facultative or microaerophilic bacteria, it should not be used alone in infections in which these bacteria may be implicated.

## Sulfonamides, Trimethoprim, and Trimethoprim-Sulfamethoxazole

### Agents to Know in this Group:
*Trimethoprim-Sulfamethoxazole (IV, oral)*

Many of the strains of both gram-positive and gram-negative bacteria originally susceptible to the sulfonamides (the first available antibiotics) have become resistant. Although many Enterobacteriaceae remain susceptible to concentrations of sulfonamides generally achieved in the urine, use of the combination of trimethoprim and sulfamethoxazole has supplanted sulfonamides alone for treatment of urinary tract infections. Trimethoprim is a synthetic antimicrobial active against many gram-positive and gram-negative bacteria, excluding *P. aeruginosa*. It is available as a single drug but is usually combined with a sulfonamide because the two drugs inhibit folic acid synthesis at sequential stages, resulting in synergistic activity against certain bacteria. The combination is effective against *Pneumocystis carinii*.

**Preparations.** Trimethoprim is available alone as an oral preparation (Trimpex, Proloprim) and in combination with sulfamethoxazole in a 1:5 trimethoprim-sulfamethoxazole ratio, both as oral and intravenous preparations (Bactrim, Septra, generic). Sulfisoxazole (Gantrisin, generic), which is highly soluble in the urine, is administered orally for urinary tract infections, and is combined with erythromycin ethylsuccinate (Pediazole) for otitis media. Sulfamethoxazole (Gantanol, generic) is used alone for the treatment of urinary tract infections.

**Pharmacology.** Trimethoprim is widely distributed in body tissues and fluids, including the normal CSF and prostatic fluid. A variable amount, usually about one half of a trimethoprim dose, is excreted unchanged in the urine, primarily by glomerular filtration. Another major portion of the drug is inactivated in the liver, and a small amount is secreted in the bile. A portion of sulfonamide drugs is acetylated in the liver to inactive conjugates. The proportion of drug thus inactivated varies with the individual and with the particular sulfonamide. Both the free and the conjugated forms are excreted in the urine, primarily by glomerular filtration.

**Side Effects and Toxicity.** Gastrointestinal side effects are unusual with lower doses of trimethoprim-sulfamethoxazole. Reversible hematologic toxicity includes hemolysis in glucose-6-phosphate dehydrogenase (G6PD)–deficient individuals as well as agranulocytosis, which is usually reversible. Thrombocytopenia, acute hemolytic anemia, and megaloblastic eythropoiesis are less common. Nephrotoxicity has been reported rarely. Allergy, particularly with rash, is relatively frequent and likely related to the sulfonamide. It is usually unclear which of the components of the combination is responsible for other adverse reactions.

**Indications.** Trimethoprim-sulfamethoxazole is indicated for the treatment of susceptible urinary tract infection, as are sulfonamides or trimethoprim alone; however, treatment with the combination is highly efficacious and economical and has become the standard of treatment. Trimethoprim-sulfamethoxazole is indicated for the treatment of shigellosis and, in high doses, for the treatment and prophylaxis of *P. carinii* pneumonia. Trimethoprim-sulfamethoxazole is used for treatment of *H. influenzae* otitis media and for treatment of bronchitis in adults. Sulfonamides alone or trimethoprim-sulfamethoxazole are used to treat nocardiosis, and in otitis media sulfisoxizole is used in combination with erythromycin.

## Quinolones

### Agents to Know in this Group:

*Ciprofloxacin* (*IV, oral*)
*Ofloxacin* (*IV, oral*)

Nalidixic acid (NegGram) was introduced in 1962 for treatment of urinary tract infections, but rapid development of resistance was noted, which limited usefulness. Additional fluorinated quinolones were subsequently developed with an extremely broad spectrum of activity, good absorption after oral administration, and effectiveness many times that of nalidixic acid. These agents inhibit DNA gyrase, which is required for DNA supercoiling.

**Preparations and Spectrum of Activity.** Nalidixic acid and norfloxacin (Noroxin) are poorly absorbed, provide low serum levels after oral administration, and are used for treatment of urinary tract infections. Norfloxacin, however, has a much broader spectrum, including *P. aeruginosa*. Ciprofloxacin (Cipro) and ofloxacin (Floxin) are better absorbed and are useful for treatment of systemic as well as urinary infections; each is also available in IV form. Lomefloxacin (Maxaquin) is available in oral form for the treatment of bronchitis and urinary tract infection and enoxacin (Penetrex) is an oral agent for urinary tract infection and gonorrhea. Ofloxacin and ciprofloxacin have high activity against Enterobacteriaceae, *P. aeruginosa, Salmonella, Shigella, Staphylococcus aureus, Moraxella catarrhalis, H. influenzae, N. gonorrhoeae, L. pneumophila, Chlamydia trachomatis,* mycoplasma, and many mycobacteria. Activity against streptococci and enterococci is moderate. Anaerobic activity is low. The spectrum of the other fluoroquinolones is not as broad as for ciprofloxacin and ofloxacin.

**Pharmacology.** The distribution of the quinolones into most extravascular sites is good, including intracellular. Ciprofloxacin does not enter CSF as well as ofloxacin. Fluoroquinolones are metabolized by the liver and excreted by the kidney. Simultaneous administration of antacids, sucralfate, bismuth, zinc, and iron with the fluoroquinolones results in binding of the fluoroquinolone in the gastrointestinal tract blocking absorption. Serum levels following oral administration of ciprofloxacin and ofloxacin are similar to those obtained IV.

**Side Effects and Toxicity.** Adverse effects of fluoroquinolones are uncommon and consist primarily of gastrointestinal effects or central nervous system toxicity (headache, dizziness, anxiety, agitation, insomnia). Seizures and psychotic reactions have been reported. Dermatologic effects, including photosensitization, are reported, but are less frequent than for doxycycline when treating traveler's diarrhea. Quinolones other than nalidixic acid are not approved for use in children under 16 years because of possible damage to developing cartilage. Ciprofloxacin causes a 20–30% increase in theophylline levels when the two are administered together and enoxacin causes a 250–350% increase in theophylline levels.

**Indications.** Use of quinolones as primary treatment is indicated for complicated urinary tract and gastrointestinal infections. They are the only oral agents effective against *P. aeruginosa* infections. Ciprofloxacin and ofloxacin also have proved effective in therapy of infections of the respiratory tract, skin, soft tissues, bone, and joint, and those associated with sexual transmission. Caution in treating *S. pneumoniae* infections with ciprofloxacin is urged because of reported treatment failures. Systemic fluoroquinolones are alternate agents for treating gonorrhea.

### Nitrofurantoin

Nitrofurantoin achieves therapeutic antibacterial levels in the urine and is used only for urinary tract infections. Many strains of *E. coli* and gram-positive cocci, such as enterococci, are susceptible to nitrofurantoin. Other Enterobacteriaceae are much less susceptible.

**Preparations.** Nitrofurantoin is available in the standard oral form (Furadantin) and in a macrocrystalline form (Macrodantin).

**Pharmacology.** Therapeutic levels of nitrofurantoin are achieved only in the urine and, perhaps, in renal tissue. Nitrofurantoin is well absorbed orally. About one third of an administered dose is excreted in therapeutically active form in the urine; the rest is inactivated.

**Side Effects and Toxicity.** Nausea and vomiting are frequent dosage-related side effects. These effects may be related to the rate of absorption of the drug and may be less severe with the less rapidly absorbed macrocrystalline form. Nitrofurantoin may precipitate acute hemolysis in patients with G6PD-deficient red blood cells. Peripheral neuritis may occur, usually in patients with decreased renal function; the drug should be stopped if paresthesias occur. Pulmonary infiltration of an acute or chronic nature is rare. Nitrofurantoin should not be used in patients with significant renal impairment. Its therapeutic activity is less, and the incidence of toxicity is high in such patients.

**Indications.** Nitrofurantoin is useful in the treatment and suppression of infections limited to the lower urinary tract due to susceptible bacteria, particularly *E. coli* and enterococci.

### Rifamycins

**Agent to Know in this Group:**

*Rifampin (IV, oral)*

Rifampin is active against many mycobacteria, against *Neisseria* species, and against many gram-positive bacteria. The possible synergistic activity of rifampin in combination with other antibiotics and with antifungal agents is being investigated in certain refractory infections. Rifampin is not indicated for the treatment of meningococcal disease but is useful for prophylaxis of potential pharyngeal carriers of meningococci or haemophilus. Emergence of resistance occurs frequently when it is used as a single agent. Therefore, when rifampin is used to treat established infection, it should be in conjunction with another agent. Rifampin is an established first-line agent for the treatment of *M. tuberculosis*. A related rifamycin, rifabutin, is available for use in advanced HIV-infected patients for the prevention of disseminated *M. avium-intracellulare* infection.

## ANTIFUNGAL AGENTS

Many circumstances in which fungi are isolated do not require therapy. When therapy is indicated, however, there are only a relatively few available agents. Antimicrobial susceptibility testing of fungi is technically difficult and is available only in specialized laboratories. Susceptibility testing is most useful when susceptibility to an antifungal agent cannot be predicted empirically.

### Amphotericin B

Amphotericin B (Fungizone) is active against most fungi that cause human disease. Intrinsic resistance to the drug is uncommon. Amphotericin B binds to fungi in two ways, a reversible binding at lower drug concentrations that causes increased permeability of fungal membranes and irreversible binding only at higher drug concentrations that accounts for fungicidal activity by the drug. Synergistic antifungal activity has been demonstrated *in vitro* by the combination of amphotericin B with several different antifungal drugs. Increased efficacy has been demonstrated clinically in cryptococcal meningitis by the combination of amphotericin B with flucytosine. In addition, amphotericin B acts as an immunoadjuvant and thus may enhance host resistance.

**Preparations and Pharmacology.** Amphotericin B is administered intravenously as a colloidal suspension. Neither its tissue distribution nor its metabolism is well understood. The drug is excreted in the urine over a period of weeks following a single dose. Serum levels are unaffected by renal function, and dosage need not be adjusted in patients with initially poor renal function. Treatment for refractory meningitis, such as that due to coccidioidomycosis, is given intrathecally. Amphotericin B may be used intraarticularly in joint infections. Liposomal amphotericin preparations may be associated with improved therapeutic ratio and are under development.

**Side Effects and Toxicity.** Caution is indicated with amphotericin B, the most toxic antimicrobial in common use today. Major toxic effects include tubular and glomerular renal dysfunction, anemia, and hypokalemia. Side effects include chills, fever, nausea, vomiting, and myalgias with the infusion, as well as phlebitis at the site of administration. The side effects appear to be ameliorated by administration of a small initial test dose with gradual increase in the daily dosage to therapeutic levels. Toxicity is less if the daily dosage is kept relatively low. Renal function, serum potassium, and hemoglobin must be monitored during therapy.

**Indications.** Amphotericin B is the standard therapy for many systemic fungal infections, including coccidioidomycosis, histoplasmosis, blastomycosis, aspergillosis, and cryptococcosis. It should be given in combination with flucytosine (5-FC) for cryptococcal meningitis.

## Flucytosine (5-Fluorocytosine)

Flucytosine (Ancobon) is active *in vitro* against most *Cryptococcus neoformans*, against about half of *Candida* species, and against some other opportunistic fungi. Increasing resistance during treatment of both cryptococcal and candidal infections is frequent when 5-FC is used alone.

**Preparations and Pharmacology.** 5-FC is available as an oral preparation. The drug is very widely distributed in body compartments, including the CSF. It is excreted unchanged in the urine.

**Side Effects and Toxicity.** The major side effects are gastrointestinal, including nausea, vomiting, and diarrhea. Thrombocytopenia, leukopenia, and anemia occur infrequently and appear to be dose related. Careful evaluation of initial renal function and monitoring during treatment, particularly when amphotericin B is used concurrently, is necessary to avoid overdosage.

**Indications.** Flucytosine is indicated in combination with amphotericin B in the treatment of cryptococcal meningitis and occasionally in the treatment of other cryptococcal or candidal infections. 5-FC is usually given in combination with amphotericin B.

## Imidazole Antifungal Agents

### Agents to Know in this Group:

*Fluconazole (IV, oral)*
*Itraconazole (oral)*

Miconazole (Monostat), now primarily a topical agent used for dermatophyte and superficial candidal infections, was the first in a promising series of new antifungal agents, the imidazoles. The agents act by inhibiting synthesis of ergosterol, an essential component of fungal membranes. Ketoconazole (Nizoral) is active against dermatophytes and has been used effectively in many systemic mycoses, including those due to *Blastomyces dermatitidis, Histoplasma capsulatum, Coccidioides immitis, Cryptococcus neoformans,* and *Candida* species. Fluconazole (Diflucan) has been used in therapy of cryptococcal meningitis and severe candidal infections. Itraconazole (Sporanox) is effective against blastomyces, histoplasma, and aspergillus.

**Preparations and Pharmacology.** Ketoconazole is well absorbed from the gastrointestinal tract in the presence of gastric acid and is available as an oral preparation. It does not enter CSF in therapeutic concentrations. Fluconazole is well absorbed from the gastrointestinal tract, independent of acidity, and achieves effective CSF levels in acute therapy and for maintenance therapy of cryptococcal meningitis. It is also available for IV use. Itraconazole bioavailability is 55% by the oral route. It is highly bound (>99%) to serum proteins and is widely distributed into lipophilic tissues. CSF levels are negligible. Ketoconazole is largely metabolized by the liver, and excretion in the urine is minimal. Fluconazole is excreted largely (80%) unchanged in the urine, and has about 11% hepatic metabolites also excreted in the urine. Itraconazole is almost completely metabolized in the liver with essentially no active drug excreted in the urine, although about 40% of parent drug is excreted in the urine as inactive metabolites.

**Side Effects and Toxicity.** Ketoconazole has been associated with rare serious hepatocellular toxicity, but is more often associated with anorexia, nausea, vomiting, and rash. The drug is not absorbed in the absence of gastric acid. It also causes a dose-dependent depression of serum testosterone and inhibited cortisol responses to adrenocorticotropic hormone (ACTH). Fluconazole does not inhibit testosterone or cortisol synthesis, but is associated with allergic reactions, drug interactions with rifamycins, and has been rarely associated with severe hepatitis. Gastrointestinal symptoms (nausea, vomiting) and allergic reactions (rash) are the most common side effects of itraconazole. Hepatitis is a rare complication.

**Indications.** Fluconazole is an alternative therapy to amphotericin B for treating cryptococcal meningitis and is used for maintenance therapy following cryptococcal meningitis in AIDS patients. It is also an alternative therapy for coccidioidomycosis and candidiasis. Itraconazole is indicated for primary treatment of blastomycosis, as primary therapy for histoplasmosis in immunocompetent patients, and as an alternate therapy for aspergillosis.

# ANTIVIRAL AGENTS

## Adamantanes

### Agent to Know in this Group:

*Rimantidine (oral)*

Amantadine (Symmetrel) and rimantidine (Flumadine) are active against influenza A virus but not against influenza B or other respiratory viruses. The drugs inhibit viral uncoating.

**Preparations and Pharmacology.** Amantadine and rimantidine are well absorbed after oral administration; amantidine is excreted unchanged in the urine, but rimantidine is extensively metabolized in the liver, with less than 25% of parent drug excreted in urine.

**Side Effects and Toxicity.** Amantidine may cause reversible neuropsychiatric symptoms such as confusion, anxiety, insomnia, and hallucinations, particularly in the elderly. Rimantidine, in contrast, has very few neurologic side effects; nausea, vomiting, and anorexia are more common.

**Indications.** Amantadine or rimantidine may be used as a supplement to an influenza immunization program for the prevention of influenza A in those who may already have been exposed and are most susceptible to its complications—the elderly and those with chronic illnesses. Both agents have been demonstrated to decrease airway resistance and to shorten the course of clinical influenza A if given within 48 h after the onset of symptoms. They are usually prescribed for high-risk individuals, and rimantidine is preferred because of its greater activity and lower side-effect profile.

## Nucleoside Analogs

### Agent to Know in this Group:

Acyclovir (*IV, oral*)

This group of antiviral agents inhibits viral DNA synthesis after they are activated by thymidine kinase to become inhibitors of viral polymerases. Host cell DNA polymerase is affected only at much higher levels. Acyclovir (Zovirax) is a purine that is effective against herpes simplex virus type 1 (HSV-1), HSV-2, and varicella-zoster virus (VZV). The activity of acyclovir against cytomegalovirus (CMV) is much less, and the drug is not clinically useful in treating CMV infections. Famciclovir (Famvir) is similar to acyclovir (it is a prodrug of penciclovir) and is also active against HSV-1, HSV-2, and VZV, but is approved in the United States for use only for VZV infections. Ganciclovir (Cytovene) is also active against the herpes viruses, but has a uniquely high activity against CMV, for which it is primarily used. Resistance to the nucleoside analogs occurs when the virus does not code for thymidine kinase or when the viral DNA polymerase is not inhibited by the drug. Herpes simplex mutants resistant by the first mechanism occur naturally and may be induced by the drugs.

**Preparations and Pharmacology.** Acyclovir is available in intravenous, oral, and topical forms. Serum concentrations of the systemic preparations are increased by renal failure. Serum levels are found to be much higher after intravenous administration than after ingestion of the oral preparation. With either preparation, the dose should be reduced and the dosage interval increased in individuals with impaired renal function. Famciclovir is available only in oral form and has a half-life of 2–3 h. Ganciclovir is administered intravenously and has a half-life of 3–4 h. An oral preparation is also available.

**Toxicity and Side Effects.** Acyclovir has caused nephrotoxicity, neurotoxicity, nausea, vomiting, and rash. Famciclovir administration has been accompanied by nausea and headache, but at no higher rate than placebo in controlled studies. Ganciclovir is much more toxic and causes granulocytopenia (40%) and thrombocytopenia (20%), which are usually reversible. Other side effects have included rash, fever, phlebitis, CNS symptoms, and abnormal liver-function tests. Ganciclovir is teratogenic, carcinogenic, and causes aspermatogenesis in animals.

**Indications.** Intravenous acyclovir is indicated for presumptive or definite herpes simplex encephalitis and for HSV and VZV infections in immunocompromised hosts. Oral acyclovir is used to prophylax against frequent HSV recurrences, to treat primary and recurrent HSV infection, and to treat herpes zoster infections in normal hosts. Famciclovir is used to treat zoster in the normal host. Ganciclovir is used to treat vision-threatening CMV retinitis and other life-threatening CMV infections in immunocompromised patients. Ganciclovir given with intravenous gamma globulin may have some efficacy in CMV pneumonitis in marrow transplant recipients, and it has been found to prevent CMV pneumonitis in CMV-infected marrow recipients. Oral ganciclovir is used for prophylaxis against CMV disease and maintenance therapy of CMV infection.

### Foscarnet

Foscarnet (Foscavir) is an analog of inorganic pyrophosphate that acts by inhibiting the pyrophosphate-binding sites on viral DNA polymerases and reverse transcriptases. It does not require thymidine kinases for activation. It is active against all of the herpes viruses, HSV-1, HSV-2, VZV, CMV, EBV, and human herpes virus 6 (HHV-6), including ganciclovir-resistant strains of CMV.

**Preparations and Pharmacology.** Foscarnet is available only in intravenous form, and has a half-life of 3 h.

**Side Effects and Toxicity.** Foscarnet is relatively toxic, particularly to the kidneys, in most patients who receive it. It also causes electrolyte and mineral abnormalities (hypokalemia, hypocalcemia, hypomagnesemia, hypophosphatemia), and may be neurotoxic, causing seizures.

**Indications.** Foscarnet is approved for the treatment of CMV retinitis but may be useful for other serious CMV and herpes virus infections in immunocompromised patients. It is the treatment of choice for acyclovir-resistant HSV-1 infection and is weakly active against HIV-1.

### Ribavirin

Ribavirin (Virazole) is a broad-spectrum antiviral drug with an unclear mechanism of action. *In vitro*, ribavirin is active against both DNA and RNA viruses. Its clinical indications, however, are quite limited at present to the inhalational treatment of respiratory syncytial virus (RSV) infection.

**Preparations.** Ribavirin is available as an aerosol requiring special nebulization equipment for treatment of certain respiratory viral agents and as an intravenous drug for Lassa fever, an arenavirus infection.

**Pharmacology.** Following aerosol administration, ribavirin is absorbed systemically to some degree, and accumulation in red blood cells (RBCs) has been documented. Metabolism and excretion are poorly understood.

**Side Effects and Toxicity.** Use of aerosolized ribavirin with a respirator can lead to malfunction secondary to drug precipitation. A normochromic, normocytic anemia can occur, and rash and conjunctivitis are reported after aerosol exposure. In animals, ribavirin is mutagenic, teratogenic, tumor-promoting, and toxic to the reproductive system. It is contraindicated in pregnancy and some recommend that pregnant health care workers be excluded from caring for patients being treated.

**Indications.** Aerosolized ribavirin is indicated for seriously ill infants or for those with underlying cardiac or pulmonary disease who develop RSV infection. Intravenous ribavirin is used for Lassa fever and other hemorrhagic viral fevers, and for hantavirus pulmonary infection.

### Antiretroviral Agents

#### Agent to Know in this Group:

*Zidovudine (IV, oral)*

Zidovudine, formerly termed azidothymidine (AZT), was the original therapy of choice for HIV-1 infections. Zidovudine (Retrovir) is a thymidine analog that is phosphorylated to a triphosphate, which interferes with HIV viral reverse transcriptase and thus with viral replication. Dideoxyinosine (ddI) (Didanosine, Videx), dideoxycytidine (ddC) (also called zalcitabine)(HIVID), stavudine (D4T), and lamivudine (3TC) are additional nucleoside analogues that are used in combination or as alternative agents to zidovudine. An additional class of antiretroviral agents, the protease inhibitors, including saquinavir (Inverase), ritonavir (Norvir), and indinavir (Crixiran) are also available for HIV therapy.

**Preparations.** Zidovudine is usually administered orally, although an intravenous preparation is also used. ddI and ddC are oral agents.

**Pharmacology.** Zidovudine is well absorbed and is rapidly glucuronidated. Both the parent drug and the glucuronide are excreted in urine. The drug is widely distributed and penetrates CSF.

**Side Effects and Toxicity.** The usual dose-limiting toxicities of zidovudine are anemia and neutropenia, usually occurring with higher doses and in those with advanced HIV disease. Recombinant erythropoietin has decreased the need for transfusions. Long-term zidovudine use may cause a toxic myopathy. Initial adverse effects include headache, myalgia, anorexia, nausea, vomiting, and insomnia. Zidovudine is carcinogenic in rodents, and its safety in pregnancy is unknown. Pancreatitis, peripheral neuropathy, bone marrow suppression, and gastrointestinal side effects occur with ddI. Peripheral neuropathy, bone marrow suppression, and gastrointestinal side effects occur with ddC.

**Indications.** Zidovudine decreases the frequency of opportunistic infections and prolongs survival in patients with HIV infection. It also delays progression of disease in HIV-infected adults with CD4 lymphocyte counts of less than $500/mm^3$ and few or no symptoms. Intolerance to zidovudine or HIV disease progression while taking zidovudine are the usual indications for use of ddI or ddC. Combination therapy with several nucleoside analogues or a nucleoside analogue with protease inhibitors appears to be the most effective current HIV therapy.

# REFERENCES

### Books

Baron, E. J., Peterson, L. R., and Finegold, S. M. *Bailey & Scott's Diagnostic Microbiology.* 9th ed. St. Louis: Mosby-Year Book, Inc., 1994.

Davis, B. D., et al. *Microbiology.* 4th ed. Philadelphia: J. B. Lippincott Co., 1990.

Galasso, G. J., Whitley, R. J., and Merigan, T. C. *Antiviral Agents and Viral Diseases of Man.* 3rd ed. New York: Raven Press, 1990.

Sherris, J. C. *Medical Microbiology.* 2nd ed. New York: Elsevier Science Publishers, 1990.

### Review Articles

Abramowicz, M., ed. The choice of antibacterial drugs. *Med. Lett. 36*:53, 1994.

Abramowicz, M., ed. Drugs for viral infections. *Med. Lett. 36*:27, 1994.

Abramowicz, M., ed. New drugs for HIV infection. *Med. Lett. 38*:35, 1996.

Baley, J. E. Pharmacokinetics, outcome of treatment, and toxic effects of amphotericin B and 5-fluorocytosine in neonates. *J. Pediatr. 116*:791, 1990.

Davies, J. Inactivation of antibiotics and the dissemination of resistance genes. *Science 264*:375, 1994.

Finegold, S. M. Mechanisms of resistance in anaerobes and new developments in testing. *Diagn. Microbiol. Infect. Dis. 12*:117S, 1989.

Murray, B. E. Problems and mechanisms of antimicrobial resistance. *Infect. Dis. Clin. North Am. 3*:423, 1989.

Neu, H. C. The crisis in antibiotic resistance. *Science 257*: 1064, 1992.

Nikaido, H. Prevention of drug access to bacterial targets: Permeability barriers and active reflux. *Science 264*:382, 1994.

Robinson, P. A. Fluconazole for life-threatening fungal infections. *Rev. Infect. Dis. 12*(Suppl. 3): S349, 1990.

Spratt, B. G. Resistance to antibiotics mediated by target alterations. *Science 264*:388, 1994.

Wolfson, J. S., and Hooper, D. C. Bacterial resistance to quinolones: Mechanisms and clinical importance. *Rev. Infect. Dis. 11*(Suppl. 5):S960, 1989.

Wood, M. J., and Geddes, A. M. Antiviral therapy. *Lancet 2*:1189, 1987.

# 39

# ANTIMICROBIAL AGENT SUSCEPTIBILITY TESTING AND MONITORING OF DRUG THERAPY

XUEDONG WANG, M.D., PH.D. and
LANCE R. PETERSON, M.D.

The clinical microbiology laboratory plays a central role in antimicrobial agent selection and use by physicians. One of the most important tasks of the laboratory is the performance of routine antimicrobial susceptibility tests on significant bacterial isolates. An obvious reasons for this is that bacteria comprise by far the most common cause of infectious diseases treated by physicians, and we have become accustomed to using specific microbial susceptibility data for directing therapy, especially in seriously ill patients. The goal of a susceptibility test is to predict by *in vitro* means the likely outcome of treating a specific patient's infection with a particular antimicrobial agent.

With some organisms, empiric therapy remains effective because significant resistance problems have not yet developed (e.g., penicillin therapy for group A, beta-hemolytic streptococci, erythromycin with or without rifampin for *Legionella*, and penicillin for *Neis-seria meningitidis* infections). In contrast, susceptibility testing is most important with species that do not have known, stable antimicrobial susceptibility patterns such as many members of the Enterobacteriaceae family, *Staphylococcus* species, and now even *Streptococcus pneumoniae* and *Neisseria gonorrhoeae*. Variation in susceptibility of microorganisms to different antimicrobial agents may be caused by mutation, transmissible episomes coding for drug resistance, or by induction and derepression of beta-lactamase enzymes. The use of *in vitro* antimicrobial susceptibility testing needs to separate resistant from susceptible organisms rapidly and reliably, thereby facilitating the selection of effective antimicrobial agents.

The selection of an antimicrobial agent for treatment of an infection depends on several factors, including the mode of action of the agent, the optimal method of administration, tissue distribution, the rate of metabolism or

594

excretion, drug-related toxicity, and cost. The site of infection, the type of microorganism involved, and the historical clinical experience with the therapeutic outcome of specific infections to guide treatment are also important factors.

## INDICATIONS FOR SUSCEPTIBILITY TESTING

Testing of all bacterial isolates for antimicrobial susceptibility is neither necessary nor desirable. For instance, alpha-hemolytic (viridans) streptococci are normally present in the throat and should not be tested for drug susceptibility unless they represent blood culture isolates and are implicated etiologically in infective endocarditis. Similarly, there is no reason to test routinely the susceptibility of group A, beta-hemolytic streptococci to penicillin, since they are invariably susceptible. Testing of identical, multiple isolates from the same patient within 24 or 48 h is also unnecessary, since it can be assumed they arise from an identical clone and have the same drug susceptibility. An exception to this rule is when an organism persists accompanied by continued evidence of clinical infection for several days. In this setting, resistance may have developed to the initial therapy, and repeat susceptibility testing can detect this reason for drug failure.

Staphylococci should be tested for susceptibility to antimicrobial agents, since resistance to penicillin and other drugs is frequent and of therapeutic importance. Members of the family Enterobacteriaceae show wide variation of susceptibility, partially due to the presence of transmissible episomes carrying drug resistance genes. The appearance of an episome-carrying variant of the infecting microorganism or replacement by a similar but drug-resistant strain (as a superinfection) can rapidly alter the course of an infection. Here "follow-up" testing can be life saving when the patient is not responding to treatment as expected clinically.

The appearance of ampicillin-resistant strains of *Haemophilus influenzae* and penicillin-resistant strains of *N. gonorrhoeae* has resulted in the development of several rapid, easily performed procedures to detect resistance due to beta-lactamase (penicillinase). In most instances, the demonstration of beta-lactamase in these organisms is all that is required to establish the need for chemotherapy with alternative antimicrobial agents. This is true for the two organisms mentioned, but laboratories need to remain alert for all types of potential resistance. Emergence of highly resistant strains of pneumococci has also caused laboratories increasingly to test the susceptibility of this organism to multiple agents. Most penicillin resistance in *Streptococcus pneumoniae* is due to altered target site affinity (penicillin-binding protein) rather than beta-lactamase production and must be detected by actual susceptibility testing.

## METHODS FOR ANTIMICROBIAL SUSCEPTIBILITY TESTING

Antimicrobial susceptibility testing is directed toward correlating *in vitro* susceptibility of a microorganism with clinically achievable concentrations of antimicrobial agents, either those found in the blood or at expected sites of infection. The susceptibility is determined by incorporating antimicrobial agents into a culture medium to ascertain whether the microorganism is inhibited from growing or, using nonroutine methods, is killed at different concentrations of the drug. Most susceptibility testing is performed either by one of the several "dilution" methods or by measuring a zone of growth inhibition surrounding paper discs containing specific amounts of the antimicrobial agent. A key to reliable testing is that the laboratory begins with an isolated, pure culture of the microbe at a known inoculum density. Mixed cultures can give unreliable results, often with false and unanticipated resistance. For example, testing *Escherichia coli* mixed with *Staphylococcus aureus* would give results indicating resistance to several agents for each microbe and could be interpreted as showing vancomycin resistance (due to the *E. coli*) in *S. aureus*, an event that has not yet happened worldwide. This is one reason testing can take a day or more beyond the first recognition that an infection is present. Accidental testing of a mixed culture should be considered when a "new" resistant pathogen is discovered.

### Selection of Antimicrobial Agents for Susceptibility Testing

In the past 30 years, numerous antimicrobial agents have been introduced that differ by only slight chemical modifications from the original member of a class of drugs. The modified forms may provide certain improvements in pharmacologic characteristics, such as superior resistance to degradation by gastric acid, improved gastrointestinal absorption, or slower renal excretion. The outcome of *in vitro* susceptibility testing to closely related antimicrobial agents is usually not affected by minor chemical modification of the compounds. For this reason, one representative agent is often chosen, since it is not considered necessary to test microorganisms against more than one tetracycline or one penicillinase-resistant penicillin, for example. Similarly, susceptibility of six to eight first-generation cephalosporins can be determined by the use of a single "class" agent such as cephalothin or cefazolin.

The organism to be tested dictates, to some degree, the appropriate antimicrobial agents selected for testing. The National Committee for Clinical Laboratory Standards (NCCLS, M7-A3, 1993) suggests the antimicrobial agents appropriate for testing of Enterobacteriaceae, *Pseudomonas aeruginosa* and other glucose non-fermenters, staphylococci, enterococci, streptococci, *Haemophilus* species, *Neisseria gonorrhoeae,* and anaerobic bacteria. The NCCLS has recently extended this listing to include recommendations regarding which agents are the most important to test routinely and those that may be tested only by special request or circumstance. Each institution may modify these suggestions depending on what agents are chosen as first-line or recommended therapy within a medical practice. These become the "formulary agents" and are crucial for the laboratory to test and report.

In summary, the final choices regarding routine antibiotic test batteries must be made by cooperative efforts of the microbiology laboratory, the infectious disease section, and the pharmacy service. This final selection is usually done through the pharmacy and therapeutics or infection-control committees. All practitioners must recognize the necessity of periodic changes to the formulary as clinical needs change and new agents are introduced or resistant microbes recognized. This also means that the microbiology laboratory's standard susceptibility testing batteries are likely to require periodic revisions.

## Broth Dilution Tests

One of the earliest methods of semiquantitative antimicrobial susceptibility testing was the macro- or tube-dilution method. This procedure is performed by making serial twofold dilutions of the test antimicrobial agent in a culture medium. Typically, eight or more dilutions of a drug may be prepared in a final volume of 1–2 mL per tube. The drug-containing tubes are then inoculated with the standardized organism suspension to yield a final inoculum density approximating $5 \times 10^5$ colony-forming units (CFUs) per milliliter in each tube. After overnight incubation at 35°C, the tubes are examined for evidence of visible growth in the form of turbidity in tubes containing subinhibitory concentrations of the antibiotic. The smallest amount of the drug that will inhibit visible growth of the microorganism is called the *minimum inhibition concentration (MIC)*. To test actual killing in this system requires subcultures from the tubes showing inhibition of growth after 18–24 h (clear tubes). These are made to fresh, drug-free medium and reincubated for an additional day to determine the minimum bactericidal concentration. The *minimum bactericidal concentration (MBC)* is defined as the lowest concentration of antimicrobial agent that on subculture either fails to show any growth, or results in an arbitrarily defined 99.9% decrease in CFUs compared to the initial inoculum. It is generally considered that antimicrobial agents with a MBC the same as, or within one dilution of, the MIC can be considered lethal or bactericidal agents, whereas antimicrobial agents showing a several-dilution difference between the MIC and the MBC are called inhibitory or bacteriostatic. The distinction between bactericidal and bacteriostatic effects of antimicrobial drugs often is relevant clinically. Bacteriostatic agents should be avoided in those who are immunocompromised, are bacteremic from endocarditis, or have meningitis.

The modification of the tube dilution test that has made broth dilution testing very popular is the miniaturization and automation seen when microtiter trays are adapted for performance of "microdilution" susceptibility tests. Instead of preparing drug dilutions in volumes of 1 mL or greater in test tubes, volumes of 100 $\mu$L are placed in the individual wells of a plastic disposable microtiter tray. Such trays ordinarily contain 96 wells, which permit 12 or more agents to be tested in a range of up to eight twofold dilutions in a single tray. Hundreds of identical microdilution trays can be prepared from a single master set of dilutions in a relatively short period. The prepared testing panels can then be stored frozen or dehydrated until needed for individual tests. Results by this testing are comparable to those obtained by the conventional broth dilution method.

Often, "chemical" modifications in the media used for these tests are made so that results correlate better with clinical outcomes determined in therapeutic trials. For example, to better simulate the *in vivo* conditions, it is recommended that the standard Mueller-Hinton broth be supplemented with $Ca^{2+}$ and $Mg^{2+}$ ions at the physiologic concentrations found in serum. When susceptibility tests are performed in this manner, the result more closely reflects the *in vivo* response of certain bacteria to the antimicrobial tested. This relationship is most apparent between *Pseudomonas aeruginosa* and the aminoglycoside antibiotics. Supplementation of the medium to physiologic concentrations of $Ca^{2+}$ and $Mg^{2+}$ results in significantly higher MICs for these drugs. When agar is used, supplementation is not usually necessary, since varying amounts of inorganic ions are present in the agar because of its derivation from seaweed.

### Agar Dilution Tests

The agar dilution susceptibility test method has nearly as long a history of use as the macrodilution broth method, and is generally considered the reference method to which all other testing is compared for accuracy. The test is performed by incorporating dilutions of antimicrobial agents into partially cooled, molten agar medium dispensed into individual covered (Petri) dishes. Although serial twofold dilutions of the antimicrobial agent can be made with agar in the same manner as with broth culture medium, it is more economical in terms of time and materials to test only several concentrations of drug that bracket the clinically useful range. Meaningful information on the MICs of a large number of microorganisms can be determined with use of only two to five concentrations of the test agent. Plates are inoculated by applying a small controlled-volume droplet of a standardized inoculum suspension onto the surface of the agar. Most often, a 1- to 1.5-$\mu$L "drop" containing approximately $1 \times 10^4$ CFUs of organism is employed. Multipoint inoculators such as a "Steers replicator" place 32–36 different isolates on each plate. Inoculated plates are incubated at 37°C in an ambient air incubator for 18 h. MICs are determined by noting on which plate (each at a specific drug concentration) visible spots of growth of each isolate disappear. An example of the results of this testing is shown in Figure 39–1.

Advantages of the agar dilution test include the ability to test a large number of isolates simultaneously at a relatively low cost, the provision of a widely accepted and highly reproducible semiquantitative result, and the ability to test some fastidious organisms that do not grow well in broth. Disadvantages of this procedure include the fact that it is very costly if only a few isolates are tested, the fact that plates must be freshly prepared and stored for only limited periods before use, and the observation that swarming organisms such as

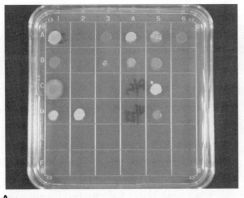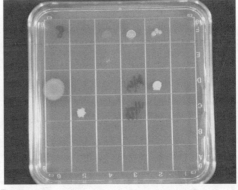

**A**                                    **B**

**FIGURE 39–1.** *A* and *B*, Agar dilution antimicrobial susceptibility plates containing different concentrations of a given drug are inoculated with several species of bacteria from a Steer's replicator. Sensitive organisms are inhibited by the concentration of antimicrobial contained in the plate, and no growth is evident at many points of inoculation; resistant organisms appear as distinct colonies of bacterial growth. MICs are determined by noting at which concentration the visible spots of growth of each isolate disappears. In this figure it is evident that *A* contains a lower concentration of drug, since there are more spots of growth on this plate than the one in *B*.

*Proteus* species can obliterate the growth of other isolates tested on the same plate. This test method detects many types of bacterial resistance mechanisms that other methods do not and is therefore accepted as the reference standard.

## Disc Diffusion Tests

One of the most reliable and popular susceptibility testing methods available is the disc diffusion or Kirby-Bauer procedure. This test consists of exposure of a pure culture of the test microorganism on an agar culture medium to a filter paper disc containing a known amount of an antimicrobial agent. Once the antimicrobial disc has been placed on the agar, diffusion of the agent from the disc produces a concentration gradient of the agent, which in turn inhibits susceptible microorganisms until a critical (low) drug concentration is reached. At this point, further bacterial multiplication is no longer inhibited. The diameter of the zone of inhibition around each antibiotic disc is semilogarithmically related to the actual MIC and is measured to the nearest millimeter (Figure 39–2). Criteria have been established to correlate the diameter of the zone of growth inhibition found on disc-agar diffusion susceptibility tests with the MIC as determined by either broth or agar dilution. An inverse relationship exists between the MIC and the zone of inhibition for rapidly growing bacteria. The larger the inhibitory zone, the lower the corresponding MIC. The results of the disc diffusion test are "qualitative," in that a category of susceptibility (i.e., susceptible, intermediate, or resistant) is derived from the test rather than an MIC. Some would argue, however, that the precision of the disc diffusion test is good enough to determine a "calculated MIC" based on comparing a particular zone size determination with standard curves of that species and drug. A modification of this test has been developed that provides quantitative MIC results. This method, called the E-test, uses strips impregnated with a gradient of antimicrobial agent and the MIC is read directly off numbers on the strip. It correlates well with other methods, but is very costly compared to Kirby-Bauer and some agar dilution approaches.

## Automated Instrument Methods

Robotic-type susceptibility testing instruments present a choice of several levels of automation. Virtually every manufacturer of broth microdilution antimicrobial susceptibility testing panels offers a view box or device to facilitate manual interpretation of results after incubation. Most manufacturers also offer an instrument-assisted reader device that permits the technologist to record the results of manual readings of the panel by use of a video display screen resembling the configuration of the tray, or alternatively, by use of a touch-sensitive template that overlays the microdilution tray. Well-designed reader devices can facilitate data recording and provide a computer-printed report, as well as data storage useful for epidemiology and formulary decisions.

The principle used in most instruments is quantitation of light scattering (comparable to visual assessment of turbidity) associated with increasing numbers of microorganisms indicating growth or, conversely, lack of growth. Cultures are monitored in small cuvettes or wells, and some instruments provide an interpretation within 6 h. Instrumentation may al-

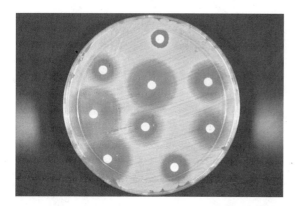

**FIGURE 39–2.** Kirby-Bauer agar diffusion test. An agar plate inoculated with *Escherichia coli* shows a series of paper discs containing different antimicrobial agents. The diameter of the zone of (growth) inhibition is measured and the susceptibility of the microorganism is determined by reference to an interpretative chart.

low the interpretation of susceptibility test end points sooner than manual readings because of the greater sensitivity of the instruments' optical systems to subtle changes in microbial growth. The only serious drawback to this "rapid" testing is that some of the most important resistance mechanisms are not phenotypically apparent until after at least 4–6 h of bacterial growth, and therefore are missed in this type of system, thus giving false-susceptible test results. All of the instruments rely heavily on microprocessor-controlled functions and utilize personal computer hardware to provide final printed reports, antimicrobial susceptibility interpretation, data storage, and information retrieval. Since these automated systems are produced for large markets, they require use of standardized batteries of tested drugs and can be more expensive to use for high-volume laboratories capable of making their own "in-house" testing media. Lately, it has also been realized that many of the automated systems fail to detect some of the newer resistance problems such as penicillin resistance in pneumococci and vancomycin resistance in enterococci, raising serious concern about their utility in larger, complex medical practices.

### Selection of a Testing System

Contemporary clinical microbiology laboratories have many options to choose from in selecting a method for routine antimicrobial susceptibility testing. In an era of great emphasis on cost containment, it is worth reemphasizing that in many settings the most economical susceptibility test method currently available is the Kirby-Bauer disc diffusion test. Its advantages include the fact it is simple to perform, is very reproducible, does not require any special equipment, provides category results readily interpreted by patient care practitioners, and offers great flexibility in selection of drugs for routine testing batteries. Despite the attributes of the disc diffusion test, many laboratories will choose instead one of the commercial microdilution or rapid automated instrument methods. These latter methods offer some real and perceived benefits to the laboratory, including the provision of more rapid or more quantitative results, improved data presentation and storage capabilities, and the possibility of automating certain tasks with satisfactory test accuracy when expertly trained medical technologists are unavailable.

## INTERPRETATION OF RESULTS

Laboratory, or *in vitro*, testing performed determines the organism's "sensitivity" to a given drug. The interpretation of the *in vitro* sensitivity tests is then done to determine if the microbe is susceptible or resistant based on defined interpretative criteria. A determination of susceptibility is typically based on the assumption that the administration of an antimicrobial agent will achieve a serum or tissue level from one- to severalfold greater than the MIC. In reporting the results of susceptibility tests by disc-agar diffusion, three basic terms are used: susceptible, intermediate, and resistant. Susceptible indicates that an infection with the test microorganism will likely respond to the usual dose of an antimicrobial agent recommended for the infection being treated. The term resistant is used for those agents that do not inhibit the test microorganism within the range of achievable blood or tissue levels. Using such an agent typically leads to a very high treatment failure rate. The term intermediate is reserved for microorganisms that may respond to an agent if large doses are used, or when the infection is in a site that usually concentrates the treatment drug (e.g., urine or bile). Some laboratories choose not to use this last term, since it can lead to confusion and inappropriate treatment choices on the part of practitioners if they are not expert in pharmacokinetics and drug–microbial interactions.

It is important to remember that there is no objective evidence supporting the reporting of an actual MIC result as any more clinically relevant than reporting of a category (susceptible, intermediate, or resistant) result in the overall outcome of therapy. Reporting of MIC results may aid an expert knowledgeable in pharmacokinetics and bacterial physiology when selecting from among a group of similar drugs for therapy of infective endocarditis or osteomyelitis, where therapy is likely to be protracted, and in the setting when multidrug resistance is present. For virtually all other infections, however, category results provide the practitioner with the necessary information to select appropriate therapy. Only those physicians specifically trained in infectious diseases or clinical microbiology are likely to be familiar with expected MICs for the multitude of antimicrobial agents presently available. Thus, if MIC results are reported, it is required by regulatory agencies for laboratories to include appropriate interpretative criteria and an interpretation with the report.

## IN VITRO STUDIES OF ANTIMICROBIAL SYNERGISM

Sometimes it is necessary to determine the susceptibility of pathogens to the synergistic action of two or more antimicrobial agents. For example, the determination of synergism is particularly useful in the treatment of patients with endocarditis caused by *Enterococcus faecalis* or *E. faecium*. Optimal treatment of endocarditis caused by these microorganisms requires the use of a cell-wall–active antimicrobial agent, such as penicillin or vancomycin, combined with an aminoglycoside, usually either streptomycin or gentamicin, that inhibits protein synthesis.

The method for studying synergism by *in vitro* tests involves a cross-titration of tube-dilution susceptibility tests, often called "checkerboard testing." This gives the minimum concentration of each agent resulting in the inhibition and killing of the microorganism. The end point may then be reported either as minimum inhibitory or lethal concentrations of the various drugs in combination. Synergy testing can also be done at a limited number of combined concentrations and measured over time in a "time–kill curve" analysis that measures the log decrease in viable microorganisms plotted against time. More killing by a combination of agents than by individual ones indicates synergy. Based on the assumption that no host defect in cellular phagocytic or immune mechanisms exists, combinations of agents sufficient to result in a 99.9% decrease in the number of inoculated microorganisms are considered sufficient to bring about a prompt clinical response. Note in Figure 39–3 that counts of viable bacteria drop significantly at 3 and 7 h with 0.5 µg/mL of ampicillin, 4 µg/mL of gentamicin, or the combination of 0.5 µg/mL ampicillin and 2 µg/mL of gentamicin. In each test, there was a significant decrease in the number of

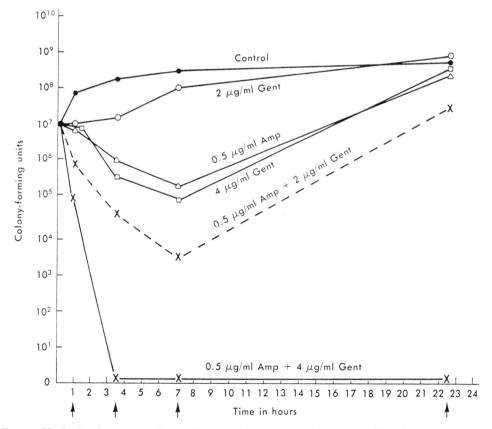

**FIGURE 39–3.** Graphic results of a test for antimicrobial synergism of ampicillin with gentamicin for *Enterococcus faecalis* from a patient with endocarditis. See text under "In Vitro Studies of Antimicrobial Synergism" for interpretation.

viable organisms detected by counts within the first 8 h. However, the counts rebound to at least the inoculated number by 22 h with 0.5 μg/mL ampicillin and 2 μg/mL of gentamicin. In contrast, the combination of 0.5 μg/mL ampicillin and 4 μg/mL of gentamicin appeared highly effective with no bacterial regrowth observed after initial killing.

## PROTEIN BINDING OF ANTIBIOTICS

Critical evaluation of existing data on binding of antibiotics to serum proteins and on pharmacokinetics provides several useful principles for administration of antibiotics. Many agents bind reversibly to serum proteins in varying amounts, resulting in free and bound components that make up the total serum level. Albumin is the major binding protein in the serum for most drugs. Protein binding is of clinical significance because only the unbound portion of the drug is the portion available for antimicrobial effect and for diffusion into interstitial tissue spaces. The free and bound portions of an antimicrobial agent are in equilibrium, and in this manner binding fulfills a storage function. Antibiotics with a high degree of binding to serum proteins are not necessarily inferior. Increasing a given drug's binding to serum proteins from 0% to 90% reduces the concentration of free drug in serum and tissue by only one half because the extravascular space, with low protein binding, is of much larger volume compared to the intravascular space containing albumin that is responsible for drug binding. In addition, the concentration of an antibiotic in extravascular fluid collections such as an abscess is essentially constant despite the marked variability of serum levels seen during intermittent administration of drug. This is because most drug reaches the extravascular space by passive diffusion and large volume-to-surface area ratios at extravascular fluid collection sites dampen the kinetic exchange of antimicrobial molecules.

An important factor in determining a successful therapeutic response is thought to be the maintenance of free drug levels at the infection site above the MIC against the infecting organism. The peak level of the drug at the site of infection never exceeds the peak level of drug in the blood and usually reaches a maximum sometime later than the peak in the serum. The effective delivery of an antimicrobial agent to the site of an infection depends on the presence of an intact blood supply. The presence of necrosis with interruption of the capillary network (abscess) may inhibit this delivery and the diffusion of the agent, offering the invading microorganism protection from effective levels of the drug. Conversely, the active inflammatory process with vascular dilation and increased permeability can aid in the delivery of agents to sites of infection.

## ASSAY OF ANTIMICROBIAL AGENTS IN SERUM AND OTHER BODY FLUIDS

Sometimes it is helpful to determine the total amount of antimicrobial agent in serum, cerebrospinal fluid (CSF), urine, or another clinical specimen to evaluate the agents effectiveness or toxicity. Assay for antimicrobial agents can be done by chemical, biologic, enzymatic, or immunologic procedures. Sulfonamide compounds are the only antimicrobial agents readily measured by chemical means.

The simplest method for measuring antibiotic concentrations is a biologic assay based on the principle of inhibition of bacterial growth by various concentrations of the test agent. In this assay, a microorganism susceptible to the antibiotic to be assayed is incorporated in an agar culture plate. A series of small paper discs impregnated with known concentrations of the antibiotic and a paper disc with the patient's serum are placed on the surface of the agar. After incubation of this type of "reverse Kirby-Bauer" test, the zones of growth inhibition of the drug are compared to reference standards on a semilogarithmic graph paper. From the curve, the serum concentration of the test agent can be easily read. The accuracy of the test is approximately 90%, well within the limits necessary for clinical usefulness.

The development of competitive binding immunoassay procedures for aminoglycosides, such as gentamicin, offers another approach for assay of antimicrobial agents. The simplicity, rapidity, and specificity of the assay have made it a popular method for measuring serum levels of gentamicin, tobramycin, and amikacin, as well as glycopeptide compounds like vancomycin.

In addition to the biologic and immunoassays, a number of other methods are available. Liquid chromatography has been adapted to the assay of a large variety of antimicrobial agents and is rapid and specific. Fluorescence polarization has also been applied successfully to the assay of antibiotics in serum. Most assay procedures are directed toward vancomycin and the aminoglycoside antibiotics due to potential renal toxicity and ototoxicity associated with their use.

## DETERMINATION OF ANTIMICROBIAL TITERS (ACTIVITY) IN SERUM AND BODY FLUIDS

The determination of the serum antibacterial activity contributed by an antimicrobial agent alone or in combination may allow the physician to determine whether they have achieved an optimal effect upon the infecting microorganism. In addition to an antibiotic, there are numerous other antibacterial substances in the blood, including opsonins, specific antibody, lysozyme, beta-lysin, and other poorly defined components, that contribute to the total antimicrobial effect of serum. For these reasons, the determination of serum levels of antimicrobial agents as a means of determining the adequacy of therapy is not always sufficient.

Some consider a more useful testing approach for monitoring patients with severe infection who are receiving antimicrobial therapy to be measurement of the inhibitory or lethal action of serial twofold dilutions of the patient's serum, CSF, urine, or other specimen against a standard inoculum of the microorganism causing the infection. This test is sometimes called the bactericidal or antimicrobial activity titer. The purpose of this test is to measure the net effect of all factors in the test specimen, such as serum or CSF, against the infecting microorganism. Serum antimicrobial activity has been used most often to monitor the treatment of patients with infective endocarditis. Empirically, it has been proposed that serum bactericidal titers of 1:8 or greater are usually associated with favorable outcomes, whereas levels lower than 1:8 may be associated with less favorable results. However, interpretation of this test is fraught with controversy and, if one uses it, an expert interpretation of the results by a practitioner familiar with use of this procedure is highly recommended.

When performing the antimicrobial activity test, one should remember that normal serum contains antimicrobial substances that may have lethal activity in dilutions of 1:4 to

1:6. To perform the test, one draws two serum samples: one within 30–60 min following the administration of the antimicrobial agent, and another just prior to the dose. This provides a "peak" and "trough" level, presumably reflecting the full therapeutic dosing range. The test sera are diluted with media, and a standard number of the patient's microorganisms are added to the diluted serum specimens. The inhibitory levels are determined after 18–24 h of incubation much like in a tube dilution MIC test. The serum bactericidal levels are determined 18–24 h later by subculture as in the MBC test.

It must be emphasized that serum assay and antimicrobial activity levels are not the only considerations when one is choosing an antimicrobial agent. The selection of any antimicrobial agent should be based on careful evaluation of the patient's needs, the likely infecting microbe(s), and the characteristics of individual antimicrobial agents. The significance of all these factors should be carefully placed in perspective.

## CASE HISTORY

### Case History 1

The patient is a newly diagnosed man with leukemia classified as AML-M1. After admission to the hospital he was given chemotherapy and developed fever on hospital day 8 while neutropenic. Amikacin and vancomycin were begun, with eventual defervescence after 4 days. On hospital day 24 he again became febrile to 103°F, and imipenem was added to his therapy because of its very broad antibacterial spectrum. Blood cultures were drawn daily and were positive each day between hospital days 24 and 29 for *Pseudomonas aeruginosa*.

There was no response after 5 days to his empiric therapeutic regimen of vancomycin, amikacin, and imipenem. The microbiology laboratory then reported that the *P. aeruginosa* cultured was resistant to gentamicin (MIC > 8 μg/mL), tobramycin (MIC > 8), piperacillin (MIC > 64), piperacillin-tazobactam (MIC > 64), aztreonam (MIC > 16), ceftazidime (MIC > 64), cefoperazone (MIC > 16), ceftizoxime (MIC > 64), imipenem (MIC > 8), and ticarcillin-clavulanate (MIC > 64).

The organism was only susceptible to ciprofloxacin (MIC < 0.5) and amikacin (MIC = 8) so ciprofloxacin replaced imipenem on day 29. His fever resolved and the bacteremia ceased within 24 h. Amikacin and ciprofloxacin were continued to complete a 4-week therapeutic course, at which time the patient was discharged to home.

## CASE 1 DISCUSSION

This case vividly demonstrates the importance of susceptibility testing, particularly in a severely immunocompromised patient infected with a virulent pathogen like *P. aeruginosa*. This is an organism that often requires two active agents for a successful outcome in patients with bacteremia or pneumonia. Since this patient's organism was highly resistant to many drugs, the empiric therapy chosen was not effective. Response was seen only after *in vitro* susceptibility test results were available and the patient's treatment was changed to include two antimicrobial agents active against his infection. Paying close attention to the laboratory results was life saving in this case.

# REFERENCES

## Books

Baron, E. J., Peterson, L. R., and Finegold, S. M., eds. *Bailey and Scott's Diagnostic Microbiology.* 9th ed. St. Louis: Mosby-Year Book Company, Inc., 1994.

Murray, B., Baron, E. J., Pfaller, M. A., Tenover, F. C., and Yolken, R. H., eds. *Manual of Clinical Microbiology.* 6th ed. Washington, DC: American Society for Microbiology, 1995.

## Review Articles

Peterson, L. R., and Shanholtzer, C. J. Tests for bactericidal effects of antimicrobial agents: Technical performance and clinical relevance. *Clin. Microbiol. Rev.* 5:420–432, 1992.

## Original Articles

Chambers, H. F. Detection of methicillin-resistant staphylococci. *Infect. Dis. Clin. North Am.* 7:425–433, 1993.

Hacek, D. M., Noskin, G. A., Trakas, K., and Peterson, L. R. Initial use of a broth microdilution method suitable for in vitro testing of fungal isolates in a clinical microbiology laboratory. *J. Clin. Microbiol.* 33:1884–1889, 1995.

Isenberg, H. D. Antimicrobial susceptibility testing: A critical evaluation. *J. Antimicrob. Chemother.* 22:73–86, 1988.

Jorgensen, J. H. Antimicrobial susceptibility testing of bacteria that grow aerobically. *Infect. Dis. Clin. North Am.* 7:393–409, 1993.

Jorgensen, J. H. Selection of antimicrobial agents for routine testing in a clinical microbiology laboratory. *Diagn. Microbiol. Infect. Dis.* 16:245–249, 1993.

Jorgensen, J. H. Selection criteria for an antimicrobial susceptibility testing system. *J. Clin. Microbiol.* 31:2841–2844, 1993.

Jones, R. N., Daniel, C., and Edson, D. C. Antimicrobial susceptibility testing trends and accuracy in the United States. *Arch. Pathol. Lab. Med.* 115:429–436, 1991.

Peterson, L. R., and Gerding, D. N. Influence of protein binding of antibiotics on serum pharmacokinetics and extravascular penetration: Clinically useful concepts. *Rev. Infect. Dis.* 2:340–348, 1980.

Peterson, L. R., Gerding, D. N., Fasching, C. E., and Costas-Martinez, C. Assay of 27 antimicrobials using a microbiological method. *Minn. Med.* 66:321–324, 1983.

Wolfson, J. S., and Swartz, M. N. Serum bactericidal activity as a monitor of antibiotic therapy. *N. Engl. J. Med.* 312:968, 1985.

# 40
# PRINCIPLES OF IMMUNIZATION

## STANFORD T. SHULMAN, M.D.

My inquiry into the nature of the cowpox commenced upwards of 25 years ago. My attention to this singular disease was first excited by observing, that among those whom in the country I was frequently called upon to inoculate many resisted every effort to give them the smallpox. These patients I found had undergone a disease they called the cowpox, contracted by milking cows affected with a peculiar eruption on their teats. On inquiry, it appeared that it had been known among the dairies time immemorial, and that a vague opinion prevailed that it was preventive of the smallpox. This opinion I found was comparatively new among them, for all the older families declared they had no such idea in their early days.

During the investigation of the casual cowpox, I was struck with the idea that it might be practicable to propagate the disease by inoculation, after the manner of the smallpox, first from the cow, and finally from one human being to another. I anxiously waited some time for an opportunity of putting this theory to the test. At length the period arrived, and the first experiment was made upon a lad of the name of Phipps, in whose arm a little vaccine virus was inserted, taken from the hand of a young woman who had been accidentally infected by a cow. Notwithstanding the resemblance, which the pustule, this excited on the boy's arm, bore to variolous inoculation, yet as the indisposition attending it was barely perceptible, I could scarcely persuade myself the patient was secure from the smallpox. However, on his being inoculated some months afterwards, it proved that he was secure. The case inspired me with confidence;

and as soon as I could again furnish myself with virus from the cow, I made an arrangement for a series of inoculations. A number of children were inoculated in succession, one from the other; and after several months they were exposed to the infection of smallpox—some by inoculation, others by variolous effluvia, and some in both ways, but they all resisted it. The result of these trials gradually led me into a wider field of experiment, which I went over not only with great attention, but with painful solicitude.

Edward Jenner, 1801

Jenner's pioneering clinical experiments in Gloucestershire in 1796, in which he showed that infection with attenuated material (cowpox) induced immunity to the dread scourge, smallpox, replaced the previous more dangerous and less effective practices of deliberate dermal inoculation with smallpox material. This marked the experimental foundation of immunology and infectious diseases and served as a pivotal event in the history of medicine, as it was based upon solid scientific demonstration of efficacy. The subsequent achievements, including the ultimate eradication of smallpox from the face of the earth in 1977 and the development of effective immunization reagents against a wide range of infectious agents, have had astounding effects upon mankind. The very impressive decline

## TABLE 40—1. GLOBAL DEATHS FROM VACCINE-PREVENTABLE DISEASES

| INFECTION | ANNUAL DEATHS |
|---|---|
| Tuberculosis | 3,000,000 |
| Measles | 1,500,000 |
| Hepatitis B | 1,000,000 — 2,000,000 |
| Neonatal tetanus | 775,000 |
| Pertussis | 500,000 |
| Rabies | 35,000 |
| Typhoid | 25,000 |
| Yellow fever | 25,000 |

Source: Data from World Health Organization, 1990.

in age-specific mortality rates in the 20th century is a result, in large part, of the successful prevention of many infectious diseases by widespread immunization programs. However, it is estimated (World Health Organization, 1990) that about 3 million children die each year (8000 each day) in the world from vaccine-preventable illness and that an additional 4 million are permanently disabled (Table 40–1). Neonatal tetanus, preventable by natural immunization and by hygienic umbilical cord care, kills about 775,000 infants yearly despite the availability of an effective tetanus toxoid vaccine for many years. Measles causes more than 1 million deaths yearly, and pertussis another half million annually. Much needs to be done to improve delivery of vaccines in the field, among both children and adults, who are very undervaccinated, even in the United States. Table 40–2 shows the extremely low cost of vaccines used in the World Health Organization's Expanded Program on Immunization. Clearly, cost of the vaccines per se is not the limiting factor. However, the actual percentages of infants surviving to their first birthday in the largest developing countries who have received immunizations remains disappointing.

In the United States, vaccine delivery in selected areas, particularly to the urban poor,

remains suboptimal. Vaccination levels for U.S. children 19–35 months old in the first quarter of 1994 ranged from 25% for hepatitis B to 71–87% for other vaccines. Table 40–3 shows the reported numbers of vaccine-preventable infections in the United States for 1993 and 1994; it is widely recognized that infections are generally significantly underreported.

## GENERAL CONCEPTS

### Natural vs. Deliberate Immunization

Following many infections, whether symptomatic or subclinical, solid long-lived natural protection against subsequent infection develops. Hepatitis A is an excellent example of an infection that is very commonly subclinical but which induces life-long natural immunity typically. In contrast, deliberate immunization, of course, refers to the medical practice of intentionally exposing individuals to a modified infecting agent (or component thereof) for the express purpose of inducing active immunity (as Jenner did) or, alternatively, to providing already formed antibody for purposes of protecting passively against infection.

### Active and Passive Immunization

Active immunization refers to the stimulation of an individual to produce an immune response (usually antibody) by the deliberate administration of an antigen (or antigens), usually prior to natural exposure to the agent. Protection is not present immediately but once it develops is usually of long duration. In contrast, passive immunization refers to the administration of preformed antibodies,

## TABLE 40–2. COST OF VACCINES IN THE EXPANDED PROGRAM ON IMMUNIZATION (WHO)*

| VACCINE | COST/DOSE ($) |
|---|---|
| Bacille Calmette-Guérin | 0.05 |
| DPT | 0.01–0.05 |
| Measles | 0.13 |
| Oral polio | 0.04 |
| Tetanus toxoid | 0.02 |

*From: Hayden, G. F. Cost of vaccines. *J. Pediatr. 114*:520, 1989. With permission.

## TABLE 40–3. REPORTED VACCINE-PREVENTABLE DISEASES IN THE UNITED STATES, 1993–1994*

| DISEASE | 1993 | 1994 |
|---|---|---|
| Congenital rubella syndrome | 5 | 8 |
| Diphtheria | 0 | 1 |
| Invasive *Haemophilus influenzae* | 1419 | 1161 |
| Hepatitis B | 13,361 | 11,534 |
| Measles | 312 | 902 |
| Mumps | 1692 | 1456 |
| Pertussis | 6586 | 3832 |
| Paralytic poliomyelitis | 3 | 1 |
| Rubella | 192 | 218 |
| Tetanus | 48 | 38 |

*From *Morbidity and Mortality Weekly Report 44*(5):99, 1995.

obtained from an immune individual or animal, to a nonimmune subject in order to provide temporary protection against an infecting agent or toxin. In this instance, protection is immediate but short-lived. The distinction between active and passive immunity was established in 1890 by the studies of Emil von Behring and Shibasaburo Kitasato related to protection against tetanus and diphtheria toxins. For this work, in 1901 von Behring was awarded the first Nobel Prize in Medicine.

### Adjuvants

Materials such as aluminum salts are included in certain vaccines for the purpose of promoting a depot effect at the vaccine site to retain the immunogen and to delay degradation and elimination, thus producing a prolonged stimulus to the immune system. This adjuvant effect is most important for achieving optimal immune responses to vaccines that contain killed microorganisms or their products.

### Local and Systemic Immunity

Systemic immunity is reflected by circulating serum antibody and is distinguished from local mucosal (generally secretory IgA) immunity. Inactivated Salk polio vaccine induces systemic immunity only, whereas live-attenuated Sabin polio vaccine administered orally induces local gastrointestinal antibody as well as systemic antibody. Mucosal antibody is important in preventing the primary gastrointestinal infection by wild poliovirus and its shedding into feces.

### Replicative and Nonreplicative Immunogens

Replicative vaccines are those live-attenuated agents (oral polio, measles, mumps, rubella, varicella, oral typhoid) that produce a subclinical infection that induces an active immune response. Nonreplicative immunogens are either killed whole organisms (pertussis, hepatitis A, killed polio vaccine), inactivated toxins (diphtheria, tetanus toxoids), or cellular constituents (pneumococcal, haemophilus polysaccharides) that induce protective immune responses.

### PASSIVE IMMUNIZATION

The most universal and physiologic form of passive immunity is the transplacental passage of IgG from mother to fetus. This is the result of an active transport process that occurs particularly during the last 2 months of gestation, resulting in IgG concentrations in full-term infants that are 100–110% of the maternal concentrations. Depending upon their gestational age, preterm infants are mildly to severely deficient in serum IgG, as compared with adult levels, because they were born prior to the period when most transplacental passage of IgG occurs, and this contributes to their enhanced susceptibility to infection. Much transplacental IgG is protective, such as against *Haemophilus influenzae* type b, measles, or varicella, whereas other IgG antibodies are clearly not protective, such as anti–human immunodeficiency virus (HIV). The half-life of transplacental IgG is 3–4 weeks, and traces are still detectable at 12 months or even later. There is sufficient transplacental antimeasles antibody still present in serum up to 12 months of age to interfere with the active immune response to live-attenuated measles vaccine in a substantial fraction of infants, necessitating delay of vaccine administration in routine (nonepidemic) circumstances to infants 12–15 months of age.

In general, passive immunization is used to achieve temporary immunity in an unimmunized exposed individual at high risk of complications (e.g., immunocompromised child exposed to varicella), or when time does not permit protection by active immunization alone after an exposure has occurred (e.g., measles, rabies, or hepatitis B). It is also employed in toxin-mediated disorders (e.g., diphtheria, botulism, tetanus), certain bites (spider, snake), or as an immunomodulator (anti-D [Rh$_o$], antilymphocyte sera). In addition, patients who are incapable of active antibody responses to immunization (e.g., B-cell deficiency) benefit from passive immunization. The forms of passive immunologic agents utilized include: (1) standard human immune serum globulin (ISG) available for intramuscular or in deaggregated preparations for intravenous use; (2) specific high-titered human globulins used in defined circumstances; and (3) antisera and antitoxins prepared in immunized animals, usually horses or rabbits. The use of reagents prepared in species other than humans is associated with a risk of hypersensitivity (serum sickness) reactions; these are related to development of antibody against the injected foreign protein. A negative scratch test or eye test followed by negative intradermal skin tests is essential before injection of an animal serum. Specific human and animal sera and antitoxins currently available are listed in Table 40–4.

Standard ISG, consisting almost exclusively of IgG (Cohn alcohol fraction II) pooled from large groups of adult donors, is used intramuscularly for the prevention of the following illnesses: (1) hepatitis A, (2) measles, (3) hepatitis B (only when hepatitis B immune globulin [HBIG] is unavailable), and (4) varicella (when varicella-zoster immune globulin [VZIG] is unavailable). It is of unproved value for prevention of hepatitis C and E. Thus, common usage relates to hepatitis A and measles prevention. ISG is also administered intramuscularly as replacement therapy in individuals with humoral immune deficiency states.

Intravenous gamma globulin (IVGG) is similar to ISG but is chemically treated to ensure deaggregation of IgG, thus obviating the complement-mediated reactions that occur when ISG is inadvertently administered intravenously. IVGG is utilized in the treatment of humoral immune deficiency states, idiopathic thrombocytopenic purpura, and Kawasaki disease (see Chapter 31), and some studies have shown its usefulness in some patients with pediatric acquired immunodeficiency syndrome (AIDS).

Specific high-titered human globulin preparations are available and are recommended for selected situations. The use of HBIG is discussed in Chapter 19. VZIG prepared from individuals convalescent from zoster (shingles) is used to prevent or ameliorate varicella in immunocompromised hosts with recent (within 96 h) exposure (see Chapter 24). Rabies immune globulin (RIG) is effective as prophylaxis when combined with active rabies immunization. RIG should be given within 24 h of exposure, infiltrated in and around the bite sites as well as intramuscularly (not in the same site as rabies vaccine). Tetanus immune globulin (TIG) contains a high concentration of tetanus antitoxin and is highly effective in prevention of tetanus when administered soon after an injury causing a major contaminated wound in an individual lacking a complete primary series of active immunization. Its value in established tetanus is unproved. Cytomegalovirus (CMV) immune globulin is now used to prevent CMV infection in seronegative renal transplant recipients and is being evaluated for treatment of CMV in protocols that combine it with ganciclovir. Pertussis immune globulin is of little or no value in treatment or prevention of pertussis. $Rh_o(D)$ immune globulin (RhoGAM) is highly effective in prevention of Rh hemolytic disease of the neonate and is indicated for Rh-negative women who have delivered an Rh-positive baby or have aborted and for Rh-negative inadvertent recipients of Rh-positive blood.

Animal sera and globulins are utilized infrequently and with the precautions noted above. Serum sickness reactions are common, including the development of rash, arthralgia or arthritis, and glomerulonephritis. Such reactions represent immune-complex–mediated events resulting from antibody produced after receipt of globulins from a nonhuman species. Tetanus antitoxin (equine) and rabies immune globulin (equine) are used only when the corresponding human preparations

## TABLE 40–4. PASSIVE IMMUNIZATION IN PREVENTION OF INFECTION

**HUMAN IMMUNOGLOBULIN**

Standard immune serum globulin (ISG)
  Hepatitis A postexposure prophylaxis: 0.02 mL/kg
  Hepatitis B prophylaxis or attenuation (only when HBIG is unavailable): 0.06 mL/kg
  Measles prophylaxis or attenuation: 0.25 mL/kg (0.5 mL/kg for immunocompromised) with maximum of 15 mL
  Varicella prophylaxis or attenuation (only when VZIG is unavailable and only for individuals at high risk of serious disease): 0.06 mL/kg
  Polio prophylaxis (rarely indicated)

Special immune globulins (all postexposure)
  Hepatitis B immune globulin (HBIG): 0.06 mL/kg (maximum: 5 mL)
  Varicella-zoster immune globulin (VZIG): one vial (125 units) per 10 kg; maximum: 5 vials
  Rabies immune globulin (HRIG): 20 IU/kg (half locally, half IM)
  Tetanus immune globulin (TIG): for treatment, 3000–6000 units; for prevention, 250 units
  Cytomegalovirus immune globulin (CMVIG): for prophylaxis in seronegative renal transplant patients; dose is 150 mg/kg every other week; efficacy for treatment is under investigation

**ANIMAL IMMUNOGLOBULINS**

For use only when human product is unavailable:
  Equine tetanus antitoxin (TAT): 50,000–100,000 units (after safety testing) in single dose (20,000 units IV, the remainder IM)
  Equine antirabies serum (ARS): 40 IU/kg (half locally, half IM) in single dose (after safety testing)

Only available preparations:
  Equine diphtheria antitoxin: 20,000–100,000 units IV (after safety testing)
  Equine trivalent (ABE) botulinum antitoxin (after safety testing)
  Equine gas gangrene polyvalent antitoxin: no longer used or available in the United States

are unavailable. Diphtheria antitoxin (equine) is effective in neutralizing non–tissue-fixed diphtheria toxin even after clinical disease is apparent; efficacy is maximal early in the disease. Similarly, equine trivalent (A, B, E) botulism antitoxin is effective in treatment of this very serious disorder by neutralizing unbound toxin. In contrast, equine gas gangrene antitoxin is of no value and is no longer available. Crotalidae antivenin is utilized in treatment of snake bites from certain poisonous species and is infiltrated locally as well as given systemically. Similarly, black widow spider antivenin is occasionally utilized. Antilymphocyte or antithymocyte globulins or sera (ALG, ALS, ATG, ATS), usually raised in horses, have been utilized for prevention of organ transplant rejection, with murine monoclonal antibodies directed against T-cell populations (e.g., OKT3) also now being used to reverse rejection.

## ACTIVE IMMUNIZATION

Active immunization programs are highly efficient in preventing viral illnesses and toxin-mediated bacterial disorders. They are clearly very cost-effective and they save lives. However, in many developing areas of the world, vaccine delivery continues to be a major challenge. Contributing to the problem of delivery of vaccines in the third world areas is the problem of maintaining the *cold chain*, which refers to the fact that many vaccines must be maintained at refrigerator or freezer temperature until just prior to administration to retain immunogenicity.

Breaks in the cold chain lead to ineffective vaccines. Vaccines composed of whole bacterial cells, rickettsiae, or mycoplasmas are only moderately effective immunogens. The goal of active immunization is to induce long-lived responses that provide protection against clinical disease. Clearly, there is a latent period between the time of immunization and the achievement of protective levels of antibody, and many vaccines require several doses to induce lasting responses. Primary immune responses are generally predominantly IgM and transient. However, secondary responses are usually predominantly IgG and long-lived. Vaccines may contain trace amounts of constituents derived from the media in which the vaccine was prepared, including tissue-culture–derived antigens, egg antigens, or serum proteins, or the vaccines may contain

preservatives or stabilizers. These contaminants serve as potential inciting agents for hypersensitivity reactions. The most common component responsible for such hypersensitivity is egg protein in vaccines prepared in embryonated chicken eggs or chicken embryo cell culture (yellow fever, mumps, measles, and influenza vaccines). Generally, those who can safely eat eggs or egg products can receive these vaccines, but those with history of anaphylaxis to eggs should not.

The formulation of vaccine schedules by public health authorities is based upon epidemiologic characteristics of the disease, age-dependent immune responses, age-specific complication risks of vaccine or of the natural disease, and duration of induced immunity. In short, policy is based upon careful risk–benefit assessments. In general, vaccines are recommended for the youngest age group both at risk and known to develop an acceptable response to vaccination. Usually, vaccine schedules call for simultaneous administration of several vaccines, often at different sites. Complications that occur at even very low frequency are significant when one deals with millions of vaccine doses yearly. An example of this is the whole-cell pertussis vaccine, which may be associated with serious adverse acute neurologic reactions with a frequency of approximately 1:300,000 doses. The cost associated with resultant litigation concerning alleged vaccine complications has led to great increases in the cost of vaccines in the United States over the past decade and has driven some vaccine manufacturers out of the field. General contraindications to active immunization include (1) moderate or severe (but not minor) illnesses with or without a fever; (2) immunocompromised state (live vaccines should be avoided); (3) recent ISG, IVGG, whole blood, or plasma administration; (4) pregnancy; and (5) anaphylaxis to a vaccine component.

*Vaccine efficacy* is established from studies of relative attack rates for a disease in vaccinated and nonvaccinated populations. For example, if 10 of 1000 vaccinated and 900 of 1000 unvaccinated exposed individuals develop infection during an epidemic, the vaccine efficacy is .90 − .01/.90 = .99, or 99% effective.

### Poliomyelitis Immunization

Vaccination against poliomyelitis has almost completely eradicated this disorder from the United States and other developed areas. It is estimated that more than 5 million cases of paralytic polio were prevented by oral vaccine in the past two decades. The phenomenal impact of international vaccine programs, mainly efforts of the Pan American Health Organization, is exemplified by the complete eradication of paralytic polio from the entire Western Hemisphere in August 1991. This was achieved by national vaccination days and intensive surveillance activities. Worldwide, great declines in incidence of paralytic polio have been achieved, with a 70% decrease from 1988 to 1993 and with 75% of countries reporting zero cases of polio in 1993. Areas of highest remaining polio activity are in sub-Sahara Africa and Asia; nearly 65% of all cases worldwide were from India, Pakistan, and Bangladesh. Outbreaks in the Netherlands in 1992 and viral excretion among unvaccinated individuals in Alberta, Canada, in 1993 highlight the need for continued high levels of protection.

Infants in the United States are now immunized routinely with Sabin trivalent, live-attenuated, oral vaccine (OPV) at 2 and 4 months of age, with booster doses administered at 12–18 months and at 4–6 years, just before entry into school. The oral vaccine replaced the Salk trivalent, inactivated (killed), parenteral vaccine in the United States because of the former's ability to induce intestinal immunity, its ease of administration, its high acceptance, and its ability to immunize some unimmunized contacts of fecally excreting vaccine recipients. The Sabin vaccine is unique in that it multiplies extensively in the intestinal tract, is widely disseminated in the family and community, and immunizes a large proportion of the unvaccinated population. However, OPV is associated with rare instances of paralysis in vaccinees and in their contacts (now about nine per year in the United States), the estimated risks being 1 per 6.8 million doses of OPV for immunologically normal vaccine recipients, and 1 per 6.4 million doses for household and community contacts. The maximal risk of paralysis occurs with the first dose of OPV (1 case of paralysis per 700,000 first doses and 1 case per 6.9 million subsequent doses), and rates are slightly greater for adults compared with children. Immunocompromised persons who are exposed to OPV virus by vaccination or by exposure to a vaccinee are at somewhat higher risk of acquiring paralytic disease.

Inactivated poliovirus vaccine (IPV), containing the three formalin-inactivated poliovirus strains, has recently been licensed in the United States as an enhanced-potency inactivated polio (E-IPV) vaccine developed in human diploid cell culture. IPV, which was responsible for the initial sharp decline from 20,000–25,000 cases yearly of paralytic polio in the United States in the 1950s, is now indicated for individuals who refuse OPV or who have a contraindication to OPV, including those with compromised immunity including AIDS, household contacts of an immunodeficient individual, partially immunized or unimmunized adult household contacts of children who will receive OPV, and unimmunized or partially immunized adults at future risk of exposure to polio. It is recommended that IPV recipients receive boosters every 5 years after their primary series of immunization at 2, 3–4, and 10–16 months of age. A full series of IPV is recommended for immunizing previously unimmunized adults. Within the next few years, it is likely that a vaccine strategy in which initial immunization with diphtheria, tetanus, and pertussis coupled with E-IPV will be recommended, then followed by OPV. It is thought that this should reduce the risk of inducing vaccine-related paralytic disease by deferring the live virus vaccine until individuals have received at least one initial immunization with E-IPV. Current indications for OPV and IPV are shown in Table 40–5.

### TABLE 40–5.  CURRENT INDICATIONS FOR POLIO VACCINE

**INDICATIONS FOR ORAL POLIO VACCINE (OPV)**

1. Healthy infants and children receiving routine immunizations
2. Unimmunized or partially immunized children at imminent risk of exposure to polio
3. Adults at future risk of polio exposure who previously received at least one dose of OPV or IPV
4. Unimmunized adults at imminent (within 4 weeks) risk of polio exposure

**INDICATIONS FOR INACTIVATED POLIO VACCINE (IPV)**

1. Unimmunized or partially immunized persons with compromised immunity
2. HIV-infected persons (with or without symptoms)
3. Household contacts of immunodeficient persons (including HIV-infected)
4. Partially immunized or unimmunized adults or other close household contacts of children to be given OPV
5. Unimmunized adults at future risk of polio exposure
6. Adults at future risk of polio exposure who have had a primary IPV series
7. Refusal of OPV immunization

## Diphtheria, Tetanus, Pertussis Immunization

Diphtheria, tetanus, pertussis (DTP) vaccine is composed of purified diphtheria and tetanus toxoids and whole killed pertussis organisms or acellular pertussis antigens. The less reactogenic acellular pertussis vaccines include cell-free pertussis toxoids that are formaldehyde-inactivated and have been licensed for the fourth and fifth DTP vaccine doses, at 15–18 months and 4–6 years. They are being tested in younger infants and may soon completely replace the whole-cell pertussis vaccine. Whole-organism pertussis vaccines are associated with relatively low efficacy and relatively frequent adverse reactions. These reactions include development of mild to moderate fever, local discomfort, local redness and swelling, drowsiness, fretfulness, and anorexia or vomiting occurring within several hours of vaccination, with spontaneous resolution. More significant adverse reactions include the following: about 1%, persistent crying lasting at least 3 h; 0.3%, very high fever ($\geq$40.5°C); 0.1%, high-pitched cry; 0.06%, seizures; and 0.06%, collapse for several hours with a peculiar hypotonic, hyporesponsive state, without long-term neurologic consequences. Because many alleged vaccine reactions actually may be caused by other factors, a temporal association with immunization does not establish a causal relationship. This has been shown to be the case with regard to the onset of infantile spasms or with sudden infant death syndrome (SIDS), both of which are relatively common in the first 6 months of life but for which a causal relationship to immunization has not been demonstrated. Pertussis vaccine has not been proved to be a cause of permanent brain damage.

Contraindications to subsequent readministration of pertussis vaccine are: (1) encephalopathy occurring within 7 days of immunization (with severe alterations of consciousness and/or focal neurologic findings), with estimated frequency of 1:140,000; (2) seizure with or without fever within 72 h; (3) persistent screaming or high-pitched cry for at least 3 h within 48 h; (4) hypotonic-hyporesponsive episode within 48 h; (5) fever greater than or equal to 40.5°C within 48 h, without other cause; and (6) anaphylactic reaction to vaccine (extremely rare). The risk of administering subsequent vaccine doses to children with these reactions is not known, but prudence

should prevail. In addition, DTP vaccine should be deferred for children with progressive neurologic conditions or progressive developmental delay, personal past history of seizures, and those with known or suspected neurologic conditions that predispose to seizures or neurologic deterioration. A family history, but not personal history, of seizures is *not* a contraindication to pertussis immunization, even though data suggest that such children are at some increased risk for simple febrile convulsions, which are considered generally benign.

Universal immunization of children is essential for control of pertussis, since there is continuing risk of pertussis in the United States, as demonstrated by large outbreaks in Chicago and Cincinnati in 1993. Experiences in other countries have demonstrated repeatedly that falling vaccine rates are associated with dramatic epidemic occurrence of pertussis, associated with fatalities and significant morbidity. As many as 500,000 preventable pertussis deaths occur each year worldwide among infants. Encephalopathy and seizures complicate the pertussis illness much more frequently than they result from pertussis immunization. DTP is recommended for infants and children at 2, 4, and 6 months of age; at 15–18 months; and at 4–6 years. Acellular pertussis vaccine is approved for the latter two doses. After the seventh birthday, DTP is replaced by Td, a vaccine that omits the pertussis component and contains a lower concentration of diphtheria toxoid to reduce reactogenicity. Boosters with Td should be given every 10 years. Children for whom pertussis immunization is deferred or contraindicated should receive DT if younger than 7 years old, and should receive four or preferably five immunizations by the time of school entry. A booster of tetanus toxoid should be given every 10 years. Since neither tetanus nor diphtheria infection necessarily confers immunity, individuals convalescent from these illnesses should receive active immunization. In contrast, those who have had culture-proven pertussis need no immunization.

Recent serologic surveys in the United States found that 20% of children 10–16 years old lack protective antitetanus levels and that only 28% of individuals 70 years or older are protected. Most cases of tetanus occur in those at least 60 years old. Clearly, vaccine delivery to adults is not optimal.

## Measles, Mumps, Rubella Immunization

Universal immunization with combined live-attenuated virus vaccines against rubeola (measles), mumps, and rubella (German measles) (MMR) is recommended at 12–15 months of age in routine circumstances, with reimmunization at 4–6 years or 11–12 years. Use of these vaccines has resulted in dramatic decreases in the frequencies of these illnesses, with concomitant decreases in the frequencies of the serious sequelae of measles, encephalitis and pneumonitis, and of congenital rubella syndrome. However, the World Health Organization indicates that 1.0 to 1.5 million children die annually from measles.

*Measles vaccine* produces a subclinical or very mild noncommunicable infection, with approximately 95% of vaccine recipients immunized at 15 months developing long-lived immunity. Vaccination in the United States between 1963 and 1967 utilized killed measles vaccine, and from 1968 to 1979 attenuated-live vaccine strains were used, sometimes with ISG, containing a less effective stabilizer than current vaccine, a procedure that commonly resulted in lack of sustained immune responses. These vaccination problems accounted for outbreaks of measles among teenage and young adult populations, such as on college campuses around 1990. Current recommendations call for reimmunization of children who were immunized at 15 months of age or older either upon entrance to middle school (junior high) or upon entrance to elementary school (4–6 years). Immunization before 12 months of age, which is indicated only in measles epidemic or highly endemic areas, frequently results in relatively short-lived antibody responses as a result of the suppressive effect of residual transplacentally acquired maternal antibody. Such children require reimmunization at approximately 15 months of age and again at age 11 or 12.

Measles vaccine can provide some degree of protection even when given up to 72 h after exposure, so that vaccine is indicated following known exposure. Adverse reactions occur in about 5–15% of measles vaccine recipients, with fever as high as 103°F for 1–2 days, beginning 7–12 days after immunization and sometimes accompanied by a mild rash. Approximately 50% of prior recipients of the killed measles vaccine used in 1963–1967 develop reactions after revaccination with live measles vaccine, usually mild local swelling and redness, sometimes with low-grade fever for 1–2 days. Rarely, more serious reactions with prolonged fever, lymphadenopathy, extensive local reactions, and rash resembling rickettsial rashes (maximal on distal extremities) may occur. However, because such individuals are more likely to develop severe reactions following exposure to wild measles virus than after live vaccine, they therefore should be reimmunized.

Live-attenuated *mumps vaccine* (Jeryl-Lynn strain) is usually given with the initial measles vaccine at 12–15 months and results in antibody in more than 95% of recipients. Vaccination results in very-long-lasting immunity, and adverse reactions to this vaccine are very rare. Postexposure mumps vaccine has not been shown to be effective.

Live *rubella vaccine* (RA 27/3 strain), also given at 12–15 months and again at 4–6 years or 11–12 years, in combination with measles and mumps vaccine, induces serum antibody in more than 98% of recipients and confers long-term (perhaps life-long) immunity (see Chapter 31). This vaccine is also recommended for susceptible adolescent and adult females to decrease the risk of the congenital rubella syndrome resulting from rubella infection early in pregnancy. Because of successful immunization programs, the congenital rubella syndrome has been reduced in the United States to only eight reported cases in 1994 and five cases in 1993. Although there is no evidence of teratogenic effects of live rubella vaccine, it is recommended that this vaccine, as well as the mumps and measles vaccines, not be given during pregnancy. Adverse reactions to primary rubella immunization include mild rash, lymphadenopathy, and arthralgias or arthritis, particularly in adult females. Unlike measles, postexposure immunization with rubella vaccine is not effective in preventing disease.

The MMR vaccine should not be given to immunocompromised or immunodeficient individuals (except for HIV-infected) and should be postponed at least 3 months after ISG or blood administration or for 11 months after high-dose IVGG therapy.

### *Haemophilus influenzae* Type b Immunization

A vaccine composed of purified *H. influenzae* type b (Hib) capsular polysaccharide was licensed in April, 1985 for children 24 months and over to prevent invasive infection by this organism. Because younger children, who are at highest risk for Hib infection, are incapable of mounting an antibody response to this T-independent antigen, conjugate vaccines in which Hib polysaccharide (polyribose phosphate) is covalently linked to a protein carrier such as diphtheria toxoid were developed (Table 40–6). The first of these T-dependent vaccines was initially licensed in the United States for children 18 months and older in December, 1987, and they are now approved for infants beginning at 2 months of age. Effective combination vaccines comprised of DPT linked to Hib have been developed and will reduce the actual number of injections needed.

The efficacy of Hib vaccination has been truly phenomenal, with the prevalence of invasive infections including meningitis caused by *H. influenzae* type b dropping by about 98% over a 5-year period in the United States.

### Pneumococcal Vaccine

At least 84 serotypes of pneumococci are known, distinguished by the antigenicity of their capsular polysaccharides, which serve as antiphagocytic virulence factors. Anticapsular antibody is opsonic and protects against invasive infection with the homologous serotype. Active immunization against pneumococci is possible because (1) a relatively limited number of serotypes account for most pneumococcal infections of humans, (2) multiple purified polysaccharides can be combined into a single injection, and (3) type-specific antibody persists for years. The current pneumococcal vaccine in the United States contains 25 $\mu$g of each capsular polysaccharide of the 23 pneumococcal serotypes responsible for 88% of bacteremic pneumococcal infections in the United States in adults, nearly 100% of those infections in children, and about 85% of acute otitis media. Children younger than 24 months do not respond well to these purified polysaccharides, which are T-independent antigens. Pneumococcal vaccine efficacy is estimated to be about 60% in high-risk populations. Pneumococcal vaccine is currently recommended for children older than 24 months with sickle cell disease, functional or anatomic asplenia, cerebrospinal fluid (CSF) leaks, nephrosis or chronic renal failure, HIV infection, and other illnesses associated with increased risk of pneumococcal infection, and for all adults 65 years or older, and adults with chronic cardiac or pulmonary disease, lymphatic malignancies, or chronic liver disease.

### Typhoid Fever Vaccine

*Salmonella typhi* has been estimated to result in 33 million infections and more than 500,000 deaths annually worldwide, particularly in areas with poor sanitation. Parenterally administered killed whole-cell vaccines (inactivated by heat and phenol or by acetone treatment) have been available since the 1960s. However, these vaccines have afforded only about 50–80% protection and are associated with a high frequency of adverse effects, including substantial fever and local reactions. Killed whole-cell vaccines administered orally are well tolerated but do not result in protection.

Two new typhoid vaccines have been developed recently and found to be safe, immunogenic, and protective in clinical trials. These are a live-attenuated strain of *S. typhi* (Ty21a) administered orally, and purified *S. typhi* capsular polysaccharide (Vi) administered parenterally. The Ty21a strain of *S. typhi* is completely deficient in the enzyme uridine diphosphoglucose-4-epimerase and harbors other mutations as well, including lacking Vi polysaccharide. Large field trials of three to four oral doses of Ty21a administered within 1 week demonstrated 42–96% efficacy for prevention of typhoid fever. This vaccine is well-tolerated and is now licensed in the United States except for children under 6 years of age. Vi polysaccharide, a capsular ma-

**TABLE 40–6.    *H. INFLUENZAE* TYPE B CONJUGATE VACCINES**

| VACCINE AND MANUFACTURER | CARRIER PROTEIN | SCHEDULE |
| --- | --- | --- |
| PRP—T (Pasteur Merieux) | Tetanus toxoid | 3 doses at 2-month intervals, 4th dose at 12–15 months |
| Hb—OC (Lederle) | CRM$_{197}$ (nontoxic mutant diphtheria toxin) | 3 doses at 2-month intervals, 4th dose at 12–15 months |
| PRP—OMP (Merck) | Outer membrane protein of *N. meningitidis* | 2 doses at 2-month intervals, 3rd dose at 12–15 months |
| PRP—D (Connaught) | Diphtheria toxoid | Recommended only for infants ≥12 months old |

terial of clinical isolates of *S. typhi*, serves as a virulence factor and has been highly purified and field-tested as a parenteral vaccine, with 72% and 64% protection against culture-proved typhoid fever. This vaccine is not yet licensed in the United States although both Ty21a and Vi vaccines are now licensed in several countries. Further efforts to develop more effective typhoid vaccines are continuing, including creation of other *S. typhi* strains with enzymatic mutations for use as attenuated-live agents, and preparation of protein-polysaccharide conjugates that include Vi conjugated to tetanus or diphtheria toxoids for enhanced immunogenicity.

### Influenza Vaccine

Influenza vaccine must be newly formulated each year because of the annual changes in the influenza A and B strains that account for epidemic disease. Influenza A of three distinct hemagglutinin subtypes (H1, H2, and H3) and two neuraminidase subtypes (N1 and N2) cause human infection, and specific antibody to these H and N antigens are important in immunity to influenza A. *Antigenic drift* refers to minor variations within the same subtype (occurring almost annually), while *antigenic shift* refers to a major change such as H1 to H2 or N2 to N1 (occurring about every 10 years). Inactivated influenza vaccine is prepared in eggs, has minimal side effects (except in those with anaphylactic reactions to egg), and contains several viral subtypes chosen to anticipate the expected prevalent viral strains for that year. Inactivated whole-cell vaccine is used for those over 12 years old, while inactivated subvirion ''split'' virus vaccine is used for children 6 months to 12 years old (see Table 40–7).

Yearly influenza vaccine is indicated in the fall for everyone over 65 years, residents of chronic care facilities, patients with chronic medical conditions and their household contacts, health care personnel, and high-risk children (asthma or chronic lung or cardiac disease, immunosuppressed, sickle cell disease, diabetes, chronic renal disease, HIV).

### Varicella Vaccine

Live-attenuated varicella vaccine was licensed for use in a single dose in the United States in early 1995 for individuals 12 months and older. Susceptibles 13 years of age and over should receive two doses 4–8 weeks apart. In clinical trials this vaccine was demonstrated to be associated with relatively few side effects (including an occasional recipient who developed a varicella-like rash with an average of five lesions), to be immunogenic, and to be 96–100% effective in preventing varicella. Insufficient data exist to assess the degree of protection against complications of varicella or to assess the duration of immunity induced. Therefore, the ultimate need for booster immunizations will be assessed as follow-up serologic data are obtained. This vaccine is not recommended now for immunocompromised hosts, those with active tuberculosis, pregnant women, or those with an active febrile infection. An experimental protocol to study administration of varicella vaccine to children and adolescents with acute lymphoblastic leukemia in remission is available.

### Other Vaccines

A large number of additional vaccines are available (Table 40–8), most being utilized for the rather selected indications outlined in the table. Hepatitis B vaccine and hepatitis A vaccine are discussed in Chapter 19.

### Current Recommendations

The schedule for routine immunizations of healthy children is shown in Table 40–9. Official vaccine recommendations are established in the United States by the Committee on Infectious Diseases of the American Academy of Pediatrics and by the Advisory Committee on Immunization Practices of the Centers for Disease Control.

### TABLE 40–7.   INFLUENZA IMMUNIZATION

| Age | Vaccine | Dose | Number of Doses |
|-----|---------|------|-----------------|
| 6–35 mo | Split | 0.25 mL | 1–2 (2 doses if first time vaccinated or if new H or N type) |
| 3–8 yr | Split | 0.5 mL | 1–2 (2 doses if first time vaccinated or if new H or N type) |
| 9–12 yr | Split | 0.5 mL | 1 |
| >12 yr | Whole or split | 0.5 mL | 1 |

TABLE 40–8.    ACTIVE IMMUNIZATION AGENTS USED SELECTIVELY

| VACCINE | TYPE | AGE | INDICATIONS | COMMENT |
|---------|------|-----|-------------|---------|
| Influenza | Killed whole or split virus | >6 mo | Chronic lung, cardiac conditions | Yearly immunization required with current vaccine |
| Yellow fever | Live-attenuated | >9 mo | Residence or travel to endemic area | Avoid in egg-sensitive individuals and infants <4 months |
| Rabies | Inactivated virus grown in human diploid cells | Any | Animal handlers or postexposure | Use with rabies immune globulin |
| Tuberculosis | BCG, attenuated-live *M. bovis* strain | Any | See Chapter 13 | Preparations vary in efficacy |
| Typhoid | Live-attenuated oral Ty21a | >6 yr | Travel or lab exposure | Moderately effective in prevention |
| Cholera | Phenol-killed *Vibrio cholerae* | >6 mo | See Chapter 17 | Marginally protective, for short period |
| Anthrax | Cell-free protein antigen | Adults | Anticipated exposure (usually occupational) | Safe and highly effective |
| Meningococcal | Four capsular polysaccharides (A, C, Y, W-135) | > 2 yr | High-risk patients, to control epidemics | Children <2 yr respond variably to individual components |
| Tularemia | Live-attenuated | >6 yr | Anticipated exposure (e.g., lab techs) | Available from CDC |
| Plague | Killed, whole bacteria | Adults | Occupational exposure | Not recommended for those living in plague-endemic areas |

TABLE 40–9.    RECOMMENDED SCHEDULE OF IMMUNIZATIONS OF NORMAL INFANTS AND CHILDREN

| AGE | IMMUNIZATION |
|-----|--------------|
| Birth | HBV |
| 1–4 mo | HBV |
| 2 mo | DTP, Hib, OPV |
| 4 mo | DTP, Hib, OPV |
| 6 mo | DTP, Hib (unless 2 doses of PRP–OMP given) |
| 6–18 mo | HBV, OPV |
| 12–15 mo | Hib, MMR (at 12 mo in high-risk area), Var |
| 15–18 mo | DTaP or DTP |
| 4–6 yr | DTaP or DTP, OPV |
| 11–12 yr | MMR, Var (if not given previously) |
| 14–16 yr | T*d* (repeat every 10 years for life) |

HBV, Hepatitis B vaccine; DTP, diphtheria, tetanus, pertussis; OPV oral polio vaccine; Hib, *H. influenzae* type b; MMR, measles, mumps, rubella; DTaP, diphtheria, tetanus, acellular pertussis; T*d*, tetanus and reduced-dose diphtheria toxoid; Var, varicella.

Six vaccines are currently recommended for routine use for adults in the United States. These include:

1. Tetanus-diphtheria toxoid booster every 10 years (after a primary series).

2. Influenza vaccine annually, particularly for those with chronic diseases, health care workers, and all persons over 65 years old.

3. Pneumococcal vaccine, for those with chronic diseases and those over 65 years of age.

4. Hepatitis B vaccine for the groups discussed in Chapter 19.

5. Measles vaccine for adults born after 1956 who have received only one dose of vaccine since their first birthday, particularly on enrolling in college, traveling to a foreign country, or entering a health care field.

6. Rubella vaccine for previously unimmunized women of childbearing age and susceptible health care personnel.

Recommended immunizations for travelers to developing countries are shown in Table

40–10. Note that more than one vaccine can be given at the same time, but that cholera and yellow fever vaccines should be given at least 3 weeks apart. Pregnancy and immunosuppression are contraindications for live virus vaccines.

## Future Vaccines

Efforts to develop new vaccines that are safe and effective are continuing. In addition to an acellular pertussis vaccine (see above), work is progressing with respect to (1) attenuated rotavirus vaccine; (2) herpes simplex vaccine; (3) malaria sporozoite vaccines; (4) HIV vaccine; (5) cytomegalovirus vaccine; and (6) group B streptococcal vaccine, among others.

Rotavirus deserves mention as the single most important etiologic agent of severe diarrhea in infants and young children, accounting for one third to one half of more than 5 million deaths each year worldwide from severe diarrhea in children under 2 years of age. Attenuated rotaviruses of bovine and rhesus origin are being evaluated as orally administered vaccines to prevent rotavirus diarrhea in infants.

Much current vaccine development is focused upon the preparation of protein-polysaccharide conjugates that result in enhanced immune responses to the polysaccharide component, particularly in young infants, as so brilliantly achieved with *H. influenzae* type b. It is probable that a number of such conjugates will be demonstrated to be effective immunogens and to result in protection against a variety of infections. Molecular biologic techniques have led to a number of new approaches to vaccine development, including synthesis of peptides or polypeptides by recombinant DNA technology or gene insertion, attenuation of pathogens by gene-segment reassortment or mutations (gene deletions or missense), and production of antiidiotypes.

## TABLE 40–10.    VACCINES FOR TRAVELERS TO DEVELOPING COUNTRIES

| VACCINE | TYPE | EFFICACY | WHEN INDICATED | DOSE* |
|---|---|---|---|---|
| Hepatitis A | Immune serum globulin or Inactivated virus | Moderate | Travel to areas with poor hygiene | 0.02 mL/kg up to 2 mL (0.06 mL/kg up to 5 mL for stay >3 mo); vaccine: Two doses |
| Hepatitis B | Purified HbsAg | High | For medical personnel, those anticipating sexual contact, or for stay >3 mo | 3 1.0-mL doses |
| Japanese encephalitis | Inactivated virus | Moderate | Travel to rural Asia in summer, especially for stay >2 wk | 3 doses, 1 wk apart |
| Measles | Live-attenuated | High | For those born after 1956 who have not received 2 doses | 1 dose (should precede ISG by ≥2 wk) |
| Meningococcal | Polysaccharide | Moderate | For travel to epidemic areas (e.g., sub-Saharan Africa) | 0.5 mL SC (1 dose) |
| Polio | IPV or OPV | High | For travel to developing countries | 1 booster of OPV or IPV; IPV if no 1° series |
| Tetanus/ diphtheria | Toxoids | High | If none in 10 years | T*d* booster every 10 years |
| Typhoid | Live oral bacteria (Ty21a) | Moderate | Travel to rural areas or where an epidemic exists or for stay >3 mo | One capsule QOD × 4 doses, at least 2 wk before departure |
| Yellow fever | Live-attenuated | Moderate | Travel to endemic areas of rural S. America or Africa | 0.5 mL SC (1 dose) |

*For children's doses, consult Report of the Committee on Infectious Diseases of the American Academy of Pediatrics, the *Red Book.*

These and other approaches should result in improved agents for use as vaccines in the future.

## CASE HISTORY

### CASE HISTORY 1

D.R. is a 5-year-old white male admitted to the pediatric intensive care unit following a rattlesnake bite on the dorsum of the right foot. This boy lives in a tent in an isolated wooded area. Neither he nor his siblings have ever seen a physician, received an immunization, or attended school. He arrived in an emergency room 15 min after the bite with rapidly progressing local inflammatory changes of the foot. He was stabilized and received (among other agents): (1) 0.5 mL tetanus toxoid intramuscularly; (2) 1.0 mL human tetanus immune globulin; (3) 140 mL horse antisnake venom intravenously and around the snakebite; (4) measles, mumps, and rubella vaccine subcutaneously; and (5) 0.5 mL trivalent oral polio vaccine. The patient steadily improved in the hospital and, although there was initial concern about possible loss of some or all of the foot, all tissue remained viable. Twelve days after admission, he developed transient painful swelling of the knees and was found to have hematuria. These findings resolved after several days.

Which of the administered agents provided active immunity and which passive? What does the episode 12 days after admission represent, and what lab test would be useful to confirm your diagnosis?

### CASE 1 DISCUSSION

This boy received both active and passive tetanus immunization, which is necessary to protect previously unimmunized individuals promptly. He received passive immunity in the form of human and equine globulins, and also was given active immunogens in the form of live-attenuated oral polio vaccine, live attenuated MMR, and a purified protein (tetanus toxoid). The symptoms of arthritis of the knees together with hematuria noted 12 days

after a large dose of equine antiserum clearly represents classic serum sickness; hypocomplementemia is present in this antigen–antibody complex–mediated illness. Serum sickness usually resolves without treatment and leaves no long-term sequelae.

## REFERENCES

**Books**

Committee on Infectious Diseases of the American Academy of Pediatrics. *Red Book.* 23rd ed. Elk Grove Village, IL: American Academy of Pediatrics, 1994.

Plotkin, S. A., and Mortimer, E. A., eds. *Vaccines.* 2nd ed. Philadelphia: W. B. Saunders Co., 1994.

**Articles**

Advisory Committee on Immunization Practices. General recommendations on immunization. *MMWR 43*: RR-1, 1994.

Anderson, D. C., Givner, L. B., and Shearer, W. T. Active and passive immunization in the prevention of infectious diseases. In: Stiehm, E. R., ed. *Immunologic Disorders in Infants and Children.* 3rd ed. Philadelphia: W. B. Saunders Co., 1989.

Gardner, P., and Schaffner, W. Immunization of Adults, *N. Engl. J. Med. 328*:1252–1258, 1993.

Gergen, P. J., et al A population-based serologic survey of immunity to tetanus in the United States. *N. Engl. J. Med. 332*:761–766, 1995.

Hayden, G. F., Sato, P. A., Wright, P. F., et al. Progress in worldwide control/elimination of disease through immunization. *J. Pediatr. 114*:520–527, 1989.

Hone, D., and Hackett, J. Vaccination against enteric bacterial diseases. *Rev. Infect. Dis. 11*:853–876, 1989.

Katz, S. L., and Gellin, B. G., eds. Measles control: Resetting the agenda. *J. Infect. Dis. 170*(Suppl. 1):S1–S66, 1994.

Livengood, J. R., Mullen, J. R., White, J. W., et al. Family history of convulsions and use of pertussis vaccine. *J. Pediatr. 115*:527–531, 1989.

Murphy, K. R., and Strunk, R. C. Safe administration of influenzae vaccine in asthmatic children hypersensitive to egg proteins. *J. Pediatr. 106*:931–933, 1985.

*Rev. Infect. Dis.* Vaccines, *11*(Suppl. 3), 1989.

Sabin, A. B. Oral poliovirus vaccine: History of its development and use and current challenge to eliminate poliomyelitis from the world. *J. Infect. Dis. 115*:420–436, 1985.

# INDEX

Note: Page numbers in *italics* indicate figures; page numbers
followed by t indicate tables.

Abdominal infection. See also *Gastrointestinal infection.*
  anaerobic, 414
  antimicrobials for, 571t
  polymicrobial, 412, 412t
  sepsis and, 476
Abortion, death from, 14, 417
Abscess, abdominal, 571t
  brain. See *Brain abscess.*
  in inflammatory injury, 44
  liver, amebiasis and, 268–270
    anaerobic, 414
  perinephric, 204–205
  peritonsillar/retropharyngeal, 82, 82t
  pulmonary. See *Pulmonary abscess.*
Acetaminophen, 150
Acid-fast bacteria, in immunocompromised host, 376
  laboratory identification of, 535–537, *537–538*
Acid-fast staining, 170–171
*Acinetobacter baumannii*, 478, 479t
Acquired immunodeficiency syndrome (AIDS). See also
    *Human immunodeficiency virus (HIV).*
  bacteremia in, 478
  candidiasis in, 119, 186
  CD4+ T lymphocytes in, 43, 346–348
  cryptococcosis in, 184–185, 190
  cryptosporidial infection in, 274–275
  dentist exposure to, 120–121
  diagnosis of, 344–345
  discovery of, 4, 344–345
  ehrlichiosis in, 440
  epidemiology of, 345–346
  Epstein-Barr virus infection in, 105, 354
  etiology of, 345
  fluconazole for, 566
  genital herpes in, 223
  giardiasis in, 272
  hematologic manifestations of, 350–351, 355–356
  histoplasmosis is, 178
  immunopathogenesis of, 346
  in child. See *Human immunodeficiency virus (HIV), in
    child.*
  Kaposi's sarcoma in, 344, 350–351
  late manifestations of, 350
  meningitis in, 184–185, 302, 485
  meningoencephalitis in, 300
  microbial mechanisms in, 8
  *Mycobacterium avium* complex in, 168, 170, 174–175,
    345
  natural history of, 347–348
  neoplastic manifestations of, 350–351, 355–356
  opportunistic infections in, 60, 349–350, 353–354

Acquired immunodeficiency syndrome (AIDS) (*Continued*)
  oral manifestations of, 119–121, 344
  pneumonia in, 345, 348–349, 359, 377
  renal disease, 355
  respiratory tract infection in, 354–355
  skin disease in, 350, 355
  syphilis in, 214
    treatment of, 215t, 217t
  treatment of, 348–350, 356–358, 592–593
  tuberculosis in, 158–159, 161, 173–174, 387
  typhilitis in, 368
Actinomycosis, in tooth decay, 11
  oral, 119–120
Acyclovir (Zovirax), for encephalitis, 338
  for genital herpes, 223–224, 224t
  herpesvirus replication and, 54
  indications for, 592
  pharmacokinetics of, 591
  side effects of, 591
Adamantane(s), 591–592
Adenovirus, defenses of, against immune system, 60
  in common cold, 99
  in gastroenteritis, 259
  in meningitis and encephalitis, 328, 328t
  in meningoencephalitis, 300
  in pharyngoconjunctival fever, 101, 107–108
  in pneumonia, 154
  morphology of, *49*
  receptor for, 50
  replication of, *52*
Adhesin, bacterial, 29, 31–33
Adrenal gland, hemorrhage in, *477*, 477–478
Adsorption, of antimicrobials, 576
Adult respiratory distress syndrome (ARDS). See *Respiratory
    distress syndrome, adult (ARDS).*
*Aeromonas hydrophila*, in diarrhea, 236, 238
  in skin abrasion, 45
Agammaglobulinemia, X-linked, 371
Agar dilution test, *597*, 597–598
  reverse, 601–602
AIDS. See *Acquired immunodeficiency syndrome (AIDS).*
Alcoholism, immune system and, 362
  lower respiratory tract infection and, 125
  *Vibrio* infection and, 253
Allergic bronchopulmonary aspergillosis, 187–188
Alpha toxin, *417*
Alphavirus, 329
Alternative pathway, in immune response, *21*, 39
Alveolar bone, 115, *115*
Amantadine (Symmetrel), 591
  for influenza, 150, 154